64066

(20)

ARCHIVES OF DISEASE IN CHILDHOOD

M. B.

VOLUME XXXIV, 1959

LONDON
BRITISH MEDICAL ASSOCIATION
TAVISTOCK SQUARE, W.C.1

CONTENTS

No. 173. *FEBRUARY 1959*

PAGE

The Surgical Importance of a Persistent Left Superior Vena Cava. ELLIOTT S. HURWITT 1

Funnel Chest: Its Effect on Cardiac Function. RUSSELL HOWARD 5

Congenital Aneurysm of the Coronary Artery. M. GROB and E. KOLB 8

Lung Hernia Secondary to Congenital Absence of Ribs. P. P. RICKHAM 14

A Subhyoid Median Ectopic Thyroid. JOHN GRIEVE 18

Pyloric Stenosis Before and After Ramstedt. SELWYN TAYLOR 20

Complications After Operation for Oesophageal Atresia. F. REHBEIN and F. YANAGISWA .. 24

Rupture of the Liver in the Newborn. ILSE WOLFROM 30

Urethral Plication in the Management of Urinary Incontinence. D. F. ELLISON NASH 33

British Association of Paediatric Surgeons: Fifth Annual Meeting 35

A Longitudinal Study of the Growth and Development of Prematurely and Maturely Born Children. Part III. Mental Development. CECIL MARY DRILLIEN 37

The Physical Development of Mongols. G. DUTTON 46

The Place of Oats in the Coeliac Diet. A. LINDSAY C. MOULTON 51

Microcephaly in One of Monozygous Twins. M. G. W. BRANDON, BRIAN H. KIRMAN and C. E. WILLIAMS 56

Oxalosis. E. KATZUNI and U. SANDBANK 60

Visceral Larva Migrans. W. DICKSON and R. C. WOODCOCK 63

Acute Pellagra in a Child Under Treatment with Isoniazid. M. G. PHILPOTT and H. P. PLAYER 68

The Diagnostic Importance of Glycosuria in Lead Poisoning in Childhood. RONALD C. ROXBURGH and LEONARD HAAS 70

Acute Haemolytic Anaemia Following the Ingestion of Para-dichlorobenzene. M. HALLOWELL 74

The Child of the Diabetic Woman. JAMES W. FARQUHAR 76

Book Reviews 97

Paediatric Societies in the British Isles 100

No. 174. *APRIL 1959*

Social and Biological Factors in Infant Mortality. VIII. Mortality in the Post-neonatal Period. S. L. MORRISON, J. A. HEADY and J. N. MORRIS 101

Nephrocalcinosis Infantum. ROBERT A. SHANKS and A. M. MACDONALD 115

A Case of Calcification of the Basal Ganglia with Osteoporosis and Other Abnormalities. P. F. BENSON 120

Sulphobromophthalein Excretion in Premature Infants. THOMAS E. OPPÉ and IRENE E. GIBBS 125

Systolic Murmurs in Children. W. MAINZER, R. PINCOVICI and G. HEYMANN 131

Sequestration of the Lung. MARY C. BUCHANAN 137

Investigation into the Aetiology and Treatment of Pica. PHILIP LANZKOWSKY 140

The Pre-eruptive Illness of Measles. M. W. PARTINGTON and J. F. P. QUINTON 149

An English Family with Waardenburg's Syndrome. M. W. PARTINGTON 154

Renal Tubular Damage in Infantile Gastro-enteritis. JOHN BLACK 158

PAGE

Idiopathic Infantile Hypoglycaemia. M. KINSBOURNE and L. I. WOOLF 166

Spontaneous Hyperinsulinism due to Benign Hyperplasia of Islet Cells. DONALD M. DOUGLAS 171

Extended Exchange Transfusion in Pre-hydropic Infants. EILEEN M. O'NEILL and RONALD R. GORDON 174

Massive Adrenal Haemorrhage in the Newborn. EILEEN E. HILL and JOHN A. WILLIAMS .. 178

Book Reviews 183

Paediatric Pathology Club 187

NO. 175. *JUNE 1959*

Editorial Note 191

Bronchiectasis in Children. Its Multiple Clinical and Pathological Aspects. HOWARD WILLIAMS and R. N. O'REILLY 192

Respiratory Stridor Produced by an Aberrant Pulmonary Artery. W. H. SCHUTT and P. M. ROBB 202

Bone Lesions of Urticaria Pigmentosa in Childhood. MARTIN H. LEES and C. ERIC STROUD .. 205

A Longitudinal Study of the Growth and Development of Prematurely and Maturely Born Children. Part IV. Morbidity. CECIL MARY DRILLIEN 210

A Case of Idiopathic Pulmonary Haemosiderosis with Myocarditis. S. CAMPBELL and C. A. J. MACAFEE 218

Congenital Heart Block. R. W. SMITHELLS and E. B. OUTON 223

Congenital Anomalies Associated with Cerebral Palsy and Mental Retardation. RONALD S. ILLINGWORTH 228

Hydranencephaly and Allied Disorders. C. S. MUIR 231

Incidence of Rheumatic Fever in Ceylon. STANLEY DE SILVA 247

Herpes Simplex Virus Infection: Dissemination in Association with Malnutrition. D. MCKENZIE, J. D. L. HANSEN and W. BECKER 250

Chronic Ulcerative Colitis in Childhood. RONALD C. KING, ARTHUR E. LINDNER and H. MARVIN POLLARD 257

Physiological Jaundice. A. A. CUNNINGHAM 262

The Diagnosis of Mental Retardation in Infancy. R. S. ILLINGWORTH and L. B. BIRCH .. 269

Congenital Hydrocephalus in Monovular Twins. V. GELLMAN 274

A Case of Rupture of the Hepatic Duct in a Newborn Infant. JOAN P. WRIGHT and HELEN E. WORSLEY 277

Book Reviews 279

NO. 176. *AUGUST 1959*

Some Respiratory and Cardiovascular Problems after Birth. G. S. DAWES 281

The Pupillary Membrane in Premature Infants. BRUNO GANS 292

Glycogen Disease. S. VAN CREVELD 298

The Syndrome of Hypoparathyroidism and Steatorrhoea. EIRIAN WILLIAMS and COLIN WOOD 302

The Treatment of Congenital Galactosaemia. NORMAN L. JONES and DAVID LEAK 307

Pregnancy Complicated by Diabetes Mellitus: A Study in Combined Obstetric and Paediatric Management. ANDREW M. CLAYE and W. S. CRAIG 312

PAGE

Varicella Encephalitis. J. D. HEPPLESTON, K. M. PEARCE and P. O. YATES 318

Neurological Sequelae of Pertussis with Particular Reference to Mental Defect. J. M. BERG 322

Cerebral Atrophy in Microcephalic Cousins. PETER E. SYLVESTER 325

The Size of Mental Defective Boys. GORDON DUTTON 331

Treatment of Tuberculous Meningitis. W. MORTON FYFE 334

Pneumocystis Pneumonia Associated with Agammaglobulinaemia. J. G. B. RUSSELL 338

Perforation of the Bowel in Henoch-Schönlein Purpura. R. BASU 342

The Natural History of the Partial Thoracic Stomach (Hiatus Hernia) in Children. I. J. CARRÉ 344

British Paediatric Association: Proceedings of the Thirtieth Annual General Meeting 354

Book Reviews 359

NO. 177. *OCTOBER 1959*

The Maintenance of Stability in the Newly Born. Part 1. Chemical Exchange. R. A. MCCANCE 361

Relationship Between Calcium-Phosphorus Metabolism, the 'Krebs Cycle' and Steroid Metabolism. ETTORE DE TONI, JR. and SERGIO NORDIO 371

Familial Vitamin D-Resistant Rickets. C. P. DANCASTER and W. P. U. JACKSON 383

Electrophoretic Studies of Serum Protein Patterns in Newborn Indian Infants. B. S. KULKARNI, R. S. SATOSKAR, M. N. PARIKH and R. G. CHITRE 392

Tetanus in African Children. A. B. TOMPKINS 398

Three Cases of Niemann Pick's Disease in Children. W. I. FORSYTHE, E. F. MCKEOWN and D. W. NEILL 406

A Study of Congenital Heart Defects in Mongolism. M. C. LIU and K. CORLETT 410

The Electrical Conductivity of Electrolytes Found in the Sweat of Patients with Fibrocystic Disease of the Pancreas. ALLAN BLOXSOM 420

The Relationship Between Decreased 5-Hydroxyindole Metabolism and Mental Defect in Phenylketonuria. C. M. B. PARE, M. SANDLER and R. S. STACEY 422

Honeycomb Lungs with Pericholangitis. S. SIVANESAN 426

Splenic Agenesis and Multilobulate Spleen. C. S. MUIR 431

Birth Trauma to the Vertebral Arteries. P. O. YATES 436

Acute Intestinal Obstruction due to Mesenteric Lymphangioma. B. M. L. UNDERHILL 442

A Description and Classification of the Common Disorders of Speech in Children. T. T. S. INGRAM 444

Book Reviews 456

NO. 178. *DECEMBER 1959*

The Maintenance of Stability in the Newly Born. Part 2. Thermal Balance. R. A. MCCANCE 459

Foetomaternal Transfusion as a Cause of Neonatal Anaemia. WILLIAM KRIVIT, ROBERT GOODLIN, NEWELL ZIEGLER and ROGER LIENKE 471

Mediastinal Duplication of the Gut. J. STANLEY ELWOOD 474

Intestinal Obstruction in a Case of Duplication of the Terminal Ileum. J. A. WILLIAMS 480

The Incidence of Inguinal Hernia in Newcastle Children. GEORGE KNOX 482

A Longitudinal Study of the Growth and Development of Prematurely and Maturely Born Children. Part V. Patterns of Maternal Care (A Study of Child Rearing in Scotland). CECIL MARY DRILLIEN 487

PAGE

Masculinization of a Female Foetus with Oestrogenic Effect. G. H. VALENTINE 495

Addison's Disease with Hypofunction of the Parathyroid Glands. H. SZCZEPAŃSKA and J. SAPIECHA 498

The Effect of Calomel on Plasma Epinephrine in the Rat and the Relationship to Mechanisms in Pink Disease. DONALD B. CHEEK and FANNIE WU 501

A Case of Arthrogryposis Multiplex Congenita with Lesions in the Nervous System. MALCOLM FOWLER 505

The Effect of a Bronchodilator Aerosol on Ventilatory Capacity in Fibrocystic Disease of the Pancreas. BRYAN GANDEVIA and CHARLOTTE ANDERSON 511

Congenital Bowing of the Long Bones: Report of a Case. A. D. BAIN and HELEN S. BARRETT .. 516

Biochemical Studies in Idiopathic Hypercalcaemia of Infancy. JOHN O. FORFAR, S. L. TOMPSETT and W. FORSHALL 525

Narcolepsy in a Child Under 7 Years Old. D. J. SALFIELD 538

Book Reviews 540

Index 543

THE SURGICAL IMPORTANCE OF A PERSISTENT LEFT SUPERIOR VENA CAVA*

BY

ELLIOTT S. HURWITT†

From the Surgical Division, the Montefiore Hospital, New York City

A left superior vena cava may be present simultaneously with a normal right superior vena cava, or, even more infrequently, as the only superior vena cava. The surgical importance of a persistent left superior vena cava varies depending on its termination into the right or left atrium, as well as the nature and severity of any associated cardiovascular anomalies.

Left Superior Vena Cava Entering Right Atrium. This is not a particularly uncommon anomaly, the vein terminating either directly into the right atrium, or indirectly by way of the coronary sinus. The embryology and frequency of this configuration have been reviewed in a previous communication (Hurwitt, Escher and Citrin, 1955). Since anomalies of the heart and great vessels tend to occur in association, one may encounter a left superior vena cava draining into the right atrium in the process of other operations, such as in the correction of a patent ductus arteriosus. Under such circumstances the anatomical course of the left superior vena cava is such that it does not interfere with the stated operation, and the vein usually has no surgical importance.

With the advent of open heart surgery, however, employing either cardiopulmonary by-pass or hypothermia, a left superior vena cava assumes real surgical significance, regardless of whether it drains into the right or left atrium. Failure to identify and mobilize this vessel, with temporary occlusion for hypothermia and cannulation or occlusion during cardiopulmonary by-pass, may seriously compromise the procedure. The necessity for this manoeuvre has been described in a number of articles, including one from this department (Robinson, Glotzer, Gilbert, Escher and Hurwitt, in press).

Left Superior Vena Cava Entering Left Atrium. As a contributing cause of cyanosis, the importance of drainage of any systemic vein into the left auricle has usually been overshadowed by the severity of associated cardiac defects. Subsequent to the summary of the reported cases (Hurwitt *et al.*, 1955), two additional such patients have come to surgery at this hospital.

Case Histories

Uncorrected Lesions

Case 1. A 4 lb. premature infant, one of male twins, was brought to the hospital on January 21, 1957, with complete ectopia cordis (Fig. 1) and severe cyanosis and dyspnoea; the twin was normal. A covering of skin was fashioned over the heart, and the baby died on the evening of the operation. A left superior vena cava entering the left atrium was only one of the eight major anomalies of the heart and great vessels found at autopsy. A normal right superior vena cava was also present. A motion picture and complete description of this case have been prepared (Hurwitt and Lebendiger, in press).

Case 2. Severe cyanosis and nearly fatal episodes of syncope were the presenting problems in this 18-month-old girl. Investigation in another hospital had established the presence of both a right and left superior vena cava and a levocardia in the presence of a situs inversus abdominalis. On June 17, 1958, an attempt was made to construct a Blalock shunt between the left subclavian artery and the left pulmonary artery, but irreversible cardiac arrest developed during mobilization of the pulmonary artery. Post-mortem examination disclosed an essentially bilocular heart, with the left superior vena cava draining into the left side of a chamber that was practically a common auricle. Splenic agenesis, described in several such cases, was not present.

Corrected Lesions

Even when severe associated anomalies of the heart are present, however, interruption of the flow of systemic venous blood into the left auricle may be beneficial, with or without attempted correction of the other lesions. Diaz and Anido (1949) reported significant improvement

* Presented at the Fifth Annual Meeting, the British Association of Paediatric Surgeons, London, July 23, 1958.

† Aided by a grant from the New York Heart Association.

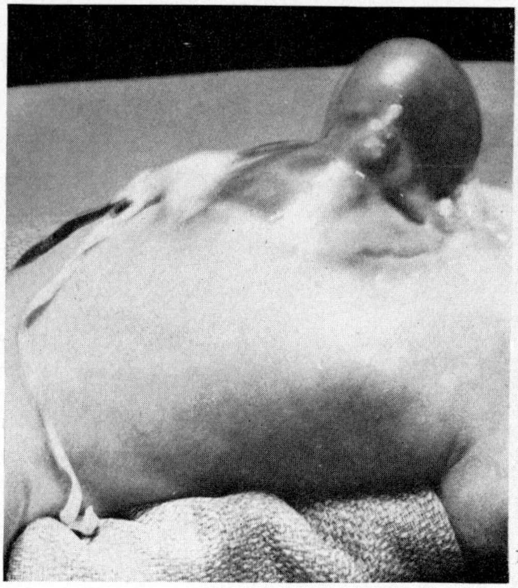

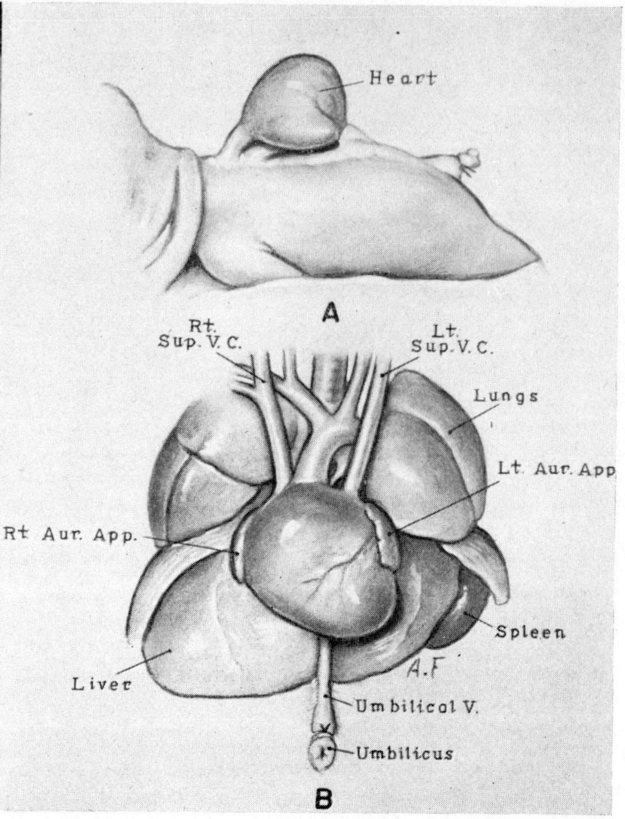

FIG. 1. Case 1. Photograph and diagram of ectopia cordis, with bilateral superior venae cavae.

in a 7-year-old tetralogy case following ligation of a left superior vena cava entering the left auricle, without any other procedure. Lessening of cyanosis was similarly described in an 8-year-old with Eisenmenger's complex, by Feindt and Hauch (1953). Ekstrom (personal communication) supplemented construction of a Blalock shunt in a 12-year-old with tetralogy of Fallot, situs inversus totalis and double superior venae cavae, by ligating the anomalous vena cava as it entered the arterial auricle.

Obviously the outlook is much more favourable when the left superior vena cava entering the left auricle constitutes the major cause of cyanosis, or when any concomitant intracardiac defects may also be amenable to correction. Examples of each of these situations have now come to operation at this hospital.

Case 3. This has previously been reported in detail (Hurwitt *et al.*, 1955). Surgical relief of cyanosis in an 8-year-old girl, due to entrance of a left superior vena cava into the left auricle, was accomplished by intrapericardial ligation of the left superior vena cava on December 29, 1954 (Fig. 2). The venous return to the heart after the procedure is depicted in Fig. 3. Post-operatively there was marked improvement in clubbing of the fingers, cyanosis. dyspnoea, appetite, and exercise performance. Slight peripheral arterial oxygen unsaturation persisted, presumably related to an atypical moderate hypoplasia of the posteriorly placed main pulmonary artery.

Case 4. A 10-year-old negro girl with acyanotic congenital heart disease was found on cardiac catheterization to have an atrial septal defect with a significant flow from left to right and a left superior vena cava. Operation, under hypothermia, was performed on July 1, 1957, through an anterior thoracic incision, entering the right pleural cavity in the fourth interspace and the left pleural cavity in the third interspace, with transverse division of the sternum. On the right there was a small superior vena cava with a normal azygos tributary. The left superior vena cava was considerably larger, was joined by a large hemiazygos vein, and entered the left atrium anteriorly to the entrance of the left pulmonary veins. Digital exploration of the right auricle confirmed the presence of a large atrial septal defect, and oxygen determinations from both auricles showed complete admixture of the blood at this level under the operative conditions (Fig. 4a).

At a body temperature of 88° F. the inferior and the two superior venae cavae were occluded for six and a half minutes while the right auricle was opened and an atrial septal defect measuring 4 cm. in length and 2½ cm. in width was repaired by a continuous silk suture. While the right auricle now contained blood with a venous oxygen saturation, blood from the left auricle at the site of insertion of the left superior vena cava was also highly

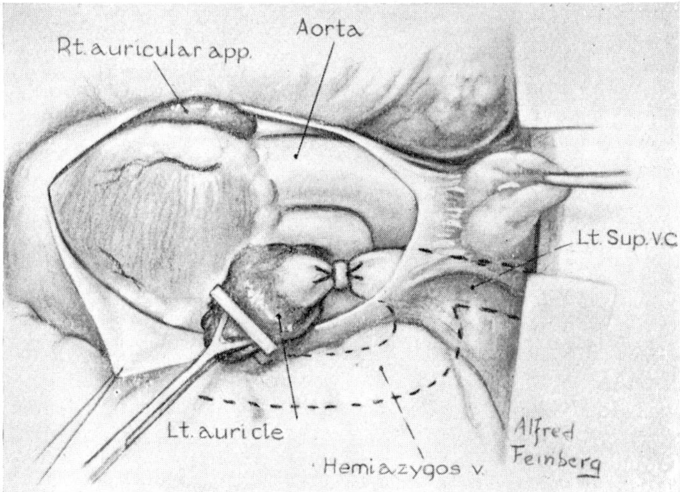

FIG. 2. Case 3. Intrapericardial ligation of left superior vena cava. Note large hemiazygos entering left superior vena cava extrapericardially. (From Hurwitt *et al.*, 1955.)

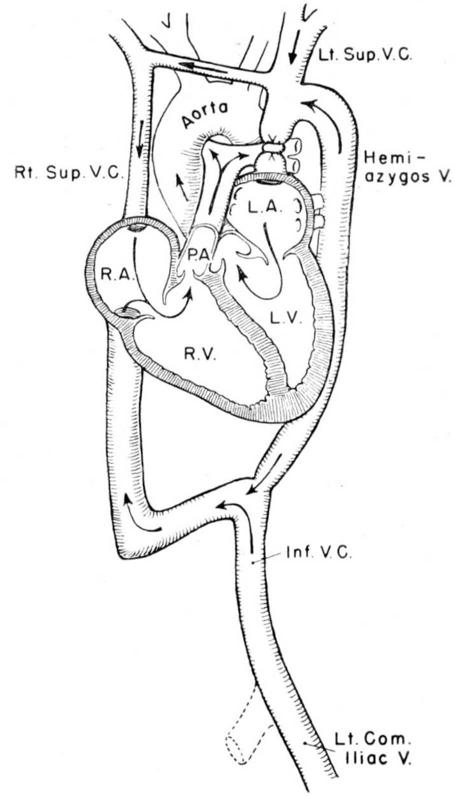

FIG. 3. Case 3. Diagrammatic reconstruction of vascular anomalies and ligation of left superior vena cava. (From Hurwitt *et al.*, 1955.) Both figures are reproduced by courtesy of C. V. Mosby Co., St. Louis, Mo.

unsaturated (Fig. 4b). Apparently the return from the left superior vena cava had been streaming practically directly through the atrial defect, and did not produce significant oxygen desaturation in the left auricle until the defect was closed.

Intrapericardial ligation of the left superior vena cava resulted in eliminating this source of systemic venous blood from the left atrium, with a restoration to normal of cardiac physiology (Fig. 4c). At no time post-operatively was there any evidence of oedema, cyanosis, or increased venous pressure, confirming the presence of adequate communicating channels between the two superior vena caval systems. The child was re-examined

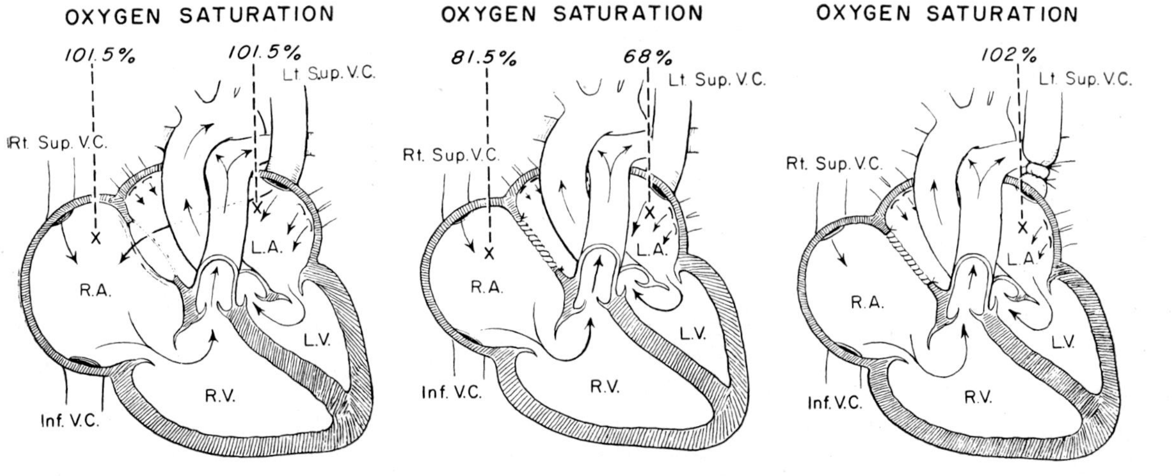

FIG. 4a, b, c.—Case 4. Status at operation: (*a*), initially; (*b*), after closure of the atrial septal defect; and (*c*), after ligation of the left superior vena cava.

one year after operation and found to be in excellent health.

Comment

Drainage of any systemic vein into the left atrium contributes to the cyanotic state, and as such merits consideration for surgical correction; the only categorical contra-indication would be atresia of the tricuspid valve. The anomalous vein will usually be a superior vena cava, although the inferior vena cava (Gardner and Cole, 1955), coronary sinus (Mankin and Burchell, 1953), and levo-atriocardinal veins (Gould, 1953) have also been reported terminating in the left auricle.

The degree of improvement following ligation of a left superior vena cava will be determined by the severity of any uncorrected associated lesions. It may be substantial, however, even in the presence of complex defects of the tetralogy type (Gould, 1953; Gardner and Cole, 1955; Hurwitt *et al.*, 1955). When the associated anomalies are also corrected, as in Case 4, or when no major concomitant abnormalities are found, the result may be excellent. Cases have been described with no associated septal defects (Potter, 1948; Gardner and Cole, 1955; Peel, Semple, Kelly and Blum, 1956; Tuchman, Brown, Huston, Weinstein, Rowe and Crumpton, 1956), and none was found in our Case 3. When the flow from the left superior vena cava is streaming almost directly through the atrial septal defect, significant arterial oxygen unsaturation may not be detected until the defect is closed, as in Case 4. Occlusion of the left superior vena cava then restores the situation to normal.

A disadvantage of approaching repair of an atrial septal defect through an incision limited to opening the right pleural cavity is the possibility of overlooking the presence of a left superior vena cava. Even in the hands of those who employ 'closed' techniques for these operations, the opportunity for correcting a left superior vena cava entering the left auricle would be missed. Most surgeons currently close atrial septal defects under direct vision with 'open' techniques. If venous inflow occlusion with hypothermia is practised, failure to take a left superior vena cava into account may result both in excessive blood loss and poor visualization of the defect, regardless of which atrium receives the anomalous vein; the same considerations apply equally to cardiopulmonary by-pass. For these reasons either a vertical sternum-splitting incision or a bilateral anterior thoracotomy with division of the sternum are preferable to right thoracotomy alone.

Interruption of a left superior vena cava entering the left auricle must be performed intrapericardially in order also to divert the flow from the hemiazygos vein to the right side (Figs. 2, 3). The interruption may be accomplished simply by ligation, as in the reported cases, or by division. If a solitary left superior or inferior vena cava were found entering the left atrium, transplantation to the right side would be necessary, either by direct suture or by a graft. One unsuccessful attempt to re-route blood in a solitary left superior vena cava from the left to the right auricle has been reported by Tuchman *et al.* (1956). When bilateral superior venae cavae are present, apparently the communicating veins across the mediastinum or through the azygos system are usually adequate, so that closure of the left superior vena cava results in shunting the blood to the right side, rather than the syndrome of superior vena caval compression. When such communications are absent, however, as suggested in the report by Peel *et al.* (1956), interruption of the left superior vena cava should be supplemented by an anastomosis to the right superior caval system.

Summary

The surgical importance of a left superior vena cava has been analysed.

Regardless of whether the left superior vena cava drains into the right or left atrium, it must be either occluded or cannulated during open heart surgery with either hypothermia or cardiopulmonary by-pass.

Any systemic vein entering the left auricle may be a major or contributing cause of cyanosis, and should be corrected, except in the presence of tricuspid atresia.

Data are presented on four cases of left superior vena cava entering the left atrium, with surgical correction in two instances, one of which has been reported previously.

Ligation of a left superior vena cava entering the left auricle and closure of a large atrial septal defect were accomplished in a 10-year-old girl.

This represents the fifth reported case of relief of cyanosis following interruption of a left superior vena cava terminating in the left auricle.

References

Ekstrom, G. (1954). Personal communication.
Feindt, H. R. and Hauch, H. J. (1953). *Z. Kreisl.-Forsch.*, **42**, 53.
Gardner, D. L. and Cole, L. (1955). *Brit. Heart J.*, **17**, 93.
Gould, S. E. (1953). *Pathology of the Heart*, pp. 491, 496. Charles C. Thomas, Springfield, Illinois.
Hurwitt, E. S., Escher, D. J. W. and Citrin, L. I. (1955). *Surgery*, **38**, 903.
—— and Lebendiger, A. *A.M.A. Arch. Surg.* In the press. Presented at the Sixth Scientific Meeting, the North American Chapter of the International Cardiovascular Society, San Francisco, June 21, 1958.
Mankin, H. T. and Burchell, H. B. (1953). *Proc. Mayo Clin.*, **28**, 463.
Peel, A. A. F., Semple, T., Kelly, J. C. and Blum, K. (1956). *Scot. med. J.*, **1**, 83.
Potter, E. L. (1948). *Arch. Path. (Chicago)*, **46**, 87.
Robinson, G., Glotzer, P., Gilbert, M., Escher, D. J. W. and Hurwitt, E. S. *Amer. J. Cardiol.* In the press. Presented in the New York Society for Thoracic Surgery, May 9, 1958.
Rodiguez Diaz, A. and Anido, H. (1949). *Dis. Chest*, **15**, 684.
Tuchman, H., Brown, J. F., Huston, J. H., Weinstein, A. B., Rowe, G. G. and Crumpton, C. W. (1956). *Amer. J. Med.*, **21**, 481

FUNNEL CHEST: ITS EFFECT ON CARDIAC FUNCTION*

BY

RUSSELL HOWARD

From the Royal Children's Hospital, Melbourne

Funnel chest, with its considerable sternal depression and obvious interference with the topography of the heart, has for some time been made the subject of the attractive paradox that, in the vast majority of cases, it has no effect on cardiac function. True, it is conceded that the deformity may in rare instances be responsible for decompensation severe enough to cause congestive failure but there exists the greatest reluctance to attribute to it any less dramatic evidences of interference with the heart's action. The all or nothing rule seems to be invoked.

There are, however, recent writers who take what seems to be a more logical stand in suggesting that diminished exercise tolerance is common in cases of funnel chest and that cardiac incompetence is its cause. Such opinions have been expressed by Lester (1950a, b, 1954), Ravitch (1951), Wachtel, Ravitch and Grishman (1956), Chin (1957) and the present author (1955). These statements are made in reporting details of large series of cases personally treated by the authors.

The essential feature of the deformity of funnel chest is a depression of the sternum, most marked at the sternoxiphisternal junction. In the funnel-chested infant this area retracts markedly on inspiration but the paradoxical movement progressively decreases until at about the age of 4 years it is replaced by orthodox movement of small amplitude. Continued chest development is characterized by the failure of the midline antero-posterior diameter to increase commensurately with the growth of the more lateral parts of the chest, i.e. the funnel becomes deeper. During this period the heart is undergoing the normal increase in size with age, with the result that eventually it may suffer compression between the sternum and the vertebral column. Although at times, this pincer action may be diminished by displacement of the organ to the left, the effect on cardiac function is similar to that of constrictive pericarditis.

* A paper read at the meeting of the British Association of Paediatric Surgeons held in London in July, 1958.

I have had the opportunity of examining and assessing over 400 patients with funnel chest but it is the 90 of these on whom I have personally operated who provide striking clinical evidence that before operation they were labouring under a physical as well as a psychological handicap. During the early post-operative period the statement is spontaneously volunteered by a high proportion of patients or parents that exercise tolerance has already greatly improved. At this time the vital capacity is still below its pre-operative level, thus rendering unlikely any explanation based on improved respiratory function. In most of these cases direct questioning before operation had failed to elicit a history of any interference with effort. This is, of course, due to failure to appreciate the effort of which a particular child should be capable, so-called normal limits being very elastic.

Ravitch (1951) reported the very convincing instance of a man, 28 years of age and suffering from severe funnel chest deformity, who developed auricular fibrillation and congestive failure with no other cause apparent. Complete recovery and return to strenuous work followed operative relief of the funnel chest.

A suggestive although uncommon symptom is precordial pain on exertion. Although many may discount the inference that this pain is of cardiac origin, the fact remains that all four cases complaining of pain were completely relieved by operation.

In an endeavour to demonstrate graphically interference with cardiac anatomy, angiocardiography has been performed on selected patients. The findings in two representative cases are given below.

Case Histories

Case 1. S.K. was a girl of 10 years with a moderately severe grade of funnel chest. A plain radiograph of the chest demonstrates the absence of cardiac displacement in the postero-anterior film (Fig. 1). The lateral view shows apparent impingement of the lower part of the sternum on the cardiac shadow (Fig. 2); as there is no displacement of the heart to the left this should indicate

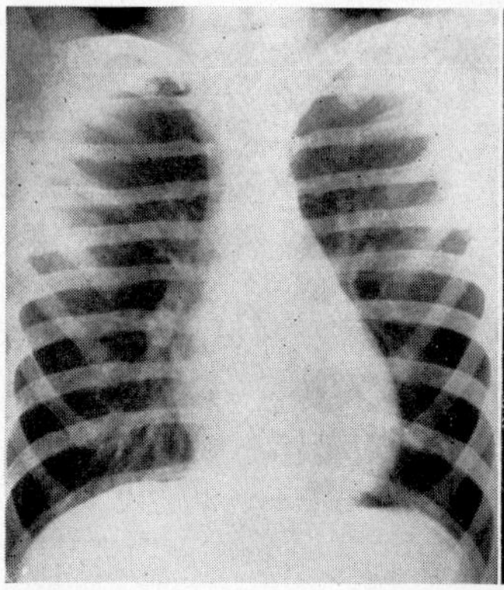

FIG. 1.

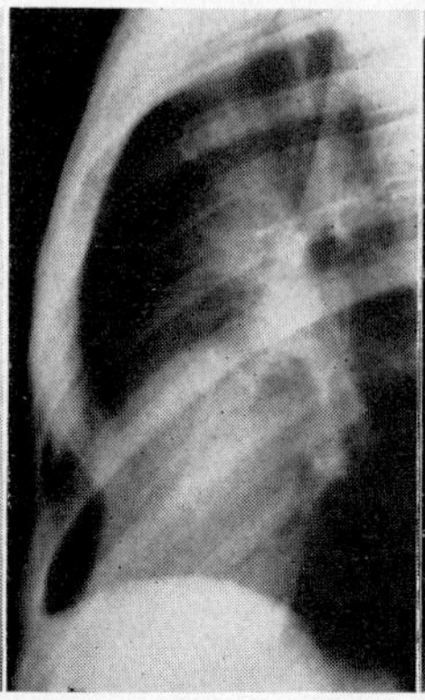

FIG. 2.

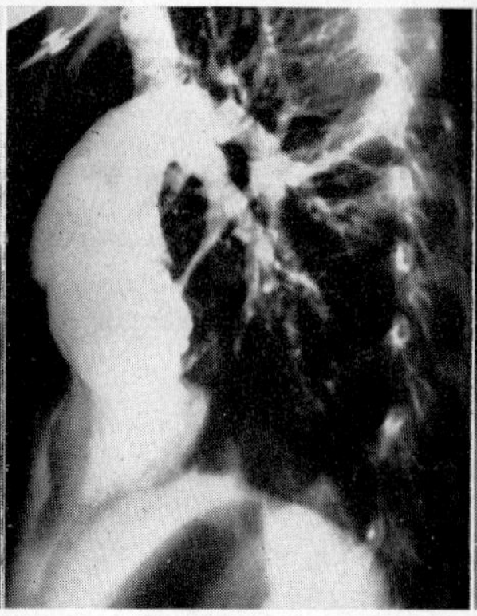

FIG. 3.

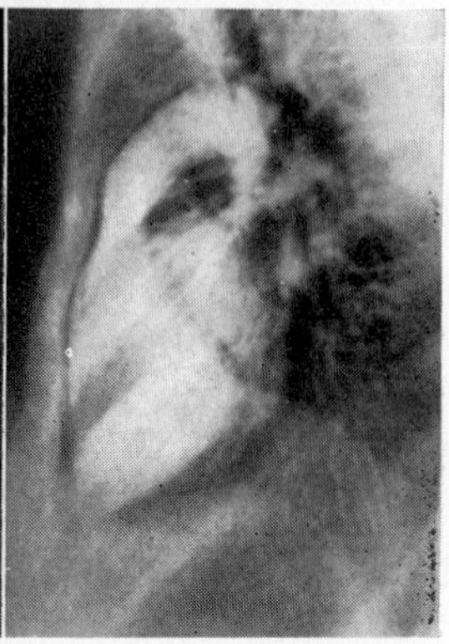

FIG. 4.

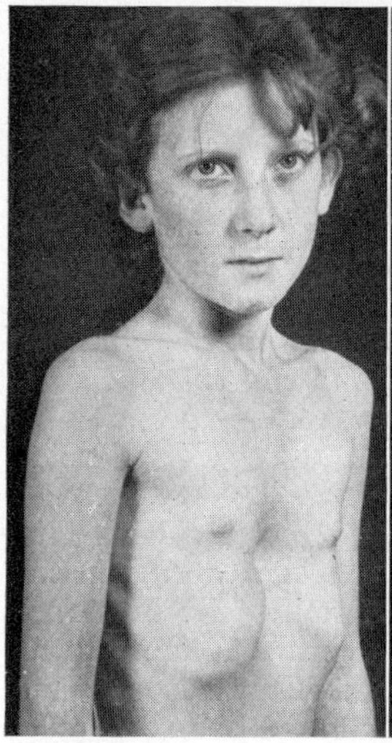

FIG. 5A.

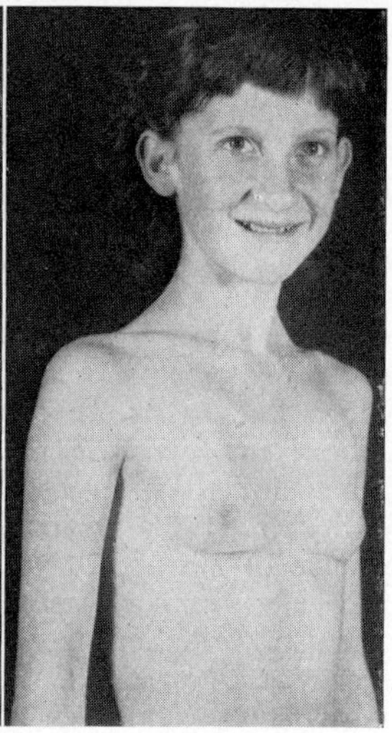

FIG. 5B.

FIG. 1.—Case 1. Postero-anterior film showing absence of lateral cardiac displacement.

FIG. 2.—Lateral film: impingement of sternum on cardiac shadow.

FIG. 3.—Pre-operative lateral angiocardiogram illustrating indentation of right ventricle.

FIG. 4.—Post-operative lateral angiocardiogram showing restoration of normal cardiac outline.

FIG. 5.—Case 1. (*a*) Moderately severe funnel chest.
(*b*) Post-operative clinical appearance.

FIG. 6.—Case 2. Postero-anterior film showing cardiac displacement to left.

FIG. 7.—Lateral angiocardiogram: 'negative shadow' of unfilled left ventricle impinges on right ventricle.

FIG. 8.—Filled left ventricle shows filling defect caused in right ventricle.

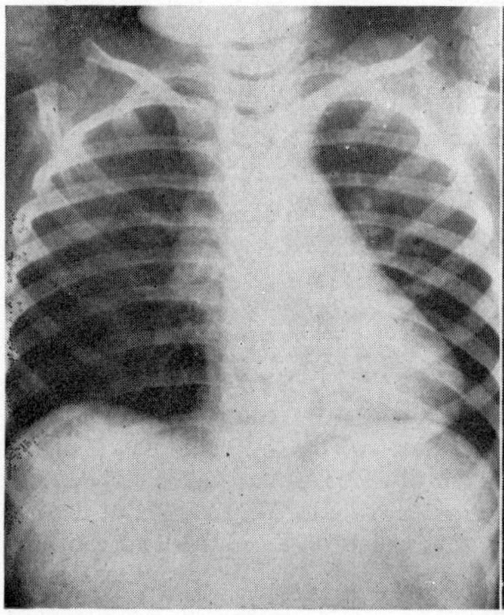

FIG. 6.

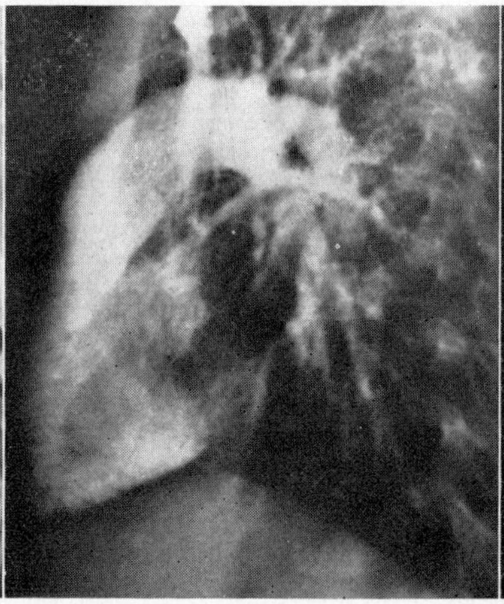

FIG. 7.

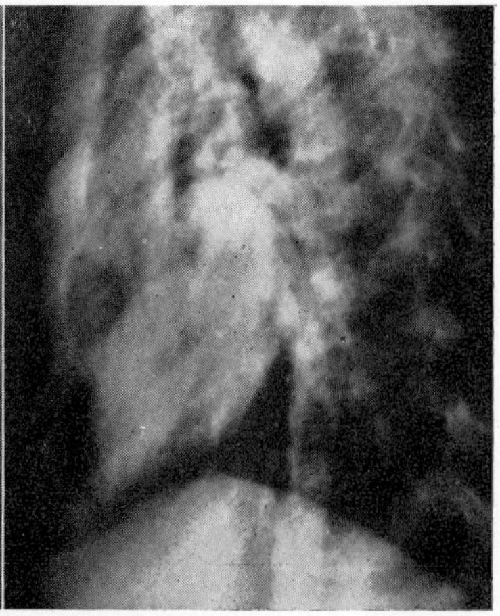

FIG. 8.

a genuine compression. Confirmation is obtained from the lateral angiocardiogram which shows the sternum deeply indenting the wall of the right ventricle (Fig. 3). Fig. 4 shows the correction of this anomaly as seen in an angiocardiogram taken some 12 months after operation whilst in Figs. 5a and b the appearance before operation and the clinical improvement in the deformity afterwards is noted.

Case 2. H.E. was a girl of 4 years with a gross funnel chest in whom the heart is displaced to the left (Fig. 6). The angiocardiogram shows how, in the rotated heart, the stouter-walled left ventricle is actually pushed into and causes a filling defect in the right ventricle. Fig. 7 illustrates the ' negative shadow ' of the *unfilled* left ventricle producing this result, whilst in Fig. 8 the *filled* left ventricle is seen to be exerting the same effect.

These considerable deformities surely must cause diminution in the capacity of the right side of the heart which, whilst not affecting the patient at rest, will take its inevitable toll of exercise tolerance. One would expect that, in response to exertion, right atrial pressure would mount and cardiac output fail to increase to a degree commensurate with requirements.

The estimation of cardiac output on exertion was performed in two cases by Wachtel *et al.* (1956). One showed no gross abnormality but the other, a patient with severe deformity and gross exercise intolerance, showed exactly the findings anticipated above (even to the extent of cardiac output actually decreasing on exertion). Post-operative readings are recorded in neither case but complete relief of symptoms was effected by operation.

The electrocardiographic findings have been far from constant in the present series. However, a number of the more severe depressions have had an inverted or flattened T-wave in Lead 11, and again the significant fact is the return to a normal pattern following operative intervention.

From the above emerge certain incontrovertible facts. These are that the heart is frequently compressed by the sternum in cases of funnel chest; that marked deformity and diminution of the capacity of the right ventricle may thereby be produced; that failure of cardiac output to increase with exercise has been demonstrated in at least one such case; and that relief of both cardiac deformity and exercise intolerance have been proved to follow operation. Surely this is sufficiently suggestive of interference with cardiac function to place the onus of proof upon those who deny its occurrence.

The important question remains as to how frequent is this occurrence. The author's firm impression, based on the clinical improvement in the early post-operative period, is that it is a common event and one which may be confidently expected to yield to the routine operation performed for funnel chest.

Summary

The question of post-operative improvement in exercise tolerance is discussed on the basis of 90 cases of funnel chest observed in pre- and post-operative phases.

The conclusion is drawn that exercise tolerance is improved in a high percentage of cases.

Proof is adduced of interference with cardiac volume caused by pressure of the depressed sternum.

It is contended that decreased exercise tolerance in cases of funnel chest is due to interference with cardiac output.

I most gratefully acknowledge the enthusiastic help of Dr. H. G. Hiller, Director of Radiology at the Royal Children's Hospital, Melbourne, in connexion with the angiocardiographic work to which so much reference is made in the text.

References

Chin, E. F. (1957). *Brit. J. Surg.*, **44**, 360.
Howard, R. N. (1955). *Med. J. Aust.*, **2**, 1092.
Lester, C. W. (1950a). *J. thorac. Surg.*, **19**, 507
—— (1950b). *J. Pediat.*, **37**, 224.
—— (1954). *J. Amer. med. Ass.*, **156**, 1063.
Ravitch, M. M. (1951). *Surgery*, **30**, 178.
Wachtel, F. W., Ravitch, M. M. and Grishman, A. (1956). *Amer. Heart J.*, **52**, 121.

CONGENITAL ANEURYSM OF THE CORONARY ARTERY*

BY

M. GROB and E. KOLB

From the Surgical Department of the Children's Hospital, Zurich, Switzerland

As compared with the totality of congenital malformations of the heart, anomalies of the coronary vessels are relatively rare. In the literature, anomalous origin of these vessels has been taken adequately into account. Less emphasis has been laid, however, on conditions such as congenital aneurysms of the coronary arteries which probably occur more frequently than is commonly believed.

The following two cases observed by us will illustrate this anomaly.

Case Histories

Case 1. She was a 7½-year-old girl, whose medical history indicated that a murmur over the heart had been noted since the age of 4 weeks. Her physical development and functional capacity, however, had been normal. She was referred to our hospital for suspected patent ductus. Physical examination revealed a loud continuous murmur, with maximum intensity in the fourth left intercostal space immediately near the apex. Roentgenograms of the thorax, electrocardiographic tracings and blood pressure readings were normal. Cardiac catheterization disclosed right heart pressures and oxygen saturation within normal limits. A patent foramen ovale was catheterized, but seemed to be without a haemodynamic significance. Angiocardiography revealed a tortuous dilated vessel on the left side of the heart, ending in a cherry-sized structure below the left ventricle (Figs. 1 and 2). These findings were easily seen to represent an aneurysmal deformation of the left coronary artery which was responsible for the continuous

* A paper read at a meeting of the British Association of Paediatric Surgeons held in London in July, 1958.

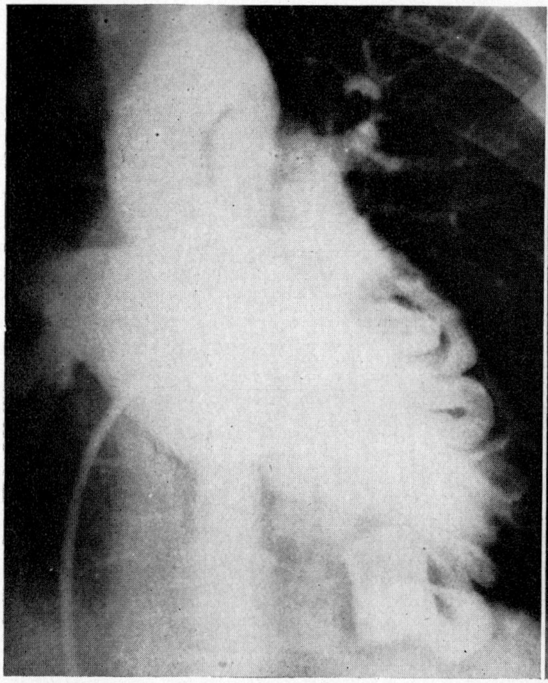

FIG. 1.—Case 1. Frontal angiocardiogram showing a tortuous vessel on the left side of the heart, ending in a saccular structure below the left ventricle.

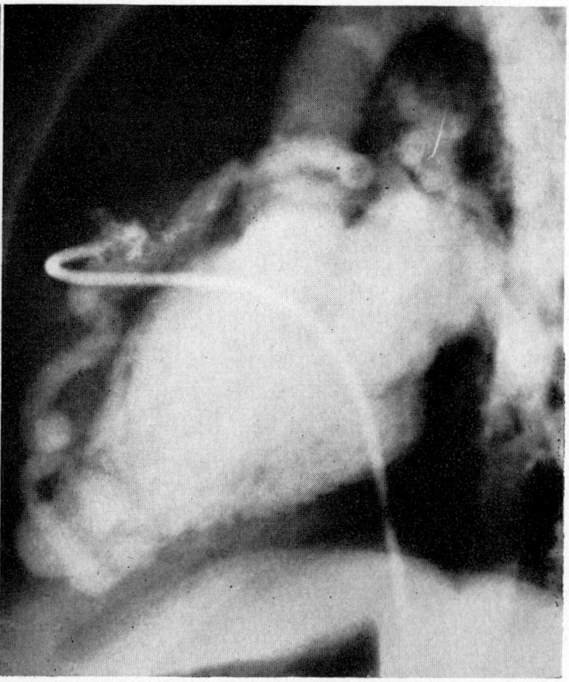

FIG. 2.—Lateral angiocardiogram. The markedly dilated left coronary artery runs down in numerous coils towards the apex and enters the aneurysm.

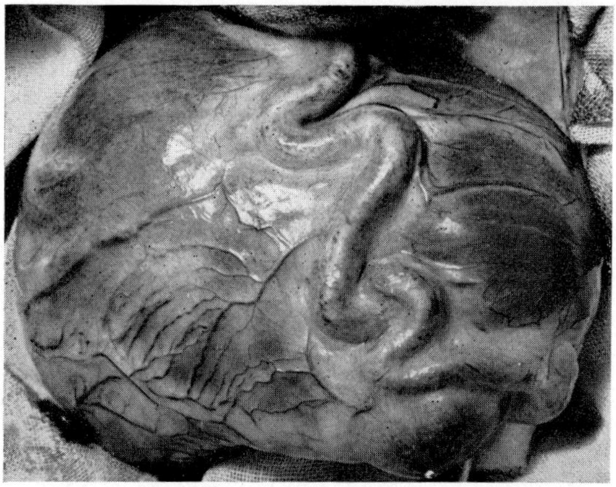

FIG. 3.—Case 1. Anterior view of the heart at operation. Serpentine dilatation of the left coronary artery. Aneurysm at the apex.

murmur. Rupture is known to occur in such aneurysms, and because of this and because the localization of the aneurysm near the apex was favourable, we decided to operate.

After a bilateral anterior incision of the thoracic wall the pericardium was opened and the condition previously mentioned was confirmed. The left coronary artery was enormously dilated down its whole course to the apex, where it turned to the right and entered a saccular aneurysm situated at the lower border of the right ventricle (Fig. 3). The dilatation involved the main stem only and not the branches. On the saccular portion of the dilated vessel a continuous thrill was palpable that disappeared after temporary clamping of the coronary artery. Since there were no signs of myocardial ischaemia at the apex due to this procedure, the coronary artery was doubly ligated at its point of entrance into the aneurysm. The previously distended sac could now easily be pressed in by the finger, but it slowly filled up again from the back. This was thought to be caused by

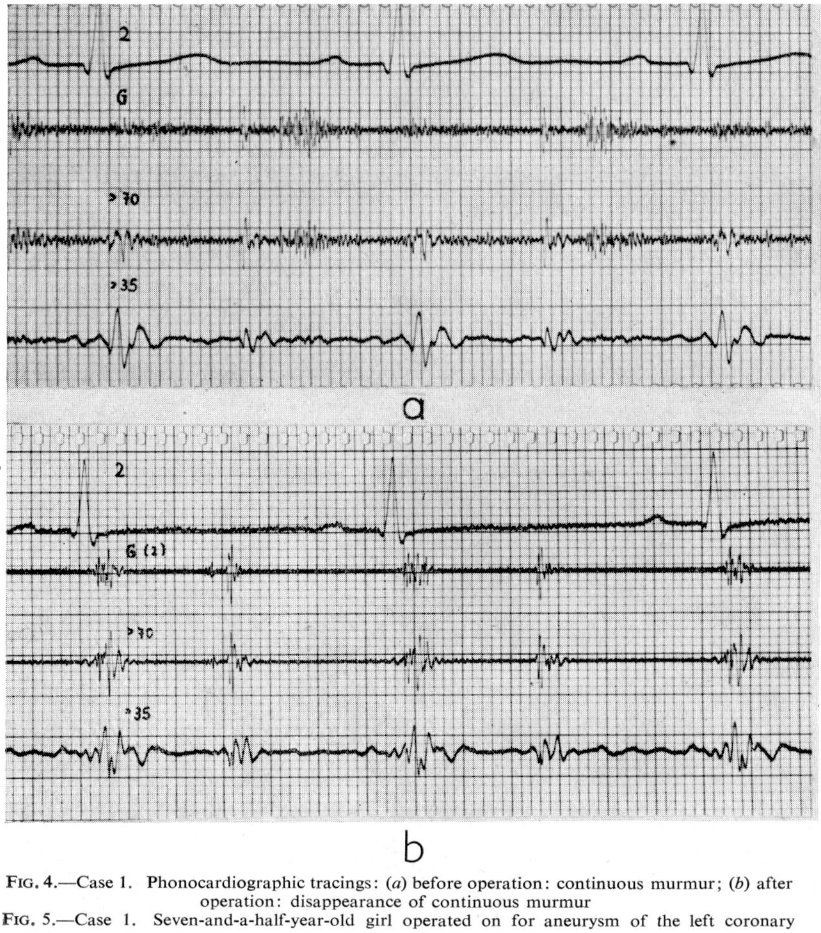

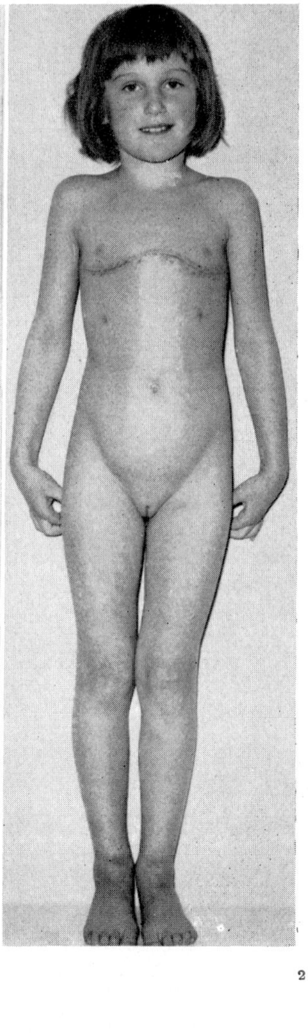

FIG. 4.—Case 1. Phonocardiographic tracings: (*a*) before operation: continuous murmur; (*b*) after operation: disappearance of continuous murmur

FIG. 5.—Case 1. Seven-and-a-half-year-old girl operated on for aneurysm of the left coronary artery.

a communication with the right ventricle, although angiocardiography failed to demonstrate this with certainty. Instead of resecting the thin-walled sac, we decided to invaginate it and to suture the margins obliquely with a row of interrupted silk sutures. The post-operative course was uneventful. Before the patient's discharge from hospital the continuous murmur could no longer be heard or demonstrated by phonocardiographic tracings (Fig. 4) and her condition was satisfactory (Fig. 5).

Case 2. A 14-year-old boy was referred to hospital owing to a precordial murmur apparent since the age of 1 year, on the basis of which a patent ductus had been assumed. His growth and development had been normal. In the last few years exercise tolerance seemed to have slightly decreased. Cyanosis and dyspnoea at rest were always absent. Physical examination revealed a continuous murmur over the heart the maximal intensity of which was located in the third intercostal space at the right sternal border. Right heart catheterization showed increased oxygen saturation of 89% in the right ventricle. Contrast visualization of the cardiac chambers performed by injection of Ioduron 70% into the right ventricle failed to reveal the lesion with clarity.

At probatory thoracotomy an obliterated Botallo's ligament was encountered. Over the heart, however, a harsh thrill was palpable which at first suggested arterio-pulmonary fistula. After incision of the pericardium we ascertained that the continuous thrill was not located in the pulmonary artery, but in an aneurysm of the right coronary artery situated immediately below the origin of this vessel. Furthermore, the left coronary artery was also anomalous, showing diffuse serpentine dilatation (Figs. 6 and 7). In view of these anatomical findings ligation of the aneurysm was not deemed advisable.

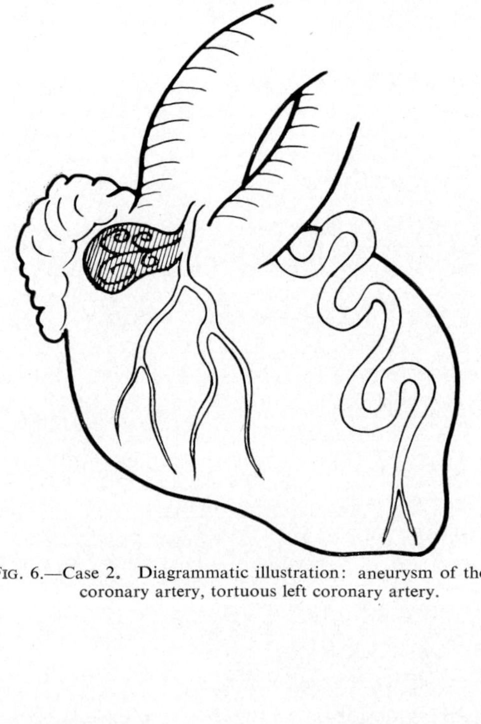

FIG. 6.—Case 2. Diagrammatic illustration: aneurysm of the right coronary artery, tortuous left coronary artery.

Discussion

In the literature of the last century we already find a few reports of similar cases (Brooks, 1886; and those of the following authors cited by Packard and Wechsler (1929): Peste, 1843; Peacock, 1846-48, 1849; Wood, 1860; Büchner, 1867; Gee, 1871; Crisp, 1871; Malet and Evans, 1887; Capps, 1899). Packard and Wechsler collected 30 cases with localized aneurysms of the coronary arteries, most of them being arteriosclerotic or mycotic in origin. These authors did not consider the possibility of congenital origin in their cases. Scott (1948), in reviewing the literature recorded a total of 48 cases, including the 30 cases mentioned by Packard and Wechsler. Ten of these cases Scott attributed to congenital anomalies. In most of them, however, the investigations were rather poor and therefore they will be omitted here. Scott himself collected 10 cases with congenital aneurysms, five of which were localized and five diffuse forms. In the others the aneurysms were thought to be acquired during later life. One of these cases (Trevor, 1912) enumerated by Scott together with the mycotic-embolic aneurysms we shall add to the congenital

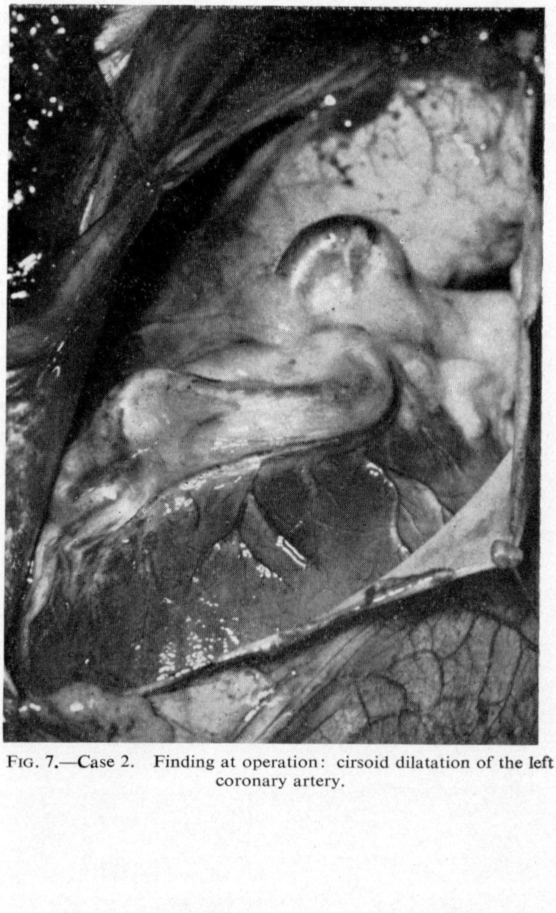

FIG. 7.—Case 2. Finding at operation: cirsoid dilatation of the left coronary artery.

aneurysms, as it presented convincing features of a congenital malformation of the coronary arteries.

Since Scott's review 21 cases of congenital aneurysms of the coronary arteries have been published, most of them showing an abnormal communication with other parts of the heart (cf. Brown and Burnett, 1949; Paul, Sweet and White, 1949; Gross, personal communication; Espino Vela, Velazquez and Fuenmayor, 1951; Baylis and Campbell, 1952; Colbeck and Shaw, 1954; Lovitt and Lutz, 1954; Davison, McCracken and McIlveen, 1955; Sondergaard, 1955; Davis, Dillon, Fell and Gasul, 1956; Knoblich and Rawson, 1956; Mozen, 1956; Apley, Horton and Wilson, 1957; Michel and Herbst, 1957; Walther, Starkey, Zervopolus and Gibbons, 1957; Edwards, Gladding and Weir, 1958; Steinberg, Baldwin and Dotter, 1958; Garomella, personal communication; Gasul, Fell and Dillon, personal communication; Morrow, personal communication). Furthermore we found four other cases reported before this review which Scott did not consider (Blakeway, 1918; Björk and Crafoord, 1947; Emminger, 1947; Valdivia, Rowe and Angevine, 1947). They raise the number of accounts of congenital aneurysms published in the last 50 years to 36.

Up to recent years the malformation in question was detected only at autopsy and was more or less of academic interest. Today cardiological investigations are able to detect the condition during life and to select the cases amenable to surgery. In a few cases the condition was discovered by chance at thoracotomy. At an operation performed for suspected patent ductus Björk and Crafoord (1947) discovered an aneurysm of the left coronary artery with a fistula to the pulmonary artery. Ligation of both the ductus and the coronary fistula was successful. Since that time there have been several case reports (Gross, personal communication; Sondergaard, 1955; Mozen, 1956; Davis, Dillon, Fell and Gasul, 1956; Walther, Starkey, Zervopolus and Gibbons, 1957) in which the diagnosis of suspected ductus led to thoracotomy. But in all these cases instead of the expected ductus, a fistulous communication between the coronary vessels and other parts of the heart was found.

In the case of Michel and Herbst (1957) a large fistula between an anomalous coronary artery and the pulmonary conus was discovered at an operation performed on a child with tetralogy of Fallot. Clamping of this vessel caused cardiac arrest, and therefore surgery was restricted to valvulotomy of the pulmonary artery.

In a patient with a continuous murmur over the heart Walther *et al.* (1957) were able to withdraw highly oxygenated blood out of the middle cardiac vein during cardiac catheterization. On the strength of this finding Walther assumed the presence of a communication between the coronary vein and a coronary artery.

In the absence of surgical intervention, however, diagnosis can only be established by angiocardiography. In Steinberg, Baldwin and Dotter's (1958) case, venous angiocardiography revealed a cluster of large coiled vessels below the left ventricle. Similarly in the case of Gasul, Fell and Dillon an aneurysm of the right coronary artery was demonstrated by contrast visualization, and at least in our first case the same technique was used with success.

Another possibility of roentgenologic investigation is offered by retrograde aortography. By means of this technique Morrow was able to demonstrate an anomalous communication between the aorta and the right atrium. Surgical exploration identified the suspected coronary aneurysm with an arteriovenous fistula, which could be closed at its right atrial aspect.

Pathological features in the 36 cases published during the last 50 years consisted either in localized, saccular, or in diffuse dilatations, involving the right coronary artery in 19 cases, the left in 15 cases; in one case both the right and the left coronary artery was affected (Rigden and Vandergriff, 1943) and in one localization was not specified (Walther *et al.*, 1957). In 32 cases a communication to other parts of the heart was demonstrated, in 10 to the right ventricle, in six to the pulmonary artery, in five to the right atrium, in four to the coronary sinus, in four to a coronary vein, in two to the left ventricle, and in one to the left atrium. The fistulous communication may be small and therefore overlooked. In the cases without any fistula, the aneurysmal dilatation may be the result of congenital defects involving especially the elastic tissue of these vessels (Forbus, 1930; Lepow, Chu and Muren, 1958).

Coronary aneurysms with fistulous connexion to the cardiac chambers or other structures of the heart have been explained aetiologically on the basis of the embryological studies by Grant and Viko (1929).

The myocardial vessels are derived from two sources. In the first foetal period blood supply to the myocardium is furnished by endothelial-lined channels protruding from the ventricular cavity into the intermuscular spaces, forming a vascular network. The other source is derived from the coronary arteries and veins growing as buds out of the truncus arteriosus and the sinus venosus during the second to the fourth week of foetal life, at the same time as the aorto-pulmonary septum is beginning to develop. First, the coronary arteries and veins expand at the surface of the myocardium to join later the intertrabecular blood spaces. Gradually this vascular network develops into capillaries, some of them, however, retaining larger communications with the ventricular cavities, known as the Thebesian orifices of the adult heart. These openings may have a diameter up to 1 mm.

Abnormal development of the vascular system may occur at different stages and involve different parts of the myocardial vessels. Abnormal localization of the buds of the coronary arteries at the common trunk will result in anomalous origin of these vessels, i.e. from the pulmonary artery. If the narrowing of the intermuscular blood spaces fails, sponge-like sinusoids in the myocardial wall, with large communications both with the coronary vessels and with the cardiac cavities, will persist (Wilson and Grant, 1926 ; Grant, 1926). If disturbance of regression is limited to one Thebesian vessel, an isolated fistula between the coronary arteries and the cardiac chambers will be the result. Blood flow from the high to the low pressure system will be increased and therefore dilatation of the affected vessel becomes more and more marked in the course of time. Given sufficient shunt-volume action over a long period of time, ventricular hypertrophy and heart failure are inevitable. In addition, blood supply to the myocardium in the area of the fistula will be decreased, as the fistulous vessel derives blood from the branches connected with it. This fact is proved by electrocardiographic tracings as well as by histological examinations of the myocardium, which in some cases exhibits signs of ischaemic injury.

The malformation, however, need not result in functional disability, especially not during pregnancy. Generally a murmur over the heart, detected by chance, is the reason for cardiac investigations. In cases with a coronary fistula a continuous murmur similar to the finding in patent ductus may be present, especially if the fistula leads to the pulmonary trunk. The site of maximal intensity, however, mostly differs from the finding in patent ductus, as it depends on the localization of the aneurysm. Therefore it may be heard best lower at the sternal border, on the sternum or even at its right margin. In phonocardiographic tracings, maximal amplitude of the continuous murmur does not occur together with the second heart sound as in Botallo's duct, but in the middle or late diastole.

Two other lesions capable of producing similar murmurs play a part in differential diagnosis : a ruptured aneurysm of the sinus of Valsalva and an aortico-pulmonary septal defect. Although cardiac catheterization may reveal the presence of a left-to-right shunt, correct non-surgical diagnosis with exclusion of other lesions accompanying shunt, is possible only with the help of angiocardiography or aortography as proved by our first case and the reports of Steinberg *et al.* (1958), Gasul *et al.* (personal communication), and Morrow (personal communication).

Summary

Two cases of aneurysms of the coronary arteries are reported. In the first case the aneurysm was localized at the left coronary artery, in the second both the right and the left coronary artery were affected.

Thirty-six cases in the literature of the last 50 years are collected, whose pathological features are summarized. In most of the cases diagnosis was established only at autopsy, and in some cases published during the last few years at thoracotomy, which was mostly performed for suspected ductus arteriosus. It must be assumed that this malformation occurs more frequently than is commonly believed.

As in many cases the main clinical finding consists of a continuous murmur over the heart, the presence of a coronary aneurysm should be taken into account simultaneously with other conditions causing a continuous murmur, especially if the localization of the murmur is unusual.

It is pointed out that modern cardiac investigations, above all angiocardiography, are able to establish a correct non-surgical diagnosis, which is illustrated by the first case reported herein.

References

Apley, J., Horton, R. E. and Wilson, M. G. (1957). *Thorax*, **12**, 28.
Baylis, J. H. and Campbell, M. (1952). *Guy's Hosp. Rep.*, **101**, 174.
Björk, G. and Crafoord, C. (1947). *Thorax*, **2**, 65.
Blakeway, H. (1918). *J. Anat. (Lond.)*, **52**, 354.
Brooks, H. St. John (1886). *Ibid.*, **20**, 26.
Brown, R. C. and Burnett, J. D. (1949). *Pediatrics*, **3**, 597.
Büchner (1867). (Cited by Packard and Wechsler.) *Aneurysma der Arteria coronaria cordis sinistra.* Vander Post, Amsterdam.
Capps, J. A. (1899). (Cited by Packard and Wechsler.) *Amer. J. med. Sci.*, **118**, 312.
Colbeck, J. C. and Shaw, J. M. (1954). *Amer. Heart J.*, **48**, 270.
Crisp, E. (1871). (Cited by Packard and Wechsler.) *Trans. path. Soc. Lond.*, **22**, 106.
Davison, P. H., McCracken, B. H. and McIlveen, D. J. S. (1955). *Brit. Heart J.*, **17**, 569.
Edwards, J. E., Gladding, T. C. and Weir, A. B. (1958). *J. thorac. Surg.*, **35**, 662.
Emminger, E. (1947). *Klin. Med. (Wien)*, **2**, 652.
Espino Vela, J., Velazquez, T. and Fuenmayor, A. (1951). (Cited by Edwards *et al.*) *Arch. Inst. Cardiol. Méx.*, **21**, 686.
Forbus, W. D. (1930). *Bull. Johns Hopk. Hosp.*, **47**, 239.
Garomella, J. J. Personal communication. (Cited by Edwards *et al.*)
Gasul, B. M., Fell, E. H. and Dillon, R. F. Personal communication. (Cited by Edwards *et al.*)
Gee, S. J. (1871). (Cited by Packard and Wechsler.) *St Bart's Hosp. Rep.*, **7**, 148.
Grant, R. T. (1926). *Heart*, **13**, 273.
—— and Viko, L. E. (1929). *Ibid.*, **15**, 103.

Gross, R. E. Personal communication. (Cited by Paul *et al.*)
Knoblich, R. and Rawson, A. J. (1956). *Amer. Heart J.*, **52**, 474.
Lepow, H., Chu, F. and Muren, O. (1958). *Amer. J. Med.*, **24**, 631.
Lovitt, W. V. Jr. and Lutz, S. (1954). *A.M.A. Arch. Path.*, **57**, 163.
Malet and Evans, A. (1887). (Cited by Packard and Wechsler.) *Lancet*, **2**, 67.
Michel, D. and Herbst, M. (1957). *Z. Kreisl.-Forsch.*, **46**, 538.
Morrow, A. G. Personal communication. (Cited by Edwards *et al.*)
Mozen, H. E. (1956). *Ann. Surg.*, **144**, 215.
Packard, M. and Wechsler, H. F. (1929). *Arch. intern. Med.*, **43**, 1.
Paul, O., Sweet, R. H. and White, P. D. (1949). *Amer. Heart J.*, **37**, 441.
Peacock (1846-48). (Cited by Packard and Wechsler.) *Trans. path. Soc. Lond.*, **1**, 227.
—— (1849). (Cited by Packard and Wechsler.) *Ibid.*, **9**, 592.
Peste (1843). (Cited by Packard and Wechsler.)
Rigdon, R. H. and Vandergriff, H. (1943). *Amer. J. Surg.*, **61**, 407.
Scott, D. H. (1948). *Amer. Heart J.*, **36**, 403.
Sondergaard, T. (1955). In *Henry Ford Hospital International Symposium on Cardiovascular Surgery*, ed. C. R. Lam, p. 490. Saunders, Philadelphia.
Steinberg, I., Baldwin, J. S. and Dotter, C. T. (1958). *Circulation*, **17**, 372.
Trevor, R. S. (1911-12). *Proc. roy. Soc. Med.*, **5**, pt. 1 (section for the study of disease in children), p. 20.
Valdivia, E., Rowe, G. G. and Angevine, D. M. (1957). *Arch. Path. (Chicago)*, **63**, 168.
Walther, R. J., Starkey, G. W. B., Zervopolus, E. and Gibbons, G. A. (1957). *Amer. J. Med.*, **22**, 213.
Wilson, J. G. and Grant, R. T. (1926). *Heart*, **12**, 295.
Wood (1860). (Cited by Packard and Wechsler.) *N.Y. med. J.*, **8**, 384.

LUNG HERNIA
SECONDARY TO CONGENITAL ABSENCE OF RIBS*

BY

P. P. RICKHAM

From Alder Hey Children's Hospital, Liverpool

It is usually assumed that lung hernia secondary to congenital absence of ribs is a great rarity. Peräsalo and Laustela (1956) describing the latest published case, of a man aged 28 years, could not find any reference to this deformity in the literature and only one of the recently published books on paediatric surgery (Swenson, 1958) mentions the malformation.

Perusal of the literature, however, does indicate that lung herniae are not so very uncommon. The earliest reported case is that by Rolland, writing in Guy de Chauliac's 'System of Surgery', in 1499. All early reports concerned lung hernias secondary to trauma or disease of the thoracic wall. The first congenital case to be reported was that of Morel-Lavallée in 1847. By 1933 Goodman was able to collect 172 cases of lung hernias of all types from the literature; about 18% of these were congenital.

In practically all the congenital herniae of the lung reported in the literature the defect in the thoracic wall was small. In some the defect was due to absence of the para-sternal ends of one or two ribs; lung hernia secondary to complete absence of ribs is uncommon. Absent ribs are, of course, frequently encountered and are often associated with spinal deformities, but it is usually the first, second, eleventh or twelfth ribs which are absent, and absence of the most proximal or distal ribs does not commonly produce lung hernia. Few of the cases reported in the literature seem to have given rise to important symptoms during early infancy. The bulging hernia and paradoxical respiration were noticed, but the infants do not seem to have been unduly distressed. In later life, however, respiratory distress, cough, recurrent bronchitis and pain are common symptoms and have often necessitated operative correction.

Various methods have been used in the treatment of congenital lung hernia. Tight bandaging of the chest wall does not appear to have been any good and has occasionally produced marked distress. Fascia lata grafts (D'Abreu, 1953) are only practicable for small defects and unsuitable for growing infants. Bone graft operations have been performed, either free bone grafts from other parts of the skeleton (Peräsalo and Laustela, 1956) or from adjacent ribs (Montgomery and Lutz, 1925).

At the time when the case described below was operated upon we were unaware of the methods of treatment reported in the literature.

Case Report

K.A., a baby girl, was born on April 18, 1957. An enormous lung hernia was easily seen and the child suffered immediate acute respiratory distress and needed to be continuously nursed in oxygen. Even in oxygen the infant had repeated severe attacks of cyanosis, and became very distressed whilst feeding. During the succeeding weeks she improved greatly and it was possible to nurse her out of oxygen, but she had recurrent attacks of bronchopneumonia, did not gain weight and became cyanosed and distressed when feeding or crying.

She was referred to Alder Hey Children's Hospital when 7 weeks old. On examination the child's state of nutrition was poor. There was a very large bulge over the left side of the thorax, which was tympanic and showed paradoxical respiratory movements. These movements were exaggerated when the child cried and she became cyanosed when crying. Clinically the patient was found to have complete absence of the left sixth, seventh, eighth, ninth and tenth ribs; this was confirmed radiologically. There was a marked right thoracic scoliosis.

Radiography of the chest confirmed the absence of five ribs of the left side, and showed the fifth rib to be broader than normal. The associated spinal scoliosis was due to wedging of the sixth to tenth thoracic vertebrae The clinical and radiographic defects are shown on p. 16.

Because of the child's failure to thrive and her repeated attacks of bronchopneumonia it was decided to attempt surgical correction of the deformity. At operation under endotracheal nitrous oxide and oxygen anaesthesia, with continuous intravenous succinyl-choline administration and controlled respiration, the thoracic wall defect was exposed through an oblique incision across the maximum convexity of the bulge. The fifth, eleventh and twelfth

* A paper read at a meeting of the British Association of Paediatric Surgeons held in London in July, 1958.

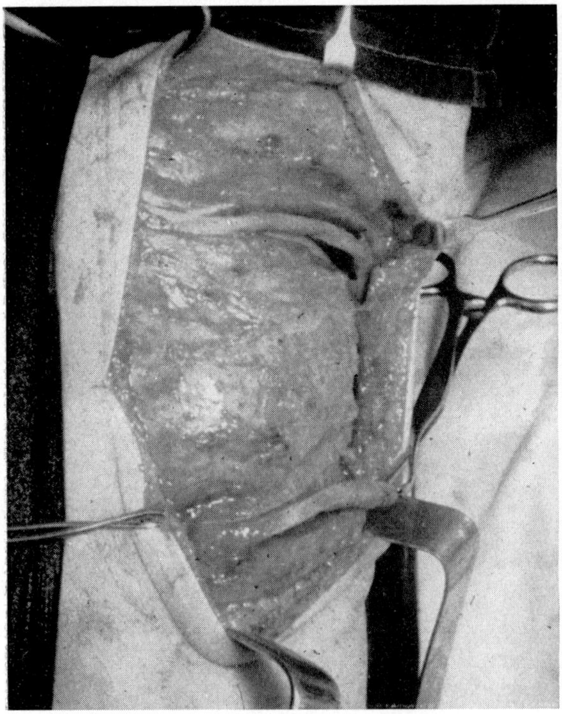

FIG. 1.—The 5th, 11th and 12th ribs are exposed.

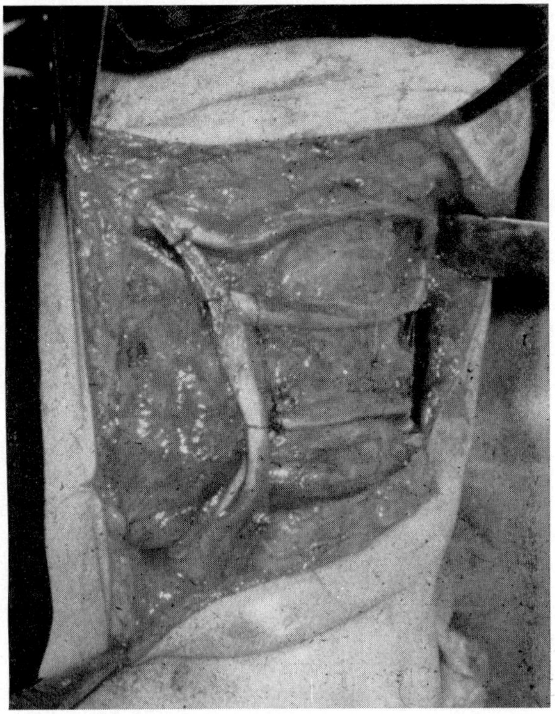

FIG. 2.—The rib grafts have been fixed to each other.

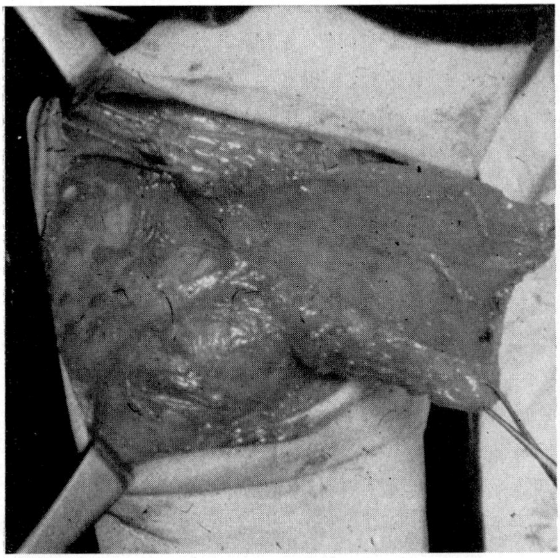

FIG. 3.—The external oblique muscle is elevated after dividing its insertion into the rectus sheath.

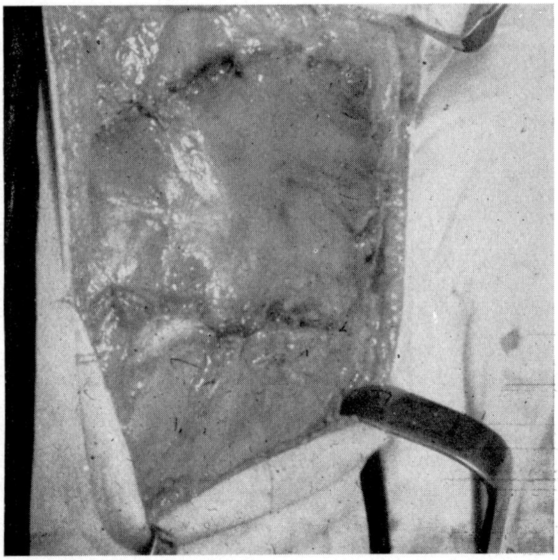

FIG. 4.—The external oblique muscle has been flapped backwards and is sewn across the defect.

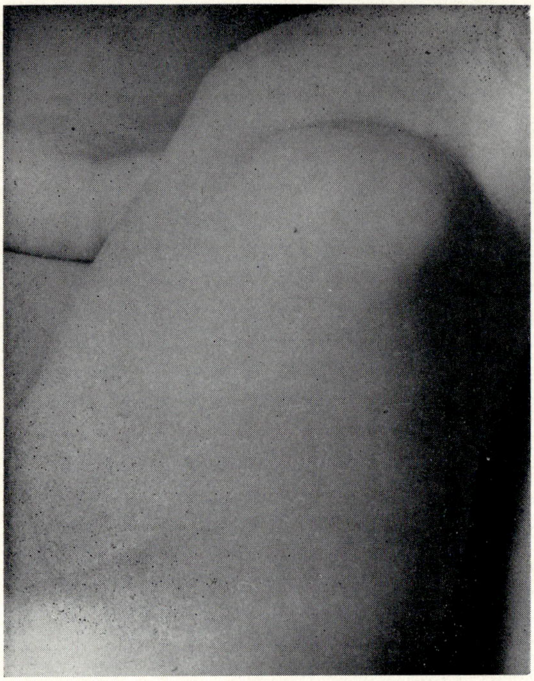

FIG. 5.—The bulging lung hernia.

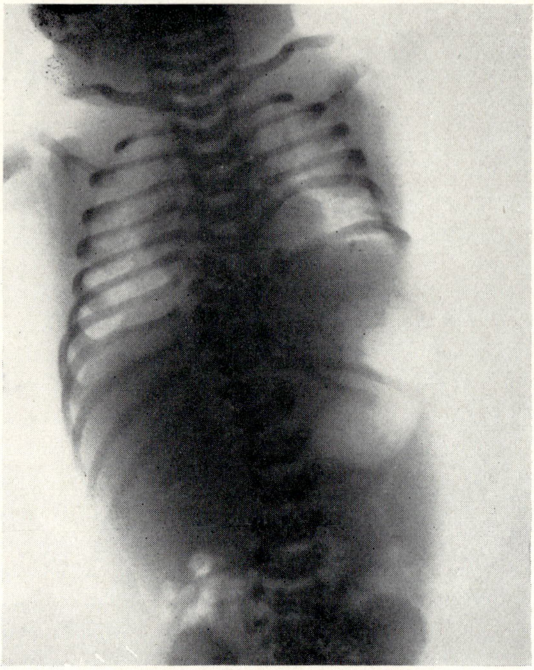

FIG. 6.—Pre-operative radiograph.

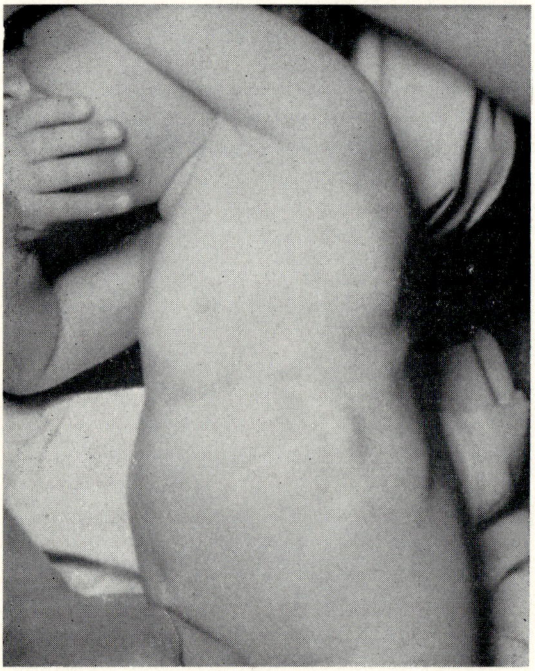

FIG. 7.—Post-operative appearance, one year after operation.

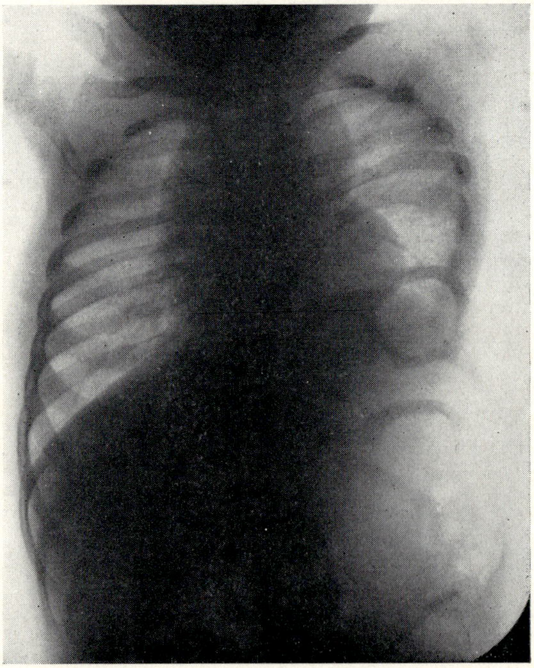

FIG. 8.—Post-operative radiograph one year after operation.

ribs were exposed (Fig. 1). Because of the great size of the defect and the youth of the patient it was decided not to attempt repair with a free fascia lata graft nor to employ any plastic materials. The fifth rib was split longitudinally with a fine saw, taking care that the periostium remained attached to both halves of the rib. The extreme anterior and posterior ends of the rib were not divided. With the aid of pericostal nylon sutures it was possible to pull the lower half of the fifth rib downwards towards the eleventh rib. The eleventh rib was similarly split, but this time the posterior end of the the upper half of the rib was divided, swung around its anterior attachment and stitched to the anterior extremity of the fifth rib thus forming a costal margin. Because of the shortness of the eleventh rib this artificial costal margin was, however, situated more posteriorly than the costal margin on the opposite side (Fig. 2). The whole insertion of the left external oblique muscle to the rectus sheath was then divided, the muscle was dissected out and reflected backwards across the whole of the thoracic wall defect (Fig. 3). It was then stitched to the surrounding muscles (Fig. 4). The wound was closed without drainage.

The child stood the operation well and there was no respiratory difficulty during the post-operative period. Since then she has developed satisfactorily and there are now no paradoxical movements on the left side of the chest. The posterior displacement of the left costal margin is, however, noticeable, and is accentuated by the thoracic scoliosis. Radiography of the chest one year after operation shows that the rib grafts have survived. Clinically the child's condition is very satisfactory. The clinical and radiographic appearances before and after operation are shown in Figs. 5, 6, 7 and 8.

There is little doubt that lung hernia secondary to congenital absence of ribs is more common than is realized. Extensive defects like the one described in this paper appear, however, to be uncommon and as they are liable to endanger the child's life during infancy, operative correction is advisable. The operative procedure reported here has produced a gratifying result.

Summary

A case of extensive pulmonary hernia secondary to congenital absence of five ribs is reported, and the surgical correction of the malformation is described. The literature is briefly reviewed.

I should like to thank Dr. Ann McCandless who referred the case to me, and Dr. G. Jackson Rees for the skilfully administered anaesthetic.

References

D'Abreu, A. L. (1953). *A Practice of Thoracic Surgery.* Arnold, London.

Goodman, H. I. (1933). *J. thorac. Surg.*, **2**, 368.

Montgomery, J. G. and Lutz, H. (1925). *Ann. Surg.*, **82**, 220.

Morel-Lavallée, J. (1847). *Mém. Soc. Chir., Paris*, **1**, 75.

Peräsalo, O. and Laustela, E. (1956). *Ann. Chir. Gynaec. Fenn.*, **45**, 303.

Rolland (1499). In Guy de Chauliac's *System of Surgery.*

Swenson, O. (1958). *Pediatric Surgery.* Appleton-Century Croft Inc., New York.

A SUBHYOID MEDIAN ECTOPIC THYROID*

BY

JOHN GRIEVE

From the Department of Surgery, Queen's College, Dundee and Dundee Royal Infirmary (University of St. Andrews)

An extensive literature exists on the anomalies of the thyroglossal duct and of lateral aberrant thyroid tissue. Apart from lingual thyroid the median ectopic gland receives little attention. The following is an example of a median subhyoid ectopic thyroid.

At intervals the boy reports and in August, 1956 (Fig. 1) he had grown normally and the thyroid had increased to 3 cm. in diameter. He continued to develop and left school at 15 to become a butcher's apprentice. The thyroid is now (June, 1958), 4 cm. in diameter (Fig. 2).

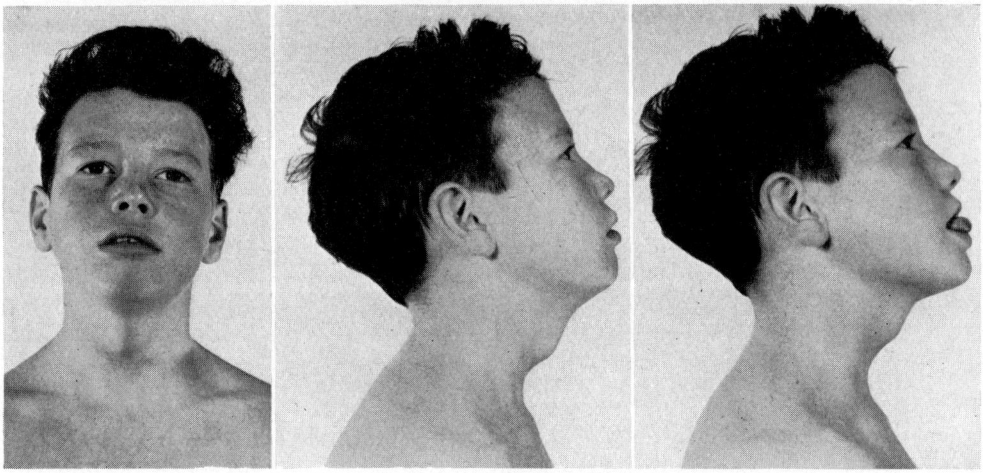

FIG. 1.—Frontal and profile views of median ectopic thyroid in August, 1956.

Case Report

In the summer of 1953 W.C.D. (born June 24, 1942) attended as a surgical out-patient. He had a midline subhyoid swelling 2 cm. in diameter, present since birth and like a thyroglossal cyst. Over the years it had increased in size in proportion to his general growth. His development was normal for an 11-year-old and his parents and older sister had no defects.

At operation on December 5, 1953, the swelling was exposed by a transverse incision. It was not a thyroglossal cyst but a normal thyroid gland and this was confirmed by vertical splitting. Behind the main swelling was a small 3 mm. gland which appeared to be a parathyroid. The normal thyroid site showed no sign of a gland and the median subhyoid swelling was left undisturbed.

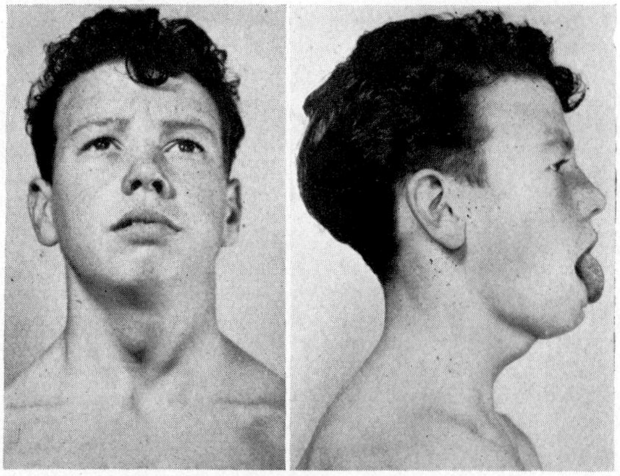

FIG. 2.—Frontal and profile views of median ectopic thyroid in June, 1958.

* A paper read at the meeting of the British Association of Paediatric Surgeons held in London in July, 1958.

Discussion

The median cervical aberrant thyroid receives little attention. Gross (1953) noted three cases in Boston Children's Hospital. All were identified as thyroglossal cysts until operation. They were left but the cosmetic result was improved by splitting the gland in half and burying the halves beneath their respective sternohyoid muscles. Werner (1955) suggested a classification of median aberrant thyroids and on this basis the present patient had a subhyoid median ectopic thyroid. That this anomaly is uncommon is shown by Levitt's (1956) experience. In his long series of normal and abnormal thyroids he saw no median subhyoid glands. The only treatment which this boy might require would be to split the gland and bury the two halves beneath the sternohyoid muscles. This would resolve any shaving difficulties !

Summary

A boy aged 11 years had a median subhyoid ectopic thyroid gland which was believed to be a thyroglossal cyst. He had no other thyroid tissue but has developed normally and the gland has increased in size in proportion to his body growth.

Mr. Murray Ettle, Department of Surgery, Queen's College, did the photography.

REFERENCES

Gross, R. (1953). *The Surgery of Infancy and Childhood.* Saunders: London.
Levitt, T. (1956). Personal communication.
Werner, S. C. (1955). *The Thyroid.* Cassell: London.

PYLORIC STENOSIS BEFORE AND AFTER RAMSTEDT*

BY

SELWYN TAYLOR

From King's College Hospital, Belgrave Hospital for Children and the Postgraduate Medical School of London

It is a remarkable fact that a condition which occurs so commonly and is so easily diagnosed as congenital hypertrophic pyloric stenosis should only have been recognized in this country about 50 years ago. There are a few isolated accounts of the condition in the earlier literature (Patrick Blair in 1717, Christopher Weber, 1758, and Williamson, of Edinburgh, in 1841). It was, however, Hirschsprung of Copenhagen (1888) who first described the disease as we know it, illustrating his account with two case histories, relating these to the post-mortem findings.

In 1898 in London, Edmund Cautley, physician to the Belgrave Hospital for Children, presented the records of two cases of pyloric stenosis to the Medico-Chirurgical Society (later the Royal Society of Medicine); for the next 20 years he was to devote a great deal of time and energy to the problem (Cautley, 1899; Cautley and Dent, 1903; Cautley, 1904, 1906, 1908). It is interesting to trace the evolution of the treatment of this condition through the methods which he employed, or which he pursuaded surgeons to employ for him, and about which he wrote so carefully. I am able to do this through the courtesy of Mr. Ramsay, lately senior surgeon at the Belgrave Hospital, who generously bequeathed me his records and papers and those of Dr. Cautley relating to pyloric stenosis.

Treatment of pyloric stenosis in those early days was of three kinds, dilatation of the pylorus, various forms of pyloroplasty and gastro-enterostomy (Mack, 1942).

Dilatation. In 1884 Loreta, in Italy, had devised an operation for treating pyloric stenosis in adults. He incised the distal stomach and forced one or two fingers through the pylorus, thus stretching it open. It was an operation attended by uncertain results, but two surgeons in this country adapted it for use in infants with some success. In Glasgow, Nicoll (1900, 1904) used a mechanical dilator introduced through the stomach, but, being dissatisfied with the results, added a gastro-enterostomy. In London Burghard (1906), of King's College Hospital, became extremely successful with this technique. He used a vertical mid-line incision to expose the stomach, held the pylorus between the fingers of the left hand and introduced a series of Hegar's dilators through an incision in the stomach until the muscle coat was felt suddenly to give way. When divulsion occurred anteriorly, this could be seen beneath the serosal layer. Probably this was the most successful surgical treatment of pyloric stenosis at that time.

Pyloroplasty. This method of treatment was introduced by Dr. Cautley's surgical colleague, Clinton Dent (Cautley and Dent, 1903) at the Belgrave Hospital using a technique previously employed in adults by von Heineke and von Mikulicz. Dent's first successful operations were on June 10 and August 19, 1902, one of the patients being a physician's son. It still surprises me how frequently the condition is encountered in doctor's families. Dent had 10 successes and two deaths in the next five years, better results than anyone else could report.

Pyloroplasty is popularly associated with the name of the French surgeon Fredet (Fredet and Guillemot, 1910; Fredet and Farret, 1912; Fredet and Tixier, 1912), and his particular contribution was incising the muscular coat, leaving the mucosa intact (extra-mucous division) since he realized the danger of soiling the peritoneal cavity. He, however, sutured the muscularis transversely, as in the classical form of pyloroplasty, his first extra-mucous pyloroplasty being performed on October 12, 1907. In Germany, Weber (1909, 1910) independently evolved an almost identical technique, his first successful operation being on December 3, 1908. Fredet was apparently never enthusiastic about his extra-mucous pyloroplasty and continued to use gastro-enterostomy as the method of choice for treating pyloric stenosis until 1921.

* Lecture to the Fifth Annual Meeting of the British Association of Paediatric Surgeons in London on July 23, 1958.

Nicoll of Glasgow, who seems never to have obtained rightful credit for his work, also evolved a form of extra-mucous pyloroplasty which he did after the V-Y fashion and described as early as 1906. He had five successes out of six patients treated by this method; he stressed the importance of not opening the mucosa, but always combined it with a Loreta dilatation (Nicoll, 1910).

Gastro-enterostomy. This operation was still being used by most surgeons in the early years of the century for treating pyloric stenosis. The mortality rate was usually 50% or more, but the patients submitted to operation were in poor condition and little was known at this time about fluid balance. It appears that the stenosis persisted in many of these patients much longer than in those who were treated by some kind of surgical attack upon the pylorus itself. There is a wealth of interesting papers published on this subject over the last 40 years.

We come now to Dr. Conrad Ramstedt of Münster, who on August 23, 1911, performed the first operation after the fashion which most of us still follow to this day. I am delighted to tell you that Dr. Ramstedt is still alive and, at the age of 91, wrote me a vigorous and interesting letter only a few months ago. Until he was 80 he was operating regularly and was only stopped then by failing eyesight. As so many accounts of the evolution of this operation have appeared, I quote now a translation of part of a letter from him, written in 1957 to Dr. Pollock, in which he describes how he came to perform pyloromyotomy. He had been invited by the paediatrician at the children's hospital in Münster to treat congenital pyloric stenosis in the first-born son of a distinguished and noble family in the district; this was the first example of the condition he had ever seen. Having reviewed the various methods available he decided to perform a pyloroplasty by the extra-mucosal method:

> 'At the laparotomy on August 23, 1911, I was astonished at the pyloric tumour as thick as my thumb. After I had split the tumour down to the mucosa for a distance of about 2 cm., I had the impression that the stenosis had been relieved. I still tried, however, to accomplish the plastic procedure by transverse suture of the muscle edges. However, the tension on the sutures was so very strong that the first one cut through immediately. Then the thought shot through my head, "A plastic alteration of the cut edges is completely unnecessary; the stenosis seems to be already relieved by a simple splitting of the pyloric muscle and coincidently the spasm as well, which is the characteristic basis of the disease." I did not complete the plastic operation on the muscle which had been originally planned, but left the cut gaping, covering it with a tab of omentum for safety's sake and ended the operation. The little one vomited a few times for the first few days which I attributed to the sutures placed at the beginning, but he recovered promptly and completely to the great joy of his parents.'

Professor Ramstedt performed this operation for the second time on June 18, 1912, and in September of that year reported these two cases to the Natural Science Assembly at Münster (Ramstedt, 1912, 1913).

It must have puzzled many who have read his papers why Professor Ramstedt spells his name with two 'm's in the early accounts of the disease and later with only one. We are indebted to Dr. Pollock of Los Angeles (Pollock and Norris, 1957; Pollock, Norris and Gordon, 1957) for the explanation. It appears that in Germany, prior to the first World War, it was usual for the family records to be part of the Church records for occasions such as births and marriages. Prior to the first World War Ramstedt had spelt his name with two 'm's, but having become interested in his own genealogy, he was surprised to discover that his grandfather had apparently made an error in the entries in the Church records and that the family name had originally been spelt with only one 'm'. He, therefore, after 1920 changed the spelling of his name to conform with the earlier records.

Ramstedt himself described his operation as a pyloromyotomy and this remains much the best word to describe what is carried out. For those who are addicted to eponymous nomenclature, I hope I have made it clear that the rightful title is Ramstedt's operation and not Fredet-Ramstedt or even Fredet-Weber-Ramstedt.

The spread of Ramstedt's operation to other parts of the world is interesting. In the U.S.A. it was adopted very quickly, enthusiastically and successfully, and quite considerable series were reported from there by 1916. In this country the 1914-1918 war delayed its adoption and it was not until the end of the war that Dr. Cautley at the Belgrave Hospital asked his surgical colleague, Mr. Ramsay, to perform the operation. As a result the first Ramstedt operation at the hospital was on July 16, 1918. The child collapsed and died a week later, although at autopsy the stenosis was shown to have been relieved. On October 29, 1918, Ramstedt's operation was performed for the second time with complete success. Subsequently Ramsay (1919, 1921) performed this operation more than 200 times at the Belgrave Hospital with remarkable success.

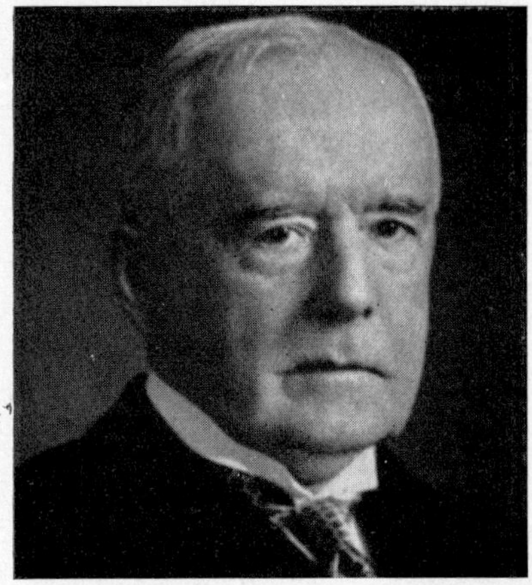

EDMUND CAUTLEY (1864-1944), Physician, Belgrave Hospital for Children, London.

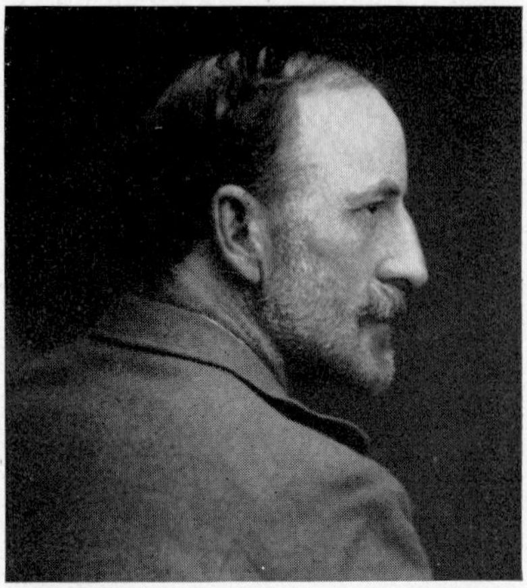

CLINTON DENT (1850-1912), Surgeon, Belgrave Hospital, London. Pyloroplasty.

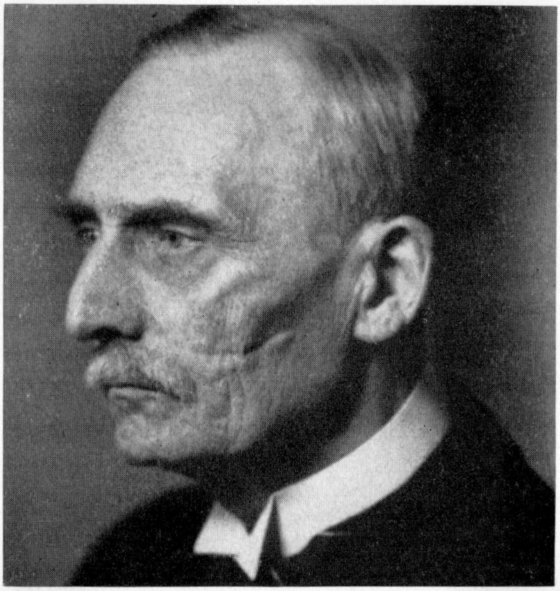

CONRAD RAMSTEDT (1867-) of Münster. Pyloromyotomy.

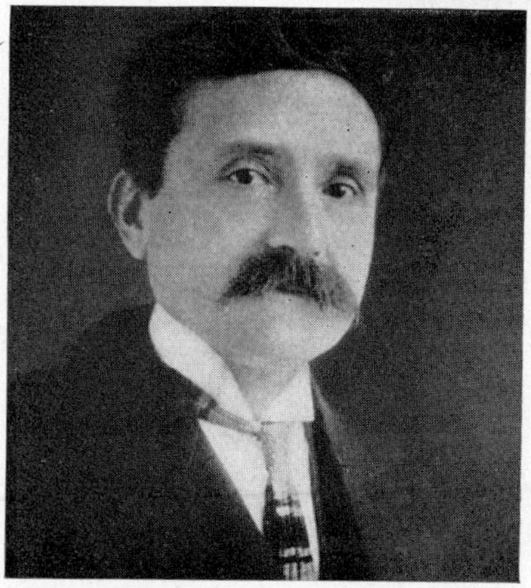

PIERRE FREDET (1870-1946) of Paris. Extramucous pyloroplasty.

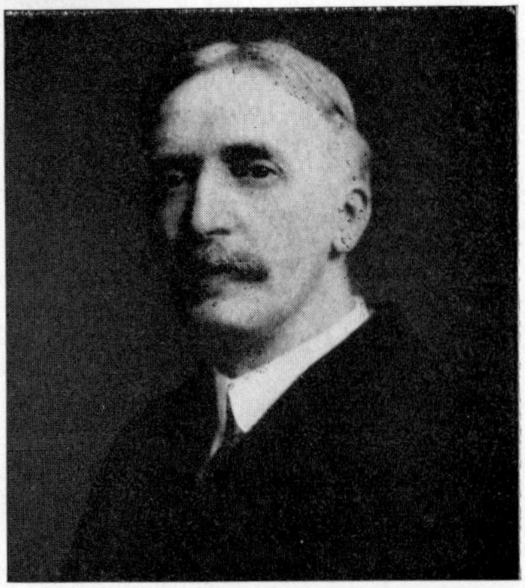

JAMES NICOLL (1864-1921) of Glasgow. V-Y pyloroplasty.

It speaks much for his skill that the notes state that he performed his first Ramstedt's operation in precisely seven minutes.

Since the cause of pyloric stenosis in infancy is unknown the treatment, whether by means of drugs or by operation, remains empirical. From the mass of papers appearing on this subject, that of Friesen, Boley and Miller (1956) in Kansas appears to offer the most rewarding approach. They studied the development of the myenteric nervous plexus in the normal human foetal pylorus and compared the findings at full term with those of biopsy carried out at Ramstedt's operation. Their findings suggest that the ganglion cells in pyloric stenosis, though present in adequate numbers, are immature. We have repeated their investigations and although we have not enough material, the present significant findings are in agreement with them. It would be in keeping with most of the observed facts if babies developed this condition because the innervation of the pylorus was 'premature'. Pooling the resources of a number of centres should make it possible to assess this theory.

REFERENCES

Blair, P. (1717). *Phil. Trans.*, **30**, 631.
Burghard, F. F. (1906). Quoted by Stiles, H. J. in *Brit. med. J.*, **2**, 943.
Cautley, E. (1899). *Med.-chir. Trans.*, **82**, 41.
—— (1904). *Brit. J. Child. Dis.*, **1**, 10.
—— (1906). *Brit. med. J.*, **2**, 939.
—— (1908). *Brit. J. Child. Dis.*, **5**, 179.
—— and Dent, C. T. (1903). *Med.-chir. Trans.*, **86**, 471.
Fredet, P. (1921). *Bull. Soc. Chir. Paris*, **47**, 451.
—— and Farret, H. (1912). *Bull. Soc. méd. Hôp. Paris*, 3 ser., **34**, 789.
—— and Guillemot, L. (1910). Congrés de Gynécologie, d'Obstétrique, et de Pédiatrie.
—— and Tixier, L. (1912). *Ibid.*, **34**, 868.
Friesen, S. R., Boley, J. O. and Miller, D. R. (1956). *Surgery*, **39**, 21.
Hirschsprung, H. (1888). *Jb. Kinderheilk.*, **27**, 1.
Loreta, P. (1884). *La divulsione digitale del piloro e la divulsione strumentale dell'esofago e del cardias invece della gastrotomia*, 2nd ed. Treves, Bologna.
—— (1887). *Gazz. Osp.*, **8**, 803.
Mack, H. C. (1942). *Bull. Hist. Med.*, **12**, 465, 595 and 666.
Nicoll, J. (1900). *Brit. med. J.*, **2**, 571.
—— (1904). *Ibid.*, **2**, 1148.
—— (1906). *Glasg. med. J.*, **65**, 253.
—— (1910). *Practitioner*, **85**, 659.
Pollock, W. F. and Norris, W. J. (1957). *Surgery*, **42**, 966.
——, —— and Gordon, H. E. (1957). *Amer. J. Surg.*, **94**, 335.
Rammstedt, C. (1912). *Med. Klin.*, **8**, 1702.
—— (1913). *Zbl. Chir.*, **40**, 3.
Ramsay, R. A. (1919). *Trans. med. Soc. Lond.*, **42**, 125.
—— (1921). *Brit. J. Surg.*, **8**, 397.
Ramstedt, C. (1922). *Zbl. Chir.*, **49**, 1329.
—— (1957). Personal communication.
Weber, C. (1758). Cited by Still, G. F. (1931). *The History of Paediatrics*, p. 400. Oxford University Press.
Weber, W. (1909). *Münch. med. Wschr.*, **56**, 1617.
—— (1910). *Berl. klin. Wschr.*, **47**, 763.
Williamson, T. (1841). *London and Edinburgh Monthly Journal of Medical Science*, **1**, 23.

COMPLICATIONS AFTER OPERATION FOR OESOPHAGEAL ATRESIA*

BY

F. REHBEIN and F. YANAGISWA

From the Surgical Department of the Children's Hospital, Bremen

Although certain advances have been made in the treatment of oesophageal atresia, there are still many problems we have to deal with. However many mistakes we learn to avoid, the possibility of complications, which may endanger a successful outcome, is still present. Gertz and Winkel Smith (1958) have already pointed out that the airing of problems is of great importance and it therefore seems justified to give a short review of the complications encountered in our patients.

It is only in the last three years that we have used the transpleural approach. In suturing we followed first the technique of Haight and Towsley (1943), Gross (1953), Swenson (1947) and others, but for two years we have preferred to use the following procedure (Fig. 1): two single stitches are inserted, and then one continuous posterior suture which is tied to the single stitches. Then the feeding tube is placed in position and the anterior wall closed with interrupted stitches. Normally we start feeding through the tube at the third day, but in cases of suture with tension we delay it till the seventh or eighth day. If tension is severe we perform a gastrostomy and also a jejunostomy.

From 1951 to 1958 we operated on 84 cases (Table 1). Eight cases which were moribund on admission or cases where only a gastrostomy was done are not included in this summary. I will come back later to the four cases without fistula, all of which died. Out of 64 anastomoses 37 survived the operation; two children died several weeks later; the remaining 35 are alive. Closure of the fistula alone without anastomosis was unsuccessful in every case. In cases where there was a wide distance between the two segments we tried to join them, using a rubber tube as a prosthesis. This technique was successful only in one case. At autopsy we could see that the distance was covered by granulation tissue, and in some cases by an epithelial layer of tissue as well. In all cases except one the tracheal-fistula had opened up. In this one case kinking of the oesophagus and fistula into the surrounding tissue had occurred (Fig. 2). Four months later this area was resected and anastomosis was performed. The latter treatment was difficult because of severe stricture.

In the recent literature mistakes and complications are often mentioned, for example by Humphreys, Hogg and Ferrer (1956), Shaw, Paulson and Siebel (1955) and particularly by Gertz and Winkel Smith (1958). Because complications in cases of anastomosis are the most interesting and also from the practical point of view the most important ones, I will only discuss our 64 anastomosed cases (Fig. 3). Out of 29 deaths 13 died of respiratory complications, 10 of suture insufficiency and recurrent fistula, and six died of other causes. This summary can only give a limited picture, because it is very rare to find that one factor alone leads to complications or death. Table 2 shows how far, for instance, the birthweight was of importance. Some of the cases died because of our lack of experience in the early years. More recently the mortality rate shows an improvement (Table 3).

The most important factors in causing death are respiratory tract complications. Quite often, on admission, atelectasis is found which can be

TABLE 1

CASES OF OESOPHAGEAL ATRESIA (1951-1958)

	Number	Survivors	Mortality (%)
With Fistula:	80	38	52
Anastomosis	64	37	43
Prosthesis (rubber tube)	9	1	89
Closure of fistula only	7	—	100
Without Fistula	4	—	100
Total	84	38	54

* A paper read at a meeting of the British Association of Paediatric Surgeons held in London in July, 1958.

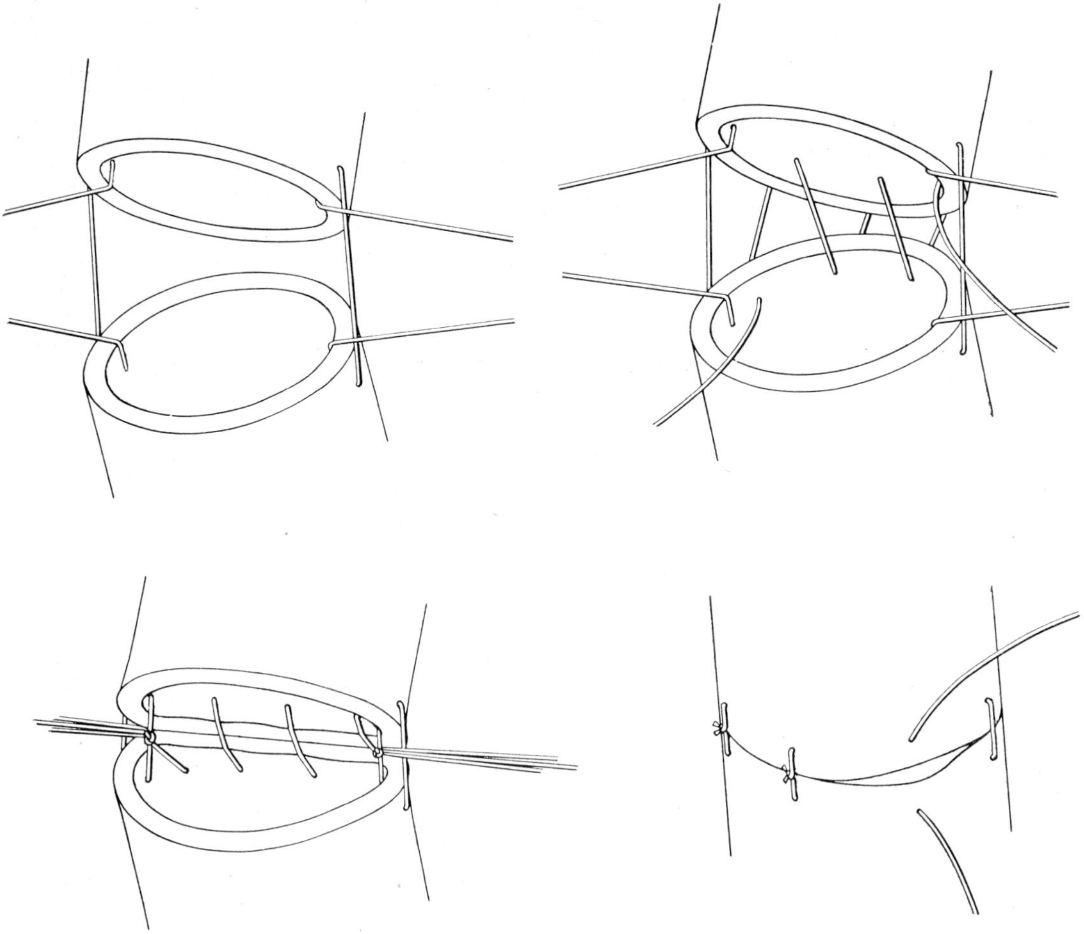

FIG. 1.—Suturing technique in oesophageal atresia.

improved or cleared up by intensive treatment. Post-operatively very often there is a large amount of secretion which leads to atelectasis and pneumonia if it is not aspirated. So it was in the majority of the 13 cases. This secretion starts on the second post-operative day and ends usually on the fourth day. Some children did not need any suction, others had to be aspirated as often as three times in 24 hours. To decide if and when suction is necessary can be done in many cases only by watching the respiration. The frequency and the type of breathing are important points as well.

TABLE 2

BIRTHWEIGHT RELATED TO RESULT OF OPERATION (64 ANASTOMOSES)

Weight (g.)	Number	Survivors	Mortality (%)
<2,000	4	—	100
2,000-2,500	27	12	56
>2,500	33	23	30

TABLE 3

CASES OF OESOPHAGEAL ATRESIA WITH TRACHEO-OESOPHAGEAL FISTULA (1951-1958)

Year	Number	Survivors	Mortality (%)
1951-1953	16	6	63
1954 ..	10	2	80
1955 ..	12	2	83
1956 ..	8	4	50
1957 ..	24	17	29
1958 ..	10	7	30
Total ..	80	38	53

Atelectasis of smaller portions of lung can usually be cleared up quite easily. A total atelectasis of one lung we could not clear up. If pneumonia was already present following atelectasis and if induration of the lung was found at operation and the lung did not collapse, the results were poor.

Tracheotomy has been performed altogether only

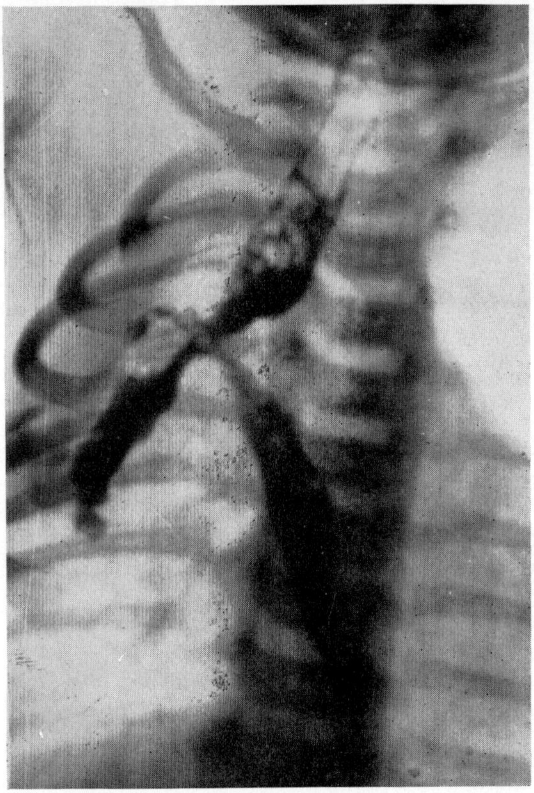

FIG. 2.—Kinking and fistula formation after approaching the oesophageal segments using a rubber tube as a guide. Healing after resection and suture.

four times in the last two years. In three cases it was necessary shortly after the operation because of severe difficulty in breathing and deep cyanosis. In spite of the stridor and cyanosis that two children showed even before operation it is presumed that endotracheal intubation caused some swelling of the mucous membranes. In one child there was so much secretion that as late as on the eleventh post-operative day a tracheotomy had to be done. All four children withstood the procedure well and we think that they were saved by it. On three occasions we had considerable difficulty in removing the tracheotomy tube. We finally succeeded after several attempts and with the help of laryngeal intubation.

Suture insufficiency and recurrent fistula can happen independently. The reopening of the tracheal fistula alone is supposedly more rare. It is due primarily in most of the cases to insufficiency of anastomosis, and local inflammation and abscess formation. This complication occurred 13 times in our 64 anastomoses. Only three of the 13 cases survived.

In one child who was operated on by the extra pleural approach we noticed leakage of air and

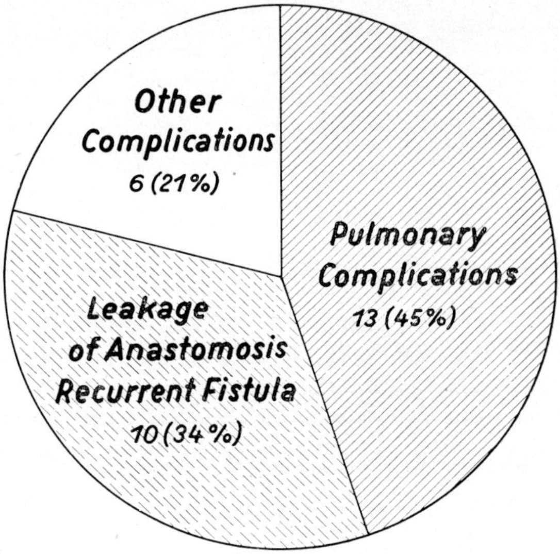

FIG. 3.—Causes of death in 29 cases (from 64 anastomoses).

contrast medium into the retropleural space on the eighth day. There was spontaneous healing.

Our first case, who is 7 years old now, had a wide suture breakdown with leakage of food into the mediastinum and then a recurrent fistula. This fistula closed up spontaneously during the next few months. Now there is still a small diverticulum in this area and the oesophagus is narrowed in one place. But the boy has no difficulty in eating and is normally developed (Fig. 4).

There were no complications at first in the third case operated on by transpleural approach. But with the start of oral feeding 14 days after the operation he suffered from coughing spells, cyanosis and abdominal distension. Radiographic examination showed a recurrent fistula. We succeeded in saving the child's life by gastrostomy and jejunal

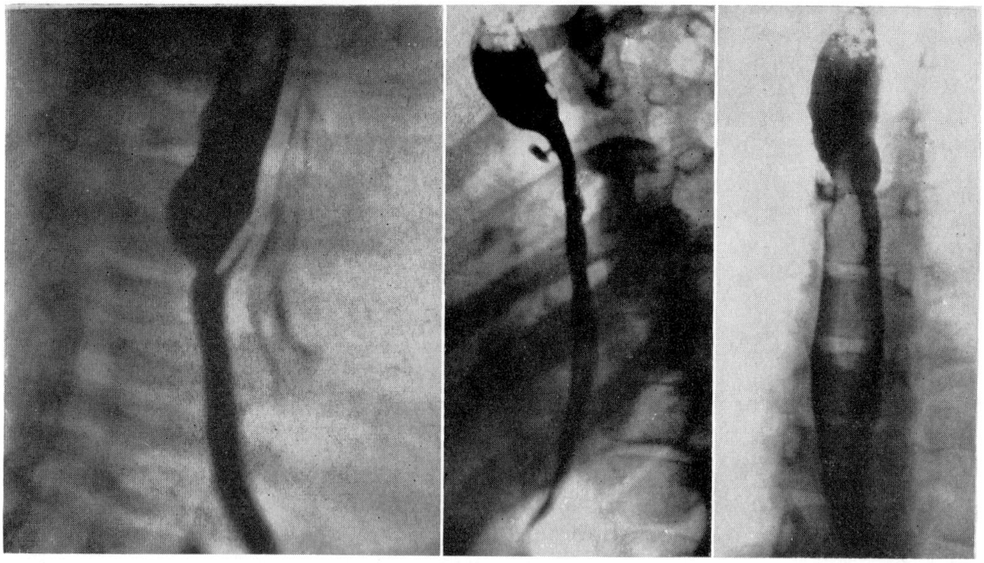

FIG. 4.—Formation of an oesophago-tracheal fistula after operation for atresia. Spontaneous healing with formation of a small diverticulum.

feeding. In spite of these measures, severe aspirations continued which retarded the child's development. Finally, at the age of 9 months, we did the second operation (Figs. 5 and 6).

A few cases where pneumothorax occurred died. Efforts to avoid aspiration by jejunal feeding in cases of insufficiency with recurrent fistula were unsuccessful except in the one case mentioned above. So we really should follow the suggestion of Shaw *et al.* (1955) and, in certain cases of suture breakdown with recurrent fistula, try as soon as possible a second suturing. According to his report Shaw was successful in a few early second operations. Success or misfortune will depend on how far there is already inflammation or abscess formation in the mediastinum. Lethal suture breakdown we only saw twice in our last 30 anastomoses. The cause of its frequent occurrence in the earlier years was probably insufficient preparation of the two parts of the oesophagus. Maybe the occurrence of suture breakdown is less dangerous when using the extrapleural approach, but in spite of that the transpleural approach is to be preferred. If there are signs of leaking at the second or third day after operation there is probably a gap between the stitches. The early leak is especially dangerous, because then no adhesions have been formed.

Among our cases we found a large number of cardiovascular defects, but in most of these cases no anastomosis could be performed. Among the 29 deaths six died of other complications (Table 4). One child died six weeks and another one 10 weeks after operation; in both cases the anastomosis had entirely healed. In the next case we diagnosed a concomitant duodenal atresia too late; here also the anastomosis was nearly healed. I just want to mention that in another child with duodenal atresia we found an extensive rupture of the stomach. In the third case a peritonitis following colostomy led to death. The last two children died of uraemia because of bilateral atresia of the ureter. Here death can only be attributed to this concomitant malformation. Three weeks after operation another child suffered from severe diarrhoea due to a necrotizing ileitis. The child's condition deteriorated rapidly, but it finally withstood the resection of the gangrenous bowel loop.

The causes of death of the four children without tracheo-oesophageal fistula are shown in Table 5.

We saw severe stenosis in two cases. These children had to stay in hospital for months and had to have intensive dilatation therapy with bougies.

TABLE 4

OTHER CAUSES OF DEATH

Osteomyelitis ..	1	Survived 6 weeks
Interstitial pneumonia	1	Survived 10 weeks
Duodenal atresia ..	1	Late diagnosis
Peritonitis	1	Imperforate anus
Uraemia	2	Congenital bilateral atresia of ureter

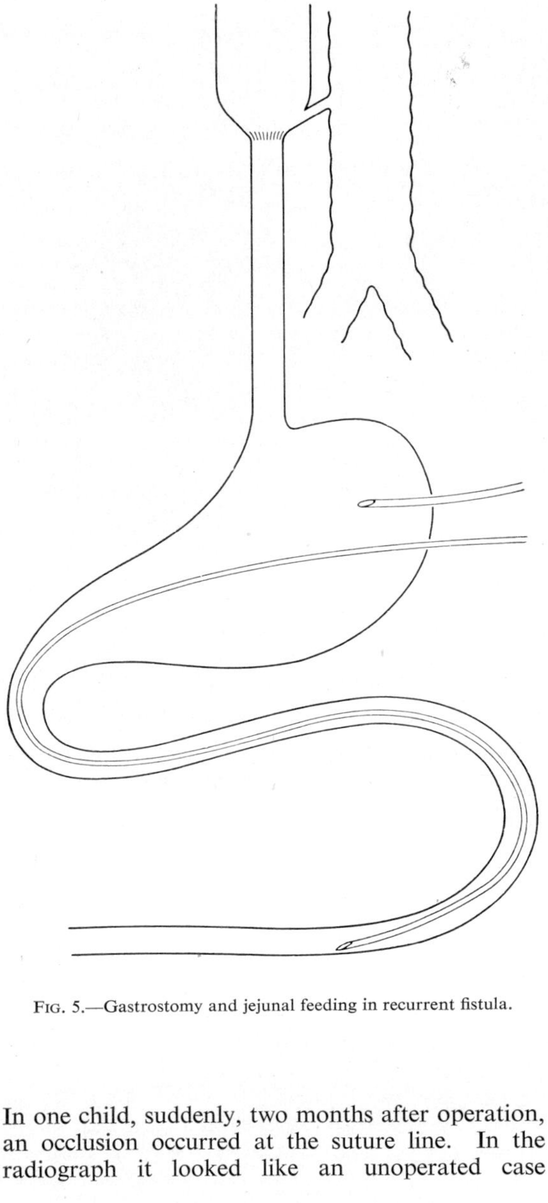

FIG. 5.—Gastrostomy and jejunal feeding in recurrent fistula.

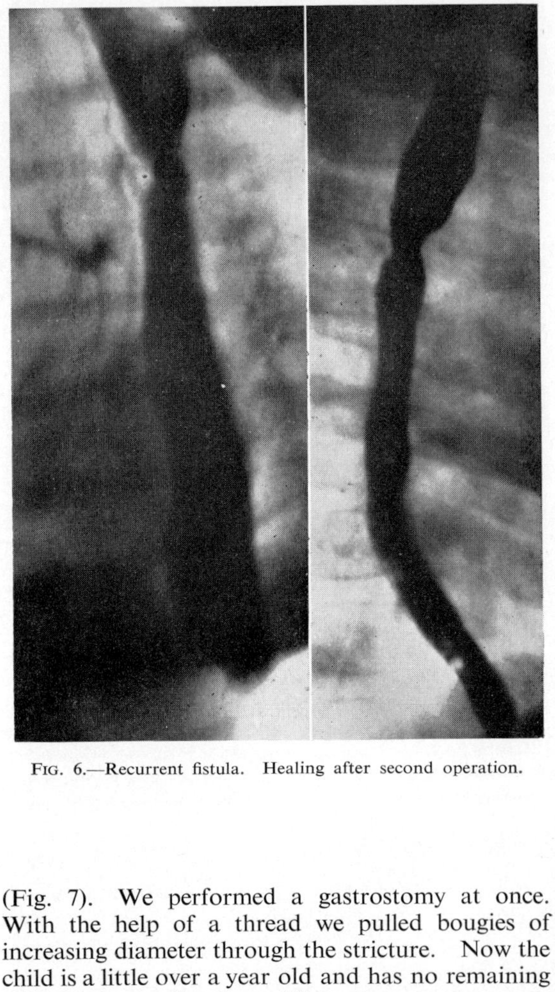

FIG. 6.—Recurrent fistula. Healing after second operation.

In one child, suddenly, two months after operation, an occlusion occurred at the suture line. In the radiograph it looked like an unoperated case (Fig. 7). We performed a gastrostomy at once. With the help of a thread we pulled bougies of increasing diameter through the stricture. Now the child is a little over a year old and has no remaining difficulty in swallowing. Slight degrees of stenosis occur more frequently, so every child gets dilatation as a routine before discharge. Frequently there are some difficulties in swallowing which can be treated easily at the age of 6 to 8 months when the food becomes more solid. In one child with recurrent aspirations a grape got stuck at the suture site and had to be removed by oesophagoscopy. In another case it was a coin that had to be removed. We have

TABLE 5

CAUSES OF DEATH IN FOUR CASES OF OESOPHAGEAL ATRESIA WITHOUT TRACHEO-OESOPHAGEAL FISTULA

(1) Peritonitis from decubitus by feeding tube
(2) Peritonitis originating from gastrostomia
(3) Death during attempt to pull stomach up to upper part of oesophagus (mongol)
(4) Arrest of breathing by compression of trachea during transposition of large bowel (age 16 months)

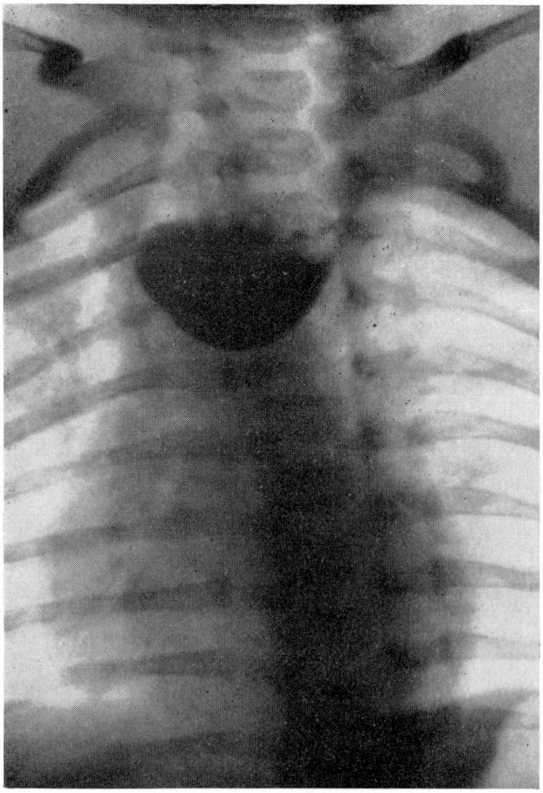

FIG. 7.—Severe stenosis two months after operation.

rarely needed to perform a gastrostomy during the last few years. In cases of severe stenosis gastrostomy is of help, as also in cases with severe aspiration.

The statistics of all those who have published the results of operating on cases with oesophageal atresia show that with growing experience the mortality rate is reduced. By improving our operative technique the number of cases in which at one time we thought joining would not be possible has become less and less. By improvement of suturing technique the number of breakdowns has also diminished. It is quite possible also that where breakdown occurs some of the cases can be saved by early repair.

Lung complications can be reduced by adequate pre- and post-operative treatment. Tracheotomy will also help to improve the final results. Deaths caused by electrolyte and fluid imbalance can be avoided.

A certain number of deaths due to inanition, cerebral bleeding, concomitant malformation and late diagnosis are inevitable and will always remain.

REFERENCES

Gertz, T. C. and Winkel Smith, C. C. (1958). *Dan. med. Bull.*, **5**, 18.
Gross, R. E. (1953). *The Surgery of Infancy and Childhood.* Saunders, Philadelphia.
Haight. C. and Towsley, H. A. (1943). *Surg. Gynec. Obstet.*, **76**, 672.
Humphreys, G. H., Hogg, B. M. and Ferrer, J. (1956). *J. thorac. Surg.*, **32**, 332.
Shaw, R. R., Paulson, D. L. and Siebel, E. K. (1955). *Ann. Surg.*, **142**, 204.
Swenson, O. (1947). *Surgery*, **22**, 324.

RUPTURE OF THE LIVER IN THE NEWBORN*

BY

ILSE WOLFROM

From the Surgical Unit, the Children's Hospital, Bremen

Rupture of the liver is a rare condition in newborn infants and most cases are diagnosed at autopsy. Only 11 instances of survival have so far been recorded, by Rogers (1934), Arden (1946, 1951), Potter (1952), Arden, Dique and Wrench (1955), Bret, Jamain and Coupé (1956), Greaves (1955), Mason Brown (1957) and Dennison, cited by Mason Brown. It therefore seems worth recording that we have encountered two cases of this condition within a period of four months. The first case was successfully treated by operation and survived, while the second died two days after operation from extensive subdural haemorrhage.

Case Histories

Case 1. (P.T.) This female infant was born spontaneously. The mother's pregnancy and labour had been uneventful. The child's birth weight was 7 lb. 6 oz. She was perfectly well during the first three days of life. At 80 hours of age, the infant suddenly turned pale and limp after being put to the breast. She was transferred to the surgical unit of the Children's Hospital at Bremen.

She was extremely pale and her breathing was shallow and irregular. One hour later the abdomen became distended. Blood picture: haemoglobin, 62%; erythrocytes, 2·8 millions; Coombs test negative. A diagnosis of intraperitoneal haemorrhage was made and the baby was given a transfusion of blood (200 ml.) preoperatively.

At operation a large quantity of fluid blood escaped from the peritoneal cavity and was found to be coming from a tear about half an inch long near the lower border of the right lobe of the liver (Figs. 1a and b). The wound was sutured with chromic catgut.

During the 24 hours after operation the child vomited small amounts of bile-stained material. She was treated by intravenous infusion and tetracycline. She then made steady progress until 1 month of age when she was discharged home. She has since been followed up and remains well.

Case 2. (S.K.) This male infant was born spontaneously after an uneventful pregnancy and labour, weighing 8 lb. 11 oz. At birth the child was asphyxiated and pale, but spontaneous breathing started after insufflation of oxygen. There were carpopedal spasms and flexion of the wrists. On the first and second day of life the child vomited small amounts of haematin-stained fluid. On the third day he suddenly became very pale, collapsed, and was transferred to our care.

On admission the child was moribund with a markedly distended abdomen. The liver was palpable about one inch below the costal margin. Blood picture: haemoglobin, 78%; erythrocytes, 3·7 millions; leucocytes, 22,000; Coombs test negative. The diagnosis of intraperitoneal haemorrhage was made, and, because of the experience and knowledge gained in connexion with Case 1, a rupture of the liver was suspected. The child's condition improved after a transfusion of blood (200 ml.) and six hours after the onset of symptoms it was decided to operate.

At operation a large quantity of blood escaped from the liver region. A tear one inch long was found in the midst of a large subcapsular haematoma on the superior surface of the right lobe of the liver. The tear was repaired by inserting three stitches of chromic catgut.

The child stood the operation quite well, but postoperatively his condition deteriorated. He was treated by intravenous fluids, tetracycline, vitamin K and

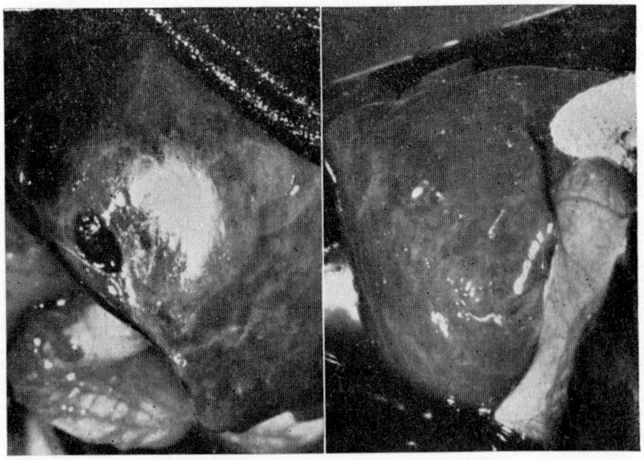

(*a*) (*b*)

FIG. 1.—Case 1. Photographs taken at operation. (*a*) Large subcapsular haematoma of the superior surface of the right lobe of the liver. The tear near the distal margin is clearly seen. (*b*) Inferior aspect of the liver with a smaller intact haematoma.

* A paper read at a meeting of the British Association of Paediatric Surgeons held in London in July, 1958.

ACC 76. He had minor convulsions and attacks of respiratory distress and two days after operation he died.

AUTOPSY. The body was that of a mature male neonate, 6 days of age, weight 8 lb. 5 oz., length 20 inches. Within the abdominal cavity was about 5 ml. of fluid blood. A large subcapsular haematoma was found on the superior surface of the right lobe of the liver. There was a tear (one inch long) near the distal margin of the right lobe. The site of the suture was intact. Another haematoma, the size of a half-crown, was found on the caudate lobe (Figs. 2 and 3). The dorsal wall of the stomach showed extensive haemorrhagic infarction of the mucosal and muscular layers. There were no abnormalities in the spleen. Both the kidneys showed a dark blue-reddish infarction of the medullary substance and papillae. There were perivascular haemorrhages and autolysis in the suprarenal glands, and broncho-pneumonia and atelectases in the lungs. A cephal-haematoma was found in the skull and there was a large subdural haematoma extending over the parietal and temporal lobe of the left cerebral hemisphere. Slight oedema of the brain was present. The anatomical diagnosis was: subcapsular haematoma of the liver with repaired rupture; haemorrhagic infarction of the stomach, both kidneys and suprarenal glands; cephal-haematoma; subdural haematoma; and broncho-pneumonia. The cause of death was subdural haematoma.

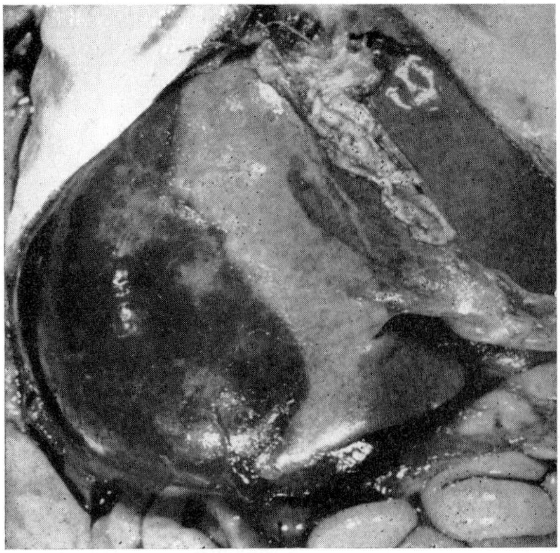

FIG. 2.—Case 2. *In situ* picture showing the huge haematoma of the right lobe of the liver.

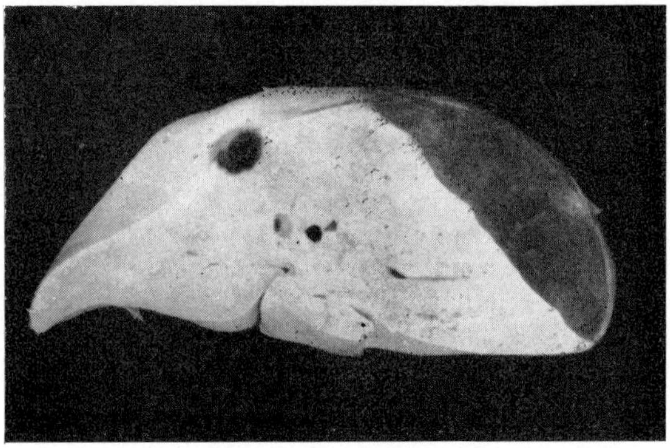

FIG. 3.—Case 2. Section of the liver. Subcapsular haematoma extending into the liver parenchyma.

Discussion

Hodge (1870) was probably the first to report a case of fatal haemorrhage from the liver in an infant 2½ days old. The question of trauma as an aetiological factor in the causation of hepatic haemorrhage has been discussed fully in the literature. Dittrich (1895) asserts that he had never known of a liver rupture without some external trauma. At that time the medico-legal aspect of the condition was widely discussed. Hedrén (1917) was the first to doubt if trauma was an aetiological factor in all cases of this condition, and he stated that hepatic rupture may be caused by physiological birth trauma.

It is impossible to discuss in full the series of events by which rupture of the liver may be brought about. Many theories have been advanced regarding the underlying cause, and the following includes some of the leading views. Gruenwald (1948) has described three possible mechanisms which may cause injury to the liver: (1) By pressure on the thorax the liver is pushed downward out of the hollow of the diaphragm which causes tension on the ligaments. He reported three cases in which the lesion was located at the coronary ligament and the hepato-duodenal ligament of the liver. (2) In cases where the lesion is found on the anterior surface of the liver, this may be caused by direct pressure of the costal margin. (3) Injuries which have no direct relationship to the ligaments or costal margin may be due to direct trauma to the liver itself.

Genell (1930) postulated that hepatic rupture may be caused by bending and compression of the foetal body. He reported a case of a woman with an oblique narrowing of the pelvis, who gave birth to two infants with hepatic rupture. Bret *et al.* (1956) collected 116 cases of hepatic haemorrhage from the literature and found a higher incidence of the condition in prematures and in infants larger than average. Henderson (1941) postulated that difficult delivery and abnormal foetal positions are the principal causes of hepatic haemorrhage in new-born infants.

In our two cases none of the above-mentioned

factors was present. Labour and delivery had been quite straightforward and the birth weights were normal.

Other factors which may play a part in the aetiology of this condition are asphyxia and increased bleeding tendency. Henderson (1941) in his series of 47 cases of hepatic haemorrhage found 35 cases which were severely asphyxiated at birth. Bělohradský (1937) and Arden (1946) implicated severe congestion of the liver in asphyxia as predisposing to rupture. The frequency of associated haemorrhages other than hepatic speaks in favour of an increased bleeding tendency, such as is present in haemorrhagic disease of the newborn. In Henderson's series 43% had associated haemorrhages. Our Case 2 showed multiple haemorrhages in other organs. Unfortunately the infant's poor condition gave no opportunity for laboratory investigations such as prothrombin estimations, determination of the bleeding time, clotting time and platelet count. During the first 48 to 72 hours of life the prothrombin and stable factor level fall sharply (Schulman and Currimbhoy, 1957). In most instances of liver rupture there is a symptom-free interval of one to seven days. This may be explained as the result of a two-stage rupture. During the first stage a haematoma arises from a contusion of the liver parenchyma, and, as all newborn infants are born with a moderate deficiency of both prothrombin and stable factor, a haematoma may arise quite easily from a trauma which otherwise has no consequences. In autopsies of newborn infants who died from other causes, a haematoma of the liver is quite often found as a secondary finding. After this symptom-free interval, when the prothrombin and stable factor deficiency is greatest, bleeding may start again with following rupture of the haematoma. In only rare instances the capsule may be torn by the original trauma and in these cases the infant dies *in utero* or immediately after birth.

It seems conceivable that hepatic haemorrhage, with and without a following rupture, belongs in the group of manifestations of haemorrhagic disease of the newborn. The symptomatology of the condition is quite characteristic. There is a sudden onset of signs of severe illness after a symptom-free interval of one to seven days. According to Bret *et al.* (1956) most ruptures occur on the third or fourth day of life. Stingl (1948) and Lundquist (1930) reported cases in which the rupture occurred on the seventh day. After this lapse of time, when the baby seems to be in perfect health, there is a sudden appearance of severe anaemia with pallor and collapse. Abdominal distension, dullness to percussion in the right flank, and hepatomegaly are also found in most cases.

The following conditions may give the same clinical picture: (1) Haemorrhage of the suprarenal gland, which is usually associated with an extreme degree of pyrexia, a palpable mass in the loin, polypnoea and convulsions. (2) Congenital haemolytic anaemia, which can be excluded by a negative direct Coombs test. (3) Rupture of the spleen, which according to Gruenwald (1948) is much less common and only occurs in luetic and leukaemic spleens. (4) Intraventricular haemorrhage, which is associated with hypothermia and neurological symptoms.

Rogers (1934) recommends abdominal paracentesis to confirm the diagnosis.

The first case which recovered after surgical treatment was recorded by Rogers (1934). Arden (1951) and Arden *et al.* (1955) reported three cases which were treated by transfusion of blood only and recovered. Montalvo, Soto Pradera, Fusté, Rodríguez Molina, Diaz Rousselot, Alfonso, Silverio and Portela (1955) in their series of 24 cases had four infants in whom internal haemorrhage was diagnosed clinically; the children were treated by blood transfusion only and all of them died.

Because the extent of the tear and the amount of bleeding cannot be determined clinically, we feel that operation is the treatment of choice and should be carried out without delay as soon as the diagnosis of intraperitoneal haemorrhage is made.

Summary

Two cases of liver rupture during the neonatal period are described, one of which survived following operation. The aetiology, symptomatology and treatment are discussed and the literature briefly reviewed.

References

Arden, F. (1946). *Med. J. Aust.*, **1**, 187.
—— (1951). *Ibid.*, **2**, 632.
——, Dique, J. C. and Wrench, D. (1955). *Ibid.*, **2**, 765.
Bělohradský, H. (1937). *Zbl. Gynäk.*, **61**, 2430.
Bret, J., Jamain, B. and Coupé, C. (1956). *Arch. franç. Pédiat.*, **13**, 1043.
Dennison, W. M. (1957). Personal communication. (Cited by Mason Brown.)
Dittrich, P. (1895). *Vjschr. gerichtl. Med.*, 3 ser., **9**, 203.
Genell, S. (1930). *Acta obstet. gynec. scand.*, **9**, 180.
Greaves, J. L. (1955). *Lancet*, **2**, 1227.
Gruenwald, P. (1948). *J. Pediat.*, **33**, 195.
Hedrén, G. (1917). *Vjschr. gerichtl. Med.*, 3 ser., **54**, 230.
Henderson, J. L. (1941). *J. Obstet. Gynaec. Brit. Emp.*, **48**, 377.
Hodge (1870). *Amer. J. med. Sci.*, **59**, 416.
Lundquist, B. (1930). *Acta obstet. gynec. scand.*, **9**, 331.
Mason Brown, J. J. (1957). *Arch. Dis. Childh.*, **32**, 480.
Montalvo, J. R., Soto Pradera, E., Fusté, F., Rodríguez Molina, D., Diaz Rousselot, J., Alfonso, J. G., Silverio, J. and Portela, J. (1955). *Rev. cubana Pediat.*, **27**, 641.
Potter, E. L. (1952). *Pathology of the Fetus and the Newborn*, p. 336. Year Book Publishers, Chicago.
Rogers, G. (1934). *Amer. J. Obstet. Gynec.*, **27**, 841.
Schulman, J. and Currimbhoy, Z. (1957). *Pediat. Clin. N. Amer.*, **4** (May), 531.
Stingl, A. (1948). *Öst. Z. Kinderheilk.*, **1**, 2.

URETHRAL PLICATION IN THE MANAGEMENT OF URINARY INCONTINENCE*

BY

D. F. ELLISON NASH

From St. Bartholomew's Hospital, London

The operation of urethral plication is based upon the procedures described by Lowsley and Kirwin (1944) and later by Millin (1947) for the treatment of post-prostatectomy incontinence. The procedure used in children (Nash, 1957) is a relatively small operation with a low risk and a very low complication rate. Three widely spaced mattress sutures of floss nylon are inserted from the ischio-cavernosus muscle on one side to that on the other in such a way that they compress from below upwards the urethra and the defective bulbo-spongiosus muscle against the triangular ligament. This manoeuvre diminishes the calibre of the bulbous urethra so that the mucosal folds may be more adequately opposed by what muscle action remains. In addition, I believe that the reduction of this large reservoir of urine in the bulb is an advantage in preventing infection. In paraplegic cases the urethra and the perineal tissues are insensitive, and if the stitches are inserted too tightly there is a risk of necrosis and fistula formation. The sites of suture contain erectile tissue and haemorrhage may be troublesome during the operation. Diathermy is essential. A No. 9E. rubber catheter is inserted for the duration of the operation, and a Gibbon's Portex catheter is left *in situ* for 24 hours post-operatively.

Application of the Operation. The operation has been performed in 21 cases of incontinence in childhood. These have been followed up for periods of two to 10 years. On six occasions the operation was performed in enuretic boys whose night incontinence was lifelong, and in whom there seemed to be no functional explanation for the disorder. One was 'cured', two were improved and the others unaffected. In one of those unaffected the bulbo-spongiosus muscle was found to be unilateral at operation.

The second group consists of 14 children with congenital spinal palsy, 13 due to spina bifida and one to sacral agenesis. This last child was cured. Of the 13 with spina bifida four had had suprapubic cystostomies, heavy infection and gross pelvic deformity. One of these boys (B.H.) had nearly died with pyelonephritis on several occasions. A life-saving suprapubic cystotomy resulted in a very good recovery in his general health, but the continuous dribbling of urine from the urethra, associated with a bilateral below-knee amputation made life very difficult. Urethral plication was performed without a catheter in position and with the sutures tight. This completely occluded the urethra and prevented any further leakage. Owing to the recurrence of pyelonephritis, with the suprapubic cystotomy, 10 years after the initial operation the perineum was explored, the sutures removed and the urethra found to be intact. Curiously enough the boy is now free from any retention, his suprapubic sinus has healed, and he can void urine satisfactorily with only a minor degree of leakage in between. For this he wears a light-weight urinal. The operation is thus a very satisfactory method of closing the urethra, permanently or temporarily in the very rare instances in which a suprapubic cystostomy is necessary. In the other three boys who have suprapubic drainage the operation was tried after the cystostomy had healed, but was unsuccessful.

Nine other boys were selected for operation on the basis of the following criteria:

Residual urine was not more than 1 oz., and there was no evidence of back pressure changes in the ureters or kidneys. Diverticulation of the bladder was not necessarily a contraindication. The bladder was capable of being distended and had a capacity of at least 3 oz.

Very few of these children have a spastic or systolic bladder, but if such a condition is present the operation is unlikely to be of any use. If the child already has some degree of control, for instance if he can pass several ounces naturally although he is incontinent as well, the operation is most likely to succeed and is always worth trying.

* A paper read at the meeting of the British Association of Paediatric Surgeons held in London in July, 1958.

Two of these boys were given complete control; in four the condition greatly improved and became manageable and in three there was no change.

The other boy who had had bladder neck resection performed twice for urinary obstruction (fibro-elastosis) had persistent incontinence following the resections. Normal control has been restored though there has been a very occasional leak during vigorous physical stress such as football.

Summary

If the operation is applied in cases selected upon the criteria outlined above, for children with incontinence arising from spina bifida, sacral agenesis or fibro-elastosis, there is a very good chance of restoring continence. In fact four out of the 11 boys were cured of their incontinence, four were improved and in three there was no change. A chance of removing this troublesome complaint from a boy who had to struggle around in double calipers was thought to be well worth taking.

References

Lowsley, O. S. and Kirwin, T. J. (1944). *Clinical Urology*. Williams and Wilkins, Baltimore.

Millin, T. (1947). *Retropubic Urinary Surgery*. Livingstone, Edinburgh.

Nash, D. F. E. (1957). *Ann. roy. Coll. Surg. Engl.*, **20**, 349.

BRITISH ASSOCIATION OF PAEDIATRIC SURGEONS

The Fifth Annual Meeting of the British Association of Paediatric Surgeons took place at The Hospital for Sick Children, Great Ormond Street, on July 24, 25 and 26, 1958. The President was Miss Isabella Forshall. During the morning sessions papers were read and on two afternoons there were ward rounds and television demonstrations at The Hospital for Sick Children. On the afternoon of July 25, the Association was invited to attend a meeting at St. Bartholomew's Hospital where members of the staff of St. Bartholomew's read papers. Dr. Willis Potts, Chicago, gave the Simpson-Smith Memorial Lecture, at The Hospital for Sick Children, on 'Oesophageal Atresia', and the Moynihan Lecture at the Royal College of Surgeons on 'Respiratory Emergencies in the New Born'.

The Annual Dinner took place on the evening of July 26, at the Apothecaries Hall. Professor Sir James Paterson Ross was the guest of honour. Paediatric surgeons from 20 different nations attended and took part in the meeting.

The following are abstracts of papers not published in full:

F. R. Edwards (Liverpool). 'Aortic Rings.' Owing to persistence of the 12 mm. embryo stage of development the oesophagus and trachea may be surrounded by vascular structures in the form of a ring. This may be in the form of a double aorta or by compression from aberrant vessels or a long ductus arteriosus passing round to a right aortic arch.

Each form of vascular ring can be explained by absorption taking place in different parts of the two aortic arches.

Severe pathological changes are produced in the trachea in the form of a chondromalacia, with narrowing of the lumen, and a secondary tracheobronchitis is often present. The oesophageal changes are temporary only. Other congenital abnormalities such as hemivertebra, spina bifida, pulmonary stenosis and tetralogy of Fallot may be present.

Only a proportion develop symptoms, depending upon the tightness of the ring.

Stridor is the main symptom, which is in part relieved by maintaining an extended state of the cervical and thoracic region. The condition may improve slowly, but the stridor tends to recur with recurrent respiratory infections. Dysphagia may be present with regurgitation into the lungs. If symptoms are present early then it suggests a double arch; if they come on at the age of 2 to 3 years it suggests a right aortic arch with a ductus.

A posterior oesophageal defect is seen on barium swallow, and angiocardiography may demonstrate the anatomical position. Bronchoscopy will demonstrate the narrowing of the trachea associated with a pulsating vessel, and oesophagoscopy will enable the retro-oesophageal vessel to be compressed against the spine. Study of the brachial and femoral pulses on the two sides will give information as to the distribution of the retro-oesophageal vessel.

Differential diagnoses are congenital oesophageal stenosis and atresia, primary laryngeal and tracheal deformities, tracheobronchitis, and enlarged bronchial and paratracheal lymph nodes.

Considerable pre-operative treatment by vapour tents, antibiotics, etc., may be required.

Operation consists of the division of the lesser arch or the individual compressing vessel, and the ligamentum arteriosum. Trial compression of the area to be divided is undertaken first to ensure that no major vessel is occluded.

Seventeen cases have been operated upon: there were 11 rings and six aberrant right subclavian arteries. All survived.

It may be some months before the tracheal deformity returns to normal and the stridor completely disappears.

W. Poradowska (Warsaw). 'Some Neonatal Problems.' Forty-nine newborn babies and infants were treated by surgery for complicated chest pathology in Warsaw over a period of three years. The cases included: (1) 32 cases of pneumothorax complicated by staphylococcal bronchopneumonia which were treated initially by suction drainage. Of these 17 did not respond and a thoracotomy, decortication and excision of the diseased segment or lobe was performed. The results in the latter group were as follows: 12 recovered completely; in three cases recovery was complicated by a pleural fistula, and two died; (2) five cases of respiratory difficulty due to congenital cysts of the lungs were operated upon and the cysts removed; (3) nine newborn babies with congenital diaphragmatic herniae were operated upon; there were two deaths, one due to other abnormalities and the second to broncho-pneumonia; (4) one case of anterior meningocoele with respiratory distress was operated on and the tumour removed, but the child died of meningitis; (5) two cases of cavernous lymph-haemangioma of the upper chest were operated upon, with one death due to massive collapse of the lung.

G. W. Taylor (London). 'Primary Lymphoedema.' An analysis of 159 patients with primary lymphoedema of the lower limb was presented. Of these patients there were 17 (11%) with lymphoedema congenita, 123 (77%) with lymphoedema praecox and 19 (12%) with lymphoedema tarda. The disease was familial in 24 patients and familial and congenital (Milroy's disease) in four patients. Lymphangiography in 139 patients revealed three main types of lymphatic abnormality. Eighty-seven (62%) patients had hypoplasia of the lymph trunks, 24 (17%) patients had varicose lymph trunks and in 21 (15%) patients there was a total aplasia of the main limb lymphatics. The prognosis was best in the patient with hypoplasia and in this group conservative treatment with elevation and support was often successful. Patients with severe lymphoedema were treated by the excisional operation of Charles. The condition of chylous reflux was described in which incompetence of the mesenteric and pelvic lymphatics allowed retrograde flow of intestinal chyle into the lower limb. These patients could be helped by retroperitoneal ligation of the incompetent lymph trunks.

A short film was also shown demonstrating spontaneous rhythmical contraction in the retroperitoneal lymphatics of patients with chylous reflux.

D. INNES WILLIAMS (London). 'Surgery of the Adrenal Cortex in Children.' Adrenal cortical tumours may produce androgenic or oestrogenic changes, Cushing's syndrome or hyperaldosteronism; or be without endocrine activity. Many of them are benign lesions for which surgery may be successfully undertaken. Operation is also required for adrenal cortical hyperplasia when associated with Cushing's syndrome and hyperaldosteronism, but not with the adrenogenital syndrome.

Eleven tumours with varying manifestations, and a case of Cushing's syndrome due to hyperplasia, were described and the diagnostic methods discussed. Consideration was given to the operative approach and to the pre- and post-operative endocrine treatment.

W. J. W. SHARRARD (Sheffield). 'Congenital Paralytic Dislocation of the Hip.' Among 57 children with myelomeningocoele and paralysis in the lower limbs, there were 58 dislocations or subluxations of the hip joint.

Twenty-six dislocations were present at birth, and occurred when there was paralysis below the third or fourth lumbar segments. It is considered that the dislocation in these cases is due to the action of strong adductor and flexor muscles acting *in utero* in the presence of paralysed gluteal muscles.

Five other dislocations and seven subluxations developed during the first 18 months of life, when there was paralysis below the second lumbar segment. This was again due to the action of adductors and flexors of the hip.

It was demonstrated that these cases require operative correction of the contracture to reduce the dislocation, and transplantation of the psoas to the greater trochanter and of the sartorius to the outer side of the knee to maintain reduction of the dislocation.

AMBROSE JOLLEYS (Manchester). 'The Value of Treatment with I.N.H. and P.A.S. in Tuberculous Peripheral Lymphadenitis.' Forty-four cases of peripheral glandular tuberculosis were divided into pairs with similar distribution, condition and progression, providing two groups for comparison. Both groups were treated by orthodox surgical means but, in addition, one received full dosage of I.N.H. and P.A.S. for three months.

The chemotherapy gave no apparent advantage when the duration of the condition, the duration of the discharge and the necessity for operative interference were compared. In fact, chemotherapy led to a delay in the institution of operative measures with a delay in the eventual cure in some cases.

Operation cannot be avoided and chemotherapy should be given for a short time before operation, in order to protect against widespread dissemination, but need not be continued for more than a fortnight afterwards.

In this series, excision of glands gave much better results than incision and curettage of abscesses, and in a third group 27 had excisions without chemotherapy with excellent results, and it appears that excision should be done whenever possible.

K. M. LAURENCE (London). 'The Natural History of Spina Bifida.' Four hundred and seven cases of spina bifida cystica born between January, 1947, and December, 1956, were followed up. All the 38 meningocoeles have survived while 185 of the remainder, classed as myelocoeles, have died. A life table, however, shows that 50% are alive at 1 year old and 36% remain living after 8 or more years.

The prognosis and features of the myelocoeles depend upon their position. The lesions in the dorsi-lumbar and lumbo-sacral regions carry the greatest risk, while sacral and purely dorsal myelocoeles fare better. A close correlation exists between prognosis and hydrocephalus which was found in 231 cases, of whom 179 cases have died. Sphincter involvement, not seen in cranial or cervical lesions, became more common down the spinal axis, while the incidence of limb paralysis, greatest in the dorsi-lumbar region, is least in the sacral and cervical.

The deaths occurred mostly in the first year of life from ascending intracranial infection (86 cases), many of the later deaths being due to hydrocephalus (49 cases), and renal failure (10 cases).

Comparison with the Registrar General's returns shows that the series is representative only for children who died after 3 months, as those dying in the first 2 months rarely get referred.

R. B. ZACHARY (Sheffield). 'Oesophago-trachea.' A fistula between the trachea and oesophagus has been reported frequently, but is usually of small dimensions. Larger communications between the two structures have occurred infrequently, and only two cases have been reported in which the entire septum was deficient. Three further cases are added to this list, two in siblings from Sheffield Children's Hospital, and one from Alder Hey Children's Hospital, Liverpool. An attempt to repair these anomalies should be made by an approach first in the right chest and then in the neck, forming two separate tubes. Two attempts have so far been made, one by Sandergaard in Sweden, and one by the author. The infants survived five and one days respectively.

A LONGITUDINAL STUDY OF THE GROWTH AND DEVELOPMENT OF PREMATURELY AND MATURELY BORN CHILDREN

PART III. MENTAL DEVELOPMENT

BY

CECIL MARY DRILLIEN

From the Department of Child Life and Health, Edinburgh

(RECEIVED FOR PUBLICATION JULY 4, 1958)

This paper describes the mental development of a group of nearly 600 premature and maturely born children from 6 months to 2 years of age. Approximately two thirds of the sample were $5\frac{1}{2}$ lb. or less at birth. The sample includes 100 pairs of twins. The composition of the sample and the method of investigation are described elsewhere (Drillien, 1958).

Mental Testing Employed

The children were visited at home at six-monthly intervals. They were given a selection of tests based on the Gesell and Amatruda (1941) and Griffiths (1954) scales. On the basis of these tests and answers given by the mothers, each child was allotted a developmental quotient at each visit. In the case of prematurely born children, weeks of prematurity have been deducted from the chronological age to give the real age.

Developmental quotient (D.Q.) is expressed as a percentage according to the following formula:

$$\text{D.Q.} = \frac{\text{Developmental age}}{\text{Real age}} \times 100.$$

The tests were selected to include locomotion, manipulation, general understanding and speech, and social adjustment. A brief description of the routine carried out is given below:

(1) **At 6 Months.** The baby is observed in the following positions: supine and pulled to sitting, sitting supported or alone, prone and standing supported. He is offered a small shining bell and his method of reaching, grasping and manipulation observed. Finally he is offered a one-inch red wooden block, and if he grasps it, a second block. The mother is questioned about age of smiling, vocalization and recognition of people.

(2) **At 12 Months.** The child is observed crawling or shuffling on the buttocks, pulling to standing, cruising and walking with one or two hands held. A minority will stand or walk a few steps alone. He is sat on the floor and offered in turn, three one-inch blocks. He is then given a metal cup containing six blocks. If he fails to return any cubes to the cup after removal this is demonstrated. Some children will attempt a tower of two blocks at this age. The mother is questioned as to any words or sounds used with meaning, whether he waves or claps his hands, and whether he responds to any simple questions (e.g. 'Where is Daddy?').

(3) **At 18 Months.** The child is observed walking, trotting or running. His method of climbing stairs and of throwing and kicking a ball is elicited by question. He is presented with six blocks and encouraged to build a tower. The mother is asked to enumerate all the words he uses and any two-word phrases. He is presented in turn with two cards containing four and six coloured pictures of common objects, and asked, 'Show me the doggie', etc. The more advanced children will first be asked to name the pictures. If he will not respond he is shown a box containing seven small objects and told to 'Take the spoon to Mummy', etc. He is asked to point out parts of the body on a doll. The mother is questioned about feeding and toilet habits.

(4) **At 2 Years.** The mother is questioned about the method of climbing stairs and ability to jump, ride a tricycle and kick a ball. It is noted whether the child is speaking in single words, two-word phrases ('Daddy away!', 'Bad boy!') or broken

sentences ('Me want out, coat Mummy', or 'Peter bad, hit baby'), and whether he uses pronouns (I, me, you) and prepositions (under, over there). It is realized that the child's speech depends to a certain extent on the type of speech heard in the home, and this has been taken into account when assessing speech development. He is presented with the same picture cards and asked to name the objects. If he fails, he is asked to point them out. Similarly the objects in the box are presented. He is given 10 blocks and encouraged to build a tower and a train of three blocks aligned. The mother is questioned as to self-feeding, co-operation in dressing and toilet habits.

Co-operation of the children is on the whole very good up to the age of 18 months. At 2 years the proportion of unco-operative children has increased. The amount of weight attached to the mother's estimation of her child's ability varies considerably with the type of mother and whether her answers have been proved reliable in the past. The testing of twins becomes difficult at the age of 2 years, as it is not often possible to separate them. The twins are either tested on alternate tests, or else one twin is tested thoroughly and the mother questioned as to differences between them. In this case an attempt is made to test the other twin at the next visit. In general, it was found that the mother's estimation of the difference in ability between twins corresponded closely with test findings. In some cases owing to lack of co-operation it was impossible to make an assessment of D.Q. at 2 years and these children have not been included in the subsequent analysis. In nearly all these cases testing has been possible at later ages.

Analysis of the Data

Developmental Ability in Different Birthweight Groups. Table 1 gives mean D.Q.s at ages up to 2 years, for male and female singletons and twins, divided into four birthweight groups. As no significant difference was found in D.Q. levels for children of different birthweights who were mature at birth, they have all been included in one group. Mean D.Q. falls steadily with decreasing birthweight in all four groups. In the group 4½ lb. or less at birth, there is a steady improvement in developmental ability, especially among female singletons, but later analysis showed that this difference between males and females is a purely fortuitous finding associated with the fact that in this sample there happens to be a greater number of mothers of apparently low intelligence in the smaller male premature groups. This will be referred to again in a later section. At all ages male and female twins show consistently lower scores than singletons of like birthweight. This finding has been recorded by other investigators (Mehrotra and Maxwell, 1949).

It is not suggested that the D.Q. ratings obtained can be considered accurate as absolute figures. A more accurate picture is probably obtained by placing the children in broader groups.

Fig. 1 shows the proportion of children by birthweight who at 2 years were considered to be : (1) grossly defective (D.Q. 55 or less), (2) mentally retarded (D.Q. 56 to 75), (3) backward or dull (D.Q.76 to 95), (4) average or good average (D.Q. 96 to 115) and (5) definitely superior in intelligence (D.Q. 116 or more). The excess in dull, retarded and grossly defective children as birthweight decreases is very striking.

Developmental Ability Related to the Intelligence of the Mother. As has been noted before in a study of the physical development of these children (Drillien, 1958), there is a predominance of poor type homes amongst the prematurely born and also of obviously less intelligent mothers. Ideally one would have liked to have obtained the I.Q.s of the parents, but the best estimation possible of the

TABLE 1

MEAN DEVELOPMENTAL QUOTIENTS BY AGE, SEX AND BIRTHWEIGHT

Birthweight (lb. oz.)	Age in months 6	12	18	24	Age in months 6	12	18	24
	Female Singletons				Male Singletons			
3·8 and under ..	73·8	80·7	88·6	90·4	77·5	79·5	88·2	81·2
3·9 to 4·8	85·8	94·0	98·3	99·4	84·0	86·9	90·6	88·9
4·9 to 5·8	99·8	102·4	102·9	102·3	97·1	96·4	96·7	97·8
5·9 and over ..	104·5	104·3	103·7	104·9	106·7	109·2	107·8	109·1
	Female Twins				Male Twins			
3·8 and under ..	66·9	69·4	72·6	75·1	74·0	74·7	78·3	79·7
3·9 to 4·8	88·6	94·9	93·7	94·7	80·1	86·2	90·8	88·3
4·9 to 5·8	96·8	95·3	97·5	99·3	91·5	96·7	94·7	93·8
5·9 and over ..	98·5	101·3	100·4	101·6	102·5	105·0	101·2	100·5

mother's intelligence has been made by dividing them into three grades: middle class and superior working class, average working class, and poor working class. It is hoped at a later date to obtain some idea of the intelligence levels of school age sibs.

Fig. 2 shows mean D.Q.s at ages up to 2 years by birthweight and grade of mother. Numbers, especially in the poor working class grade, were not large enough to subdivide further into male and female singletons and twins, though what analysis was possible showed that the differences for maternal grades were similar in all four groups. For all maternal grades, mean D.Q. at 2 years rises steadily with increasing birthweight. In the smaller premature groups (i.e. those 4½ lb. or less at birth) there is an improvement in developmental ability up to the age of 18 months in children born to the more intelligent mothers. Those who were over 4½ lb. at birth show little variation in mean D.Q. at different ages in any maternal grade group except in the mature controls where children in the worst homes score higher at 1 year than at 2 years. This is due to backwardness in speech in this group and will be referred to later. Children who were 3½ lb. or less at birth in the average and poor working class groups show no improvement comparable to that in the best maternal grade, the differences at 2 years between the three maternal grade groups being much more marked in the smaller prematures than in those over 4½ lb. at birth. In spite of the improvement noticed in the prematurely born children of the more intelligent mothers, they still appear to have some handicap at the age of 2 as compared with the mature control group.

Fig. 3 illustrates this point in another way and shows the proportion of children considered to be of average or above average intelligence at 2 years, by birthweight and maternal grading.

Fig. 4 divides the children at 2 years by birthweight and maternal grading, into the broad groupings given above, and again shows the striking excess in the proportion of dull, retarded and grossly defective prematurely born children found where the mother's intelligence appears to be average or poor. In the mature control group there is an excess of children of obviously superior ability in the best maternal group, but the differences by maternal grade are not nearly so obvious. It seems likely that a combination of inferior genetic endowment and a poor environment with restricted opportunities has a more marked effect on early development in those who were small at birth than on maturely born children from a similar background. It will be interesting to see whether at a later age the differential between the children of the best and worst mothers in the smaller premature groups will approximate more nearly to that found in the mature group.

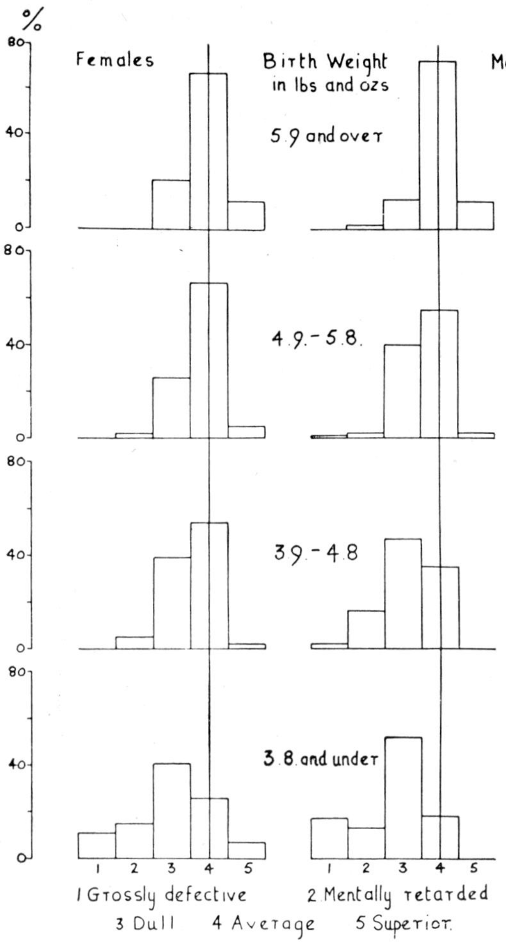

FIG. 1.—Developmental grading at 2 years. By sex and birthweight.

Milestones of Development. Table 2 gives the proportion of children of different birthweights who, at certain ages, had reached six milestones of development. The milestones recorded are as follows: (1) Sitting unsupported on a hard surface for 10 minutes. (2) Standing unsupported for 30 seconds. (3) Walking alone across a room. (4) Five definite words used with meaning, apart from Mamma, Dadda and Ta-ta. (5) At least 20 meaningful words and several two-word phrases. (6) Speaks in broken sentences.

Children in the smallest weight group are more than 6 months retarded at 2 years as compared with

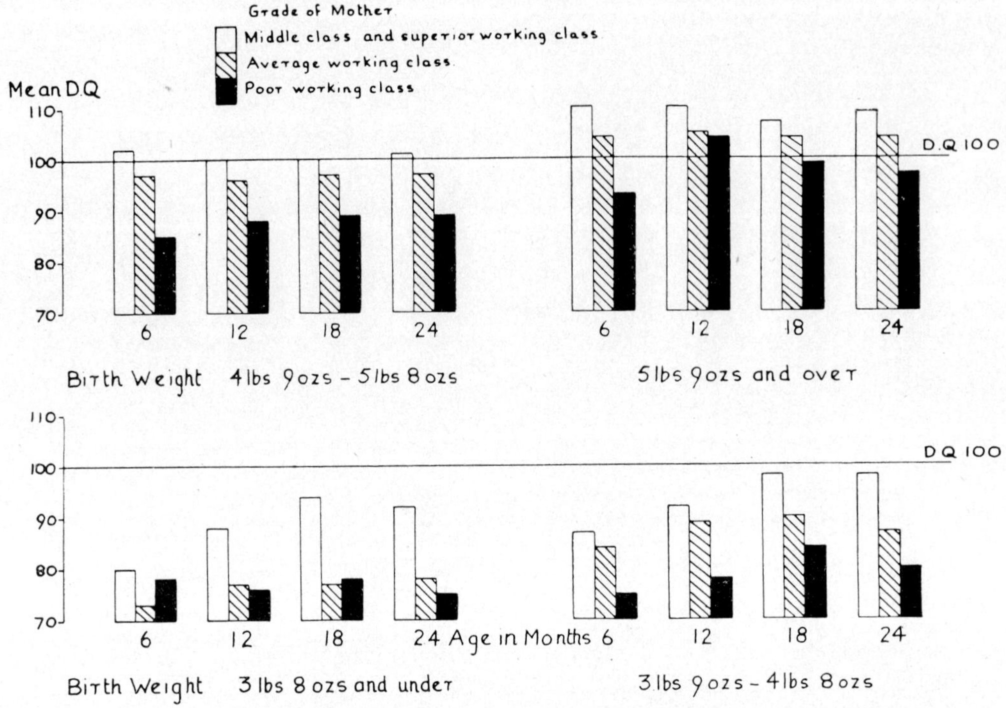

FIG. 2.—Mean development quotients by age, birthweight and grade of mother.

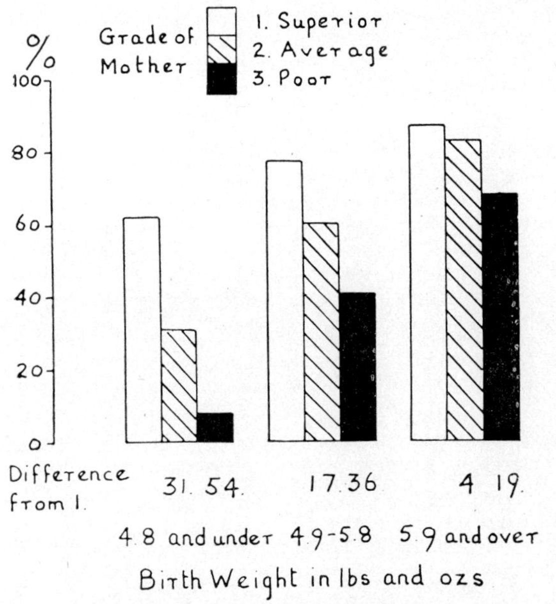

FIG. 3.—Proportion of children of average intelligence at 2 years by birthweight and grade of mother.

maturely born children. Prematurely born boys appear to be especially retarded as regards speech, but this again seems to be due to an excess of poor type mothers. It seems impossible to devise developmental tests, the results of which are unaffected by opportunity and environment. Perhaps at 6 months of age the infant's reactions are least affected by his upbringing, but even at that age frequent illness, which is much more common in poor homes, may produce an apparent retardation.

The attainment of these milestones has been tested in relation to birthweight and maternal grading, and the results are shown in Table 3. Males and females have been combined to provide bigger numbers. Milestones have been selected for the ages at which about one-half of the children might be expected to have reached this stage. It is obvious that in locomotor activities, the children from the worst homes are not retarded to anything like the degree that they are in speech. It seems likely that as soon as the child reaches the age when verbal testing becomes important, the D.Q. gradings of those in the best homes are being artificially boosted by the fact that they are spoken to frequently, and shown books, whereas children from the worst homes are

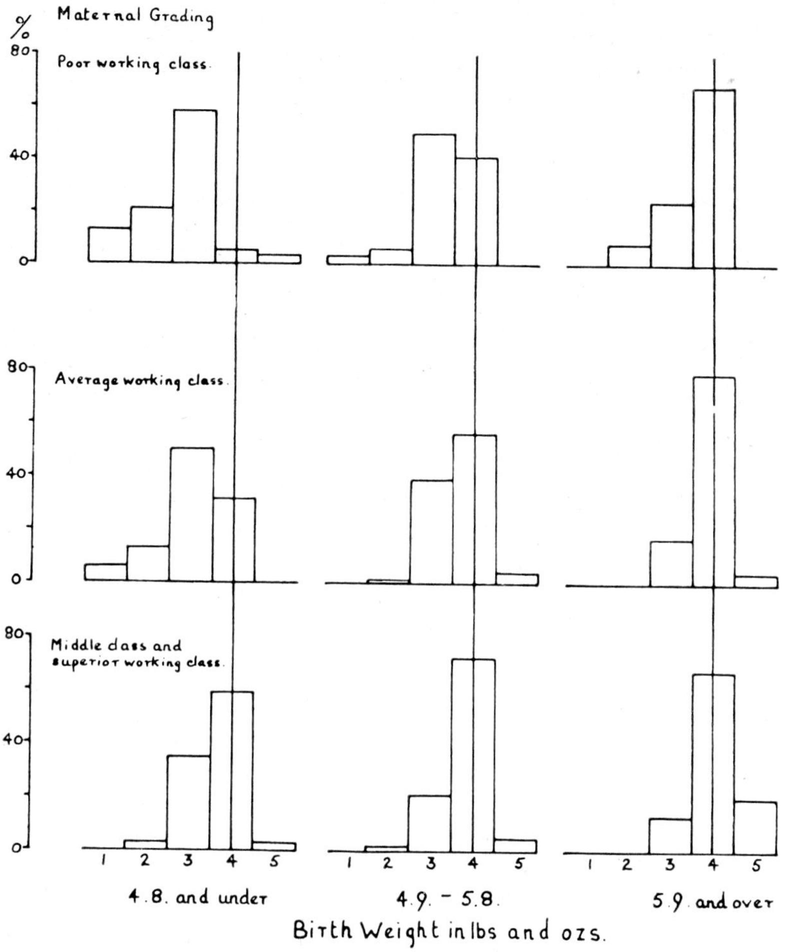

FIG. 4.—Developmental grading at 2 years by birthweight and grade of mother.

given a D.Q. grading which is too low, owing to their lack of opportunity.

The Relation of Developmental Ability to Family Placing. It is well known that firstborn children obtain higher scores on intelligence tests than later born children (Scottish Council for Research in Education, 1949; Burt, 1950). Table 4 gives mean D.Q. scores at 2 years, according to place in family, for premature and maturely born children.

Table 5 further subdivides the children according to grade of mother. Here family placing is given as first or later born, as there are not sufficient numbers to divide into the four family placing groups given in Table 4. The difference between first and later born children is greatest in the smallest premature group, except for those with the least intelligent mothers where the difference between first and later born children is as high, or higher in those over 4½ lb. at birth. The proportion of first births decreases with grade of mother in all birthweight groups, and this may account for some of the difference in mean D.Q. levels for different maternal grades shown in Fig. 2.

In Table 6 the mean D.Q. levels at 2 years are shown for different birthweight and maternal grades that would be expected if the parity distribution of all groups were the same as that found in the total sample. This standardization reduces the difference between maternal grade groups, but not to any great extent.

TABLE 2

MILESTONES OF DEVELOPMENT BY SEX AND BIRTHWEIGHT

Birthweight (lb. oz.)	Months	Locomotion			Speech			No. Cases
		Sit	Stand	Walk	5 Words	Phrases	Sentences	
				Girls				
3·8 and under ..	12	70·4	3·7	—	—	—	—	27
	18	88·9	70·4	40·7	51·9	7·4	—	
	24	96·3	81·5	81·5	81·5	40·7	14·8	
3·9 to 4·8 ..	12	95·7	21·3	4·3	—	—	—	47
	18	97·9	91·5	78·7	78·7	19·1	—	
	24	97·9	95·7	93·6	95·7	68·1	21·3	
4·9 to 5·8 ..	12	98·1	40·0	8·7	4·9	—	—	103
	18	100·0	97·1	93·2	82·5	28·2	—	
	24	100·0	99·0	99·0	98·1	80·6	39·8	
5·9 and over ..	12	100·0	36·8	12·6	8·4	1·1	—	95
	18	100·0	98·9	96·8	83·2	38·9	1·1	
	24	100·0	100·0	100·0	100·0	90·5	44·2	
				Boys				
3·8 and under ..	12	56·0	4·0	—	—	—	—	25
	18	92·0	44·0	36·0	24·0	—	—	
	24	100·0	84·0	84·0	64·0	20·0	4·0	
3·9 to 4·8 ..	12	78·1	7·3	—	—	—	—	55
	18	98·2	72·7	61·8	36·4	3·6	—	
	24	98·2	94·5	90·9	85·5	49·1	14·5	
4·9 to 5·8 ..	12	96·7	17·4	6·5	—	—	—	92
	18	98·9	89·1	85·9	67·4	10·9	—	
	24	98·9	98·9	97·8	97·8	66·3	26·1	
5·9 and over ..	12	99·0	58·4	21·8	9·9	—	—	101
	18	100·0	98·0	97·0	95·0	35·6	1·0	
	24	100·0	100·0	100·0	99·0	85·1	48·5	

TABLE 3

MILESTONES OF DEVELOPMENT BY BIRTHWEIGHT AND GRADE OF MOTHER

Birthweight (lb. oz.)	Maternal Grading	Standing Alone	Walking	5 Words	20 or More Words 2-3 Word Phrases	Broken Sentences	No. Cases
		Percentage reaching milestones at: 12 months	18 months		24 months		
4·8 and under	1		65	70	54		57
	2		60	44	39		57
	3		50	30	20		40
4·9 to 5·8 ..	1	31	89	86	82		66
	2	25	90	77	73		91
	3	18	87	55	68		38
		12 months			18 months	24 months	
5·9 and over ..	1	45			47	55	100
	2	48			34	42	65
	3	58			13	8	31

TABLE 4

MEAN DEVELOPMENTAL QUOTIENTS BY FAMILY PLACING AND BIRTHWEIGHT

Birthweight (lb. oz.)	Place in Family: 1st		2nd		3rd		4th or later	
	Number	Mean D.Q.	Number	Mean D.Q.	Number	Mean D.Q.	Number	Mean D.Q
5·8 and under ..	191	99·2	70	89·0	44	89·4	33	89·8
Over 5·8	98	106·9	39	102·3	20	103·5	21	98·3

TABLE 5

MEAN DEVELOPMENTAL QUOTIENTS BY FAMILY PLACING, GRADE OF MOTHER AND BIRTHWEIGHT

Birthweight (lb. oz.)	Maternal Grading	First Births (%)	Family Placing: First	Family Placing: Later	Difference in Mean D.Q.
			Mean D.Q.		
4·8 and under	1	58	101·9	91·4	10·5
	2	51	93·1	85·4	7·7
	3	41	84·3	75·0	9·3
4·9 to 5·8	1	70	104·6	98·0	6·6
	2	62	100·7	96·6	4·1
	3	43	100·6	87·5	13·1
5·9 and over	1	65	108·3	105·1	3·2
	2	46	104·8	101·0	3·8
	3	40	104·0	94·7	9·3

TABLE 6

MEAN DEVELOPMENTAL QUOTIENTS BY BIRTHWEIGHT AND GRADE OF MOTHER STANDARDIZED FOR FAMILY PLACING

Birthweight (lb. oz.)	Maternal Grading	Mean D.Q. Standardized for Parity	Difference in D.Q. from Maternal Grade 1	Mean D.Q. not Standardized for Parity	Difference in D.Q. from Maternal Grade 1
4·8 and under . .	1	96·7		97·0	
	2	89·7	− 7·0	89·3	− 7·7
	3	80·2	−16·5	78·8	−18·2
4·9 to 5·8	1	101·7		102·7	
	2	98·8	− 2·9	99·0	− 3·7
	3	94·8	− 6·9	93·2	− 9·5
5·9 and over . .	1	106·9		107·1	
	2	103·1	− 3·8	102·7	− 4·4
	3	99·9	− 7·0	98·4	− 8·7

TABLE 7

INCIDENCE OF POST-NATAL SYMPTOMS BY BIRTHWEIGHT

Birthweight (lb. oz.)	No. of cases	Post-natal Symptoms: None	1	2	3
3·8 and under . .	49	71·4	10·2	12·2	6·1
3·9 to 4·8 . .	100	79·0	10·0	9·0	2·0
4·9 to 5·8 . .	187	85·0	8·6	3·2	3·2
5·9 and over . .	192	93·7	3·1	0·5	2·6

The Importance of Birth Injury on Later Mental Development. On the basis of the later examination of mental development in 69 of a group of 102 surviving premature infants who were considered to have suffered intracranial injury at birth, Hess (1934) stated that 'premature birth unassociated with intracranial injury does not affect mental development'. This opinion has been repeated frequently, e.g. Brander (1937); Beskow (1949); Alm (1953).

A reliable post-natal history was obtained of about 528 of the total sample of 595 infants. Post-natal symptoms which Hess suggested might be attributed to intracranial injury were classified as follows: (1) Poor condition at birth, shocked, cyanosed or slow to breathe. No further complications after the first 24 hours. (2) Cyanotic or apnoeic attacks after the first 24 hours. (3) Suspected intracranial injury, cerebral crying, twitching, irritability or convulsions.

The incidence of these symptoms in infants of different birthweight is shown in Table 7. Where the baby exhibited more than one of the groups of symptoms the case is classified under that considered most serious in prognostic significance. The incidence of these symptoms increases with decreasing birthweight.

Only 3% of the total sample and 3·3% of the total premature sample were considered to show definite signs of cerebral damage which is much lower than Hess's figure of 10·4%. If those who were shocked at birth, or later had cyanotic attacks, are included the percentage of possible cerebral damage is raised to 14·2% which is comparable with Hess's figure, considering that his sample contained fewer very small babies.

Table 8 gives mean D.Q. at 2 years for prematurely born children who showed these post-natal symptoms compared with those of similar birthweight whose progress was uncomplicated. The numbers are small, but there is little to suggest that

TABLE 8

MEAN DEVELOPMENTAL QUOTIENTS AT 2 YEARS BY BIRTHWEIGHT AND PRESENCE OR ABSENCE OF POST-NATAL SYMPTOMS

Birthweight (lb. oz.)	Post-natal Symptoms None	1, 2 and 3
3·8 and under ..	72·6	82·7
3·9 to 4·8	92·9	90·3
4·9 to 5·8	99·8	92·2

birth injury has been a major factor in determining later mental development in this sample of children. The incidence of complications of pregnancy and delivery in the premature group was not significantly different in those who showed or did not show these symptoms. Six maturely born children, four with difficult deliveries showed cerebral signs or had cyanotic attacks. The mean D.Q. at 2 years for these cases was 105.

It is probable that premature babies are more likely to sustain cerebral damage as a result of birth injury, and that in some cases mental retardation and cerebral palsy may result, but it also seems likely that in more cases post-natal symptoms which are commonly attributed to cerebral damage are, in fact, due directly to the immaturity of the baby.

Discussion

There are few published studies of mental development in prematurely born children of pre-school age. Knobloch, Rider, Harper and Pasamanick (1956) examined a group of children of different birthweights at 40 weeks, using the Gesell scale, and found that the proportion of mentally retarded or defective infants was 17·6% in those less than 3·3 lb. at birth compared with 1·8% in the larger premature group, and 1·6% in the mature control group. The percentage of children of above average ability in these birthweight groups was 5·3, 16·3 and 21·8.

Douglas (1956a) concluded that prematurely born children were not retarded in the pre-school period if allowance were made for the degree of prematurity. This opinion was based on the mother's estimation of the age of walking, elicited when the child was 2 years old. Children who were not walking at that age were excluded. Douglas divided his prematurely born children by estimated gestation time, into three groups. In the present survey no great weight has been attached to the mother's timing of milestones of development given in retrospect; however, they were all asked the age at which the child first walked unaided. To check the accuracy of these reports after an interval of one to two years, a number of mothers in the sample have been asked again at a later date to give the age at which their child first walked alone. The answers obtained bore little relation to information recorded earlier. Mothers of premature and retarded infants were particularly liable to be inaccurate.

A comparison of mean walking ages for singleton births in this investigation and that carried out by Douglas, is given in Table 9. Children who were not walking at 2 years have been excluded in both groups to make the results comparable, although if those cases had been included, average age of walking in the Edinburgh sample would have been even later in the prematurely born. The average age of walking in both the mature control groups is identical, but there is a marked disparity in the premature groups. Although these are not strictly comparable because of different methods of classification it is still obvious that either the children in the present survey are more retarded than prematurely born children in general, or else that there has been a tendency on the part of mothers of premature infants in the National Survey to overestimate their children's ability. More information is available about school age children (e.g. Beskow, 1949; Knehr and Sobol, 1949; Douglas, 1956b).

The general opinion seems to be that prematurely born children score lower on intelligence tests and do less well at school in academic subjects than their maturely born contemporaries. In many of these studies children who are educationally subnormal are excluded, and the estimation of mental ability in prematurely born children is assessed in those that remain, thus seriously underestimating the real effect of premature birth on later mental development.

TABLE 9

AVERAGE AGE OF WALKING IN EDINBURGH AND NATIONAL SURVEYS

Birthweight (lb. oz.)	Edinburgh Survey: Average walking age (months)	Edinburgh Survey: No. not walking	National Survey (Douglas): Months of prematurity	National Survey (Douglas): Average walking age (months)	National Survey (Douglas): No. not walking
3·8 and under ..	18·4	6	2 or more	14·8	8 (2 or more; 1 to 2; 0 to 1)
3·9 to 4·8 ..	16·1	6	1 to 2	14·1	
4·9 to 5·8 ..	14·7	2	0 to 1	13·4	
5·9 and over ..	13·4	–	Mature	13·4	1

Summary

A group of children of different birthweights has been tested on the Gesell developmental scale at six-monthly intervals up to the age of 2 years. The following conclusions were reached:

Mean developmental quotient falls steadily with decreasing birthweight, at all ages, and twins show consistently lower scores than single born children. At 2 years there is a striking excess of dull, retarded and grossly defective children in the smaller premature groups (i.e. those of $4\frac{1}{2}$ lb. or less at birth).

Developmental ability is related to the apparent intelligence of the mother. At 2 years, for all birthweights, children born to the more intelligent mothers obtain higher D.Q. scores. The difference between scores of children in the best and worst maternal grades is much greater in those who were less than $4\frac{1}{2}$ lb. at birth than in the mature control group. A steady improvement in developmental ability is shown by the smaller premature infants in the best maternal grade. No comparable improvement is seen in those with the least intelligent mothers.

Prematurely born children are slower in learning to walk and talk. Children whose mothers are apparently of low intelligence are more retarded in speech than in locomotor activities.

Firstborn children show higher scores on developmental testing than later born children. The difference between first and later born children is greater for prematurely born children and for children from a poor background.

The incidence of certain post-natal symptoms suggestive of cerebral injury increases with decreasing birthweight. At 2 years there was little to indicate that mental ability differed in those of like birthweight who had, or had not, exhibited these symptoms.

It is a pleasure to thank Professor R. W. B. Ellis for his help and encouragement throughout.

This investigation is being supported by a grant from the Scottish Hospital Endowments Research Trust.

REFERENCES

Alm, I. (1953). *Acta paediat. (Uppsala)*, 42, Suppl. 94.
Beskow, B. (1949). *Acta paediat. (Stockh.)*, 37, 125.
Brander, T. (1937). *Acta psychiat.*, **12**, 313.
Burt, C. (1950). Papers of the Royal Commission on Population, Vol. V. Memoranda. H.M.S.O., London.
Douglas, J. W. B. (1956a). *Brit. med. J.*, **1**, 1210.
—— (1956b). *Med. Offr*, **95**, 33.
Drillien, C. M. (1958). *Arch. Dis. Childh.*, **33**, 423.
Gesell, A. and Amatruda, C. (1941). *Developmental Diagnosis*. P. B. Hoeber, New York.
Griffiths, R. (1954). *The Abilities of Babies*. University of London Press.
Knehr, C. A. and Sobol, A. (1949). *J. Psychol.*, **27**, 355.
Knobloch, H., Rider, R., Harper, P. and Pasamanick, B. (1956). *J. Amer. med. Ass.*, **161**, 581.
Mehrotra, S. N. and Maxwell, J. (1949). *Popul. Stud.*, **3**, 295.
Scottish Council for Research in Education (1949). *The Trend of Scottish Intelligence*. London.

THE PHYSICAL DEVELOPMENT OF MONGOLS

BY

G. DUTTON

From St. Lawrence's Hospital, Caterham

(RECEIVED FOR PUBLICATION JULY 7, 1958)

Because it is a well differentiated and common form of mental defect, mongolism has been exhaustively studied. Most of the studies, however, have been directed at the possible aetiology of this condition. This paper is not concerned with aetiological problems but is a discussion of two purely physical findings in mongol boys, height and skeletal age. Some findings in adult male mongols have been included for reasons that will be apparent.

Material

The material is derived from the wards of a large hospital dealing with mental defectives. All cases are typical mongols, in whom diagnosis is without question, and cases that require close study to determine that they are mongols have been excluded since the value of this work was thought to depend on the homogeneity of the material. Both adult and child male mongols were selected on the known physical characteristics: eyes, epicanthus, tongue, etc. The survey has been limited to male mongols because the bed allocation at the hospital is such that it was not possible to obtain a worthwhile group of female mongol children.

Methods

Height. This was measured in the erect position in bare feet with a conventional stadiometer. The 'standard erect posture' of Krogman (1950) was used throughout the measurements. The figures for full height so obtained have been used as the raw figures and also converted to a height age by reference to the tables for normal children of Sutcliffe and Canham (1950). These tables have been chosen because they are comparatively recent, referring to a survey in 1947, and also because they were obtained on English children.

The height age so obtained has been converted to a percentage by dividing by the life age and multiplying by 100. This has the advantage of allowing comparisons to be made irrespective of age (Talbot, Sobel, Burke, Lindemann and Kaufman, 1947), and also of a direct comparison with skeletal age.

Skeletal Maturation. The skeletal age has been assessed by the inspectional method from a radiograph of one hand and wrist, comparisons being made with the standards in the atlas of Greulich and Pyle (1950). Each film was assessed by me, blind, on three separate occasions, the mean being taken as the skeletal age. The raw figures so obtained have been used for comparison with the mean and standard deviations given by Greulich and Pyle.

The figure for skeletal age has also been accorded the same treatment as that for the height age and a developmental quotient obtained for the purpose of comparison.

The data from these investigations have been used throughout in a cross-sectional manner although they have been obtained from both cross-sectional and longitudinal surveys carried out on the children at this hospital.

Results

These are given diagramatically in the following figures.

Height. Fig. 1 is a comparison between the height of mongol boys in inches and their life age in years. The mean for normal boys and two standard deviations below the mean (London County Council, 1955) are given.

The figure demonstrates how far behind the normal in height the mongol boy is, for no case in this series falls within the normal range and the larger number of them are well below minus two standard deviations.

When height quotients are considered (height quotient is height age multiplied by 100 and divided by life age) it is found that the peak incidence is at

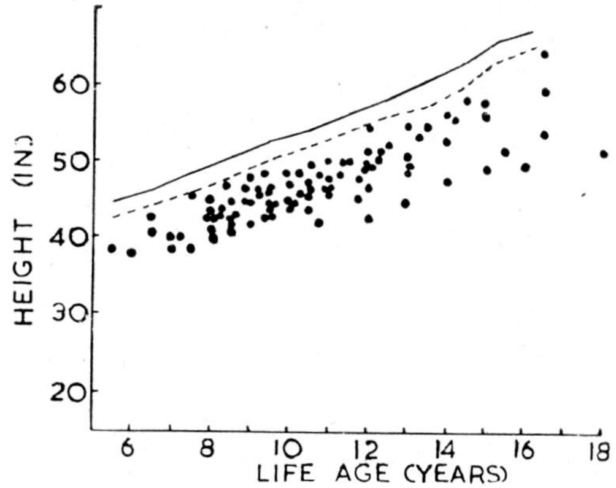

FIG. 1.—The relation of the heights of mongol boys to their life age. ——— = mean for normal boys; – – – – = 2 S.D. below the mean. (Mean and S.D. from London County Council, 1955).

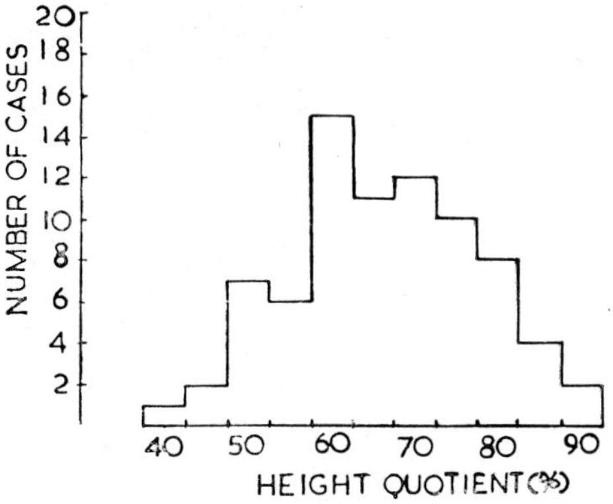

FIG. 2.—The distribution of the height quotient in mongol boys. (Height quotient is height age divided by life age and multiplied by 100.)

about the 60% level. This is demonstrated in Fig. 2. The mean height quotient of 78 assessments was found to be 67·8%. The normal range quoted by Talbot *et al.* (1947) for height quotients is 80-120%.

Skeletal Development. Skeletal age compared with life age is shown in Fig. 3. The mean for normal boys and two standard deviations above and below the mean (Greulich and Pyle, 1950) are included for purposes of comparison.

This picture is very different from that obtained when height was being considered, for now we find that mongol boys are predominantly normal as far as their skeletal maturation is concerned.

Fig. 4 demonstrates the frequency of the developmental quotients as far as the skeletons of mongol boys are concerned. This shows that the peak incidence is around the 100% level. In fact the arithmetic mean for the skeletal quotient on these cases was found to be 94·5%. This accentuates the difference between the height and the skeletal development and for comparison both developmental quotients are given in Table 1.

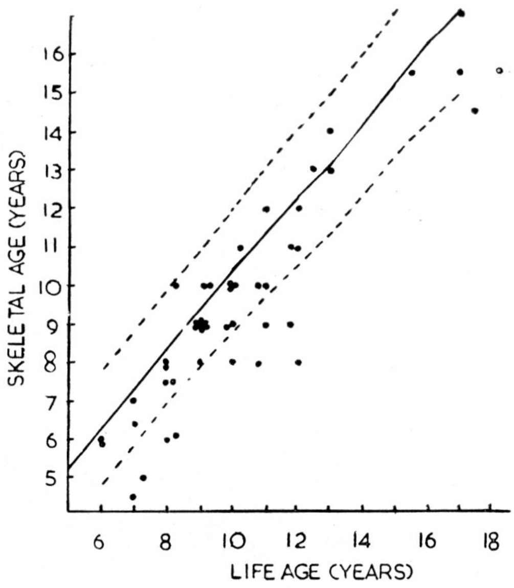

FIG. 3.—Skeletal age compared with life age in mongol boys. ——— = mean for normal boys; – – – – = 2 S.D. above and below the mean (from Greulich and Pyle, 1950).

TABLE 1

MEAN DEVELOPMENTAL QUOTIENTS OF MONGOL BOYS

$\frac{\text{Height Age}}{\text{Life Age}} \times 100$	$\frac{\text{Bone Age}}{\text{Life Age}} \times 100$
67·8%	94·5%

Mongols appear to present a failure of linear growth without a concomitant failure of skeletal development. It was necessary to examine the failure in linear growth more closely from a developmental angle. Bayley and Pinneau (1952) from a longitudinal study of the growth of a group of children have produced figures for the mean and standard deviations of percentage of mature height reached for the life age. But to compare the height of mongols with that of normal adults seemed unreasonable and it is fairer to compare the growing mongol boy with adult male mongols. It was therefore necessary to determine what was the mean

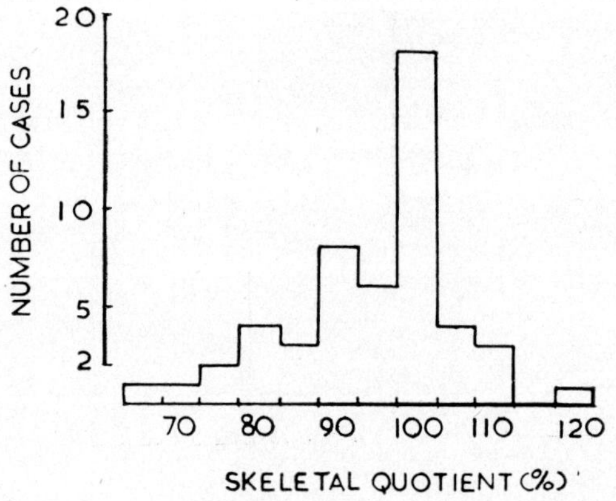

FIG. 4.—The distribution of skeletal quotients in mongol boys. (Skeletal quotient is skeletal age divided by life age and multiplied by 100.)

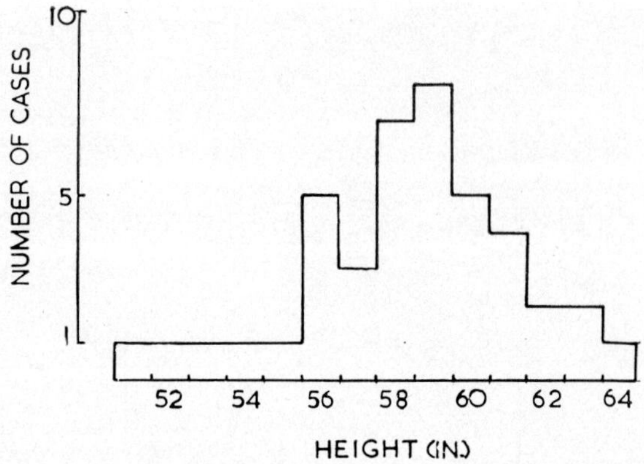

FIG. 5.—The distribution of heights of adult male mongols.

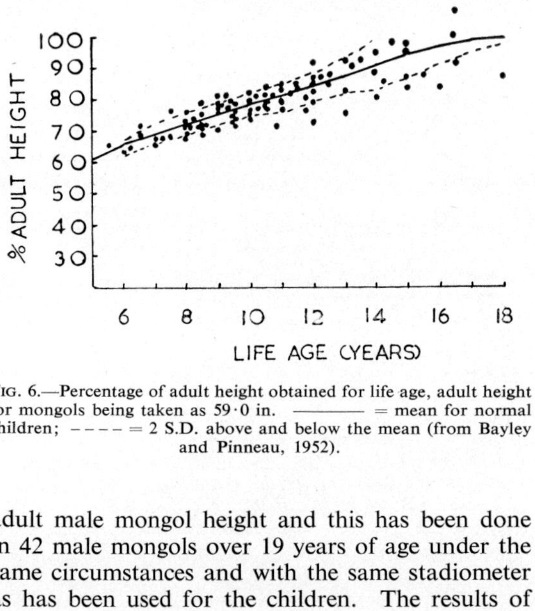

FIG. 6.—Percentage of adult height obtained for life age, adult height for mongols being taken as 59·0 in. ——— = mean for normal children; - - - - = 2 S.D. above and below the mean (from Bayley and Pinneau, 1952).

adult male mongol height and this has been done in 42 male mongols over 19 years of age under the same circumstances and with the same stadiometer as has been used for the children. The results of this assessment are given in Fig. 5, which shows the peak incidence occurring at 59·0 in. This is actually the arithmetic mean of the group. This result compares with the figures quoted by Benda (1949), in which the mean height of 12 male mongols over 19 years is 58·8 in., whilst the mean obtained from the figures of Brousseau (1928) on 22 mongol men is 57·5 in. For the purpose of comparison the figure of 59·0 in. as the adult male mongol height has been used.

Fig. 6 has been derived using the adult height of mongols as above and converting the actual height to a percentage of this. The percentage so obtained has been plotted against the life age. The normal and two standard deviations above and below the mean have been given and are taken from the work of Bayley and Pinneau (1952). From this graph it is seen that the height of mongol children develops towards their adult height in a similar manner to normal children.

Discussion

It is often stated that mongols are examples of the unfinished child. Kirman (1957) says 'Mongolism is essentially a picture of delayed physical and mental development', and Penrose (1954) 'The clinical and pathological signs of mongolism can be summarized by saying that almost all of them are indications of retarded development'. There is, however, one aspect of their development that has been shown in this paper to be essentially normal: the maturation of the skeleton.

The maturation of the skeleton has often been referred to in works on mongolism but there is quite a discrepancy in the results. Brousseau (1928) says that there is retarded development but admits later that opinions differ and points out that whilst there may be delay in ossification in mongolism it is not so marked as in cretinism. Engler (1949) is of the opinion that there is no appreciable delay in the appearance of centres of ossification and suggests that this may be used to differentiate mongolism from cretinism. Kirman (1957) makes no direct reference to the skeletal age at all. Benda (1949) does not give any details but states that the appearance of ossification centres is frequently retarded and resembles the picture of cretinism. Hefke (1940) in his paper on the anomalies to be found radiographically in the hands of mongols has reviewed the literature and quotes very divergent opinions as regards the skeletal age. He goes on to describe his findings in 72 mongols between the ages of 2 months and 15 years. He found osseous development was normal in 79%, advanced in 14% and delayed in 7% but he does not say what constitutes normality in relation to standard deviations in his series. In my series, and assuming that cases falling between plus and minus two standard deviations are normal, I found no cases to be hypermature and 20·8% were delayed as regards their skeletal maturity. In mongols, then, from this series it can be said that nearly 80% have a normally developing skeletal maturation. At one time it was thought that the short stature of adult mongols was due to a hypermature skeleton that had resulted in the premature fusion of epiphyses, but this hypothesis is not tenable on the evidence of skeletal maturation presented here.

When height alone is considered mongol children are found to be very retarded in linear growth, no cases coming up to the normal expectation. This has been reported before but when one considers the development of linear growth towards normal adult *mongol* height the maturation is surprisingly normal. A comparison between the height and expected height for age shown in Fig. 1 and Fig. 6 showing the percentage of adult height obtained for age shows this difference very well. From this it seems fair to say that in mongol boys, although the absolute height is depressed when compared with that of normal boys, the development of height is normal for mongols and that this is yet another aspect of maturation which proceeds normally.

To differentiate between growth and development is important since these two aspects are under different control. The maturation of the skeleton is influenced by the thyroid; in cretinism there is a marked delay in skeletal maturation and the administration of an active thyroid principal brings about a remarkable skeletal advancement (Zondek, Kaatz, Leszynsky, Margoliash and Stein, 1958).

Linear growth, on the other hand, is under the control of the anterior pituitary growth hormone and this has little influence on maturation. There are, of course, other factors which are integrated in the hormonal control of growth (Hubble, 1957), but as regards the differentiation between growth and development the growth factor and the thyroid hormone appear to be the prime movers. Even so it would be incorrect to isolate these two factors since it is necessary for other hormones to be present as well as an adequate supply of the necessary building materials for normal growth and development to occur.

Since the problem is one of growth failure it is permissible to look at the problem from the aspect of protein metabolism and, if one accepts the equations given by Hubble, the two possibilities are a diminution of the anabolic hormones (the left hand side of the equation) or an increase in the catabolic hormones (the right hand side of the equation). In the pre-steroid phase of growth in mongols I have found the daily excretion of total 17-ketosteroids and 17-ketogenic steroids to be essentially normal and this would appear to exonerate the adrenals. These findings, which are as yet unpublished, are in agreement with the results of Bixby and Benda (1944) who found that the adrenal androgens were normal in mongols but that there was a failure of testicular androgens.

The evidence presented here supports the contention that in mongols thyroid function is normal and this is in agreement with the findings of Sobel, Strazzulla, Sherman, Elkan, Morgenstern, Marius and Meisel (1958) who were unable to detect a significant difference in the levels of protein-bound iodine in mongols and controls. Benda, on the other hand, considers that mongols show an increase in blood cholesterol and a low B.M.R. Sobel *et al.* (1958) did not confirm the alteration in the level of cholesterol.

When carbohydrate metabolism is considered as an indirect method of assessing insulin secretion there is a difference of opinion between Sobel *et al.* (1958) and Benda (1949), the former finding normal levels of fasting blood sugar and the latter an increased sugar tolerance with flat curves and an inability of adrenalin to raise the blood sugar significantly. The evidence offered by Benda does not suggest an abnormality of insulin metabolism but rather a primary abnormality of glycogen storage and release by the liver.

Returning then to the equations for hormonal growth, during the pre-steroid phase in mongols, three of the principal protein anabolizers and the principal catabolic hormone are exonerated and all that is left is the growth factor on the anabolic side of the equation. This hormone is not as easily assessed as the others, and in fact there is no direct assay available, but the evidence suggests that it is this aspect of the endocrine system that is at fault in mongols if the disorder is of a hormonal nature.

Summary

Two aspects of the physical development of mongol boys are discussed, height and skeletal maturation. It is shown that skeletal maturation is normal in 80% of cases and that mongols although deficient in linear growth mature normally towards mongol adulthood.

The possible significance of these findings is discussed in relation to endocrine imbalance.

I wish to express my thanks to Dr. J. M. Crawford, Physician Superintendent at Botleys Park Hospital, Chertsey, for his encouragement and for his permission to undertake the survey. I am also grateful to the nursing staff and patients for their willing co-operation and to Mr. E. Comer, the hospital radiographer, who took all the radiographs.

References

Bayley, N. and Pinneau, S. R. (1952). *J. Pediat.*, **40**, 423.
——, —— (1952). *Ibid.*, **41**, 371.
Benda, C. E. (1949). *Mongolism and Cretinism*, 2nd ed. Grune and Stratton, New York.
Bixby, E. M. and Benda, C. E. (1944). *Amer. J. ment. Defic.*, **49**, 138.
Brousseau, K. (1928). *Mongolism: A Study of the Physical and Mental Characteristics of Mongolian Imbeciles.* Williams and Wilkins, Baltimore
Engler, M. (1949). *Mongolism.* J. Wright, Bristol.
Greulich, W. W. and Pyle, S. I. (1950). *Radiographic Atlas of Skeletal Development of the Hand and Wrist.* Stanford, California.
Hefke, H. W. (1940). *Amer. J. Dis. Child.*, **60**, 1319.
Hubble, D. (1957). *Brit. med. J.*, **1**, 601.
Kirman, B. H. (1957). In L. T. Hilliard and B. H. Kirman's *Mental Deficiency*, p. 308. Churchill, London.
Krogman, W. M. (1950). *A Handbook of the Measurement and Interpretation of Height and Weight in the Growing Child.* Monogr. Society for Research in Child Development. Serial No. 48, vol. 13, no 3.
London County Council (1955). *Report on the Heights and Weights of School Pupils in the County of London in 1954.*
Penrose, L. S. (1954). *The Biology of Mental Defect*, 2nd ed Sidgwick and Jackson, London.
Sobel, A. E., Strazzulla, M., Sherman, B. S., Elkan, B., Morgenstern S. W., Marius, N. and Meisel, A. (1958). *Amer. J. ment. Defic.*, **62**, 642.
Sutcliffe, A. and Canham, J. W. (1950). *The Heights and Weights of Boys and Girls.* Murray, London.
Talbot, N. B., Sobel, E. H., Burke, B. S., Lindemann, E. K. and Kaufman, S. B. (1947). *New Engl. J. Med.*, **236**, 783.
Zondek, H., Kaatz, A., Leszynsky, H. E., Margoliash, E. and Stein, J. A. (1958). *Brit. med. J.*, **1**, 546.

THE PLACE OF OATS IN THE COELIAC DIET

BY

A. LINDSAY C. MOULTON

From the Department of Paediatrics and Child Health, University of Birmingham, and Birmingham Children's Hospital

(RECEIVED FOR PUBLICATION JUNE 21, 1958)

Since the discovery by Dicke (1950) that remarkable benefit followed the withdrawal of wheat and rye from the diet of the coeliac child, much work has been done on the significance of these and other foodstuffs in the coeliac syndrome. Few of these studies, however, involved oats, a food containing a prolamin similar to the gliadin of wheat which was proved to be injurious by van de Kamer, Weijers and Dicke (1953).

In 1955, van de Kamer and Weijers suggested that the effects of various foodstuffs on the coeliac patient are related to their amide:non-amide nitrogen ratios and they compiled a list of foods arranged according to this ratio. In many respects their series agrees with the known effects of the foods in coeliac disease. Oats and oatflakes are of interest as they are placed on the margin between the harmful and non-harmful foods.

Previous workers on oats, Dicke, Weijers and van de Kamer (1953), and van de Kamer *et al.* (1953), who fed the same child 140 g. oatmeal per day, and Hansted (1955), who gave one child 150 g. oatmeal per day, claim that such large intakes have some harmful effect. However, in another patient, 75 g. oatmeal per day produced only a slight increase in fat excretion (Hansted, 1955). The effect of still smaller amounts on two groups of three patients each was investigated by Sheldon (1955). The first group received 2 oz. (56 g.) oatmeal per day and the second 1 oz. (28 g.). Despite the short duration of his experiments, he concludes that oatmeal, at these more normal levels, has no ill effect on coeliac children. Frazer (1956) reports that his team found no deleterious effect of oats, but details are not given.

Hansted (1956a) suggests that either a high intake of oats for a short time or a small intake over an extended period is necessary to cause an increase equivalent to that produced by wheat in the fat excretion of coeliac children. Attention has been focused on this suggestion in the present investigation. Four cases only have been studied as the continuous fat balances necessary to demonstrate any resulting slight upward trend in fat excretion are very time consuming. A further problem is that high intakes of oats are not easily maintained, as the child becomes tired of the flavour and overwhelmed by the bulk of the food.

The possibility of using oat protein itself was explored but, although several methods of preparation were attempted, considerable difficulties were encountered. Oats do not yield a gluten, although they contain a gliadin and a glutelin similar to those found in the gluten of wheat. Thus preparation of protein by merely washing gluten free from starch is not feasible. No concentrated oats in the form of protein have been used in the present investigation, though dry separation of oat protein particles by means of a micronizer would appear to be the most suitable method of preparation. If in future experiments large quantities of oats prove too much for a child's appetite, replacement with equivalent amounts of this oat protein could be attempted.

Methods and Patients

Continuous fat balance studies over relatively long periods were carried out, fat being estimated daily in the stools by the method of van de Kamer, Huinink and Weijers (1949). Any uneaten food was weighed, analysed for fat and its oat content calculated. Three-day sliding means of the faecal fat excretion and the percentage fat absorption were calculated. In addition, seven-day means of fat intake, fat excretion, percentage fat absorption and oat intake were obtained as these figures show more clearly the general trend of the results. Both for this reason and because of the rather lengthy results in certain cases, only the seven-day means have been charted (Figs. 1-4).

Four coeliac children, diagnosed according to the criteria described by Smellie (1956), were fed on a diet which was gluten-free apart from the content of Three Bears Oats (quick porridge oat flakes: fat content 6·3%; amide: non-amide nitrogen ratio = 14). As the nitrogen content of oats varies considerably (Moir, 1946), one batch of oatflakes was used throughout. The quantities of oatflakes fed were 46, 70, 163 and 169 g. per day, the lengths of the trials being 45, 96, 22 and 23 days respectively.

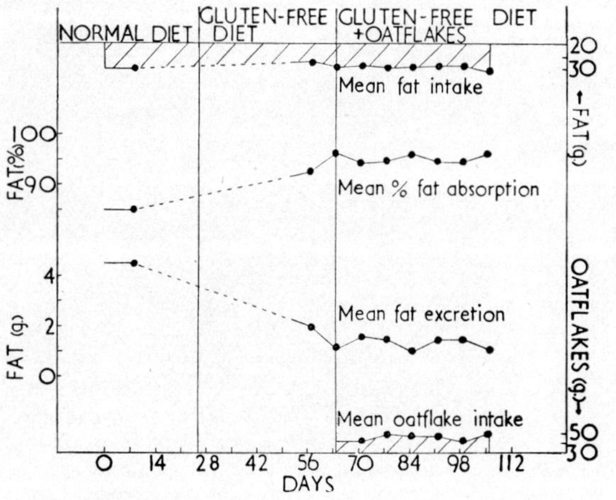

FIG. 1.—Seven-day means of fat excretion and percentage fat absorption in Case 1.—Average oatflake intake 46 g. per day.

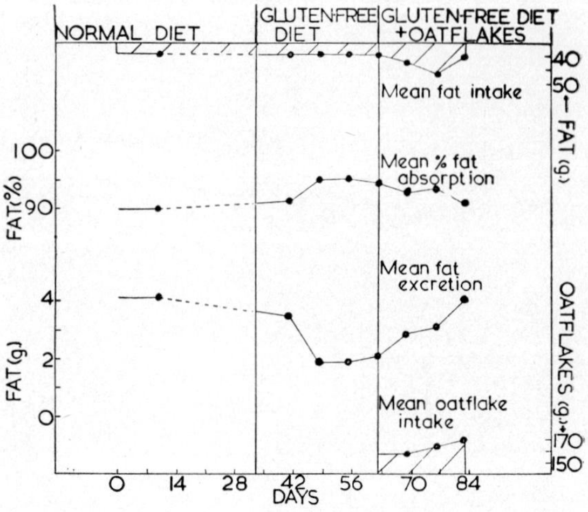

FIG. 3.—Seven-day means of fat excretion and percentage fat absorption in Case 3. Average oatflake intake 163 g. per day.

Results

The results are presented in Figs. 1 to 4 and Tables 1 and 2. In Table 1 are shown the average quantities of fat excreted during normal diets containing gluten, together with the low values to which the patients' faecal fat excretions fell when they were given gluten-free diets. Consumptions of small quantities of oatflakes (46 and 70 g. per day), added to the previous gluten-free diet, caused no rise in fat excretion, but increases up to seven-day mean values of 4·0 and 4·1 g. fat per day during the trial period resulted when 169 and 163 g. per day were eaten.

Discussion

Barley (Hansted, 1956b), wheat and rye (Dicke, 1950) are considered harmful to coeliac children; in the case of wheat, the prolamin or gliadin is thought to be responsible (van de Kamer *et al.*,

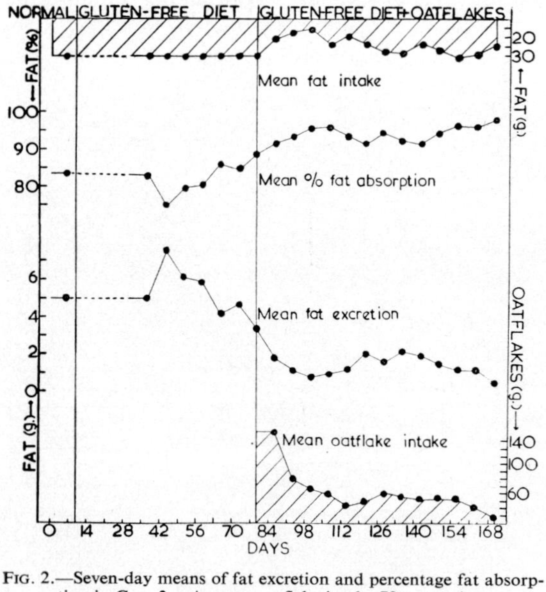

FIG. 2.—Seven-day means of fat excretion and percentage fat absorption in Case 2. Average oatflake intake 70 g. per day.

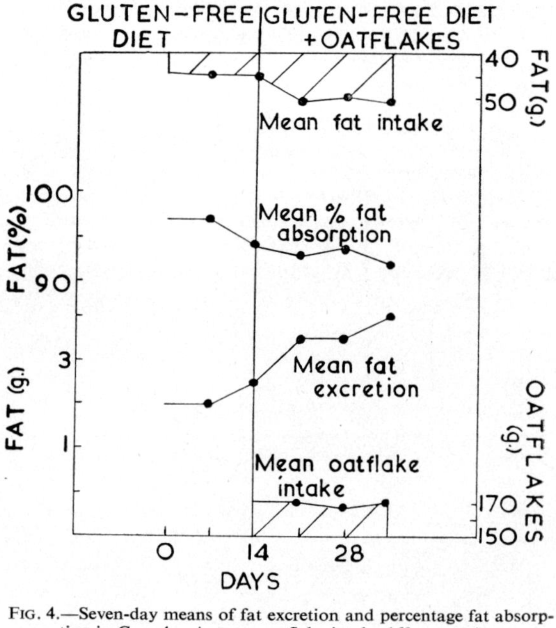

FIG. 4.—Seven-day means of fat excretion and percentage fat absorption in Case 4. Average oatflake intake 169 g. per day.

TABLE 1
CASE HISTORIES

Patient	Age (yr.)	Presenting Symptoms	Normal Diet (before treatment)			Gluten-free Diet			Gluten-free Diet + Oatflakes			
			Days (averaged)	Mean Fat Excr. (g./d.)	Mean Fat Absorp. (%/d.)	Duration (days)	Fat Excr. (g./d.)	Fat Absorp. (%/d.)	Mean Oatflake Intake (g./d.)	Duration (days)	Fat Excr. (g./d.)	Fat *Absorp. (%/d.)
1	2 9/12	Anaemic. Pale and easily tired since birth	8	4·5	85	39	≮1·1	≯96·3	46	45	≯1·6	≮94·5
2	15/12	Stools frequent and bulky for 1 m. before admission. Distended abdomen. Weight loss	6	5·0	83·5	71	≮3·4†	≯88·7†	70	96	≯2·2	≮92·3
3	10	Thin, pale child. Recurrent diarrhoea over previous 4 yr.	10	4·1	90	30	≮2·0	≯95	163	22	≯4·1	≮91
4	11	Diarrhoea attacks since 7 m. old. Diagnosed as coeliac at 18 m. On home gluten-free diet since 3½ yr.	5	5·0	?‡	19§	2·2	95·1	169	23	≯4·0	≮92

* Seven-day means.
† Although the child was not fully equilibrated on a gluten-free diet at this stage, oatflakes were given on the assumption that the fat excretion would not rise if they were harmless.
‡ Record lost.
§ Strict gluten-free diet in hospital, as opposed to gluten-free diet at home.

1953). It is therefore of interest that, in a list of the quantities of prolamins in the dry grains of several cereals, in which the total protein contents are approximately equal, Brohult and Sandegren (1954) give wheat, rye and barley prolamins as 40-50%, 30-50% and 35-45% respectively of total protein, and oats as only 10-15%. That of rice is low. Thus, large quantities of prolamin are found in all three of the harmful cereals mentioned above, smaller amounts in oats, possibly correlated with their less detrimental effect, and very little in rice which can be safely eaten by coeliac children.

The prolamin content of maize, however, is stated to be 50-55% of the total protein. If all cereals containing large quantities of prolamin are to be considered detrimental to the coeliac patient this high value for maize prolamin requires consideration. It is approximately equal to the figures of

TABLE 2
COMPARISON OF PUBLISHED RESULTS WITH PRESENT FINDINGS

	Age (yr.)	Oat Intake (g./d.)	Duration of Oat Supplement (days)	Gluten-free Diet Fat Excr. (g./d.)	Gluten-free Diet Fat Absorp. (%/d.)	Gluten-free Diet+Oats Fat Excr. (g./d.)	Gluten-free Diet+Oats Fat Absorp. (%/d.)
Dicke *et al.* (1953) . . } Above authors; also van de Kamer *et al.* (1953) }	9	140?	3-4 w.	4·3*	91·3*	7·3*	85·3*
		140	52†	2·4	95·5	5·2	89·6
Hansted (1955)	9	150	1 m.†	3·5‡	89·9‡	5·2‡	85·1‡
"	4	75	1 m.†	1·4‡	95·9‡	2·3‡	93·6‡
Sheldon (1955)	1 9/12	28	18	—	—	—	93
	5 10/12	28	22	—	87	—	87
	7 2/12	28	34	—	93	—	93
	4 3/12	56	15	—	95·5	—	97
	4 2/12	56	15	—	91	—	88
	10 4/12	56	22	—	91	—	89
Present Study	10	163	22	2·2	94·5	3·5	91·9
	11	169	23	2·3	95·1	3·7	93
	1 6/12	70	96	5·2	82·7	1·4	94·2
	3	46	45	1·5	94·7	1·3	95·5

* These values are high as they were obtained just after the patient was changed from a normal diet for the first time. The second set of figures probably indicates the patient's true reactions.
† Approximately.
‡ Hansted has presented these data in the form of graphs only; approximations from these are given.

Hansen, Brimhall and Sprague (1946), but wide ranges for the prolamin content of maize, 25-60% and 28-57% of total protein, are given by Doty, Bergdoll, Nash and Brunson (1946) and Showalter and Carr (1922) respectively, as the prolamin content of the maize grain rises with increasing maturity (Zeleny, 1935) and nitrogen content (Showalter and Carr, 1922; Hansen, Brimhall and Sprague, 1946). Despite this variation, if maize prolamin is similar in structure and action to that of wheat, it is reasonable to suppose that maize would be detrimental to coeliac children. Hansted (1956b), without giving details, claims that maize, as such, is well tolerated, but in the majority of trials including those of van de Kamer *et al.* (1953), Dicke *et al.* (1953) and Hansted (1955), the only forms of corn (maize) investigated were cornstarch, or cornflour which consists almost exclusively of cornstarch (Ford, 1946). Thus although cornstarch like wheatstarch is harmless to the coeliac patient, the maize prolamin, zein, does not appear to have been tested and may, therefore, be injurious both by itself and in the form of the maize grain.

When placed in order of magnitude, the various cereal prolamin contents, quoted above, correspond to a series of foods similar, apart from maize, to that given by van de Kamer and Weijers (1955). In this latter series, rice, maize, oatflakes, oats, barley flour, rye flour, wheat flour and gliadin, among other foods, are arranged according to their amide:non-amide nitrogen ratios which are 11, 11, 12, 13, 14, 17, 23 and 30 respectively. Thus, without suggesting a precise quantitative relationship between either of these sets of figures and the effect of the foods on the coeliac, it is obvious that, should the prolamin be responsible for the deleterious effect, much greater quantities of oats than wheat could be eaten with safety by coeliac children.

If large quantities of oats or oatflakes are likely to have harmful effects, the three levels of intake fed in the present experiments ought to result in a progressive increase in fat excretion Such an increase is shown in Table 2 in which the lowest level of oatflake feeding (46 g. per day) corresponds to a fat excretion of 1·3 g. per day and the highest (169 g. oatflakes per day) to 3·7 g. faecal fat per day. The fat excretion during the 70 g. oatflake diet, though slightly higher, resembles that corresponding to the 46 g. oatflake diet. It should be noted that in Table 2 the results of the present study are given in the form of averages of all the fat excretion and percentage fat absorption values obtained during each particular dietary period, without allowance being made in the calculations for the children's fat excretions to become equilibrated on each new diet. Since the child having 70 g. oatflakes per day was not fully equilibrated on a gluten-free diet, an average of all available figures gives a falsely high fat excretion. Reference to Fig. 2 shows that her final fat excretion on a gluten-free diet was much lower than 5·0 g. per day.

In Table 2, the results of other workers are given for comparison. They seem to follow the same general trend, although the varying lengths of the studies complicate their appraisal. The first three sets of figures are the results of feeding large quantities of oatmeal over long periods. They demonstrate a rise in fat excretion to values just above the upper limits of normal. In the present investigation, the figures obtained during the feeding of even greater amounts of oatflakes have not reached such high levels. Possibly if we could have persuaded our children to eat large quantities of oatflakes for a longer period, their excretion of fat would have risen even further. Indeed, the mean values for the third seven-day periods had reached 4·1 and 4·0 g. per day on 163 and 169 g. oatflakes respectively (Figs. 3 and 4). The fact that oatflakes were fed in the present experiments, whereas oatmeal was investigated by the other authors, may have some significance, for according to the list of amide-non-amide nitrogen ratios of van de Kamer and Weijers (1955) oatflakes with a ratio of 12 ought to be slightly less harmful than oatmeal at 13. However, the ratio in our particular batch of Three Bears Oats was 14. Variations in nitrogen content, etc., may frequently be caused by changes in weather and soil conditions. The value 14 still does not approach wheat flour at 23 or wheat gliadin at 30.

Our results give some indication of the intake of oatflakes which can be given to the coeliac with safety. Thus, one patient receiving 70 g. oatflakes per day for 90 days and another receiving 46 g. per day for 45 days showed no increase in fat excretion. Hansted (1955) found that a child fed on 75 g. oatmeal per day for one month did show a slight increase in fat excretion (Table 2). This might appear to conflict with our findings but the increase, noted by Hansted, is well within normal limits. Thus, it seems that 1-2 oz. (28-56 g.) oatflakes per day may be given to the coeliac with safety, a conclusion which is supported by Sheldon's (1955) shorter studies when feeding 1 oz. (28 g.) oatmeal per day (Table 2). Two of his three cases who received 2 oz. (56 g.) oatmeal per day did suffer a slight deleterious effect, although he does not consider the change in fat absorption of importance. This view is probably justified as, in England at least, oats are unlikely to be eaten every day, though a trial of a foodstuff suspected of having only a slight effect should be continued for a considerable time, especially when only small amounts are eaten. The increase in fat excretion, produced by the largest intakes which have been given, are still within normal limits and, in our experience, it was almost impossible for the patients to consume even this bulk of oats daily.

Summary

The effects of giving 46, 70, 163 and 169 g. oatflakes per day to four coeliac children for 45, 96, 22 and 23 days respectively have been studied and the results compared with those of other workers. It is concluded that, at least in some coeliac patients, amounts up to 2 oz. (56 g.) oatflakes per day may be fed without ill effect. Even the highest quantities of oatflakes given (169 g. per day for three weeks, an amount almost impossible to consume) only produced an increase in faecal fat excretion up to the verge of normal limits.

I would like to express my gratitude to Professor J. M. Smellie, Mr. H. B. Salt and Dr. O. H. Wolff for their interest and valuable criticism, to Miss J. E. Tilley for skilful management of the oatflake diets, to the nursing staff of the Birmingham Children's Hospital for their unfailing co-operation and to J. and J. Colman, Ltd., for the gift of Three Bears Oats used throughout the investigation.

My thanks are also due to Dr. N. Blakebrough, Department of Chemical Engineering, Birmingham University and the Scottish Co-operative Wholesale Society Cereal Laboratory, Glasgow, for helpful advice on the preparation of oat protein and to Reckitt & Colman, Ltd., Norwich, A. & R. Scott, Ltd., Edinburgh, and Henry Simon, Ltd., Stockport, for practical aid in this problem.

References

Brohult, S. and Sandegren, E. (1954). In *The Proteins*, ed. G. Neurath and K. Bailey, Vol. 2, part A, p. 487. New York.

Dicke, W. K. (1950). *Coeliakie.* M. D. Thesis. Utrecht.

——, Weijers, H. A. and Kamer, J. H. van de (1953). *Acta paediat.* (*Uppsala*), **42**, 34.

Doty, D. M., Bergdoll, M. S., Nash, H. A. and Brunson, A. M. (1946). *Cereal Chem.*, **23**, 199.

Ford, W. P. (1946). In *The Nation's Food*, ed. A. L. Bacharach and T. Rendle, p. 196. London.

Frazer, A. C. (1956). *Proc. roy. Soc. Med.*, **49**, 1009.

Hansen, D. W., Brimhall, B. and Sprague, G. F. (1946). *Cereal Chem.*, **23**, 329.

Hansted, C. (1955). *Ugeskr. Laeg.*, **117**, 481.

—— (1956a). Personal communication.

—— (1956b). 8th International Congress of Paediatrics, exhibition 137. Copenhagen.

Kamer, J. H. van de, Huinink, H. ten Bokkel and Weijers, H. A. (1949). *J. biol. Chem.*, **177**, 347.

—— and Weijers, H. A. (1955). *Acta paediat.* (*Uppsala*), **44**, 465.

——, —— and Dicke, W. K. (1953). *Ibid.*, **42**, 223.

Moir, H. C. (1946). In *The Nation's Food*, ed. A. L. Bacharach and T. Tendle, p. 205. London.

Sheldon, W. (1955). *Lancet*, **2**, 1097.

Smellie, J. M. (1956). *Med. ill.* (*Lond.*), **10**, 279.

Showalter, M. F. and Carr. R. H. (1922). *J. Amer. chem. Soc.*, **44** 2019.

Zeleny, L. (1935). *Cereal Chem.*, **12**, 536.

MICROCEPHALY IN ONE OF MONOZYGOUS TWINS

BY

M. G. W. BRANDON, BRIAN H. KIRMAN and C. E. WILLIAMS

From the Fountain Hospital, London

(RECEIVED FOR PUBLICATION JULY 15, 1958)

Twin studies have frequently been carried out by those interested in the causation of mental deficiency. Some of the work on this subject is summarized by Böök, Schut and Reed (1953). It is assumed that if the twins are monozygous then hereditary factors will be identical; it is often assumed that the intra-uterine environment will likewise be identical. Though this may be true in general, there are important exceptions the study of which may throw light on the intra-uterine origin of abnormalities. Considerable differences in weight between 'identical' twins are well recognized. Penrose (1937) described syphilis in one of monovular twins and Hinden (1956) reported microcephaly in one of a monozygotic twin pair.

The object of this paper is to give an account of two more pairs of monozygous twins, one member of each pair being healthy, the other being mentally defective and having a head circumference within the microcephalic range. Microcephaly is here defined as a head circumference of less than three standard deviations from the mean for age and sex (Böök *et al.*, 1953). The normal standards used are those of Westropp and Barber (1956).

Case Reports

Case 1. The father is a motor mechanic and the mother was a factory worker before marriage. They were aged 22 and 19 respectively at the birth of the patient and were in good health generally. The maternal great grandmother is said to have had two sets of twins, one being a blind child; a maternal aunt also has twins. The patient and his brother were the result of the first pregnancy, which, according to the hospital where the twins were born, lasted eight months. The mother is said to have had pneumonia at the fourth month and pyelitis at the sixth. The delivery was uneventful, the patient was born first. The mother was affected by eclampsia for several days after the delivery and has a blank in her memory for this period. The patient weighed 3 lb. 3 oz. and his skull circumference was 12 in.; the brother weighed 4 lb. 2 oz., but unfortunately his skull circumference was not measured. The placenta was noted to be uniovular in type and no further details are available from the hospital although the mother says that she understood that the patient's cord came from the side of the placenta whilst that of his brother was centrally attached.

The patient was slightly cyanosed at birth with bruising of the face, forehead, left shoulder, right wrist and some oedema of the lower limbs. Marked jaundice began on the second day lasting till the twenty-fourth, the serum bilirubin being 11 mg. % on the ninth day. On the fifteenth day there was hiccuping but no neck rigidity or hypertonia although some twitching of the face was noted. Subsequent progress was described as satisfactory and the infant was discharged from hospital at the seventh week weighing 4 lb. 11 oz. The brother had

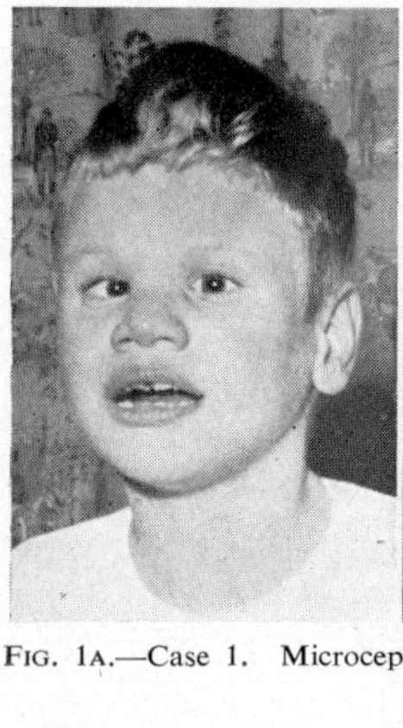

FIG. 1A.—Case 1. Microcephalic twin.

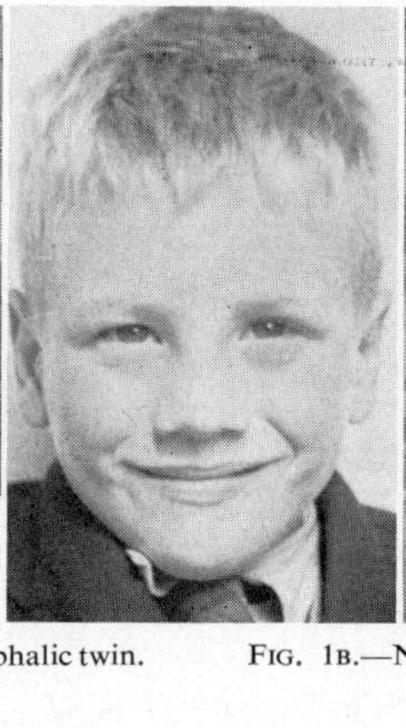

FIG. 1B.—Normal twin.

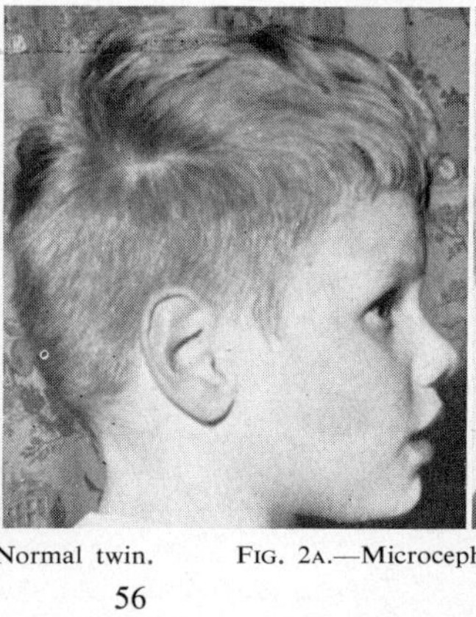

FIG. 2A.—Microcephalic twin.

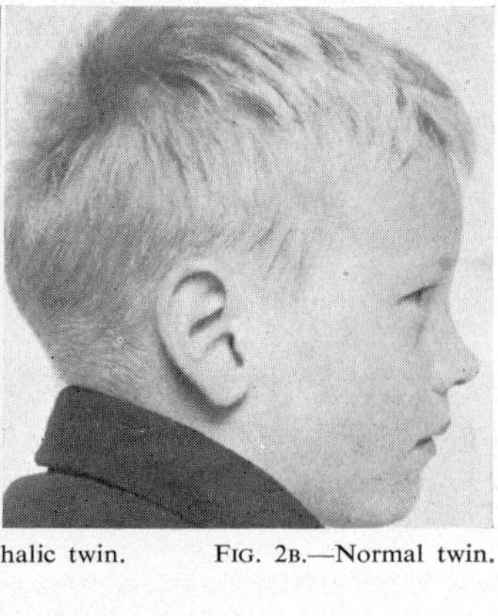

FIG. 2B.—Normal twin.

some slight bruising of the vertex after delivery and developed a slight transient jaundice on the sixth day.

By contrast with his brother the patient failed to take notice and at 8 months when examined under anaesthetic was found to have optic atrophy, a finding which was confirmed at the age of 1 year. At 3 years he still did not walk and was thought at hospital not to have light perception. The small head was then noted. On admission to the Fountain Hospital aged 3 years and 4 months he was described as an imbecile with a developmental quotient of 22. The Vineland social maturity scale was used: this is very similar to a developmental scale at the early age ranges. He could see, followed objects with his eyes, but would not grasp them. He could not stand, walk or talk except to say ' Hallo '. His weight was 21 lb. and height 32½ in. The cranial circumference was 16½ in. (41·9 cm.); the length 5½ in. (14·0 cm.); breadth 4 in. (10·2 cm.); cranial index 0·73.

He made little progress and at the age of 5 years and 9 months he could still only crawl and appeared almost blind with occasional nystagmus, scoring a social quotient of 13 (Figs. 1A and 2A). The head circumference at 7 years was 17¾ in. (45·1 cm.). The mean for boys of 7 years is 52·7 cm. and the patient is between five and six standard deviations less than the mean for his age and sex in this respect. The head length is 6 in. and the breadth 4⅝ with a cranial index of 0·77.

The brother (Figs. 1B and 2B) is now a normal boy of 7 years with a vocabulary level of 9 years and an intelligence quotient of 108 on the Terman-Merrill scale, of 113 on the Progressive Matrices and of 116 on the Goodenough. The cranial circumference is 20 in. (50·8 cm.) which is between one and two standard deviations below the mean for his age and sex. The length of the head is 18·1 cm. (7 1/10 in.); the breadth is 13·5 cm. (5 3/10 in.); the cranial index 0·75.

He presents no physical or mental abnormalities.

The twins were noted to be very similar at birth and at the present time, despite the difference in head size, they look very like each other, they have the same blue eyes and hair colour. The blood groups of the family are as follows:

Father: A1, MSMs, P−, R_1r, Lu(a−), K−, Le(a+), Fy(a+), Jk(a+b+).

Mother: A2, MsMs, P+, $R^w{}_1R_1$, Lu(a−), K−, Le(a−), Fy(a+), Jk(a+b+).

Patient: A2, MsMs, P−, R_1R_1, Lu(a−), K−, Le(a−b+), Fy(a+), Jk(a+b+).

Brother: A2, MsMs, P−, R_1R_1, Lu(a−), K−, Le(a−), Fy(a+), Jk(a+b+).

Dr. Ruth Sanger concluded on the basis of these results that the probability of dizygosity was 0·76%. Palm prints of the twins were also studied and the patterns on the fingers were in agreement. The palmar patterns were not very similar superficially but the difference in the sum of the Atd angles was only 4 degrees. Combining the two sets of data Professor Penrose concluded that the probability of dizygosity was 0·213%, i.e. 1/476. The present measurements of the twins are set out as follows:

	Patient	Patient's Brother
Head circumference	45 cm.	51 cm.
Biparietal diameter	12·2 cm.	13·5 cm.
Occipito-frontal diameter	15·3 „	18·1 „
Weight	34 lb. 6 oz.	50 lb. 11 oz.
Total height	41 in.	46·5 in.
Height from feet to top of symphysis	19·5 in.	23 „
„ „ head „ „ „	21·5 „	23·5 „
Span	42·5 „	48·5 „

Case 2. The father is an engineer and the mother was a dressmaker before marriage; they were aged 35 and 33 respectively at the patient's birth. There is no report of any mental or physical defect, mental illness or fits in the family and the parents are in good health. The patient and her twin sister were the result of the fifth pregnancy. The first child was stillborn and is said to have been ' strangled by the cord ' and to have weighed 8 lb. The second was also stillborn at 7 months and there was said to have been no movement for three months prior to the delivery. The mother is said to have had toxaemia during that pregnancy. The third and fourth pregnancies resulted in normal boys, the former of whom weighed 10 lb. 7 oz. The mother was well during the twin pregnancy but suffered from swollen feet towards term. Labour was precipitate and occurred at home whilst the mother was sitting on a chair. The first and normal twin was born as the water broke and the patient ' shot out ' 10 minutes later. She was taken to hospital because she did not cry and she was put into an oxygen tent. The birth weight was 4 lb. 10 oz. The baby was said to have fallen on the floor when she was born. She was admitted to a premature unit where she was found to be collapsed and to show signs of ' cerebral irritation '. There were episodes of twitching during the first 4 days of life and she had to be fed by oesophageal tube for the first 10 days. Her progress was satisfactory as far as feeding went but when seen at a year she was a microcephalic idiot. She could not sit, could not feed herself, there were repetitive movements and she seemed unable to focus. The birth weight of the normal twin was 7 lb. No difficulty was experienced with her during the post-natal period and she weighed 8 lb. 3 oz. when discharged from hospital.

The patient was seen again in hospital at 16 months for examination of the eyes under anaesthesia. Both discs were pale but not definitely pathological. There was a right internal strabismus and the head circumference was 15¾ in. (40·0 cm.). She could still not sit up, was definitely backward and there was no evidence of cerebral palsy. The normal twin appeared very much like the patient apart from the shape of the head, which in her case measured 18 in. in circumference.

The child was first admitted to the Fountain Hospital at 28 months. She weighed 22 lb. and the height was 33½ in.; cranial circumference 16½ in. (41·9 cm.); length 5 in. (12·7 cm.); breadth 4 in. (10·2 cm.); cranial index 0·80. She frequently assumed an opisthotonic position. She could not assume or maintain the sitting position. She could not stand, walk, talk or feed herself. She was spoon-fed with difficulty and could not chew. She did not appear blind and seemed to fix objects,

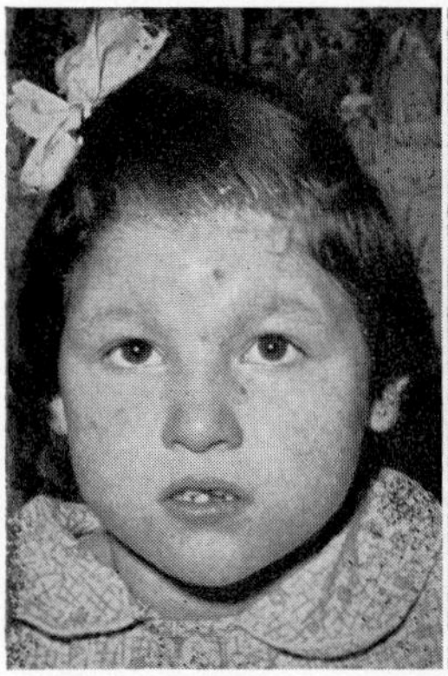

FIG. 3A.—Case 2. Microcephalic twin.

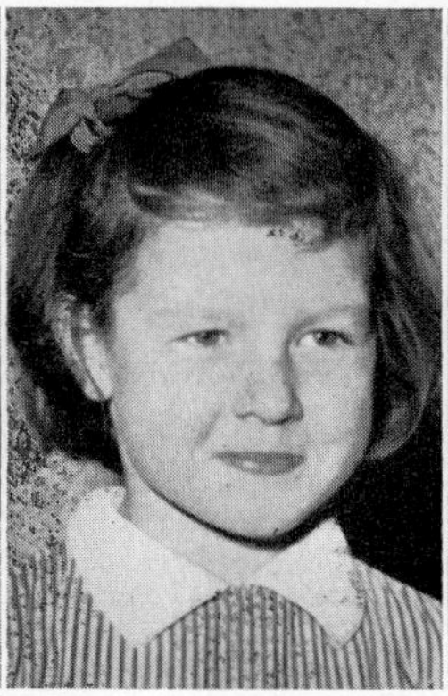

FIG. 3B.—Normal twin.

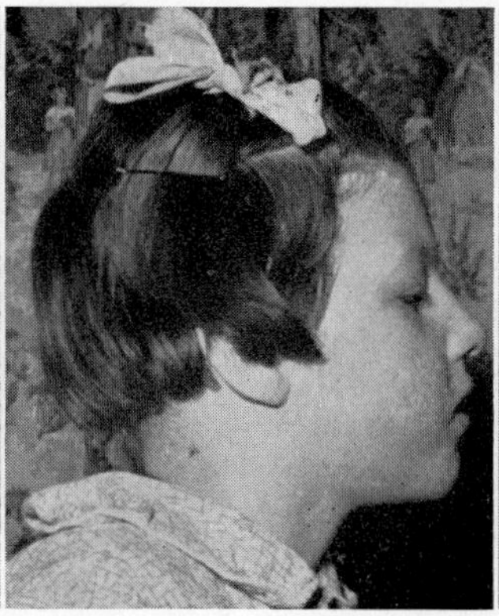

FIG. 4A.—Microcephalic twin.

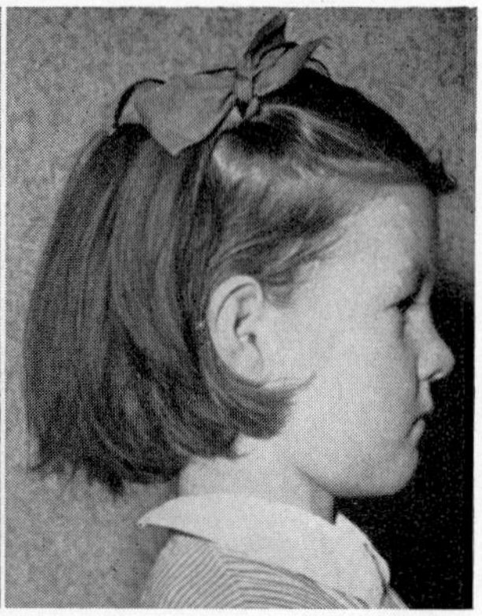

FIG. 4B.—Normal twin.

though her squint made assessment of this difficult. She smiled when a bell was rung, but she made no attempt to take objects. Her social quotient on the Vineland scale was then 9.

Very little progress was made and when the child was examined at the age of 6 years, the quotient on the same scale was 10 which was almost identical (Figs. 3A and 4A). Although interested and responsive she would only grasp toys when they touched her hand and retained them for only a few seconds. She could not stand, walk or talk and could not feed herself. She was doubly incontinent. Two major epileptic fits had been recorded during the last year. The head circumference was 17⅝ in. (44·8 cm.). The mean for girls of 6 years is 51·7 cm. and the patient is between four and five standard deviations less than the mean for her age and sex in this respect. The head length is 5⅝ in. (14·3 cm.), and the breadth 4⅝ in. (11·7 cm.), with a cranial index of 0·82.

The sister (Figs. 3B and 4B) is now a normal girl of 6 years with a good vocabulary and memory for verbal items. She achieved a score of 109 on the Terman-Merrill scale and of 112 on the Goodenough ' draw a man ' test. She is considered above average in ability. The cranial circumference is 20 in. (50·8 cm.) which is within the standard deviation from the mean for her age and sex. The length of the skull is 6 7/10 in. (17·0 cm.) and the breadth 5 3/10 in. (13·5 cm.), cranial index 0·79. She presented no physical or mental abnormalities, apart from a contracture of the little finger which she has in common with the patient.

Although the twins were similar in other respects the patient was distinguished from birth by her oddly shaped head which was flat at the back and had a sloping forehead, also by her slow development. The eye colour appears identical but the normal girl's hair is fairer with blond streaks in front (? influence of extraneous factors). The blood groups of the family are as follows:

Father: B, MSMs, P+, R_1r, Lu(a+), K−, Le(a−), Fy(a−), Jk(a+).
Mother: O, MSNs, P−, R_1R_2, Lu(a−), K−, Le(a+b−), Fy(a+), Jk(a−).
Patient: O, MsNs, P+, R_1R_1, Lu(a−), K−, Le(a−), Fy(a−), Jk(a+b+).
Sister: O, MsNs, P+, R_1R_1, Lu(a−), K−, Le(a−), Fy(a−), Jk(a+).

Dr. Ruth Sanger who kindly provided this information estimated the chance of dizygosity as 0·40 %, i.e. 1/250. This was improved by Professor Penrose to 0·25%, i.e. 1/400, by consideration of finger ridge counts and atd angles.

Discussion

From the evidence presented it may reasonably be assumed that these two twin pairs were each identical. One child in each pair is both mentally defective and microcephalic.

In Case 1 there was some evidence of birth trauma in the affected twin. In this case, however, the child's head was already 3·5 standard deviations below the mean at birth. This is a greater reduction than might be expected merely because of prematurity. This child also had jaundice, but the serum bilirubin, though raised to 11 mg. %, did not reach the critical level of 18 mg. % (Crosse, Meyer and Gerrard, 1955) at which kernikterus is likely to ensue, nor was transfusion required. Optic atrophy, which was present in this case, has not, in our experience, been a feature of the post-kernikteric syndrome (Crome, Kirman and Marrs, 1955).

In Case 2 the affected twin was distinguished by her flattened occiput and sloping forehead. The head circumference at 16 months was 40·0 cm., which corresponds to the mean for a 3-month-old baby and is more than four standard deviations below the mean for age and sex. Despite the history of precipitate labour and neonatal distress, it is improbable that such a reduction in size was due solely to birth injury.

The balance of the evidence, therefore, in both cases, favours the view that the microcephaly was due to factors operating during pregnancy, though it is admittedly difficult to exclude 'birth injury' in the broad sense of the term, as a causal factor.

Since, in each case, the other twin is normal it becomes difficult to assign the defect to the influence of hereditary factors, although there is a strong tendency to do this in regard to microcephaly. Indeed Komai, Kishimoto and Ozaki (1955) state that ' the evidence for the production of microcephaly by non-genetic agents other than irradiation is not convincing'. There is no history of irradiation in these two cases and it seems difficult to escape the conclusion that the small size of the head is due to unknown adverse factors operating during pregnancy.

The potentially adverse effects of twinning may be considered as a factor in these cases. It is well recognized that twins tend to have a low birth weight and are more subject to the hazards which beset premature infants. There is also a certain association between very low birth weights and congenital abnormality. Thus, in cases of rubella embryopathy (Director-General Public Health Services, New South Wales, 1945) the birth weight is low, averaging 5 lb. 15 oz. in 130 cases. In 99 cases of microcephaly at the Fountain Hospital the average birth weight was 6 lb. 1 oz. It may be argued that in, for example, genetically determined cases of microcephaly it is the brain defect which produces the smallness of the foetus. On the other hand, in cases such as those reported here it may be that adverse factors, including multiple pregnancy, tend to produce both low birth weight and brain defect.

Certain difficulties of definition arise in considering this problem. If a baby has a low birth weight, then is it correct to assess the head size on the basis of standards derived from babies most of whom had a normal birth weight? Experience suggests that, although this procedure may seem illogical, it will afford a rough guide as to the baby's prospect of normal development and that a marked reduction below the norm indicates a probability of permanent microcephaly.

A related problem concerns the definition of 'true' microcephaly which is usually equated with forms of the condition which are thought to be genetically determined. A critique of the concept of 'true' microcephaly is contained in a separate communication. Although many authors suggest that it is possible to recognize the condition clinically there is little general agreement on the signs although long-headedness ('Aztec form') is the one on which there is best accord. The cranial index in the present cases was 73 and 77 in Case 1 and 80 and 82 in Case 2. These measurements compare with Penrose's (1954) figure of 73, being an average for 10 cases of microcephaly, a figure which is in the dolichocephalic range. The present cases therefore do not provide evidence against the view that genetic cases of microcephaly can be distinguished by dolicocephaly.

Summary

Two pairs of uniovular twins are described. In each case one member of the pair was microcephalic and the other normal. The cause of the abnormality was not apparent from the history but appears to have been operative during pregnancy. These cases suggest that environmental causes of microcephaly may be important in the absence of a history of irradiation or rubella.

References

Böök, J. A., Schut, J. W. and Reed, S. C. (1953). *Amer. J. ment. Defic.*, **57**, 637.
Crome, L., Kirman, B. H. and Marrs, M. (1955). *Brain*, **78**, 514.
Crosse, V. M., Meyer, T. C. and Gerrard, J. W. (1955). *Arch. Dis. Childh.*, **30**, 501.
Director-General Public Health Services, N.S.W. (1945). *Med. J. Aust.*, **2**, 122.
Hinden, E. (1956). *Brit. med. J.*, **1**, 333.
Komai, T., Kishimoto, K. and Ozaki, Y. (1955). *Amer. J. hum. Genet.*, **7**, 51.
Penrose, L. S. (1937). *Lancet*, **1**, 322.
—— (1954). *The Biology of Mental Defect*, 2nd ed., pp. 84 and 134 Sidgwick and Jackson: London.
Westropp, C. K. and Barber, C. R. (1956). *J. Neurol. Neurosurg. Psychiat.*, **19**, 52.

OXALOSIS

BY

E. KATZUNI and U. SANDBANK

From the Paediatric and Pathological Departments, Kaplan Memorial Hospital, Rehovot, Israel

(RECEIVED FOR PUBLICATION JUNE 16, 1958)

Oxalosis is a metabolic disturbance manifested by hyperoxaluria and leading to the deposition of calcium oxalate crystals in the parenchyma of the kidneys as well as in many other organs.

Until the end of 1957 only 22 cases of oxalosis had been reported: eight cases in adults and 14 in children. Le Poutre (1925) found calcium oxalate crystals in a renal biopsy taken from a child 4½ years old. Lass (1941) reported a similar finding in a man dying accidentally at the age of 25 years.

Davis, Klingberg and Stowell (1950) described the case of a 12-year-old boy who suffered from nephrolithiasis and died as a result of renal failure. Calcium oxalate crystals were found in the kidneys and in the bones. Chou and Donohue (1952) reported on a 7-year-old boy who suffered from nephrolithiasis and died of renal failure. Calcium oxalate crystals were found scattered throughout the bones, the heart, thymus, spleen and the pituitary gland. These authors were the first to consider the disease as an inborn error of the metabolism of the oxalates. Dunn (1955) termed the disease 'oxalosis', and because he found calcium oxalate crystals in the bone marrow advised diagnosis by sternal puncture. The relation of the disease to primary hyperoxaluria was demonstrated by Newns and Black (1953), by Aponte and Fetter (1954) and later by Archer, Dormer, Scowen and Watts (1957).

We present a case of oxalosis which slightly differs from the other cases reported because of extreme youth and the presence of calcium oxalate crystals in many different organs in addition to those already described.

Case History

A girl, 3 months old, was admitted to hospital because of convulsions lasting a few minutes, accompanied by vomiting. The parents and five other children were all in good health. The patient was born at home, the delivery being normal. Her weight at birth is not known. In addition to breast milk she was given buttermilk (Eledon) from birth. Her weight on admission was 2·9 kg., her temperature was 39° C., her general condition was poor and she was pale and dehydrated. At times she was very restless, and this phase was followed by general convulsions lasting a few minutes. Afterwards the child became apathetic.

Physical examination revealed nothing relevant. The cerebrospinal fluid, which was examined immediately after her admission, was normal in all respects. Haemoglobin was 8·1 g. %, erythrocytes 2,720,000, leucocytes 12,000. The urine contained albumin +++, leucocytes were 20 per field, erythrocytes 3-7 and there were many calcium oxalate crystals; the *p*H was 5·8. Urine culture was sterile, Because of the small amount of urine excreted daily (about 20 ml.), the total excretion of calcium, phosphates and oxalates could not be determined.

The blood chemistry on admission showed: urea 178 mg. %, calcium 5·3 mg. per 100 ml. serum, phosphorus 13·4 mg. per 100 ml., alkaline phosphatase 19·4 BU. The CO_2 content was 20 vol. %.

The urea went up within seven days to 206 mg. % and rose to 275 mg. % before death.

The CO_2 content dropped to 14 vol. % after 12 days. Calcium was 3·7 mg. % after 12 days and 4·1 mg. % after 18 days, and phosphorus 14·0 mg. per 100 ml. serum. Potassium on the eighteenth day (one day before death) rose to 28·4 mg. per 100 ml. (7·3 mEq./1). At the same time sodium values were 290 mg. % (126 mEq./1.) and chlorides 294 mg. % (83 mEq./1.). Total proteins on admission were 5·85 g. %, albumin 4·45 g. %, globulin 1·4 g. %. Electrophoresis of the proteins showed increase of α_2-globulin, and decrease of γ-gobulin.

Radiographs of the bones were normal. Intravenous urography was not performed owing to the severely impaired renal function, but a plain radiograph of the abdomen did not show any pathological condition of the kidneys.

During her stay in the hospital the child vomited several times a day and later developed diarrhoea. A stool culture was negative. Treatment included infusions, sedatives and appropriate diet. Her condition deteriorated gradually and she died on the twenty-third day after admission.

Autopsy Findings. Macroscopically the kidneys were small, weighing 10 g. (normal 22 g.); the capsules, which stripped easily, revealed a smooth surface. On cross section the differentiation between cortex and medulla was obvious, the normal ratio being maintained. The pelves were of normal size, shiny and smooth. The ureters were normal and so was the renal pedicle. Three parathyroid glands were detected: two upper and one lower. They were dark brown in colour, the size of a pin head. None of the other organs showed pathological macroscopic findings.

Microscopically most of the tubules in the medulla

and the cortex of the kidneys were dilated and filled with bright yellowish polygonal crystals, arranged in a rosette formation (Fig. 1). The lining epithelium of the tubules

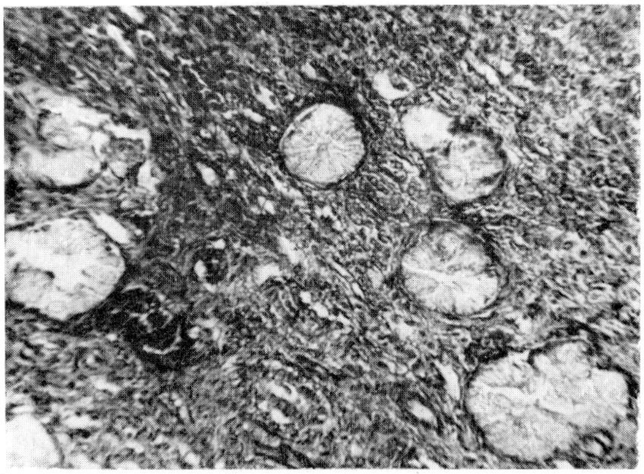

FIG. 1.—Kidney. Crystals arranged in rosette formation in dilated renal tubules. H. and E. × 320.

was flat, and, because of the pressure of the dilated full tubules on the unaffected ones, it was impossible to tell which part of the tubules was affected. The glomeruli were normal, free from crystals; so were the pelves and the ureters. The blood vessels of the kidneys were normal.

Crystals, similar to those found in the tubules, were detected in the myocardium, in the lungs, brain, thymus, thyroid, bone and cartilage. In the myocardium (Fig. 2) the crystals were seen in the muscle fibres, and in the lungs they were found in the septa between the alveoli. In the brain (Fig. 3) they were equally dispersed in the white and in the grey matter. Crystals were found also in the cerebellum. In the thyroid gland they were seen within the colloid only, and not in the interstitial tissue. They were also found in the bones and cartilages, especially concentrated at the osteochondral junction (Fig. 4).

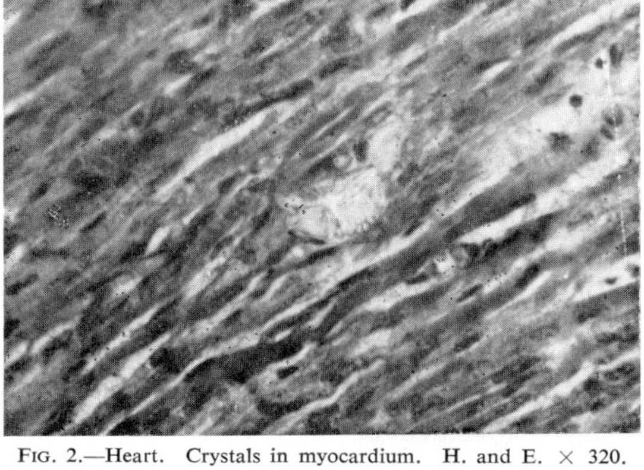

FIG. 2.—Heart. Crystals in myocardium. H. and E. × 320.

Microscopic examination of the parathyroid glands showed a uniform cellular structure, with no fat seen; many dilated vessels were apparent. The cells contained

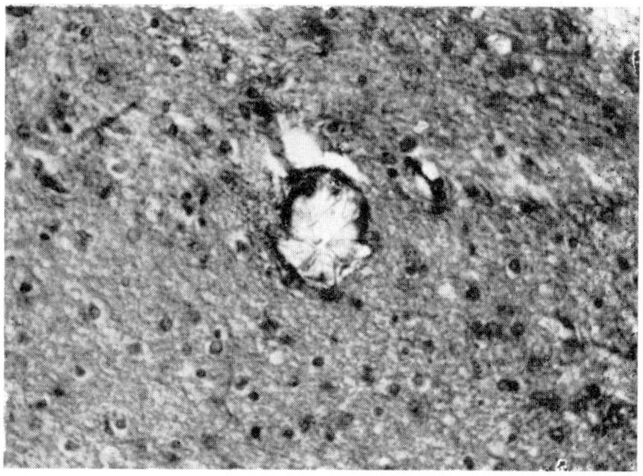

FIG. 3.—Brain. Crystals in white matter. H. and E. × 320.

round nuclei, surrounded by clear protoplasm, presenting the typical appearance of water clear cells.

Sections of the kidneys were treated with various chemical agents in order to determine the solubility of the crystals. These were found to be soluble in concentrated hydrochloric and in sulphuric acids. In the latter, careful examination revealed needle shaped crystals presumably calcium sulphate crystals. Furthermore, the crystals were found to be insoluble in alcohol, ether, glacial acetic acid, lithium carbonate and ammonium hydroxyde. With Von Kossa-reaction they stained black, but did not stain with the alizarin-red-S-stain.

Quantitative analysis for calcium in the kidney showed 188 mg. of calcium per 1 g. of net weight of renal tissue. With polarized light the crystals demonstrated birefringency. The Johnson incineration method gave a positive reaction.

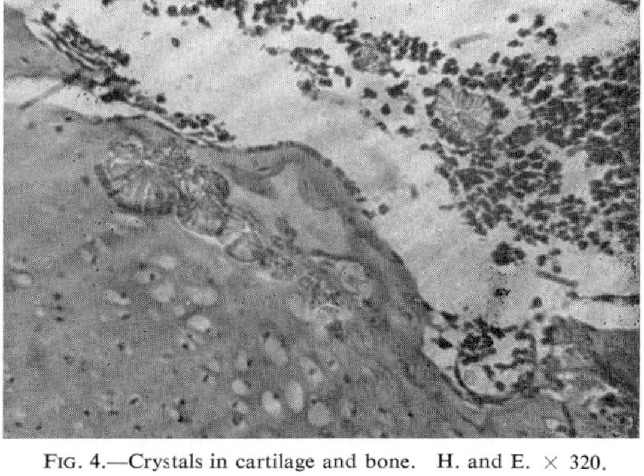

FIG. 4.—Crystals in cartilage and bone. H. and E. × 320.

Discussion

Discussing oxalate metabolism, Jeghers and Murphy (1945) stated that the source of the oxalates may be either exogenous (from food intake) or endogenous. Very little is known of the metabolism of oxalates from endogenous sources. The congenital defect which is supposed to exist in oxalosis is said to be unassociated with calcium metabolism, for it is not always calcium oxalate that is found, but other forms of oxalates. Origin from the Krebs citric acid cycle is not proven. Breakdown of ascorbic acid has been suggested as a possible source. Recently Archer *et al.* (1957) emphasized the production of oxalic acid from glycine as a result of the failure to degrade this amino acid normally via glyoxalate to formate and carbon dioxide.

As our patient was fed on breast milk and buttermilk only, an exogenous source of the oxalate could thus be easily ruled out. It is, however, still to be decided whether the deposition of the oxalates is the result of insufficient kidney excretion or of excessive production of oxalates. Archer *et al.* (1957) in a series of examinations of oxalate excretion in the urine, conclude that it does not appear to result from a low renal oxalate threshold, but rather from metabolic over-production. Simkó (1957) suggested that oxalosis is initiated by a lesion of the distal portion of the renal tubuli. It is worth while to note that in our case a marked hypoplasia of the kidneys was found. However, it is impossible to decide in retrospect whether the hypoplasia was primary, causing failure of oxalate excretion, or secondary, caused by the large accumulation of oxalates leading to decreased activity of the kidneys.

We mention the severe metabolic disturbances of calcium, phosphorus and alkaline phosphatase, and the autopsy findings of marked hyperplasia of the parathyroid glands, which may be diagnosed as secondary hyperplasia of the parathyroids due to renal failure. In the case of Hollósi (1957) the clinical manifestations were osteoporosis, renal rickets and osteodystrophy, accompanied by parathyroid hyperplasia. The patients described so far have been between the ages of 4½ months (Carson, 1951) and 57 years (Zollinger and Rosenmund, 1952). In Carson's case the symptoms continued for 10 days and the child died of renal insufficiency. Calcium oxalate crystals were found in the kidneys only. Oxalate crystals in such large quantities and in so many organs as in our case were found only by Chou and Donohue (1952) in a child of 7, and by Hollósi (1957) in a 4½-year-old girl. The fact that the symptoms in our case became manifest as early as the third month led us to think that the metabolic disturbance might have already begun during intra-uterine life. Otherwise it is difficult to imagine such a massive and widespread deposition of crystals within three months of birth. We are also of the opinion that Dunn's (1955) recommendation of sternal puncture as an aid to diagnosis is appropriate. In our case, too, a large number of crystals were found in the sternum. Because several cases have been reported in one family, the urine of our patient's family was examined, but no oxalate crystals were found.

Summary

A case is described of a child, 3 months old, who died of renal failure. Autopsy showed calcium oxalate crystals in kidneys, heart, brain, thyroid, thymus, lungs, bones and cartilage. The accepted views on the aetiology and course of oxalosis are discussed.

We wish to thank Dr. W. Jonas (Paediatric Department) and Dr. A. Reif (Pathological Department) for their permission to publish this case. We also thank Mrs. E. Bielsky for technical aid.

References

Aponte, G. E. and Fetter, T. R. (1954). *Amer. J. clin. Path.*, **24**, 1363.
Archer, H. E., Dormer, A. E., Scowen, E. F. and Watts, R. W. E. (1957). *Lancet*, **2**, 320.
Carson, M. J. (1951). *J. Pediat.*, **39**, 251.
Chou, L. Y. and Donohue, W. L. (1952). *Pediatrics*, **10**, 660.
Davis, J. S., Klingberg, W. G. and Stowell, R. E. (1950). *J. Pediat.*, **36**, 323.
Dunn, H. G. (1955). *A.M.A. J. Dis. Child.*, **90**, 58.
Hollósi, K. (1957). *Zbl. allg. Path. path. Anat.*, **96**, 220.
Jeghers, H. and Murphy, R. (1945). *New Engl. J. Med*, **233**, 208.
Lass, E. (1941). *Frankfurt., Z. Path.*, **55**, 265
Le Poutre (1925). *J. Urol. méd. chir.*, **20**, 424.
Newns, G. H. and Black, J. A. (1953). *Gt Ormond Str. J.*, No. 5, p. 40.
Simkó, I. (1957). *Ann. paediat. (Basel)*, **189**, 1.
Zollinger, H. U. and Rosenmund, H. (1952). *Schweiz. med. Wschr.*, **82**, 1261.

VISCERAL LARVA MIGRANS

BY

W. DICKSON and R. C. WOODCOCK

From the Bolton District General Hospital, Farnworth, Lancashire

(RECEIVED FOR PUBLICATION JULY 15, 1958)

There are many causes of persistent eosinophilia in children, but Perlingiero and György (1947) described a case in which there was also hepatic enlargement, anaemia and fever. Two years later Zuelzer and Apt (1949) described eight similar cases and suggested that they formed a definite syndrome. Since then several more have been reported and it has been shown that this syndrome is frequently caused by invasion of the viscera by the larvae of the dog or cat ascarid. We would like to describe a further case and review the progress that has been made in the study of this syndrome.

Case Report

Marjorie was admitted to hospital as an urgent case on September 14, 1956, because she had had a severe convulsion.

She was nearly 2 years of age, the third child of healthy parents. Her first year was free from illness and she made good physical progress, sitting up at 6 months of age and standing at 9 months. When she was 11 months old she was allowed to crawl about in her grandmother's back yard and it was then observed that she was a dirt eater. Shortly after her first birthday she developed an acute febrile illness with wheezy respirations. She was treated with penicillin and in about five days the fever subsided but the noisy respirations persisted for about one month. After this illness her disposition began to change; she became irritable, miserable and unfriendly and would speak only to her mother and grandmother. Her appetite became poor and she failed to gain weight. These rather indefinite symptoms were still present when she was admitted to hospital.

No other member of the family had had convulsions but the following additional history was obtained about Marjorie. Since the age of 1 month she had what her mother described as mild fits in which she would go unconscious for a few seconds and then lie limp for about 15 minutes. She was then having about two attacks a week but they had become more frequent recently. When she was 6 months of age she had four major convulsions in three days and since then she has had three major attacks.

There was no family history of allergic disease. The family had a cat and a dog; the dog was killed in an accident the night after Marjorie's admission to hospital.

Examination on admission: she was pale, restless and miserable. Her temperature was 103° F. The only abnormal findings were injection of the throat, enlargement of the tonsillar glands and a few moist sounds in her lungs. Her liver was enlarged three fingers below the costal margin and it was smooth and firm.

She was thought to have had a febrile convulsion following an upper respiratory infection and further investigations were carried out to find the cause of the enlarged liver.

The results of laboratory investigations were as follows: Hb 8·5 g. %, R.B.C. 4,440,000 per c.mm., C.I. 0·68; W.B.C. 23,000 per c.mm.; eosinophils, 67%; platelets, 272,000 per c.mm.; B.S.R., 31 mm. in the first hour, 61 mm. in the second hour; serum proteins, 8·6 g. %; albumin, 4 g. %; globulin, 4·6 g. %; electrophoresis γ globulin fraction markedly increased. Liver function tests showed serum alkaline phosphatase, 31 units (K.A.); serum bilirubin, within normal limits; thymol turbidity, 2 units; thymol flocculation, normal; zinc turbidity, 9 units; serum cholesterol, 115 mg. %; urine, no abnormalities; W.R. and Kahn tests negative.

Radiographs of the skull were normal; in those of the chest there was mottling in both upper lobes. A Mantoux test 1:1,000 was negative.

No ova or parasites were seen on repeated examination of the patient's stools, the cat's faeces or the dirt from the back yard.

Iliac marrow puncture showed an eosinophilia but most of the cells were mature and the picture was not that of an eosinophilic leukaemia.

The blood of the father, mother and sibs was tested; the W.B.C. and differential count were normal.

Liver Biopsy. At operation, the liver was enlarged and its appearance most striking. It was studded with firm greyish nodules which varied slightly in size but were all a few millimetres in diameter.

A small, wedge-shaped fragment of liver tissue about 1 cm. in diameter, containing some of the nodules, was removed and fixed in formol saline.

Serial sections of all the tissues were made and they showed inflammatory foci separated by normal liver tissue. In some fields the liver cells had been destroyed

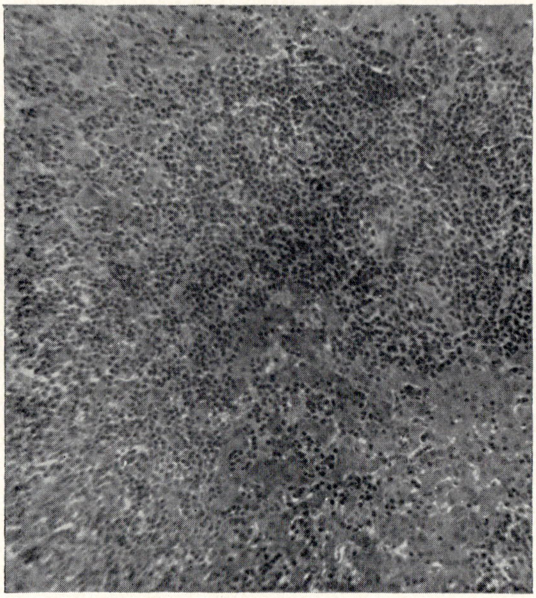

FIG. 1.—Liver. An early lesion. The section shows a focus of inflammatory infiltration consisting mainly of eosinophils. The eosinophils permeate between the liver cells at the periphery of the lesion. In the right hand corner a heavy concentration of eosinophils is shown infiltrating some amorphous debris.

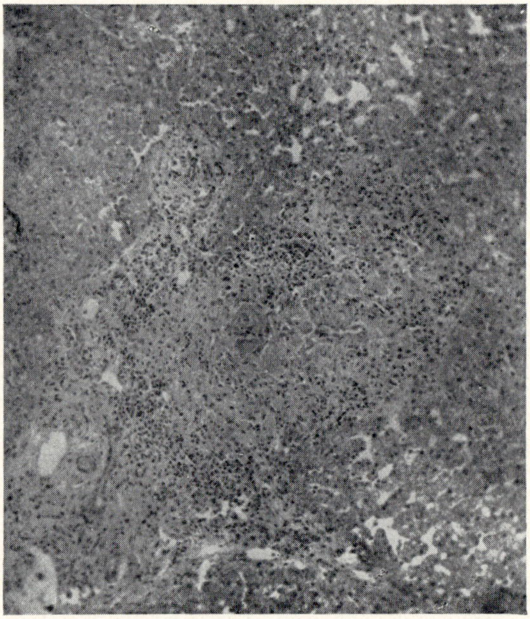

FIG. 2.—Liver. A late lesion—low power. A discrete granuloma consisting of epithelioid cells and giant cells with a zone of lymphocytes and plasma cells surrounding them.

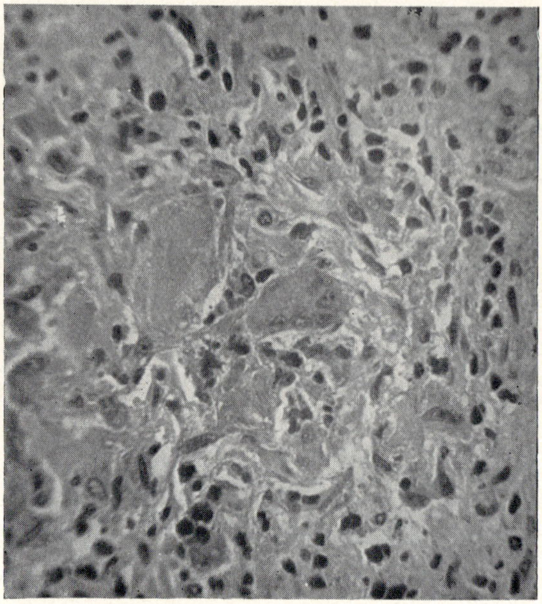

FIG. 3.—Liver. A late lesion—high power. The foreign body giant cells surrounding a clump of amorphous debris are demonstrated.

and replaced almost exclusively by eosinophils. These areas varied in size, were irregular in shape and merged into the surrounding liver tissue. Several distinct clumps of eosinophils invading amorphous débris were seen (Fig. 1) and the appearances strongly suggested that the débris was derived from degenerated fragments of larvae.

There was an inflammatory reaction around and within the portal tracts. In some places most of the cells were eosinophils but in others there was a large proportion of lymphocytes and plasma cells.

Several discrete granulomas were seen. They consisted of ephithelioid cells and giant cells of the foreign body type with a zone of lymphocytes and plasma cells surrounding them (Fig. 2). No foreign body was detected in any of these lesions but some contained fragments of unidentifiable necrotic débris (Fig. 3).

Other similar lesions were undergoing fibrosis and the gritty feel of some of the nodules at operation suggested that calcification may have occurred. This has been reported in the literature in visceral larva migrans.

Jung (personal communication) and his colleagues in New Orleans have examined the sections and agree that the appearances are typical of visceral larva migrans.

Progress. Marjorie has now been observed for nine months and, apart from a course of oral and intramuscular iron, she has had no treatment. The disease has followed a benign course. She has not had any further convulsions or pulmonary symptoms. Her irritability and anorexia have gradually improved and now she is back to normal health. Her eosinophil count

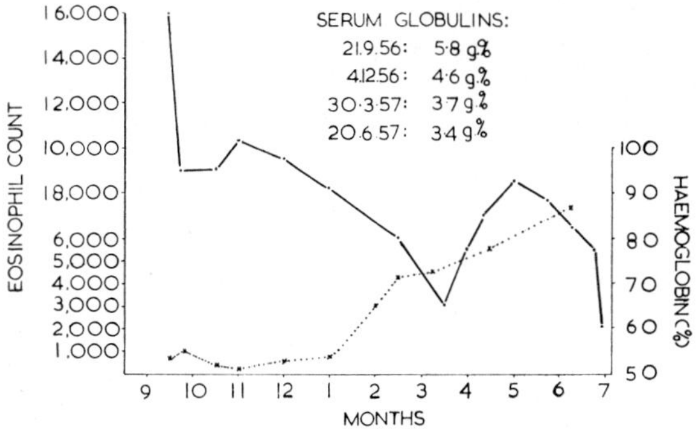

FIG. 4.—Marjorie. Eosinophil count, serum globulins and haemoglobin levels in a case of visceral larva migrans.

has varied but has remained well above normal for more than one year. Her haemoglobin and serum globulin have very slowly returned to more normal levels (Fig. 4).

Review of Literature

Several reports of a syndrome like the one described have appeared in the American literature. Zuelzer and Apt (1949) were the first to report a group of eight cases which appeared to have a common aetiology and demonstrate a syndrome.

The syndrome occurs in young children and is characterized by pica, pulmonary symptoms with a low grade pyrexia, an enlarged liver studded with eosinophilic granulomas, chronic blood eosinophilia, anaemia and hyperglobulinaemia.

The histology of the liver lesions suggested that the inflammation had an allergic basis but the aetiology was obscure until nine years ago, when Mercer, Lund, Bloomfield and Caldwell (1950) found the larva of an ascarid in a liver lesion. Later Behrer (1951) made a similar finding in another case. They thought that the larvae were those of the human ascarid, but a year later Beaver, Snyder, Carrera, Dent and Lafferty (1952) described three cases and in one a larva was identified as that of the dog ascarid, *Toxocara canis*. They named the syndrome 'visceral larva migrans' and considered that, like the commoner cutaneous larva migrans, it was due to the migration of nematode larvae through the tissues of an infected person.

A year later Milburn and Ernst (1953) described a further case in which the larva was identified. This case followed the typical benign course, but in the same year Brill, Churg and Beaver (1953) described a fatal case in which granulomas were found in the lungs, heart, liver and kidneys, and the toxocara was again demonstrated. In 1956 Dent, Nichols, Beaver, Carrera and Staggers described the post-mortem findings in a case which died from homologous serum jaundice. Again the characteristic lesions, some containing parasites, were widely scattered in numerous organs, including the brain. It is interesting to note that Beautyman and Woolf (1951) found an encapsulated ascarid in the thalamus of a child dying of poliomyelitis. Further cases have been reported by Heiner and Kevy (1956) and Gault and Webb (1957), writing from South India, described five cases and suggested that invasion of the liver and lungs by nematode larvae is the cause of tropical eosinophilia.

Discussion

(*a*) **Pathogenesis.** The human ascarid, *Ascaris lumbricoides*, has a rather complicated life cycle. The adult worms live in the small intestine where they feed on its contents and lay eggs. After being discharged in the faeces, the eggs may remain dormant for several years or may embryonate in damp soil in two to four months. Infection is by ingesting the embryonated eggs. The larvae escape from the eggs in the small intestine; they penetrate the wall and are carried to the liver in the portal blood stream. There they rest for a few days before resuming their journey through the right heart to the lungs. During this period they grow considerably in size. After about eight days they are carried up the trachea to the mouth and are swallowed a second time. On this occasion they remain in the bowel and develop to maturity.

The different species of ascarids only complete their life cycles if they are in the correct hosts. The first part of the cycle, that is the larval migration, is not specific. Human ascarids migrate in mice and other animals but none reach sexual maturity. Similarly cat and dog ascarids will migrate in human beings but the larvae will be destroyed in the viscera before they can return to the gut. Thus no eggs will be passed in the faeces as no adult worms are present in the gut. The larvae are destroyed in the viscera of a foreign host and so may not be seen in liver biopsies in all cases. In fact they have been found only in six cases. The inflammatory reaction will be more severe than with the homologous ascarid and thus the signs and symptoms of the disease will be more marked. Beaver *et al.* (1952) have suggested that patients who develop this syndrome have an allergic diathesis and this may enhance the response to the infection.

Salient Features. PICA. Infection of dogs and cats with toxocara is widespread. The animals may even be infected *in utero*. Examination of the soil from places frequented by them often reveals large numbers of ova.

A history of pica was obtained in over 90% of cases and ingestion of the ova of the toxocara in the dirt is the source of the infection.

Age Group. The cases belong to a very definite age group: 1 to 3 years.

The reason for this may be that pica is uncommon after 3 years of age or that, in older children, owing to the larger size of the liver capillaries, the toxocara may pass more easily into the lungs. This may account for some of the cases of Loeffler's syndrome, which belongs to an older group and is not associated with hepatomegaly.

Pulmonary Symptoms. Pulmonary symptoms caused by invasion of the lungs by the larvae occur early in the course of the disease and may precede, by a few months, the development of the eosinophilia and hepatomegaly. Common symptoms are cough, coryza and frequently a wheezing type of breathing, often associated with pyrexia. They vary in severity and are often accompanied by radiological changes in the lungs which may resemble miliary tuberculosis. Usually these lung changes are of short duration.

Convulsions. Convulsions and rather obscure cerebral symptoms have been reported in several cases. Zuelzer and Apt (1949) thought that an encephalopathy due to vascular sensitization was possibly part of the syndrome. However, it now appears that infiltration of the brain by larvae may be the cause of the symptoms, for larvae have been found in the brains of mice which have been fed with toxocara ova.

In our case, if the parents' observations are correct regarding the age of onset of the convulsions, it is unlikely that they were caused by the infection. Nevertheless, it is interesting that, as the child's general condition has improved, the convulsions have ceased without treatment.

Hepatomegaly. This is a constant feature in all cases. The liver is usually firm, smooth and regular and may be enlarged as much as five fingers below the costal margin. It seems possible that the parenchymal damage may account for the anorexia, irritability and lassitude. The liver function tests are indicative of parenchymal damage in about 30% of cases.

Anaemia. This is also a fairly constant finding. It is of the iron deficiency type but it responds only slowly to oral or intramuscular iron. The average haemoglobin at the height of the symptoms was about 8 g.

Leucocytosis. Leucocytosis with a high percentage of eosinophils was present in all cases at some time in the illness. Counts as high as 120,000 W.B.C. per c.mm. with 87% eosinophils in the differential count have been recorded, but the average count is about 30,000 W.B.C. per cm. with 50% eosinophils.

These blood changes may not appear until two to three months after the onset of the respiratory symptoms. Behrer (1951) suggests that the cause of the eosinophilia is the keratin which the larva sheds when it moults in passing through the various stages of its life cycle. Keratin can be demonstrated in liver sections and it is a very powerful eosinophilic stimulant.

Hyperglobulinaemia. A raised serum globulin, due to an increased gamma globulin, has been found in all cases in which it was estimated. This suggests that foreign larvae stimulate a powerful antibody response and that hypersensitivity or serological reactions may prove helpful in diagnosis. This is desirable as the larvae can only be demonstrated with difficulty in liver biopsies, which in children of this age are best obtained by laparotomy. Heiner and Kevy (1956) have described an agar diffusion precipitation reaction between the patient's serum and an antigen prepared from the toxocara larvae. The test gives promise of providing a specific diagnosis in the near future.

Jung (personal communication) and his associates performed the test on our patient's serum one year after the onset of symptoms. The serum showed no significant titre of antibodies against toxocara or ascaris, so it is possible that this patient may have been infected with a larval worm other than the two mentioned. Jung states that two groups of parasites have been shown in experimental animals to produce symptoms similar to visceral larva migrans: some hookworms and spirurids.

Liver Biopsies. Characteristic lesions have been found in the liver in all cases in which biopsy has been performed. On naked eye examination the presence of numerous small greyish white plaques arranged indiscriminately is strongly suggestive of the diagnosis. Microscopic examination reveals numerous inflammatory foci of varying ages which have been caused by migrating parasites. The younger lesions consist of aggregates, mainly of eosinophils, which have replaced liver cells. The more mature ones are granulomas consisting of epithelioid cells and foreign body giant cells surrounded by a zone of lymphocytes and plasma cells. The oldest lesions are granulomas undergoing fibrosis or even calcification.

Larvae are rarely seen in the lesions but small and often degenerate fragments are occasionally found. The very early lesions are most likely to contain a parasite. When they are present the opinion of an expert parasitologist is necessary for their complete identification. The important diagnostic features are as follows: (1) *T. cati* measures 350μ in length and 17μ at its greatest diameter. *T. canis* is a little larger. (2) There is a simple oesophagus 120μ long terminating distally in an elongated bulb 8μ in diameter, which contains a conspicuous nucleus 3μ in diameter. (3) In a cross-section larval crests or alae, 1μ long, may be seen.

Marjorie's progress is typical of the usual course of the disease. The ultimate prognosis is good, although many of the children go through a long period of ill health. No form of treatment has any effect either on the duration of symptoms or the course of the disease.

Summary

A case of visceral larva migrans is described.

The literature is reviewed and the important signs and symptoms are discussed.

The disease may be an important cause of chronic eosinophilia in childhood and may account for many of the cases considered to be Loeffler's syndrome or tropical eosinophilia.

The disease may be more common in this country than is realized because of the high incidence of toxocara infection in cats and dogs. It is suggested that other parasites of domestic pets, such as hookworms, may produce this condition.

The authors would like to thank Dr. R. C. Jung for examining the serum and sections, Professor W. F. Gaisford for his helpful advice and criticism and Mr. J. Parker, Mr. D. Hart and Miss E. Barton for technical and secretarial assistance.

References

Beautyman, W. and Woolf, A. L. (1951). *J. Path. Bact.*, **63**, 635.
Beaver, P. C., Snyder, C. H., Carrera, G. M., Dent, J. H. and Lafferty, J. W. (1952). *Pediatrics*, **9**, 7.
Behrer, M. R. (1951). *J. Pediat.*, **38**, 635.
Brill, R., Churg, J. and Beaver, P. C. (1953). *Amer. J. clin. Path.*, **23**, 1208.
Dent, J. H., Nichols, R. L., Beaver, P. C., Carrera, G. M. and Staggers, R. J. (1956). *Amer. J. Path.*, **32**, 777.
Gault, E. W. and Webb, J. K. G. (1957). *Lancet*, **2**, 471.
Heiner, D. C. and Kevy, S. V. (1956). *New Engl. J. Med.*, **254**, 629.
Jung, R. C. Personal communication.
Mercer, R. D., Lund, H. Z., Bloomfield, R. A. and Caldwell, F. E. (1950) *Amer. J. Dis. Child.*, **80**, 46.
Milburn, C. L., Jr. and Ernst, K. F. (1953). *Pediatrics*, **11**, 358.
Perlingiero, J. G. and György, P. (1947). *Amer. J. Dis. Child.*, **73**, 74.
Zuelzer, W. W. and Apt, L. (1949). *Ibid.*, **78**, 153

ACUTE PELLAGRA IN A CHILD UNDER TREATMENT WITH ISONIAZID

BY

M. G. PHILPOTT and H. P. PLAYER

From the Victoria Hospital for Sick Children, Hull

(RECEIVED FOR PUBLICATION JULY 23, 1958)

Toxic manifestations during isoniazid therapy are encountered in less than 5% of cases treated, and we have been able to trace little mention of them in children in the literature. The drug is now widely used in the treatment of tuberculosis and is universally prescribed as an adjuvant to streptomycin in tuberculous meningitis. The following case report concerns a child who developed pellagra late in the treatment for tuberculous meningitis.

Case Report

Betty S., aged 8 years 11 months, was admitted to Victoria Hospital for Sick Children, Hull, in October, 1956, with a week's illness characterized by fever, headache and some vomiting. She had been seen first on the third day of symptoms. On admission she was fully conscious, but had spinal rigidity, early papilloedema, and weakness of the left internal rectus. A diagnosis of tuberculous meningitis was confirmed by examination of the cerebrospinal fluid and the tuberculin reaction (Heaf) was strongly positive. No primary complex was located, and no tuberculous contact was known. The girl, living in the country, may have had access to raw milk. A full course of treatment was commenced on the day of admission, consisting of streptomycin, 10 mg./lb. 12-hourly, intramuscularly; para-amino-salicylic acid, 250 mg./lb. daily, in four-hourly doses; and isoniazid, 5 mg./lb. daily in eight-hourly doses orally. Her weight was 59 lb. and for working out the doses, the figure of 60 lb. was used initially. She was also given 60 mg. of streptomycin intrathecally every day for six days a week. Progress was satisfactory but slow. The intrathecal injections were reduced to two a week after two months, and were not discontinued until January 21, 1957. The intramuscular streptomycin was discontinued on April 8 and the girl was discharged home on May 8. At that time she was extremely well and the C.S.F. had returned to normal. Para-amino-salicylic acid and isoniazid were continued, the doses having been adjusted for weight increase. At an out-patient attendance in May she was still very well.

The girl was seen at home on May 27 owing to the development of a rash on her face, hands and shins two days previously. Intellect was normal. By June 4, when she was next examined, there was weakness of all four limbs. The skin of the face, the backs of the hands, and the shins were glazed, dull red and pigmented, and the skin of the right hand had been easily broken by a football (Fig. 1). There were sordes around the mouth

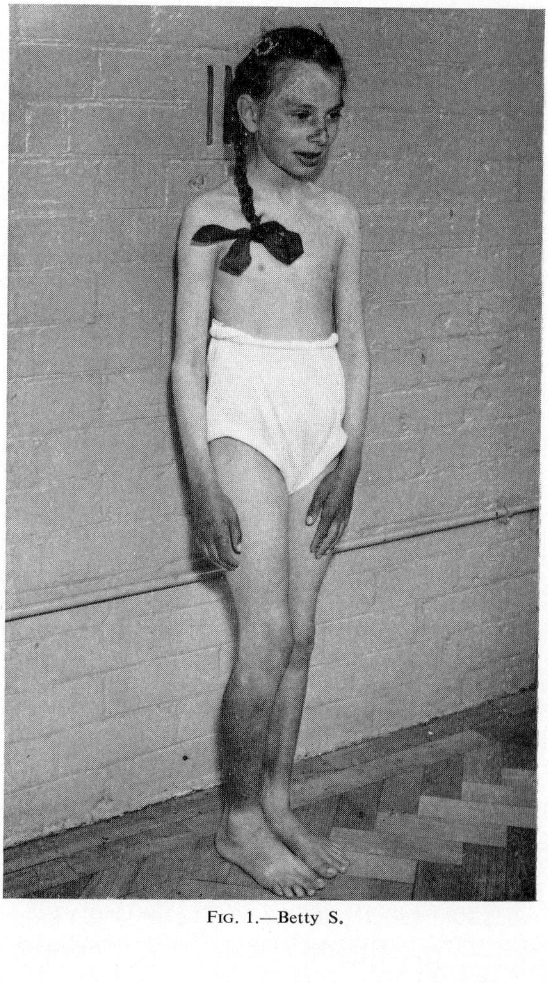

FIG. 1.—Betty S.

and the tongue was glazed and sore. The reflexes were all diminished. Bowel function was normal. The picture suggested pellagra and the girl was readmitted to hospital. All treatment was discontinued and she was given 2 dr. eight-hourly of a vitamin B complex containing aneurine hydrochloride, 10 mg.; nicotinamide, 40 mg.; riboflavine, 10 mg.; pyridoxine, 10 mg.; and d/calcium pantothenate, 10 mg. per fluid oz. The child improved rapidly, and all signs and symptoms had cleared by June 16, when she was discharged home again. The vitamin B complex was continued until July 23 and the para-amino-salicylic acid and isoniazid were never reintroduced. The girl has remained in the best of health ever since.

Discussion

It seemed unlikely that this picture of acute pellagra was due to para-amino-salicylic acid, but reports of similar toxic effects from isoniazid in adults had been made. Pegum (1952) described a patient with 'burning feet'. McConnell and Cheetham (1952) and Harrison and Feiwel (1956) reported cases of acute pellagra. Interference with nicotinic acid metabolism was indicated as the cause of the symptoms in these cases. Biehl and Vilter (1954) have shown that disorganization of pyridoxine metabolism occurs during isoniazid medication and Ungar, Parkin, Tomich and Muggleton (1954), experimenting with mice, came to similar conclusions. It is of interest, however, that the case of Harrison and Feiwel (1956) was receiving added pyridoxine during isoniazid therapy and yet developed symptoms. Wood (1955) reported pellagra in ill-nourished tuberculous patients treated with isoniazid which was difficult to control with added vitamin B complex. A review of the neurotoxic effects of isoniazid was made in a recent leading article (*British Medical Journal*, 1958).

While in hospital our patient was taking a full diet and vitamin supplements providing approximately aneurine 1 mg., riboflavine 1 mg., pantothenic acid 0·5 mg. and nicotinic acid 6 mg. daily. After discharge no vitamin preparations were given and the diet may not have been as well regulated. There had been a week of very sunny weather during the time the symptoms developed, but the child denied going out of doors very much.

From the clinical point of view some interference with nicotinic acid metabolism seems to be probable in this case although pyridoxine, and possibly riboflavine, were also affected. Certainly there was a most dramatic response to vitamin B complex therapy, and it would behove those treating children with isoniazid to ensure a satisfactory dietary intake and prescribe vitamin B supplements.

Summary

A case of acute pellagra is reported occurring in a girl aged 9 years 8 months after commencing treatment for tuberculous meningitis. The condition cleared in less than two weeks on discontinuing isoniazid therapy and introducing vitamin B complex. To avoid toxic manifestations from isoniazid it seems reasonable to administer vitamin B supplements during treatment with this drug.

Our thanks are due to Dr. R. J. Pugh who commented on this paper.

REFERENCES

Biehl, J. P. and Vilter, R. W. (1954). *J. Amer. med. Ass.*, **156**, 1549.
British Medical Journal (1958). Leading article, **1**, 880.
Harrison, R. J. and Feiwel, M. (1956). *Brit. med. J.*, **2**, 852.
McConnell, R. B. and Cheetham, H. D. (1952). *Lancet*, **2**, 959.
Pegum. J. S. (1952). *Ibid.*, **2**, 536.
Ungar, J., Parkin, K. R., Tomich, E. G. and Muggleton, P. W. (1954). *Ibid.*, **2**, 220.
Wood, M. M. (1955). *Brit. J. Tuberc.*, **49**, 20.

THE DIAGNOSTIC IMPORTANCE OF GLYCOSURIA IN LEAD POISONING IN CHILDHOOD

BY

RONALD C. ROXBURGH and LEONARD HAAS

From the Queen Elizabeth Hospital for Children and The London Hospital

(RECEIVED FOR PUBLICATION JULY 24, 1958)

In 1926, McKhann described three cases of lead poisoning in small children; he noticed, among other symptoms and signs, that marked but transient glycosuria was present in two of the three cases. Seven years later McKhann and Vogt (1933) reviewed all the case notes of children with lead poisoning admitted to the Boston Infants and Children's Hospitals between the years 1924 and 1933. These amounted to 89 cases, and the presence of glycosuria had been noted 'frequently' especially in the presence of encephalopathy. In a similar review from New York Goettsch and Mason (1940) collected records of 39 cases of lead poisoning between 1923 and 1938; in this series the incidence of glycosuria was 20%. In one of the cases glycosuria persisted for five weeks. More recently Ennis and Harrison (1950) found glycosuria in four out of 10 cases of lead poisoning. Burrows, Rendle-Short and Hanna (1951) reported that glycosuria was commonly found in such cases. Six years ago, one of us (R.C.R.) in conjunction with Millichap and Llewellin (1952) reported five cases of lead poisoning in young children due to ingestion of paint. It was noticed at that time that two of the cases had had glycosuria for a short period at the onset, but the diagnosis in those cases had been established on other evidence.

Further reports of childhood lead poisoning have come from Zak and Finkelstein (1952), Gianattasio, Bedo and Pirozzi (1952), Wilson, Thomson and Dent (1953), Byers, Maloof and Cushman (1954), Marsden and Wilson (1955), Tanis (1955), and O'Donohoe (1956). In many of these cases it had been noticed that glycosuria was present.

However, it had apparently been an incidental finding and the purpose of this paper is to show the diagnostic value of glycosuria, especially in the cases of lead poisoning without encephalopathy. In the following three cases, seen consecutively, it was the presence of marked glycosuria in the absence of a raised blood sugar level that led to a search for other evidence of lead poisoning.

Case Reports

Case 1. J.A. was a boy, aged 1½ years. He had been unwell for about two weeks with malaise and vomiting. Anorexia had been marked, there had been obvious weight loss and he was very constipated. It had been noticed that he had become very pale.

He was admitted to the Queen Elizabeth Hospital on August 13, 1957, for investigation. On examination, he was a pale listless child weighing 21 lb. 5 oz. (9·5 kg.). He was fully conscious. There were no abnormal physical signs in the cardiovascular, respiratory or central nervous systems. The spleen tip was palpable. The urine showed a moderate amount of sugar, giving a yellow reduction of Benedict's reagent. Rothera's test was also positive and a trace of protein was found.

Laboratory investigations gave the following results: Blood haemoglobin, 50% (7·4 g.); R.B.C., 4·98 million per c.mm.; W.B.C., 8,200 per c.mm.; blood sugar, 92 mg. %. Microscopic examination of the urine showed the presence of 20 red and 20 white blood cells per high power field. On August 20, while the blood sugar level was 88 mg. %, the urine contained 470 mg. % of glucose.

In view of the persistence of glycosuria in an ill, listless and anaemic child, it was considered that the underlying cause might be lead poisoning. Further investigations showed that marked punctate basophilia of the red blood cells was present, radiographs of the radius and ulna showed a dense heavy metal band at the distal metaphysis, urinary coproporphyrins were greatly increased, and the urinary lead concentration was 0·56 mg./l.

In view of these findings, the parents were further questioned about possible exposure to lead. They at once confirmed that the child had for the past three months been in the habit of chewing the paint off the edges of the window-sills and doors. Analysis of some of the paint scrapings showed a high lead content.

PROGRESS AND TREATMENT. In view of the relatively mild course of the illness, it was at first decided to withhold specific E.D.T.A. therapy and the acute symptoms subsided gradually, though the anaemia persisted. Glycosuria persisted for three weeks from the time of admission. Paper chromatography of the urine three months later showed a normal amino-acid excretion pattern and no evidence of glycosuria. Treatment with calcium di-sodium versenate was commenced orally on

November 22 in a dosage of 1·75 g. daily and following this the urine lead concentration rose from 0·03 to 6·0 mg./l. No side effects were noticed nor was there any recurrence of evidence of tubular damage. Now, nine months after the onset, there is no sign of mental deterioration. Treatment with versenate has been continued orally for five months and the urine lead concentration is still raised (1·28 mg./l.).

Case 2. L.L., a girl, aged 6¼ years, whose father is a house painter, was admitted to the Queen Elizabeth Hospital on August 30, 1957, on account of vomiting and malaise for two weeks, and abdominal colic for three days. It was later discovered that she had had pica at the age of 2 years. She was an ill afebrile child weighing 37 lb. (16·65 kg.). She was fully conscious, but was very irritable and was slightly dehydrated. There were no abnormal physical signs in the cardiovascular, respiratory or alimentary systems. Neck stiffness and papilloedema were absent, but there was marked muscular hypotonia despite normal tendon reflexes. The urine was found to contain a trace of protein, gave a yellow reduction of Benedict's solution and a strongly positive Rothera's test. Laboratory investigation confirmed that the sugar was glucose. On microscopy there were eight W.B.C.s and moderate numbers of granular casts per one-sixth field.

Because of these findings, further investigations for lead poisoning were undertaken. In the blood, the haemoglobin was 55% (8·14 g.) and punctate basophilia was present. Radiographs of the radius and ulna showed the presence of a dense heavy metal line at the distal metaphysis and this sign was also present at the costochondral junctions as seen on the routine chest film. The urinary coproporphyrin output was greatly increased, as was the amino-acid output on paper chromatography. The urine lead concentration in a 24-hour specimen was 0·4 mg./l. The blood sugar level, in the presence of glycosuria, was 82 mg. %. The blood urea was 52 mg. %. Cerebrospinal fluid was not examined. The glucose tolerance curve was normal. In view of these conclusive findings, the parents were further questioned on the possible sources of lead at home, but apart from her father being a house painter, it was not possible to discover how lead had been ingested.

Progress and Treatment. The child rapidly lost her acute symptoms following rehydration and at first no treatment with versenate was given. Moderate glycosuria persisted for the first three weeks in hospital. Specific therapy with oral calcium di-sodium versenate was started on October 14, 1957, six weeks after admission. Dosage was 1·2 g. daily at first, later increased to 6·0 g. daily. The urine lead concentration rose from 0·6 to a maximum level of 3·5 mg./l. There were no ill-effects from this treatment but slight diarrhoea occurred when 6·0 g. daily was being given, so this was reduced to 3·0 g. daily, which was well tolerated. The child's general condition and mental state improved considerably after a week of treatment with versenate, suggesting that de-leading was of benefit to her metabolic processes. By the end of four months on this treatment she had gained 14 lb. (6·3 kg.) in weight and the haemoglobin had risen to 90% (13 g.).

Case 3. Philip E., aged 4 years 8 months, was admitted in deep coma to the London Hospital on September 20, 1957.

He had been lethargic, moody, disinterested and lacking in appetite for some weeks. On the previous day he had complained of abdominal pain and had vomited. On the afternoon of admission he collapsed whilst playing in the street. He was admitted to another hospital, where he was found to be extremely drowsy and confused; his pupils were dilated and barely reacted to light; there was a flaccid left-sided hemiparesis. During the course of a few hours he sank into deep coma, and was transferred to the London Hospital for a neurosurgical opinion.

On admission the pupils were fixed, dilated and did not react to light. All limbs were flaccid and the deep tendon reflexes were absent. Both plantar responses were extensor. Firm supra-orbital pressure produced only faint response. The optic fundi appeared normal. The weight was 30 lb. (13·5 kg.).

He was considered to have rising intracranial pressure and, under local anaesthesia, burr holes were made. The ventricles could not be located. The cortex looked congested and plum-coloured; it was normal on biopsy.

Post-operatively, he had several epileptiform convulsions. He was given rectal hypertonic saline with a view to reducing intracranial pressure. On the morning after admission his condition had improved. He was conscious, though still confused and irrational, and was moving all his limbs. The tendon reflexes, all present, were brisker on the right and there was definite weakness of that side. The right plantar response was extensor, the left flexor. At this stage the urine was found to contain a considerable amount of sugar, being orange to Benedict's test. The blood sugar level was 85 mg. per 100 ml. The blood picture was as follows: haemoglobin, 49% (7·3 g./100 ml.); W.B.C. 13,300, polymorphs 50%, lymphocytes 44%, monocytes 5%, metamyelocytes 1%. There was moderate anisocytosis and poikilocytosis of unequally staining red cells. Platelets were plentiful.

Twenty-four hours later he appeared to have fully recovered. He was well orientated, alert and intelligent. There were no abnormal neurological signs. An air encephalogram was carried out. The ventricles on this occasion were located with ease, and were found to show a normal radiological pattern.

Thereafter, his clinical condition remained good. However, heavy glycosuria continued for three weeks. A normal sugar tolerance curve showed that this was due to a lowering of the renal threshold. This fact, considered together with the hitherto unexplained encephalopathy and the hypochromic anaemia, appeared to us highly suggestive of lead poisoning. The following investigations were therefore carried out: radiographs of the long bones showed increased density along the lines of the metaphyses; staining of a blood film with methylene blue showed many stippled cells; further examination of the urine revealed an excess of coproporphyrins; its total lead content was 0·65 mg./l.

Oral calcium di-sodium versenate was commenced on October 15, 1957, in a dosage of 1 g. daily, increased gradually until 3 g. daily were given. The urinary output of lead excreted rose to figures between 0·6 and 1·6 mg./l. In addition three doses of 1 g. of intravenous versenate were administered at weekly intervals. These caused the amount of lead in the urine to rise to 8·4, 8 and 3·67 mg./l. respectively. No side effects were noted and there was no evidence of further renal damage at any time. Glycosuria and excess coproporphyrinuria disappeared three and eight weeks after admission respectively. He was discharged after 12 weeks in hospital weighing 38 lb. (17 kg.) and out-patient treatment with oral versenate was continued. He was re-admitted on three occasions in January, April and July, 1958, for short periods of observation, and each time was given a further intravenous infusion of versenate. These led to lead excretions of 2·5, 1·8, and 1·5 mg./l. At present he is well and free from symptoms. The dense line on the radiograph has receded proximally from the metaphysis by several mm.; the blood picture is normal with a haemoglobin of 90% (13 g.) and there is no evidence of basophil stippling. Treatment was discontinued on July 10. However, lead excretion in the urine is still raised and fluctuates between 0·2 and 0·52 mg./l.

Sources of Lead

The commonest cause of lead poisoning in small children is the ingestion of paint flakes containing lead (Chisolm and Harrison, 1956), and this proved to be the source in Case 1 of the present series. This child was in the habit of nibbling paint off the window sills and doors. In Case 2 of the series, the source of lead could not be determined. The father was a house painter but any connexion between this and the child's illness was denied. In Case 3 of the series a somewhat unusual source was incriminated. He always chewed objects within his grasp but never cot-sides or windowsills. His favourite occupation was drawing with coloured crayons. It was pointed out to us that the colours ranging from pale yellow to orange were made with lead chromate (Bonnell, 1957). Samples of the patient's crayons were therefore analysed in the Department for Research in Industrial Medicine at the London Hospital. This confirmed that the 'leads' of the yellow and the orange pencils have a lead content of 5%. Furthermore the paints used to colour the outside of the crayons were also found to contain 5% of lead. This potential source of lead poisoning does not seem to have been reported in this country hitherto. As coloured pencils are present in every home it seems important to draw attention to their potential danger.

Discussion

It has been shown in these three cases of lead poisoning that glycosuria was occurring in the presence of a normal blood sugar level. There was also evidence of renal damage in Cases 1 and 2. All these abnormalities were transient; the glycosuria persisted for approximately three weeks in each case from the time of admission. In two of the cases the acute symptoms subsided after admission to hospital without the supervention of encephalopathy; it is possible that this type of case may be occurring in children without being diagnosed. It is significant that it was not only the severe case that was associated with glycosuria.

It is known from animal experiments that lead poisoning damages the renal tubule (Blackman, 1936). Marsden and Wilson (1955) found microscopic evidence of damage to the proximal convoluted tubule in two children who died of lead poisoning; both cases had exhibited glysosuria and amino-aciduria in life. The histological changes were those of intranuclear inclusions, giant nuclei, and fatty vacuolation of the cytoplasm.

According to Anderson (1954) the glycosuria that may accompany lead poisoning in childhood is apparently of renal origin since the blood sugar level is unaffected; it probably results from tubular damage. It must be concluded that the effect of the lead is to interfere with the intracellular enzyme systems which normally facilitate the re-absorption of glucose and amino-acids from the proximal tubules. It appears that this is a special feature of lead poisoning in childhood, since the occurrence of glycosuria is not a recognized pathological finding in adults with chronic lead poisoning.

However, glycosuria and amino-aciduria have been described in other metallic poisonings, e.g. mercury, in uranium toxicity in animals (Voegtlin and Hodge, 1949) in Wilson's hepato-lenticular degeneration, and in ferrous sulphate poisoning (Brown and Gray, 1955). A case of special interest was described by Chisolm, Harrison, Eberlein and Harrison (1955) in which, following lead poisoning in a child, transient glycosuria, amino-aciduria, hypophosphataemia and rickets occurred; this syndrome closely simulated the findings in the de Toni-Fanconi syndrome.

Conclusions

It is probable that glycosuria is present to some degree in most cases of childhood lead poisoning and this fact should be more widely appreciated. In any case of persistent renal glycosuria occurring in a child who is otherwise unwell, the diagnosis of lead poisoning must always be considered.

The experience gained during the treatment of the cases with oral calcium di-sodium versenate leads us to suggest that prolonged courses are without danger to the patient and, in addition, continue to enhance the renal excretion of lead in increased amounts. That the excretion of lead should be as complete as possible is shown by Henderson (1954) from Queensland, Australia, who gives evidence of the danger of chronic renal disease occurring in young adults who had been afflicted with lead poisoning in childhood. So far, no such series of cases has been reported in this country.

Summary

Three further cases of lead poisoning in children are described. The diagnosis of the condition was reached at an early stage after admission to hospital because of the discovery of glycosuria, which led to further tests for lead poisoning. The glycosuria persisted for three weeks. There was no evidence of residual renal damage at the end of six months. All three cases were treated with prolonged courses of oral calcium di-sodium versenate resulting in prolonged excretion of lead in the urine.

Evidence is put forward to suggest that coloured crayons of the yellow and orange ranges may be a danger to children on account of their content of lead chromate.

We are grateful to Dr. Helen Mackay, to Dr. C. T. Potter, and to Dr. Richard Dobbs for permission to publish these cases which were under their care: to Dr. J. A. Bonnell for much assistance, advice and many urine-lead estimations carried out in the Department for Industrial Medical Research at the London Hospital; to Dr. B. Levin for numerous laboratory investigations at the Queen Elizabeth Hospital.

References

Anderson, J. A. (1954). In *Textbook of Pediatrics*, 6th ed. Ed. W. E. Nelson, p. 630. Philadelphia.
Best, C. H. and Taylor, N. B. (1955). *The Physiological Basis of Medical Practice*, 6th ed. London.
Blackman, S. S. Jr. (1936). *Bull. Johns Hopk. Hosp.*, **58**, 384.
Bonnell, J. A. L. (1957). Personal communication.
Brown, R. J. K. and Gray, J. D. (1955). *Canad. med. Ass. J.*, **73**, 192.
Burrows, N. F. E., Rendle-Short, J. and Hanna, D. (1951). *Brit. med. J.*, **1**, 329.
Byers, R. K., Maloof, C. A. and Cushman, M (1954) *A.M.A. Amer. J. Dis. Child.*, **87**, 548.
Chisolm, J. J. and Harrison, H. E. (1956). *Pediatrics*, **18**, 943.
——, Harrison, C., Eberlein, W. R and Harrison, H. E. (1955). *A.M.A. Amer. J. Dis. Child.*, **89**, 159.
Ennis, J. M. and Harrison, H. E. (1950). *Pediatrics*, **5**, 853.
Gianattasio, R. C., Bedo, A. V. and Pirozzi, M. J. (1952). *A.M.A. Amer. J. Dis. Child.*, **84**, 316.
Goettsch, E. and Mason, H. H. (1940). *Amer. J. Dis. Child.*, **59**, 119.
Henderson, D. A. (1954). *Aust. Ann. Med*, **3**, 219.
Marsden, H. B. and Wilson, V. K. (1955). *Brit. med. J.*, **1**, 324.
McKhann, C. F. (1926). *Amer. J. Dis. Child.*, **32**, 386.
—— and Vogt, E. C. (1933). *J. Amer. med. Ass.*, **101**, 1131.
Millichap, J. G., Llewellin, K. R. and Roxburgh, R. C. (1952), *Lancet*, **2**, 360.
O'Donohoe, N. V. (1956). *Arch. Dis. Childh.*, **31**, 321.
Tanis, A. L. (1955). *A.M.A. Amer. J. Dis. Child.*, **89**, 325.
Voegtlin, C. and Hodge, H. C. (1949). *Pharmacology and Toxicology of Uranium Compounds*. McGraw-Hill, New York.
Wilson, V. K., Thomson, M. L. and Dent C. E. (1953). *Lancet*, **2**, 66
Zak, F. G. and Finkelstein, W. E. (1952). *J. Mt Sinai Hosp.*, **19**, 352.

ACUTE HAEMOLYTIC ANAEMIA FOLLOWING THE INGESTION OF PARA-DICHLOROBENZENE

BY

M. HALLOWELL

From the Children's Hospital, Birmingham

(RECEIVED FOR PUBLICATION JULY 21, 1958)

Reports of cases of haemolytic anaemia after the ingestion of moth-balls are scanty. Nash (1903) briefly records a case of a boy of 13 who developed black urine after eating a single moth-ball in mistake for a sweet, but no haematological data are given. Zuelzer and Apt (1949) describe the case histories of four young negro children who developed acute haemolytic anaemia and haemoglobinuria following the ingestion of moth-balls containing naphthalene. Gidron and Leurer (1956) report a girl of 16 who developed an acute haemolytic anaemia with haemoglobinuria after swallowing 6 g. of naphthalene in an attempt to commit suicide. The following is a report of a child who developed an acute haemolytic anaemia with methaemoglobinuria after the ingestion of another demothing agent, para-dichlorobenzene.

Case History

Paul S., aged 3 years, was admitted to the Birmingham Children's Hospital on March 9, 1958, with a history of a cough for a few days. The day before admission he seemed listless, his sclera became yellow and the urine he passed was almost black in colour. There was no family history of jaundice or anaemia. On examination he was jaundiced and his mucous membranes were pale. His temperature was 97°F., pulse rate 100 per minute and blood pressure 95/70. The liver and spleen were not enlarged. He had a dry cough, but the lung fields were clear. A blood count showed haemoglobin 56% (8·25 g./100 ml.), reticulocytes 5%, leucocytes 14,700, predominantly granulocytes. The blood group was O, Rhesus positive, the serum bilirubin 2·6 mg. % and the blood urea 53 mg. %. As he had not passed urine for 15 hours before admission he was catheterized and 4 oz. of dark, port wine coloured urine were obtained. Spectroscopic examination showed the characteristic bands of methaemoglobin and Schumm's test for methaemalbumen was positive. On microscopy there were no red cells.

The next day the Coombs test was carried out by three independent haematologists and reported by each as being negative. The blood was fully investigated for the presence of antibodies but none was found. There were no cold agglutinins. A chest radiograph was normal. His haemoglobin had now fallen to 36% (5·4 g./100 ml.), his pulse rate had risen to 150 per minute and his blood pressure had dropped to 80/50. He was transfused with one pint of blood, which produced a brief and transient increase in the methaemoglobinuria, and then given intravenous fluids for the succeeding 36 hours.

During the third day in hospital the methaemoglobinuria ceased. His urinary output was markedly reduced during the first two days but subsequently improved and by the sixth day his blood urea had fallen to 17 mg. %.

When the haemolytic phase had subsided the following investigations were carried out. Red cell fragility: haemolysis commenced at 0·45% and was complete at 0·32%. No sickling of the red cells was demonstrable and no target cells were seen. The Wasserman and Kahn reactions were negative.

Following the blood transfusion his haemoglobin rose to 74% (11·0 g./100 ml.) but gradually fell over the next five days to 53% (7·8 g./100 ml.). On the seventh day in hospital his reticulocyte count reached 17%. He was discharged home on March 26, 1958, on an oral iron preparation. When last seen on April 14, 1958, he was clinically well and his haemoglobin had risen to 78% (11·6 g./100 ml.).

Discussion

On admission it was considered that this child was probably suffering from an acute haemolytic anaemia secondary to a virus pneumonia, but the negative Coombs test and absence of cold agglutinins in the blood made this unlikely. Enquiries were then directed to poisons and drugs. The family doctor had not prescribed any medicine other than Mist. ipecac et opii pro infant., but his interview with the mother revealed that the child had been playing with a small canister labelled 'Demothing Crystals'. These crystals, which contain para-dichlorobenzene had been given away with a vacuum cleaner which the mother had purchased some months ago. His mother said that during the four to five days before the onset of jaundice and methaemoglobinuria she had seen him playing with the crystals, sprinkling them over the floor, spreading them out with his hands, then replacing them one by one in the canister, all the time playing with a comforter in and out of his mouth.

The first specimen of urine was examined biochemically. After precipitation of the methaemoglobin the deproteinized urine gave an intense naphthoresorcinol reaction and did not contain any inorganic sulphate. By paper chromatography, spots suggestive of four abnormal phenols were observed. At this time appropriate reference compounds for their identification were not available.

The other specimens of the dark urine passed during the first three days in hospital were pooled and kept in the refrigerator for six days. By this time the colour had changed to a very dark red and spectroscopic examination no longer showed methaemoglobin; it had been reduced to haemoglobin.

Synthetic specimens of 2:5 dichlorophenol and 2:5 dichloroquinol were available at the end of the six days. A 24-hour specimen of urine collected when the child had practically recovered was used as a normal control. This specimen and the above mentioned pooled specimen of urine were hydrolyzed and examined for phenols by paper chromatography. The abnormal urine revealed traces of 2:5 dichloroquinol and at least two other phenols not present in the control, but 2:5 dichlorophenol was not found.

Para-dichlorobenzene metabolism has been studied in rabbits by Azouz, Parke and Williams (1955). The chief metabolites to be expected after the ingestion of para-dichlorobenzene are 2:5 dichlorophenol and 2:5 dichloroquinol. Phenols and quinols are conjugated with glucuronic acid and sulphuric acid and then excreted. The finding in this case of an intense naphthoresorcinol reaction and the conversion of practically all the inorganic sulphate into ethereal sulphate is in keeping with the formation of these metabolites. This, together with the finding of traces of 2:5 dichloroquinol and other abnormal phenols is strong presumptive evidence that the child must have ingested some of the para-dichlorobenzene crystals.

The urine was several days old at the time of the second examination and the methaemoglobin had been reduced; 2:5 dichloroquinol may have been responsible for this reduction, and if this were so it would explain the fact that only traces were present.

According to Browning (1953) the chief toxic effects of para-dichlorobenzene in animals are liver and kidney damage. No toxic effects have been reported in man. Methaemoglobin formation has not been observed in the rabbit, but this animal does not form methaemoglobin as readily as man.

Benzene itself is a recognized haemolytic agent. Erf and Rhoads (1939) described the case histories of nine industrial workers who were exposed to benzene fumes. They developed a chronic haemolytic anaemia. Nabarro (1948) described a case of acute haemolytic anaemia occurring six days after the ingestion of another benzene compound mononitrobenzene. He stated that haemolysis is found in all moderately severe cases of mononitrobenzene poisoning.

Demothing crystals which contain para-dichlorobenzene are freely available to the general public and are sold in vast quantities each year, particularly during the spring season. The importance of keeping them out of the reach of children cannot be over emphasized.

Summary

A case of acute haemolytic anaemia occurring in a child of 3 years after the ingestion of para-dichlorobenzene is reported. The haemolysis was severe and necessitated a blood transfusion. Complete recovery occurred. The biochemical findings in the urine are fully reported and the metabolism of para-dichlorobenzene is discussed.

My thanks are due to Professor J. M. Smellie for permission to publish this case and for his advice and also to Professor J. M. Webster, to Dr. W. Weiner, Dr. K. B. Rogers and Dr. J. N. M. Chalmers for the haematological investigations, to Dr. G. D. H. McQuitty the family doctor, and to Dr. W. V. Thorpe who carried out the biochemical studies.

References

Azouz, W. M., Parke, D. V. and Williams, R. T. (1955). *Biochem J.*, **59**, 410.
Browning, E. (1953). *Toxicity of Industrial Organic Solvents*, p. 189. *Med. Res. Coun. Industr. Hlth Res. Bd.* Rep. No. 80 (rev. ed.). H.M.S.O., London.
Erf, L. A. and Rhoads, C. P. (1939). *J. industr. Hyg.*, **21**, 421.
Gidron, E. and Leurer, J. (1956). *Lancet*, **1**, 228.
Nabarro, J. D. N. (1948). *Brit. med. J.*, **1**, 929.
Nash, L. F. (1903). *Ibid.*, **1**, 251.
Zuelzer, W. W. and Apt, L. (1949). *J. Amer. med. Ass.*, **141**, 185.

THE CHILD OF THE DIABETIC WOMAN*

BY

JAMES W. FARQUHAR

From the Department of Child Life and Health, University of Edinburgh, and the Simpson Memorial Maternity Pavilion, Royal Infirmary, Edinburgh

(RECEIVED FOR PUBLICATION JULY 28, 1958)

Over a century ago Bennewitz (1828), when delivering a diabetic woman, observed that the giant foetus whose head had been born but whose shoulders were stuck fast 'seemed anxious and sighed with a clear voice'. In this depressed state the infant died, as so many of his kind have done since.

Pregnancy complicating diabetes and the development of children born to diabetic women became problems only with the development of insulin. Before the dawn of the insulin era diabetes mellitus was associated with female infertility, possibly as a consequence of poor nutrition (Sinden and Longwell, 1949), and when pregnancy did occur the foetal mortality ranged from 40% (Duncan, 1883) to 70% (Eshner, 1907). With insulin, however, the infertile diabetic woman is now exceptional in the extensive experience of White (1952), and Stevenson (1956) found that in his Belfast series 70% were pregnant within one year of marriage and that over 90% were pregnant within two years. Although maternal mortality in diabetic pregnancy has been almost entirely eliminated, a distressing foetal loss persists. Until recently pre-viable abortions were included in the over-all foetal mortality figures. No evidence exists, however, to prove that abortions are any commoner among diabetic than among non-diabetic women (Peel and Oakley, 1950). A figure of 6·4% found by Pedowitz and Shlevin (1955) was well within the normal range in their experience, 10% of abortions were reported by Stevenson (1956), and Barns and Morgans (1949) discovered a diabetic abortion rate of 10·9% and a non-diabetic rate of 11·8%. Because of this only viable foetal loss rates are customarily compared.

The perinatal mortality for all booked pregnancies at the Simpson Memorial Maternity Pavilion has been less than 40 in 1,000 births in recent years, and this contrasts with the figure of 166 in 1,000 births for those diabetic women who were adequately supervised from not later than the twentieth week of gestation, and upon whom, or upon whose babies, exceptional and co-ordinated care was lavished by a team composed of an obstetrician, a physician and a paediatrician. These results are compared in Table 1 with other American and European series. The Danish and Belfast figures have been calculated for roughly the same years as this series but later improvement was noted in both. The neonatal death rate is given only where this could be calculated from the figures given.

The purpose of this paper is to describe the morphology of infants born to diabetic women, their clinical progress in the first month of life, their metabolic disorders, the possible links between maternal diabetes and the embryopathy, the management of the newly born and their further development up to the age of 10 years.

Clinical Description and Progress of the Newborn.

The children of diabetic men do not differ discernibly at birth from those born to non-diabetic men (Babbott, Rubin and Ginsburg, 1958). Those born to diabetic mothers, however, commonly exceed both the mean body weight and crown-heel length for their gestational age (Cardell, 1953; Pedersen, 1954). Because of their gigantism and because of a strong tendency toward intra-uterine death after the thirty-sixth week, caesarean birth some weeks before term is commonly practised, and most of the babies in this series were so delivered.

The infants are remarkable (Fig. 1) not only because, like foetal versions of Shadrach, Meshach and Abednego, they emerge at least alive from within the fiery metabolic furnace of diabetes mellitus, but because they resemble one another so closely that they might well be related. They are plump, sleek, liberally coated with vernix caseosa, full-faced and plethoric. The umbilical cord and the placenta share in the gigantism. During their first

* A Honyman-Gillespie Post-graduate Lecture delivered at the University of Edinburgh on May 22, 1958.

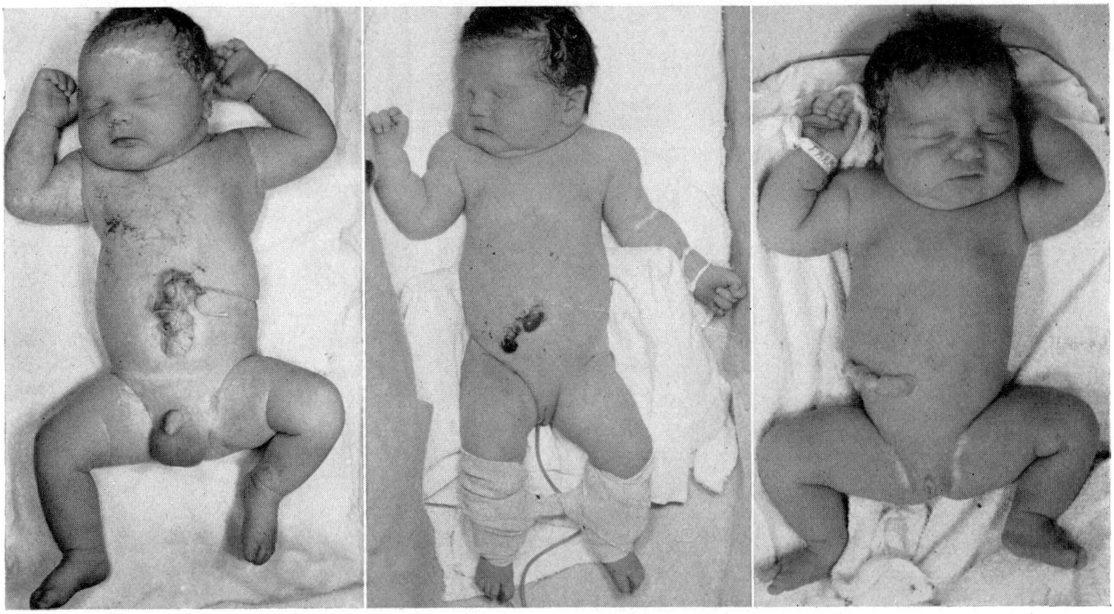

FIG. 1.—Unrelated infants of diabetic women.
'. . . for some of us are out of breath
And all of us are fat.' (*Lewis Carroll.*)

24 or more extra-uterine hours they lie on their backs, bloated and flushed, their legs flexed and abducted, their lightly closed hands on each side of the head, the abdomen prominent and their respiration sighing. They convey a distinct impression of having had such a surfeit of both food and fluid pressed upon them by an insistent hostess that they desire only peace so that they may recover from their excesses. And on the second day their resentment of the slightest noise improves the analogy while their trembling anxiety seems to speak of intra-uterine indiscretions of which we know nothing.

Of the 123 viable pregnancies in the series, occurring in women who were known to have diabetes mellitus, 96 resulted in the birth of a live child, and of these, 57 (59·4%) survived the newborn period without serious incident. Most of them showed prolonged Moro embrace responses which were elicited so easily that even a light footfall in the room, a hand laid gently on the cot, or the movement of a camera shutter was sufficient to evoke a series of movements which have been described by the inexperienced as twitchings or convulsions.

Those infants whose first feed is delayed until the fourth day, for reasons which will be given later, will certainly become restless before then and will show some evidence of dehydration. Physiological jaundice is common and, as in infants of comparable gestational age, it may be quite deep and prolonged. Infection of the skin occurs easily unless strict precautions are taken. Very little breast tissue is apparent during the first two weeks.

Those babies whose clinical progress was abnormal may be grouped together as the 'dyspnoeic' and the 'cyanotic attack' infants. Loose as such descriptive terms may be, insufficient evidence exists as yet to support the adoption of others.

Dyspnoea (Fig. 2). Difficult respiration was observed in 21 babies (21·9%). In some, respiration was established slowly, occasionally only with assistance, and breathing then remained distressed. In others the baby cried immediately on removal head first from the uterus, quickly became pink, and then after a few minutes or an hour or more dyspnoea gradually developed. In only two cases did respiratory difficulty make its first appearance after the first day, and one of these infants had pneumonia.

The duration of dyspnoea varied from a few hours to more than three days and is indicated in Fig. 2. Cyanosis of varying degree accompanied the forcible respirations, the sternal and costal indrawing and the strange tremulous expiratory whine which is known to the midwives as 'murmuring'. Seriously affected babies became very limp, and the Moro response,

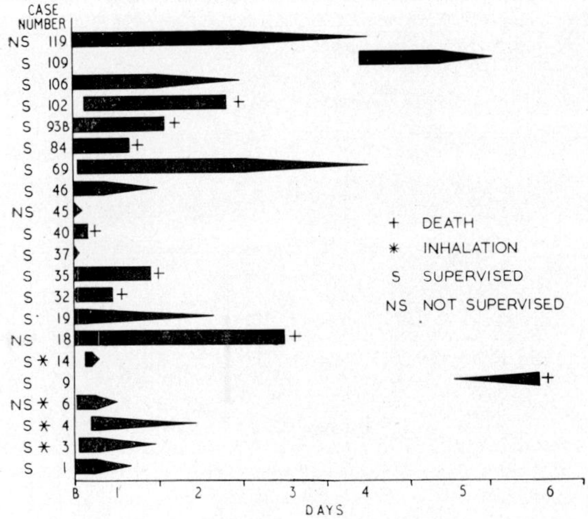

FIG. 2.—The duration of dyspnoea. Inhalation of glucose solution occurred in some cases. Supervision refers to ante-natal obstetric care.

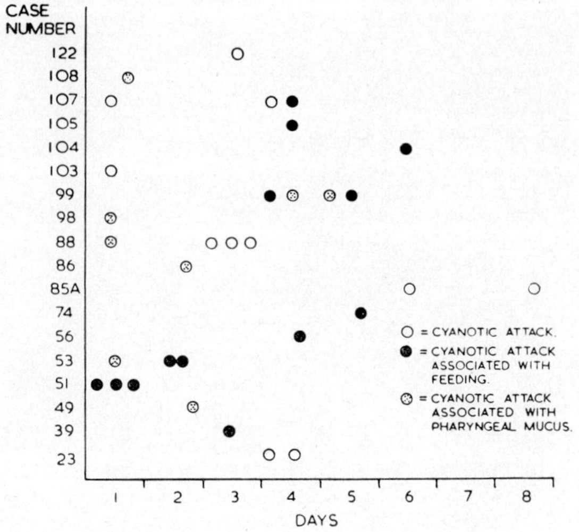

FIG. 3.—The time incidence of cyanotic attacks.

so very active in the well offspring of the diabetic woman, was lost at least temporarily. All the deaths in this series were preceded by dyspnoea, and in all cases acute cyanotic attacks were superimposed upon the distress and were often the terminal event. The survivors showed gradual improvement over periods of up to 24 hours, and where dyspnoea became progressively less noticeable over six to nine hours the baby's recovery could be expected.

Cyanotic Attacks (Fig. 3). Cyanotic attacks were observed as unaccompanied abnormalities in 18 babies (18·8%). Such incidents were unheralded and dramatic, and were characterized by infrequent or temporarily interrupted respiration and profound cyanosis. They were almost always already well established when observed by the nurse and unless the physician is spending much time simply observing premature babies, he may never see such an attack. The attacks were quite unlike that which is superimposed upon respiratory distress and more nearly resembled an exaggeration of the common irregular respiratory pattern of the small immature newborn infant (Boutourline-Young and Smith, 1950). It was as if the centre which inhibits respiration in pre-natal life (Barcroft, 1947) were temporarily to re-establish control. At one moment the infant was pink and well and then before the observer's eyes the pink skin gave way to grey and then to deepening shades of cyanosis. Respiration might be infrequent or even absent for a minute or longer. The infant became toneless and, in severe cases, apparently lifeless. Bradycardia was profound and was often found as soon as cyanosis was obvious. It was, however, not necessarily the result of the same central discharge which arrested respiration, because hypopnoea or apnoea always existed for an undetermined space of time before the changing colour attracted the observer's attention.

Such attacks may occur at any time in the first week, they may be single or multiple and they are usually brief (Fig. 3). Some are associated with small accumulations of mucus which can be aspirated from the pharynx and others occur when premature attempts are made to feed the baby. Most of them cannot be explained at present. The isolated cyanotic attack has never been lethal in my experience. Although treatment may be unnecessary the infant's appearance is so alarming that action is always taken. A clear airway is assured and then sensory or chemical stimulation of respiration is added and oxygen is given temporarily. Such treatment is about as scientific as shaking a clock which has stopped, but fortunately the mechanism is intact and requires no more drastic remedy.

Some Factors which Influence Progress

Birth Weight. (Fig. 4). The influence of birth weight upon the progress of the live-born baby of the diabetic woman is apparent from Fig. 4. The curve of mean birth weight at varying gestational ages, the latter based on the date of the last menstrual period, is derived from the figures of Ellis (1951). Dyspnoea and death were commoner among the lighter babies at any gestational age, or among babies of 1,700 g. birth weight or less. Uncom-

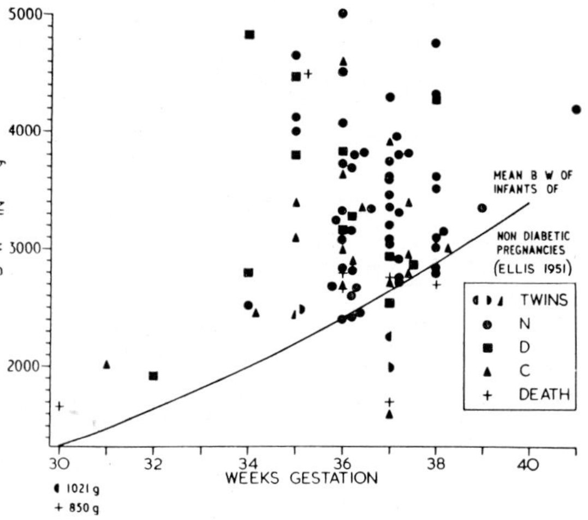

FIG. 4.—Birth weight, maturity and clinical behaviour. N = Normal. D = Dyspnoea. C = Cyanotic attack(s).

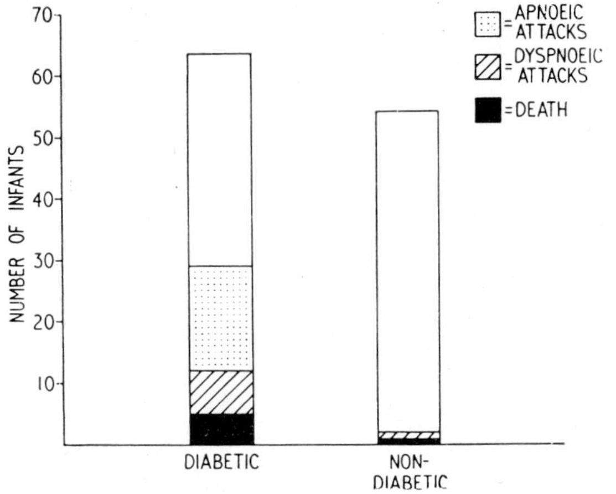

FIG. 5.—Mortality and morbidity among babies born prematurely at 35-38 weeks by caesarean section to women not in labour.

plicated cyanotic attacks were also commoner among the lighter babies. Only one baby of over 3,000 g. (6·6 lb.) birth weight died.

Influence of Caesarean Section (Fig. 5). A higher morbidity and mortality exists among infants born to non-diabetic women by caesarean section than among infants of comparable maturity born spontaneously. This may result from the maternal or foetal illness which dictated the need for section or from circulatory stresses imposed by the method of delivery. A comparison was made between infants of the same maturity born by elective caesarean section to groups of diabetic and non-diabetic women who had not been in established labour. Both groups of women were patients in the same hospital between 1948 and 1955. Three infants born to diabetic women died, but of these one had suffered pre-natal exsanguination and another had very severe erythroblastosis foetalis and kernikterus. They have been excluded from consideration in Fig. 5 as in neither case was death a result of diabetes mellitus or caesarean section. The third child died of pulmonary haemorrhage. Mortality and certainly morbidity were significantly higher among the infants of diabetic women than among those of the control group. The former were, however, observed more carefully and some cyanotic attacks may have passed unnoticed among the normal babies (Fig. 5). The comparison strongly suggests that diabetes and *not* caesarean section is the principal harmful influence.

Diabetic Control and Severity (Figs. 6 and 7). Control of the mother's diabetes has been graded for me by the two physicians concerned during the eight-year period. Good control implies that the patients were free from symptoms, were not ketotic at any time and that the blood sugar determined weekly three hours or more after a meal never exceeded 140 mg. %. Control is classed as bad if the patient had two or more ketotic episodes of 24 hours' duration or longer during the pregnancy or if the weekly blood sugar taken three hours or more after a meal exceeded 250 mg. % on more than one occasion. Fair control describes those who were to be found somewhere between the two other

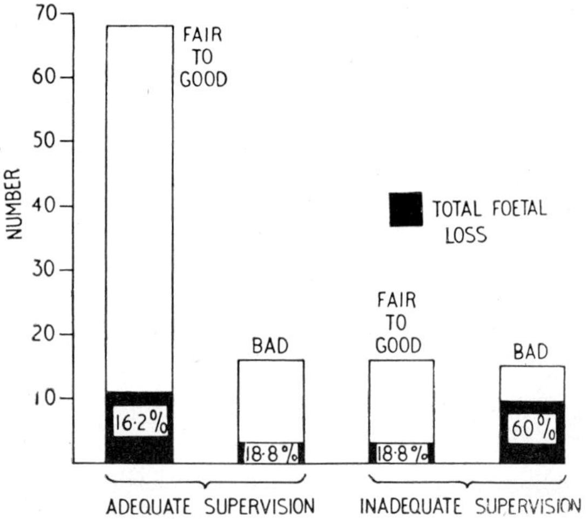

FIG. 6.—The influence of diabetic control upon foetal loss. The 115 cases are divided into two groups according to the standard of diabetic control, 'fair to good' and 'bad'. These are further subdivided according to the adequacy of ante-natal obstetric supervision.

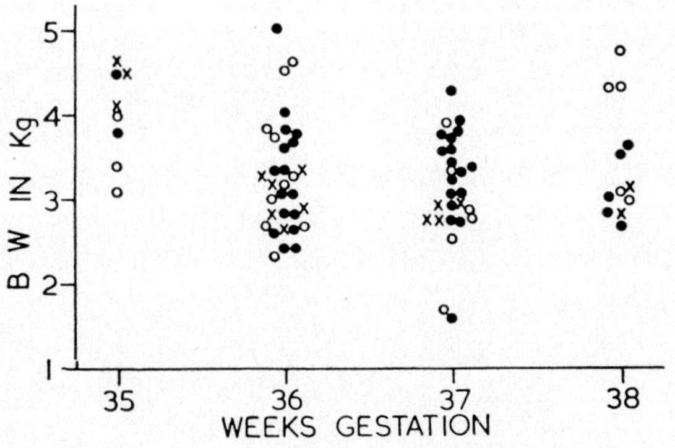

FIG. 7.—The influence of diabetic control upon birth weight. *Control:* O = Good. ● = Fair. × = Poor.

groups. In the present series poor control carried an increased risk to the foetus (Fig. 6) which became disastrous when linked with inadequate antenatal obstetric care.

From the data available in this study no clear influence of diabetic control on birth weight is apparent (Fig. 7) but a suggestion exists that as pregnancy proceeds toward term poor control adversely influences foetal growth. Certainly the large recent study of White Class F diabetic mothers (those with nephropathy) by Oppé, Hsia and Gellis (1957) quoted a viable foetal mortality exceeding 50% for such as compared with the 18% loss for the less severely affected women (Table 1) and the babies of the Class F group were found to be smaller.

Family Birth Weight (Fig. 8). The birth weights and the maturity of all sibs of the children in this series were ascertained wherever the information was available, and these were grouped in families. In order that the diagram may be more easily understood it has been subdivided into 12 small graphs with three or four families on each. The number allotted to each family is the number of the first case in that family to be included in the present series. The point at which the mother was found to have diabetes mellitus is indicated on the horizontal axis of each small graph and the years before and after read to the left and right from there.

The horizontal broken line on each graph indicates 4·0 kg. (8·8 lb.) birth weight. The only children of diabetic women are naturally excluded.

The birth of heavy babies during the pre-diabetic years is as apparent here as it was in the series studied by Miller, Hurwitz and Kuder (1944), Gilbert (1949) and Futcher and Long (1954). Many of these large babies in the present series are shown to be sibs.

Maternal Build (Fig. 9). The birth weight group of only children in the series has been plotted against the maternal height and weight prior to the onset of pregnancy. In the case of families composed of more than one child the average birth weight in all the children has been plotted against the height and weight prior to the onset of the last pregnancy. The weaknesses in this comparison are acknowledged. The infants vary in maturity, but the only children are mostly in the 36-38 week range and the majority of babies of multiparous diabetic women were delivered at term. The build of mothers of only children was in fact the build at the time of the child's birth, but in the case of multiparous women their weight when the last child was born does not necessarily represent their weight when child-bearing began. These points and the small size of the groups make impossible an analysis of such other possibly important factors as birth rank, maternal age and social group of the father.

No clear relationship exists between foetal birth weight and maternal build except that with some

TABLE 1
FOETAL MORTALITY IN THE DIABETIC PREGNANCY

Series	Place	Number of Cases	Mortality* Perinatal	Mortality* Neonatal	Comment
White, Gillespie and Sexton (1956)	Boston	628	111	—	
Oppé, *et al.* (1957)	Boston	736	180	110	Excluding all diabetic women with nephropathy
M.R.C. (1955)	U.K.	70	243	114	Treated
		66	258	152	Untreated
Pedowitz and Shlevin (1955)	New York	73	82	27	
Adams (1955)	Oregon	101	158	79	
Richardson, Snaith and Sibley (1955)	Newcastle	71	155	70	
Peel (1955)	London	298	270	149	
Clayton (1956)	London	201	280	149	
S.M.M.P. (1955)	Edinburgh	115	226	69	
		84	166	83	Adequately supervised
Pedersen and Brandstrup (1956)	Copenhagen	265	218	—	
		92	80	—	1953-55 on long-term treatment
Stevenson (1956)	Belfast	49	200	20	Pregnancies occurring 1951-55

* Expressed in terms of per 1,000 viable pregnancies.

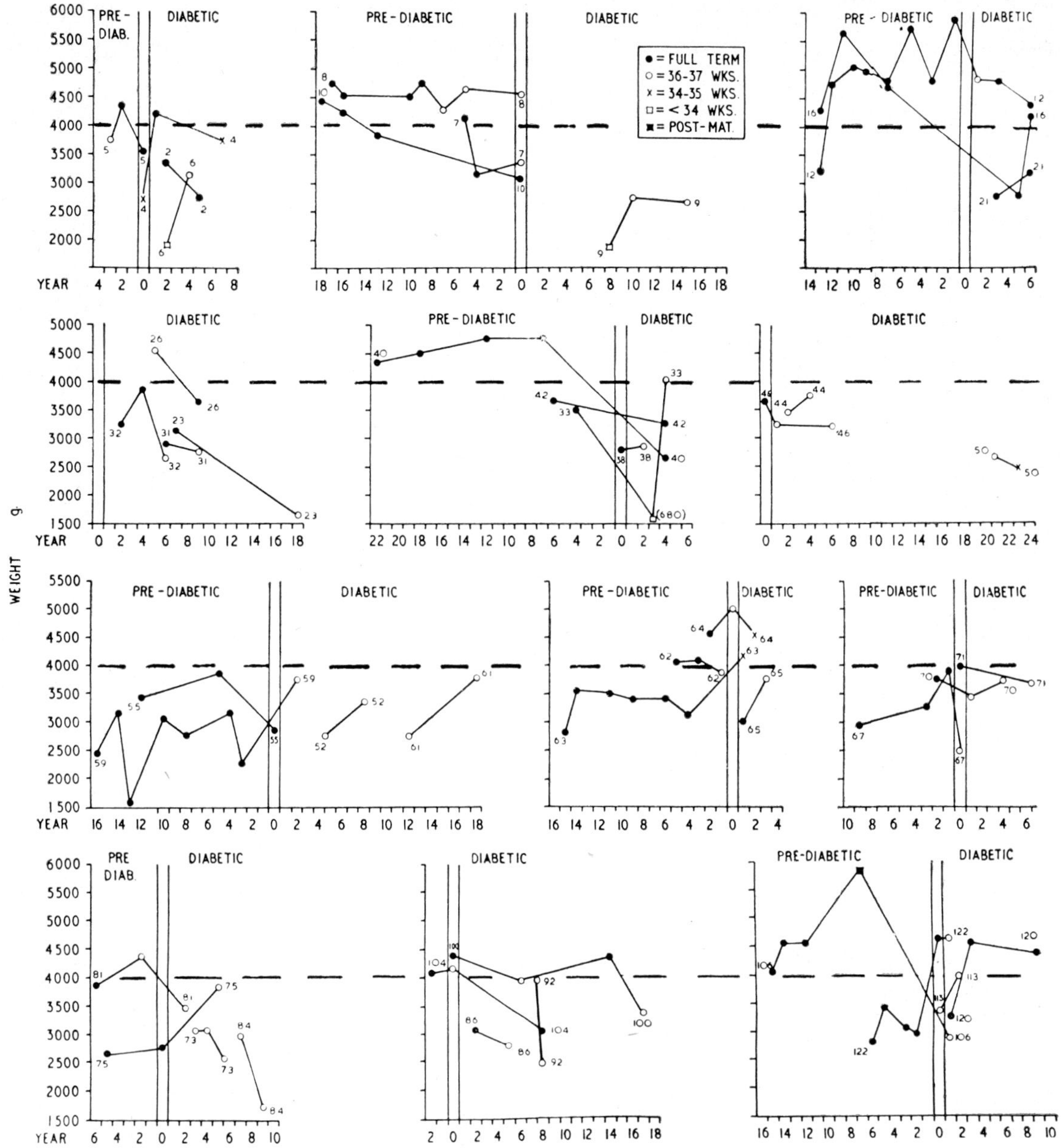

FIG. 8.—Family birthweights and the duration of maternal diabetes.
(The case numbers allow comparison with Fig. 10.) The figure 680 in the middle chart of the second line refers to a birthweight of 680 g.

exceptions infants of less than 3·0 kg. at birth appear to be commoner among lighter mothers. The birth of babies exceeding 4·0 g. to short light diabetic women is unusual.

Family Mortalities (Fig. 10). In this figure the families are arranged in horizontal lines. The pre-diabetic and diabetic years of the mother's life are again indicated. The fate of the foetus is shown by symbols. The viable foetal loss of 121 per 1,000 during the pre-diabetic years compares with 195 per 1,000 after the establishment of clinical diabetes. The neonatal death rates* of 61 and 69 per 1,000

* Neonatal deaths are expressed here not in terms of per 1,000 live births but of per 1,000 viable pregnancies.

viable pregnancies are less obviously different. Neonatal deaths among diabetic primipara, however, number 77 per 1,000. These figures suggest that mortality rises with the development of clinical diabetes, and when the 23 multiparous mothers who were diabetic in each pregnancy are considered, the viable foetal loss is 236 per 1,000 and the neonatal deaths are 73 per 1,000. These figures are contrasted in turn with the results of 54 viable pregnancies among eight women whose child-bearing began at least 10 years before the development of diabetes mellitus. Only six of these babies died, and of these five were neonatal deaths, which give a viable foetal loss of 111 per 1,000 and the neonatal death rate is 93 per 1,000. The very low incidence of intra-uterine death contrasts with the situation after clinical diabetes appears. The high neonatal death rate occurred at a time when the rate was significantly higher than now among the general newborn population. The families were mostly big ones and social conditions may have been adverse.

Mortality and Foetal Birth Weight in the Pre-Diabetic Group (Table 2). The groups of mothers whose child-bearing life began at least 10 years before diabetes was diagnosed, bore a remarkable number of large babies. The birth weights of 52 of them are known, and of these, 32 weighed 4·0 kg. or more at birth.

TABLE 2

BIRTHWEIGHTS OF CHILDREN BORN TO PRE-DIABETIC WOMEN

Family	No. of Children: Weights Known	No. of Children: 4·0 kg. or more	Birthweight Trend
8	7	7	Sustained
10	4	2	Downward
12	11	10	Sustained
16	5	4	Only 4th less than 4 kg.
40	5	4	Only last below 4 kg.
59	8	0	Upward
63	7	1	Only last below 4 kg. (35 wk.)
106	5	4	Only last below 4 kg. (37 wk.)
Total	52	32	

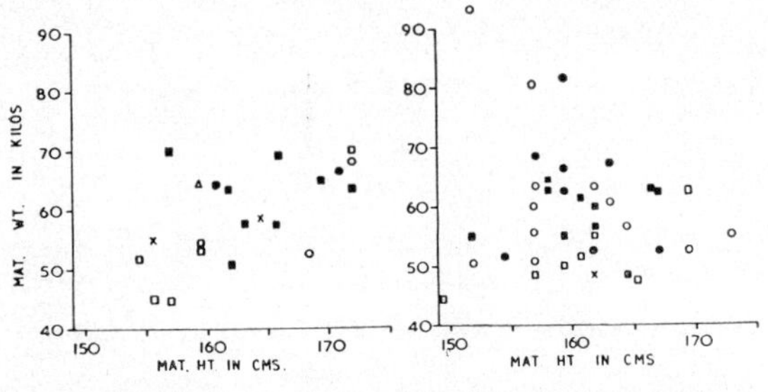

FIG. 9.—The relationship of maternal build to foetal birthweight. *Foetal birthweights:* ● = 4 kg. or more. ○ = 3·5 kg. but less than 4. ■ = 3 kg. but less than 3·5. □ = 2·5 kg. but less than 3. × = 2 kg. but less than 2·5. ▲ = less than 2 kg.

Thus those mothers who developed diabetes after their first child was at least 10 years old not only produced the typical large babies of diabetic women but they did so at the cost of comparatively few lives and with less than 2% of intra-uterine deaths. This fact is complementary to that apparent in Fig. 3, i.e. that death and dyspnoea are commoner among the smaller infants at any gestational age. The growth promoting and the lethal influences upon the foetus are not therefore necessarily identical.

Pathology

Infants born to diabetic women show anatomical and histological abnormalities which have been described in detail by Cardell (1953). These include gigantism, visceromegaly and significant changes in

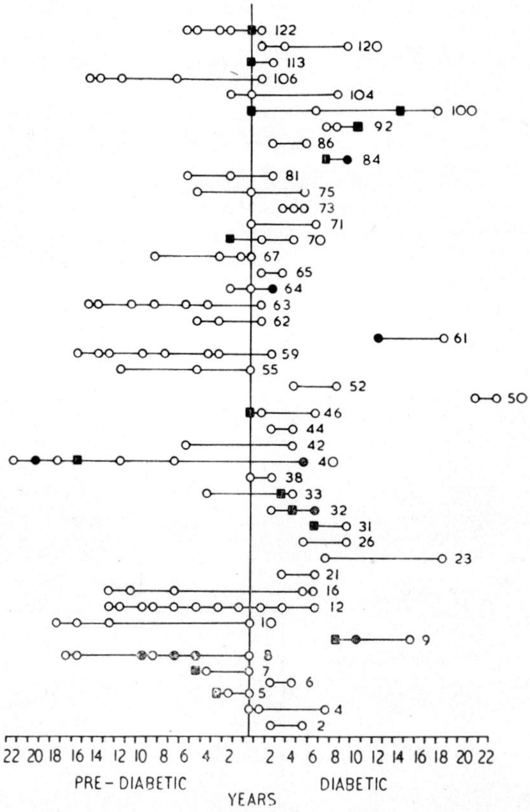

FIG. 10.—Family mortalities and the duration of maternal diabetes. ○ = survival. ● = N.N.D. ■ = I.U.B. (The case numbers allow comparison with Fig. 8.)

TABLE 3
PRINCIPAL AUTOPSY FINDINGS

Case No.	Maturity (weeks)	Birthweight (g.)	Nature of Delivery	Principal Autopsy Finding
9	37	2,764	C/S	Pneumonia. Terminal inhalation
18	36	2,807	Breech. Forceps to head	Massive adrenal haemorrhage
32	36	2,651	C/S	Hyaline membrane
35	30	1,644	Assisted breech	Intracranial haemorrhage
40	38	2,693	C/S	Signs of asphyxia
84	37	1,701	C/S	Massive cerebral haemorrhage. Hyaline membrane
93B	30	850	Spontaneous twin breech	Atelectasis. Prematurity
102	35	4,508	C/S	Renal thrombosis

endocrine glands. Over 20 reports of pancreatic islet hyperplasia in such babies are quoted by Pedersen (1952), and these have been substantiated by the quantitative studies of Tejning (1947), Beek (1952) and by Cardell who showed that the beta cells are chiefly involved and that a positive direct correlation exists between the volume of islet tissue and the size of the baby. Enlargement of the adrenal glands involves principally the cortex, and cardiomegaly, with some increase in myocardial glycogen, is common. The commonest autopsy finding in most series is pulmonary hyaline membrane. Renal vein thrombosis occurs rarely (Tveterås and Rudström, 1956; Avery, Oppenheimer and Gordon, 1957).

Autopsies have been carried out by Dr. Agnes Macgregor on all eight deaths in this series and the principal findings are given in Table 3. Only the pneumonic death was preventable. Extreme prematurity cannot always be avoided, but breech delivery was not permitted after 1949. Islet hyperplasia was reported in the pancreas of each case by Dr. R. F. Ogilvie.

Metabolic Abnormalities of the Foetus

The problems relating to the collection of specimens increase the difficulty of metabolic investigation at this age. The principal abnormalities described concern potassium, calcium and glucose.

Potassium. According to Björklund (1953) the serum potassium of babies born to diabetic women is low, and he found 'suppression or sagging' of the S-T segment, pathological negative T and U waves and prolongation of the QT interval on their electrocardiograms, but no such changes in a control group. They existed whether the baby showed clinical disturbance or not, but in no abnormal baby was the E.C.G. normal. Such E.C.G. changes in adults have been ascribed to potassium deficiency.

Depression or sagging of the S-T segment was apparent in nine of 11 E.C.G. tracings obtained from babies in the present series. Some of the infants were asymptomatic and others who were dyspnoeic showed no other evidence of potassium deficiency. The T wave abnormalities at this age are not believed to be specific of hypokalaemia but may represent a metabolic disorder. Depression or inversion of the T waves is more likely to relate to intracellular potassium levels than to serum levels and McCance (1955) does not believe that they truly reflect potassium lack. No evidence exists for giving such infants potassium and it may be dangerous. In one clinic where parenteral potassium has been given the neonatal mortality is higher than in the Edinburgh series.

Calcium. Low serum calcium levels in infants born to diabetic women and in premature babies of non-diabetic women have been reported by Craig and Buchanan (1958). The babies in the diabetic group were mostly prematurely born. The levels recorded are certainly below the accepted normal range and the authors suggest that the neuromuscular irritability of these infants on the second and later days of life may be hypocalcaemic tetany, a condition which bears little resemblance to tetany in the more mature subject (Talbot, Sobel, McArthur and Crawford, 1952; Wilkins, 1957). Unfortunately the series includes no proper control study so that there is no real evidence that the low calcium levels are directly responsible for symptoms. No suggestion has been made that dyspnoea or cyanotic attacks are of hypocalcaemic origin. The infants studied by Farquhar and Smith (1958) during exchange transfusion for haemolytic disease did not show increased neuromuscular irritability even at very low levels of calcium ion. Calcium was not found by Craig and Buchanan (1958) to relieve the neuromuscular irritability of the babies of diabetic women and better results were obtained with chloral hydrate.

No serum calcium determinations were made on the infants in the present series.

Glucose. The blood sugar falls more consistently, more rapidly and further in infants born to diabetic mothers than in normal babies of non-diabetic mothers. This hypoglycaemia is at its height at 2-3 hours and it is corrected spontaneously in 4-6 hours. No correlation exists between the speed of fall, the lowest level reached, the development of symptoms or later progress (Farquhar, 1954, 1956a). The minute volume of expired air, measured in a small number of babies, did not vary significantly in the first few hours. During the years 1948-51 glucose was given by mouth or by injection to infants of diabetic mothers in doses roughly equivalent to those used in glucose tolerance tests, in an attempt to prevent hypoglycaemia. Even with this precaution the blood sugar tended to fall (Table 4).

Maternal Diabetes and Foetal Abnormality

Morphology of the Foetus. The diabetic woman exerts influences upon her baby which accelerate growth, stimulate hypertrophy of the pancreatic islets and particularly of the beta cells, provoke increased formation of glycogen in at least some infants and a sharp fall in blood sugar beyond the normal range in almost all. The increased pancreatic beta cells can reasonably be expected to produce increased amounts of insulin. They do not appear to be a different 'foetal tissue' analogous to the foetal adrenal cortex with activities confined only to pre-natal life. If they do not secrete more insulin then it is difficult to imagine what other function such specialized cells can perform or to believe that the insulin mechanism is the victim of an intrinsic metabolic block similar to the enzyme defects existent in some forms of goitrous cretinism.

The impression gained in the present study is that these babies tolerate glucose abnormally well in the first few hours but that the situation rapidly alters. Against this may be set the apparently definite conclusions of Read (1951) but serious faults are present in his study. Enough circumstantial evidence exists to justify the belief that the immediate post-natal hypoglycaemia of infants born to diabetic women results from increased foetal insulin secretion and that separation of the infant from the maternal circulation ends the pancreatrophic influence. Moreover, although the pancreatic islet hyperplasia has been shown only in fatal cases, these babies did die of causes other than hypoglycaemia, and almost all surviving babies have been hypoglycaemic so that pancreatic hyperplasia at birth can be assumed to exist among survivors.

Foetal hyperinsulinism may be stimulated by maternal hyperglycaemia, pituitary growth hormone or corticosteroids or by the baby's adrenocortical response to maternal corticotrophin. The occurrence of gigantism and pancreatic islet hyperplasia in babies of pre-diabetic women means that high maternal blood sugar levels are not responsible for these abnormalities by themselves. The suspected role of pituitary growth hormone (P.G.H.) in the production of human diabetes mellitus has received support from the observations of Luft, Ikkos, Gemzell and Olivecrona (1958) that such material purified from human pituitary glands provokes rapid hyperglycaemia and ketosis in young hypophysectomized diabetic human adults. This hormone, in amounts insufficient to cause maternal acromegaly, may very well stimulate the foetal pancreas and accelerate the growth of already rapidly growing foetal tissue. According to Ikkos, Luft and Gemzell (1958) P.G.H. may also cause some increase in salt retention and in the extracellular volume. It could explain, therefore, the slight fluid retention suspected in babies of diabetic women.

Adrenal corticosteroids may also stimulate the pancreatic islets, as in Cushing's syndrome, and cause fluid retention. Their production is increased in young diabetics (Klein, Papadatos, Fortunato and

TABLE 4

BLOOD SUGAR LEVEL RESPONSE IN INFANTS OF DIABETIC WOMEN TO THE ADMINISTRATION OF GLUCOSE IN THE FIRST 6 HOURS OF LIFE

Case	Weight in Kg.	Blood Sugar Levels and Doses of Glucose Given *						
		Hours After Birth						
		Birth	1	2	3	4	5	6
3	4·5	66 (2)	(15) 50		(15) 70			100
4	3·8	180	(4)		(6) 34			
7	3·4	120 (1)	78		(8·5) 60			70
8	4·5	60 (5)	74	(7·5)	74	(7·5)		(10) 64
14	2·9	182 (2·5)	124	72	(7·5)		138	
18	2·8	254 (1)	180	180 (1)	86	52		
19	2·8	(2) 522	132	66 (1)	74		74 (1) 78	
23	1·6	153 (2)	88 (0·5) 70		58 (0·5)	56 (0·5)	56	
29	4·7	102 (2·5)	94		104			44
30	2·8	94 (2·5)	72		50		62	66
32	2·7	108 (2·5)	98		80			
33	4·1	102 (2·5)		58				
39	3·7	114 (1)	117	48	57			60
40	2·7	43	(1) 51	57	62			
42	3·3	76 (2·5)		69		55 (1·5)		
44	3·5	90 (1)	53 (1·5)	42			53	
45	4·3	55 (1)	46	54				
46	3·3	53 (1)	60	62	60			
48	2·4	70 (2)	82	69				
49	3·3	49 (1)	42	34				
50	2·6	150 (1) 117 74	43	36	31 (1)		74 67	
53	—	51 (1) 47	49		60			
55	2·8	40 (1) 20 46	56			52 (0·5)	59	43
59	3·7	56 (1) 42 35	57			86		
61	3·8	92 (1) 100 78	71			78		
62	3·8	84 (1) 82 85		92		89		100
69	3·8	62 (1) 60 54	48			79		74
70	3·7	51 (0·5) 24 21		18 (1·5)	43			60

* The figures in brackets represent grammes of glucose given. Where underlined once the oral route of administration was used, where underlined twice the dose was intravenous. Otherwise the glucose was given by intramuscular injection.

Byers, 1955; Klein, Weigand, Iunes and Greenman, 1956; Grayzel, Warshall, Elkan and Sternberg, 1957) and in pregnancy (Cope, Boysen and McCrae, 1951). There is some evidence, however, that they may not pass the placental barrier, whereas corticotrophin may do so (Farquhar, 1956b). If such is the case then maternal corticotrophin may increase the pancreatrophic influence by stimulating the foetal adrenal cortex.

Evidence for foetal hyperadrenocorticism has been sought in studies of post-natal weight loss, urine volume and formaldehydogenic steroid excretion. The post-natal weight loss is proportionate to the delay in allowing the baby to feed but is no different in infants of diabetic and non-diabetic women (Farquhar and Sklaroff, 1958). The babies of the present series did, however, excrete rather more urine during the first 24-48 hours of life than infants born either by caesarean section or spontaneously to non-diabetic women (Table 5).

Eosinophil studies have provided no positive evidence of foetal hyperadrenocorticism (Farquhar, 1954, 1955, 1956b). The babies in the present series delivered by caesarean section to diabetic women excreted more urinary acid-stable formaldehydogenic steroids than normal infants of almost comparable maturity born by the same route or by the vagina (Fig. 11) The method of Tompsett and

TABLE 5

TWENTY-FOUR HOUR URINE VOLUMES OF BABIES BORN TO DIABETIC AND NON-DIABETIC WOMEN

Group	Case	Day 1 (ml.)	Day 2 (ml.)	Day 3 (ml.)
Normal (vaginal birth) ..	g	18	30	37
	h	19	16	—
	i	5	7	—
	j	10	34	30
	k	5	6	17
	l	5	16	43
	m	12	12	15
Normal (caesarean section) ..	n	28	63	—
	o	38	—	—
	p	24	47	—
	q	36	15	11
	r	11	37	28
	s	15·5	9·5	—
	t	7	29	52
	u	32·5	44	28
Diabetic	99	36	31	—
	100	60	40	—
	102	40	45*	—
	103†			
	104	45	97	—
	105	19	40	34
	106	7	28	37
	107	60	83	22
	108	67	73	80
	110	60	33	40
	113	12	45	—
	119	60	35	—
	122	30	95	82
	123	60	20	35

* In 16 hours (baby died).
† Record lost.

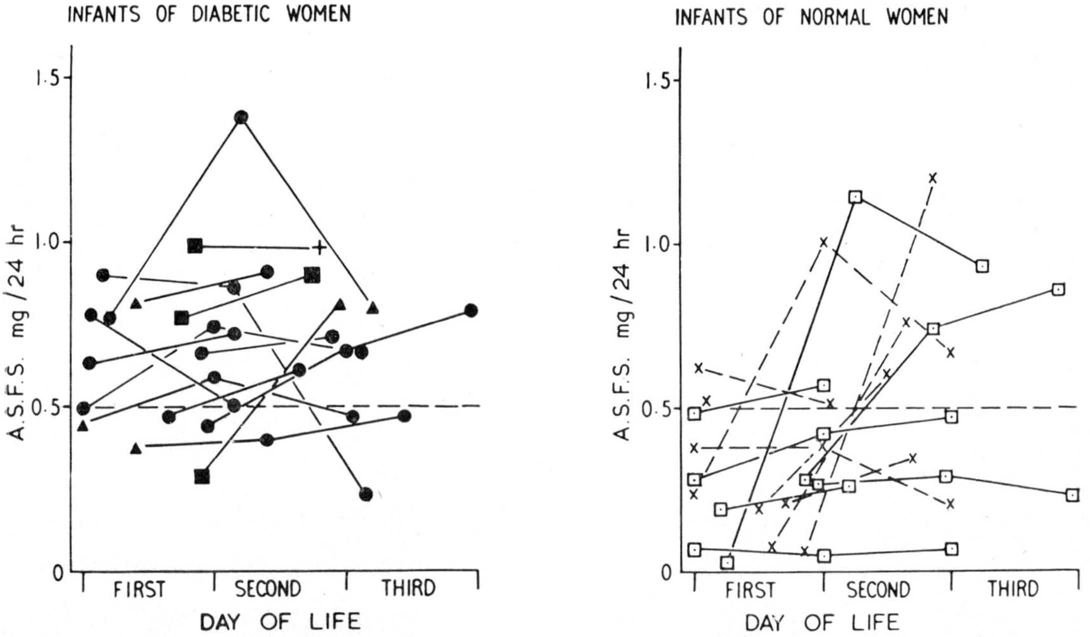

FIG. 11.—Serial daily urinary excretion of acid-stable formaldehydogenic steroids.
Diabetic: ● = Normal. ■ = Dyspnoea. ▲ = Cyanotic attacks. + = Death.
Normal: □ = Vaginal deliveries. × = Caesarean sections.

Smith (1954) was used. The principal limitation of formaldehydogenic steroid methods appears to be their failure to measure all the urinary corticosteroids (Marrian, 1951). This finding is in accord with the observations of Hoet (1954) who believes that hyperadrenocorticism plays some part in the morphology and morbidity of such babies.

Pathology of the Foetus. Pulmonary hyaline membrane, although found in only two of the eight (25%) autopsies performed in this series, occurred in 80% or more of neonatal deaths in the large diabetic series of White (1952), Peel (1955) and Clayton (1956). A reversible degree of this abnormality may be the explanation of dyspnoea with survival in other babies. It is so common a finding that a knowledge of its cause may shed light on the whole problem of perinatal and neonatal morbidity in infants of diabetic women and on diabetes mellitus itself. The work done recently in a number of fields may indicate this. Migration of up to 25% of the plasma from the capillaries into the extravascular space in the first hours after delivery is physiological in the normal newborn baby (Gairdner, Marks, Roscoe and Brettell, 1958) and in the premature (Baar, 1956). The pulmonary resistance in newborn lambs is high before the lungs expand, and may be increased by tying the cord before respiration is established (Dawes, Mott, Widdicombe and Wyatt, 1953; Born, Dawes, Mott and Widdicombe, 1954). The electron-microscopy studies of Van Breemen, Neustein and Bruns (1957) have confirmed that the hyaline membrane consists of blood plasma which has leaked from the vascular compartment, and that this is made possible by visible changes in the epithelial linings of ducts and alveoli and in the endothelial lining of capillaries. The infant of the diabetic woman is usually born prematurely and his cord is commonly clamped before the onset of respiration. If perinatal hypoxia could be proved this might represent the cause of capillary damage in the lungs and elsewhere. and it would contribute toward pulmonary hypertension.

Placental Dysfunction. The placenta of the diabetic woman is not obviously abnormal on inspection. It has been described as large by White (1952) and Peel (1955) believes that intra-uterine death is due to the foetus outgrowing the efficiency of the placenta. The ratio of placental to foetal weight is normal in the present series (Fig. 12). If the foetus is large for gestational age so is the placenta, and no relationship can be found between the ratio and the clinical state of the foetus. Much has been said by White and her colleagues about hormonal changes associated with placental failure in the diabetic pregnancy, and good results have been claimed by them for hormone replacement therapy, but these have not been confirmed consistently in other American clinics nor by any in the United Kingdom. Most of those who have examined the histology of diabetic placentae have failed to demonstrate abnormalities which do not occur with equal frequency in the placentae of non-diabetic women (Reis, De Costa and Allweiss, 1950). Abnormal stromal oedema in diabetic placentae was observed, however, by Mackay of the Joslin Clinic (reported by White, 1952) when the tissue was carefully fixed within 30 minutes of birth. The oedema was not found in the placentae of non-diabetic women.

The vigorous erythropoiesis and the normoblastaemia of babies born to diabetic women led Berglund and Zetterström (1954) to believe that these infants suffered from pre-natal hypoxia and their investigation of the oxygen saturation of cord blood seemed to confirm this. Much attention has been paid recently to the dwindling supply of oxygen available to the foetus in late normal or in abnormal pregnancy (Walker and Turnbull, 1953; Walker, 1954; Turnbull and Baird, 1957; MacKay, 1957). The oxygen available to a number of babies in the present series was determined by MacKay (1955) and the results have been plotted in Fig. 13 with an indication of the anaesthetic employed at caesarean section and of the mean values found by her for normal pregnancies. No obvious relationship exists between the oxygen saturation per cent. and the later clinical behaviour of the foetus. Such oxygen levels

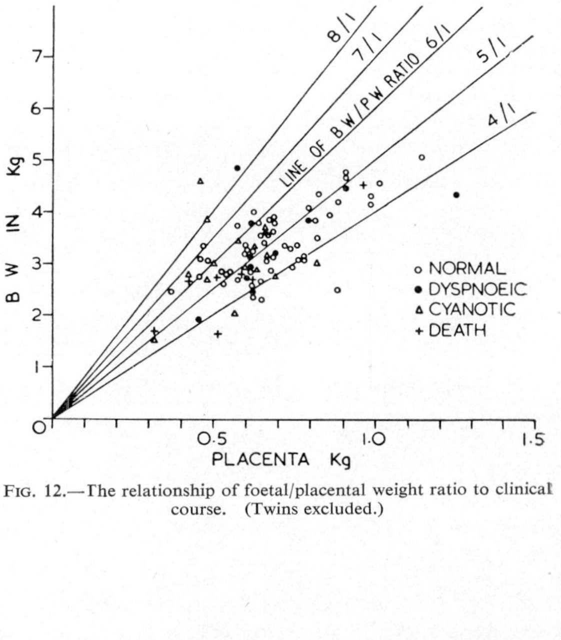

FIG. 12.—The relationship of foetal/placental weight ratio to clinical course. (Twins excluded.)

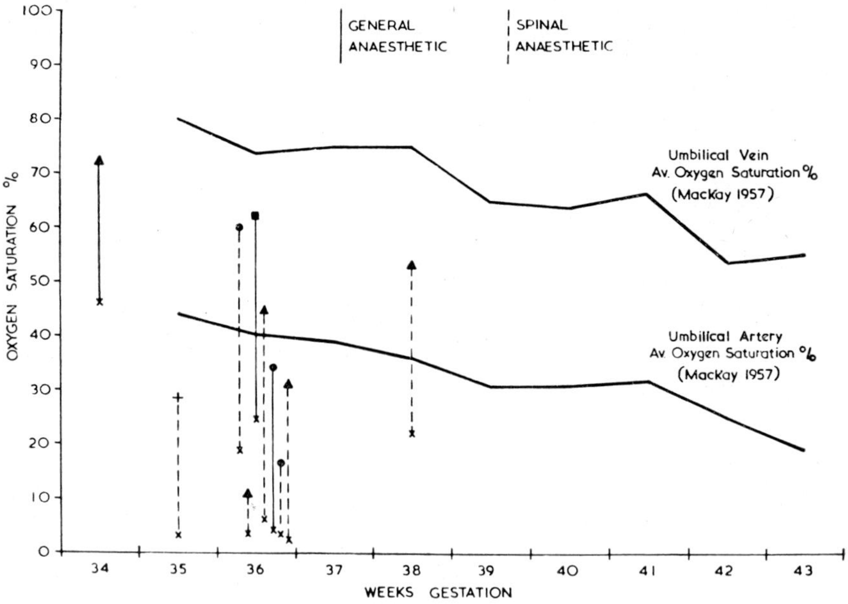

FIG. 13.—Oxygen saturation of umbilical cord blood at delivery of diabetic women. (The average values refer to normal pregnancies.) *Umbilical vein:* ● = Normal. ▲ = Cyanotic attacks. ■ = Dyspnoea. + = Death. *Umbilical artery:* = ×.

may not represent the true situation, however, but only the conditions prevailing after delivery of the foetus. The oxygen pressure gradient across the haemochorial human placenta may indicate the infant's available oxygen more accurately, and Prystowsky (1957) has shown that it falls significantly in abnormal, including diabetic, pregnancy. These observations strongly suggest that perinatal hypoxia exists in diabetic pregnancy and that this may cause intra-uterine or neonatal death, or respiratory distress with survival.

The chorionic villi, which share a common origin with the foetus, respond in the same way to the growth-promoting influence. In many pregnancies the larger placenta supplies a larger foetus, but in others it becomes unhealthy at about the thirty-second week with resulting retardation of foetal growth and increased risk. When it fails later the foetus is already large and sudden intra-uterine death may result from the relatively greater deficiency. P.G.H. may accelerate the life of the placenta and so shorten its limited span, but the lower mortality among the large babies of pre-diabetic mothers does not support this. Microscopic degenerative changes have been shown by Ditzel and Moinat (1957) to develop in the conjunctival capillaries of diabetic women in later pregnancy and these can be related to inadequacy of diabetic control. Can the premature placental degeneration of diabetes mellitus be related to the vascular degeneration of this disease? That the latter may be caused by adrenal corticosteroids has been suggested by Becker (1952) Becker, Maengwyn-Davies, Rosen, Friedenwald and Winter (1954), Williams (1955), and, with less certainty, by Maengwyn-Davies, Lerman, Pogell, Stone and Friedenwald (1956). This suggestion has received no support from the work of Rifkin, Solomon and Lieberman (1958) but further work on the possible role of individual normal or abnormal corticosteroids continues. The infants of this series seemed to excrete increased amounts of formaldehydogenic steroids. The occurrence of classical vascular degeneration in cases of pure pancreatic diabetes (Lawrence, 1950; Duncan, MacFarlane and Robson, 1958) supports the belief that it may result from the metabolic disorder caused by insulin deficiency and that an inherited vulnerability or dyspituitarism are not necessarily involved. Insulin deficiency, however, is unlikely to be responsible for the foetal deaths during the mother's pre-diabetic years, and it is interesting to recall that in Fig. 10 intra-uterine deaths are less common before the development of clinical diabetes. Strict diabetic control is now advocated as the only way in which vascular degeneration may be prevented or delayed (Dunlop,

1954) and whether similar changes in the placenta are the result of insulin deficiency, corticosteroids or an as yet undetermined factor, strict diabetic control in pregnancy and good obstetrics are the only ways by which the foetal mortality can be reduced (Pedersen and Brandstrup, 1956).

Treatment of the Newborn

The treatment of the newborn consists of gentle resuscitation and continuous observation in a warm room for four days or more. Although routine gastric aspiration at birth has been practised, the large volumes of gastric content reported by Gellis, White and Pfeffer (1949) have not been found in our series (Fig. 14). Feeding should be delayed until the morning of the third day and possibly till later in small infants. Clear fluids only are given during the first day of feeding. Antibiotics and oxygen play no part in routine management. The hypoglycaemia does not require correction, the giving of potassium salts is probably both unnecessary and dangerous, and calcium has little effect on the neuromuscular irritability. Sedation is probably undesirable. Nursing supervision must be conscientious or dramatic cyanotic attacks may be missed by an inattentive nurse even sitting by the cot. The baby's pharynx should be gently aspirated before respiration is stimulated by flicking the baby's foot. Oxygen may be given for a few minutes. Chemical stimulation is rarely necessary.

The treatment of the dyspnoeic syndrome is unsatisfactory. Oxygen may be given in concentrations not exceeding 35%, but water-vapour mists have been shown to be ineffective (Hsia, Peterson and Gellis, 1957). The babies should not be disturbed unless to aspirate mucus. Assisted respiration by mechanical means may help but it is less important than trying to prevent the hypoxia which precedes the membrane's formation. Strict diabetic control alone is the most effective preventive so far, particularly when it permits vaginal delivery at term. Minor skin infections, to which the babies seem predisposed, should be treated with aqueous gentian violet or, in severe cases, by the systemic use of the effective antibiotic.

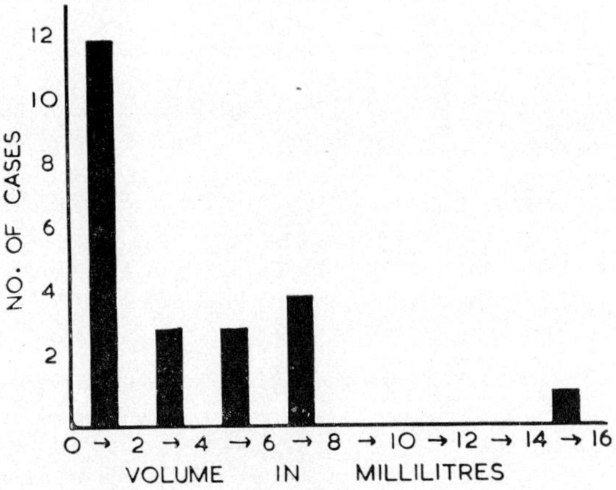

FIG. 14.—The volume of gastric contents at birth.

Lactation

Normal lactation in diabetic women has been reported by Wilder and Parsons (1928), Merkler (1929) and Peckham (1931) but it is more commonly described as poor. It was deficient in all the cases reported by McIlroy, Hill and Pillman-Williams (1931), and in the experience of Peel (1951) only half these mothers are able to breast feed adequately. Lactation may start normally and then fail (Barns and Morgans, 1952) or it may be established only with difficulty but remain adequate afterwards (Peel and Oakley, 1950).

Inadequate maternal nutrition was held to be responsible by Skipper (1933) and to be partly responsible by Sheumack (1949). Not all such mothers are obviously malnourished now and the improvement in diabetic nutrition is the recognized explanation for the altered fertility among such women. Premature delivery may be partly responsible (Peel 1951; Barns and Morgans, 1952; Rolland, 1954). An immature baby certainly may provide poor stimulation for the breast even if suckling were permitted during the first few days. The lactation even of non-diabetic women, however, is established more slowly after caesarean than after spontaneous delivery. Prolactin deficiency is suspected by Sheumack (1949) and a pituitary abnormality by Peel (1951).

The breast feeding history of 60 non-diabetic women who were delivered by caesarean section has been studied (Fig. 15, inset). Half of them were breast feeding their babies fully at discharge from hospital and only a third had failed completely. The composition of this group of infants has already been described (Farquhar and Sklaroff, 1958) and differs mainly by being rather more mature than the diabetic group. In contrast to this the breast feeding history of diabetic women, most of whom had been delivered by caesarean section, in the present series is poor (Fig. 15). Considerably more than half the women either abandoned the attempt in the first week, or less commonly no attempt was made. A further large group failed during the first 4 to 6 weeks. Some, however, were fully or partly success-

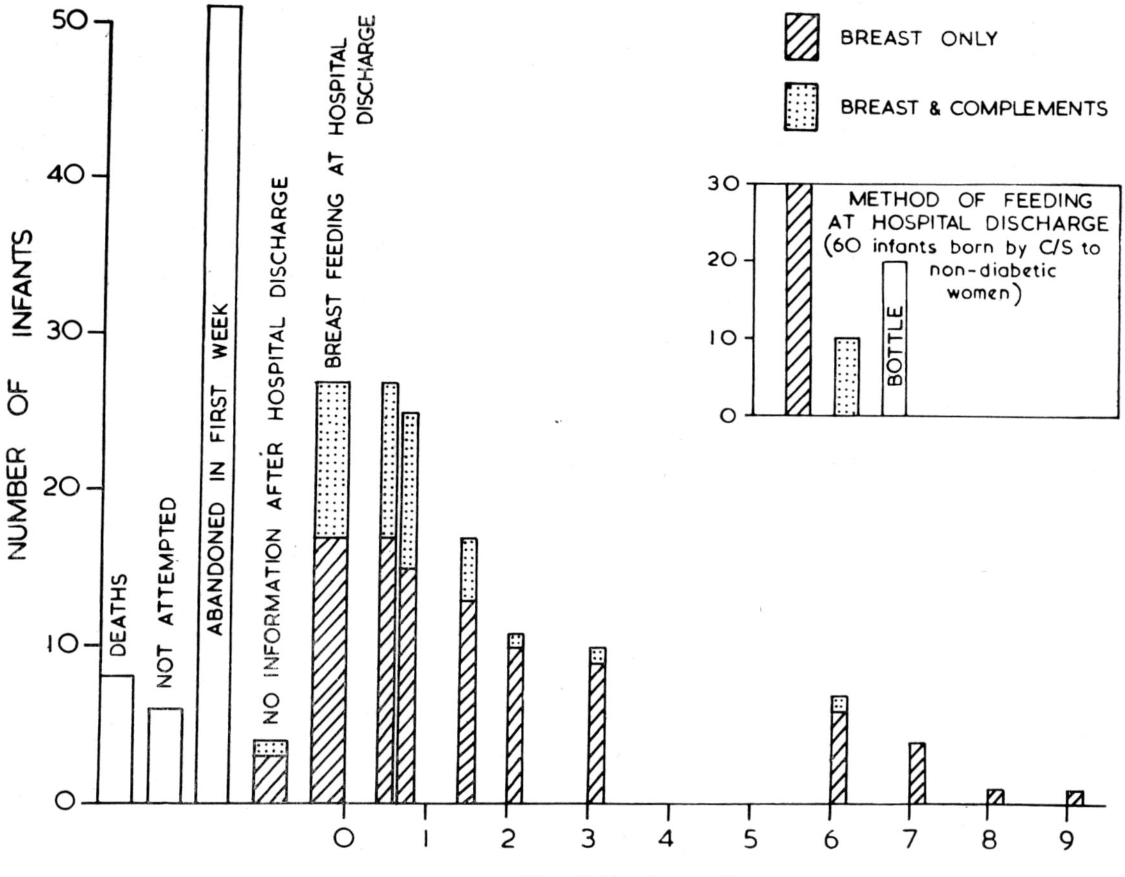

FIG. 15.—The breast feeding history of 96 infants born to diabetic women.

ful until weaning was established at 6 to 9 months of age. More detailed information about these groups is available from Table 6. No consistent relationship has been found between the pre-diabetic and diabetic obstetric histories of the mothers or the size of the babies and the success or failure of breast feeding. Although the hypothesis that inadequate lactation is but one facet of a complicated metabolic disorder involving the pituitary no convincing evidence for this has been advanced so far. Almost certainly more diabetic women could breast feed if every encouragement were provided. That she should do so is not, however, a matter of great consequence nowadays.

Congenital Malformations

Early this century, Herman (1902) referring to diabetic pregnancy stated that 'the chances are two to one that the child will die *in utero*. Its life is therefore not of much account'. With the improved survival rate, however, the fate of the survivors assumes greater importance.

The incidence of congenital malformations in those series which include 40 or more cases ranges from none (Patterson and Burnstein, 1949; Hall and Tillman, 1951) to 80% in the large Boston series (White, 1952). Most published series quote an incidence of from 2 to 3% but Barns and Morgans (1949) claimed 10%, Peel and Oakley (1950) 63% and Hagbard (1956) 62%. Fredrikson, Hagbard, Olow and Reinand (1957) found only one of 123 cases derived from a larger group of which they thought that many probably died earlier of malformation. Few of these authors examined a control group of babies born to non-diabetic women, and where they did so no description of the control material was given. Of all of these quite the most extraordinary contrast lies in White's claims of 80 and 1·8% of congenital malformations in babies born to diabetic and non-diabetic women respectively. Her statement (1949) that these anomalies were severe in only 10% and lethal in only 2% raises doubt as to whether she looked for the same range of abnormalities in the control group.

Several explanations can be found for these wide variations in incidence. Some authors may have included every trivial abnormality found on clinical examination, whereas others used technical aids to diagnosis or recorded only the lethal malformations discovered at autopsy. Some have mentioned only those anomalies which are obvious in the first week whereas others have followed their cases and have added those malformations which were discovered later. The nearest approach to a properly controlled study so far is probably that of Cardell (1953) who found incidences of 25% and 20·2% at autopsy in babies of diabetic and non-diabetic women respectively. The difference was not considered significant. Abnormalities of the eye, such as congenital cataract, and of other systems may not always be apparent at autopsy.

Almost all of the surviving children in this series have been re-examined personally and compared with the same number of children who were born in the same hospital and whose non-diabetic mothers had been matched for the month and year of conceiving the child and for age and parity with the mothers in the diabetic group. A medical history was taken in each case and the children were submitted to a standard clinical examination. Technical investigations such as radiography were undertaken only if some positive lead existed, e.g. recurrent urinary infections, scoliosis. Only those malformations which were considered to be

TABLE 6

FEEDING RECORD OF 88 SURVIVING BABIES OF DIABETIC WOMEN

Group	Total	Duration: Months	Duration: Weeks	Reasons for Failure or Interruption	
Breast feeding not attempted	6	—	—	Diabetes	2
				Tuberculosis	1
				Previous failure	2
				Maternal refusal	1
Breast feeding abandoned in first 7-10 days	51			Inadequate lactation	28
				Breast abnormalities	6
				Puerperal infection	1
				Maternal non-infective illness	4
				Prematurity	5
				Refusal to fix	3
				Poor sucking	1
				Illness of baby	2
				Mongolism	1
Breast feeding only	17		2	Maternal refusal	1
				Inadequate lactation	1
			3	Maternal fatigue	1
				Mother 'too busy'	1
			6	Maternal fatigue	1
				Failing lactation	1
				Husband's advice	1
		2		Failing lactation	1
		3		Insulin reactions	1
				Failing lactation	2
		6		Breast abscess	1
				Failing lactation	1
		7, 8, 9		Weaning (abundant lactation)	4
Breast feeding with complement	10		2	Inadequate lactation	2
				Breast abnormalities	1
				Disinterest in breast	1
			4	Failing lactation	1
				Medical advice (reason unknown)	1
			6	Failing lactation	1
				'Crying baby'	1
			7	Failing lactation	1
		6		Failing lactation	1
Incomplete information*	4	3 were fully and 1 was partly breast fed at time of hospital discharge.			
Total	88				

* Contact lost because of death of mother or child, or because of emigration or adoption.

TABLE 7
PHYSICAL ABNORMALITIES PRESENT SINCE BIRTH*

Diabetic Group (93)		Non-diabetic Group (93)	
Sacral agenesis	1	Club foot	1 }
Congenital cataracts	1	Hypertrophic pyloric stenosis	1 }
Patent ductus arteriosus	1	Coarctation of aorta	1
Hydronephrosis	1	Cardiac murmurs, 'organic'	4
Mongolism	1	Mental defect, mild diplegia	1
Mental defect	2	Short oesophagus	1
Scoliosis (hemivert.)	1	Inguinal hernia	2
Extra thumb	1	Mod. funnel sternum	1
Fused central incisors	1	Cong. absence one nail	1
		Epidermolysis bullosa	1
	10	(13 children)	14

* Groups matched for maternal age and parity and for month and year of delivery at S.M.M.P.

disabling, potentially disabling, in need of surgical correction, or disfiguring were included, and such trifling deformities as mild plagiocephaly, small pilonidal sinuses, prominent ears or small naevi normally covered by clothing were excluded. Little difference in incidence emerged between the two groups (Table 7) but in this comparatively small study the abnormalities in the diabetic group may be rather more severe. The recorded cardiac murmurs in the non-diabetic group were considered to be organic but, because the children were asymptomatic, no further investigation was undertaken except in the case of the child with aortic coarctation.

Later Development

Relationship of Neonatal Condition to Later Health. Almost all the surviving children in the series have been re-examined on at least one occasion at ages ranging from 2 to 10 years. Their progress is shown in Fig. 16 in relation to their neonatal condition. In each group the absolute figures are given and these are then expressed in percentages. Those groups of infants who were originally dyspnoeic or affected by cyanotic attacks contain a relatively greater number of abnormal babies than the group whose neonatal course was uncomplicated.

Growth. Reports concerning the physical progress made by children of diabetic women have, until recently, emanated mainly from Boston. From the large numbers available to White, Koshy and Duckers (1953) 105 children were selected because they lived near the Joslin Clinic. The children were

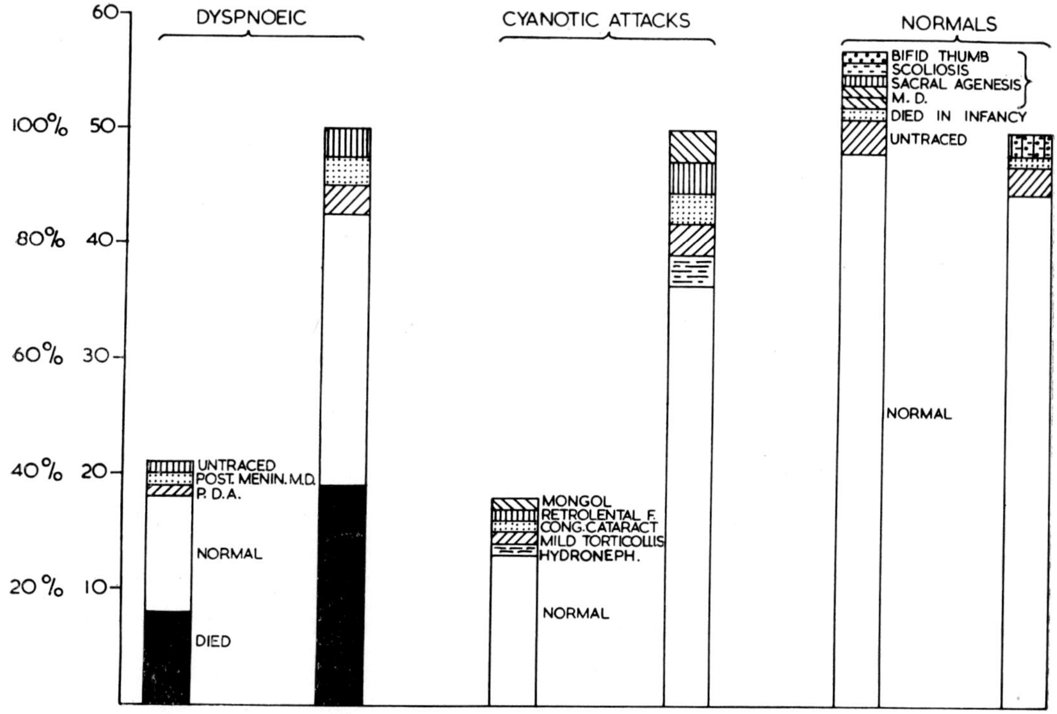

FIG. 16.—Neonatal condition and later development.

stated to be commonly above average height and weight, but the information given does not constitute proof that, as a group, they were necessarily abnormal.

Selecting their cases only by response to their invitation to them to submit to examination, Fredrikson *et al.* (1957) examined 123 surviving children from a much larger group born to both pre-diabetic and diabetic women. When the heights and weights were compared with Swedish normal values, the children who were born before the onset of maternal diabetes were found to be below average and the difference was claimed to be significant statistically. Those born after the onset of the disease were on average slightly taller than normal but the difference was small and statistically not significant. The weights of the children did not differ from the normal.

The surviving Edinburgh cases were re-examined in 1955 and again in 1957. Almost all were examined and measured personally. The very few exceptions were mostly overseas where they were examined by doctors employing the same techniques. The same measuring rod and beam balance were used for all except the overseas children. The standing height was measured with the child stripped and erect against a wall, and the naked weight was measured by an Avery beam balance of checked accuracy. In the case of children of 18 months or less the total length, rather than the standing height, was measured with the apparatus devised by Thomson (1956). The heights at one or both examinations are shown in Fig. 17. The heights of the group of matched controls (see Congenital Malformations) are also recorded. The unbroken line represents the mean height derived from cross-sectional data

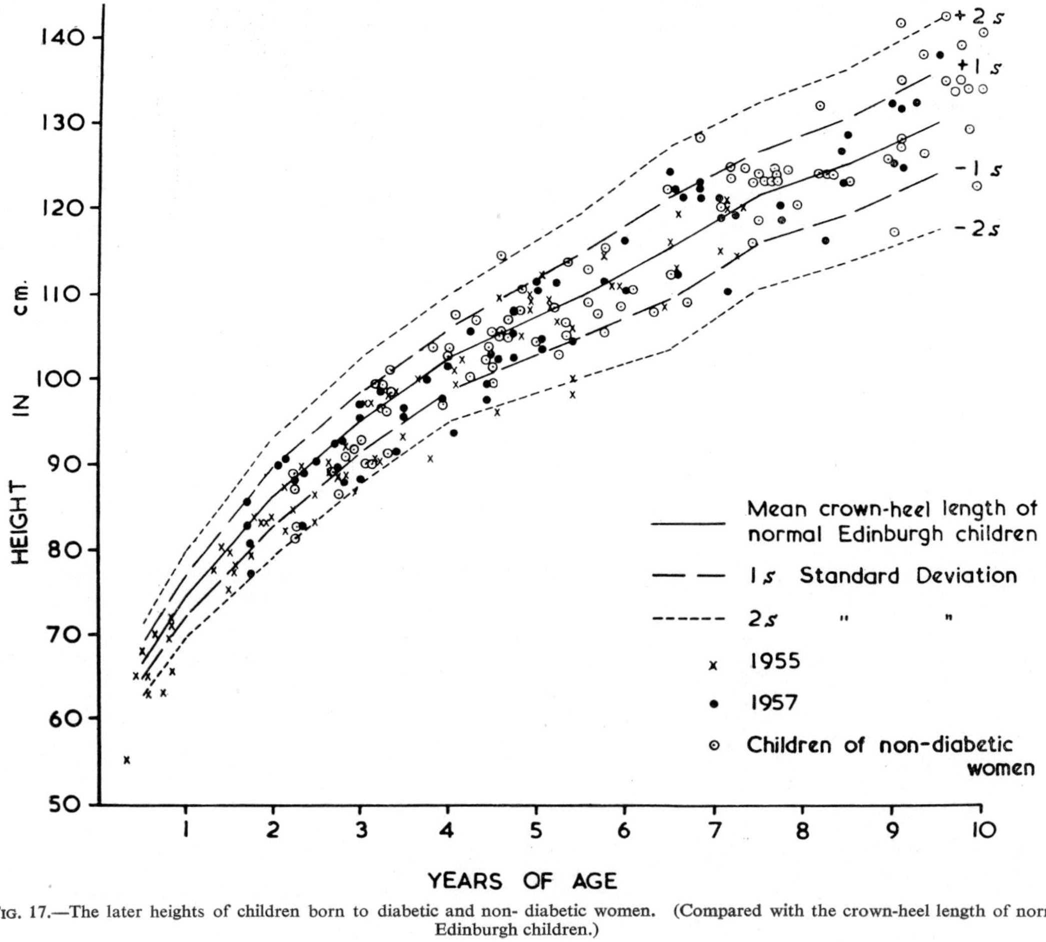

FIG. 17.—The later heights of children born to diabetic and non- diabetic women. (Compared with the crown-heel length of normal Edinburgh children.)

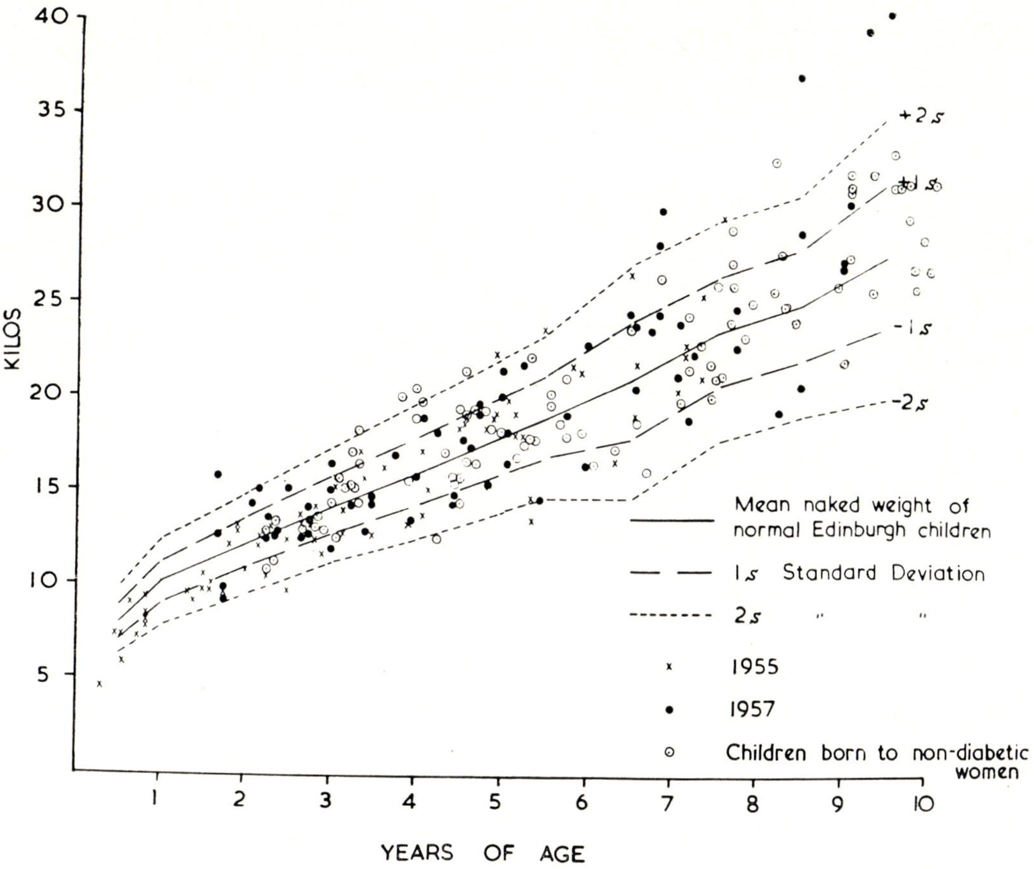

FIG. 18.—The later naked weights of children born to diabetic and non-diabetic women. (Compared with the naked weights of normal Edinburgh children.)

for Edinburgh pre-school (Thomson, 1956) and school-age children (Provis and Ellis, 1955) of the present decade. The broken lines represent ± 1 and ± 2 standard deviations (S.D.) about the mean at each year. No abnormality of linear growth is so far detectable in the diabetic group.

The weights of children in the diabetic group at one or two examinations and those of the children in the control group are shown in Fig. 18. The normal mean and standard deviations for weight from the same Edinburgh studies are recorded. A few children lie above or below the ± 2 S.D. lines, but four lie above + 3 S.D. and three of these are in the ninth or tenth years of age.

Birth Weight and Later Height. The birth weight, which is subject to the limitations previously mentioned, is recorded against the later height and age in Fig. 19. Those children who weighed 4 kg. or more and who were weighed on two later occasions are linked on the graph. The only child to gain weight steeply in the interval between examinations is indicated. He was of lower birth weight. There is no indication that those babies who are very big at birth 'grow away' from the others with the passage of years. They do tend to remain among the taller children, but there are exceptions and some of the lighter babies at birth are later found among the taller children.

Birth Weight and Later Weight. The birth weight is recorded against the later weight and age in Fig. 20. There is no indication that those babies who exceeded 4 kg. at birth are excessively heavy later. There is perhaps instead a tendency for them to be of average weight by the age of 7 years. Of

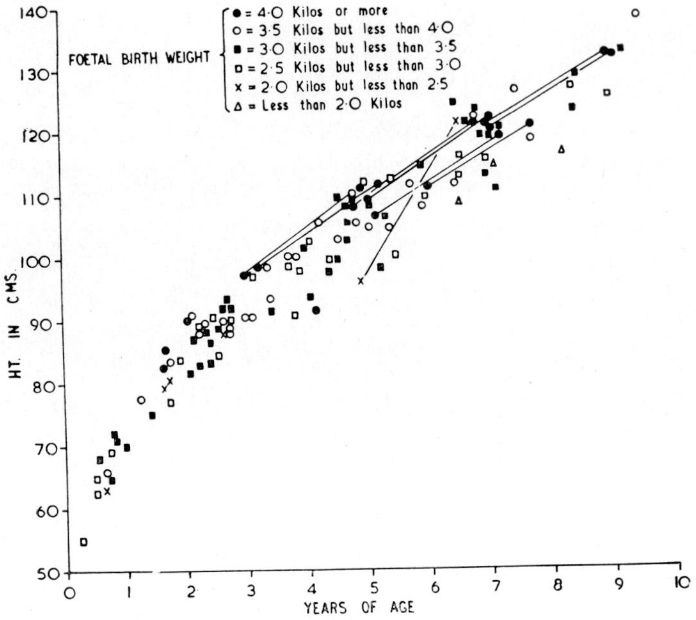

FIG. 19.—The relationship between birthweight and later height.

of diabetic parents would probably develop the disease and that the presence of diabetes in the families of both parents increases the risk of diabetes in the child even if the parents themselves are unaffected. The development of the disease in one in four children born to diabetic women was forecast by Reis *et al.* (1952). A study of 1,241 diabetic propositi (Harris, 1950-51) showed that of the 1,418 children born to them only 10 became diabetic, and he estimated that about 1·4% of children of a diabetic parent may be expected to develop the disease by the age of 40 years.

By means of oral glucose tolerance tests Ditzel, White and Duckers (1954) found that of 75 children of diabetic mothers seven were already diabetic and a further 13 were 'borderline' diabetics. This incidence is surprising even when taking into consideration the fact that two thirds of the diabetics and less than half the suspects were over the age of 10 years. The chances of the offspring of a single diabetic parent eventually developing diabetes were

the three children whose weight exceeded + 3 S.D. of the mean in the ninth and tenth years, none exceeded 4 kg. at birth and two weighed 3·5 kg. or less. These three had shown a sharp increase in weight in two years but other children of comparable birth weight were of average or low weight later.

Development of Diabetes Mellitus. The previous sections indicate that if the infants of diabetic women survive the newborn period then they are likely to be as healthy and to grow as normally as the children of non-diabetic women at least until the age of 10 years. But the possibility exists that a population is being salvaged which will live to develop and to propagate diabetes mellitus.

There is little doubt that the predisposition to diabetes mellitus is often inherited (Pincus and White, 1933; Harris, 1950-51; Bartels, 1953; Steinberg, 1955). The child of the diabetic woman was not considered by Skipper (1933) to be especially liable to the disease, but Peel and Oakley (1950) believed that the child

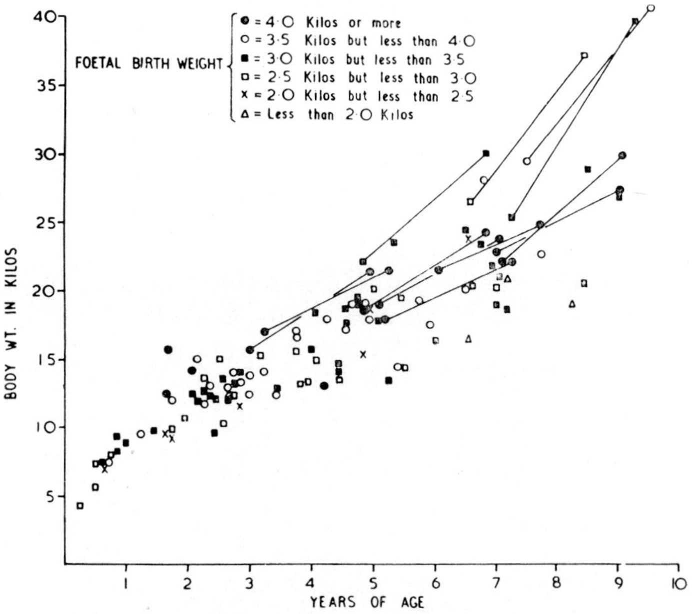

FIG. 20.—The relationship between birthweight and later weight.

later estimated to be 22% for their whole life span (White, 1957). In contrast, of the 123 children studied by Fredrikson *et al.* (1957) only one was found to be diabetic. The children of the present series have not been subjected to glucose tolerance tests, but none has developed diabetes so far and none shows glycosuria after oral loading with glucose. None of them has developed the precocious growth described by Ditzel *et al.* (1954) as being associated closely with reduced glucose tolerance and vascular changes. The numbers of course at each age are relatively small, but the total is no smaller than the Boston group and it has the virtue of being unselected. Selection of cases from the area conveniently placed to a famous diabetic clinic could introduce considerable bias into the results. It may favour particular social or racial groups or diabetic parents who live there so that their own surveillance might be made easier.

The prediction of diabetes mellitus in the present series by using the steroid-glucose tolerance test (Fajans and Conn, 1954) has not been attempted so far. The obese children in a small series investigated in this way by Komrower (1957) showed no evidence of being pre-diabetic, and West (1957), using prednisolone, found that positive results were less commonly found in younger than in older subjects, and he suggested that the test was of only limited ability in the prediction of eventual diabetes mellitus.

The chances of inheritance when both parents are diabetic may be high, but the risk when only the mother is diabetic is still uncertain. Time will provide the answer more effectively and with less likelihood of making mothers anxious and children unhappy than the purely mechanical use of laboratory prediction methods with the associated need for explanation and hospital admission.

Summary

Although the development of insulin improved the fertility of diabetic women it created the problem of the diabetic pregnancy in which the viable foetal loss rate is still high.

The latter may be reduced by combined management of the pregnancy by a small team consisting of obstetrician, physician and paediatrician.

Even then, however, the foetus may still die *in utero* in the last month or less commonly, in the first few days of extra-uterine life.

The majority of babies are both heavy and long for their gestational age.

Many babies suffer from prolonged dyspnoea or from cyanotic attacks during the first few days of life. Of these, those with dyspnoea have the poorest prognosis.

The mortality and morbidity are highest among the smaller babies at any gestational age.

No clear relationship exists between maternal build and foetal birth weight but the latter varies with maturity. The birth weight may be remarkably consistent in families, however, and some women almost consistently give birth to giant offspring, among whom there is no increase in the mortality rate.

Conversely the risk of foetal death is greater in some women than in others, and their babies are not necessarily large. Gigantism and foetal death do not apparently result from the same maternal disorder.

The most frequent findings at autopsy are pulmonary hyaline membrane and hyperplasia of the pancreatic islets.

Circumstantial evidence exists of foetal hyperinsulinism.

Hyperinsulinism may result *in utero* from stimulation by maternal P.G.H. or corticotrophin.

There is evidence that the health of the foetus is influenced adversely by functional degeneration of the placenta. This may result from poor diabetic control, from acceleration of the placental life-span or from the influence of adrenal steroids. Of these only the first can be influenced at present.

The treatment of the foetus is briefly outlined.

Breast feeding is infrequently successful, but to any possible maternal endocrine cause for this may be added many extrinsic factors which interfere with the feeding situation.

The incidence of important congenital malformations may be no higher among children born to diabetic women than in normal children.

Those infants whose neonatal course is uneventful are less likely than others to show evidence of malformation later.

The heights and weights of children of various ages up to 10 years in this series differ very little from those for children born to non-diabetic mothers in the same city.

The size of the baby at birth bears no consistent relationship to its later growth.

None of the 88 babies who survived the newborn period has so far developed clinical diabetes mellitus. None shows glycosuria after oral glucose loads. No steroid-glucose tolerance tests have been undertaken.

The newborn child of the diabetic woman has been influenced in its intra-uterine development not only by genetic constitution but by the diabetic environment. His excessive growth may very well result from maternal P.G.H., but another factor, possibly adrenal steroid, is responsible for placental degeneration and foetal distress or death.

I wish to thank Dr. G. Douglas Matthew and Professor R. W. B. Ellis for their original invitation to take paediatric responsibility for the infants born to diabetic women, and for their advice on various matters during the 10 years since. I am grateful to Mr. Clifford Shepley and his staff for the illustrations, to Mr. G. R. Pendrill and Miss B. Newton, Librarian and Assistant Librarian respectively of the Royal College of Physicians of Edinburgh, for help with the literature and for translations, to Miss A. Brown and Miss D. Trench for help with various parts of the work, and to Miss E. Meikeljohn for most efficient secretarial assistance. Finally, I wish to thank the Committee of the Honyman Gillespie Trust for their invitation to deliver this lecture.

References

Adams, T. W. (1955). *Obstet. Gynec.*, **5**, 160.
Avery, M. E., Oppenheimer, E. H. and Gordon, H. H. (1957). *New Engl. J. Med.*, **256**, 1134.
Baar, H. S. (1956). Discussion following Paper 106. VIIIth International Congress of Paediatrics, Copenhagen.
Babbott, D., Rubin, A. and Ginsburg, S. J. (1958). *Diabetes*, **7**, 33.
Barcroft, J. (1947). In *Child Health and Development* by R. W. B. Ellis. Churchill, London.
Barns, H. H. F. and Morgans, M. E. (1949). *Brit. med. J.*, **1**, 51.
——, —— (1952). *Ibid.*, **1**, 1058.
Bartels, E. D. (1953). In *Clinical Genetics*, ed. by A. Sorsby. Butterworth, London.
Becker, B. (1952). *Ann. intern. Med.*, **37**, 273.
——, Maengwyn-Davies, G. D., Rosen, D., Friedenwald, J. S. and Winter, F. C. (1954). *Diabetes*, **3**, 175.
Beek, C. van (1952). Report on the 1st International Congress of the International Diabetes Federation, Leyden, Netherlands. 1952, p. 28 (abstract).
Bennewitz, H. G. (1828). *Edinb. med. surg. J.*, **30**, 217.
Berglund, G. and Zetterström, R. (1954). *Acta paediat. (Uppsala)*, **43**, 368.
Björklund, S. I. (1953). *Ibid.*, **42**, 526.
Born, G. V. R., Dawes, G. S., Mott, J. C. and Widdicombe, J. G. (1954). *Cold Spr. Harb. Symp. quant. Biol.*, **19**, 102.
Boutourline-Young, H. J. and Smith, C. A. (1950). *Amer. J. Dis. Child.*, **80**, 753.
Cardell, B. S. (1953). *J. Obstet. Gynaec. Brit. Emp.*, **60**, 834.
Clayton, S. (1956). *Scot. med. J.*, **1**, 138.
Cope, C. L., Boysen, X. and McCrae, S. (1951). *Brit. med. J.*, **2**, 762.
Craig, W. S. and Buchanan, M. F. G. (1958). *Arch. Dis. Childh.*, **33**, 505.
Dawes, G. S., Mott, J. C., Widdicombe, J. G. and Wyatt, D. G. (1953). *J. Physiol. (Lond.)*, **121**, 141.
Ditzel, J., White, P. and Duckers, J. (1954). *Diabetes*, **3**, 99.
—— and Moinat, P. (1957). *Ibid.*, **6**, 307.
Duncan, J. M. (1883). *Trans. obstet. Soc. Lond.*, 1882, **24**, 256.
Duncan, L. J. P., MacFarlane, A. and Robson, J. S. (1958). *Lancet*, **1**, 822.
Dunlop, D. M. (1954). *Brit. med. J.*, 2, 383.
Ellis, R. W. B. (1951). *Arch. Dis. Childh.*, **26**, 411.
Eshner, A. A. (1907). *Amer. J. med. Sci.*, **134**, 375.
Fajans, S. S. and Conn, J. W. (1954). *Diabetes*, **3**, 296.
Farquhar, J. W. (1954). *Arch. Dis. Childh.*, **29**, 519.
—— (1955). *Ibid.*, **30**, 133.
—— (1956a). *Ibid.*, **31**, 203.
—— (1956b). *Ibid.*, **31**, 483.
—— and Sklaroff, S. (1958). *Ibid.*, **33**, 323.
—— and Smith, H. (1958). *Ibid.*, **33**, 142.
Fredrikson, H., Hagbard, L., Olow, I. and Reinand, R. (1957). *Nord. Med.*, **57**, 669.
Futcher, P. H. and Long, N. W. (1954). *Bull. Johns Hopk. Hosp.*, **94**, 128.
Gairdner, D., Marks, J., Roscoe, J. D. and Brettell, R. O. (1958). *Arch. Dis. Child.*, **33**, 489.
Gellis, S. S., White, P. and Pfeffer, W. (1949). *New Engl. J. Med.*, **240**, 533.
Gilbert, J. A. L. (1949). *Brit. med. J.*, **1**, 702.
Grayzel, H. G., Warshall, H. B., Elkan, B. and Sternberg, A. (1957). *Diabetes*, **6**, 480.
Hagbard, L. (1956). *Acta obstet. gynec. scand.*, **35**, Suppl. 1.
Hall, R. E. and Tillman, A. J. B. (1951). *Amer. J. Obstet. Gynec.*, **61**, 1107.
Harris, H. (1950-51). *Ann. Eugen. (Lond.)*, **15**, 95.
Herman, G. E. (1902). *Edinb. med. J.*, n.s. **11**, 119.
Hoet, J. P. (1954). *Diabetes*, **3**, 1.
Hsia, D. Y-Y., Peterson, H. G. and Gellis, S. S. (1957). *Pediatrics*, **20**, 234.
Ikkos, D., Luft, R. and Gemzell, C. A. (1958). *Lancet*, **1**, 720.
Klein, R., Papadatos, C., Fortunato, J. and Byers, C. (1955). *J. clin. Endocr.*, **15**, 215.
——, Weigand, F. A., Iunes, M. and Greenman, L. (1956). *Pediatrics*, **17**, 214.
Komrower, G. (1957). Personal communication.
Lawrence, R. D. (1950). *Brit. med. J.*, **2**, 107.
Luft, R., Ikkos, D., Gemzell, C. A. and Olivecrona, H. (1958). *Lancet*, **1**, 721.
McCance, R. A. (1955). Personal communication.
McIlroy, L., Hill, G. and Pillman-Williams, E. C. (1931). *Postgrad. med. J.*, **6**, 159.
Mackay, D. G. (1952). Reported by P. White in *Treatment of Diabetes Mellitus* by E. P. Joslin *et al.*, 9th ed.
MacKay, R. B. (1955). M.D. Thesis. University of Edinburgh.
—— (1957). *J. Obstet. Gynaec. Brit. Emp.*, **64**, 185.
Maengwyn-Davies, G. D., Lerman, S., Pogell, B. M., Stone, H. H. and Friedenwald, J. S. (1956). *Bull. Johns Hopk. Hosp.*, **99**, 16.
Marrian, G. F. (1951). *J. Endocr.*, **7**, proc. lxix.
Medical Research Council (1955). *Lancet*, **2**, 833.
Merkler, D. (1929). *Med. Klin.*, **25**, 1468.
Miller, H. C., Hurwitz, D. and Kuder, K. (1944). *J. Amer. med. Ass.*, **124**, 271.
Oppé, T. E., Hsia, D. Y-Y. and Gellis, S. S. (1957). *Lancet*, **1**, 353.
Patterson, M. and Burnstein, N. (1949). *Arch. intern. Med.*, **83**, 390.
Peckham, C. H. (1931). *Bull. Johns Hopk. Hosp.*, **49**, 184.
Pedersen, J. (1952). *Diabetes and Pregnancy*. Danish Science Press, Copenhagen.
—— (1954). *Acta endocr. (Kbh.)*, **16**, 330.
—— and Brandstrup, E. (1956). *Lancet*, **1**, 607.
Pedowitz, P. and Shlevin, E. L. (1955). *Amer. J. Obstet. Gynec.*, **69**, 395.
Peel, J. H. (1951). *Practitioner*, **166**, 143.
—— (1955). *Brit. med. J.*, **2**, 870.
—— and Oakley, W. (1950). *Trans. 12th Brit. Congr. Obstet. Gynaec.* London.
Pincus, G. and White, P. (1933). *Amer. J. med. Sci.*, **186**, 1.
Provis, H. S. and Ellis, R. W. B. (1955). *Arch. Dis. Childh.*, **30**, 328.
Prystowsky, H. (1957). *Bull. Johns Hopk. Hosp.*, **101**, 48.
Read, C. H. (1951). Trans. int. and 4th Amer. Congr. Obstet, Gynec. *Amer. J. Obstet. Gynec.*, **61A**, 392.
Reis, R. A., DeCosta, E. J. and Allweiss, M.D. (1950). *Ibid.*, **60**, 1023.
Richardson, G. O., Snaith, L. and Sibley, J. C. (1955). *J. Obstet. Gynaec. Brit. Emp.*, **62**, 262.
Rifkin, H., Solomon, S. and Lieberman, S. (1958). *Diabetes*, **7**, 9.
Rolland, C. (1954). *Edinb. med. J.*, **61**, 257.
Sheumack, D. R. (1949). *Med. J. Aust.*, **2**, 553.
Sinden, J. A. and Longwell, B. B. (1949). *Proc. Soc. exp. Biol. (N.Y.)*, **70**, 607.
Skipper, E. (1933). *Quart. J. Med.*, **26** (n.s. **2**), 353.
Steinberg, A. G. (1955). *Eugen. Quart.*, **2**, 26.
Stevenson, A. E. M. (1956). *Brit. med. J.*, **2**, 1514.
Talbot, N. B., Sobel, E. H., McArthur, J. W. and Crawford, J. D. (1952). *Functional Endocrinology. From Birth through Adolescence.* Harvard University Press, Cambridge, Mass.
Tejning, S. (1947). *Acta med. scand.*, suppl. 198.
Thomson, J. (1956). Quoted by R. W. B. Ellis in *Child Health and Development*, 2nd ed. (1956). Churchill, London.
Tompsett, S. L. and Smith, D. C. (1954). *J. clin. Endocr.*, **14**, 922.
Turnbull, E. P. N. and Baird, D. (1957). *Brit. med. J.*, **2**, 1.
Tveterås, E. and Rudström, P. (1956). *Acta paediat. (Uppsala)*, **45**, 545.
Van Breemen, V. L., Neustein, H. B. and Bruns, P. D. (1957). *Amer. J. Path.*, **33**, 769.
Walker, J. (1954). *J. Obstet. Gynaec. Brit. Emp.*, **61**, 162.
—— and Turnbull, E. P. N. (1953). *Lancet*, **2**, 312.
West, K. M. (1957). *Diabetes*, **6**, 168.
White, P. (1949). *Amer. J. Med.*, **7**, 609.
—— (1952). In *Treatment of Diabetes Mellitus* by E. P. Joslin. 9th ed.
—— (1957). *Diabetes*, **6**, 523.
——, Gillespie, L. and Sexton, L. (1956). *Amer. J. Obstet. Gynec.*, **71**, 57.
——, Koshy, P. and Duckers, J. (1953). *Med. Clin. N. Amer.*, **37**, 1481.
Wilder, R. M. and Parsons, E. (1928). *Colo. Med.*, **25**, 372.
Wilkins, L. (1957). *The Diagnosis and Treatment of Endocrine Disorders in Childhood and Adolescence*, 2nd ed. Thomas, Springfield, Illinois.
Williams, R. H. (1955). *Textbook of Endocrinology*, 2nd ed. Saunders, Philadelphia.

BOOK REVIEWS

Pediatric Index. By Edwin F. Patton. (Pp. 639. 101s. 6d.) London: Henry Kimpton. 1958.

The preface of this book states that it is an 'alphabetical systematization of pediatric thought'. It is in three sections. The first lists under symptoms, signs or parts of the body, the problem which confronts the doctor. Each subsection is divided up into three arbitrary age groups: 'birth to age two weeks', 'two weeks to two years' and 'almost any age'. To take an example: under the heading—'Vomiting, two weeks to two years', 25 possible diagnoses are listed, one of which reads, 'Beginning at from birth to two or three weeks, increasing in frequency, violence and amount, with visible gastric peristaltic waves, olive pyloric tumour palpable when abdomen relaxed, malnutrition, dehydration, extreme hunger; *Obstruction, alimentary tract, in stomach, at pylorus, by stenosis, hypertrophic, congenital*' (italics in original). The next entry reads: 'With head retraction, dysphagia, dyspnoea, cyanosis, barking cough, hoarseness, wheezing: *Obstruction, respiratory tract, in trachea, by thymus, hypertrophic*'.

Having found the probable diagnosis, the reader may then search in Section 2 for further details of the condition. Each disease is described under three headings. The first is 'Rule out'. In the case of pyloric stenosis this includes a differential diagnosis of nine conditions. The second heading is 'Confirmation'. Here radiological and laboratory investigations are mentioned, followed by the clinical features. The third heading is 'Treatment'.

In Section 2 the information given about the various diseases is often very scanty and frequently misleading. Thus, while one of the classifications of cerebral palsy is given as: (1) spastic, (2) athetotic, (3) ataxic, (4) tremorous, (5) aphonic (*sic*), the paragraph describing the condition makes no attempt to differentiate these types. 'Increase in reflexes' apparently occurs in all. The possibility of associated mental deficiency is not mentioned. When considering prematurity, we are asked to 'rule out small baby because of small or poorly attached placenta'. Under 'confirmation' the book states: 'All babies under 250 gm. (5 lb.) or 37 wks. or less gestation arbitrarily classified as premature.' This is not the usual teaching. Twenty-eight pages are devoted to the signs, symptoms and treatment of different types of poisons. This is probably the best feature of the book.

Section 3 contains miscellaneous data such as laboratory special tests. Under this heading three only are described: the estimation of urine calcium by Sulkowitch's method, urine bilinogen by the use of Ehrlich's reagent, and the test for the detection in the stool of swallowed adult blood.

The preface states that the book should be useful to students, but it is clearly not accurate enough for them. A general practitioner confronted with an obscure case might possibly be reminded of a diagnosis which had previously eluded him.

Pediatric Index is a large book which has obviously cost the author much in time and effort. Unfortunately the result is so poor that the book cannot be recommended.

Häufigkeit und Art meteorotroper Erscheinungen im Kindesalter. By Wolfgang Menger. (Pp. 131; 21 figures. Sw. fr. 20.80.) Basel and New York: S. Karger. 1958.

That the weather may influence disease is a supposition founded in folklore, but appearing to some to be akin to quackery. The scientific study of the problem is in its infancy. Dr. Menger has reviewed some of the literature, confining himself almost entirely to German and Swiss sources. (There is no mention, for instance, of the work of Sir Leonard Rogers, nor of the Khamsin.)

The variables in the weather (temperature, pressure, humidity, wind force) are difficult to study separately and to assess graphically. Moreover they are but measurements of the results of what is happening in the air. They do not in themselves constitute the weather. We speak of a depression when in fact it is merely a man-made measurement which is depressed. Menger prefers to deal with different types of air-mass, such as polar continental, cold maritime and continental tropical. He recorded them from hour to hour, and has devised a method of plotting them on a diagram like a compass dial. He noted the times of incidence of various diseases in the Mainz University Children's clinics and inserted these on the same diagram. He also studied the power of concentration in school children, infants' sleep and premature births. He concludes that sea air rather than polar continental is favourable to concentration, but promotes disturbances of sleep. (Mouriquand and Charpentier, two other authors whom he ignores, found quite a different effect.) Premature births were more common in warm moist air-streams, though cold fronts were also effective. Exacerbations of tuberculosis were noted in the spring (maritime tropical air). Haemorrhage in meningococcal disease seemed to depend on the weather rather than the severity of the infection, polar air being held responsible. Epidemic meningitis was also found to follow the influx of polar air.

On cyclical vomiting the author appears to be 20 years out of date as he considers it to be the result and not the cause of acetonaemia. It follows the appearance of maritime tropical air. He has no sound explanation for these phenomena, and the criticism might be made that the exact hour at which a disease starts is very difficult to determine and may not coincide with the time at which the cause is active. Nor has he explored the possibility of intermediary factors between the weather and the disease, as for instance the shutting of windows in cold weather, vitamin lack in early spring or river bathing in hot weather. Nevertheless this monograph is interesting and should be read by all who are exploring this attractive by-way of medicine.

Leukämie im Kindesalter, Vol. 4. By J. OEHME, W. JANSSEN and CH. HAGITTE. (Pp. viii+169; 57 figures, 7 colour plates. DM 38.25.) Leipzig: Georg Thieme. 1958.

In their introduction the authors say that theirs is the first exhaustive monograph on leukaemia in childhood since that of Willi in 1936. In tackling their subject they have followed the accepted handling of the condition, discussing the pathological anatomy, the clinical manifestations, the effect on particular organs, biochemistry and therapy. The section on the aetiology is, as might be expected, lamentably short. A noble attempt is made to reduce the enormous literature on leukaemia in children to some sort of order in that the various papers are grouped together in sections dealing with prognosis, leukaemia and infection and so forth. In a short monograph the authors have assembled a vast store of factual knowledge but they have found it difficult to say anything which everybody does not already know. As long as the book is used as a basis for further work it will serve a useful purpose and it will also have a place in the library of those seldom called upon to manage cases of leukaemia.

L'Enfant Physiquement Handicapé: Rôle Médico-social du Médecin. By CLEMENT LAUNAY and D.-J. DUCHE. (Pp. 196. Fr. fr. 2,600.) Paris: G. Doin. 1958.

The authors of this interesting book take the now widely held view that medical care of physically handicapped children is essentially an educative process, leading the child to develop effectively the function he has. There is a basic need for the doctor's socio-medical guidance and understanding when a child is defective, for a child is a member of a family which also needs help; the young patient cannot be treated as an isolated medical problem. The writers consider under three headings physical handicaps of children, (1) sensory, e.g. blindness, (2) motor, e.g. infantile palsies and epilepsies, (3) somatic, e.g. diabetes. Adjunctive measures, if used at all, should be subordinated to the general plan of habilitation, that is training for life. Many physically handicapped children are also mentally retarded and even those of good intelligence may become 'retarded' by deprivation of the educative processes of ordinary home life if they are segregated in institutions. Surprisingly, the authors give much information about institutions in France for the segregation of handicapped children and no practical suggestions for their education within the family circle; surprisingly, because these doctors have evidently made a profound study of the needs of children in their three groups and have laid stress on the educative nature of their medical care.

Family Guide to Teenage Health. By EDWARD T. WILKES. (Pp. xvii+244; illustrated. $4.00.) New York. Ronald Press Co. 1958.

This is one more book about the trials and difficulties which beset children of both sexes on their hard road to adulthood. In clear language and the avoidance of technical mumbo Dr. Wilkes explains the ordinary facts of growth of the body and the development of sexual characteristics. Adolescent psychology and maturation into a grown-up are dealt with at length and with considerable sympathy.

It is possible that there is a public for this book in this country; but most parents who studied biology to G.C.E. level at school will already know most of the contents; perhaps the non-medical parent would appreciate a reference book where the difficulties of growing-up are dealt with authoritatively and yet understandingly, and to them this book can be recommended without cavil.

Ciba Foundation Colloquia on Ageing, Vol. 4. **Water and Electrolyte Metabolism in Relation to Age and Sex.** Edited by G. E. W. WOLSTENHOLME and M. O'CONNOR. (Pp. xii+327; 85 figures. 45s.) London: J. and A. Churchill. 1958.

This fourth volume of the *Ciba Colloquia on Ageing* contains a great deal which is of interest to the paediatrician. The standard of the papers is extremely high and the discussion at the end of each contribution makes stimulating reading for those who have previously grappled with some of the problems which are considered.

The description by Fourman and Leeson of hypernatraemia and hyponatraemia in cerebral disturbances offers a rational explanation of many of the electrolyte disturbances which occur after brain injury or craniotomy. Thaysen's study of the electrolyte secretion by the sweat and salivary glands provides some basic facts about the variables involved, though none of the participants was able to offer an explanation, for the dysfunction of the sweat glands in mucoviscidosis.

Perhaps the most important papers for the paediatrician are those on the effect of variable protein and mineral intake upon the body composition of the growing animal (Wallace, Weil and Taylor) and Widdowson and McCance's exposition of the development of acid-base control in the infant and young animal. The first of these papers should be read by the medical advisers to all firms which produce proprietary milks, to help them to resist their own sales talk.

Talbot and Richie contribute an extremely thoughtful paper on the body's tolerance for varying intakes of water and electrolytes, a matter of concern to all who review from time to time their schedules for the treatment of gastro-enteritis.

The content as a whole reflects great credit on the chairmanship of Professor McCance and the organizing and editorial abilities of Dr. Wolstenholme and his staff.

It is perhaps worth the attention of paediatricians that British medicine, though ably represented at this Colloquium, did not include a single practising paediatrician. We should do well to think long and deeply over this absence of basic paediatric research in Great Britain.

Einführung in die Kinderheilkunde, 4th ed. By PROFESSOR E. GLANZMANN. (Pp. xi+1068; 31 figures. £6 7s. 6d.) Vienna: Springer-Verlag. 1958.

Pädiatrie. Ein Lehrbuch für Studierende und Arzte. Edited by H. OPITZ and B. DE RUDDER. (Pp. xvi+1220; 527 figures. No price given.) Berlin-Göttingen-Heidelberg: Springer-Verlag. 1957.

These two massive single volume textbooks in the German language epitomize the change that has taken place in medical writing over recent years. Their very titles and use of words emphasize these changes: *Einführung in Die Kinderheilkunde* versus *Paediatrie: Dysporia Entero-broncho Pancreatica Congenita Familiaris* versus *Mucoviscidosis*.

Professor Glanzmann's book is a monument to a lifetime spent in the study of practice in the art of paediatrics and is an erudite *tour de force*, the like of which we shall surely never see repeated. The basis of this massive book is the lecture demonstration and Professor Glanzmann is at his best with a case to show around which he can build up a picture of the disease being studied.

This approach is old-fashioned as are many of the basic ideas and assumptions. But for anyone not in a hurry, the Professor's yesteryear outlook, fine didactic teaching, his thumbnail sketches of disease as it was, his delight at the successes achieved by antibiotics and his evident awe at the approach of the steroid age, all join to give the reader an understanding of the art rather than the science of medicine and have a charm and informed delight which takes one back to Osler's original descriptions or Robert Hutchison's lectures.

The other is a contemporary collective work, with two editors and thirty-three contributors, giving an authentic up-to-date account of paediatrics with percentile growth charts, diagrams, mille equivalents, standard deviation and all the paraphernalia of a standard book of reference. The field is carefully and intelligibly covered, up to and including hyperelectrolytaemia. For a busy house physician or registrar wanting a quick, reliable answer to an immediate clinical problem or an up-to-date summary of facts with which to impress an impending clinico-pathological conference, this is clearly the book of choice.

Each book is over 1,000 pages long, illustrations are profuse, and both are elegantly produced by Springer-Verlag in almost identical styles. They look fine on the reviewer's shelf but at £6 each would be expensive to anyone not reading German fluently.

Hearing Therapy for Children, 2nd ed. By ALICE STRENG, WARING J. FITCH, LEROY D. HEDGECOCK, JAMES W. PHILLIPS and JAMES A. CARRELL. (Pp. v+353; illustrated. $6.75.) New York and London: Grune and Stratton. 1958.

This is a good book. In the first half the authors explain the general problems of deafness in children, causes, possible medical treatment, detection, hearing tests, and all about hearing aids. The other half gives details of the educational treatment of children with moderate impairments and the education of the severely deaf.

The outline of the problems of deaf children equals, or even excels, anything written on the subject in this country. The authors combine the best ideas evolved in the U.S.A. and here. It is rightly emphasized that psychologically there is a difference between a child with five senses and one with four. It is difficult for such a child to keep in touch with his environment and to know it fully.

The effects of deafness of various types is explained with great understanding. The problems centred round a hearing defect are not limited to a faulty hearing equipment. It is a disorder of communication which has far reaching consequences on every aspect of life. The effects on the parents are emphasized. 'Serious responsibility rests with the physician in interpreting the problems of deafness realistically and hopefully. Referral by him to an appropriate agency in or near the community may be the first step in building hope and assurance for the parents.'

Screening tests in schools are clearly described and practical instructions are given on how to conduct these tests. The fundamental principles of clinical audiometry are explained, and the necessity for correct interpretation of audiograms stressed.

There are a few mistakes. For example, the statement that a virus infection, such as rubella, during pregnancy may cause both deafness and cerebral palsy is incorrect. It is stated that 'the child is not ready for an accurate audiometric test between the age of four to six'. Reliable audiometric tests can be carried out at some centres in this country from the age of $3\frac{1}{2}$.

The book is well set out and easy to read. It seems to be intended primarily for the intelligent parent and teacher, but is free from the usual 'popular' approach which so often allows inaccuracies for the sake of simplification. It contains much valuable information which should be very useful to doctors who are or should be interested in the problems of deafness in children.

The IXth International Congress of Paediatrics will take place in Montreal, Canada, from July 19-25, 1959.

Further information may be obtained from the Secretary General, P.O. Box 215 Westmount, Montreal 6, Canada.

PAEDIATRIC SOCIETIES IN THE BRITISH ISLES

The following is a list of paediatric societies and their principal officers at the time of compilation. Alterations when they occur, information on new societies or any omissions from this list should be passed to the Secretary of the British Paediatric Association.

I: National

British Paediatric Association

President: Dr. J. Forest Smith
Secretary: Dr. P. R. Evans
Institute of Child Health,
The Hospital for Sick Children,
Great Ormond Street, London, W.C.1.

The Royal Society of Medicine, Section of Paediatrics

President: Dr. Charles Pinckney
Secretaries: H. H. Nixon, Esq., F.R.C.S.
Dr. Hugh Jolly
The Royal Society of Medicine,
1, Wimpole Street, London, W.1.

The British Association of Paediatric Surgeons

President: Miss Isabella Forshall, F.R.C.S.Ed.
Secretary: R. B. Zachary, Esq., F.R.C.S.
Children's Hospital,
Sheffield.

The Scottish Paediatric Society

President: Dr. Agnes Macgregor
Secretary: Dr. R. G. Mitchell
Department of Child Health,
Queen's College, Dundee.

Scottish Surgical Paediatric Society

President: Matthew White, Esq., F.R.F.P.S.G., F.R.C.S.Ed.
Secretary: Wallace M. Dennison, Esq., F.R.F.P.S.G., F.R.C.S.Ed.
13, Ashton Road,
Glasgow, W.2.

Paedriatic Pathology Club

Secretary: Dr. J. L. Emery
Department of Pathology,
Children's Hospital,
Sheffield 10.

Ulster Paediatric Society

President: Professor F. M. B. Allen
Secretary: Dr. W. A. B. Campbell
19 Adelaide Park,
Belfast.

Irish Paediatric Association

President: Dr. Anna M. E. McCabe
Secretary: Dr. J. P. R. Rees
18, Fitzwilliam Square,
Dublin.

Welsh Paediatric Club

Secretary: c/o Professor A. G. Watkins
Department of Child Health,
Llandough Hospital,
Penarth, Glam.

II: Regional

The Aberdeen Child Health Society

President: Professor John Craig
Secretary: Dr. Mark Fraser
8, Queen's Terrace,
Aberdeen.

Caernarvonshire and Anglesey Paediatric Club

President: Dr. Gwyn Griffith
Secretary: Dr. Margaret Slater
Bryniau,
Belmont Road, Bangor, North Wales.

Kent Paediatric and Child Health Society

President: Dr. Wilfrid Sheldon
Chairman: Dr. S. D. V. Weller
Secretary: Miss H. E. Caunce,
(Almoners Department),
Farnborough Hospital, Kent.

Leicester Paediatric Club

President: Dr. J. V. Braithwaite
Secretary: Dr. F. E. B. Kelly
78, Letchworth Road,
Leicester.

The Leeds Regional Paediatric Club

President: Dr. M. Philpott
Secretary: Dr. M. W. Arthurton
Bradford Children's Hospital,
St. Mary's Road, Bradford 8.

The Liverpool Paediatric Club

President: Professor N. B. Capon
Secretary: Dr. H. Angelman
147 London Road,
Stockton Heath, Cheshire.

Manchester Paediatric Club

President: Dr. Margaret Egan
Secretary: Professor Wilfrid Gaisford
Department of Child Health,
St. Mary's Hospital, Manchester 13.

Midland Regional Paediatric Society

President: Dr. Jean M. Mackintosh
Secretaries: Dr. W. H. P. Cant
Dr. B. S. B. Wood
Department of Paediatrics and Child Health,
The Children's Hospital, Ladywood Road,
Birmingham 16.

The North of England Paediatric Society

President: Dr. W. J. Pierce,
Secretary: Dr. J. M. Stansfeld,
Hillcrest,
Farnley Hey Road, Durham.

Paediatric Society of the South-East Metropolitan Region

Chairman: Dr. R. C. Mac Keith
Secretary: Dr. David Morris
7, Wimpole Street,
London, W.1.

Sheffield Regional Paediatric Society

President: Dr. C. C. Harvey
Secretary: Dr. T. Wright,
Woodlands,
75, Doddington Road, Lincoln.

South West Paediatric Club

President: Professor A. V. Neale
Secretary: Dr. John Apley
Children's Hospital
St. Michael's Hill
Bristol 2.

SOCIAL AND BIOLOGICAL FACTORS IN INFANT MORTALITY*

VIII. MORTALITY IN THE POST-NEONATAL PERIOD

BY

S. L. MORRISON, J. A. HEADY and J. N. MORRIS
From the Social Medicine Research Unit of the Medical Research Council, London Hospital

(RECEIVED FOR PUBLICATION AUGUST 13, 1958)

This paper reports further results from the inquiry into the social and biological background of all the stillbirths and infant deaths that occurred among the 1½ million children born in England and Wales during 1949 and 1950. The method of the inquiry was described in the first paper of the series (Morris and Heady, 1955a) as follows:

> 'The present inquiry, which is an epidemiological exercise in the vital statistics of infant mortality, uses the documents of birth and death registration of England and Wales, and for the first time brings them together. Information about the mother's age, the number of her children, the duration of her marriage before the birth, and whether the birth was single or multiple, is obtained at birth registration (but not for the public record); while other data, such as the age of the infant, and the cause of death, are obtained when the death is registered. Information on the social circumstances surrounding the birth or death, such as the father's occupation, the community in which the family lived, and the infant's legitimacy is also available. All this material will be brought together for the two years 1949-50, and for the whole of England and Wales. Since similar information for stillbirths was easily available at the same time they are also included in the inquiry. In addition, mortality in the second year of life of children born in 1949 is being studied.'

The factors considered here in relation to deaths occurring between the end of the fourth week of life and the end of the first year, the post-neonatal period, are: the age of the mother at delivery, the birth rank of the child,† the duration of the mother's marriage, the occupation and social class of the father, the region of the country where the parents were living at the time of the birth; the age of the infant at death, the cause of death, and the place of death, that is, whether the death occurred in hospital or not. Part I of the paper is concerned mainly with the relationship between the mother's age, the birth rank of the child, and mortality in the post-neonatal period; Part II is concerned with the certified causes of that mortality.

Material

The figures given here relate to all the 1,322,150 single legitimate live births that occurred in England and Wales in 1949 and 1950; illegitimate and multiple births are not considered in this paper. For technical reasons, some of the tables and diagrams are based on births which occurred only in 1949 or only in 1950.

Presentation

The basic data are presented in Tables 1 and 2 and Appendix Table A. The main diagrams present the mortality rates given in the tables in the form of mortality ratios calculated from these rates. In each part of the diagrams the overall mortality rate for the infants of mothers of all ages and parities is taken as 100 and the mortality rate for infants of mothers of a particular age and parity group is represented as a percentage of this overall rate. For example, in Fig. 1, the overall mortality rate for all infants in the period 4 weeks to 6 months is 7·8 per 1,000. For the second and third children

---

* A series of articles reporting an inquiry made jointly by the Social Medicine Research Unit (Medical Research Council) and the General Register Office. These articles (see References) were prepared by the Unit in collaboration with the General Register Office, and have been approved for publication by the joint working party responsible for the inquiry.

† Birth rank is defined here as the number of children borne by the mother, surviving, dead or stillborn, including the present one. The terms 'parity' and 'family size' are also used with precisely the same meaning.

of mothers aged 20-24 years the rate is 13·7 per 1,000. If 7·8 is taken as 100, 13·7 becomes 176 and this is the ratio plotted in the figure.* Similarly, in the first section of Fig. 3 the mortality rate for all infants in social classes I and II is 5·5 per 1,000 and this rate is taken as 100. The mortality ratio is used rather than the rate because attention is paid here to the variation of mortality within each part of the diagrams. If crude rates were used the scale would obscure even large proportionate variations in the smaller rates.

To make the diagrams more easily read, birth ranks have been combined into three groups: first children, second and third children, and fourth and subsequent children. This grouping summarizes the main trends.

The vertical scale of the principal diagrams is a logarithmic one in order to give equal proportionate differences between ratios the same importance. For example, a mortality ratio of 50% is the same distance below the 100% base line as one of 200% is above it; on an arithmetic scale, 50% would be only half the distance below the base line of 100% that 200% would be above it.

Part I: Effects of Birth Rank and Mother's Age

Fig. 1 illustrates the pattern of stillbirth and infant death ratios for five periods from birth to the end of the second year of life, in relation both to the birth rank of the infant and the mother's age.†

It can be seen that there are two periods with distinctive patterns; stillbirths, and deaths during the period 4 weeks to 6 months. The stillbirth pattern is well known, the rates increasing sharply with increasing maternal age in each birth rank group, from, for example, 17·8 per 1,000 births for first infants of mothers aged 16-19 years to 55·8 per 1,000 for first infants of mothers aged 40-44 years.

* The ratios plotted in the figures cannot be precisely checked from the tables since these ratios were calculated from rates worked to two decimal places.

† The numbers and rates on which this figure is based are given in the seventh paper of the series (Heady and Morris, 1959).

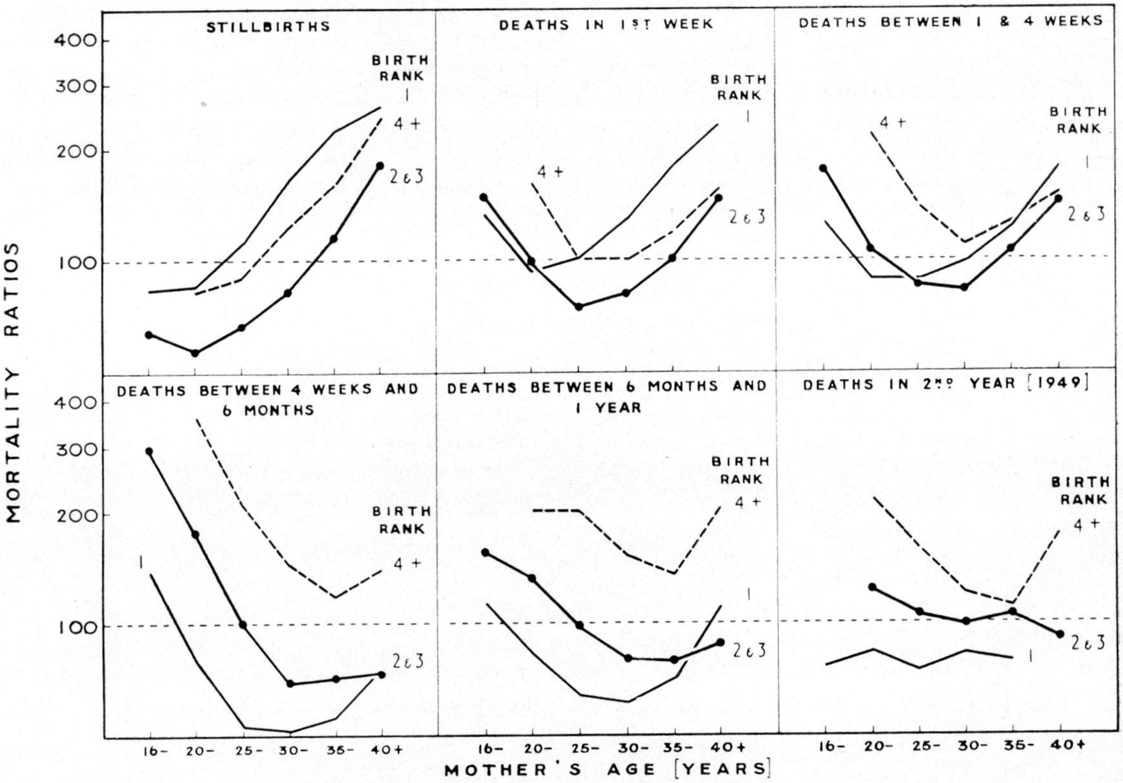

FIG. 1.—Variation of mortality with birth rank of infant and the mother's age: stillbirths, infant mortality and deaths in the second year of life. The date '1949' in the last section indicates 'births of 1949'. The single, legitimate births of England and Wales, 1949-50.

In the first part of the post-neonatal period (from the age of 4 weeks to 6 months), ratios are lowest for mothers aged 30-39 years in each of the birth rank groups. There is a slight rise for mothers aged 40 and above and a steep rise of ratios with decreasing age from 30-34 to 16-19 years. The highest ratios in each birth rank group, therefore, are found in the youngest mothers. In Fig. 1a the ratios for the same period are shown with three maternal age groups plotted against birth rank. For mothers in each age group, the ratios rise sharply with increasing birth rank, the increase being greater for young than for older mothers. In sum, the larger the family the greater is the risk for the baby; with similar size of family, the baby of the younger mother is at a higher risk of death than that of the older mother.

In the second half of the post-neonatal period (6 months to 1 year), the variation in ratios is less but a similar pattern is present. There are differences, however, the two most noticeable ones being the now more U-shaped curve for first children, and the much smaller rise in ratios for later children of young mothers, i.e. the effect of mother's age is less important than in the earlier period. In the second year of life, mortality ratios no longer show a very distinct pattern in relation to the mother's age.

In Fig. 2 the post-neonatal period is shown in more detail.* There are slight differences between the periods 4 weeks to 3 months and 3 months to 6 months, but it is clear that the main difference

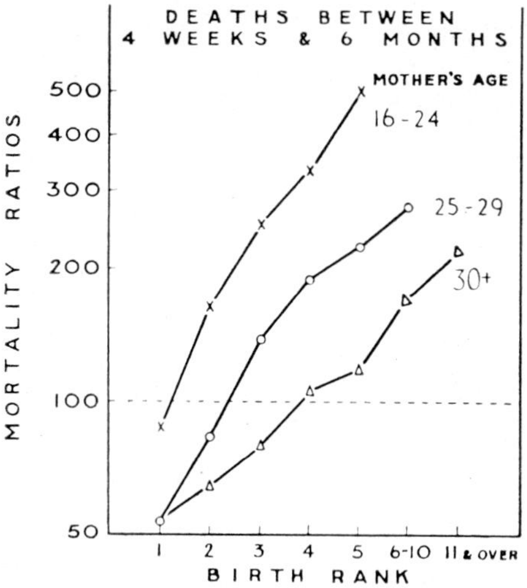

FIG. 1a.—Variation of mortality between 4 weeks and 6 months with birth rank of infant: mothers of different ages compared. The single, legitimate live births of England and Wales, 1949-50.

occurs between the periods 4 weeks to 6 months and 6 months to 1 year. Fig. 2 also shows that, because the majority of post-neonatal deaths occur in the period 4 weeks to 6 months, the pattern of mortality in the whole period is very similar to that of the first part of it. Thus, while the other figures given in this paper refer to the whole post-neonatal period, the pattern they show is predominantly that of its first half.

In the post-neonatal period (4 weeks to 12 months)

* Numbers of deaths and rates for four stages of the post-neonatal period are given in Appendix Table A.

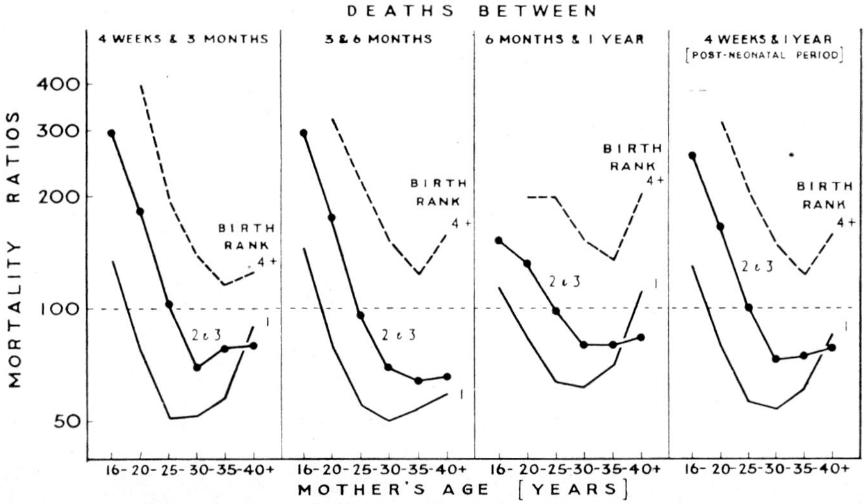

FIG. 2.—Variation of mortality with birth rank of infant and the mother's age: three stages of the post-neonatal period and the whole period. The single, legitimate live births of England and Wales, 1949-50.

then, we have shown that there are large variations in infant death rates according to the age and parity of the mother. For example, the third children of mothers under 25 years of age have death rates three times those of third children of mothers over 30 years of age.

Social Class.* It is well known that post-neonatal mortality rates rise steadily from social class I to social class V. In Table 1 death rates are given by birth rank and maternal age for three social class groupings and it can be seen that the expected social class trends occur in each maternal age—birth rank compartment, i.e. for mothers of a particular age and infants of a particular birth rank, the classical picture of steadily rising rates from classes I and II to classes IV and V appears. Fig. 3 presents these rates in the form of mortality ratios. Very similar patterns appear in each of the three social class groupings, with the highest ratios in the same 'vulnerable' group in each class, i.e. the later infants of young mothers. The mortality ratio (though not, of course, the actual mortality rate) for fourth and later children is in fact higher in classes I and II than in the other classes. It is clear, therefore, that the relatively high mortality rates among infants of young mothers with large families are not a phenomenon peculiar to any one social class due to some simple poverty factor. It is also true that the higher death rates in classes IV and V cannot be

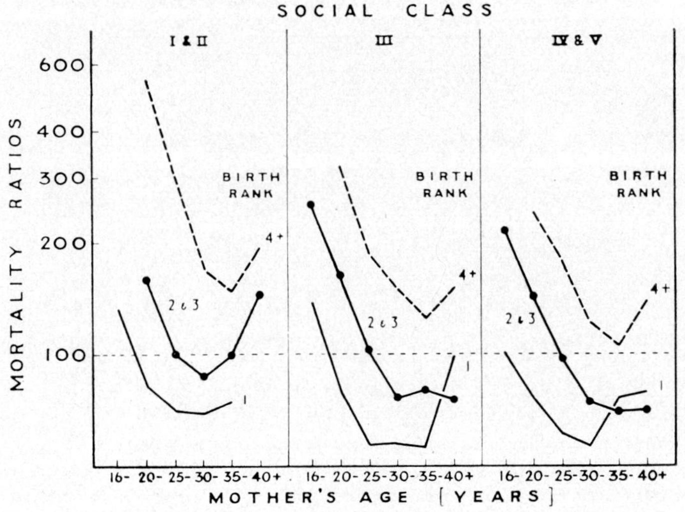

FIG. 3.—Variation of post-neonatal mortality with birth rank of infant and the mother's age: three social class groupings. The single, legitimate live births of England and Wales, 1949-50.

* The Registrar General allocates occupations to social classes according to the following scheme: class I—leading professions and business, class II—'lesser' professions etc., class III—clerks and skilled workers, class IV—semi-skilled workers, class V—unskilled labourers. Infants are allocated to social classes according to the occupation of the father.

TABLE 1

POST-NEONATAL MORTALITY IN THREE SOCIAL CLASS GROUPINGS IN RELATION TO BIRTH RANK AND MOTHER'S AGE
DEATHS OF INFANTS AGED 4 WEEKS TO 1 YEAR AND RATES PER 1,000 LIVE BIRTHS*

Single, Legitimate Live Births, England and Wales, 1949 and 1950

	Social Class of Father																	
	I and II						III						IV and V					
	Birth Rank 1		Birth Rank 2, 3		Birth Rank 4 and over		Birth Rank 1		Birth Rank 2, 3		Birth Rank 4 and over		Birth Rank 1		Birth Rank 2, 3		Birth Rank 4 and over	
Mother's Age (yr.)	D	R	D	R	D	R	D	R	D	R	D	R	D	R	D	R	D	R
16–19	16	7·7	1				365	13·9	83	24·9			255	15·6	90	33·0		
20–24	121	4·4	90	8·4	7		1,122	8·2	1,232	16·5	108	34·1	688	11·4	992	21·9	101	35·3
25–29	138	4·0	219	5·6	37	13·2	537	5·8	1,495	10·5	427	20·1	282	9·2	889	14·7	417	26·3
30–34	55	3·8	170	5·0	53	9·0	183	6·0	633	7·8	421	15·1	82	8·2	328	10·8	369	18·6
35–39	25	4·0	110	5·6	55	8·3	70	5·6	333	8·0	360	12·9	57	12·1	170	10·7	323	15·6
40+	11	7·6	33	7·3	32	10·0	26	9·4	73	8·0	199	15·8	16	13·9	38	10·1	218	20·6
All Ages and Birth Ranks†	Deaths (D) 1,177			Rate (R) 5·5			Deaths 7,690			Rate 10·3			Deaths 5,327			Rate 15·1		

* Rates are not shown where there are fewer than 10 deaths.

† Including the few cases where either the mother's age or the birth rank was not stated.

Mother's age refers to age attained on her last birthday before the present birth.

Birth rank refers to the number of children, surviving, dead and stillborn (and including the present birth), by the mother's present and any previous husband. Abortions before 28 weeks of pregnancy are excluded.

The absence of an entry for deaths indicates that there were none.

explained by the concentration of young mothers with large families in these classes.

Geographical Distribution. In addition to social class differences in post-neonatal mortality, regional differences have long been recognized, in particular the higher rates in the North of England and in Wales. However, analysis of the mortality rates by mother's age and parity in four regional groupings (South-East England, Midlands and South-West, Northern England, and Wales), showed that the typical pattern of mortality ratios appeared in each regional group. It was not possible to make a similar analysis for smaller areas.

Duration of Marriage. Another factor apparently related to post-neonatal mortality is the duration of the mother's marriage. This, together with parity, can give an indication of birth spacing and it is possible to compare the mortality rates of infants born shortly after a previous child with those where there has probably been a longer gap. (The measure used is an indirect one, since a woman of 30 who has been married for five years before having her second child may have had the first one only shortly before. However, there is more likely to have been a longer period between the children than if she had had her second child within two years of marriage.) Fig. 4a compares the mortality rates of 'closely spaced' births (defined as second and third births in less than two and three years of marriage respectively) with all other second and third births in three age groups of mothers. In each age group, the 'closely spaced' births have higher mortality rates than the others.

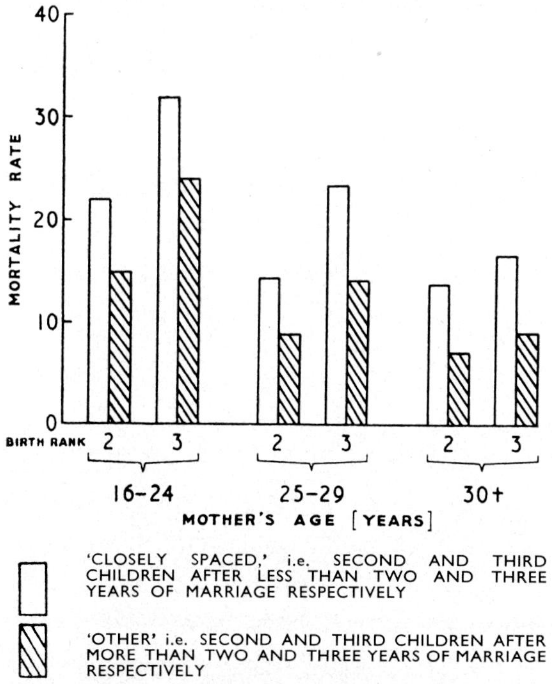

FIG. 4a.—Comparison between post-neonatal mortality of 'closely-spaced' and other births: three maternal age groups. The single, legitimate live births of England and Wales, 1949-50.

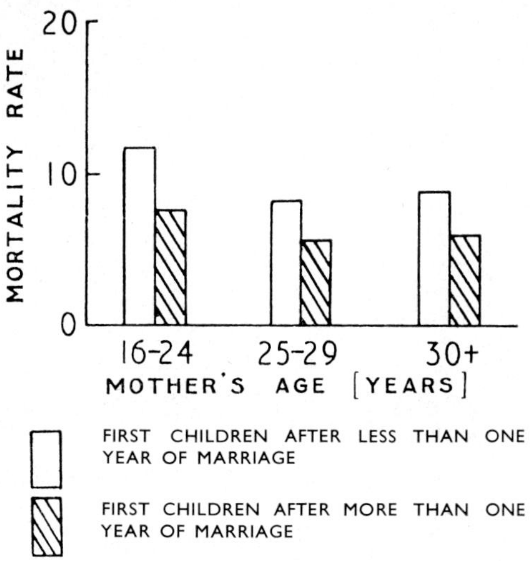

FIG. 4b.—Comparison between post-neonatal mortality of first children born in less than one year of marriage and after more than one year of marriage: three maternal age groups. The single, legitimate live births of England and Wales, 1949-50.

In Fig. 4b the mortality rates of first children born after less than one year of marriage are compared with those for first children born after a longer period. In the three maternal age groups, those born after less than one year are at a disadvantage. 'Duration of marriage', then, apparently reflects something in addition to birth spacing, since first children are also affected by it. 'Rapidity of breeding' cannot be the explanation.

Figs. 5a and b show the same phenomena in the three social class groupings. Once again, it is clear that this finding occurs within each social class group, and therefore cannot be 'explained' by social class differences, i.e. by assuming that most 'closely spaced' births occur in social classes IV and V, in the families of unskilled and semi-skilled labourers.

Other Factors. The social class and regional differences in mortality have long been known. The fact that the same patterns of mortality according to birth rank and mother's age are found in each of these classes, and in each of the regional groups indicates that there are also factors cutting across social class which affect the survival of infants in all social classes and regions. It is interesting that in

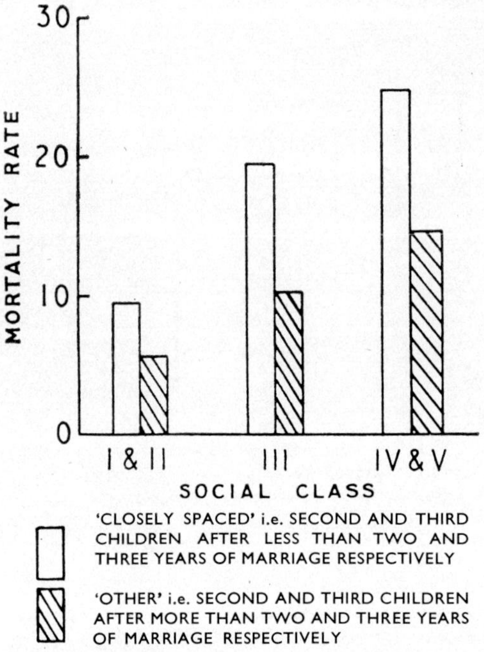

FIG. 5a.—Comparison between post-neonatal mortality of 'closely spaced' and other births: three social class groupings. The single, legitimate live births of England and Wales, 1949-50.

one group of infants, fourth and later children of mothers aged 20 to 24 years, the most vulnerable group, the differences between the classes is almost obliterated (Table 1). The rates for these infants are as follows: classes I and II—26·3*, class III —34·1, classes IV and V—35·3. In other words, the babies of young mothers with three or more other children are at an almost equally high risk of dying whether their fathers are professional men or unskilled labourers.

Part II: The Cause of Death

Fig. 6 illustrates the maternal age and birth rank pattern of mortality in the post-neonatal period for the six main groups of registered causes of death. The numbers and rates on which the diagram is based are given in Table 2, and the detailed composition of the cause groups in Table 3. Respiratory infections are the main cause of death in this period.

It will be noticed that the basic pattern shown in Part I for all causes of mortality (Fig. 2) appears in each of the cause groups of Fig. 6 except congenital malformations. For these latter deaths the differences between infants of mothers of various ages and of different parities are much less than in the other groups.† In deaths attributed to 'accidents' the pattern is most striking, with the highest ratio twenty times that of the lowest. The highest mortality rate is 5·9 per 1,000 for fourth and later children of mothers aged 20-24 years, and the lowest is 0·3 per 1,000 for first children of mothers aged 25-34. That is to say, while one out of 3,333 first children of mothers aged 25-34 years died from an 'accident' in the post-neonatal period, the comparable figure for fourth and later children of mothers aged 20-24 years was one death out of every 169 such children born.

It appears, then, that variations in mortality with maternal age and parity cannot be explained in terms of any single cause of death; all the major causes (with the exception of congenital malformations) show the same pattern. Of these causes only 'accidents' appears at first glance to be unrelated to infection and since 'accidents' also show the most striking variations in rates, it may be worth looking more closely at them.

'Accidents.' There has been considerable interest recently in the problem of accidental death in infancy. The hypothesis has been advanced in this country (Davison, 1945), in Australia (Bowden,

* This figure does not appear in Table 1 as it is calculated from less than 10 deaths.

† The numbers of deaths in the post-neonatal period due to congenital malformations are too small to enable maternal age—parity patterns to be shown for individual malformations since more than 60% of the deaths certified as due to congenital malformations occur in the neonatal period.

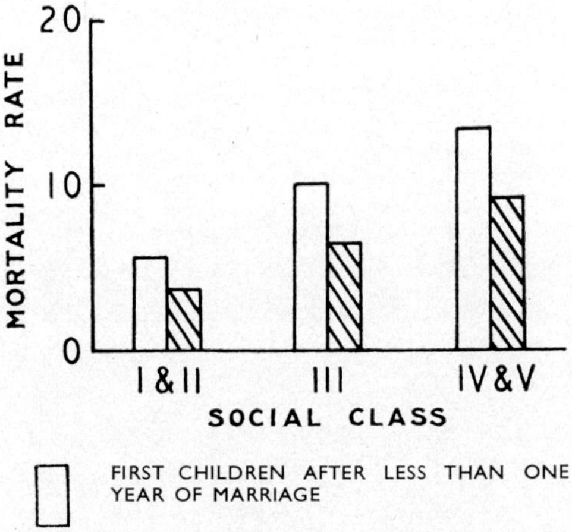

FIG. 5b.—Comparison between post-neonatal mortality of first children born in less than one year of marriage and after more than one year of marriage: three social class groupings. The single, legitimate live births of England and Wales, 1949-50.

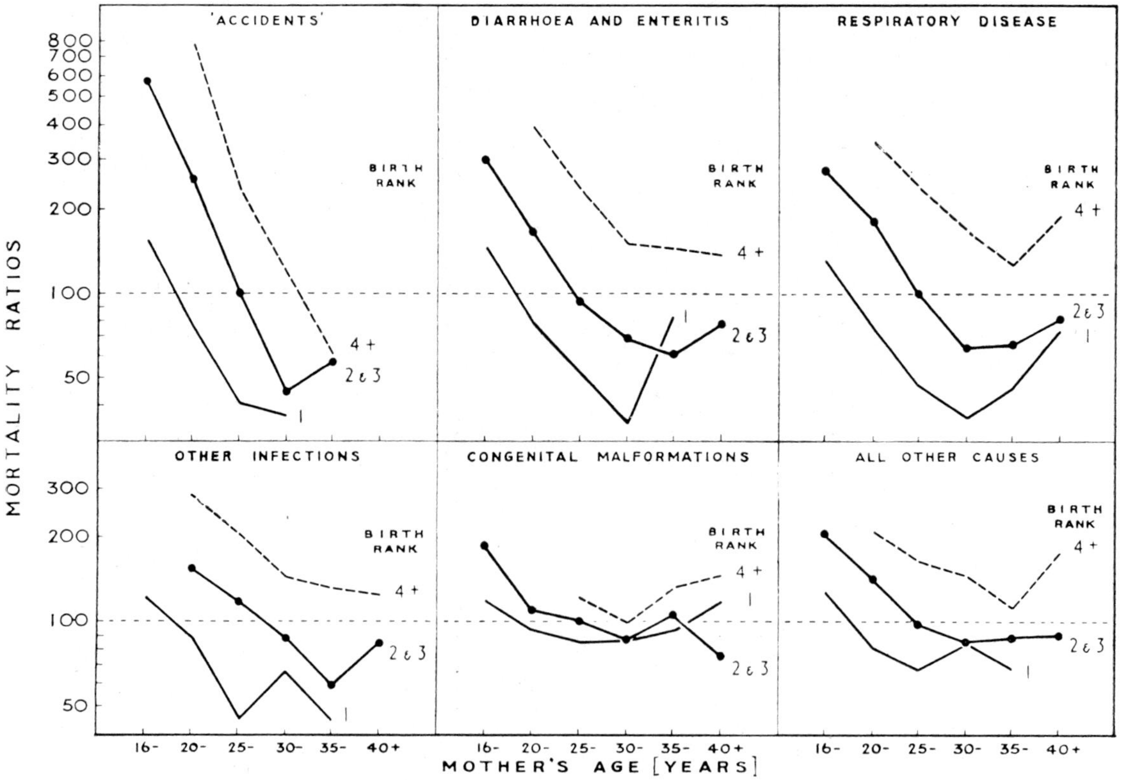

FIG. 6.—Variation of post-neonatal mortality with birth rank of infant and the mother's age: six cause groups. The single, legitimate live births of England and Wales, 1949-50.

1950) and in the United States (*J. Amer. med. Ass.*, 1950), that many of these deaths are due to a fulminating respiratory infection. For infants born in 1950, it is possible to subdivide the accidental deaths that occurred into two groups. The first, which contains only 12% of all the deaths attributed to 'accidents', includes falls, burns and traffic accidents. The second group, containing 88% of these deaths, comprises 'accidental inhalation and ingestion of food' (E921,922)* and 'accidental mechanical suffocation' (E924), and it is this group that includes most of the sudden, unexpected deaths in the post-neonatal period. Fig. 7 illustrates the death rates in the second group according to the season of birth of the infants, expressed as percentages of the rate for the whole year. The variation of the death rates is very similar to that of bronchopneumonia, with the highest rates amongst children born in the last two quarters of the year. That is to say, infants aged between 1 and 6 months during the winter months were at a much higher risk of

* An explanation of these international code numbers is given in the footnote of Table 3.

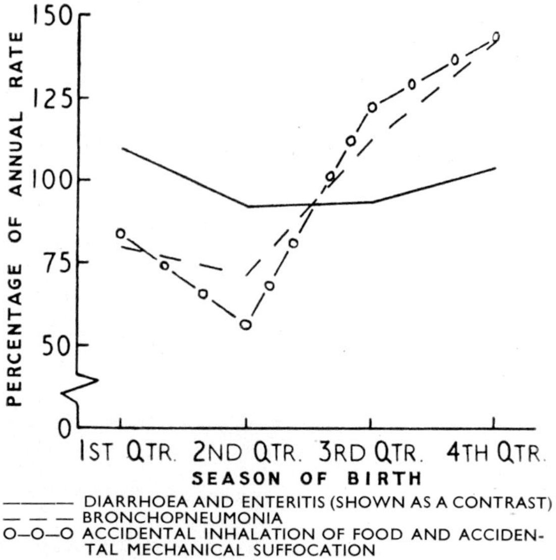

FIG. 7.—Variation of post-neonatal mortality for various causes according to season of birth. The single, legitimate live births of England and Wales, 1950.

TABLE 2

POST-NEONATAL MORTALITY IN SIX CAUSE GROUPS IN RELATION TO BIRTH RANK AND MOTHER'S AGE
DEATHS OF INFANTS AGED 4 WEEKS TO 1 YEAR AND RATES PER 1,000 LIVE BIRTHS*

Single, Legitimate Live Births, England and Wales, 1949 and 1950

Cause Groups†

'Accidents'

Mother's Age (yr.)	Birth Rank 1 D	1 R	2, 3 D	2, 3 R	4 and over D	4 and over R
16–19	52	1·2	27	4·3		
20–24	125	0·6	254	1·9	37	5·9
25–29	49	0·3	179	0·7	71	1·8
30–34	15	0·3	50	0·3	47	0·9
35–39	3		33	0·4	25	0·5
40+	3		4		8	
All Ages and Birth Ranks‡	Deaths (D) 987	Rate (R) 0·7				

Diarrhoea and Enteritis

Mother's Age (yr.)	Birth Rank 1 D	1 R	2, 3 D	2, 3 R	4 and over D	4 and over R
16–19	94	2·1	27	4·3		
20–24	266	1·2	325	2·5	37	5·9
25–29	122	0·8	337	1·4	138	3·5
30–34	28	0·5	148	1·0	118	2·2
35–39	29	1·2	68	0·9	117	2·1
40+	7		20	1·2	54	2·0
All Ages and Birth Ranks‡	Deaths 1,939	Rate 1·5				

Respiratory Diseases

Mother's Age (yr.)	Birth Rank 1 D	1 R	2, 3 D	2, 3 R	4 and over D	4 and over R
16–19	253	5·6	72	11·4		
20–24	706	3·1	998	7·6	94	14·9
25–29	314	2·0	1,028	4·2	404	10·1
30–34	87	1·6	396	2·7	382	7·1
35–39	47	2·0	219	2·8	300	5·4
40+	17	3·2	60	3·5	212	8·0
All Ages and Birth Ranks‡	Deaths 5,604	Rate 4·2				

Other Infections

Mother's Age (yr.)	Birth Rank 1 D	1 R	2, 3 D	2, 3 R	4 and over D	4 and over R
16–19	51	1·1	7			
20–24	188	0·8	183	1·4	17	2·7
25–29	68	0·4	264	1·1	77	1·9
30–34	35	0·6	121	0·8	74	1·4
35–39	10	0·4	43	0·6	70	1·3
40+	4		14	0·8	31	1·2
All Ages and Birth Ranks‡	Deaths 1,262	Rate 1·0				

Congenital Malformations

Mother's Age (yr.)	Birth Rank 1 D	1 R	2, 3 D	2, 3 R	4 and over D	4 and over R
16–19	83	1·9	18	2·9		
20–24	328	1·5	225	1·7	8	
25–29	211	1·3	379	1·6	75	1·9
30–34	75	1·4	198	1·4	85	1·6
35–39	34	1·5	128	1·7	115	2·1
40+	10	1·9	20	1·2	60	2·3
All Ages and Birth Ranks‡	Deaths 2,058	Rate 1·6				

All Other Causes

Mother's Age (yr.)	Birth Rank 1 D	1 R	2, 3 D	2, 3 R	4 and over D	4 and over R
16–19	104	2·3	23	3·7		
20–24	326	1·5	333	2·6	23	3·6
25–29	197	1·2	417	1·7	118	3·0
30–34	79	1·5	221	1·5	141	2·6
35–39	29	1·2	123	1·6	112	2·0
40+	9		28	1·6	85	3·2
All Ages and Birth Ranks‡	Deaths 2,372	Rate 1·8				

* Rates are not shown where there are fewer than 10 deaths.
† The detailed composition of the groups is given in Table 3.
‡ Including the few cases where either the mother's age or parity was not stated.

TABLE 3

COMPOSITION OF CAUSE GROUPS

(1) 'Accidents'	All deaths attributed to an accident (E800-965)*.
(2) Diarrhoea and enteritis ..	Enteritis and diarrhoea (571, 764).
(3) Respiratory diseases ..	Pneumonia (490-493, 763), bronchitis (500-502), other diseases of respiratory system (470-483, 510-527)
(4) Other infections	Tuberculosis (001-008, 010-019), whooping cough (056), measles (085), other infective and parasitic diseases (020-055, 057-084, 086-138)
(5) Congenital malformations	All congenital malformations (750-759)
(6) All other causes ..	All other causes of death

* Numbers in brackets refer to the code numbers of the International Statistical Classification of Diseases, Injuries and Causes of Death, 6th Revision. (World Health Organization, 1948.)

dying from an 'accident' than were those infants aged between 1 and 6 months during the summer. It has been shown before (Registrar General, 1954) that total infant mortality rates from 'accidents' are higher in the winter than in the summer.

It may be, therefore, that the majority of 'accidental' deaths in the post-neonatal period are due to infection and that infection in its broadest sense is the predominant cause of all deaths in this period.

We have shown, then, that the infants of young mothers, and especially of those with more than one child, are particularly liable to die of infection in the first part of the post-neonatal period, i.e. from 4 weeks to 6 months. Thereafter, this special vulnerability is less noticeable. This vulnerability is found in relation to other infants in the same social class and living in the same geographical area and it is increased if the mother has been married for only a relatively short time before the child is born (i.e. less than one year for the first child, less than two years for the second, less than three years for the third). In addition, these 'vulnerable' infants are, like others, exposed to increased risk with descending social class and with residence in the North of England or in Wales.

Once variations in mortality have been demonstrated between the infants of mothers of differing parities and ages, and in different social classes, three possibilities arise: either there are variations in the incidence of disease, or in the case fatality, or in both. This inquiry provides no evidence about the incidence of disease; it does provide indirect evidence about case fatality in so far as it may be assumed that infants who have had more attention from the medical services suffer a lower case fatality than others. The indirect evidence is found in the comparison of deaths occurring in hospital and at home.

Place of Death. To consider first the social class differences, it can be seen from Table 4 that the percentage of deaths in the post-neonatal period occurring in hospital in 1950 fell from 70% in class I to 52% in class V. (The striking difference is between class I and the rest.) In class I, therefore, probably 70% of those children who died had been under the care of paediatricians in hospital while in class V (whose total mortality was nearly four times that of class I) only 52% of such children could have had that care. Either a much larger proportion of deaths in class V were sudden, or there was a failure to admit the seriously ill child to hospital. Although 'where the average standard of housing is relatively good . . . the paediatrician and family doctor . . . can often treat serious illness partly or wholly in the home' (Gairdner, 1956), it seems highly unlikely that deliberate selection of this kind would lead to more labourers' children than children of professional people being treated at home. It is more likely that a considerable proportion of the serious illness in infants of all classes except class I in 1950 was not under the care of specialists at all. In the most important cause of death in this period, respiratory infections, less than half the deaths in classes II to V occurred in hospital.

Fig. 8 shows the relationship between the mortality rate of maternal age—parity groups and the percentage of deaths in the group occurring in hospital. Like the social class distribution, the groups with the highest death rates, later children of young mothers, have the lowest percentage of deaths in hospital. From this point of view also, it appears that in 1950 infants at the greatest risk did not come under the care of paediatricians.

These differences in the amount of medical care provided suggest that some of the variations in mortality rates between social classes and between maternal age—parity groups may be attributable to differences in case fatalities arising from differences in the quality of the medical care received.

Douglas (1951) and Grundy and Lewis-Faning (1957) have shown that the incidence of disease increases with descending social class. Thus probably both factors (incidence and case-fatality) vary with social class and may account for the different mortality rates between classes. The only evidence we can find about variations of incidence with maternal age and birth rank is given by Lowe and McKeown (1954). Their figures apply to 'infectious episodes in the first three years of life' and they show that in equivalent housing conditions, the number of such episodes increases with increasing birth rank and, for the same birth rank, is higher for children of mothers under 30 than over 30. The high mortality rates of later infants of young mothers may reflect, therefore, both a higher incidence of disease and a higher case fatality.

TABLE 4

PLACE (HOSPITAL OR ELSEWHERE) WHERE POST-NEONATAL DEATHS OCCURRED: BY SOCIAL CLASS
England and Wales, 1950

Social Class of Father	Deaths			
	In hospital (no.)	Elsewhere (no.)	In hospital (%)	Elsewhere (%)
I .	78	34	70	30
II .	240	200	55	45
III .	1,993	1,607	55	45
IV .	698	653	52	48
V .	608	553	52	48
All classes*	3,623	3,054	54	46

* Including the few where the social class was not stated.

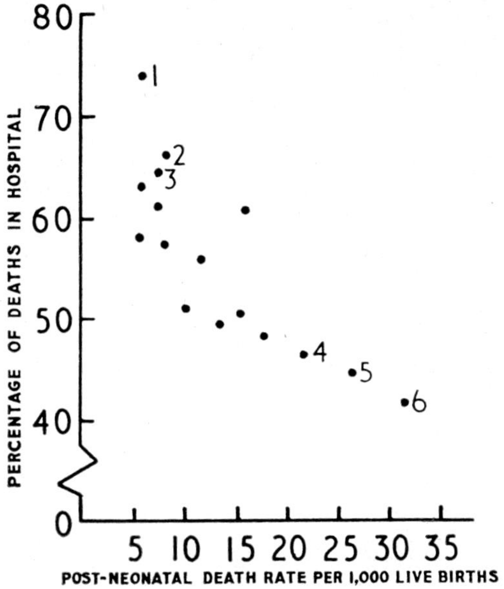

		Mother's Age	Birth Rank
AGE-BIRTH RANK GROUPS WITH HIGHEST % DEATHS IN HOSPITAL	1	30–34	1
	2	40+	1
	3	35–39	2, 3
AGE-BIRTH RANK GROUPS WITH LOWEST % DEATHS IN HOSPITAL	4	25–29	4+
	5	16–19	2, 3
	6	20–24	4+

FIG. 8.—Relation between post-neonatal death rates of maternal age and birth rank groups and percentage of post-neonatal deaths in hospital. The single legitimate live births of England and Wales, 1950.

Comment

Social class differences in post-neonatal mortality rates have long been recognized; these differences, and also those between occupations in the same social class (for example, miners and clerks in class III), appear to have remained relatively constant from 1911 until 1950 (Morris and Heady, 1955b). Regional differences are also well known but these now appear to be diminishing.* The closing of the social class gap is obviously going to be a long-term process. The finding of the same vulnerable groups of infants, later babies of young mothers, and the similarity of the patterns of mortality by maternal age and birth rank within social classes seem to merit attention for two main reasons. First, because the special attention of the medical services to these vulnerable groups may be a way of speeding the reduction of the overall post-neonatal mortality rates; and second, because it is possible that variations in mortality by maternal age and birth rank will become of increasing importance if and when differences between classes diminish.

We have shown that infant death rates are closely related to birth rank and mother's age and also that the majority of deaths in the post-neonatal period are probably due to infection. In other words, the pattern of mortality may reflect the impact of infection. It is interesting to look back to Fig. 1 in the light of this suggestion. The patterns of mortality ratios for stillbirths and for post-neonatal deaths are radically different but the neonatal pattern can be described as a mixture of these two patterns. The neonatal pattern may be a combination of two quite different patterns, that of the pre-natal period (due to pre-natal causes), and that of the post-neonatal period (due predominantly to infection). In Fig. 1, then, the curves are consistent with the idea that during the neonatal period the infant is still exposed to the effects of some pre-natal causes of disease and is also meeting external infection for the first time.

There are two independent findings to consider: first, that in the same birth rank, the babies of younger mothers have higher death rates; second, that for the same maternal age, babies of higher birth ranks have higher death rates.

To take first the infants of mothers of the same age, we have shown an increase in mortality with increasing birth rank in each maternal age-group, the greatest increase being for infants of mothers under 25 years of age. In addition the death rates of infants born after a relatively short duration of marriage were higher than those of other infants. Taken together, these facts suggest that the difficulty of looking after a larger family where, especially if there are other very young children, there is a greater risk of infection, increases the risk of death for babies in such families. Badger, Dingle, Feller, Hodges, Jordan and Rammelkamp (1953) have shown that the incidence of respiratory infections in pre-school children rises with increasing size of family, while Brimblecombe, Cruickshank, Masters, Reid, Stewart and Sanderson (1958) have shown that crowding within the family is an important factor in the spread of acute respiratory infection, and such crowding is more likely in the larger families. However, an increased risk also applies to a first child born within a year of marriage compared to those born after a longer interval, which suggests that some less obvious factor also plays a part. Table 5 provides further evidence against the hypothesis that the greater difficulties of rearing a larger family account for all the observed differences in mortality rates. The mortality rate for infants of mothers who have lost a previous child from any cause are higher than for other infants, that is, the higher rates are in the families that are smaller by at least one child. Deaths from diarrhoea and enteritis, from bronchopneumonia and from 'other respiratory diseases' have been selected for this comparison to obviate the possibility that previous loss of a child may have some purely medical bearing on the loss of the present one; it seems unlikely that previous loss would lead directly to increased risk of dying from gastro-enteritis or respiratory disease of a later infant.

Variations in the mortality rates of infants of the same birth rank with maternal age cannot be explained by any obvious hypothesis. For instance, the rates for first children rise from 5·7 per 1,000 for mothers aged 30-34 years to 14·2 per 1,000 for mothers of 16-19 years. It will be remembered that similar variations occurred within social classes

TABLE 5

POST-NEONATAL MORTALITY RATE FROM VARIOUS CAUSES PER 1,000 LIVE BIRTHS IN RELATION TO DEATH OF PREVIOUS CHILDREN

BIRTH RANKS 2, 3 AND 4

England and Wales, 1950

Cause of Death	All Previous Children Living (rate)	One or More Previous Children Dead (rate)
Diarrhoea and enteritis	1·2	1·3
Broncho-pneumonia	3·1	3·9
Other respiratory infections	1·5	1·8

* In the third paper of this series (Daly, Heady and Morris, 1955) it was shown that in 1949 post-neonatal death rates ranged from 7·0 in the Eastern Region to 17·9 in the Northern. In 1956, the range was from 5·3 in the South Western Region to 8·4 in the North Western Region (Registrar General, 1958).

(Fig. 3) and are therefore independent of social class.

It appears, then, that factors other than mere family size and the environmental factors such as income which are fairly directly reflected by the father's occupation must be sought to explain the patterns of mortality by maternal age and parity. There is no evidence from this inquiry about any variation of the incidence of disease by maternal age and parity or direct evidence about variations of case fatality rates. However, evidence that infants in the 'vulnerable group' may be failing to reach the care of paediatricians has been presented (Fig. 8) and it was suggested that this may influence the case fatality rates of these infants. The reason for this failure could be either that the standard of general practitioner care available to them was below average, or that the mothers of this group failed to call for medical aid as promptly as did other mothers. It is unlikely that variations in the standard of general practitioners are responsible since the same 'vulnerable group' is found amongst mothers in social classes I and II as well as amongst those in classes IV and V. The second possibility is supported by the facts shown in Fig. 9. Since autopsies of patients dying at home are usually performed on a coroner's order, it may be presumed that in these cases either there has been some doubt in the attending doctor's mind about the cause of death, or that he has not attended the patient during the last illness. The higher percentage of autopsies on infants in the 'vulnerable group' who died at home may be an indication, therefore, that a higher proportion of the mothers of this group have not called in their general practitioners at a sufficiently early stage.

An interesting relationship has recently been demonstrated between the proportion of infant deaths in hospital and the use of medical services by mothers. Douglas and Blomfield (1958), in their survey of children born in the first week of March, 1946, were able to identify a group of 558 mothers who made 'good use' of the ante-natal services (that is, had attended in the first three months of pregnancy) and to match this group (for sex, social group, birth rank of the child, and geographical area) with a similar number of 'poor users' (who attended in the last three months). They found that, out of five deaths in the post-neonatal period among infants of 'good use' mothers, four occurred in hospital, while out of 10 deaths among infants of 'poor users', only one occurred in hospital. Douglas and Blomfield (1958) write: 'We can infer that . . . "poor users" sought medical care at a later stage in their children's illnesses than did . . . "good users". Whether this was because they failed to recognize serious illness or because they relied upon the advice of someone other than the doctor, we cannot say.'

There is other evidence that the mothers of infants in the vulnerable groups do not use the 'extra' medical services, child welfare clinics, as fully as do other mothers. For example, in Newcastle (Spence, Walton, Miller and Court, 1954) the percentage of attendances at Welfare Clinics dropped from 71% of first children to 60% of fourth and subsequent children. The same picture was found in a new housing estate in Hertfordshire (McDonald, 1957).

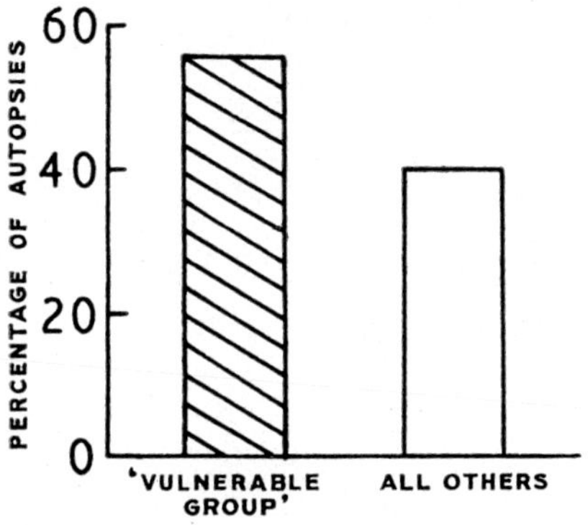

FIG. 9.—Percentage of autopsies among deaths at home for later infants of young mothers, the 'vulnerable group', and for all other infants. The single, legitimate live births of England and Wales, 1950.

In addition McDonald found that there was a tendency for Health Visitors to visit the homes of attenders at the clinics more often than the homes of non-attenders. It has also been noted (Douglas, 1951) that there may be a considerable delay before the Health Visitor makes her first call, and the young mother may be left to her own devices at perhaps her most difficult time, the first weeks following her return from hospital, or, in a home confinement, after the midwife has stopped visiting.

The hypothesis suggested by these facts is that young mothers are slower to seek medical advice about their infants, possibly because they are less able to recognize serious illness. This may be an indication of generally lower standards of maternal care. In other words, the factor which may be responsible for the higher mortality rates of infants of young mothers is poor maternal care. Maternal care is of recognized importance in the prevention of infant deaths but efforts to grade mothers according to their capability have not been very successful. For example, two recent studies (Spence *et al.*, 1954; Grundy and Lewis-Faning, 1957) placed mothers on a scale of capability retrospectively and it is difficult to escape the conclusion that such facts as the size of the family and the baby's health influenced the judgment.

Investigations in Aberdeen on a prospective basis may be relevant to this problem. A series of studies of married women during their first pregnancy were carried out by Professor Baird and his colleagues together with the Social Medicine Research Unit. Some of their findings may help to throw light on the variations in post-neonatal mortality rates recorded here and the relevant information is summarized below.

(1) Older mothers tended to make more use of sources of information about pregnancy and labour and 'irrespective of social class, give the impression of being more careful in their planning and preparation' (Baird and Scott, 1953).

(2) The successful use of contraception is associated with a higher intelligence test grading of the wife within each social class (Baird and Scott, 1953).

(3) Within social classes the mother's consumption of milk and vitamin concentrates rose steadily as maternal age increased (Marr, Hope, Stevenson and Thomson, 1955).

The overall suggestion is that the younger mothers in each social class take less care during pregnancy and may well provide poorer care for their infants in the post-neonatal period.

The link between these findings relating to women having their first baby and the higher mortality rates of later infants of young mothers may be provided by another Aberdeen study which found that the younger the mother and the shorter the interval between marriage and the first birth, the greater the number of subsequent children (Baird, 1946).

It appears, then, that the relatively high post-neonatal mortality rates of both first and later infants of young mothers in all social classes may be related to a lower standard of maternal care. In other words, the 'biological' factors of maternal age, parity and duration of marriage, may, in the post-neonatal period, reflect social factors, i.e. standards of maternal care.

This is not to say that the standard of maternal care is the whole answer to this question of differential post-neonatal mortality rates within social classes. It is possible that real biological factors affect the vitality of the baby and its capacity to meet environmental stresses. It has been shown that the post-neonatal mortality rates of premature infants are considerably higher than those of mature infants (Gibson and McKeown, 1951); it is possible that variations in the mortality rates of mature infants may be related to poor nutrition or 'pregnancy stress' in the mother (Stott, 1957). The work of Drillien (1957) and Illsley (1955) suggests that the childhood environment of the mother herself may play a part in this problem.

Epidemiology and Clinical Paediatrics. The inquiry reported here is an epidemiological approach to the problems of infant mortality. The uses of epidemiology (Morris, 1957) may be described at three levels. First, it aims at providing a total or representative picture of a situation, in the present instance the relationship between infant mortality rates and maternal age and the birth rank of the child. Patterns become obvious that could not be seen by the individual clinician; it is one way of 'completing the clinical picture' and 'identifying syndromes'. Secondly, it discovers problems; by locating vulnerable groups it shows empirically, regardless of the stage of understanding of aetiology, where health services should be concentrated. Lastly, by demonstrating differences between the death rates of various groups of infants it provides clues to aetiology.

An illustration of these three uses of epidemiology is provided by the analysis of 'accidental' deaths. At the first level, no clinician could see enough children with and without accidents to recognize the very striking relationship between the mother's age, the birth rank of the child, and post-neonatal death rates from accidents. At the second level, it can be shown (from Table 2 and Appendix Table A) that 40% of the 'accidental' deaths occurred amongst a group of infants who comprised less than one-sixth of the births. This is the 'vulnerable group', the later infants of young mothers, and it provides a manageable target for Public Health and clinical services. If special attention were to be paid to this small group of infants (small in relation to all births), and their death rate brought down to that of other babies, there would be a reduction of 25% in the total post-neonatal deaths due to 'accidents'.

At the third level, in the search for causes, the data given here support the hypothesis that many 'accidental' deaths are due to respiratory infections. Barrett (1954) doubts the validity of the fulminating infection theory and the data given here showing the concentration of accidental deaths amongst the later infants of young mothers does suggest that failure to recognize illness may be more important in these cases than a sudden overwhelming infection. Another epidemiological study on a smaller scale (Emery and Crowley, 1956) throws light on the causation of these deaths. Emery and Crowley investigated 50 'sudden unexpected deaths' and found that there were often symptoms in the infants for a few days before death. Unfortunately they did not give the maternal age and parity, but their study does confirm the hypothesis that the mothers of infants dying from 'accidents' are less able to recognize the symptoms of serious illness.

Although the post-neonatal mortality rate for England and Wales has fallen from 11·1 per 1,000 in 1950 to 6·9 per 1,000 in 1956 (Registrar General, 1958), there is no reason to believe that the differences in rates according to maternal age and parity presented here have disappeared. It must, therefore, be important for the medical services to pay particular attention to these young mothers and to try to reduce the differential mortality within social classes as well as between them.

Summary

A distinctive pattern of mortality by maternal age and birth rank has been demonstrated in the post-neonatal period. This pattern shows relatively high death rates for the infants of young mothers, with particularly high rates for the later children of such mothers; they form a vulnerable group of infants. The same pattern was found within the social classes and within geographical regions. It has also been shown that, independently of social class, the post-neonatal mortality rate is higher for the infants of mothers whose duration of marriage is short in relation to the number of children they have borne.

The same pattern of mortality rates was found for all the major causes of death except congenital malformations. The seasonal distribution of deaths due to 'accidents' provides another indication that infection may play a part in such deaths.

The proportion of post-neonatal deaths which occurred in hospital declined from social class I to social class V; in addition, this percentage was smaller for the vulnerable group of infants, that is, the later infants of young mothers. It appears possible that paediatricians in 1949-50 were not treating much more than half the cases of the most serious illness in babies aged between 1 month and 1 year.

Some relationships between epidemiology and clinical paediatrics are considered.

We are grateful to the staff of the General Register Office for professional, technical, and computing help; to Dr. R. H. Dobbs and Dr. F. J. W. Miller for valuable criticism and advice; and to colleagues in the Social Medicine Research Unit, in particular to Mr. C. Daly, Miss M. A. Ireland (secretary) and Mrs. V. P. Hall (computer).

References

Previous papers in this series:

I Morris, J. N. and Heady, J. A. (1955a). *Lancet*, **1**, 343.
II Heady, J. A., Daly, C. and Morris, J. N. (1955). *Ibid.*, **1**, 395.
III Daly, C., Heady, J. A. and Morris, J. N. (1955). *Ibid.*, **1**, 445.
IV Heady, J. A., Stevens, C. F., Daly, C. and Morris, J. N. (1955). *Ibid.*, **1**, 499.
V Morris, J. N. and Heady, J. A. (1955b). *Ibid.*, **1**, 554.
VI Heady, J. A. and Morris, J. N. (1956). *Brit. J. prev. soc. Med.*, **10**, 97.
VII Heady, J. A. and Morris, J. N. (1959). *J. Obstet. Gynaec. Brit. Emp.* In the press.

Badger, G. F., Dingle, J. H., Feller, A. E., Hodges, R. G., Jordan, W. S., Jr. and Rammelkamp, C. H. Jr. (1953). *Amer. J. Hyg.*, **58**, 31.
Baird, D. (1946). *Lancet*, **2**, 41.
—— and Scott, E. M. (1953). *Eugen. Rev.*, **45**, 139.
Barrett, A. M. (1954). In *Recent Advances in Paediatrics*, edited by D. Gairdner, p. 301. Churchill, London.
Bowden, K. M. (1950). *Med. J. Aust.*, **1**, 65.
Brimblecombe, F. S. W., Cruickshank, R., Masters, P. L., Reid, D. D., Stewart, G. T. and Sanderson, D. (1958). *Brit. med. J.*, **1**, 119.
Davison, W. H. (1945). *Ibid.*, **2**, 251.
Douglas, J. W. B. (1951). *Lancet*, **2**, 440.
—— and Blomfield, J. M. (1958). *Children Under Five*, p. 104. Allen & Unwin, London.
Drillien, C. M. (1957). *J. Obstet. Gynaec. Brit. Emp.*, **64**, 161.
Emery, J. L. and Crowley, E. M. (1956). *Brit. med. J.*, **2**, 1518.
Gairdner, D. (1956). *Proc. roy. Soc. Med.*, **49**, 974.
Gibson, J. R. and McKeown, T. (1951). *Brit. J. soc. Med.*, **5**, 177.
Grundy, F. and Lewis-Faning, E. (1957). *Morbidity and Mortality in the First Year of Life.* Eugenics Society, Cardiff.
Illsley, R. (1955). *Brit. med. J.*, **2**, 1520.
Journal of American Medical Association (1950). **142**, 1296.
Lowe, C. R. and McKeown, T. (1954). *Brit. J. prev. soc. Med.*, **8**, 24.
McDonald, A. D. (1957). *Publ. Hlth.* (*Lond.*), **70**, 122.
Marr, J. W., Hope, E. B., Stevenson, J. D. and Thomson, A. M. (1955). *Proc. Nutr. Soc.*, **14**, 7.
Morris, J. N. (1957). *Uses of Epidemiology.* Livingstone, Edinburgh.
Registrar General (1954). *Statistical Review of England and Wales*, 1950. *Text, Medical.* H.M.S.O., London.
—— (1958). *Statistical Review of England and Wales*, 1956. *Part III, Commentary.* H.M.S.O., London.
Spence, J., Walton, W. S., Miller, F. J. W. and Court, S. D. M. (1954). *A Thousand Families in Newcastle upon Tyne.* Oxford University Press, London.
Stott, D. H. (1957). *Lancet*, **1**, 1006.
World Health Organization (1948). *Manual of the International Statistical Classification of Diseases, Injuries, and Causes of Death.* Geneva.

See next page for Appendix Table A.

APPENDIX TABLE A

MORTALITY RATES PER 1,000 LIVE BIRTHS AT FOUR STAGES IN THE POST-NEONATAL PERIOD IN RELATION TO BIRTH RANK AND MOTHER'S AGE*

Single, Legitimate Live Births, England and Wales, 1949 and 1950

Birth Rank	Stage	Mother's Age (years) 16–19		20–24		25–29		30–34		35–39		40–44		45+		Not Stated		Total All Ages	
		D†	R†	D	R	D	R	D	R	D	R	D	R	D	R	D	R	D	R
1	Deaths between																		
	4 wk.–3 mth.	260	5·8	752	3·3	349	2·2	123	2·2	58	2·5	20	3·9	1		1		1,564	**3·0**
	3–6 mth.	224	5·0	626	2·8	306	1·9	95	1·7	44	1·9	10	2·0	1		2		1,308	**2·5**
	6–9 mth.	94	2·1	351	1·6	182	1·1	61	1·1	32	1·4	12	2·3					732	**1·4**
	9 mth.–1 yr.	59	1·3	210	0·9	124	0·8	40	0·7	18	0·8	6						457	**0·9**
	Live Births	44,840		225.096		159,519		55,153		23,499		5,140		254		754		514,255	
2	Deaths between																		
	4 wk.–3 mth.	75	12·7	741	7·1	629	3·7	256	2·8	138	3·2	21	2·5	5		2		1,867	**4·4**
	3–6 mth.	57	9·7	542	5·2	473	2·8	189	2·1	76	1·8	18	2·2	1		4		1,360	**3·2**
	6–9 mth.	19	3·2	235	2·3	283	1·7	97	1·1	51	1·2	9		1				695	**1·6**
	9 mth.–1 yr.	6		141	1·4	157	0·9	82	0·9	38	0·9	13	1·6					437	**1·0**
	Live Births	5,892		104,487		169,727		90,461		43,092		8,258		378		884		423,179	
3	Deaths between																		
	4 wk.–3 mth.	6		276	10·5	455	6·3	181	3·3	121	3·5	34	4·1			2		1,075	**5·4**
	3–6 mth.	7		236	9·0	332	4·6	160	2·9	96	2·8	20	2·4	1		1		853	**4·3**
	6–9 mth.	4		95	3·6	165	2·3	95	1·7	54	1·6	13	1·6			1		427	**2·2**
	9 mth.–1 yr			52	2·0	110	1·5	74	1·3	40	1·2	9		1		1		287	**1·5**
	Live Births	407		26,366		72,828		55,261		34,458		8,371		402		458		198,551	
4	Deaths between																		
	4 wk.–3 mth.			88	16·9	204	7·8	138	5·1	88	4·2	27	4·2			2		547	**6·3**
	3–6 mth.			49	9·4	179	6·8	104	3·9	66	3·1	23	3·6			4		425	**4·9**
	6–9 mth.			20	3·9	90	3·4	52	1·9	38	1·8	20	3·1	2		2		224	**2·6**
	9 mth.–1 yr.			10	1·9	52	2·0	46	1·7	31	1·5	12	1·9	3		1		155	**1·8**
	Live Births	28		5,194		26,234		26,946		21,171		6,416		396		246		86,631	
5	Deaths between																		
	4 wk.–3 mth.			17	18·4	88	9·6	75	5·7	46	3·7	19	4·0					245	**6·0**
	3–6 mth.			19	20·6	73	8·0	72	5·5	42	3·4	28	5·9	2		1		237	**5·8**
	6–9 mth.			5		38	4·2	44	3·4	37	3·0	16	3·4	2				142	**3·5**
	9 mth.–1 yr.			1		22	2·4	22	1·7	19	1·5	3						67	**1·6**
	Live Births	2		922		9,165		13,147		12,544		4,769		343		123		41,015	
6–10	Deaths between																		
	4 wk.–3 mth.			3		45	9·8	108	8·1	129	6·4	76	6·9	5		1		367	**7·3**
	3–6 mth.			2		54	11·7	100	7·5	114	5·6	64	5·8	8				342	**6·8**
	6–9 mth.			2		30	6·5	47	3·5	55	2·7	36	3·3	7		1		178	**3·5**
	9 mth.–1 yr.					8		33	2·5	43	2·1	31	2·8	7				122	**2·4**
	Live Births			187		4,605		13,275		20,251		11,016		1,122		196		50,652	
11+	Deaths between																		
	4 wk.–3 mth.							1		16	11·4	13	6·6	3				33	**8·1**
	3–6 mth.							3		12	8·6	19	9·6	2				36	**8·8**
	6–9 mth.							2		2		13	6·6	4				21	**5·2**
	9 mth.–1 yr.									1		3		2				6	
	Live Births					11		269		1,403		1,971		409		17		4,080	
Not Stated	Deaths between																		
	4 wk.–3 mth.			1		1				1						4		7	
	3–6 mth.					1		1								2		4	
	6–9 mth.							1								1		2	
	9 mth.–1 yr.																		
	Live Births	89		982		1,095		595		331		95		5		595		3,787	
Total All Birth Ranks	Deaths between																		
	4 wk.–3 mth.	341	**6·7**	1,878	**5·2**	1,771	**4·0**	882	**3·5**	597	**3·8**	210	**4·6**	14	**4·2**	12	**3·7**	5,705	**4·3**
	3–6 mth.	288	**5·6**	1,474	**4·1**	1,418	**3·2**	724	**2·8**	450	**2·9**	182	**4·0**	15	**4·5**	14	**4·3**	4,565	**3·5**
	6–9 mth.	117	**2·3**	708	**2·0**	788	**1·8**	399	**1·6**	269	**1·7**	119	**2·6**	16	**4·8**	5		2,421	**1·8**
	9 mth.–1 yr.	65	**1·3**	414	**1·1**	473	**1·1**	297	**1·2**	190	**1·2**	77	**1·7**	13	**3·9**	2		1,531	**1·2**
	Live Births	51,258		363,234		443,184		255,107		156,749		46,036		3,309		3,273		1,322,150	

* Rates are not shown where there are fewer than 10 deaths. † D=Deaths R=Rates

NEPHROCALCINOSIS INFANTUM

BY

ROBERT A. SHANKS and A. M. MacDONALD

From The Royal Hospital for Sick Children, Yorkhill, Glasgow

(RECEIVED FOR PUBLICATION SEPTEMBER 10, 1958)

Since Lightwood's description in 1935 of six cases of renal calcinosis encountered in a series of 850 autopsies this condition has attracted widespread attention and has been recorded in association with many different diseases including renal acidosis, idiopathic hypercalcaemia, hypophosphatasia, hyperoxalaemia and sarcoidosis. In addition to the cases in which the clinical diagnosis would suggest such a lesion, nephrocalcinosis has been found at autopsy in several infants dying in this hospital of apparently unrelated diseases. The purpose of this paper is to describe the results of a survey of all cases of nephrocalcinosis encountered at autopsy in the Royal Hospital for Sick Children, Glasgow, during the past three decades.

Until the middle of 1949, kidneys were examined histologically only when there was some indication to do so; figures for the incidence of nephrocalcinosis before this date will therefore be incomplete but may perhaps be presumed to include those macroscopically obvious. After this period the kidneys were examined in every autopsy and in most cases re-examined in order to ensure that none was missed. In the period under review (1928-57) there were 84 cases in all, of which 60 occurred during the decade 1949-57. Excluding the first five months of 1949 the figures for this latter decade can be taken as representing the true incidence of this lesion in children coming to autopsy (Table 1).

TABLE 1

INCIDENCE OF NEPHROCALCINOSIS AT AUTOPSY

Year	No. of Autopsies	Kidneys Examined	No. of Cases
1928-37 ..	2,673	187	9
1938-47 ..	2,672	251	15
1948-57 ..	1,751	1,475	60

The detailed histology of the lesion of nephrocalcinosis has already been described by Rhaney and Mitchell (1956) who had access to some of our material. On closer examination of our series, however, it became evident that what appeared to be various stages in the production of the fully developed picture could be identified in the same tissue including an early lesion in which deposition of calcium had not yet occurred. Thereafter on a further survey of the histological sections in this series a number of cases were found in which this early lesion occurred alone. Such cases have been included in our series in the conviction that they are indications of the same pathological process and the apparent illogicality of including lesions without demonstrable calcium under the term nephrocalcinosis was thought preferable to deviating from a term now firmly established in the medical literature.

For the purpose of description we have classified the histological appearances according to the following criteria.

Type I. Scanty Precalcinotic Lesions. These are small and obviously early lesions characterized by the distension of a single tubule which sometimes contains a hyaline cast. The epithelium shows minor damage such as blurring of the cell outline, pyknosis of the nuclei and loss of definition of the basement membrane which is replaced by acellular granular debris and occasionally accompanied by a giant cell (Fig. 1).

Type II. Abundant Precalcinotic Lesions. These lesions are larger than those of Type I and involve several adjacent tubules (Fig. 2). The number of tubules involved varies from lesion to lesion while the degree of distortion may be such as to make them barely recognizable. In some a giant cell may be seen but in none can calcium be demonstrated. The connective tissue surrounding the lesion is condensed; later there is an increase in fibrous tissue which eventually obliterates the lesion to become a fibrous node (Fig. 3). The lesions are irregularly distributed along the affected tubules which may be obstructed at several levels (Fig. 4). Depending upon the chance cut of the histological section examined, a cystic or granulomatous appearance may then appear in the same field.

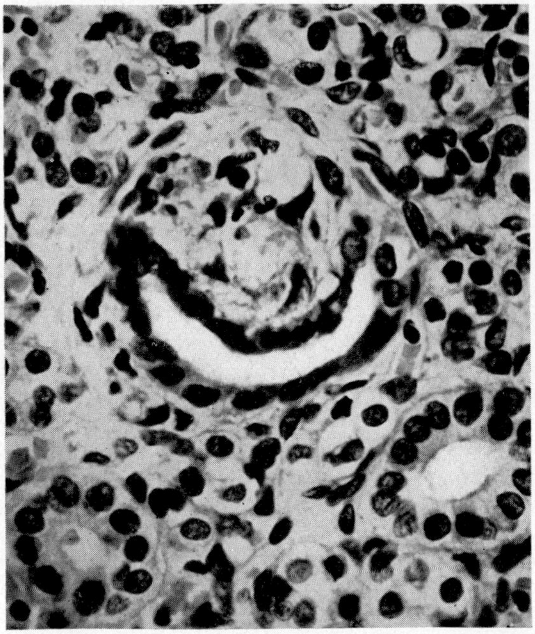

FIG. 1. Type I. Scanty precalcinotic lesion. A single tubule distended and showing nuclear pyknosis and early deposition of acellular granular debris adjacent to it. H. and E. × 580.

Type III. Renal Medullary Calcinosis. These lesions are almost completely confined to the renal medulla and some but not all show demonstrable calcium. For convenience three sub-types are described: (*a*) infrequent lesions found near the cortex differing from Type I in the presence of deposited calcium. (*b*) Abundant lesions of the renal medulla with occasionally a few minimal cortical lesions as well; the renal damage is as extensive as in Type II from which it is distinguished by a heavy deposit of stainable calcium (Fig. 5): this is always recognizable to the naked eye. These, too, may become fibrotic (Fig. 6). The characteristic position near the cortex suggests involvement of Henle's loop. All in all this group may be taken as the picture of renal medullary calcinosis at its height, a picture which has already been amply described (Rhaney and Mitchell, 1956). (*c*) These are scanty lesions differing from Type IIIa in their position which is in the papilla rather than the juxta-cortical zone. They have been found in association with pyelonephritis and pelvic calculi and are probably unrelated to the other types described. They account for only two of the total of 84 cases seen in the period under review.

Type IV. Renal Medullary and Cortical Calcinosis. The only histological criterion for this group is the presence of calcinotic lesions not only in the renal medulla but to a considerable extent in the cortex also; the glomeruli, however, are not affected. The medullary lesion is usually more extensive. The example illustrated is a severe lesion (Fig. 7).

Type V. Renal Cortical Calcinosis. These lesions are nearly entirely confined to the cortex and any medullary lesions present are very scanty and small.

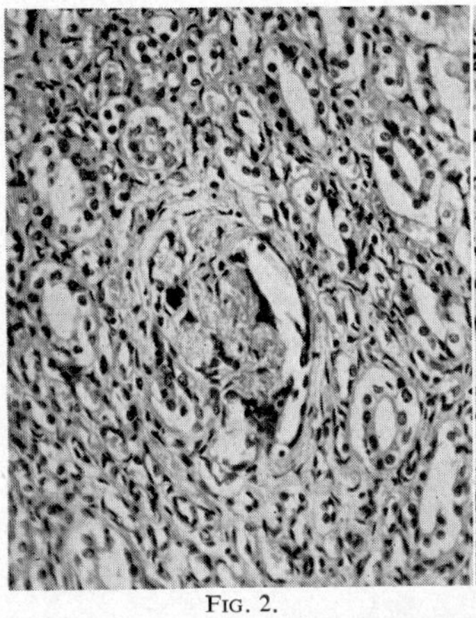

FIG. 2.

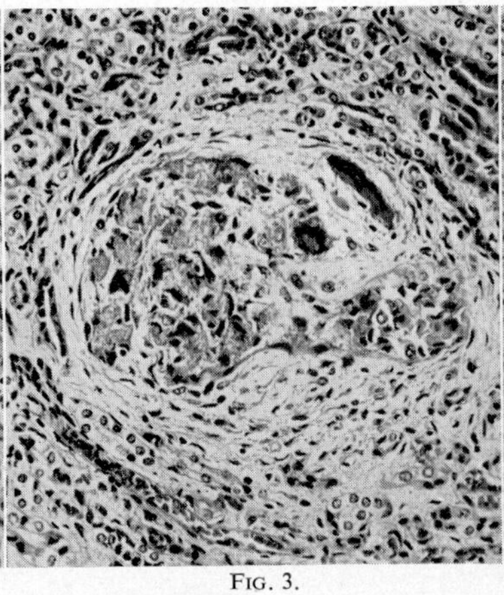

FIG. 3.

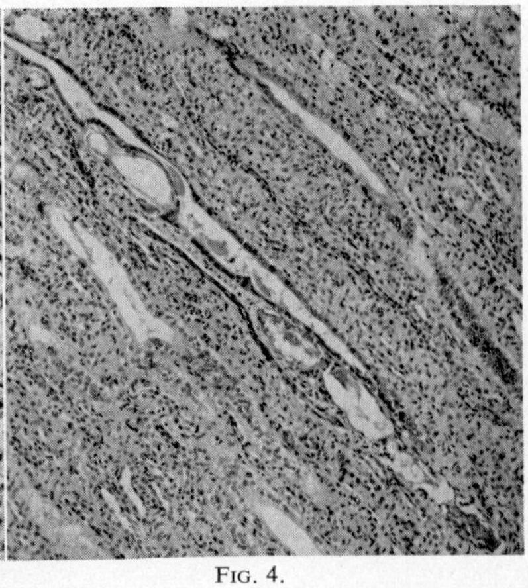

FIG. 4.

FIG. 2. Type II. Abundant precalcinotic lesions. Several adjacent tubules involved in a granulomatous mass. Early 'giant cell' formation is shown. Many such lesions are found. H. and E. × 170.

FIG. 3. Type II. Abundant precalcinotic lesions. Evidence of early fibrosis around the lesion. H. and E. × 170.

FIG. 4.—Type II. Precalcinotic lesion. Longitudinal section of tubules to show obstruction at different levels and pressure collapse of adjacent tubules. The cystic appearance is considered to be artefact. In life debris lay in the space which is outside the tubule in the site of the basement membrane. H. and E. × 75.

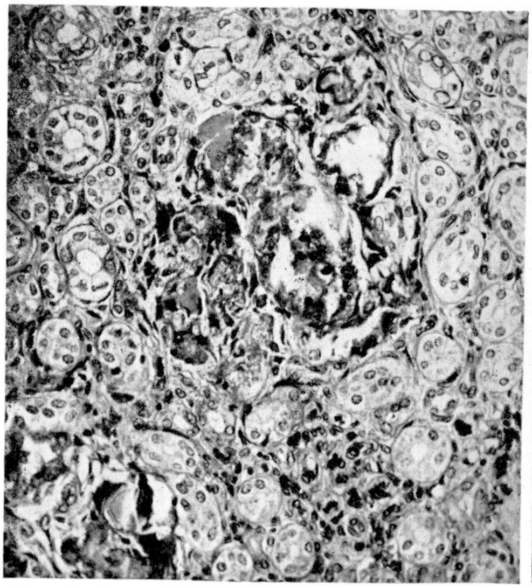

FIG. 5.—Type IIIb. Medullary calcinosis. Mass of calcium replacing group of adjacent tubules in varying stages of distension and obliteration. H. and E. × 190.

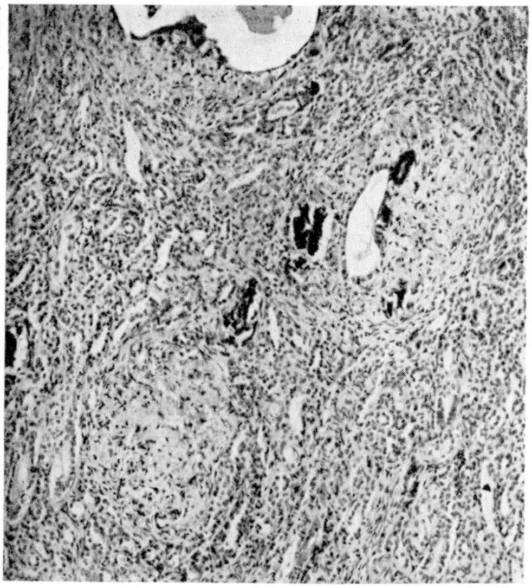

FIG. 6.—Type IIIb. Medullary calcinosis. Fibrous nodes, some containing calcium. The healing lesion. H. and E. × 85.

They have been found only in the first two decades under review.

Type VI. Unclassified. Two lesions have been included merely because the presence of stainable calcium brings them into the category of nephrocalcinosis; they are clearly not related to any of the foregoing, one being the end result of a venous thrombosis, the other calcification of a renal vein in a child with extensive pyelonephritis.

Results

The general incidence of these lesions at autopsy is seen in Table 1. The incidence of the several types is shown in Table 2. For the reasons

TABLE 2

INCIDENCE OF RENAL LESION ACCORDING TO TYPE

Year	Type							
	I	II	IIIa	IIIb	IIIc	IV	V	VI
1928-37	1	0	1	3	1	0	3	0
1938-47	2	1	4	3	0	2	2	1
1948-57	12	13	4	20	3	7	0	1

mentioned above, only the figures for the most recent decade can be regarded as comprehensive. Nevertheless, if we accept the suggestion that severe medullary calcinosis is unlikely to be missed at autopsy, we can conclude that for Type IIIb at least, the earlier figures, too, provide an index of its occurrence and a suggestion that the greatly increased numbers of cases of nephrocalcinosis found in the period 1948-57 reflect a true increase in its incidence. Nevertheless, the figures for the first two decades are so small that detailed con-

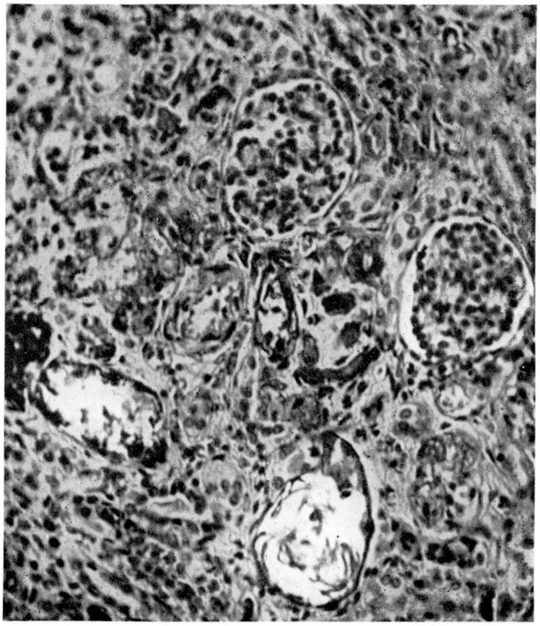

FIG. 7.—Type IV. Renal medullary and cortical calcinosis. Calcium deposition in the tubules in the cortex. Glomeruli not affected. H. and E. × 230.

sideration will be confined to the figures for 1948-57.

The age incidence is shown in Table 3 and it is clear that nephrocalcinosis is primarily a disorder of infancy and rarely occurs over the age of 2 years. Of the 47 infants in the last decade there were 10 in the first three months, 19 in the second, 10 in the third and eight in the last. Thus almost half the total 60 cases were under 6 months of age at death and it follows that the condition has its origin during this period in an even larger proportion.

TABLE 3

AGE INCIDENCE

Year	Age in years			
	0–1	1–2	2–3	Over 3
1928-37 ..	3	1	0	5
1938-47 ..	9	1	2	3
1948-57 ..	47	10	0	3

Clinical Diagnosis. A retrospective clinical appreciation of each case was undertaken in order to determine as far as possible the associated clinical condition and symptomatology which might be related to the kidney lesion. It became abundantly clear that only a few of the children with post-mortem nephrocalcinosis were recognized in life to be suffering from one of the known causes of this lesion. Of the 60 cases only 12 belonged to what we may call the 'renal acidosis' group. Four were diagnosed as hyperchloraemic renal acidosis, seven as idiopathic hypercalcaemia while an additional child had both. Table 4 shows the distribution of clinical and pathological diagnoses under fairly general headings. It will be appreciated that as several children had more than one pathological condition, the total number of diagnoses exceeds the number of cases.

Symptomatology. A detailed analysis of the symptoms and in particular of such symptoms as vomiting and constipation which are frequently associated with the clinical syndrome of idiopathic hypercalcaemia was unprofitable. Vomiting in fact occurred in 40 cases and constipation in 21 but in most cases this could easily be attributed to the associated disease from which the child died.

Vitamin D. Information regarding vitamin D intake was not complete in all records. In 52 there was a history of prolonged administration of fortified milk and/or vitamin D supplements. In two infants there was no history of administration of vitamin D in significant amounts. One who died of fibrocystic disease of the pancreas had been given cod liver oil for one week only and received milk fortified with vitamin D_2 only during her fortnight's stay in hospital: the lesion found at autopsy was Type II. The other who died of hyperchloraemic renal acidosis and enteritis had been given fortified milk for three weeks and cod liver oil in moderate doses for two weeks.

Discussion

It is apparent that a wide variety of pathological conditions, in themselves sufficient to cause death, have been found in association with the lesion of nephrocalcinosis. Indeed the distribution of diagnoses in our series is merely one that would be expected in any selection of autopsies of this age group. The first and most obvious explanation for these findings is that nephrocalcinosis is a casual autopsy finding, seldom related to the cause of death. The virtual absence of the condition in children over the age of 2 years likewise suggests that not only is it usually not lethal, it normally proceeds to complete resolution. Clearly no group of lesions which may be produced by such widely different causes as hypophosphatasia and hyperoxaluria can be regarded as homogeneous. Nevertheless, the implications are that most of them belong to a benign disorder of infancy without severe symptoms and with an excellent prognosis.

TABLE 4

DIAGNOSES OF 60 CASES OF NEPHROCALCINOSIS SEEN DURING 1948-57

	Congenital Abnormality	Infection	Miscellaneous	Total	Percentage Total Cases
System:					
Alimentary ..	5	14	8	27	45
Respiratory ..	—	16	—	16	26
Cardiovascular ..	6	—	—	6	10
Central nervous ..	10	4	4	18	30
Genito-urinary (excl. nephrocalcinosis) ..	1	1	1	3	5
Miscellaneous Conditions:				20	33
Renal acidosis ..			5		
Hypercalcaemia ..			8		
Hypophosphatasia ..			1		
Others ..			6		

This brings it into line with the condition of idiopathic hypercalcaemia of infancy which is known to be relatively benign and known also to produce renal medullary calcinosis in those few that have come to autopsy. In this hospital there have been 40 cases of idiopathic hypercalcaemia recognized during the past seven years and of these four died (McBean, 1958). Three came to autopsy and renal medullary calcinosis was found in all.

A simple theory which would appear to satisfy the facts at our disposal is that symptomless hypercalcaemia is a more widespread condition than has been appreciated and that renal lesions thereby produced are only detected when the child happens to die of some other condition. When hypercalcaemia is more severe or prolonged, symptoms are produced which lead to a clinical diagnosis. During the second year of life the lesions presumably resolve leaving no scar. It is tempting to regard this as yet another pointer to the association between idiopathic hypercalcaemia, nephrocalcinosis and vitamin D for it is at this age that children usually cease to be given milk and cereals which are fortified with synthetic vitamin D.

Summary

Eighty-four cases of nephrocalcinosis infantum have been encountered during the thirty-year period 1928-57 and of these 60 occurred in the last decade. It is thought that this indicates a true increase in the incidence. Most cases (70%) were found in the first year of life.

An early lesion in which calcium has not yet been deposited can be recognized.

Nephrocalcinosis infantum appears to be a benign lesion and unrelated to the cause of death. It is concluded that the lesion resolves spontaneously during the second year of life and is probably related to symptomless hypercalcaemia however caused.

We are grateful to our senior colleagues for permission to report cases under their care.

References

Lightwood, R. (1935). *Arch. Dis. Childh.*, **10**, 205.
Rhaney, K. and Mitchell, R. G. (1956). *Lancet*, **1**, 1028.
McBean, M. S. (1958). Personal communication.

A CASE OF CALCIFICATION OF THE BASAL GANGLIA WITH OSTEOPOROSIS AND OTHER ABNORMALITIES

BY

P. F. BENSON*

From the Children's Department, University College Hospital, London

(RECEIVED FOR PUBLICATION SEPTEMBER 2, 1958)

Introduction

Calcification of the basal ganglia is often found microscopically in normal adult brains. It is no longer believed to represent the end result of inflammation or other disease process (Foley, 1951). Cases where this calcification is gross enough to be visualized radiologically are much more rare. In most instances these have been associated with hypoparathyroidism, either idiopathic or post-operative. It is also found in pseudo-hypoparathyroidism where the target organs are believed to be refractory to parathyroid hormone which is normally produced (Albright, Burnett, Smith and Parson, 1942; MacGregor and Whitehead, 1954). Toxoplasmosis is another cause (Sutton, 1951). The intracranial calcification of the Sturge-Weber syndrome may also involve the basal ganglia.

There remains a group of adult cases with calcification of the basal ganglia visible radiologically, which is often familial and is frequently associated with a progressive neurological disorder. The only child in the literature with this abnormality is one of two brothers described by Neill and Dingwall (1950). In the case to be described, calcification of basal ganglia was associated with other bizarre findings to make a symptom complex not previously reported.

Case Report

J.C., aged 12 years (Figs. 1 and 2) was admitted to University College Hospital on June 17, 1957, for investigations of spinal osteoporosis detected on a lateral radiograph of the chest.

She was born two weeks prematurely after a normal pregnancy and delivery. Her birth weight was 5·0 lb. There were no neonatal disturbances and apart from being below average weight and stature, she progressed normally.

Her milestones were a little delayed, she sat up unaided at 9 months, stood alone at 15 months, and said a few single words at 2 years.

At the age of 2 years when she weighed 15 lb. 8 oz. (below the third percentile: Stuart, Anthropometric chart), she was seen at another hospital where the presence of dwarfism led to the diagnosis of hypopituitarism. From about 2 years of age she was subject

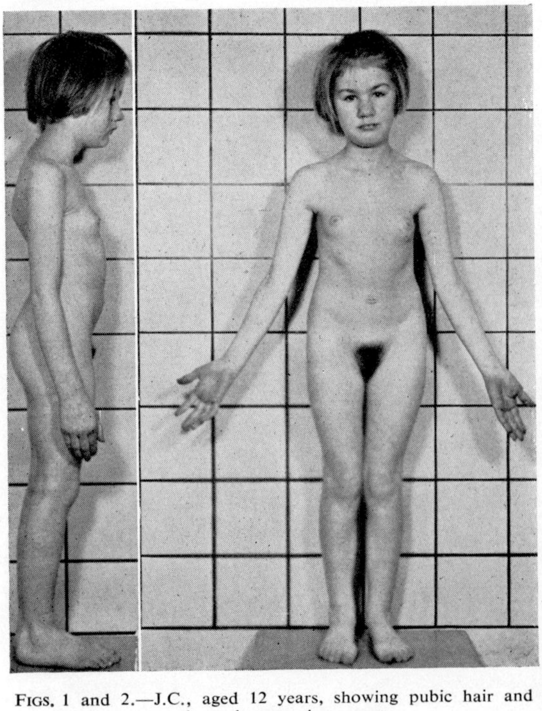

FIGS. 1 and 2.—J.C., aged 12 years, showing pubic hair and moderate breast enlargement.

* Now at The Harriet Lane Home, The Johns Hopkins Hospital, Baltimore, U.S.A.

to recurrent attacks of bronchopneumonia. A systolic cardiac murmur was detected at 5 years of age by the school doctor. At the age of 8 years she was admitted to a second hospital with severe enteritis, in a semi-conscious, collapsed state requiring a blood transfusion of two pints. She recovered within a week after chemotherapy. A lateral radiograph of the chest taken at this time already showed a moderate degree of osteoporosis of the spine with biconcave vertebrae.

Following an attack of pneumonia she was admitted to the City General Hospital, Sheffield (under a Dr. Brown) for cardiac investigation, including catheterization and angiography. A diagnosis of ventricular septal defect was made.

At 12 years 8 months regular menstruation started. At this time she still wet her bed about three times a week.

Several records of her height and weight after the age of 8, showed these all to be below the third percentile (Stuart, Anthropometric chart). Her parents and her only sibling, a 14-year-old sister, were well and of average height: father, 5 ft. 11 in.; mother, 5 ft. 6 in.; sister, 5 ft. 6 in.

Physical Examination. She was a cheerful but emotionally immature girl, retarded mentally with an I.Q. of 63 (Dr. K. Soddy). She was small and slender with a dorsal kyphosis and a short neck.

Her measurements at 12 years of age were as follows:

Height	46 inches
Upper segment	$22\frac{1}{2}$,,
Lower segment	$23\frac{1}{2}$,,
Head circumference ..	18 ,,
Arm span	$49\frac{1}{2}$,,

There was therefore proportional dwarfism with microcephaly. She had pubic and axillary hair with moderate breast enlargement. There was no skin pigmentation, cyanosis or clubbing.

Her heart apex beat was at the fifth left intercostal space in the anterior axillary line. There was a loud blowing systolic murmur, without a thrill, maximal at the third interspace at the left sternal border. The peripheral pulses were normal and the blood pressure was 105/70.

On walking up four flights of stairs slowly, she became pale, slightly cyanosed and breathless. Her chest movements were symmetrical and moderately good, with a prolonged expiratory phase. The percussion note was normal but there were coarse crepitations over both lungs.

No abnormality was found in the nervous system. Her sight and hearing were quite normal. Her fundi appeared normal. There was no evidence of a cerebellar or other motor disorder. Her tendon reflexes were normal and her plantar responses flexor.

The liver, spleen and kidneys were not palpable and a normal sized uterus could be felt rectally. Her external genitalia appeared normal. Her teeth were in good condition and normal for her age and size.

Investigations. BIOCHEMICAL. A calcium balance was performed in the Metabolic Ward with the usual full precautions (Fig. 3). The child was given a constant normal diet throughout which approximated to her previous home diet. After six days' equilibration, six-day faecal specimens were collected between carmine markers, and also three-day urines. These, together with the diet, were analysed for total calcium. After the first two six-day control periods pure dihydrotachysterol (DHT) was given orally as indicated in Fig. 3. Professor Dent reports on the results as follows: 'It was unfortunate that a capricious appetite led to slightly inconstant intake as shown. In addition the most important balance period (the fourth) at the height of the vitamin D intoxication had to be scrapped owing to vomiting. The control balance is less positive than it should be for a child of her age. The sudden rise and fall in plasma and urine calcium coinciding with giving and stopping the DHT are clear and unequivocal. They indicate an excessive, sudden vitamin D-like action. The balance changes are more ambiguous but there was no markedly positive balance induced by the DHT. The unusual clinical and biochemical sensitivity to the DHT is fully consistent with the diagnosis of severe osteoporosis and definitely excludes any possibility of there being any form of dietary or metabolic rickets. It also means that she cannot benefit from administration of large doses of vitamin D in any of its forms.'

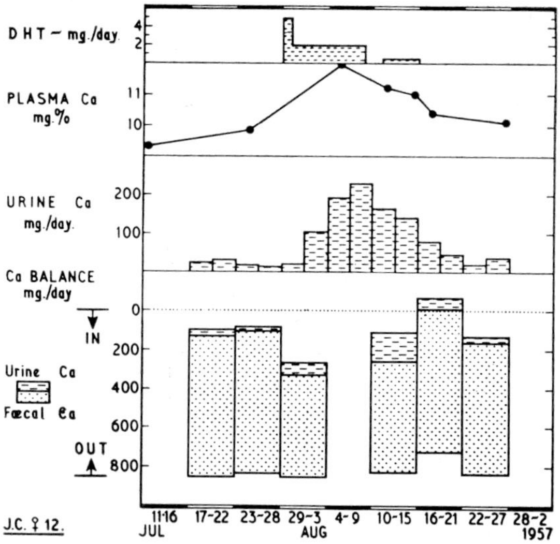

FIG. 3.—Calcium balance.

Vitamin A absorption was normal. Five-day fat balance: absorption 94·5%. Glucose tolerance: blood sugars fasting 105 mg. %, then half-hourly after 23·5 g. glucose, 135, 152, 125, 110 mg. % (normal). Plasma values are shown in Table 1.

Urinary gonadotrophin was 10 units/24 hr. and urinary oestrone 1·9 g./24 hr., oestradiol 1·5 g./24 hr., and oestriol 1·0 g./24 hr.

A urinary amino-acid chromatogram was normal. Serum proteins: total 7·4 g. %; albumin: 4·7 g. %;

TABLE 1

PLASMA VALUES

Date	Plasma Calcium (mg./100 ml.)	Plasma Phosphate (mg./100 ml.)	Plasma Alkaline Phosphatase (K.A. units/100 ml.)	Plasma Urea (mg./100 ml.)
18.6.57 ..	9·3	5·3	16·5	30
25.7.57 ..	9·8	5·0	14·0	54
26.8.57 ..	10·1	4·6		48

globulin: 2·7 g. %, A/G 1·7. Plasma electrophoresis was normal. Plasma cholesterol was 149 mg. % and plasma bicarbonate: 24·2 mEq./l. Plasma chloride: 103 mEq./l., plasma sodium: 139 mEq./l., plasma potassium: 4·3 mEq./l. Renal function tests showed a maximum urea clearance of 34·6%, 43%; a urine concentration test 1,020 (5 specimens after 8-14 hr. dehydration) and a urine dilution test of 1,003.

HAEMATOLOGICAL. Hb 67%, 84%, 82%, 80%. W.B.C., 19.7.57: 27,000/c.mm. (neut. 82·5%, lymph. 11·5%, monos. 6%); 20.8.57: 16,000/c.mm. (neut. 95·0 %, lymph. 4·0%, monos. 1%). E.S.R. 35, 40, 30, 40 mm./hr.

OTHER INVESTIGATIONS. Routine urine tests were normal. Chromosomal sex: (buccal smear) chromatin positive. Complement fixation test for toxoplasmosis: negative; dye test for toxoplasmosis: 1:8 (Dr. I. A. B. Cathie). Deciduous teeth: (Professor Prophet) teeth small, structure and histology normal. E.C.G. and E.E.G. were normal. Radio iodine uptake: 40·1%, normal. Sweat electrolytes: not increased (Shwachman palmar plate method).

Radiographs (Dr. C. J. Hodson) showed: bilateral calcification of the basal ganglia of the skull not seen on skull radiographs done in 1951 (Figs. 4 and 5); a moderate osteoporosis of the spine with biconcave vertebrae (Fig. 6); moderate osteoporosis of the long bones; probably a stone in the right kidney (straight radiograph) I.V.P.: normal. No definite signs of stone seen. Chest: marked cardiac enlargement, probably affecting mainly the right side, with some evidence of increased vascularity. Bone age: 11 years.

Discussion

The unusual finding of radiologically demonstrable symmetrical calcification of the basal ganglia with osteoporosis and the subsequent discovery of a probable renal calculus, suggested the possibility of gross disorder of calcium metabolism. Studies were therefore undertaken by Professor Dent in the Metabolic Ward. They confirmed the radiological diagnosis of osteoporosis as distinct from rickets (or osteomalacia), and at the same time excluded any possibility of the presence of true or pseudo-hypoparathyroidism.

The low levels obtained in the maximum urea clearance test (34·6% and 43%) may indicate a diminished renal functional reserve in spite of a nearly normal blood urea.

Radiologically demonstrable calcification of the basal ganglia was first reported by Fritzsche (1935) in two brothers and a sister examined in the third decade. They had been retarded since childhood.

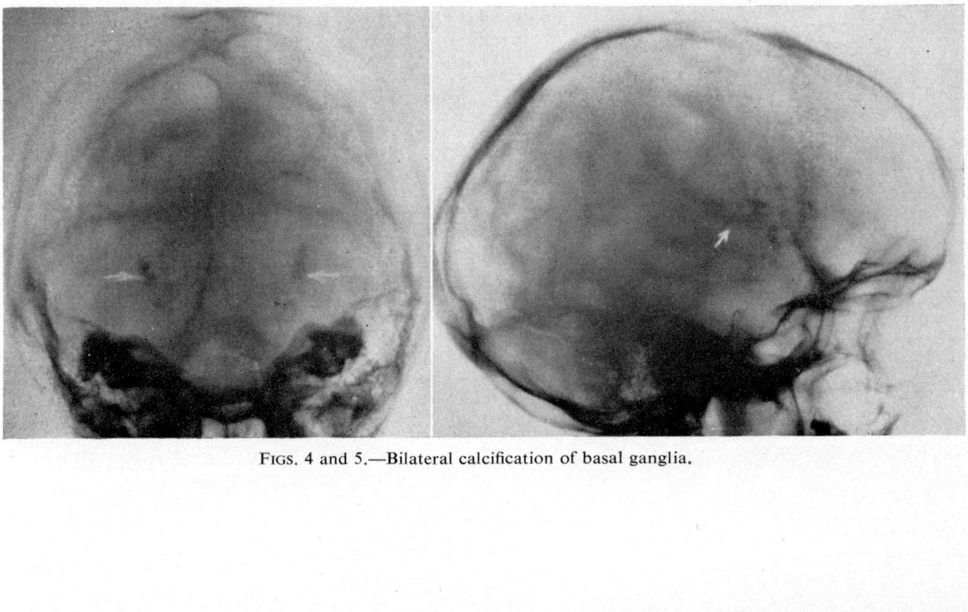

FIGS. 4 and 5.—Bilateral calcification of basal ganglia.

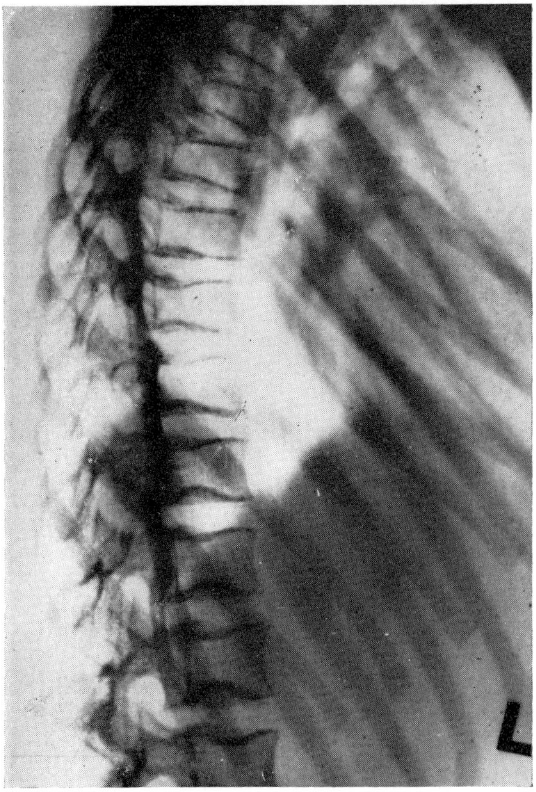

FIG. 6.—Moderate osteoporosis of spine with biconcave vertebrae.

Two had fits and two had a progressive muscular rigidity without tremor. The parents were consanguinous and inheritance by a recessive gene was suggested by the author. Kasanin and Crank (1935) described a male, aged 32 years, who had a 10-year history of convulsions. He became mentally retarded and developed a progressive spasticity. At necropsy, extensive cerebral calcification was found. The fundamental lesion was degeneration of the finer blood vessels, with the production of an iron-containing albuminoid matrix on which calcium was precipitated. Eaton, Camp and Love (1939) reported six cases of calcification of the basal ganglia. Of these, Cases 1, 2 and 6 were probably due to hypoparathyroidism. Case 3 was a 55-year-old female with syphilis and thyrotoxicosis. Case 4 was a male, aged 31 years, who presented with a hemiplegia. Case 5 was a female of 40 years with 'obvious mental retardation' and a basal metabolic rate of +39%. Rand, Olsen and Courville (1943) described a 24-year-old female who had always been a problem child. She also suffered from epilepsy and hypertension, but showed no evidence of hypoparathyroidism. Neill and Dingwall (1950) described two brothers, aged 16 years and 11 years, with microcephaly, optic atrophy and retinal degeneration. They were mentally retarded and had an unsteady gait, gross tremor and dysarthria. Radiologically they had calcification of the basal ganglia and osteoporosis. The elder became almost completely deaf. The authors considered that these signs resembled those present in the syndrome of progeria. Retinal changes and ataxia were also present in the cases described by Strobos, De la Torre and Martin (1957). Foley (1951) described a female, aged 60 years, who four years earlier developed a progressive illness characterized by slow movements, failing memory and frequent attacks of vertigo. She was mentally retarded with an I.Q. of 79. Her lower limbs were spastic. Her daughters, aged 28 and 21 years, though symptomless, both showed calcification of the basal ganglia. Sammet and Bucy (1951) described a male, aged 43 years, with calcification of the basal ganglia. He was a dipsomaniac but had no mental or neurological disturbance. Strobos *et al.* (1957) described two brothers, aged 48 and 44 years, with dysarthria, ataxia and heavy pigmentation of both maculae, showing calcification of the basal ganglia. Twenty-eight other members of the family were examined but no other cases of calcification were found. The authors include arteriosclerosis, encephalitis, tuberous sclerosis and toxic adenoma of the thyroid as causes of radiologically visible calcification of the basal ganglia. Matthews (1957) described a family of three sisters, aged 54, 61 and 59 years, who showed a slowly progressive neurological disorder resembling Parkinsonism. The two elder sisters showed calcification of the basal ganglia. The youngest had not been radiographed. The blood chemistry was normal but as no response was obtained to parathyroid hormone administered intravenously, the author suggested that these cases may represent a 'different fraction' of pseudo-hypoparathyroidism.

The presence of dwarfism, congenital heart disease and osteoporosis in a patient with female configuration, suggested the diagnosis of gonadal dysgenesis (Turner's syndrome). The absence of anomalies such as neck webbing or valgus elbow, or the presence of pubertal changes, or even the occurrence of menstruation is compatible with the diagnosis (Hoffenberg and Jackson, 1957). However, the present case was not thought to be an example of this condition. The urinary excretion of gonadotrophic hormone was normal and the chromosomal sex was female (Dr. G. I. M. Swyer). Direct inspection of the gonads at laparotomy was not thought justified, especially as some authorities believe that both complete gonads must be examined histologically before gonadal dysgenesis can be ruled out.

In conclusion, the metabolic studies failed to reveal a cause for the osteoporosis or calcification of the basal ganglia, or the probable presence of a renal calculus. A genetic aetiology is suggested by the presence of multiple, apparently unconnected abnormalities.

Summary

A 12-year-old girl is described with dwarfism, mental retardation, and a ventricular septal defect. Radiologically she showed calcification of the basal ganglia, generalized osteoporosis and probably a renal calculus. Her blood chemistry was normal. There was no evidence of a hereditary disorder.

The diagnosis of hypoparathyroidism and gonadal dysgenesis were considered, but discarded. No similar case has been found described in the literature on idiopathic symmetrical calcification of the basal ganglia.

I am grateful to Dr. R. E. Bonham Carter for permission to publish this case which was under his care. Acknowledgments are due to Professor Dent for allowing me to publish the results of the calcium balance and for reading the text. I should like to thank Dr. N. R. Butler for many helpful suggestions and all those mentioned in the article for the special investigations.

References

This case was published briefly in the proceedings of The Royal Society of Medicine (1958), **51**, 736.

Albright, F., Burnett, C. H., Smith, P. H. and Parson, W. (1942). *Endocrinology*, **30**, 922.

Eaton, L. M., Camp, J. D. and Love, J. G. (1939). *Arch. Neurol. Psychiat. (Chicago)*, **41**, 921.

Foley, J. (1951). *J. Neurol. Neurosurg. Psychiat.*, **14**, 253.

Fritzsche, R. (1935). *Schweiz. Arch. Neurol. Psychiat.*, **35**, 1.

Hoffenberg, R. and Jackson, W. P. U. (1957). *Brit. med. J.*, **2**, 1457.

Kasanin, J. and Crank, R. P. (1935). *Arch. Neurol. Psychiat. (Chicago)*, **34**, 164.

MacGregor, M. E. and Whitehead, T. P. (1954). *Arch. Dis. Childh.*, **29**, 398.

Matthews, W. B. (1957). *J. Neurol., Neurosurg. Psychiat.*, **20**, 172.

Neill, Catherine A. and Dingwall, Mary M. (1950). *Arch. Dis. Childh.*, **25**, 213.

Rand, C. W., Olsen, C. W. and Courville, C. B. (1943). *Bull. Los Angeles neurol. Soc.*, **8**, 118.

Sammet, J. F. and Bucy, P. C. (1951). *Amer. J. Roentgenol.*, **66**, 880.

Strobos, R. R. J., Torre, E. de la and Martin, J. F. (1957). *Brain*, **80**, 313.

Stuart, H. C. *Anthropometric Chart*, The Children's Medical Center, Boston, Mass.

Sutton, D. (1951). *Brit. J. Radiol.*, **24**, 31.

SULPHOBROMOPHTHALEIN EXCRETION IN PREMATURE INFANTS

BY

THOMAS E. OPPÉ and IRENE E. GIBBS*

From the Department of Child Health, University of Bristol, and the Departments of Paediatrics and Pathology Southmead General Hospital, Bristol

(RECEIVED FOR PUBLICATION OCTOBER 6, 1958)

It is probable that 'physiological' jaundice of the newborn is due primarily to the inability of certain immature and fullterm infants to synthesize glucuronides efficiently. Glucuronides are formed by the transfer of glucuronic acid from uridine di-phosphate glucuronic acid (U.D.P.G.A.) to acceptor substances such as bilirubin. This reaction is enzymic and is carried out largely by the liver, although other organs may participate. It has been shown by experiments *in vitro*, using both human and animal liver tissue, that the activity of the liver in performing glucuronide synthesis is absent until about mid-gestation, rises slowly up to birth and then increases quite rapidly until adult values are reached at 14-20 days of post-natal life.

It is of fundamental interest to know whether the development of these enzyme systems is a function of chronological maturity or whether it is largely an adaptive process brought about by the necessities and opportunities of extra-uterine life. In the premature infant failure to acquire bilirubin homeostasis may result in kernikterus which renders the problem of more than academic concern. It seemed worth while, therefore, to examine the ability of the premature infant to clear sulphobromophthalein (B.S.P.), a substance which is believed to undergo excretion by the liver as a glucuronide. This dye is in general use as a test of 'liver function' and has been applied previously to infants, although not in an endeavour to obtain evidence concerning glucuronide synthesis.

Materials and Methods

The B.S.P. excretion curve was obtained in 34 premature infants. Three groups were selected: (1) Infants aged 0-24 hours (14 infants); (2) infants aged 5 days (10 infants); (3) Infants aged 14 days (10 infants). Apart from post-natal age no special selection took place and infants were tested as available. The test was not performed on babies whose low birth weight might have been due to placental insufficiency nor were ill infants investigated. Jaundice was not regarded as a contra-indication if there was no evidence of haemolytic disease. Some tests were attempted but failed for technical reasons, and these are not included in the results. The infants received routine premature care which included the administration of potassium menaphthosulphate (Vikastab) 2 mg. soon after birth. In order to ensure that this vitamin K analogue did not affect the B.S.P. test, it was not given to three of the 1-day-old babies.

The B.S.P. excretion test was modified in order to reduce venepuncture to a minimum and to allow estimation of B.S.P. on small samples of blood. The following procedure was adopted. At the beginning of the test at least 1 ml. of whole blood was drawn by heel prick to provide a serum blank and for micro-estimation of serum bilirubin (Evelyn and Malloy). The test dose of sulphobromophthalein, 5 mg. per kg. body weight diluted in 1 ml. of sterile normal saline, was injected slowly into an antecubital or superficial ankle vein. Following the injection of B.S.P., 0·5 ml. samples of capillary blood were obtained by heel prick at five, 15, 30 and 45 minutes and at one hour. These times were accurately recorded. No local or general reactions were observed in any of the infants.

Estimation of B.S.P. The blood was collected into small centrifuge tubes without anti-coagulant. The samples were incubated at 37° C. for one to two hours before centrifuging in order to aid clot retraction. The serum was drawn off and the test solutions made up as follows: Serum 0·1 ml. Buffer 0·1 ml. (Sorënsen glycine buffer (*p*H 10·48) made up to molar strength). Water 0·8 ml. Each test solution was read in the spectrophotometer against its own blank which comprised serum 0·1 ml. and 0·9 ml. isotonic Na_2SO_4. The optical density readings were obtained with the Hilgar 'Spekker' instrument with filter No. 606 (corresponding to 580 mμ), and the 1 cm. micro cell was used for the solutions.

* Research assistant with a grant from the South Western Regional Hospital Board.

A calibrations curve was made using a standard solution of B.S.P., 10 mg. per 100 ml. in serial dilutions as follows:

Standard Solution of B.S.P. (ml.)	Serum (ml.)	Buffer (ml.)	Water (ml.)	B.S.P. (mg./100 ml.)
0·1	0·1	0·1	0·7	2
0·2	0·1	0·1	0·6	4
0·3	0·1	0·1	0·5	6
0·4	0·1	0·1	0·4	8
0·5	0·1	0·1	0·3	10

These solutions were read in the same instrument against a blank solution containing serum 0·1 ml.; isotonic Na_2SO_4 0·9 ml.

The B.S.P. excretion curve was drawn for each infant by plotting the amount of B.S.P. in mg. % remaining in the serum against time after injection of B.S.P. At least five points were obtained for each infant. If the amount of B.S.P. remaining in the serum is converted into logarithms the B.S.P. excretion is transformed into two straight lines whose slopes can be measured. The first rapid phase of B.S.P. removal we have termed Slope I, the second slower phase, Slope II. As we have modified the standard B.S.P. excretion test in order to use capillary blood, it was necessary to perform our test on adults. Altogether 23 adult volunteers without liver disease were tested. In six, parallel samples of venous and capillary blood were used for estimation of B.S.P. We were satisfied that the method used with infants was comparable with standard methods.

Results

The results are most conveniently expressed in terms of the two phases of B.S.P. excretion as measured by Slopes I and II of the semi-log plot: and also conventionally as the percentage of B.S.P. retained in the blood at 45 minutes. These results for individual babies are given in Tables 1, 2 and 3, together with correlations for sex, birth weight and incidence of jaundice. It should be noted that the 1-day-old babies (Table 1) have been classified according to the presence or absence of hypoxia. Although no infant was sick at the time the estimation was performed, some infants had undergone a period of respiratory difficulty marked by dyspnoea, apnoeic attacks or intermittent cyanotic spells. Except for Case 12, this was not serious, but it nevertheless appears to have markedly affected the results of the B.S.P. excretion test in the 1-day-old babies.

Jaundice was marked present or absent on clinical grounds. It applied to the neonatal course of the baby as well as to conditions existing at the time of the B.S.P. test. A baby was classified as 'jaundiced' if the icterus was sufficient to justify estimating the serum bilirubin. In the cases so classified serum bilirubin values of more than 10 mg. % (Malloy and Evelyn) were found. It can

TABLE 1

FOURTEEN PREMATURE INFANTS UNDER 1 DAY OF AGE WITH AND WITHOUT RESPIRATORY DISTRESS

No.	Sex	Gestational Age (weeks)	Weight (g.)	Slope I	Slope II	% B.S.P. Retention at 45 min.	Jaundice
1	F	39	2,240	0·02	—	18·6	—
2	M	38	1,814	0·04	0·013	11·5	—
3	F	35	2,353	0·05	0·004	11·2	—
4	F	34	1,729	0·03	0·006	17·4	—
5	F	34	1,588	0·04	0·002	20·8	+
6	F	37	2,410	0·04	0·008	17·0	—
7	M	37	2,041	0·02	0·011	10·7	—
Means			2,025 Infants 4-23 hours age	0·03	0·006 No respiratory distress	15·3	
8	M	38	2,410	0·03	0·001	14·6	—
9	M	38	2,155	0·02	0·001	18·6	+
10	M	37	1,724	0·02	0·002	23·9	—
11	F	36	2,155	0·06	0·005	8·1	+
12	F	38	2,126	0·02	0·001	33·1	Died
13	M	35	1,588	0·02	0·009	23·9	—
14	M	36	1,899	0·01	0·006	36·3	—
Means			2,008 Infants 4-23 hours age	0·03	0·004 Respiratory distress	22·6	

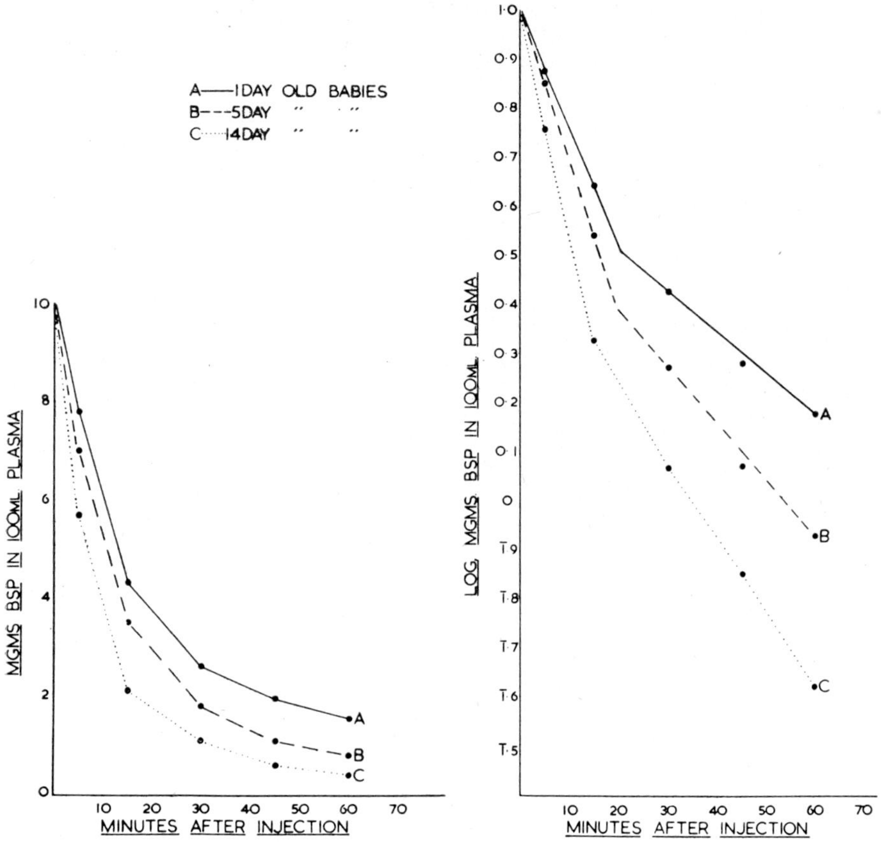

FIG. 1.—Mean B.S.P. excretion curves in three groups of babies after intravenous injection of B.S.P. 5 mg. per kg. body weight.

TABLE 2

TEN PREMATURE INFANTS 5 DAYS OF AGE

No.	Sex	Gestational Age (weeks)	Weight (g.)	Slope I	Slope II	% B.S.P. Retention at 45 min.	Jaundice
15	M	34	2,013	0·03	0·012	12·3	+
16	M	36	2,183	0·03	0·006	9·3	+
17	M	32	1,871	0·02	0·015	7·1	+
18	F	36	1,814	0·04	0·020	5·6	+
19	M	37	1,928	0·02	0·001	18·6	+
20	M	38	2,410	0·04	0·010	10·9	+
21	M	37	2,182	0·02	0·013	13·2	—
22	M	37	1,984	0·04	0·010	15·8	—
23	F	38	2,353	0·03	0·008	13·8	+
24	M	35	2,296	0·04	0·010	15·5	—
Means			2,103	0·03	0·011	12·2	

be seen by inspection of the tables that jaundice did not correlate with poor ability to excrete B.S.P.

Mean excretion curves for the three groups of infants are shown in Fig. 1. It is apparent that there is a progressive trend toward adult excretion of B.S.P. from the 1-day to the 14-day-old infants. Although both stages of B.S.P. excretion are slower in the youngest infants, the most marked differences are in the excretory phase (Slope II) and in the 45-minute retention values. The difference in 45-minute retention between the 1-day and 14-day-old babies is statistically highly significant (P = 0·005).

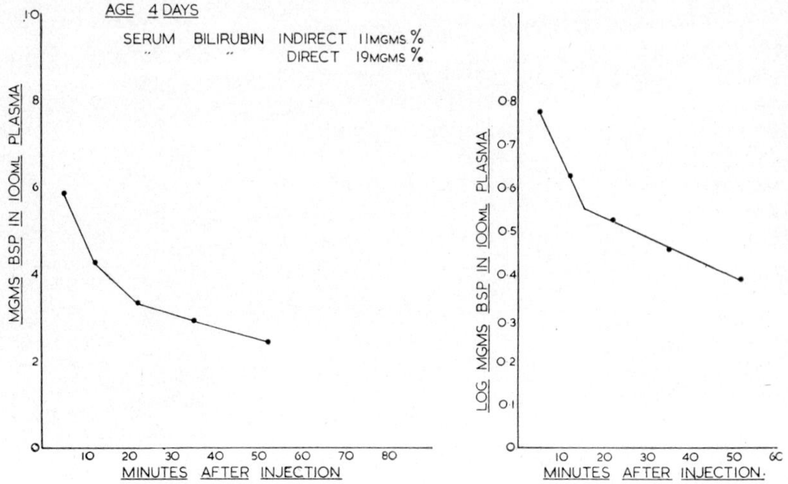

FIG. 3.—B.S.P. excretion curve of infant aged 4 days with 'inspissated bile syndrome'.

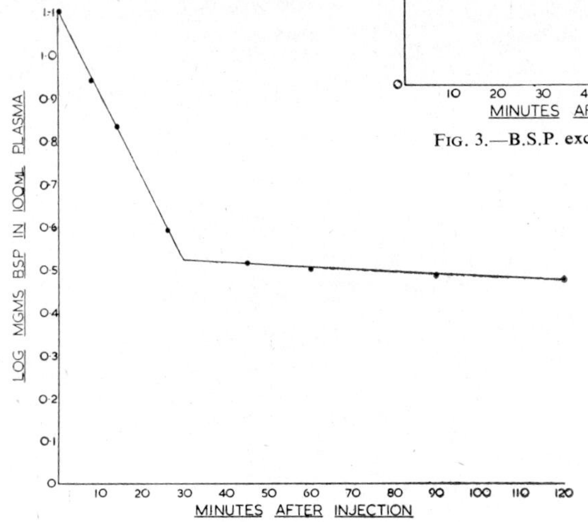

FIG. 2.—B.S.P. excretion curve in infant with atresia of bile ducts.

As an aid to the interpretation of the excretion curves the opportunity was taken to perform the test on infants known to have obstructive jaundice. The curves of two such infants, a case of congenital atresia of the bile ducts (Fig. 2) and a case of haemolytic disease with obstructive jaundice ('inspissated bile syndrome') (Fig. 3) are shown. In the case of the latter infant it is noteworthy that the abnormal curve is due to the biliary obstruction not to the haemolytic disease as two cases of severe haemolytic disease without direct reacting bilirubin in the serum gave normal curves.

TABLE 3

TEN PREMATURE INFANTS 14 DAYS OF AGE

No.	Sex	Gestational Age (weeks)	Weight (g.)	Slope I	Slope II	% B.S.P. Retention at 45 min.	Jaundice
25	F	37	1,871	0·06	0·031	2·1	—
26	F	38	2,381	0·06	0·009	6·5	+
27	M	34	1,474	0·06	0·009	7·5	+
28	F	36	2,155	0·04	0·012	13·3	+
29	M	33	1,474	0·03	0·020	7·9	+
30	M	38	2,265	0·04	0·014	9·8	—
31	M	37	2,070	0·05	0·009	10·0	—
32	M	38	1,474	0·04	0·020	5·1	—
33	F	36	1,304	0·04	0·008	10·0	—
34	M	36	1,389	0·03	0·020	8·9	—
Means			1,786	0·05	0·015	8·1	

Discussion

Sulphobromophthalein (B.S.P.) has been used by several investigators to test 'liver function' in newborn infants. There is general agreement that during the first few days of life B.S.P. is inadequately cleared by both fullterm (Mollison and Cutbush, 1949; Yudkin, Gellis and Lappen, 1949) and premature infants (Obrinsky, Denley and Brauer, 1952). Direct comparison of our results with those of previous workers is not possible because of differences in method, and selection of cases. However, it is clear that a progressive improvement in the ability of infants to remove B.S.P. from the circulation takes place during the first 21 days of post-natal life. The impairment of B.S.P. clearance noted in the first few days of life is not clearly related to gestational age, birth weight or the incidence of jaundice. It seems likely, therefore, that the development of the excretory mechanism for B.S.P. is part of the physiological process of adaptation to extra-uterine life rather than a function only of maturity. We have, in addition to confirming these facts, showed that perinatal hypoxia of even mild degree can result in demonstrable further impairment of B.S.P. clearance.

Sulphobromophthalein is an unphysiological substance which is excreted almost exclusively in the bile (Rosenthal and White, 1925). Following intravenous injection it disappears rapidly from the blood at a rate which is influenced by several factors, including hepatic blood flow, metabolism within the liver cell and the patency of the bile ducts. Although the metabolism of B.S.P. is incompletely understood, its chemical relationship with other phenolic compounds, such as phenolphthalein, leads one to expect it to be excreted as a glucuronide. There is *in vitro* evidence that this is so (Brown and Burnett, 1957). For this reason it is permissible to regard the metabolism of B.S.P. as similar in some respects to that of bilirubin which is also excreted in the bile as a glucuronide (Schmid, 1956).

There is now much direct experimental evidence that the enzyme systems concerned with glucuronide formation have only limited activity in foetal and early neonatal life. Lathe and Walker (1957) demonstrated poor bilirubin conjugation by newborn human liver slices and Dutton (1958) has shown only negligible amounts of glucuronide formation in human foetal liver and kidney. Brown and Zuelzer (1958), working with the microsomal fractions of guinea pig liver, have demonstrated increasing conjugating activity from almost zero at mid-gestation to near adult at 14-20 days of post-natal life. At least two enzymes, uridine-diphosphate-glucose dehydrogenase and glucuronyl transferase, are concerned in this reaction and it is the diminished activity of these enzymes which is responsible for the restricted conjugation ability of foetal and neonatal tissues. It is of interest to note that other enzyme systems essential in post-natal life, but not required in foetal life, also show negligible activity in foetal and early neonatal life, as has been demonstrated by Kenney, Reem and Kretchmer (1958) for phenylalanine hydroxylase and glucose-6-phosphatase.

It is tempting to ascribe the defect in B.S.P. excretion, which we have shown, to a conjugation deficiency. Were this so it is clear that the events of post-natal life are more important than gestational age and birth weight in bringing the process to maturity. This suggests strongly that during foetal life the conjugation mechanism is dormant and is either excited by the stimulus of birth or released from inhibition. Whether birth acts as a stimulus because of the cessation of placental function forcing the baby to conjugate its own bilirubin and other substances or whether the change in the *milieu interieur* of the liver in regard to temperature and oxygenation is the main factor is uncertain. Both factors may be of consequence. Stempfel, Broman, Escardó and Zetterström (1956) have shown that infants with severe haemolytic disease of the newborn may be born with significant amounts of conjugated (direct-reacting) bilirubin in the cord blood. This suggests that hepatic conjugation takes place during intra-uterine life if massive haemolysis creates a large enough bilirubin overload. On the other hand, our results showing the effects of even mild hypoxia in post-natal life suggest that changes in the internal environment of the liver are of equal importance. Some of the effects of anoxia on liver blood flow and function have been reviewed by Andrews (1957) and it is clear that the metabolism of the liver is extremely susceptible to changes in oxygenation.

However, we cannot assume with confidence that B.S.P. excretion is identical with that of bilirubin. There is no direct relationship between poor B.S.P. elimination and the presence of jaundice. Some babies who clear B.S.P. rapidly become jaundiced and some of the poor B.S.P. excretors maintain effective bilirubin homeostasis. Furthermore, it has been reported that humans suffering from congenital hyperbilirubinaemia due to defective conjugation have normal B.S.P. excretion (Crigler and Najjar, 1952); the same is true of congenitally jaundiced rats (Axelrod, Schmid and Hammaker, 1957). While we have not succeeded in showing that the degree of chronological maturity is of importance in determining B.S.P. clearance, there is abundant evidence that prematurity is of importance in relation to hyperbilirubinaemia (Billing, Cole and Lathe, 1954; Meyer, 1956). In this connexion it is noteworthy that environmental factors, such as aceto-menaphthon (Synkayvit) (Bound and Telfer, 1956; Meyer and Angus, 1956); and sulphafurazole (Gantrisin) (Silverman, Andersen, Blanc and Crozier, 1956), do exert a profound effect on the incidence and severity of neonatal jaundice. In spite of these inconsistencies in the parallel between bilirubin and B.S.P. metabolism we feel that the demonstrated impairment of B.S.P. clearance is related to a conjugation defect, but other explanations must be discussed.

It is possible that some form of biliary obstruction might explain the abnormal B.S.P. curves and it is therefore of interest to compare the infants in the first days of life with those with obstructive jaundice. In both instances the initial phase of B.S.P. removal (Slope I) is rapidly accomplished. This is probably related to liver blood flow. The most marked changes are in the second phase. The completely obstructed infant, P.D., showed a flat Stage II slope (Fig. 2) while an infant with neonatal 'hepatitis' and the infant with 'inspissated bile syndrome' (Fig. 3) showed curves not dissimilar to the normal first-day infants. We reject, however, the interpretation that the first day curves are due to biliary obstruction. If retention or regurgitation of bile occurred regularly in the first few days of life evidence of conjugated bilirubin would be expected in the blood and urine, but none is found. If this absence of conjugated bilirubin is ascribed to lack of conjugation, then hyperbilirubinaemia should always occur. Most often it does not. Biliary obstruction cannot explain the impaired B.S.P. clearance in non-jaundiced infants. Obrinsky *et al.* (1952) thought that post-natal circulatory adjustments consequent upon birth and affecting the blood flow to the liver were an important factor. If this were so, alterations in the first phase of B.S.P. removal would be prominent. We were unable to show marked alterations in Slope I and in this are at variance with Obrinsky and his colleagues. However, their data do not show that complete excretion curves were obtained on each baby and it is only by obtaining adequate early samples that deductions as to the first stage can be made. The clearance of B.S.P. is related to its concentration in the hepatic arteries and the metabolic activity of the bile ducts (Andrews, 1955). We can offer no evidence on these points, although they may well be of significance in regard to the interpretation of our findings.

Summary

The B.S.P. excretion test has been applied to three groups of premature infants aged 1 day, 5 days and 14 days respectively.

The curves obtained show a progressive change towards adult values related to post-natal age but not gestational age, birth weight or jaundice.

Mild hypoxia produces a further impairment of B.S.P. excretion in the infants less than 24 hours old.

The relationship between these findings and hyperbilirubinaemia of prematurity is discussed.

This work was made possible by a grant from the South Western Regional Hospital Board to Dr. Irene Gibbs. We are grateful to Professor A. V. Neale and Dr. Beryl Corner for much encouragement. Dr. F. J. W. Lewis, Director of the Department of Pathology, Southmead Hospital, gave generously of laboratory facilities and advice. Dr. J. Tovey helped at all stages of the investigation and helped perform many of the tests on adults. We are especially grateful to Sister Luffman of the Premature Baby Unit for her co-operation, without which the work would not have been possible.

References

Andrews, W. H. H. (1955). *Lancet*, **2**, 166.
—— (1957). *Brit. med. Bull.*, **13**, 82.
Axelrod, J., Schmid., R. and Hammaker, L. (1957). *Nature* (*Lond.*), **180**, 1426.
Billing, B. H., Cole, P. G. and Lathe, G. H. (1954). *Brit. med. J.*, **2**, 1263.
Bound, J. P. and Telfer, T. P. (1956). *Lancet*, **1**, 720.
Brown, Audrey K. and Burnett, H. (1957). *A.M.A. J. Dis. Child.*, **94**, 510.
—— and Zuelzer, W. W. (1958). *J. clin. Invest.*, **37**, 332.
Crigler, J. F. and Najjar, V. A. (1952). *Pediatrics*, **10**, 169.
Dutton, G. J. (1958). *Lancet*, **2**, 49.
Kenney, F. T., Reem, G. H. and Kretchmer, N. (1958). *Science*, **127**, 86.
Lathe, G. H. and Walker, M. (1957). *Biochem. J.*, **67**, 9P.
Meyer, T. C. (1956). *Arch. Dis. Childh.*, **31**, 75.
—— and Angus, J. (1956). *Ibid.*, **31**, 212.
Mollison, P. L. and Cutbush, Marie (1949). *Ibid.*, **24**, 7.
Obrinsky, W., Denley, M. L. and Brauer, R. W. (1952). *Pediatrics*, **9**, 421.
Rosenthal, S. M. and White, E. C. (1925). *J. Amer. med. Ass.*, **84**, 1112.
Schmid, R. (1956). *Science*, **124**, 76.
Silverman, W. A., Andersen, Dorothy H., Blanc, W. A. and Crozier, D. N. (1956). *Pediatrics*, **18**, 614.
Stempfel, R., Broman, B., Escardó, F. E. and Zetterström, R. (1956). *Ibid.*, **17**, 471.
Yudkin, S., Gellis, S. S. and Lappen, P. (1949). *Arch. Dis. Childh.*, **24**, 12.

SYSTOLIC MURMURS IN CHILDREN

A SURVEY OF 240 CASES

BY

W. MAINZER, R. PINCOVICI and G. HEYMANN

From the Western Galilee District of Kupat-Holim, Workers' Sick Fund of Israel

(RECEIVED FOR PUBLICATION AUGUST 27, 1958)

The general practitioner has to deal almost daily in his work with the problem of systolic murmurs. He finds such murmurs often in apparently healthy children during a routine check and is then confronted by the question whether to consider these murmurs as of no importance, or to investigate further.

There exists a wide discrepancy among publications on the incidence of systolic murmurs in children in general, the percentage varying from 20% to more than 90% (Lessof and Brigden, 1957). Also on the prevalence of what are termed 'innocent' systolic murmurs, Fogel (1957) quotes a range of 8% to 86·6% from various studies.

In order to throw further light on the problem the authors have surveyed the child population of 13 rural settlements and two educational institutions in the Haifa area with regard to the finding of systolic cardiac murmurs.

Material and Methods

The material consists of all cases in which systolic murmurs were found among a total of 2,035 children up to the age of 15 years during the year 1957. Each child with a systolic murmur was investigated with regard to history, physical examination, fluoroscopic, electrocardiographic and related laboratory findings. In all cases blood counts were made in order to exclude anaemia as the cause of a systolic murmur, and sedimentation rates were determined in a search for signs of rheumatic fever or other active processes. To narrow down the margin of subjective error in auscultation, each child was examined by all three investigators. From the results obtained, a survey was made of the incidence and clinical significance of the murmurs heard, considering also sex, age, familial occurrence, occurrence among siblings, and ethnic origin. The children were divided into three age groups: from birth to 5 years, from 5 to 10 years, and from 10 to 15 years. As to their ethnic origin, three sections of the population were distinguished: (1) children of western origin, whose parents came from Europe or North-America; (2) children of Mediterranean origin, including Greece, Turkey, North-Africa and also Iraq, though the latter does not border immediately on the Mediterranean Sea; and (3) children from India.

Concerning their clinical significance, the murmurs were classified into four types: (1) innocent murmurs; (2) murmurs indicating possible heart disease; (3) murmurs indicating probable heart disease; and (4) organic murmurs in heart disease. The following standards were applied:

(1) **Innocent Murmurs.** Murmurs in children who did not show any signs of heart disease, either with regard to history, or to physical, laboratory, fluoroscopic or electrocardiographic findings. Wells (1957) writes: 'The decision that a systolic murmur is innocent depends not only on the character of the murmur itself, but also on the absence of any evidence of organic heart disease.'

(2) **Possible Heart Disease.** Murmurs with signs referable to heart disease but not conclusive of structural changes, such as, for instance, an incomplete right bundle branch block in the electrocardiographic pattern, or a slight prominence of the pulmonary conus silhouette.

(3) **Probable Heart Disease.** Murmurs in children with pathological evidence referable to structural changes at the heart, where, however, diagnosis of cardiac disease was still uncertain. Within this category were counted fluoroscopic or electro-

cardiographic evidence of heart hypertrophy, and also left axis shift, which, according to Katz (1949), is not a normal finding in children. A combination of an incomplete right bundle branch block with a prominent pulmonary conus, too, was considered as probably due to heart disease (atrial septal defect) (Wagner and Graham, 1957).

(4) **Heart Disease.** Murmurs in children, where a definite diagnosis of heart disease could be made according to accepted standards.

The quality of the murmurs was defined with relation to intensity, continuity, and, location according to the point of maximum audibility. To indicate the intensity of systolic murmurs, Luisada (1954) recommends the six gradations of Levine. For practical purposes, however, the authors of this paper found it sufficient to use only the three grades of 'faint', 'moderate', and 'loud', as accepted by the Criteria Committee of the New York Heart Association (1955), thereby disregarding the finer distinctions of 'very faint' and 'very loud', which have been added in the latest edition of the nomenclature. This is also in accordance with the opinion of Leopold (1957), quoting Levine and Harvey, that the system of six gradations, when used by different clinicians, may, anyhow, differ by one gradation. When the continuity of the murmurs was considered, a distinction was made between 'constant' and 'inconstant'. Murmurs which could always be heard, regardless of the posture of the patient or of time, were called 'constant', while the term 'inconstant' was given to murmurs which disappeared with a change in posture or could be heard only occasionally during the course of several weeks.

Results

Among 2,035 children examined 240 cases of systolic murmurs were found, i.e. an incidence of 11·8% (Table 1).

TABLE 1

INCIDENCE ACCORDING TO AGE.

0-5 years		5-10 years		10-15 years	
Cases		Cases		Cases	
(No.)	(%)	(No.)	(%)	(No.)	(%)
61	30	106	51	39	19

In this comparison the children of the two educational institutions have not been taken into consideration, as they were only of one age group, namely 10 to 15 years.

A graphic representation of the age-incidence of systolic murmurs shows that the percentage increases from early childhood until it suddenly reaches its peak after the age of 5. It remains highest at the age group from 5 to 10 years and then decreases again towards the age of 15 (Fig. 1).

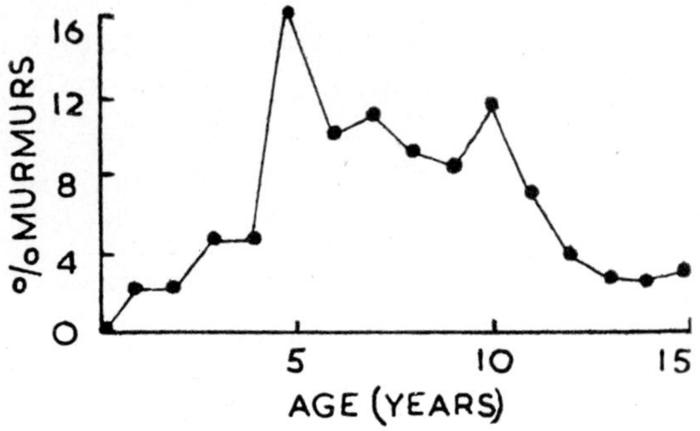

FIG. 1.—Age incidence of systolic murmurs.

More male children were found to have systolic murmurs (56%) than females (44%), this proportion remaining approximately the same at all age groups (Table 2).

TABLE 2

INCIDENCE OF SYSTOLIC MURMURS IN RELATION TO SEX

	0-5 years		5-10 years		10-15 years		Total	
	M.	F.	M.	F.	M.	F.	M.	F.
Cases (No.)	33	28	59	47	34	25	126	100
(%)	54	46	56	44	57	43	56	44

In this compilation the results of one boarding school, at which only boys are received, had, of course, to be omitted. In the course of the analysis of the results in the 13 settlements an interesting fact was encountered, namely that 40% of all systolic murmurs occurred among siblings, i.e. among two or more children of the same parents (Table 3).

TABLE 3

FAMILIAL OCCURRENCE OF SYSTOLIC MURMURS

Murmurs (Total no.)	Familial Cases	
	(No.)	(%)
206	83	40

Among ethnic groups, the Mediterranean had the highest incidence (13%) though only slightly higher

TABLE 4

INCIDENCE WITH REGARD TO ETHNIC ORIGIN

	Children (No.)	Systolic Murmurs (No.)	Systolic Murmurs (%)
Western	986	113	11·5
Mediterranean . .	898	115	13
India	151	12	8

than the Western with 11·5%, while children from India had the lowest rate with 8% (Table 4).

Clinical Significance. Of all systolic murmurs 64·2% were innocent and in only 3·3% of children with systolic murmurs could a definite diagnosis of heart disease be established. About one-third of all murmurs could not be regarded outright as innocent, but many of these showed only slight pathological results after further investigations, while in about 13% there was still doubt as to the diagnosis in spite of significant clinical signs (see Table 5).

TABLE 5

INCIDENCE OF SYSTOLIC MURMURS WITH REGARD TO CLINICAL SIGNIFICANCE

I Innocent Murmurs		II Possible Heart Disease		III Probable Heart Disease		IV Heart Disease	
(No.)	(%)	(No.)	(%)	(No.)	(%)	(No.)	(%)
154	64·2	47	19·5	31	13	8	3·3

A survey of the electrocardiographic findings (Table 6) showed a normal E.C.G. in almost 78% of the children with systolic murmurs.

TABLE 6

MAIN ELECTROCARDIOGRAPHIC PATTERNS

Normal E.C.G.		Left Axis Deviation		Incomplete Right Bundle Branch Block		Left Ventricular Hyper-trophy		Right Ventricular Hyper-trophy	
(No.)	(%)	(No.)	(%)	(No.)	(%)	(No.)	(%)	(No.)	(%)
186	77·5	14	6	30	12·5	8	3	2	1

The results of fluoroscopy are shown in Table 7. Since sometimes more than one change could be found in the same child there are more fluoroscopic findings than there were cases of systolic murmur.

As to the location of systolic murmurs, five different sites of maximum audibility could be discerned in this investigation: (1) parasternal murmurs, which were located at the third or fourth thoracic interspace at the left sternal border; (2) murmurs heard at the so-called 'Erb's point', that is at the third or fourth left interspace, midway between the lateral margin of the sternum and the axillary line, also known as 'secondary aortic area' (Pullen, 1945); (3) murmurs heard over the apex; (4) pulmonic murmurs; and (5) aortic murmurs.

TABLE 7

FLUOROSCOPIC FINDINGS

Normal		Pulmonary Prominence		Aortic Prominence		Mitral Configuration	
(No.)	(%)	(No.)	(%)	(No.)	(%)	(No.)	(%)
201	84	19	8	3	1·2	3	1·2

Aortic Configuration		Left Ventricular Hypertrophy		Right Ventricular Hypertrophy		Global Hypertrophy	
(No.)	(%)	(No.)	(%)	(No.)	(%)	(No.)	(%)
2	0·8	10	4	8	3·4	3	1·2

From Table 8 it can be seen that by far the greatest number of systolic murmurs were parasternal (77% of the total and 80% of all innocent murmurs). Then followed the precordial murmurs at Erb's point and the apical murmurs with 10% and 9% respectively. Pulmonic murmurs were only about 4%, and only one case of a systolic murmur over the aortic valve was found, which, incidentally proved to be innocent.

Table 8 also represents the results as to intensity of the murmurs. Most of the murmurs were faint or moderate and only a comparatively small number of loud murmurs were heard (about 4%). However, among the group of heart diseases proper (Table 8*e*) the percentage of loud murmurs was 25%.

The following conditions were distinguished among the eight cases of definite heart disease:

Diagnosis	No. of Cases
Rheumatic heart disease . .	4
Mitral insufficiency . .	3
Patent ductus arteriosus . .	1

Most of the murmurs were constant. Only 19 inconstant murmurs were registered (8%). Eleven of these were innocent murmurs, four indicated possible heart disease, two probable heart disease, and in two cases of heart disease there were also inconstant murmurs (Table 9). As to their location, 12 of the inconstant murmurs were parasternal, four could be heard at Erb's point and three were pulmonic in location. Most of them were faint, one was moderate and one was loud (Table 10).

TABLE 8

QUALITY OF MURMURS IN RELATION TO INTENSITY AND SITE OF MAXIMAL AUDIBILITY

(*a*) TOTAL NUMBER OF SYSTOLIC MURMURS

	Faint		Moderate		Loud		Total	
	(No.)	(%)	(No.)	(%)	(No.)	(%)	(No.)	(%)
Para-sternal	99	41·1	83	35·1	2	0·8	184	77
Erb's point	15	6·3	8	3·2	2	0·8	25	10
Apex ..	3	1·2	15	6·3	3	1·2	21	9
Pulmonic	6	2·4	1	0·4	2	0·8	9	3·6
Aorta ..					1	0·4	1	0·4
Total ..	123	51	107	45	10	4	240	100

(*b*) INNOCENT MURMURS

	Faint		Moderate		Loud		Total	
	(No.)	(%)	(No.)	(%)	(No.)	(%)	(No.)	(%)
Para-sternal	65	42	57	37·3	1	0·7	123	80
Erb's point	6	4	5	3·3	1	0·7	13	8
Apex ..	2	1·4	9	5·2	1	0·7	12	7·3
Pulmonic	4	2·6	1	0·7	1	0·7	6	4
Aorta ..					1	0·7	1	0·7
Total ..	77	50	72	46·5	5	3·5	154	100

(*c*) POSSIBLE HEART DISEASE

	Faint		Moderate		Loud		Total	
	(No.)	(%)	(No.)	(%)	(No.)	(%)	(No.)	(%)
Para-sternal	20	42	15	32			35	74
Erb's point	5	10·5	1	2·5			6	13
Apex ..			4	8			4	8
Pulmonic	1	2·5			1	2·5	2	5
Total ..	26	55	20	42·5	1	2·5	47	100

(*d*) PROBABLE HEART DISEASE

	Faint		Moderate		Loud		Total	
	(No.)	(%)	(No.)	(%)	(No.)	(%)	(No.)	(%)
Para-sternal	11	36	10	32	1	3	22	71
Erb's point	3	10	2	7	1	3	6	20
Apex ..	1	3	1	3			2	6
Pulmonic	1	3					1	3
Total ..	16	52	13	42	2	6	31	100

(*e*) HEART DISEASE.

	Faint		Moderate		Loud		Total	
	(No.)	(%)	(No.)	(%)	(No.)	(%)	(No.)	(%)
Para-sternal	3	37·5	1	12·5			4	50
Apex ..			1	12·5	2	25	3	37·5
Erb's point	1	12·5					1	12·5
Total ..	4	50	2	25	2	25	8	100

TABLE 9

INCONSTANT MURMURS WITH RELATION TO CLINICAL SIGNIFICANCE

	Faint	Moderate	Loud	Total
Innocent	10		1	11
Possible heart disease ..	3		1	4
Probable heart disease ..	1	1		2
Heart disease	2			2
Total	16	1	2	19

TABLE 10

INCONSTANT MURMURS, LOCATION AND INTENSITY

	Faint	Moderate	Loud	Total
Parasternal	11	1		12
Erb's point	3	1		4
Pulmonic	2		1	3
Total	16	2	1	19

Discussion

The incidence of 11·8% systolic murmurs in this survey is relatively low compared to the incidence in most other similar reports, in which it varied from 20% to over 90%. However, Szabo and Ross (1957), who investigated the occurrence of heart diseases among school children of the three major cities of Israel, were struck by the comparatively low incidence, especially of innocent murmurs, in this country; they give a rate of 9% for Haifa. Nevertheless, the age distribution of systolic murmurs corresponds with that found by other authors. The diagram of age-incidence (Fig. 1) follows in principle that given by Epstein (1948), the difference being not the relative incidence at the various age groups, but the absolute numbers, which Epstein found considerably higher. A new fact, of which we found no mention in the literature, is the high percentage of systolic murmurs among siblings. Though only children up to the age of 15 years have been taken into consideration, many other cases are known to the authors in which at least one parent, or another brother or sister above the age group investigated, had a systolic murmur. This would put the familial occurrence of systolic murmurs even higher than the 40% reported. It appears, therefore, that a familial factor is involved in the problem of systolic murmurs. The nature of such a factor is not known. A possible explanation, in accordance with the theory that innocent murmurs arise from eddy currents caused by a difference in the size of the outlet from the ventricles into the great vessels, would be that the individuals of a family have a similar anatomical cardiac structure.

The question of so-called 'functional', 'accidental', 'haemic' or 'innocent' murmurs has been much discussed among clinicians. The authors have accepted the term 'innocent', originally coined by Evans (1947), generally recommended in recent publications and also adopted by the American (New York) Heart Association (1955). This investigation confirmed the conception that there is no physical criterion for an 'innocent' murmur, with regard either to quality or location. The incidence of innocent murmurs in this survey was 64·2% of all systolic murmurs. This coincides approximately with the percentage by Fogel (1957) of 60·4%.

The group classified as 'possible heart disease' comprised 19·5% of all cases with systolic murmurs. It included those with only slightly abnormal findings on further investigation.

The group of 'probable heart diseases' comprises children with pathological signs referable to structural changes in the heart, but in whom special investigations like angiocardiography or heart catheterisation were not undertaken either because of their general well-being, or because the risks were not considered justifiable. The incidence of these cases was 13%. Systolic murmurs in children with diagnosed heart diseases constituted 3·3%. Altogether the three groups of 'not innocent' murmurs represented 35·8%.

The great importance of the electrocardiographic and fluoroscopic investigations (see Tables 6 and 7) in the differentiation between innocent and not innocent murmurs needs to be especially emphasized.

Most of the recent publications agree that innocent systolic murmurs are loudest at the left sternal border in the third and fourth intercostal spaces (Rhodes, 1955; Stuckey, 1955; Fogel, 1957). The authors can verify this in the present paper not only for innocent murmurs, but for all systolic murmurs (Table 8). Of the innocent murmurs the site of maximal intensity was parasternal (at the left sternal border in the third or fourth intercostal space) in 123 out of 154 cases, that is 80%; Fogel (1957) reports 76%. Among the systolic murmurs indicating possible heart disease 74% were parasternal, of the murmurs of probable heart disease 71%, and of the murmurs in patients with definite heart disease the parasternal location of the murmurs was still preponderant, though its proportion was lower (50%). From these facts it is evident that no conclusion can be drawn from the parasternal location of a systolic murmur regarding either its nature or its clinical significance. The same holds true for the other sites of maximal intensity as can be seen from Table 8.

Similarly, the intensity itself was not of diagnostic significance. In all four groups (Table 8) most of the systolic murmurs were faint in intensity (50% and 55%). A lesser, but still considerable, number of murmurs was moderate. In the first three groups there was only a comparatively small number of loud murmurs (from 3·5% to 6%), but in the fourth group of murmurs, representing structural changes in the heart or heart disease, the number of loud murmurs equalled those of moderate intensity. Blake and Goodale (1957) draw attention to the danger of drawing conclusions from the intensity of a murmur, in view of the loud systolic murmur that can emanate from a small, insignificant ventricular septal defect and the very faint murmur of pulmonary atresia.

No significance could be attached to the constancy or inconstancy of a murmur. Tables 9 and 10 show that the inconstant murmurs comprised only a small number (8%) of all systolic murmurs and were present in all four groups in about equal proportions. There was no relation, either, between inconstancy and location of the murmur.

Summary

Among 2,035 children up to the age of 15 years, examined during the year 1957, 240 were found to have systolic murmurs, that is 11·8%. The incidence was highest in the age group from 5 to 10 years. More male children had murmurs than females, the proportion remaining approximately the same in all age groups. Forty per cent of all murmurs occurred among siblings, but more cases were known to the investigators, amongst the parents or older siblings, which puts the familial incidence even higher. The hypothesis is advanced that perhaps particular identical anatomical construction of the ventricular outlet among members of the same family may be responsible for this phenomenon.

The highest proportion of systolic murmurs were found among the so-called Mediterranean group, followed by the children of Western origin, whilst the lowest percentage was discovered among the children from India.

Out of 240 systolic murmurs, 64·2% were innocent and 35·5% were considered to be pathological. However, only in eight cases could a definite diagnosis of heart disease be established ; the rest showed either only minor pathological findings as a result of further investigations and were therefore classified as 'possible heart disease', or, as in 31 cases (13%), in spite of pathological evidence referable to heart disease, a definite diagnosis was not made. This latter group was called 'probable heart disease'.

No physical criterion could be found by which to distinguish an innocent murmur, either in relation to intensity, location, or continuity of the murmur. A thorough clinical examination, including relevant laboratory tests, electrocardiogram and fluoroscopy, is necessary in each case in order to arrive at the proper distinction. Even so, there is no warrant that a murmur, at first considered innocent, may not indicate a structural disposition to develop a serious heart condition at a later time.

References

Blake, J. R. and Goodale, W. T. (1957). *Med. Clin. N. Amer.*, **41**, 1224.

Epstein, N. (1948). *J. Pediat.*, **32**, 39.

Evans, W. (1947). *Brit. Heart J.*, **9**, 1.

Fogel, D. H. (1957). *Pediatrics*, **19**, 793.

Katz, L. N. (1949). *Electrocardiography*, p. 180. Lea and Febiger, Philadelphia.

Leopold, S. S. (1957). *The Principles and Methods of Physical Diagnosis*, 2nd ed., p. 308. Saunders, Philadelphia.

Lessof, M. and Brigden, W. (1957). *Lancet*, **2**, 673.

Luisada, A. A. (1954). *Heart*, 2nd ed., p. 83. Williams and Wilkins, Baltimore.

New York Heart Association (1955). *Nomenclature and Criteria for Diagnosis of Diseases of the Heart and Blood Vessels*, p. 26.

Pullen, R. L. (1945). *Medical Diagnosis*, p. 372. Saunders, London and Philadelphia.

Rhodes, P. H. (1955). *Bull. Denver rheum. Fever diagn. Serv.*, **12**, 69.

Stuckey, D. (1955). *Med. J. Aust.*, **2**, 841.

Szabo, M. and Ross, L. (1957). *Dapim Refuiim*, **16**, 134.

Wagner, J. and Graham, G. R. (1957). *Brit. Heart J.*, **19**, 318.

Wells, B. (1957). *Ibid.*, **19**, 129.

SEQUESTRATION OF THE LUNG

BY

MARY C. BUCHANAN

From the Queen Elizabeth Hospital for Children, London

(RECEIVED FOR PUBLICATION SEPTEMBER 15, 1958)

The condition of an abnormal pulmonary artery supplying a sequestrated segment is not well known although more than 30 cases have been described. The fact that these cases have come from a few centres (Pryce, 1946; Pryce, Sellors and Blair, 1947; Butler, 1947; Douglass, 1948; Bruwer, Claggett and McDonald, 1950; McDowell, Robb, Hinds and Nicks, 1951; Kergin, 1952; McDowell, Robb and Indyk, 1955) suggests that the condition may not be as rare as is believed. Once infected the sequestrated lobe is the cause of a chronic and disabling illness which can be completely cured by surgery and therefore merits attention.

Pryce (1946) and Pryce, Holmes Sellors and Blair (1947) fully described the condition and were first to publish eight cases successfully treated by surgery. The condition consists of a large artery arising from the abdominal or thoracic aorta, and entering the lung in the region of the diaphragm to supply a sequestrated or dislocated portion of the lung. The tissue in this ectopic piece of lung consists of normal pulmonary elements, with bronchi which are not in continuity with the bronchi of the normal lung. In some cases there are infective changes present with associated bronchiectasis. In others the tissue is largely cystic. The abnormal artery may (1) supply normally connected lung, (2) supply the sequestrated mass and normal lung, and (3) supply only the mass. The artery is elastic and is a pulmonary artery. Because of its origin from the aorta the pressure in this vessel is higher than in a normal pulmonary artery and arteriosclerotic changes are not infrequent even when the normal pulmonary vessels show no such change. Infective changes in the tissue supplied may predispose toward this sclerosis. Apart from this abnormal artery the cardiovascular system is normal. The blood leaves the abnormal segment by the pulmonary veins.

In the articles by Pryce (1946) and Pryce *et al.* (1947) the development of the ectopic tissue is discussed: the abnormal vessel is the primary malformation and Pryce and his fellow workers suggest that sequestration is the result of traction exerted through the capillaries of the adventitious blood supply in the developing lung. In their opinion infection of the mass probably occurs by direct spread from a pneumonic process in the adjacent lung, perhaps occasionally from the blood stream. The persistence of infection, which sometimes proceeds to suppuration, appears to be due to lack of adequate bronchial drainage.

Cases usually present as recurrent pneumonia, empyema, cysts or bronchiectasis. The abnormal vessel, especially if arising from the abdominal aorta, may not be easily seen at operation, and, if unsuspected, fatal haemorrhage may result.

The present case is described as it shows some interesting features.

Case History

Joyce W., aged 8 years 3 months, attended the Queen Elizabeth Hospital, London, in January, 1952, with vague symptoms of ill health. She tired readily and had occasional headaches and pains in the limbs. She had had a cough for two weeks. Clinically there was no abnormality. A Mantoux 1:1,000 tuberculin test was negative and her E.S.R. was 7 mm./hour. A chest radiograph then taken showed no evidence of a pulmonary lesion except basal emphysema on both sides. After six weeks' convalescence she was better in every way.

She remained well for about two years. Then she was admitted to the Queen Elizabeth Hospital, London, in November, 1955, aged 11 years 1 month. The history obtained was similar to that of the previous episode. She had been unwell for two weeks. For seven days headaches were severe and she was giddy on taking exercise. She had one epistaxis. For two weeks she had had a hard, dry cough. On admission she was a sallow, tired-looking girl, but cheerful. Her temperature was 103° F. Respiratory rate varied between 20/25 per minute. Movement of the right base was slightly diminished and the vocal resonance was decreased. There were a few rales at both bases. Mantoux 1 : 1,000 was repeatedly negative. The blood showed a polymorph leucocytosis in the region of 18,000 total W.B.C. with 85% segmented cells. The haemoglobin was 90% (13·46 g. %). On admission a radiograph of the chest showed a partial collapse of the right middle lobe and the anterior segment of the lower lobe. Dr. Hodson suggested that there 'might be underlying changes' (Fig. 1).

Treatment with full doses of sulphadimidine was ineffective in controlling the symptoms and pyrexia. After three days penicillin was added with no effect. Two days later this treatment was discontinued and she was treated with aureomycin. She began to feel much better and the pyrexia settled in two weeks from admission. During this time she had pyrexial episodes, with return of headache lasting from three to four days. Serial radiographs showed some resolution of the lesion at the right base, but there was a considerable degree of residual damage. A tomogram on December 20, 1954, showed cyst-like cavitation in the periphery of the right lower lobe, irregular consolidation and bronchial wall thickening.

After 13 weeks in hospital the cough had cleared and the E.S.R. had been normal for two weeks. There was still diminished movement and decreased vocal resonance over the right lower zone, but no adventitious sound. She was discharged home to be admitted for a bronchogram about one month later if the lesion persisted.

Three weeks later in March, 1955, she was re-admitted with anorexia and recurrence of cough. The physical findings were as on discharge. She had a moderate pyrexia (100° F.). The E.S.R. was raised and there was a polymorph leucocytosis. On this occasion treatment with sulphadimidine was successful in controlling the symptoms. Two weeks later she was apyrexial and her blood tests were normal in all respects. A bronchogram was done and Dr. Hodson reported 'all the major segments were identified in the left lower lobe. The diseased area lies medial to the lower lobe behind the heart and causes a spreading out and arching of the right lower bronchi round it. It itself seems to have no communication with the bronchial tree. The whole behaviour, site and appearance of this lesion suggests sequestrated lung segment' (Figs. 2 and 3).

Excision of the right lower lobe was performed by Mr. Holmes Sellors on May 16, 1956. The lung was free except for a few recent adhesions between the lower lobe and the diaphragm. There was a small mass in the posterior basal segments. Entering this mass from the region of the diaphragm was a vessel about 3 mm. in diameter. Dissection lobectomy was quite straightforward.

The size of the right lower lobe was 9 by 11 by 8 cm.

ON SECTION. In the posterior subapical area there was a small abscess cavity about 0·5 cm. in diameter. In the posterior basal region there was an area of lipoid pneumonitis containing what appeared to be a number of small abscesses. In the antero-medial portion of the lobe there was a tube-like structure which extended laterally and divided into a number of branches. This was thought to be an ectopic bronchus. There was emphysema of the basal segments.

HISTOLOGY. The abscess in the posterior subapical area was lined by fibrous tissue, with a single layer of low cuboidal epithelium in places. This could have originally been a bronchiectatic cyst. In the posterior basal area the small abscesses were destroyed small bronchi. There was also a larger bronchiectatic cavity with ulceration of its surface, and loss of its ciliated epithelium. This was surrounded by areas of chronic pneumonitis with the alveoli filled in places with lipoid phagocytes. Many of the ulcerated bronchi were filled with pus. The 'pipe-like' structure proved to be a thin-walled ectopic bronchus with rudimentary cartilage. The wall contained no glands or muscle. Laterally, the wall was broken up by abscess fragmentation, the abscess perforating into an adjacent small bronchus.

After operation the patient was very well. Her appetite was excellent and she had plenty of energy: 'quite a different child; has never been known to be so lively.' Previously she had been easily irritated and easily tired.

Discussion

The main interest in the case described above is the apparently normal chest radiography taken two

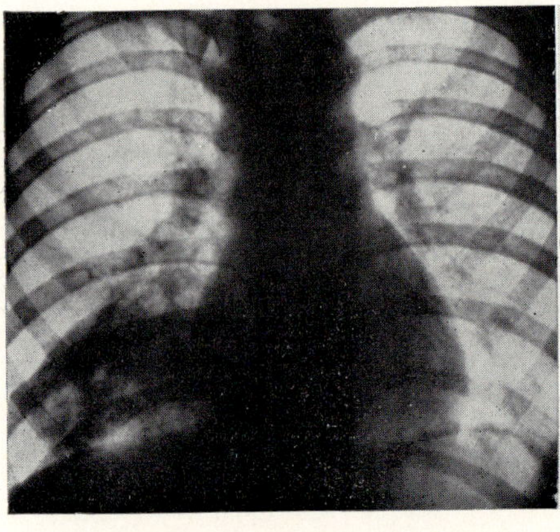

FIG. 1.—Joyce W. Partial collapse of right middle lobe and anterior segment of lower lobe.

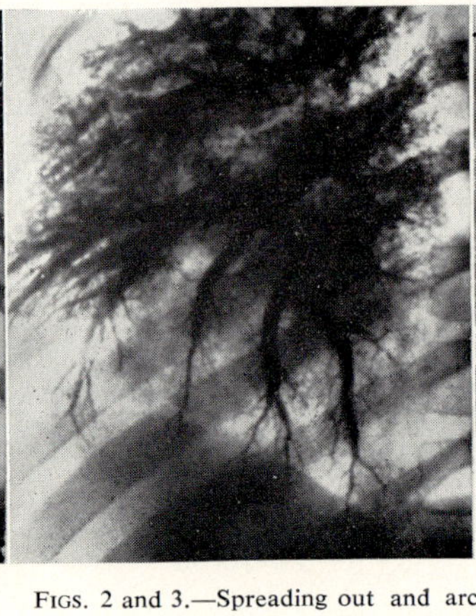

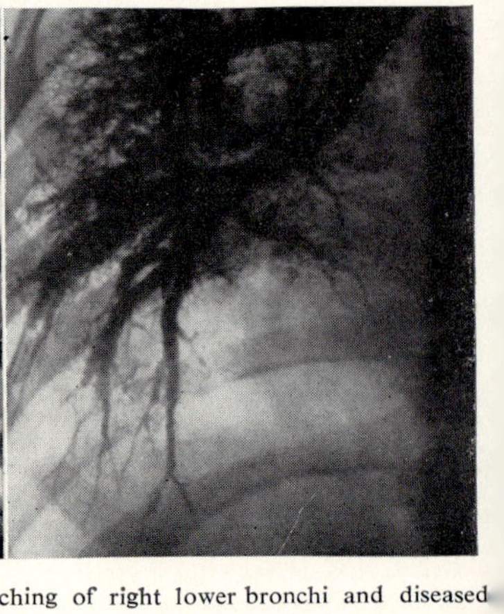

FIGS. 2 and 3.—Spreading out and arching of right lower bronchi and diseased area.

years before the series of illnesses which culminated in lobectomy. There appear to be three explanations for this: (1) The sequestrated segment was unaerated and uninfected and in this state occupied such a small volume that it cast no shadow on the radiograph. (2) The segment contained air but was without infective changes and disturbed the normal pulmonary markings so little that again it cast no peculiar shadow. (3) Sequestration of the segment occurred in the following two years, i.e. was postnatal.

Against (1) is the unlikelihood that even a small collapsed segment in this region would fail to produce some kind of irregularity in a good quality film.

Against (3) is the rudimentary structure of the ectopic bronchial tissue found in the abnormal segment after excision. Were this bronchus amputated well after birth it would be likely to retain a more or less normal structure.

The second explanation seems the most likely: that there was a small communication between the air contained in the surrounding normal lung and the air spaces in the ectopic tissue, which was sufficient to aerate the latter, but which was insufficient to drain the products of infection once the latter had occurred.

Summary

The syndrome of sequestrated lung segment is probably not as rare as is generally believed. The condition is disabling. It is cured by operation. There are few symptoms referable to the lungs, minimal physical signs but gross radiological changes. The condition once suspected can be diagnosed before operation. The anatomical lesion is again described and the presence of an abnormal vessel from the abdominal aorta is foreseen. Comment is made on the probable aetiology of the condition.

I wish to thank Dr. C. T. Potter for his permission to publish an account of this case; also Dr. C. J. Hodson for the radiographic prints and for helpful criticism.

REFERENCES

Bruwer, A., Claggett, O. T. and McDonald, J. R. (1950). *J. Thorac. Surg.*, **19**, 957.
Butler, E. F. (1947). *Ibid.*, **16**, 199.
Douglass, R. (1948). *Ibid.*, **17**, 712.
Kergin, F. G. (1952). *Ibid.*, **23**, 55.
McDowell, C., Robb, D. and Indyk, J. S. (1955). *Thorax*, **10**, 73.
——, —— Hinds, W. R. and Nicks, R. (1951). *Brit. J. Surg.*, **39**, 87.
Pryce, D. M. (1946). *J. Path. Bact.*, **58**, 457.
——, Sellors, T. Holmes and Blair, L. G. (1947). *Brit. J. Surg.*, **35**, 18.

INVESTIGATION INTO THE AETIOLOGY AND TREATMENT OF PICA*

BY

PHILIP LANZKOWSKY†

From the Department of Child Health, University of Cape Town and Red Cross War Memorial Children's Hospital, Rondebosch, Cape Town, South Africa

(RECEIVED FOR PUBLICATION OCTOBER 6, 1958)

The name pica is derived from the Latin word meaning magpie. In reviewing the literature no adequate definitions are to be found. Those of Hubrigkt (1562) and Schrey (1719), as quoted by Cooper (1957), are antiquated and of historical interest only. Pica could be described as a perversion of appetite with persistent and purposeful ingestion of unsuitable substances, seemingly of no nutrient value. It is associated with the passage of these substances unchanged in the stool, and with radiological evidence of their presence in the gut when they are radio-opaque.

Pica is world-wide in distribution, and occurs at all ages. Each individual or local group seems to specialize in one direction, eating only a particular type of material. Many small children, at some time in early life, put in their mouths and occasionally swallow inedible matter, but this is so well recognized that it causes only the mildest of domestic upsets. Even if an occasional individual does so repeatedly, medical advice is not sought unless the performance in this respect becomes spectacular.

The purpose of this paper is to report on a series of children suffering from pica.

My attention was drawn to pica by a casual remark passed by the mother of a boy who was being treated for hypochromic anaemia, that since the commencement of iron medication the boy had stopped eating dirt.

For centuries writers have recorded observations on pica, but the most recent reports, however, still left the matter of therapy an unsolved problem. The earliest writers centred their attention on the condition as it affected pregnant women.

Boezo (1638), Hancock (1831), Nouverre (1833), Segond (1833), Cragin (1835), Gould (1876), Kovatsch (1879), Gros (1903), Tosatti (1907), Major (1935), all quoted by Cooper (1957); Livingstone as cited by Waller (1874); Duprey (1900); Orr and Gilks (1931); Dickins and Ford (1942); and De Castro (1952) all mentioned an association between pica and minerals; some of them suggested iron for treatment. Hancock attributed pica to 'paucity of good blood and lack of proper nutrition'. Segond, Cragin, Duprey, Gros, and Tosatti all indicated that anaemia was part of the picture and Gould recorded a cure after iron therapy. According to Waller, the explorer Livingstone commented on clay and earth-eating and stated that it was 'the cause of bloodlessness' amongst the African tribes in Zanzibar. Orr and Gilks and De Castro realized that the 'edible earths' were rich in sodium, iron and calcium, and Dickins and Ford suggested that negro children might eat dirt to make up for an iron deficiency in their diet.

Unfortunately, many of these observers clouded the issue by introducing simultaneously other feasible explanations for the pica. Lack of proper nutrition was incriminated by Hancock. Duprey admitted that his subjects had a meagre diet. Rake (1884) thought that economic reasons, with the idea of saving food, might be a basic cause amongst the Hindus in Trinidad. Gelfand (1945) noted that pica was common in Kenya amongst the African tribes (Kikuyu) living mainly on a vegetarian diet as contrasted with its absence in the high-protein-eaters (Masai). Dickins and Ford (1942) confirmed this observation in rural Negro school children in the Mississippi area, where they found the incidence of pica significantly higher in children consuming fewer iron-rich foods. Cooper (1957) found a greater incidence of nutritional problems in children suffering from pica and thought that poor nutrition might be the underlying factor. Debilitating disease such as tuberculosis and malignant or tropical disease was thought by Gelfand to be at the root of the inanition and death which had been known as

* Paper presented at the Postgraduate Seminar, Red Cross War Memorial Children's Hospital, Rondebosch, Cape Town, September, 1958, and at the South African Paediatric Congress, Pretoria, October, 1958.

† Recipient of a Dr. C. L. Herman Research Grant, University of Cape Town Staff Research Fund.

'cachexia Africana', previously thought to be a pathological form of geophagy.

Other possible explanations have been advanced. A depraved appetite was alleged by Nouverre (1833) to be at the root of the trouble. Livingstone agreed and stated that both slaves and rich men were affected and the condition was called 'safura' by the Africans. Duprey described it as a craving so strong that the coolies of Carriacou carried gravel around on their person and would cry and beg for the dirt which they cherished so much. Butterworth (1909) described as a habit the somewhat allied disorder of swallowing hair.

Mental deficiency was invoked by Kanner (1948) who found that 16 out of 30 children with pica studied by him were severely retarded and almost all were below average intelligence. As additional causes he added faulty habit training and parental neglect. Still had denied this in 1915 but stated that such children had a 'nervous temperament' and Cooper's finding, in 1957, that the I.Q. of her pica-group was 87·2% supports Still's contention.

Infestation by intestinal parasites has been commonly suspected to be an associated factor and, though ankylostomiasis was frequently incriminated, many different types of worms have been mentioned. Duprey favoured ankylostomiasis. Gelfand (1945) was emphatically opposed to this view. Kovatsch and Dukes (1884) associated pica with ascaris; Gros (1903) with ascaris and oxyuris; Mathieu (1927) as quoted by Cooper, with ascaris, oxyuris, trichuris, and hymenolepis, and Major (1935) with oxyuris.

Causes of a more abstruse nature have been suggested. Gelfand pointed out that pica is common practice in the Rhodesias, Nyasaland, Portuguese East Africa, the Congo, East, West and North Africa. Earth-eating is frequently closely associated with the religious or magical beliefs of the natives and is not a subject for discussion with the white man. There is a presumed personal and spiritual bond between the land and the tribe or clan living on it who pay homage, and in some instances make yearly sacrifices, to the land. On entering alien soil an African may, as an act of homage, eat a little of it. His wife, children, and even the baby must also partake in this rite. Furthermore, in recognizing the fertile powers of the earth it is assumed that if a woman eats earth she will be more fertile before pregnancy and by continuing to eat it will increase her powers of lactation. Her children are brought up in that belief from the day they are born. This aspect of the problem has nothing to do with the universally recognized cravings of pregnant women.

Mothers may withhold information as to the occurrence of pica in their children and this makes an assessment of its incidence more difficult. Dickins and Ford (1942), however, found that 26% of boys and 25% of girls in Mississippi ate dirt, and De Castro (1952) found that geophagy was common amongst school children in Bahia, Brazil. Cooper (1957) stated that 21·9% of children referred to the Mothers' Advisory Service Clinic at Baltimore had a history of pica.

Although children with pica may have a craving for a variety of substances it is fortunate that most of these are inert and, although they occasionally lead to minor ailments do not cause any serious disturbance to the health of the child. There is, however, one type of poisoning which these pica children may acquire, and that is lead poisoning. Ruddock (1924), McKhann (1926), Stetson (1947), Tanis (1955), Williams, Kaplan, Couchman and Sayers (1955) as quoted by Cooper, have each recorded a series of cases of lead poisoning due to ingestion of paint and they state that pica is an important aetiological factor in lead poisoning. Nims (1842), and Peak (1857), as quoted by Cooper (1957) and Rake (1884), a century ago recorded deaths from intestinal perforation or obstruction caused by the ingestion of gravel, stone or sand. Even with modern surgery, ingestion of inedible material can produce major hazards in the shape of bezoars from the perpetual swallowing of hair (trichobezoar), rags, threads or fibrous plant roots (phytobezoar) and by such unlikely material as wellington boots, india rubber, and rubber doorstops (Butterworth, 1909; Kanner, 1948; Ford, 1958).

From this welter of possibilities no rational line of thought seems to have emerged. Iron deficiency has been mooted and iron therapy suggested as an aid to treatment but it has not been shown that iron alone could stop the perversion. Malnutrition is not uncommonly associated with pica but there is no evidence to prove that malnutrition is essential for the development of this condition. Worm infestation has been blamed but the indictment left unproven. All these should be susceptible to clinical testing; factors beyond human control such as mental deficiency, depraved appetite, religious and tribal customs might take on a new significance or lose entirely the hypothetical place which they at present occupy in the problematical aetiology of pica.

Present Investigation

Children attending the Red Cross Hospital out-patient department who presented either with pica, or where pica was part of the history, were investigated. During a five-month period there were 12 such patients seen at the hospital, 10 of them

CLINICAL FEAT

Case No.	Age, Sex, Race, Birthweight	Symptoms, Duration, Type	Severity	Worms
1	4 7/12. M. Col.	Pica. Over 2 yr. Black soil. Pieces of brick	Daily. Pockets of sand carried. Scratched walls to get brick	Ascaris
2	6 7/12. M. Col. 13 lb. 3½ oz.	Pica. 3½ yr. Sand at first. Pebbles only, 3 yr.	Daily. Attended every hospital in town and several physicians	Ascaris
3	2 4/12. F. Col.	Pica. 1 yr. Sand	Intermittently	Ascaris
4	3 8/12. F. White. 8 lb. ½ oz.	Abdominal pain. Pica. 2½ yr. Small stones. Pieces of brick. White sand, soil. Pieces of wood. Anorexia	Daily	Ascaris
5	2 1/12. F. Col. 6 lb. 3 oz.	Worms. Pica over 1 yr. Sand. Anorexia	Daily. Child had to be restrained. Scratched walls to get brick	Ascaris Tapeworm
6	1 8/12. F. Col. 8 lb. + Control	Pica. 1 yr. Sand. Little stones. Coal. Pieces of wood Diarrhoea Anorexia Restless	Daily. Removed spoons from table to eat sand with	No
7	2 2/12. M. Col. 7 lb.	Diarrhoea. Pica over 1 yr. Sand, earth. Ash Worms Anorexia	Daily. 'Handfuls every day. It was his diet' states mother. Licked sand off boots and off the floor. Required restraint. Mother left work on account of the severity of his condition	Ascaris
8	2 yr. F. Col. 6½ lb.	Pica 6 m. Sand. Small stones. Diarrhoea	Daily. Restrained	Ascaris
9	3 9/12. F. Col. 5 lb.	Pica 2 yr. Sand. Stones. Clay Diarrhoea	Daily. Restrained	Ascaris
10	1 10/12. M. White. 9 lb. 3 oz.	Pica over 1 yr. Sand. Pebbles stones Anorexia	Daily. 'Was never without a stone or sand in the mouth'. Amount of sand eaten was incredible. Restrained	No
11	3 4/12. F. Col.	Diarrhoea. Pica, ?. Sand Cough	Daily	Ascaris *Trichura tr*
12	4 yr. M. Col. 8 lb. 5 oz.	Abdominal mass. Pica 3 yr. Sand	Daily	Ascaris

were Cape Coloured and two were white. There were seven girls and five boys and their ages ranged from 1 year, 8 months to 6½ years. The duration of pica was from a minimum of six months to a maximum of three and a half years, in children of 2 and 6½ years respectively. In one case the pica was intermittent, with periods of a few weeks' respite, but in the remainder it was persistent and an almost daily occurrence. Of the 12 patients, seven sought advice because of pica, two for diarrhoea, and one of the others for each of the following complaints: abdominal pain, worms, and an abdominal mass with anaemia. Other associated complaints were anorexia and restlessness.

In most cases pica was so severe that the mothers had taken active steps to restrain the children. Most of them had been locked up indoors, for varying periods of time, away from a source of dirt. Under these conditions some would scratch at the walls in order to get access to pieces of brick and plaster. One constantly carried sand in his pockets in order to have a supply readily available all day. Another would lick sand off the boots of visitors and off the floor. One mother stated that the quantity of sand eaten was almost incredible. Most of the children were known to pass sand in their stools.

A wide variety of substances, depending upon their availability, was ingested. As white sand is common in the Cape it was eaten in nearly every

'A GROUP

Intelligence	Behaviour	Appearance	Radiography	Response to Treatment
, Normal milestones. states 'bright lad'	Good	Well-nourished	Opaque material compatible with sand in colon	Cured. Played in sand but did not eat any. Appetite greatly improved
average. Normal mile-	Temper tantrums	Well-nourished	Opaque material in bizarre sizes and shapes in G.I. tract, mainly in colon	Cured
Normal milestones	Well-behaved	Well-nourished	—	Cured. Appetite greatly improved. More energetic. Less restless
verage. Normal mile- Mother states 'cleverer :r brother of 5 yr.'	Good	Well-nourished	No opaque material	Cured Appetite greatly improved Mother states 'more alive'
verage. Normal mile- Very good memory	Good	Well-nourished	—	Cured. Dramatic improvement in appetite
verage. Normal mile- Good memory. Mother :leverest child of five	Good	Well-nourished. Pallor	No opaque material	I.M. sterile water: No change in behaviour. I.M. Iron-dextran: Cured. Less irritable. Appetite improved
verage. Normal mile- Speaks two languages counts very well	Good	Well-nourished	—	Cured. Appetite and general behaviour improved
Normal milestones	Good	Well-nourished Pallor +	—	Cured. Appetite greatly improved. Not so restless, more lively
	Good	Well-nourished. Pallor +	Opaque material compatible with sand in large bowel more on R.	Cured. 'Skoon verandering'.* Played and ate better
Normal milestones	Temper tantrums. Spiteful, difficult child	Well-nourished	Opaque material in large bowel	Cured. Vast improvement. Mother stated 'a different child' in appetite and less irritable. Refused an orange which fell on to sand whereas before treatment deliberately rubbed most of food in sand before eating it
	Good	Miserable, malnourished Severe pallor	No opaque material in G.I. tract	Transfusion: no change. Only cured after I.M. Iron-dextran
Normal milestones	Good	Well-nourished. Pallor. Abdominal mass. Histology: lymphosarcoma	Opaque material in G.I. tract	Died from primary disease without discharge from hospital

nge'.

case, either alone or in combination with other substances. Black soil, pieces of brick, stones (Fig. 1), pieces of wood, black coal, and clay were taken in addition to sand in varying combinations and amounts.

The appearance of the children was not conspicuously abnormal. There was no tell-tale appearance which would lead an observer to suspect the condition. The general standard of physique appeared to be normal (Fig. 2). Only one child showed overt clinical signs of undernutrition. Five showed clinical evidence of anaemia with pallor of the mucosae. One patient had a palpable abdominal mass, and a diagnosis of lymphosarcoma was made on biopsy. In the remaining cases all the systems were normal on physical examination. In no case was splenomegaly found. The clinical features for each individual are shown in Table 1.

One of the main reasons for this investigation was to determine whether an iron-deficiency existed. Haemoglobin, P.C.V. and M.C.H.C. estimations were done and peripheral smears were examined (Table 2). Unfortunately in the earlier cases haematological examination was incomplete.

The haemoglobin level ranged from 3·0 g. % to 10·9 g. % with a mean of 7·89 g. % and a standard deviation of 2·64. The haemoglobin estimation was done by the oxyhaemoglobin method using a Klett-Summerson colorimeter.

The mean P.C.V. was 29·5% with a range from

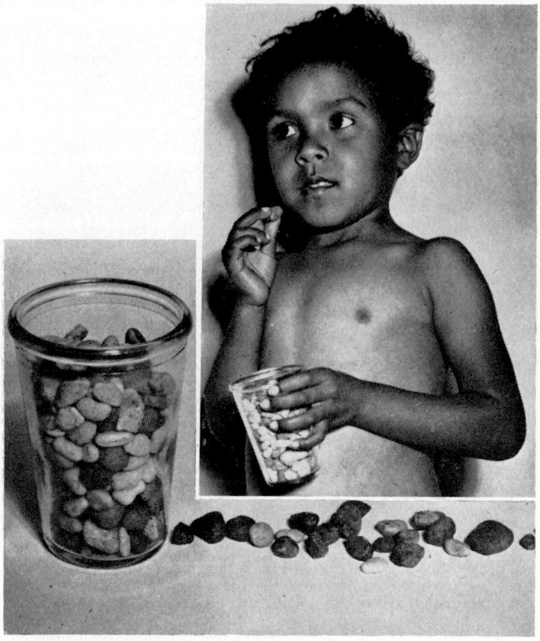

FIGS. 1 and 2.—Case 2. Daily diet of pebbles taken for three years by a coloured boy aged 6 years 7 months, with pica. Note normal physique.

19% to 37% and a standard deviation of 6·68.

The mean M.C.H.C. was 27·5% with a range from 21% to 32% and a standard deviation of 3·96.

Peripheral smears showed marked hypochromasia, anisocytosis and poikilocytosis in cases where the anaemia was of a severe degree, and all gradations of an iron deficiency pattern to normal red blood cells.

Serum protein estimations were done on 11 cases, by the Weichselbaum biuret method. Results showed a mean of 7·19 g. % for total serum proteins, 3·87 g. % for serum albumin and 3·32 g. % for serum globulin (Table 3).

Ten children (83%) gave a history of ascaris infestation. One child had tapeworm and another *Trichuris trichiura* in addition to ascaris. Confirmatory evidence of worm infestation was looked for. Peripheral blood smears were obtained in five cases. These showed an eosinophilia of 5, 7, 8, 8, and 10% respectively and all had passed roundworms.

The mentality of the subjects was scrutinized. Contrary to expectation, the intelligence of the children as a whole in this survey was average, and, in a few instances, considered to be distinctly above average. No formal intelligence tests were applied but the intelligence was assessed by the author in conjunction with the parents and on the basis of developmental data, language, and social adjustment. While it is fully realized that this is only a rough guide to the I.Q., it is sufficient for this purpose to indicate that these children with pica were for practical purposes mentally normal.

The children did not appear to suffer from behaviour disorders. Ten of these children could be described as normally well-behaved children. Two, however, had temper tantrums.

Radiological examinations were done on eight cases. Five showed opaque material interpreted as sand or stones in the large bowel, and to a lesser extent in the small bowel (Figs. 3-6). In one of these the appendix was outlined and filled with sand (Fig. 7). None had a previous history of roentgenographic contrast studies and none had taken any medicines containing radio-opaque materials, e.g.

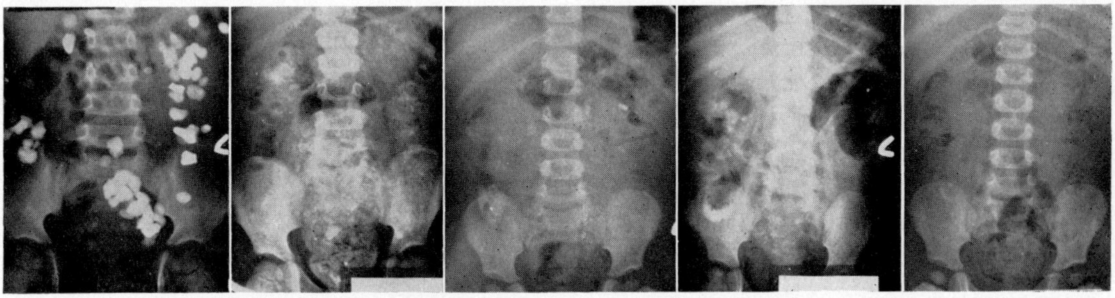

3 4 5 6 7

FIG. 3.—Case 2. Radio-opaque material of bizarre sizes and shapes compatible with stones in small and large intestine in coloured boy with pica.

FIG. 4.—Case 1. Radio-opaque material compatible with sand in colon in coloured boy with pica.

FIG. 5.—Case 10. Radio-opaque material compatible with sand in colon in white boy with pica.

FIG. 6.—Case 9. Radio-opaque material compatible with sand in caecum and ascending colon of coloured girl with pica.

FIG. 7.—Case 10. Radio-opaque material compatible with sand in the appendix in white boy with pica.

TABLE 2
HAEMATOLOGICAL VALUES IN PICA GROUP

Case No.	Hb. (g. %)	P.C.V. (%)	M.C.H.C. (%)	Morphology Red Blood Corpuscles	Eosinophil Count (%)
1	8·6	32	30	Hypochromasia slight	—
2	10·9	37	29	Normal	7
3	8·9	28	32	—	—
4	10·6	34	31	Normal	—
5	9·7	—	—	Hypochromasia slight	8
6	7·9	32	24	Hypochromasia slight	—
7	9·5	—	—	Hypochromasia slight Poikilocytosis slight	10
8	4·1	20	21	Hypochromasia ++ Anisocytosis + Polychromasia slight	8
9	4·6	19	24	Hypochromasia +++ Anisocytosis slight Polychromasia slight	—
10	9·7	34	29	—	—
11	3·0	—	—	Hypochromasia +++ Anisocytosis ++ Poikilocytosis ++ Target cells few	—
12	7·0	—	—	Hypochromasia + Anisocytosis +	5
Total cases	12	8	8	—	5
Mean	7·89	29·5	27·5	—	8
Standard deviation	2·64	6·68	3·96	—	—

bismuth or barium. Of the three cases in which there was no radiographic evidence, two had a history of diarrhoea in addition to pica.

Once the foregoing investigations had been completed therapy was commenced (Table 4). Intramuscular iron-dextran compound (Imferon) in doses varying from 200-400 mg. was given in nine cases. The total dose of intramuscular iron-dextran compound (Imferon) was given in one injection and calculated, in each case, according to the original haemoglobin level and the body weight.* One of

*The formula used was $9W + \frac{W}{6}(100 - Hb\%) =$ mg. of iron.
Where W = Weight of patient in pounds.
Hb% = Observed haemoglobin percentage.

TABLE 3
SERUM PROTEIN ESTIMATIONS IN PICA GROUP

Case No.	Total Serum Proteins (g. %)	Serum Albumin (g. %)	Serum Globulin (g. %)
1	7·80	3·53	4·27
2	7·38	4·54	2·84
3	6·08	3·38	2·70
4	8·40	3·74	4·66
5	7·49	4·65	2·84
6	6·96	3·80	3·16
7	6·60	3·60	3·00
8	7·50	3·74	2·76
9	7·42	3·77	3·65
10	6·92	4·85	2·07
11	7·58	2·96	4·62
12	—	—	—
Mean g. %	7·19	3·87	3·32
Standard deviation	0·66	0·55	0·82

TABLE 4
RESPONSE TO TREATMENT IN PICA GROUP

Case No.	Haemoglobin Before (g. %)	Haemoglobin After (g. %)	Treatment I.M. Iron-Dextran Compound (mg.)
1	8·6	11·7	400
2	10·9	10·9	300
3	8·9	11·9	200
4	10·6	11·3	Ferrous gluconate 150 mg. b.d.
5	9·7	11·8	200
6 (Control)	7·9	10·8	Sterile water 2 ml. 300 mg. later
7	9·5	12·2	200
8	4·1	10·5	300
9	4·6	10·9	400
10	9·7	11·6	200
11	3·0	9·0	Transf. 330 ml. 300 mg. later
12	7·0	14·5	Transf. 600 ml.
Mean	7·89	11·43	278 mg.
Standard deviation	2·64	1·29	—

these nine cases was initially used as a control and given 2 ml. of intramuscular sterile water. This did not cause any change in the child's behaviour and the severity of the pica persisted unchanged. He was subsequently given 300 mg. intramuscular iron-dextran compound (Imferon) and responded dramatically with complete cessation of the pica.

Two patients who were admitted to hospital, one with a diagnosis of lymphosarcoma and the other with diarrhoea and severe iron deficiency anaemia, received blood transfusions. The one with lymphosarcoma died without being discharged from hospital and does not figure in these comments. The other was only seen again two months after her discharge. The mother then reported that she had continued eating sand and dirt. On examination her haemoglobin had fallen from 9 g. % on discharge to 5 g. %. She was then given intramuscular iron-dextran compound and her pica ceased dramatically within 10 days.

One white patient was given oral ferrous gluconate.

The results of treatment on the whole, were highly gratifying. In one child only (Case 2), there was no change in the haemoglobin level. The remaining children showed a marked rise in haemoglobin level after treatment. The mean haemoglobin on completion of treatment was 11·43 g. %, showing a mean rise of 3·54 g. %.

All the children showed a complete cure of their pica, usually within one to two weeks of commencement of treatment and in some instances in a shorter time. Several of the children who had eaten sand for many years continued to play with sand and stones, but had no inclination to eat these substances. The mothers were instructed not to restrict their activities. All the children showed the usual beneficial effects of iron therapy on behaviour, appetite and sense of well-being. Many cases have now been followed for over a year without a recurrence of pica.

The five cases which before treatment had shown radio-opaque material in the bowel all showed complete radiographic clearing within 10 days.

Discussion

In the course of this study some details complementary to the main issues have been noted. Although the alleged major factors in the production of pica have been examined there are other possibilities which cannot be entirely ignored. It is often reported that pica occurs more frequently in children coming from a poor socio-economic background. The present series, however, did not show this. The mean weekly income, assessed on a *per capita* basis, amongst the Cape Coloured children in this series was 26·13 shillings, as compared with 13·08 shillings for a control group of 50 unselected out-patients. This shows a statistically significant difference between the weekly income of the two groups. The pica group are apparently better off financially. The reason for this marked discrepancy in socio-economic status may be that the mothers of low socio-economic status are too occupied to attend to what they consider to be a mere aberration in the child's eating habits.

The birth weights of these children were investigated, since it had been shown by Cooper (1957) that the percentage of the premature-born amongst children suffering from pica was abnormally high. The mean birth weight of the children in this series was 7 lb. 15½ oz. with a range from 13 lb. 3½ oz. to 5 lb. The mean birth weight for Cape Coloured children in a control group of 74 normal births studied by the author was found to be 6 lb. 15½ oz. This demonstrates that the children suffering from pica in this series had a statistically significant higher birth weight as compared with the birth weights of a random sample of normal infants.

The present series of cases confirms the reported frequency of worm infestation in pica. The Cape Coloured children of this area are known to be commonly affected in this way and in a random sample of the hospital's out-patients 25 of 120 children (21%) gave a history of worm infestation. The proportion of infestations in the pica group (83%) is significantly higher. Nevertheless, no steps were taken to alter this situation during the trial of iron therapy. Worm ova were not looked for, but this in no way invalidates this observation as the same criteria (viz. history and eosinophilia) for determining the incidence were used in both the pica and the control groups. Any hypothetical bearing of the presence of intestinal worms on the aetiology of pica appears therefore, to have no substantial foundation in fact.

The somewhat indefinite evidence in the literature, namely Cooper's average I.Q.of 87%, against the association of mental deficiency with pica was confirmed in the present series of cases.

The main factors appear to be nutrition and anaemia. The nutritional state of the children in this series was good in comparison with other children of similar age and background. The serum protein levels were significantly higher than those of a control group of 77 anaemic out-patients of comparable age and background. These latter showed a mean total serum protein of 5·67 g. %, serum albumin 3·39 g. % and serum globulin of 2·28 g. %. The mean for the pica group was

7·19 g. % for total serum proteins, 3·87 g. % for serum albumin and 3·32 g. % for serum globulin.

While the total protein in the pica group is entirely adequate, it is apparent that the albumin levels are relatively low and the globulin fractions rather high (see Table 3). The reason for this is not apparent.

All the children showed iron deficiency anaemia to a greater or lesser extent. The haemoglobin levels were significantly lower than those in a control group of 70 unselected out-patients of comparable age and background. These latter, varying from 1 to 7 years in age, showed a mean haemoglobin of 10·52 g. % with a standard deviation of 1·70. The mean for the pica group was 7·89 g. %. The morphology of the red blood cells (as judged from the smear), the haemoglobin, P.C.V. and M.C.H.C., coupled with the response to therapy, indicated that the anaemia was of the iron deficiency type. The M.C.H.C., which is regarded as the most sensitive index of iron-deficiency anaemia (Latsky, 1943), was below normal in every patient, confirming the presence of an iron-deficient state.

The logical result of the above findings was to treat all these patients with iron. It must be emphasized that at the time of treatment of the pica no other medicaments (e.g. vermifuges or antibiotics) were employed. No psychological advice was given and the condition was treated purely as anaemia. Intramuscular iron was chosen in preference to oral iron in most cases, because previous experience had shown that the oral administration of medicines was not reliable in the type of population under consideration. Parenteral iron therapy was the only way of ensuring that the patient received the drug. The response to intramuscular therapy is quicker than to oral iron and, consequently, the number of hospital visits was reduced to a minimum. Previous writers have insisted that these cases were very resistant to medical treatment. Through the ages discouraging measures such as whipping or restraint of some sort have been the sheet anchor of therapy, and more recently the services of an energetic nanny (Sheldon, 1955) have been advocated. No such adjuvants to iron therapy were employed in this investigation.

'The effort to maintain a constant internal environment, or homeostasis, constitutes one of the most universal and powerful of all behaviour urges or drives' (Richter, 1943). Adrenalectomized rats, in a laboratory, consume unusual amounts of salt solution. Patients with Addison's disease crave salt and thereby provide an early and significant indication of the nature of their illness. Parathyroidectomized rats prefer calcium lactate solution to water and children with parathyroid deficiency show a craving for chalk and plaster. Diabetics drink excessive amounts of water and they and patients with thyrotoxicosis compensate for their increased metabolic needs by polyphagia. Davis (1928) showed that a child, given free choice of selection of food, would maintain itself in excellent nutrition in all respects without adult guidance. She reported on a rachitic child who voluntarily consumed cod-liver oil until about the time the blood calcium and phosphorus reached normal levels, and radiographs showed the rickets to be healed. Theiler, Green and Du Toit (1924), as quoted by Cooper (1957), described osteophagia in cattle as a herbivore's response to osteomalacia. The feeding of phosphorus-rich substances to the cattle resulted in the eradication of the pica.

If these children with pica do, in fact, feel an instinctive need for iron to restore their haemoglobin levels to normal a slight difficulty arises as to the child in this series who was given a blood transfusion yet continued to have pica. A similar query may be directed at the child who lost his pica without showing a rise in haemoglobin level. A possible explanation would be that the transfused blood although it corrected the anaemia contained an insufficient amount of iron (35 mg./100 ml.) to meet the needs of restoration and iron storage, and that in the other child it was really the storage-iron deficiency which was responsible for his condition. This is analogous to the presence of glossitis, dysphagia (sideropenic dysphagia) and koilonychia as a result of marked epithelial changes occurring in tissue-iron deficiency without anaemia (Waldenström and Kjellberg, 1939; Waldenström, 1946; Henderson, 1954; Bothwell and Glyn Thomas, 1958). This is a state of delicate metabolic equilibrium and blood transfusion restores the haemoglobin to normal but is insufficient to satisfy tissue needs. Thus treatment in pica must be adequate enough to correct anaemia, when present, and to refill the iron stores. Since it is extremely difficult to replenish body stores by the oral route (Finch, Haskins and Finch, 1950) it may be necessary in some instances, in addition to the reasons given above, to use parenteral iron in the treatment of this condition.

Since this paper was prepared eight further cases of pica have been seen. They all showed the typical clinical features already described, and all were cured by intramuscular iron-dextran compound (Imferon).

Finally, it must be admitted that the commonest mineral deficiency in children throughout the world is almost certainly iron, and a subconscious craving for it might well be expected.

Conclusions and Summary

The literature on the subject of pica is briefly reviewed. An investigation of 12 children suffering from pica is described. The main abnormality found was an iron deficiency anaemia. Treatment of this with iron was invariably followed by the rapid disappearance of pica. The conclusion is drawn that iron deficiency is the major cause of pica and that iron therapy is curative.

I am indebted to Professor F. J. Ford, Head of the Department of Child Health, University of Cape Town, for his constant guidance, advice and criticism in the preparation of this paper, to Dr. J. D. L. Hansen and Dr. W. Emdin for their advice, and to Dr. J. F. Mostert, Medical Superintendent of the Red Cross War Memorial Children's Hospital, for permission to publish this work. Thanks are also due to the honorary physicians and colleagues who referred cases of pica to me, to Mr. T. Turner for technical assistance in the serum protein estimations, and Mr. B. Todt for the photography.

References

Boezo, M. H. (1638). (Quoted by Cooper, M.) *De Pica*. Sm., Lipsiae.
Bothwell, T. H. and Thomas, R. Glyn (1958). *S. Afr. med. J.*, **32**, 614.
Butterworth, W. W. (1909). *J. Amer. med. Ass.*, **53**, 617.
Castro, J. de (1952). *Geography of Hunger*, p. 80. Gollancz, London.
Cooper, M. (1957). *Pica*. Charles C. Thomas, Springfield, Illinois.
Cragin, F. W. (1835). (Quoted by Cooper, M.) *Amer. J. med. Sci.*, **17**, 356.
Davis, C. M. (1928). *Amer. J. Dis. Child.*, **36**, 651.
Dickins, D. and Ford, R. N. (1942). *Amer. Soc. Rev.*, 7, 59.
Dukes, C. (1884). *Lancet*, **2**, 822.
Duprey, A. J. B. (1900). *Ibid.*, **2**, 1192.
Finch, S., Haskins, D. and Finch, C. A. (1950). *J. clin. Invest.*, **29**, 1078.
Ford, F. J. (1958). Personal communication.
Gelfand, M. (1945). *E. Afr. med. J.*, **22**, 98.
Gould, A. N. (1876). (Quoted by Cooper, M.) *Boston med. Surg. J.*, **94**, 417.
Gros, H. (1903). (Quoted by Cooper, M.) *La Caducée*, **3**, 248.
Hancock, J. (1831). (Quoted by Cooper, M.) *Edinb. med. surg. J.*, **35**, 67.
Henderson, I. D. (1954). *Lancet*, **1**, 493.
Hubrigkt, J. F. (1562). (Quoted by Cooper, M.) *De Appetitu Depravato Pica Dicto*. Altdorff.
Kanner, L. (1948). *Child Psychiatry*, 2nd ed., p. 475. Charles C. Thomas, Springfield, Illinois
Kovatsch, W. (1879). (Quoted by Cooper, M.) *Memorabilien*, **24**, 97.
Latsky, J. M. (1943). *An experimental investigation into the blood in Cape Peninsula school children in relation to their nutritional state*. Ph.D. Thesis. University of Cape Town.
McKhann, C. F. (1926). *Amer. J. Dis. Child.*, **32**, 386.
Major, W. (1935). (Quoted by Cooper, M.) *Un. Méd. Can.*, **64**, 1424.
Mathieu, J. (1927). (Quoted by Cooper. M.) *Arch. Méd. Enf.*, **30**, 591.
Nims, H. (1842). (Quoted by Cooper, M.) *Boston med. surg. J.*, **25**, 114.
Nouverre, M. G. (1833). (Quoted by Cooper, M.) *J. Méd. prat.*, **13**, 65.
Orr, J. B. and Gilks, J. L. (1931). *Spec. Rep. Ser. med. Res. Coun. (Lond.)* No. 155.
Peak, H. (1857). (Quoted by Cooper, M.) *New Orleans med, surg. J.*, **13**, 299.
Rake, B. (1884). *Brit. med. J.*, **1**, 994.
Richter, C. P. (1943). *Harvey Lect.*, 1942-43. Series 38, **63**.
Ruddock, J. C. (1924). *J. Amer. med. Ass.*, **82**, 1682.
Schrey, W. H. (1719). (Quoted by Cooper, M.) *De Appetitu Erroneo quem Vulgo Picam Vocunt*. Dissertation. Literatis Immanuelis Titii, Leipsig.
Segond, A. (1833). (Quoted by Cooper, M.) *Tr. Med. Paris*, **13**, 156.
Sheldon, W. (1955). *Diseases of Infancy and Childhood*, 7th ed., p. 613. J. & A. Churchill. London.
Stetson, C. A. (1947). *J. Maine med. Ass.*, **38**, 10.
Still, G. F. (1915). *Common Disorders and Diseases of Childhood*, 3rd ed. p. 779. Henry Frowde, London.
Tanis, A. L. (1955). *A.M.A. Amer. J. Dis. Child.*, **89**, 325.
Theiler, A., Green, H. H. and Du Toit, P. J. (1924). (Quoted by Cooper, M.) *Phosphorus in the Live Stock Industry* (*re* Osteophagia in S.A. cattle). Department of Agriculture, Union of South Africa.
Tosatti, C. (1907). (Quoted by Cooper, M.) *Gazz. Osp. Clin.*, **28**, 154.
Waldenström, J. and Kjellberg, S. R. (1939). *Acta radiol. (Stockh.)*, **20**, 618.
—— (1946). *Acta med. scand.*, Suppl. **170**, p. 252.
Waller, H. (1874). *The Last Journals of David Livingstone, in Central Africa from 1865 to his Death*, Vol. 2, p. 83. John Murray, London.
Williams, H., Kaplan, E., Couchman, C. and Sayers, R. (1955). (Quoted by Cooper, M.) *Publ. Hlth Rep. (Wash.)*, **167**, 3.

THE PRE-ERUPTIVE ILLNESS OF MEASLES

BY

M. W. PARTINGTON* and J. F. P. QUINTON

From the Jenny Lind Children's Hospital, Norwich

(RECEIVED FOR PUBLICATION SEPTEMBER 11, 1958)

According to Sydenham (1717), the rash of measles appears on the fourth, or sometimes the fifth, day of the illness. This has remained the standard teaching of most of the authorities on infectious diseases and paediatrics (e.g. Sheldon, 1948; Banks, 1949; Harries and Mitman, 1951; Top, 1955). However, Panum (1847), in his classic report of a measles epidemic, states that although the prodromal illness usually lasts two to four days it can last up to eight days. Some modern writers agree and allow that on occasion the prodromal illness may be as long as six to eight days (e.g. Joe, 1947; Stimson and Hodes, 1956; Ellis, 1956). Recently Christensen, Schmidt, Bang, Andersen, Jordal and Jensen (1953), observing a very similar epidemic in Southern Greenland to that described by Panum in the Faroe Islands, also found that the prodromal illness may be as long as eight days. Two cases with a prodromal illness lasting nine and 11 days respectively were recorded by Selby (1936), and Spence, Walton, Miller and Court (1954), in their 1,000-family survey, found two patients who were ill throughout the incubation period.

A relatively unknown feature of the pre-eruptive period of measles is the 'illness of infection', first described by Goodall (1925). Despite at least 25 cases reported in the literature (Erdheim, 1926; Abercrombie, 1929; Meyer and Greenthal, 1930; Smith, 1944), and a reasonable theoretical basis (Grist, 1950), it has received scant attention.

* Present address: The Department of Child Health, University of Sheffield.

Personal observation suggested that both a long prodromal illness and the illness of infection are not at all uncommon in measles and so we thought it of interest to review our own material.

Methods and Material

The case notes were scrutinized of all patients with the diagnosis of measles admitted to the Norwich Isolation Hospital between July 1, 1952, and April 1, 1958, and to the Jenny Lind Hospital between January 1, 1951, and April 1, 1958. A large proportion of these patients had been seen by one or both of us in the acute phase. Cases were allowed into the series if they satisfied the following conditions: (1) The patient was thought to have measles by the physician in charge of the case at the time. (2) There were reasonably precise indications in the case notes of the time of onset of the illness (e.g. 'Ten days ago . . .', 'A week ago . . .', a definite date or fever on a temperature chart). (3) There were equally clear indications of the day an unmistakable measles rash appeared. (4) The patient had both fever and a morbilliform rash. (5) Each patient had in addition at least one of the following: (*a*) Koplik's spots, (*b*) conjunctivitis, (*c*) respiratory catarrh.

Over 120 case notes were available and 82 fulfilled these requirements.

Results

Table 1 shows the cases distributed according to the day of the illness on which the morbilliform rash

TABLE 1

CASES DISTRIBUTED ACCORDING TO THE DAY OF THE ILLNESS ON WHICH THE MEASLES RASH CAME OUT

	Group I							Group II								
Day of illness	1	2	3	4	5	6	7	8	9	10	11	12	13	14	15	16
Number of cases	0	5	14	7	9	16	6	3	4	5	3	1	3	3	1	2
	57							25								

Division of cases into Groups I and II (see text).

appeared. In 35 patients the rash had come out on or before the fifth day and by the end of the week in another 22. These cases have been called Group I. In the remaining 25 patients, nearly one-third of the series, the rash appeared on or after the eighth day of the illness, and these have been called Group II. Some general data on the whole series is shown in Tables 3, 4 and 5.

Group I (57 cases). Nineteen patients in this group developed a measles rash on or before the third day of the illness.

Case 1. Glynn E., aged 22 months. Nine days previously his brother developed a measles rash. Day 1: Without warning he had a generalized convulsion and three further fits in the next two hours. On admission to hospital he was found to have fever, irritability, bilateral conjunctivitis, and Koplik's spots in each side of the mouth. Day 2: Characteristic measles rash appeared.

In 38 patients the rash came out on the fourth to the seventh day of illness.

Case 2. Tanji B., a girl, aged 4 years. In contact with measles at school. Day 1: Became irritable with a fever of 104° F. and an inflamed throat. Day 2-3: Passed eight watery stools with much mucus. Day 4: Onset of cough. Day 5: Began to vomit with her cough. Admitted to hospital and found to have fever, a running nose, injected fauces, a harsh cough and many palpable cervical glands. Day 6: Koplik's spots and a measles rash appeared. Her sister, admitted with her, also developed measles.

Group II (25 cases). In this group the measles rash appeared on or after the eighth day of the illness. The group can be sub-divided into (*a*) those in whom the pre-eruptive illness was a long, continuous, but otherwise characteristic, prodromal illness (17 cases), and (*b*) those in whom the illness was diphasic (eight cases). Case 3 is an example of the first kind of illness.

Case 3. Jennifer W., aged 5 years. In contact with measles at school. Day 1-6: Developed a persistent cough. Day 7-11: Stayed away from school, had a runny nose, complained of episodic abdominal pain, was off her food and vomited several times. Day 12: Conjunctivitis, photophobia and fever. Day 13: Rash noticed in the morning which faded. Day 14: Rash reappeared. Admitted to hospital with fever, misery, conjunctivitis, confluent morbilliform rash on the face and upper trunk, injected fauces, enlarged cervical glands and rapid breathing.

The next patient's illness lasted 14 days before the measles rash came out. The illness was severe at the onset, then remitted, although it did not subside completely, and again became severe a few days before the rash appeared.

Case 4. Doreen B., aged 6 years. Day 1-3: Cough, fever and vomiting diagnosed as influenza. Day 4-11: Better, but still had anorexia, malaise and a cough. Day 12-13: Started to vomit again, was feverish and apathetic. Day 14: Admitted to hospital. Found to have fever, a loose cough, enlarged cervical glands and rales at both lung bases. Day 15: Widespread measles rash.

In eight patients in this group the pre-eruptive illness was diphasic with a distinct period of apparently normal health separating the first phase from the second.

Case 5. Susan B., aged 2 years. Two weeks previously admitted to hospital with bronchopneumonia which responded to treatment with penicillin. In contact with measles in the ward. Day 1: Evening temperature of 100° F. Day 2-5: Appeared in good health. Day 6-10: Slight malaise and fever. Day 11-13: Fever, rales at the left lung base; penicillin restarted. Day 14: Measles rash on face, limbs and trunk (Fig. 1).

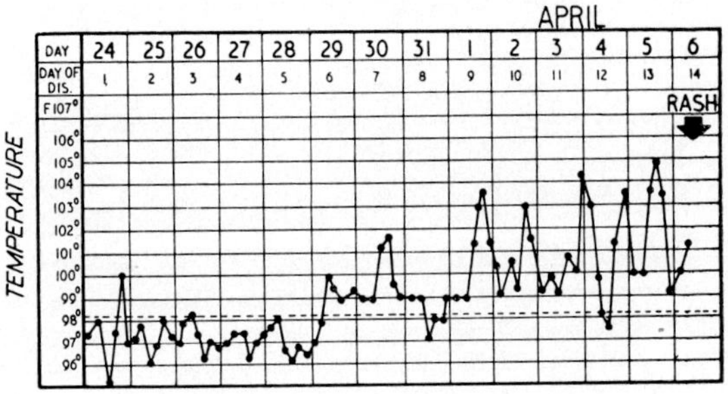

FIG. 1.—Temperature chart of Case 5 showing both a brief febrile illness of infection and a long prodromal illness.

In this last patient the first illness was no more than a spike of fever on a temperature chart, but in others it was more dramatic.

Case 6. James A., aged 4 years. Day 1-3: Anorexia, enlarged cervical glands and a 'pin-head' rash on the neck and behind the ears which spread to the trunk on Day 4. Day 5-8: Rash disappeared, felt completely well. Day 9: Malaise. Day 10: Conjunctivitis, running nose and a cough. Day 11: Measles rash on face and trunk. Day 14: Admitted to hospital with an extensive morbilliform rash, Koplik's spots, rhinorrhoea, a harsh cough and conjunctivitis.

Case 7. Christopher B., aged 5 years. Day 1-7: Developed a 'cold' with a loose cough and repeated vomiting. Day 8-9: Began to improve. Day 10-11: Up and about, apparently well. Day 12-13: Malaise. Day 14: Started vomiting again. Day 15: Admitted to hospital with fever, a loose cough, enlarged cervical glands, a nasal discharge, inflamed fauces and rales in the lungs. Day 16: Widespread measles rash.

In Fig. 2 these seven cases are presented schematically. The histories are all reduced to the same time scale by assuming that in every case the interval between infection and the appearance of the rash is 14 days. Each case history is meant to represent a different type of pre-eruptive illness and the number of cases of each type in this series is shown in the figure. In Type 1 the rash comes out on or before the third day of the illness (or on the eleventh to the fourteenth day of the incubation period). In Type 2 the rash appears after four to seven days of illness and in Type 3 on or after the eighth day. In other words these three types form a series of increasingly long prodromal illnesses.

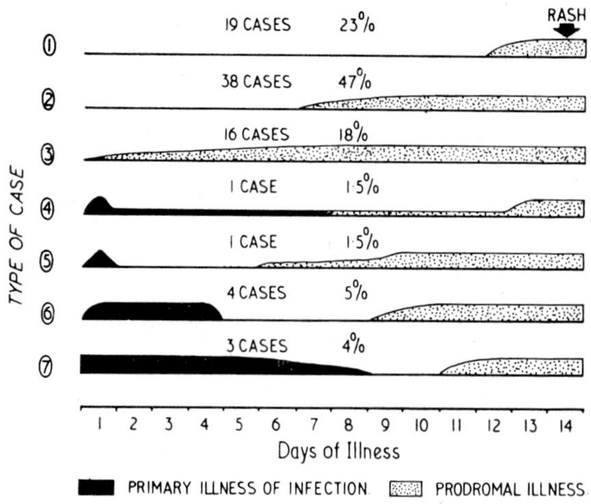

FIG. 2.—Schematic presentation of various types of pre-eruptive illness in measles. Number of cases of each type in this series is shown. Type 5 represents Case 5 (see Fig. 1 and text).

The fourth case may be regarded as a transitional type between those patients with a long prodromal illness and those with a distinct diphasic onset. The pre-eruptive illness lasted 14 days but it was severe at its onset then partially remitted and again became severe just before the rash came out.

The last three types of illness are all diphasic with an increasingly long first phase or primary illness of infection (Type 5 lasting one day, Type 6, two to four days and Type 7 longer than four days). These are associated with a shorter or longer second phase, prodromal illness (two to eight days) and a distinct intervening period of apparently normal health (two to four days).

Table 2 lists the clinical features of the illness of infection. Any of these may also be found in the prodromal illness. Although these two types of illness have been represented differently in Fig. 2

TABLE 2

CLINICAL FEATURES OF THE ILLNESS OF INFECTION

Patient	Clinical Features	Duration (days)
S.B.	Fever	1
M.S.	Fever, lethargy	2
S.C.	Vomiting	3
J.A.	Anorexia, cervical lymphadenopathy, 'pin-head' rash	4
W.E.	Fever, vomiting, lethargy, cervical lymph-adenopathy, splenomegaly	4
P.S.	Fever, cough, delirium	8
C.B.	Cough, vomiting	9
E.S.	Fever, vomiting, abdominal pain, rhinor-rhoea	9

it seems probable that the only essential differences between them are their severity and their timing in relation to the initial infection (see discussion).

Groups I and II were compared with regard to sex, age and year of onset. The differences in sex and age distribution (Tables 3, 4) are not significant. Although fluctuations in the number of cases of measles occurred from year to year there was no obvious difference between the two groups in this respect (Table 5).

TABLE 3

SEX DISTRIBUTION

	Male	Female	Total
Group I ..	31	26	57
Group II ..	10	15	25
Total	41	41	82
	$\chi^2 = 0 \cdot 92$	$p \simeq 0 \cdot 4$	

TABLE 4

AGE DISTRIBUTION

	Age (years)			
	0–2	3–5	6+	Total
Group I ..	25	19	13	57
Group II ..	5	15	5	25
Total	30	34	18	82
	$\chi^2 = 4 \cdot 46$ $0 \cdot 2 > p > 0 \cdot 1$			

TABLE 5

YEAR OF ONSET

	Year of Onset						
	1951/2	1953	1954	1955	1956	1957/8	Total
Group I ..	13	8	19	2	8	7	57
Group II ..	8	1	8	3	3	2	25
Total ..	21	9	27	5	11	9	82

Discussion

This series shows a greater variation in the length of the pre-eruptive illness of measles than those reported by others. Thus Hermann (1914) found that in 84% of his patients the rash appeared on the third to the fifth day of illness. In the series reported by Christensen *et al.* (1953), the comparable figure is 66·7% whereas in our own it is 36·5%.

In 17 patients (about 20%) the rash came out on the eighth to the sixteenth day of continuous illness. Apart from a few of Christensen's patients whose rash appeared on the eighth day and the four patients cited previously (Selby, 1936; Spence *et al.*, 1954), no comparable cases have been found in the literature.

Smith (1944) estimated that at least 10% of patients with measles have an illness of infection. Our figures (eight out of 82) agree well with this.

It cannot be claimed that this series is an unbiased sample of measles if only for the fact that all the cases were hospital admissions. This factor might possibly increase the likelihood of a long prodromal illness, but there is no way of assessing this from our data.

In an attempt to explain our results the patients with a diphasic onset and those with a long prodromal illness were grouped together and compared with the rest of the series. There were no significant differences in sex or age distribution or year of onset. This last finding suggests that the high frequency of a long pre-eruptive illness in this series was not due to a peculiar set of conditions obtaining in one particular epidemic.

Except for their duration the clinical features displayed by those patients with a prodromal illness longer than a week were no different from those usually described in measles. It has already been pointed out that the clinical features of the illness of infection (Table 2) are similar to those of the prodromal illness. Other workers have noted this similarity and even a morbilliform rash has been reported in the first phase (Goodall, 1925; and possibly Case 6 above). This may explain some relapses in measles and second attacks occurring within two or three weeks of the first (Smith, 1944).

Grist (1950) has applied the work of Burnet (1946) and Fenner (1948) to the pathogenesis of measles. It is suggested that after the initial infection, probably by way of the respiratory tract, the virus gains access to the blood stream and a viraemia ensues. After this invasion, which may take several days, the virus settles in the reticulo-endothelial system for the rest of the incubation period. Here it multiplies and then emerges in a second viraemia which is responsible for the customary clinical features of measles. It follows that if the first viraemia causes symptoms at all they might well be similar to those of the second phase illness; furthermore they might be less severe if only because the amount of circulating virus is less (Fenner, 1948). Our findings fit in well with this concept.

Fenner thought that this hypothesis might prove applicable to other acute infections. However, it is only in measles that an illness of infection has been clearly recognized. In poliomyelitis the onset is diphasic in 40% of cases with a minor illness followed by a period of health before the major illness develops (Russell, 1956). Whilst it is reasonably certain that the virus is present in the bloodstream at the time of the minor illness, it is not clear whether this corresponds with either Fenner's first or second viraemia.

Lymphocytic choriomeningitis may also have a diphasic onset. A minor illness with either influenzal or upper respiratory catarrhal features precedes the major illness by 10 days in at least 35% of patients (Adair, Gauld and Smadel, 1953). This could be an illness of infection. Clinically a similar diphasic onset may occur in sporadic, primary pyogenic meningitis. In a recent series of 74 cases we found that 18 (25%) had a catarrhal or influenzal illness in the 10 days prior to the major illness with an intervening period of normal health.

It seems likely that many preceding minor illnesses are overlooked in these (and possibly other) diseases especially since the two phases of the illness are separated by a period of apparent health. Further work is needed to clarify these observations but it does seem reasonable to distinguish this kind of diphasic onset from that occurring in acute nephritis, rheumatic fever and acute disseminated encephalomyelitis where the continued presence of the infective organism is not necessary for the second phase illness to develop.

As Smith (1944) points out, it is really more surprising that 'the incubation of a virus in a body almost always occurs in a quiescent phase' than that symptoms should occur during this period. Our observations suggest that at least in measles the incubation period is less quiescent than is commonly supposed.

Summary

The onset of measles was studied in 82 patients. It was found that in 17 patients (20%) the rash came out on the eighth to the sixteenth day of the illness. A further eight patients (10%) had an illness of infection.

These findings are discussed. It is argued that there is little essential difference between the illness of infection and the prodromal illness except in time-relationship to the initial infection. This agrees with Fenner's (1948) hypothesis.

It is concluded that both an illness of infection and a long prodromal illness are commoner in measles than is usually reported.

We wish to thank Dr. R. M. Mayon-White and Professor R. S. Illingworth for criticizing the manuscript and Derek Martin of the Department of Medical Illustration, The Hospital for Sick Children, Great Ormond Street, for the figures. We should also like to thank the many house physicians at the Jenny Lind and Norwich Isolation Hospitals whose case notes contained enough information to make this study possible.

REFERENCES

Abercrombie, G. F. (1929). *Brit. J. Child. Dis.*, **26**, 15.
Adair, C. V., Gauld, R. L. and Smadel, J. E. (1953). *Ann. intern. Med.*, **39**, 675.
Banks, H. S. (1949). *The Common Infectious Diseases.* Arnold, London.
Burnet, F. M. (1946). *The Background of Infectious Diseases in Man.* Melbourne Permanent Postgraduate Committee, Melbourne.
Christensen, P. E., Schmidt, H., Bang, H. O., Andersen, V., Jordal, B. and Jensen, O. (1953). *Acta med. scand.*, **144**, 430.
Ellis, R. W. B. (1956). *Disease in Infancy and Childhood*, 2nd ed. Livingstone, Edinburgh.
Erdheim, S. (1926). *Brit. J. Child. Dis.*, **23**, 240.
Fenner, F. (1948). *Lancet*, **2**, 915.
Goodall, E. W. (1925). *Clin. J.*, **54**, 69.
Grist, N. R. (1950). *Glasg. med. J.*, **31**, 431.
Harries, E. H. R. and Mitman, M. (1951). *Clinical Practice in Infectious Diseases*, 4th ed. Livingstone, Edinburgh.
Herrman, C. (1914). *Arch. Pediat.*, **31**, 885.
Joe, A. (1947). *The Acute Infectious Fevers.* Churchill, London.
Meyer, P. R. and Greenthal, R. M. (1930). *Arch. Pediat.*, **47**, 399.
Panum, P. L. (1847). *Observations made during the Epidemic of Measles on the Faroe Islands in the Year 1846*; Eng. trans. by A. S. Hatcher (1940). Published by Delta Omega Society, New York.
Russell, W. Ritchie (1956). *Poliomyelitis*, 2nd ed. Arnold, London.
Selby, R. (1936). *Brit. med. J.*, **1**, 262.
Sheldon, W. (1948). *Diseases of Children.* Churchill, London.
Smith, R. E. (1944). *Guy's Hosp. Rep.*, **93**, 8.
Spence, J., Walton, W. S., Miller, F. J. W. and Court, S. D. M. (1954). *A Thousand Families in Newcastle upon Tyne.* Oxford University Press, London.
Stimson, P. M. and Hodes, H. L. (1956). *A Manual of the Common Contagious Diseases*, 5th ed. Kimpton, London.
Sydenham, T. (1717). *The Whole Works of that Excellent Practical Physician*, 7th ed. Wellington, London.
Top, F. H. (1955). *Communicable Diseases*, 3rd ed. Mosby, St. Louis.

AN ENGLISH FAMILY WITH WAARDENBURG'S SYNDROME

BY

M. W. PARTINGTON*

From the Jenny Lind Children's Hospital, Norwich

(RECEIVED FOR PUBLICATION OCTOBER 8, 1958)

In 1951 Waardenburg first described a syndrome consisting of (1) lateral displacement of the inner canthi of the eye and of the inferior lacrimal punctae (dystopia canthorum), (2) a high broad nasal root, (3) confluence of the eyebrows with hypertrichosis of their medial parts, (4) partial or total heterochromia iridum, (5) a white forelock, and (6) unilateral or bilateral congenital deafness. From his extensive material Waardenburg concluded that the syndrome has a dominant autosomal inheritance but that each of its components shows a variable penetrance. Thus out of his 161 affected individuals from 14 families, 99% had dystopia canthorum, 78% the broad nasal root, 45% the confluent eyebrows, 25% heterochromia iridum, 20% congenital deafness and 17% a white forelock. He estimated that in the Netherlands this syndrome accounts for about 1·43% of all deaf mutes, and that in whole or in part it occurs in 1 in 42,000 persons.

Except for one Swiss subject all Waardenburg's cases were Dutch. From the literature he recognized two probable American cases and possible German and Italian examples. Keizer (1952) described another Dutch family and Wildervanck (1957) reported a further five cases also from Holland. Mackenzie (1958) has described an example from Scotland. On the other hand, Klenka (1956) examined 374 deaf mutes in Prague and was unable to find a single typical case. No other examples have been found in the literature. It seemed, therefore, that the present pedigree was worth recording.

Family History

The Family. The family pedigree is shown in Fig. 1. The propositus was brought to hospital because of obvious congenital deafness. Her parents (IV-1 and 2, see pedigree) provided much of the family history. The maternal grandfather (III-5) and his second wife (not shown in the pedigree) were also interviewed and several photographs were available. The white forelock is well recognized by them as an inherited feature. The family all live in Norfolk and have done so for many generations.

I-2. This lady probably showed part of the syndrome but the evidence is meagre. She is remembered as having had a similar appearance around the eyes and nose to other affected persons in the family but a good full-face photograph shows only thick eyebrows and a high, wide nasal root.

II-4. The grandmother was clearly affected. She had a small white forelock, one iris was blue and the other brown. As judged from three photographs she had dystopia canthorum and a broad nasal root. She died, probably from pneumonia, in her early forties.

II-6. A sister of the above had no white forelock but from a good photograph she seems to have had dystopia canthorum and the typical nasal root. She never married and died at the age of 50 from cancer (site unknown).

III-6. The only daughter of II-4 had a white forelock as a child and as a young woman, but did her best to hide it. At the age of about 23 years her hair went completely grey. Her eyebrows tended to grow together in the midline but her eyes were both the same blue colour. She is also remembered as having had the characteristic appearance of the eyes and nose but this is not obvious from the one available photograph. She died at the age of 40 from hypertension.

IV-2 (Fig. 2). The mother of the propositus has a broad white forelock (which as a child her mother had tried to hide). She has dystopia canthorum with lateral displacement of the inferior lacrimal punctae so that they lie opposite the inner edge of the cornea. The distance between the inner canthi is 40 mm., the interpupillary distance is 60 mm., and the outer canthal distance is 100 mm. The irises are blue with a hazel tinge and are of the same colour. The nose root is broad and the eyebrows tend to grow together in the midline. (This latter trait is not seen in Fig. 2 because the eyebrows are plucked). At the age of 6 years she had measles and after this was found to be deaf in the right ear. She was

* Present address: Department of Child Health, University of Sheffield.

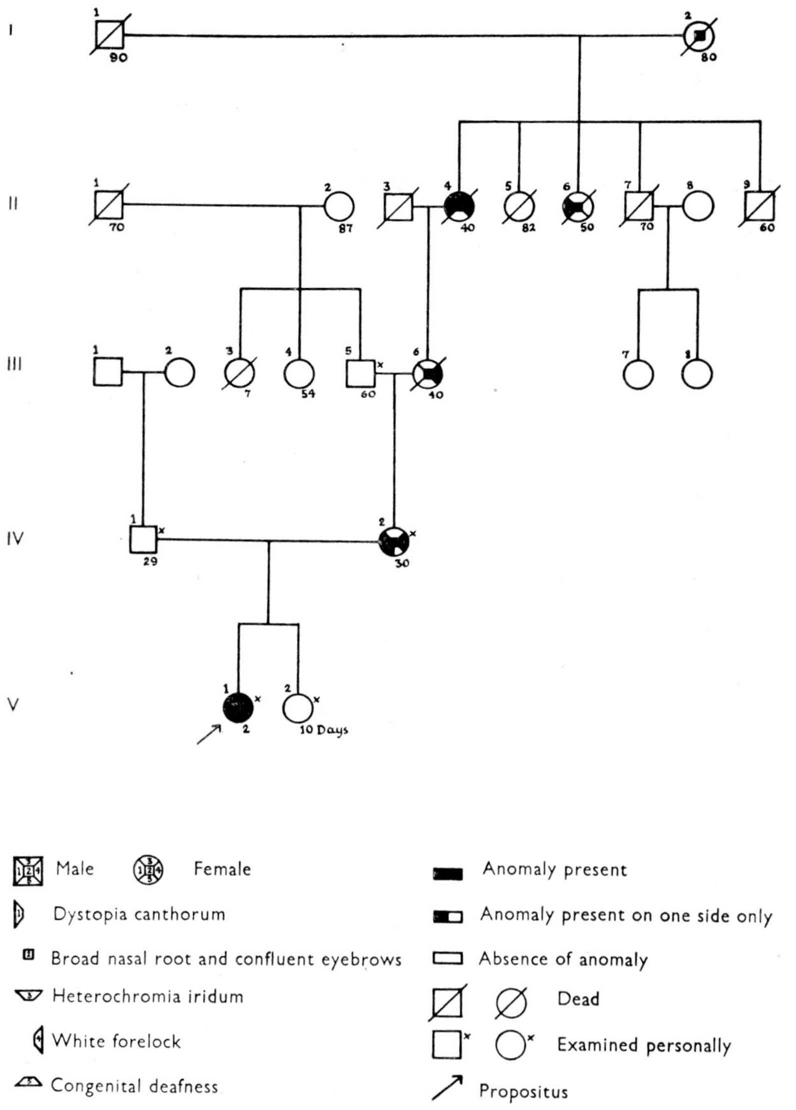

FIG. 1.—The pedigree (Waardenburg's symbols).

seen by an aural specialist who said that the ' nerve had been destroyed '. She is completely deaf on that side. She has a patch of albino hairs about 3 cm. across on the left leg. She is in good health.

V-1. The propositus is now aged 2 years. She was born at full term after a normal pregnancy. The white forelock was noticed at birth. The inner quarters of the eyebrows and the inner halves of the eyelashes are also white. The nasal root is broad and the eyebrows grow together in the midline (this is not obvious in Fig. 2 because the hairs are white). The eyes are intensely blue but at 10 o'clock in the right iris there is a light brown patch about 3 mm. across. There is dystopia canthorum and the inferior lacrimal punctae lie opposite the inner edge of the cornea. The inner canthal distance is 32 mm., the interpupillary distance 55 mm., and the outer canthal distance 90 mm. She appears to be totally deaf, only responding to loud vibratory noises. She babbles and mouths words. She is not retarded except in speech. There is an irregular patch of skin on the inner arm which fails to pigment in sunlight and a similar streak runs down the middle of her forehead. She has had no major illnesses and is in good general health.

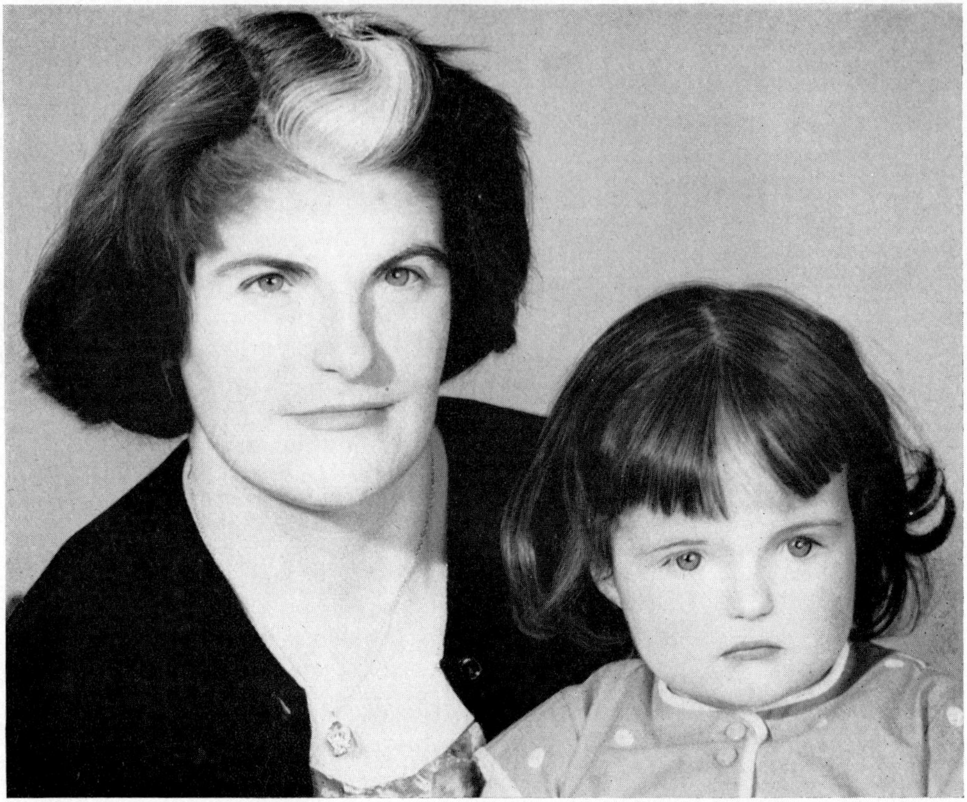

FIG. 2.—Mother and daughter (IV-2 and V-1) showing the white forelock, dystopia cathorum and broad nasal root.

There is little to note about the other members of the family. II-1 had numerous white spots on the skin of his arms for many years which was thought to be vitiligo. III-3 died at the age of 7 years from diphtheria. III-5 at the age of 60 has grey hair. IV-1 has brown isochromic eyes and no sign of dystopia canthorum (inner canthal distance 30 mm., interpupillary distance 60 mm., outer canthal distance 110 mm.). V-2, the sister of the propositus, at the age of 10 days seemed a normal healthy baby. There is no white forelock, dystopia or confluent eyebrows and she reacts to sounds.

Discussion

This family history illustrates many aspects of Waardenburg's syndrome. The mode of inheritance is consistent with an autosomal dominant gene of variable penetrance. The most important feature of the syndrome, congenital deafness, may be unilateral or bilateral and this is shown in mother and daughter (IV-2 and V-1). These subjects also show dystopia canthorum. Dystopia was present in two of their forebears (II-4 and 6), and, though the evidence is not very good, probably in two others as well (I-2 and III-6). This anomaly is far easier to see in the living person than in photographs. It is frequently mistaken for hypertelorism (and was so mistaken at the first interview in the present case). Waardenburg gives as the extreme normal adult limits for the inner canthal distance 24 to 39 mm., and 54 to 75 mm. for the interpupillary distance; in women the distances are shorter than in men. In dystopia canthorum the inner canthal distance is 40 mm. or more and the interpupillary distance is normal whereas in hypertelorism both measurements are increased.

As Waardenburg points out his figures for the incidence of the other components of the syndrome are almost certainly under-estimates. Heterochromia iridum is conspicuous if complete (II-4) but easy to miss if only partial (V-1). Confluent eyebrows are not readily remembered and may be disguised (IV-2). The white forelock may be inconspicuous, forgotten in later life or deliberately concealed as it was by one of the present family (III-6) both in herself and in her daughter. (The mother shown in Fig. 2 has been accused on more than one occasion of bleaching her own and her daughter's hair.) Premature greying of the whole head of hair occurred in one individual who had previously had a white forelock (III-6) which supports Waardenburg's contention that this is probably another expression of the syndrome equivalent to the white forelock. Wildervanck (1957) reports that in one of his cases two of the forebears had white patches at the back of the head. It is also possible that albino spots of skin (V-1) or body hair (IV-2) may be associated with the syndrome.

In other recorded cases there has been no obvious sex-linkage so that there is probably no significance in the fact that all the affected persons in this pedigree are female.

It is of interest to speculate where the gene may have come from in this family. It could have arisen by mutation as seemed to have happened in some of Waardenburg's cases. It could have been brought over here from the Netherlands. There have been two waves of Flemish immigration to this part of England, one in the fourteenth and one in the sixteenth century. (One of the unaffected persons (III-5) has the name of Williment and is of remote Dutch descent.) Yet again the syndrome may be as common in other peoples as in the Dutch but it has not yet been sufficiently recognized and reported.

Summary

An English family with Waardenburg's syndrome is described. Five members showed various parts of the syndrome and in the sixth it was complete.

I would like to thank Dr. J. F. P. Quinton for permission to publish this case and Dr. A. S. Robertson for referring the family to me. I would also like to thank Dr. A. E. Bashford for Fig. 1.

References

Keizer, D. P. R (1952). *Ned. T. Geneesk.*, **96**, 2541.

Klenka, L. (1956). *Čsl. Ofthal.*, **12**, 270. Cited in *Excerpta med. (Amst.)*, (1957). Section 12 (Ophthalmology), **11**, 54.

Mackenzie, J. (1958). *Arch. Dis. Childh.*, **33**, 477.

Waardenburg, P. J. (1951). *Amer. J. hum. Genet.*, **3**, 195.

Wildervanck, L. S. (1957). *Ned. T. Geneesk.*, **101**, 1120.

Addendum

Since this paper was accepted for publication it has been brought to the author's notice that an exhibit of this syndrome was shown by the Royal National Throat and Ear Hospital, London, to the Annual Conference of the British Medical Association in 1958. This included an account of some histological findings indicating complete absence of the organ of Corti and the vestibular membrane. (*Brit. med. J.* (1958) **2,** 322.)

RENAL TUBULAR DAMAGE IN INFANTILE GASTRO-ENTERITIS

BY

JOHN BLACK

From The Hospital for Sick Children, Great Ormond Street, London

(RECEIVED FOR PUBLICATION AUGUST 17, 1958)

Introduction

The natural history of acute tubular necrosis in adults has been well documented, but accounts of the condition in infants and children are rare. Most of the descriptions of tubular necrosis in the paediatric literature refer to older children (Riddell, 1951; Kaplan and Fomon, 1953; Wagner, 1954), but Pratt (1948) described two cases due to sulphonamides, aged 10 months and 18 months, and Jonsson (1951) published three fatal cases of severe asphyxia neonatorum with oliguria and raised blood urea, but at autopsy in Jonsson's cases there were haemoglobin casts in the distal tubules with no degeneration of the tubular epithelium. Doxiadis (1947) described tubular changes in some fatal cases of gastro-enteritis, but the details of the renal histology given are insufficient to make it clear whether he was dealing with acute tubular necrosis or with some type of nephrocalcinosis. The pathological aspect of renal disorders in early life associated with circulatory disturbances has been fully reviewed by Zuelzer, Charles, Kurnetz, Newton and Fallon (1951) who showed that various types of acute renal failure not uncommonly develop in severely dehydrated children. They described a range of vascular complications affecting the kidney, including 'lower nephron nephrosis' (acute tubular necrosis). In many of their cases diarrhoea and vomiting appeared to have been the precipitating symptoms. Carré and Squire (1956) published three cases of anuria with tubular necrosis, which were studied in great detail. The cause of the anuria was uncertain in the first case, and was thought to be due to sulphonamides and a penicillin reaction respectively in the other two cases.

Recent work (Oliver, MacDowell and Tracy (1951) and Van Slyke (1954)) has indicated that, apart from certain poisons, renal ischaemia is the probable cause of most cases of acute tubular necrosis, and that the ischaemia is itself a response to certain circulatory disorders associated with severe shock. In children, acute gastro-enteritis is probably the commonest cause of dehydration and shock, and it is surprising that there have been no reports of the clinical recognition of tubular damage in this condition. The only observations on this subject are those of Calcagno and Rubin (1951) and of Kerpel-Fronius, Varga, Kun and Vönöczky (1954). Calcagno and Rubin (1951) produced evidence of failure of water reabsorption during the acute phase of dehydration and shock in two severe cases, but found that complete recovery occurred within 24 hours and five days respectively. Kerpel-Fronius *et al.* (1954) stated that it was often some days or even weeks before complete restoration of renal function occurred.

Two cases with evidence of tubular damage are here reported in full, together with a retrospective survey showing that minor degrees of renal damage are not uncommon in gastro-enteritis.

Case Reports

Case 1 (G.B.). On December 19, 1950, an 18-month-old male child was admitted to hospital with a two-day history of severe diarrhoea and vomiting. He was comatose and very dehydrated (Table 1). There was slight stiffness of the neck and back, but the limbs were hypotonic.

TABLE 1
INVESTIGATIONS ON ADMISSION: CASE 1

(1) Blood Chemistry
Serum chlorides: 580 mg. % as NaCl (99·1 mEq./l.)
Serum potassium: 9·5 mg. % (2·4 mEq./l.)
Serum protein: 6·5 g. %
Blood urea: 152 mg. %
(2) Cerebrospinal Fluid
Cells: 4 per c.mm.
Protein: 80 mg. %
Sugar: 125 mg. %
Chlorides: 840 mg. % as NaCl (143 mEq./l.)
(3) Urine
Highly concentrated
Reaction: acid
Protein: 50 mg. %
No reducing sugar detected
Microscopy: an occasional white cell

Progress and Treatment. Half-strength Hartmann's solution in 2½% glucose was given immediately, followed by half-strength plasma. There was a temporary improvement but by the third day he was still hypotonic and uninterested in his surroundings, though his hydration appeared quite normal. By the eighteenth day he seemed to have made a complete recovery from the gastro-enteritis and was discharged. On his return home his apathy did not improve, he was difficult to feed and did not speak. He was therefore readmitted for further investigation (Table 2).

TABLE 2

INVESTIGATIONS ON RE-ADMISSION: CASE 1 (13.1.51)

(1) Blood chemistry
- Serum chlorides: 577 mg. % as NaCl (98·7 mEq./l.)
- Plasma bicarbonate: 37·5 vols. CO_2 % (16·7 mEq./l.)
- Serum potassium: 16 mg. % (4·2 mEq./l.)
- Blood urea: 23 mg. %

(2) Urine
- Reaction: alkaline
- Protein: 170 mg. %
- Microscopy: numerous epithelial cells

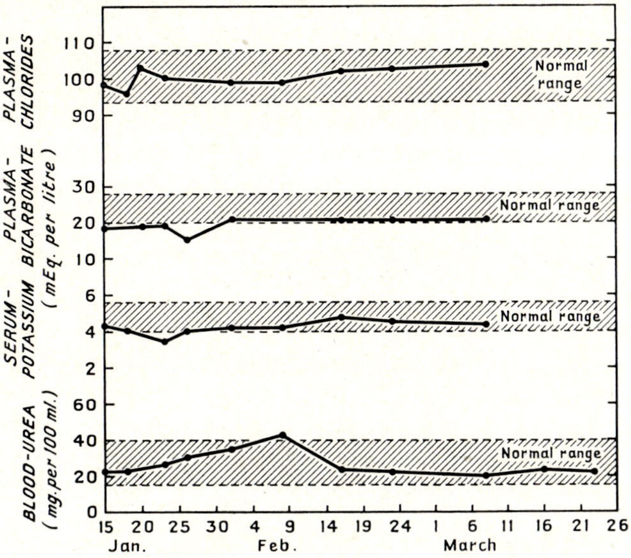

FIG. 1.—Case 1. Blood chemistry during second admission. A mild acidosis and transient hypokalaemia were found. With treatment, the blood chemistry became normal and remained normal after treatment was stopped.

Progress During Second Admission. (Fig. 1.) There was now evidence of a bilateral pyramidal lesion probably due to thrombosis of the sagittal sinus. The blood chemistry showed a moderate acidosis with normal serum potassium and blood urea (Table 2). A few days later the serum potassium fell to 15·4 mg. % (3·9 mEq./l.) and then to 13·8 mg. % (3·5 mEq./l.).

As there was no diarrhoea to account for the acidosis the urine was investigated for evidence of a tubular defect causing failure of acidification of the urine. The urinary *p*H varied between 6·5 and a definitely alkaline reaction

TABLE 3

URINE TESTS: CASE 1

Date	Reaction or *p*H	Specific Gravity	Urea (mg. %)	Protein (mg. %)	Amino Acids	Deposit	Remarks
19.12.50	Acid	—	—	50	—	Occasional W.B.C.	
16. 1.51	Alkaline	—	—	170	—	E.C.* ++	
17. 1.51	Neutral	—	—	150	—	E.C. ++	
18. 1.51	6·5	'Dilute'	—	—	++	E.C. +	Slight reduction of Benedict's solution. Acidotic
22 1.51	Acid	—	—	50	—	E.C. +	
23. 1.51	6·49	1,027	2,900	0	—	E.C. +	After 12-hour fluid restriction. Acidotic
23. 1.51	6·47	1,017	3,000	Trace	Slight increase above normal	E.C. +	Amino acids added to feeds. Acidotic
24. 1.51	Alkaline	1,026	—	30	—	Addis count normal	
27. 1.51	5·7	1,027	3,300	Trace	—	—	NH_3 coeff. 6·3 %
29. 1.51	—	—	—	—	—	—	Slight reduction of Benedict's solution
12. 2.51	Alkaline	—	—	—	Normal	E.C. +	
19. 2.51	6·07	—	—	—	+	—	Galactose 10-15 mg % No amino acids in feeds
5. 3.51	—	—	—	0	—	Occasional R.B.C., W.B.C., E.C.	
27. 3.51	Acid	—	—	0	Normal	—	

* E.C. = Epithelial cells.

(Table 3) in spite of the acidosis. On one occasion there was some reduction of Benedict's solution and chromatography of this specimen showed marked amino-aciduria. Amino-aciduria was found in a lesser amount five days later. Proteinuria was also present (170 mg. %) and this persisted for eight days. On microscopy a large number of epithelial cells was found.

Treatment was started with a sodium citrate-citric acid mixture (Albright's solution) and potassium chloride. The blood chemistry gradually returned to normal and remained normal when the alkali and potassium chloride were stopped after 36 days treatment.

By the fourteenth day after readmission the urine was quite normal apart from the persistence of epithelial cells on microscopy, and renal function appeared to have completely recovered, as shown by a specific gravity of 1,026 after a 12-hour fluid restriction (though there was no evidence of defective water reabsorption at any time). An Addis count and a combined inulin and urea clearance were also normal (Table 4).

TABLE 4

RENAL FUNCTION TESTS: CASE 1

Date	Procedure	Result	Comment
23.1.51	12-hr. fluid restriction	S.G.: 1027	Normal response
24.1.51	Addis count 12-hr. overnight urine collection	Volume: 190 ml. S.G.: 1026 Protein: 30 mg. % R.B.C.: 114,000 W.B.C.: 1,444,000 Casts: Nil	
25.1.51	Combined urea and inulin clearance*	Urea clearance Period I: 119%† Period II: 188%† Period III: 210%† All maximum clearances	Normal
		Inulin clearance Period I: 111 ml./min. Period II: 74 ml./min. Normal for age: 110 ml./min. Surface area: 0·51 sq. metres	Normal
		Case 2	
19.2.52	Urea clearance*	Single period (4 hours) 94·1% average	Normal
		Surface area: 0·30 sq. metres	Normal

* Clearances have been recalculated as for a surface area of 1·73 sq. metres.
† Of average normal.

Comment. There was severe dehydration with azotaemia on admission, and it seems fairly certain that the cerebral damage was sustained at this time: this aspect of the case has been considered fully by Schlesinger and Welch (1952). The urine on admission showed nothing abnormal apart from a slight excess of protein, and renal damage was not suspected until the second admission. It is curious that no thirst or polyuria was noticed at any time and that the tubular damage apparently affected only the H-ion exchange mechanism, and the reabsorption of amino acids and glucose. The exact significance of the proteinuria in terms of glomerular or tubular damage will be discussed later. That structural damage to the tubular epithelium did occur was confirmed by the large number of epithelial cells found in the urine. Recovery of renal function appeared to be complete.

Case History

Case 2 (G.A.). On January 27, 1952 a 12-week-old male infant was admitted to hospital from a residential nursery. No history of diarrhoea or vomiting could be obtained, but it was stated that he had not been taking his feeds well for some days. During his stay of three weeks in the nursery he had lost one pound in weight. On admission he was very shocked and dehydrated, with peripheral cyanosis. There was dyspnoea from gross abdominal distension. His lips and mouth were bile-stained and he was vomiting spontaneously small quantities of bilious fluid. After rectal examination a small amount of bright yellow fluid faeces was passed. As there was no clinical or radiological evidence of an organic obstruction it was considered that he was suffering from gastro-enteritis with ileus, probably due to hypokalaemia. His blood chemistry (Table 5) confirmed this.

TABLE 5

INVESTIGATIONS ON ADMISSION: CASE 2

(1) Radiograph of Abdomen
Great distension of small and large intestine with numerous fluid levels. No evidence of organic obstruction

(2) Blood Chemistry
Plasma bicarbonate: 28·0 vols. CO_2 % (12·5 mEq./l.)
Plasma chlorides: 729 mg. % as NaCl (124·6 mEq./l.)
Serum potassium: 7·7 mg. % (1·97 mEq./l.)
Serum protein: 4·8 g. %
Blood urea: 36 mg. %

(3) Urine
(Small concentrated specimen)
*p*H: 5·0
Protein: 40 mg. %
Urine chlorides: 911 mg. % as NaCl (155·7 mEq./l.)
Microscopy: 1-10 red blood cells per H.P.F.; occasional granular cast
Culture: Sterile

(4) Blood Culture
Sterile

Progress and Treatment. Treatment was with continuous gastric suction and intravenous fluids, using half-strength Hartmann's solution in 2½% glucose. Later 1/6th M sodium lactate was given with additional potassium chloride intravenously at first and then by mouth. Because of the persistent hypokalaemia (Fig. 2) the potassium chloride was continued till the seventeenth day. On the second day oedema developed and lasted for eight days. Vomiting persisted until the eleventh day, after which oral feeding was gradually established. The diarrhoea, however, continued for three weeks. Though gastric suction was necessary during the first five days the abdominal distension decreased gradually and had disappeared by the twelfth day. On the fifth day there was a deterioration in the child's condition and he appeared to be slightly dehydrated in spite of the oedema of the hands and feet. At the same time polyuria was noticed and there was a loss of 1 lb. in weight during the next 24 hours, with only a slight decrease in the oedema. In spite of the dehydration the urine was dilute. The fluid intake was therefore increased to 46 oz. (1,288 ml.) daily in order to keep pace with the urinary losses. At this time also the haemoglobin was found to be 50% (Sahli), and a total of 125 ml. of blood was given in two transfusions. In view of the polyuria the urine and renal functions were investigated and definite evidence of renal tubular damage was found (see below).

Apart from one short episode of diarrhoea there was now a gradual improvement: the potassium chloride was stopped on the eighteenth day and oral feeding without intravenous supplements was established at the same time. Thereafter the feeds were increased and there was a gradual gain in weight. He was finally discharged after eight weeks in hospital. When seen again two months later he appeared well and had gained 2 lb. 4 oz. in weight.

Blood Chemistry. (Fig. 2.) On admission there was a severe acidosis with hyperchloraemia almost certainly due to diarrhoea, though this had apparently passed unnoticed. The blood urea on admission was normal (36 mg. %) in spite of the gross dehydration; this may have been due to a very rapidly developing dehydration.

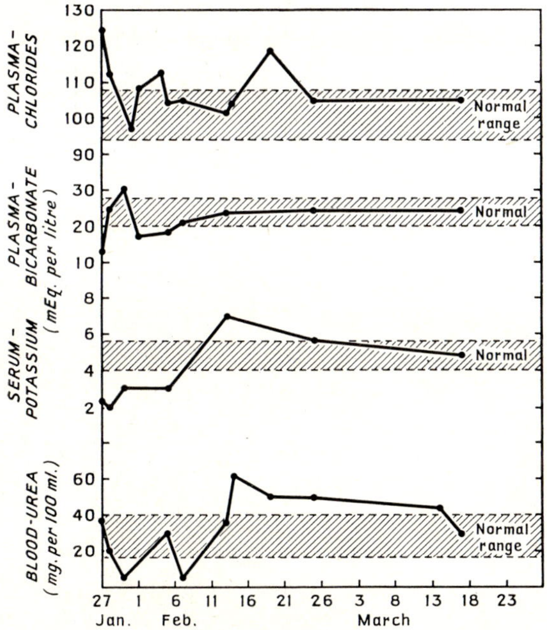

FIG. 2.—Case 2. Blood chemistry. On admission there was a marked hyperchloraemic acidosis with hypokalaemia. This was followed by an alkalosis for a short period. The first raised blood urea and serum potassium may have been due to an episode of dehydration combined with the giving of excess oral potassium chloride. The high blood urea values which persisted may well have been due to a high protein intake, as the urea clearance was normal when the blood urea was still raised.

After treatment with sodium lactate a slight alkalosis developed (plasma bicarbonate 57·6 vols. CO_2% or 25·7 mEq. per l.) which had increased on the fifth day (plasma bicarbonate 67·2 vols. CO_2% or 30 mEq. per l.) and was accompanied by oedema. The hypokalaemia found on admission persisted for 12 days. No additional potassium was given during the first 12 hours while there was still considerable dehydration. The changes in blood urea were carefully followed throughout the illness. After the initial normal value on admission the level fell to 20 mg. % on the second day and to 6 mg. % three days later. At this stage the protein intake was very small as most of the fluid requirement was being given intravenously. By the nineteenth day the blood urea had risen to 61 mg. %; this rise coincided with a rise in the protein intake and was not associated with dehydration nor did it appear that glomerular insufficiency was responsible, as a urea clearance five days later was quite normal (94·1% of average normal) when the blood urea was still 50 mg. %. It was only at the end of the seventh week that the blood urea finally became normal.

Urinary Findings (Table 6 and Fig. 3) and Renal Functions (Table 4). The routine examination of the urine on admission did not show any unusual features apart from a slight proteinuria (40 mg. %) and a few red blood cells and granular casts on microscopy. These findings are not uncommon during a state of dehydration (see Table 7). It was not until the fifth day that any unusual degree of renal damage was suspected. At this time there was definite polyuria in the presence of slight dehydration, when oliguria would normally be expected. The urine was found to be dilute (S.G. 1,007) with a *p*H of 7·5, a protein content of 50 mg. % and a chloride content of 580 mg. % as NaCl (99·1 mEq. per l.). The slightly alkaline urine was not considered remarkable in view of the alkalosis, but the levels of chloride in the urine and serum were almost identical, indicating failure to absorb the chloride contained in the glomerular filtrate (Fig. 3). Next day the urine was examined by chromatography and a marked amino-aciduria was found. There was now considerable proteinuria (reported as '++' on the boiling test) and a slight rise in the specific gravity to 1,012 (no allowance for the proteinuria was made). The *p*H was now 8·3 in spite of a moderate acidosis, and the urinary chloride level remained almost the same as that in the serum (urinary chlorides 608 mg. % as NaCl. or 104 mEq. per l., serum chlorides 632 mg. % as NaCl. or 108 mEq. per l.). The urinary urea was very low (190 mg. %). There was thus evidence of failure of reabsorption of water and chloride (Fig. 6) (and presumably of sodium also) and of amino acids. There was also a failure of acidification of the urine. The significance of the proteinuria will be discussed later.

Recovery occurred rapidly. By the ninth day the specific gravity of the urine had risen to 1,026 and the chloride content had fallen to 465 mg. % as NaCl (79·5 mEq. per l.). On the nineteenth day the urinary urea concentration had risen to 1,440 mg. % and the *p*H had fallen to 6·4, though there was still a considerable degree of proteinuria (450 mg. %). Six days later a urea

TABLE 6

URINE TESTS: CASE 2

Date	Reaction or pH	Specific Gravity	Urea (mg. %)	Chlorides (mg. % as NaCl)	Chlorides (mEq./l.)	Protein	Amino Acids	Deposit	Remarks
27.1.52	5·0	—	—	911	155·7	40	—	1-10 R.B.C. per H.P.F.	Small 'concentrated' specimen
30.1.52	Alkaline	—	—	—	—	50	—	5-10 R.B.C. per H.P.F.	Alkalotic
31.1.52	7·5	1,007	240	580	99·1	—	—	—	Alkalotic
1.2.52	8·3	1,012	190	608	104·0	++	++	—	Acidotic
3.2.52	7·3	1,005	—	436	74·5	++	±	—	Acidotic
4.2.52	6·8	1,026	—	465	79·5	++	+	—	Acidotic
14.2.52	6·4	1,012	1,440	262	44·8	450	—	Nil	
19.2.52	6·4	1,010	900	360	61·5	80	—	Nil	
25.2.52	6·5	1,014	1,450	474	81·0	100	—	—	
14.3.52	—	1,006	—	238	40·7	20	—	—	
17.3.52	Alkaline	—	—	—	—	20	—	Nil	
19.3.52	—	—	—	—	—	—	Nil	—	

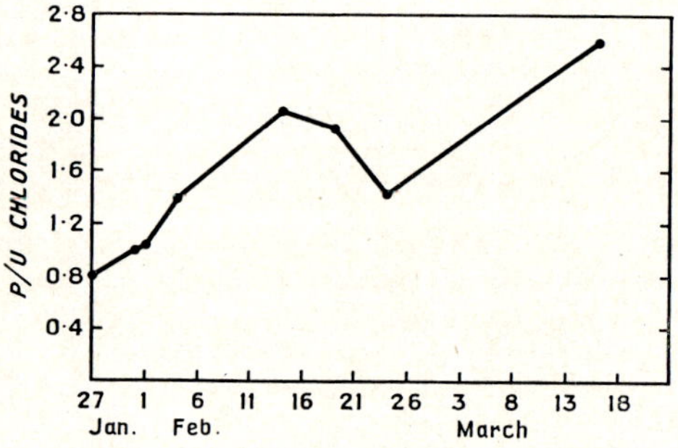

FIG. 3.—Case 2. During the first five days after admission the ratio of plasma chloride levels to those in the urine (P/U) remained in the region of one, indicating the passage of a urine similar in composition to the glomerular filtrate. With recovery the P/U ratio rose.

clearance of 94·1% of average normal (Table 4) was obtained. The proteinuria continued for another week (200 mg. %) but later specimens of urine showed only traces of protein (20 mg. %) and were normal in every other respect.

Comment. This child was very ill on admission to hospital and initial treatment was concerned with the dehydration and abdominal distension; these aspects of the case have been considered more fully elsewhere (Schlesinger, Payne and Black, 1955). Examination of the urine from the fifth day onwards showed a definite degree of tubular damage, which rapidly improved. Though it was not possible to test all the functions of the renal tubules it was clear that there was impairment of H-ion exchange and of the reabsorption of water, chlorides and amino-acids. Proteinuria was considerable and persisted for longer than any of the other urinary abnormalities. By the twenty-fourth day a urea clearance gave a normal result and complete clinical recovery appeared to have taken place.

Retrospective Survey (Table 7). During a survey of potassium metabolism in gastro-enteritis (Schlesinger *et al.*, 1955) a record was made of all cases showing significant urinary abnormalities. Routine examination of the urine was done as soon after admission as possible and consisted of culture, microscopy and estimation of protein. Only those cases with a proteinuria of 40 mg. % or more have been considered, but it was noticed that traces of protein (less than 40 mg. %) and a few granular casts were very frequently present if the urine were examined immediately after admission, when dehydration was at its maximum. Of 653 cases reviewed, 21 had proteinuria of 40 mg. % or more. From Table 7 it appears that there is a rough correlation between the clinical estimate of dehydration and the amount of protein in the urine, though it must be emphasized that the cases recorded in Table 7 are only a few of those admitted in comparable states of dehydration. In most of the 21 cases the proteinuria was found on the first or second day and persisted for two to three days only. In a few instances it continued for longer (M.G. 12 days, B.W. 15 days, Mary R. 25 days).

In this group there were four fatal cases, all of which showed some histological changes in the nephron.

(1) **G.T.**, age 6 weeks. Admitted with a history of four weeks of diarrhoea and vomiting. On the sixth day the urine showed 40 mg. % of protein and a few leucocytes. Death on the fourth day probably from hyperkalaemia. At autopsy the kidneys were congested and the convoluted tubular epithelial cells were somewhat swollen.

(2) **R.F.**, age 1 year. Admitted with a three-week history of vomiting. On admission the urine was normal, but by the twelfth day a trace of protein was present, with numerous red cells and a few leucocytes. A week later, the protein had increased to 200 mg. % and then gradually decreased. The red cells decreased in number but the number of epithelial cells increased until death at 24 days. At autopsy the kidneys contained numerous pyaemic abscesses. There were also widespread degenerative changes involving the whole length of the tubules, including the collecting tubules. Death was due to pyaemia.

(3) **R.B.**, age 4 months. Admitted with diarrhoea and vomiting for one week. The urine was normal on admission but by the fifteenth day contained 100 mg. % of protein, numerous epithelial cells and some leucocytes and red cells. Death on the twenty-eighth day was due to osteomyelitis and septicaemia. At autopsy the glomeruli were swollen and Bowman's capsules and the tubules were filled with an albuminous fluid. The tubular epithelial cells were vacuolated and the tubules were dilated throughout their length.

(4) **M.R.**, age 4 months. Admitted with a three-day history of diarrhoea and vomiting. On the third day after admission the urine contained 100 mg. % of protein, a moderate number of epithelial cells and a few leucocytes, red cells and granular casts. Death occurred next day with oedema and fits. The blood urea on the day before death was 148 mg. % but no oliguria was noted at any time. At autopsy the kidneys were congested and there was interstitial oedema. Bowman's capsules contained an albuminous fluid. The convoluted tubules showed evidence of severe damage and were filled with an albuminous fluid and red cells. The collecting tubules showed similar changes.

TABLE 7

PROTEINURIA IN GASTRO-ENTERITIS

Name	Sex	Age	Degree of Dehydration	Maximum Blood Urea (mg. %)	Maximum Proteinuria (mg. %)	R.B.C.	W.B.C.	Casts	Comments
S.L. ..	F	15/12	+++	N.R.	800	0	+	Cellular +	
R.F. ..	F	1 yr.	+++	N.R.	200	Occas.	+	Occas. granular	Died
M.R. ..	M	4/12	++	160	100	Occas.	Occas.	Occas. granular	Died
J.C. ..	M	6/12	+	44	100	0	Occas.	Granular +	
R.B. ..	M	4/12	+	N.R.	100	Occas.	5–10 E.C.++	0	Died
J.M. ..	M	6/12	+	80	100	0	1–2 E.C.	Occas.	
Mary R. ..	F	10/52	+	N.R.	100	0	0	0	
E.T. ..	M	2/12	++	N.R.	70	0	4-5	0	
I.L. ..	M	3/52	+	38	70	Occas.	Occas.	0	
A.T. ..	M	4/12	+	N.R.	70	0	0	Occas.	
R.P. ..	M	6/12	+	N.R.	65	0	0	Granular +	
J.C. ..	M	7/52	0	N.R.	60	0	0	Occas.	
W.M. ..	M	5/12	+	22	50	0	+	Occas.	
B.W. ..	F	4/12	+	34	48	0	0	0	
C.H. ..	M	2/12	++	148	45	0	0	0	
M.V ..	M	7/12	++	14	45	0	0	0	
M.G. ..	F	2/12	+	N.R.	45	0	Occas.	Occas.	
M.L. ..	M	4/52	+	35	40	0	0	0	
G.T. ..	M	6/52	+	83	40	0	Occas.	0	Died
D.F. ..	M	4/52	++	31	40	15-20	5	0	
R.G. ..	F	7/12	+	N.R.	40	Occas.	Occas.	0	

N.R. = Not recorded. E.C. = Epithelial cells. Occas. = Occasional.
R.B.C. and W.B.C = figures indicate number of cells per H.P.F. in centrifuged specimen

Comment. Of the four cases G.T. showed the least histological changes and death was probably due to hyperkalaemia. The other three cases showed varying degrees of proteinuria with epithelial cells, which probably indicated desquamation of the tubular epithelium.

It is of interest that Cases R.B. and M.R. showed an albuminous fluid in Bowman's capsules, which apart from the possibility of reflux, suggested that the protein in the urine originated in an increased permeability of the capsular epithelium.

Discussion

Acute tubular necrosis may vary greatly in severity. In mild cases there is suppression of urine for only a few hours without the blood urea rising above normal (Bull, Joekes and Lowe, 1955). Nevertheless, the diuretic phase even in such cases requires careful management if dehydration and electrolyte depletion are to be avoided. When the anuria or oliguria is of short duration the patient may pass into the diuretic phase without renal damage being suspected. This is particularly liable to happen in infantile gastro-enteritis where attention is focused on the gastro-intestinal tract. If the diagnosis is suspected when the diuretic phase has already developed (see Case 2) a timed specimen of urine should be collected for as long a period as possible in order that an estimate of the urinary output can be made. The specific gravity of the urine should be measured and also the urinary chloride content, as the chloride levels in the urine or serum tend to be approximately the same during the diuretic phase, the urine coming to resemble a glomerular filtrate. Other tubular functions are also affected. The H-ion exchange mechanism appears to be damaged so that the urine tends to remain constantly neutral or slightly alkaline even in the presence of an acidosis. Transient glycosuria and amino-aciduria sometimes occur (Burch and Ray, 1949; Bull, Joekes and Lowe, 1950; Lowe, Moodie and Thomson, 1954; Carré and Squire, 1956), but normal blood levels should be demonstrated before these findings can be taken as unequivocal evidence of tubular damage. Of the two cases described here, polyuria was found in Case 2, failure of acidification of the urine and amino-aciduria in both cases, and glycosuria in Case 1. In Case 2 there was also the tendency for the urinary chloride levels to approximate to those of the serum. Proteinuria persisted until the fifth week in both cases. The significance of proteinuria in tubular necrosis has not been determined, but it has been recognized in many papers on the subject (Swan and Merrill, 1953; Lowe *et al.*, 1954; Wagner, 1954; Bull *et al.*, 1955). The proteinuria could be caused by a defect in tubular reabsorption of a normal load from the glomerular filtrate, assuming that the glomerular filtrate in man does indeed contain protein (Oliver, 1948; Rather, 1952; Sellers, Griggs, Marmorston and Goodman, 1954; Hardwicke and Squire, 1955). Alternatively, if the amount of protein in the glomerular filtrate were greatly increased by altered permeability of the glomerular membrane the mechanism for tubular reabsorption of protein could become overloaded, and proteinuria would result. There is good evidence of glomerular damage in the early stages of the syndrome of tubular necrosis (Bull *et al.*, 1950; Oliver *et al.*, 1951) and it is possible that an abnormal permeability to plasma proteins may persist for some time after all the tests of glomerular filtration rate have returned to normal (see Cases 1 and 2). Such a mechanism of abnormal permeability has been suggested in tubular necrosis (Oliver *et al.*, 1951) and in nephrosis (Hardwicke and Squire, 1955). At present there is no evidence as to the exact cause of the proteinuria in tubular necrosis, but further information might be obtained from electrophoresis of the urinary proteins, as in the studies already made in other renal conditions (Rigas and Heller, 1951; Wolvius and Verschure, 1957). Whatever the cause of the proteinuria in tubular necrosis, its presence in a patient recovering from severe shock or dehydration is a good indication to investigate the renal functions more fully. It has been recently pointed out, however, that in severe potassium deficiency many of the functions of the tubule are affected and that proteinuria may occur (Milne, Muehrcke and Heard, 1957), so that potassium deficiency must always be considered as a contributory or even the sole cause of tubular dysfunction in the presence of electrolyte disturbances. Milne *et al.* (1957) have pointed out that defective function of the proximal tubule is rare in potassium deficiency and therefore glycosuria and amino-aciduria are unlikely to occur in such circumstances. The cellular content of the urine in tubular necrosis has received only passing mention in a few of the descriptions (Burch and Ray, 1949; Swann and Merrill, 1953). In Case 1 there was a considerable number of epithelial cells in the urine from the thirty-seventh day (and probably earlier) until the forty-ninth day. In view of the histological findings in such cases it is probable that these cells represent epithelium shed from the necrotic tubules. Further investigation of the cellular output by improved methods (Houghton and Pears, 1957) may help to evaluate the frequency with which minor degrees of tubular damage occur in states of shock or dehydration.

The management of adults with tubular necrosis has been ably covered by Bull and his co-workers (Bull, 1955; Bull *et al.*, 1955). Carré and Squire (1956) have described the treatment of three children with tubular necrosis and there is little to add to their general scheme of treatment. However, when diarrhoea is present, variable and usually unknown amounts of fluid and electrolytes are lost in the stools so that analysis of the urine no longer gives an adequate guide to the daily requirements. Probably the best control under such circumstances is by daily weighing and repeated estimations of the blood chemistry. In the two cases presented here the replacement of electrolytes was not difficult. In Case 1 the acidosis was easily rectified by sodium citrate-citric acid mixture and the hypokalaemia by potassium chloride. In Case 2 the fluid intake had to be increased during the diuretic phase, but there was no chloride depletion, probably because the fluid supplied at this time was in the form of half-strength Hartmann's solution which contains 0·3% of sodium chloride. In this case also the serum potassium was kept normal without difficulty in spite of the diarrhoea. Recovery was rapid in both cases and normal glomerular filtration rates were obtained in Case 1 in the sixth week of the illness and in Case 2 in the fourth week. Though all tubular functions were not tested separately, there appeared to be recovery of all the previously defective renal functions. The subsequent progress of these two cases, from the renal point of view, was normal.

Summary

Renal tubular damage is described in infantile gastro-enteritis. The importance of detecting this complication is emphasised.

I wish to thank Dr. B. E. Schlesinger and Dr. W. W. Payne for their help in the preparation of this paper, and Dr. Martin Bodian for his reports on the histology.

References

Bull, G. M. (1955). *Lancet*, **1**, 731, 777.
——, Joekes, A. M. and Lowe, K. G. (1950). *Clin. Sci.*, **9**, 379.
——, ——, —— (1955). *Lancet*, **2**, 1152.
Burch, G. E. and Ray, C. T. (1949). *Ann. intern. Med.*, **31**, 750
Calcagno, P. L. and Rubin, M. I. (1951). *Pediatrics*, **7**, 328.
Carré, I. J. and Squire, J. R. (1956). *Arch. Dis. Childh.*, **31**, 512.
Doxiadis, S. A. (1947). *Ibid.*, **22**, 180.
Hardwicke, J. and Squire, J. R. (1955). *Clin. Sci.*, **14**, 509.
Houghton, B. J. and Pears, M. A. (1957). *Brit. med. J.*, **1**, 622.
Jonsson, B. (1951). *Acta paediat. (Uppsala)*, **40**, 401.
Kaplan, S. A. and Fomon, S. J. (1953), *A.M.A. Amer. J. Dis. Child.*, **85**, 633.
Kerpel-Fronius, Ö., Varga, F., Kun, K. and Vönöczky, J. (1954). *Acta med. Acad. Sci. hung.*, **5**, 27.
Lowe, K. G., Moodie, G. and Thomson, M. B. (1954). *Clin. Sci.*, **13**, 187.
Milne, M. D., Muehrcke, R. C. and Heard, B. E. (1957). *Brit. med. Bull.*, **13**, 15.
Oliver, J. (1948). *J. Mt Sinai Hosp.*, **15**, 175.
——, MacDowell, M. and Tracy, A. (1951). *J. clin. Invest.*, **30**, 1305.
Pratt, E. L. (1948). *Amer. J. Dis. Child.*, **76**, 14.
Rather, L. J. (1952), *Medicine (Baltimore)*, **31**, 357.
Riddell, H. I. (1951). *J. Urol. (Baltimore)*, **65**, 513.
Rigas, D. A. and Heller, C. G. (1951). *J. clin. Invest.*, **30**, 853.
Schlesinger, B. and Welch, R. G. (1952). *Gt Ormond Str. J.*, No. 3, p. 14.
——, Payne, W. and Black, J. (1955). *Quart. J. Med.*, **24**, 33.
Sellers, A. L., Griggs, N., Marmorston, J. and Goodman, H. C. (1954). *J. exp. Med.*, **100**, 1.
Swann, R. C. and Merrill, J. P. (1953). *Medicine (Baltimore)*, **32**, 215.
Van Slyke, D. D. (1954). *Ann. intern. Med.*, **41**, 709.
Wagner, J. (1954). *Gt Ormond Str. J.*, No. 7, p. 66.
Wolvius, D. and Verschure, J. C. M. (1957). *J. clin. Path.*, **10**, 80.
Zuelzer, W. W., Charles, S., Kurnetz, R., Newton, W. A. and Fallon, R. (1951). *A.M.A. Amer. J. Dis. Child.*, **81**, 1.

IDIOPATHIC INFANTILE HYPOGLYCAEMIA

BY

M. KINSBOURNE* and L. I. WOOLF†

From The Hospital for Sick Children, Great Ormond Street, London

(RECEIVED FOR PUBLICATION OCTOBER 10, 1958)

Occasionally an infant presents with the sudden onset of frequent epileptic seizures in whom the only finding of diagnostic significance is a persistently low blood sugar level.

The many causes of hypoglycaemia are discussed by Conn and Seltzer (1955), but in practice the possibilities in such a case are:

(1) Syndrome of 'idiopathic infantile hypoglycemosis' (McQuarrie, 1954), divisible in the first instance into 'leucine sensitive' and 'leucine insensitive' types (Cochrane, Payne, Simpkiss and Woolf, 1956). In the leucine sensitive type the hypoglycaemia is sharply aggravated by the oral ingestion of leucine, or of protein containing this amino acid. (2) 'Hyperinsulinism', pancreatic islet cell adenoma (Sherman, 1947) or hyperplasia, either macroscopic (Bickerstaff, Dodge, Gourevitch and Hearn, 1955), or microscopic (Engelhardt, Kraayenbrink and Villeneuve, 1955). (3) A rare presentation of some other endocrine defect, e.g. of pituitary, adrenal or thyroid function, or of a disorder of carbohydrate metabolism such as glycogen storage disease or galactosaemia.

The clinical and biochemical features of Group 3 are well known. The differential diagnosis of Groups 1 and 2 is less familiar, and the pathogenesis of Group 1 has hardly been explored.

The present paper describes a severe case of leucine insensitive idiopathic infantile hypoglycaemia. Biochemical findings, some of which seem not previously to have been described, are discussed in relation to pathogenesis.

Case History

A female infant, aged 4 months, was admitted to The Hospital for Sick Children, Great Ormond Street, on December 2, 1957, having become suddenly subject to frequent, uncontrollable, generalized fits without focal features three weeks earlier. The fits, which occurred at any time of day or night, were accompanied by a progressive deterioration of her previously normal mental function. Her family history was of no significance, except perhaps that her brother's rate of weight gain had been high: 8 lb. 1 oz. at birth, 23 lb. at 5 months and 79 lb. at 7 years. After a normal birth (birth weight: 7 lb. 8 oz.) the patient was breast fed for three weeks, then bottle fed, gaining weight very rapidly all the time.

On examination, she was obese (weight 17 lb.) with extreme hypotonia of the limbs and depressed reflexes. She sucked well, but seemed unaware of her environment, and responded only to pain with a high pitched cry. The head circumference was 16¼ inches; there were no other abnormal signs.

There was no protein, reducing substance or ketone bodies in the urine. Blood examination showed Hb. 82%, W.B.C. and differential count were normal. Serum electrolytes were normal, except serum potassium 3·1 mEq./l. Blood sugar, during a fit was 35 mg./100 ml. (Folin and Wu estimation). Cerebrospinal fluid showed protein, 120 mg./100 ml.; sugar, 16 mg./100 ml.; chloride, 720 mg./100 ml. A W.R. was negative. Liver function tests were normal. There was no excess of blood galactose.

An E.E.G. (Dr. Pampiglione) showed 'An excess of slow activity over the two hemispheres with occasional paroxysmal changes. Isolated sharp waves suggest the presence of discharging areas.' A radiograph of the skull was normal.

Further blood sugar estimations confirmed a severe fasting hypoglycaemia.

Oral and intragastric glucose had failed to abolish the hypoglycaemia at a time when the infant suddenly developed diarrhoea and became acutely dehydrated. A rapid intravenous infusion of 5% dextrose restored normal hydration; three hours after the infusion was started the blood sugar had risen to 470 mg./100 ml.; and in another one and a half hours to 700 mg./100 ml., although very little glucose was given in the meantime.

The blood sugar dropped back to hypoglycaemic levels in the next 24 hours, and then could not be raised even by further intravenous 5% dextrose. Therefore ACTH gel was given intramuscularly, 8 units 12-hourly, with an immediate dramatic rise in blood sugar concentration, and complete cessation of fits. After one month it was possible to reduce the ACTH to 8 units daily, and after another month prednisolone 2 mg. eight-hourly was successfully substituted.

The hypotonia soon disappeared. The rate of weight

* Present address: Bellevue Hospital, 550 1st Avenue, New York 16, N.Y., U.S.A.

† Present address: M.R.C. Population Genetics Research Unit, Warneford Hospital, Oxford.

gain diminished almost to zero in the early months of treatment; then was resumed at a more normal level (Fig. 1).

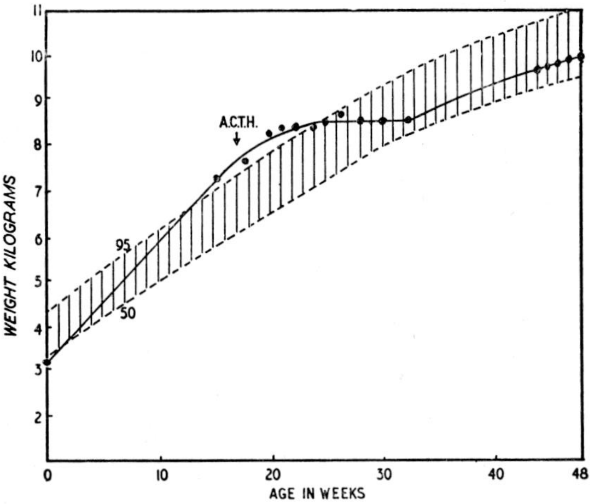

FIG. 1.—The patients' weight at different ages. The time of starting ACTH (and, later, steroid) therapy is indicated. The 50th and 95th percentiles for the weight of girls at different ages are shown and the area between shaded (Sundal, 1957; Tanner, 1958).

At 10 months of age and six months after starting treatment she was more alert than before, but was still grossly retarded (G.Q. 22, Griffiths scale), with a head circumference of 17¼ inches.

Methods of Investigation

Blood was collected, by heel prick, in bottles containing fluoride and oxalate. True blood sugar and non-sugar reducing substances were determined as described by Cochrane *et al.* (1956). Glucose was determined using glucose oxidase (Huggett and Nixon, 1957) and the biodeminrolit-treated tungstic acid blood filtrate. Urine for adrenaline estimation was collected over timed intervals in bottles containing 6N HCl. Adrenaline in urine was determined by a modification of the method of Euler and Orwen (1955); Snaith and Woolf (in preparation). In two specimens of urine catecholamines were also determined by Dr. M. Mann using a biological method.

Phenolic acids in urine were also analysed by a paper chromatographic method (cf. Armstrong, Shaw and Wall, 1956).

Results

Leucine Tolerance Test. The true blood sugar, initially 105 mg./100 ml., did not drop within 90 minutes of feeding leucine (0·15 g./kg. body weight). The non-sugar reducing substances (Cochrane *et al.*, 1956) were ≡13 mg. glucose per 100 ml. blood, which is normal.

This test was carried out under ACTH cover since it would have been potentially dangerous to feed leucine if the blood sugar were below about 30 mg. per 100 ml., and the results would have been difficult to interpret; there is no evidence that ACTH modifies sensitivity to leucine.

Serial Blood Sugars. (Before treatment with ACTH or steroids.) After being fed at 2.0 p.m. her blood sugar concentrations (Folin-Wu method) were:

Time (p.m.)	2.40	3.0	4.0	5.0	6.0
Blood sugar (mg./100 ml.)	42	37	31	26	24

Glucose Tolerance Test. The results are shown in Fig. 2.

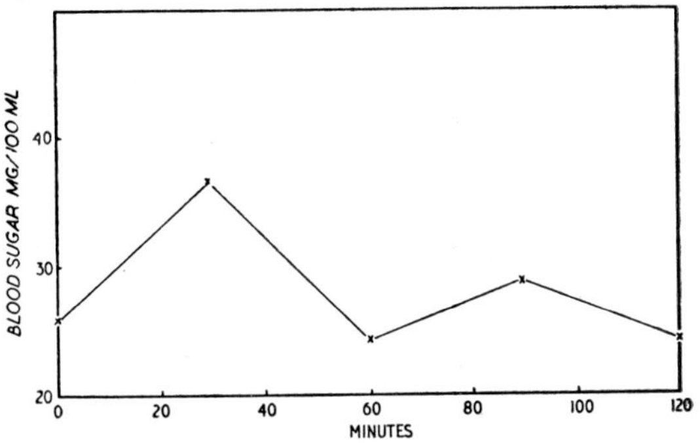

FIG. 2.—Glucose tolerance curve. 13 g. of glucose was fed at time 0.

Plasma Insulin-like Activity. This was determined twice by Dr. J. Vallance-Owen. Before treatment with ACTH he found 120 micro-units of insulin-like activity per ml. of plasma, the blood glucose concentration being 6 mg./100 ml. This is near the upper limit of the normal range. After ACTH therapy was instituted he found 45 micro-units of insulin-like activity per ml. of plasma, the blood glucose concentration being 106 mg. per 100 ml.

Insulin Tolerance Test. The results of four tests, all carried out under cover of ACTH or prednisolone, are shown in Fig. 3.

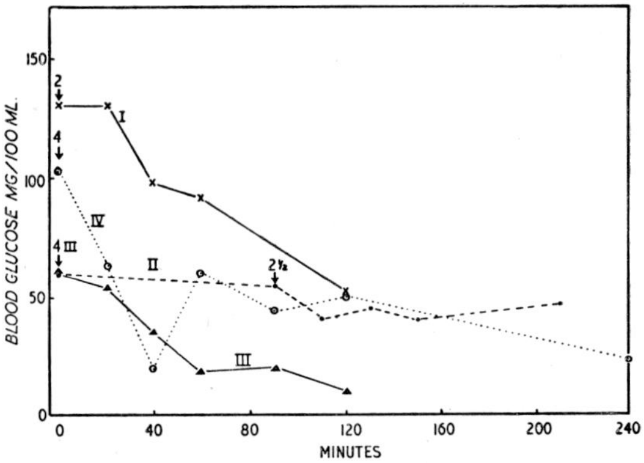

FIG. 3.—Insulin tolerance tests. Test I: 30.12.57. Test II: 20.6.58. Test III: 13.3.58. Test IV: 7.3.58. The indicated number (2, 2.5, 5 and 4 respectively) of units of insulin was injected intradermally at the time marked by the arrow.

Adrenaline Tolerance Tests. The results of four tests are shown in Fig. 4.

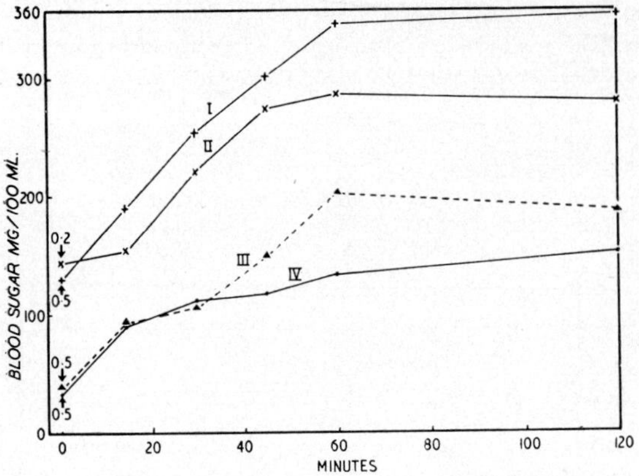

FIG. 4.—Adrenaline tolerance tests. Test I: 3.1.58. Test II: 20.1.58. Test III: 10.1.58. Test IV: 18.6.58. The indicated number of ml. of 1:1,000 adrenaline was injected subcutaneously at the time marked by the arrow (0·2 ml. for curve II, 0·5 ml. for the rest).

Glucagon Tolerance Test. The results of two tests are shown in Fig. 5.

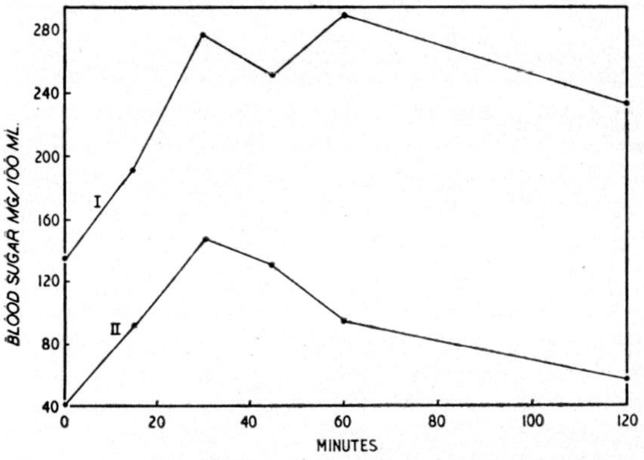

FIG. 5.—Glucagon tolerance tests. Test I: 21.1.58. Test II: 21.7.58. 0·2 mg. of glucagon was injected at time 0 in each case.

Urinary Adrenaline. The first two specimens of urine examined apparently contained large amounts of adrenaline:

Specimen	1	2
Cat assay of urine	14·7	30 μg./12 hr.
Cat assay of urine concentrate ..	29·4	90 ,, ,,
Chromatography urine concentrate	200-300	170 ,, ,,

Unfortunately the techniques of adsorbing the catecholamines on alumina and of chromatography had not at that time been perfected and these two results must be considered doubtful. ACTH was withheld during the 24 hours of this test, but at the end the blood sugar concentration was 94 mg./100 ml.

In all subsequent urine specimens examined, no trace of adrenaline could be found. This in spite of the fact that hypoglycaemia was induced (*a*) by twice withholding prednisolone for up to 25 hours and (*b*) by giving insulin on two occasions, when blood sugar levels dropped to 35, 22, 20, 10 mg./100 ml. respectively.

3-Methoxy-4-hydroxymandelic acid, probably the major urinary metabolite of adrenaline (Armstrong, McMillan and Shaw, 1957) was not increased in amount in any of these specimens of urine as compared with control specimens passed before the onset of hypoglycaemia.

Discussion

Diagnosis. There was no evidence of pituitary dwarfism, Addisonian pigmentation or cretinism in this case. There was no hepatomegaly or ketonuria, and there was a good glycaemic response to adrenaline which excluded glycogen storage disease. Blood and urine examination excluded galactosaemia. The great rarity of hyperinsulinism in infancy and the normal plasma insulin level justified treating the case in the first instance as idiopathic without resorting to laparotomy and pancreatic biopsy.

Thus the present case resembles the cases described by McQuarrie as infantile idiopathic hypoglycaemia in which there was a severe hypoglycaemia causing convulsions uncontrolled by dietary measures, but responding to ACTH or gluco-corticoids. The result of the leucine tolerance test puts the infant into the leucine insensitive group.

Treatment. McQuarrie (1954) found ACTH superior to cortisone. In the present case prednisolone which can be given orally proved effective at a reasonably low dose. The response to ACTH or prednisolone is not only far greater than that normally elicited, but exceeds that found in infantile hypoglycaemia of various causation (Sherman, 1947; Geppert, Spencer and Richmond, 1950; Ulstrom, Ziegler, Doeden and McQuarrie, 1952; Engelhardt *et al.*, 1955; Cochrane *et al.*, 1956).

When the glucose supply to cells exceeds their oxidative requirements, the excess enters other metabolic pools involving fat formation in particular. This effect is inhibited by adrenal cortical steroids (Boutwell and Chiang, 1954). This may be the basis of the infant's very rapid weight gain, and its striking suppression by ACTH.

The very high blood glucose levels when the infant was first given intravenous fluid are difficult to explain. The continued rise in blood sugar level from 470 to 700 mg./100 ml., while little more dextrose was given, suggests an outpouring of glucose from depots into the blood, which could possibly be due to gluco-corticoids released in response to the stress of acute dehydration and of cutting down on a vein for infusion.

Judging by her present backwardness and the microcephaly, presumably secondary to brain damage, this infant, though she had fits for less than four weeks, has suffered some irreversible mental impairment. This illustrates the urgency in diagnosing and treating this condition.

Investigations. The rapid drop in the blood sugar level during the fasting state suggests too rapid a loss of glucose from the blood to the tissues. The oral glucose tolerance test supports this impression which is confirmed by the failure even of intravenous glucose to produce normal sugar levels.

The value of plasma insulin-like activity, obtained before treatment, was a high normal, as found in an adult after a carbohydrate meal and was far less than that found in organic hyperinsulinism in infancy (Engelhardt *et al.*, 1955; Cochrane *et al*, 1956). In normal adults the plasma insulin-like activity varies inversely with the blood sugar level (Vallance-Owen and Hurlock, 1954); at so low a level of blood glucose as 6 mg. % it is surprising to find any insulin-like activity at all. The 'low normal' figure after treatment is further evidence against hyperinsulinism, but is difficult to interpret, since ACTH may raise the plasma level of insulin antagonist (Vallance-Owen and Lukens, 1957).

The initial response to intradermally administered insulin was normal, thus excluding tissue hypersensitivity to the hormone. The continued drop in blood sugar concentration, over several hours after administration of insulin, is seen in some normal infants (Daniel, 1941).

Unlike older children (Snaith and Woolf, unpublished) and adults (von Euler and Luft, 1952), this infant did not excrete increased urinary adrenaline in response to hypoglycaemia, whether induced by administration of insulin or by withholding steroid. We have no way of deciding whether this was due to a failure to produce adrenaline or a failure to release it into the blood stream in response to hypoglycaemia. Each test was preceded by several days of adequate therapeutic control, which excluded the possibility of exhaustion of the adrenal medulla by over-stimulation. Cortico-steroid treatment as such has no effect on the secretion and release of adrenaline (Luft and von Euler, 1952).

The enormous rises in blood sugar level elicited by adrenaline and glucagon are unprecedented in 28 years' experience at Great Ormond Street (Payne, personal communication) and apparently also in the literature (Desmond, 1953, in normal neonates; Livingston and Bridge, 1942, in normal infants; McQuarrie, 1954, in idiopathic infantile hypoglycaemia; Cochrane *et al.*, 1956, in leucine sensitive hypoglycaemia). Although adrenaline is said to release ACTH from the anterior pituitary (Gershberg, Fry, Brobeck and Long, 1950) the initial response to adrenaline was in this case too rapid for this to make an important contribution, and there is no evidence that glucagon causes release of ACTH. This hypersensitivity is unlikely to be due to previous lack of circulating adrenaline since an adrenalectomized child had a normal response to injected adrenaline (Payne, personal communication). Nor does long-term treatment with ACTH or cortisone cause hypersensitivity to adrenaline.

Pathogenesis. In the normal subject, glucose is continuously transferred from the blood to the cells at a rate that depends, among other things, on the concentration of insulin in the plasma which is itself dependent on the blood sugar level. In the fasting state the blood sugar concentration is maintained from tissue stores under the control of a number of hormones: adrenaline, glucagon, gluco-corticoids and, hence, ACTH. Yet deficiency of each of these hormones is not alone sufficient to cause hypoglycaemia (Zucker and Berg, 1937; Goldner, Volk and Lazarus, 1952; Lazarus and Volk, 1953; Staehelin, Labhart, Froesch and Kägi, 1955; Ginsberg and Paton, 1956; von Euler, 1956).

The failure to maintain normal blood sugar levels on amounts of oral or intravenous glucose that should have been adequate in an infant of this size suggests that there is an excessive loss of glucose to the tissues. This is associated with a moderately high level of blood 'insulin', which cannot alone account for the hypoglycaemia, but suggests a failure to inhibit the secretion of insulin. It further appears that the body has lost the power to respond to hypoglycaemia, even though each hormone in turn, adrenaline, glucagon and ACTH, has been shown to produce an adequate glycaemic response. In other words, there was a failure in the mechanisms that limit the passage of glucose into the cell, and also a failure in the mechanism guiding the release of hormones homeostatic for blood sugar. The latter must itself be a cellular function and may be another aspect of the former.

Summary

A case of severe leucine insensitive idiopathic infantile hypoglycaemia is presented and biochemical tests are discussed in relation to its pathogenesis. A complex disturbance of hormonal and cellular factors controlling blood sugar level is revealed, perhaps based on a single fundamental cellular defect.

We should like to thank Dr. G. H. Newns for permission to study and report this case, Dr. W. W. Payne for much helpful advice and for carrying out many of the estimations, Dr. J. Vallance-Owen for estimating plasma insulin-like activity, the nursing staff for their untiring care and assistance, and the Research Committee of The Hospital for Sick Children for a research fellowship awarded to one of us (L.I.W.).

REFERENCES

Armstrong, M. D., McMillan, A. and Shaw, K. N. F. (1957). *Biochim. biophys. Acta*, **25**, 422.
——, Shaw, K. N. F. and Wall, P. E. (1956). *J. biol. Chem.*, **218**, 293.
Bickerstaff, E. R., Dodge, O. G., Gourevitch, A. and Hearn, G. W. (1955). *Brit. med. J.*, **2**, 997.
Boutwell, R. K. and Chiang, R. (1954). *Arch. Biochem.*, **50**, 461.
Cochrane, W. A., Payne, W. W., Simpkiss, M. J. and Woolf, L. I. (1956). *J. clin. Invest.*, **35**, 411.
Conn, J. W. and Seltzer, H. S. (1955). *Amer. J. Med.*, **19**, 460.
Daniel, W. A. Jr. (1941). *J. Pediat.*, **19**, 789.
Desmond, M. M. (1953). *Ibid.*, **43**, 253.
Engelhardt, J., Kraayenbrink, K. and Villeneuve, V. H. de (1955). *Maandschr. Kindergeneesk.*, **23**, 85.
Euler, U. S. von (1956). *Noradrenaline*, p. 287. (American Lecture Series No. 261.) Charles C. Thomas, Illinois.
—— and Luft, R. (1952). *Metabolism*, **1**, 528.
—— and Orwen, I. (1955). *Acta physiol. scand.*, **33**, Suppl. 118, p. 1.
Geppert, L. J., Spencer, W. A. and Richmond, A. M. (1950). *J. Pediat.*, **37**, 1.
Gershberg, H., Fry, E. G., Brobeck, J. R. and Long, C. N. H. (1950). *Yale J. Biol. Med.*, **23**, 32.
Ginsberg, J. and Paton, A. (1956). *Lancet*, **2**, 491.
Goldner, M. G., Volk, B. W. and Lazarus, S. S. (1952). *Metabolism* **1**, 544.
Huggett, A. St. G. and Nixon, D. A. (1957). *Lancet*, **2**, 368.
Lazarus, S. S. and Volk, B. W. (1953). *Metabolism*, **2**, 500.
Livingston, S. and Bridge, E. M. (1942). *J. Amer. med. Ass.*, **119**, 117.
Luft, R. and Euler, U. S. von. (1952). *Metabolism*, **1**, 179.
McQuarrie, I. (1954). *A.M.A. Amer. J. Dis. Child.*, **87**, 399.
Payne, W. W. (1958). Personal communication.
Sherman, H. (1947). *Amer. J. Dis. Child.*, **74**, 58.
Staehelin, D., Labhart, A., Froesch, R. and Kägi, H. R. (1955). *Acta Endocr.* (*Kbh.*), **18**, 521.
Sundal, A. (1957). *The Norms for Height* (*Length*) *and Weight in Healthy Norwegian Children from Birth to 15 Years of Age.* Griegs, Bergen.
Tanner, J. M (1958). In *Modern Trends in Paediatrics* by A Holzel and J. P. M. Tizard, p. 325. Butterworth, London.
Ulstrom, R. A., Ziegler, M. R., Doeden, D. and McQuarrie, I. (1952). *Metabolism*, **1**, 291.
Vallance-Owen, J. and Hurlock, B. (1954). *Lancet*, **1**, 68.
—— and Lukens, F. D. W. (1957). *Endocrinology*, **60**, 625.
Zucker, T. F. and Berg, B. N. (1937). *Amer. J. Physiol.*, **119**, 539.

SPONTANEOUS HYPERINSULINISM DUE TO BENIGN HYPERPLASIA OF ISLET CELLS

BY

DONALD M. DOUGLAS

From the Department of Child Life and Health, University of Edinburgh, and the Royal Hospital for Sick Children Edinburgh

(RECEIVED FOR PUBLICATION OCTOBER 21, 1958)

Since Cushing (1930) reported the first successful operation on a patient with an insulin-secreting adenoma, over 400 cases, found to have symptoms associated with tumours of the islet cells, have been reported in the world literature; but there have also been cases in which the diagnosis has been made clinically, but examination of the pancreas, either at operation or autopsy, has failed to reveal anything in the nature of a tumour. In some of these cases the pathologist has reported a generalized hyperplasia of the islets, the cells being increased both in size and number. The subject has been well reviewed by Howard, Moss and Rhoads (1950). These authors found reports in the literature of 81 patients diagnosed as suffering from hyperinsulinism, in whom no tumour was discovered at operation. In 10 of these no histological report was available. Of the remaining 71, 48 were reported as having normal pancreatic tissues, four showed 'chronic inflammation', one hypoplasia, and 18 hyperplasia of the islet cells. Two of the latter group were children. One (Callaway, 1946) was a boy of 8 years, who had a history of 'faints' and convulsions for a year; on one occasion his blood sugar was found to be 23 mg. %. Subtotal resection of the pancreas was performed, after which the symptoms did not recur during the following five years and subsequent blood sugar levels were within normal limits. The other case was a girl of 4½ months (Agustsson, Tudor and Chisholm, 1947), with a six-weeks' history of convulsions. On one occasion a blood sugar level of 18 mg. % was found. Subtotal resection of the pancreas was carried out with clinical and biochemical cure. She was followed up for eight months after operation. In reporting this case the authors emphasized the importance of early diagnosis and treatment if serious neurological sequelae were to be avoided. The criteria they accepted as indicating the need for surgery were those propounded by Whipple (1938). They are as follows:

(1) There should be proof of a persistent or a frequent recurring hypoglycaemia by blood analysis. (2) It should be shown that the symptoms expected to be relieved by surgery can be relieved by dextrose administration. (3) It should be shown that the symptoms cannot be relieved by conservative measures of diet regulation.

Case Report

Baby W. F., the third child of healthy parents, was admitted to the Royal Hospital for Sick Children, Edinburgh, in July, 1951, because of recurrent fits. He had been born at full term and weighed 7¼ lb. When he was 6 weeks old his weight gain was considered unsatisfactory, so breast feeding was discontinued and he was put on to a modified cow's milk formula. This he evidently took satisfactorily. One morning, when 7 weeks old, he was found in his cot, unconscious and twitching. This turn lasted a few minutes only and then he appeared well, but he had further similar attacks seven and 10 weeks later, and thereafter each morning before being given his first feed of the day. He was given phenobarbitone, gr. ¼ t.d.s. with apparent benefit, for the fits became less frequent, only recurring about once a week. This state of affairs continued till he was 8 months old, when he commenced having fits about twice a day. It was then that he was admitted to hospital for fuller investigation. It was noted on admission that he was a well nourished infant, weighing 20 lb. 10 oz. He could not sit up unaided and appeared very lethargic. No other abnormality was discovered on physical examination. Many investigations were carried out but no abnormality was discovered. However, a lumbar puncture revealed a clear cerebrospinal fluid, normal cytologically and biochemically except that the sugar level was only 20 mg. %. A glucose tolerance test was therefore carried out. The result was as follows:

	(mg. %)
Fasting blood sugar ..	40
After ½ hour	52
After 1 hour	60
After 1½ hours	74
After 2 hours	56

Essentially similar results were obtained when the test was repeated on three occasions.

The blood sugar levels were estimated on a number of occasions that coincided with the onset of the convulsive episodes. These levels varied from 32 to 42 mg. %. An attempt was made to control the seizures by the administration of large quantities of sugar; this was partially successful but it was found necessary to give over 100 g. of sugar per day to be effective. This was clearly impracticable as a long term dietetic measure. An insulin sensitivity test produced no untoward reaction (1 unit of soluble insulin injected intravenously) and so on October 23, 1951, laparotomy was carried out by Mr. Mason Brown. An apparently normal pancreas was found and about two thirds of it were resected. The child made a satisfactory recovery from the operation, took normal feeds for his age, and the fits did not recur during the post-operative period. He also appeared more alert and vigorous. Seventeen days after operation a further glucose tolerance test was carried out. The result was as follows:

	(mg. %)
Fasting blood sugar	70
After ½ hour	112
After 1 hour	123
After 1½ hours	109
After 2 hours	80

Six months later the test was repeated and found to be essentially unchanged, the occasion being a further admission to hospital on account of an isolated convulsion. He was then aged 18 months, weighing 26 lb., and looking very fit. He was not walking or saying any words but no other abnormality could be discovered and he was discharged home. During the next year he had four further isolated fits and he was therefore given phenobarbitone, gr. 1 daily, and the fits did not recur. When seen at the age of 7½ years, it was noted that he was mentally retarded. He was walking well and his mother claimed that he understood most of what was said to him, but his vocabulary consisted of only about three or four words. There was some slight stiffness of his right arm and hand and he tended to use his left hand more willingly. The reflexes of both the right arm and leg were rather more brisk than those of the left. It was considered that he had a right hemiplegia. In other ways his condition was satisfactory.

Pathological Report on the Pancreas (Dr. Agnes Macgregor). The entire specimen, comprising about half the length of the pancreas and including the tail and the left part of the body, was divided into eight blocks and all of these were serially sectioned, producing nearly 4,000 sections. About 800 of these were stained and examined. No islet cell adenoma was present in the specimen. The islets of Langerhans showed certain abnormalities. (1) There was probably some increase in the average size of the islets as compared with normal controls from infants of the same age (Fig. 1). (2) The shape of many islets was irregular; often lateral projections or buds were present, suggesting active growth. (3) Many islets contained an unusual number of cells, the nuclei being packed close together, especially at the periphery of the islets. (4) Many other islets showed remarkable irregularity in the size of the cells (these islets were not, as a rule, those that had an increased number of cells). The nuclei of the large cells were much increased in size and sometimes irregular in shape, being lobulated. Sections stained by Gomori's method indicated that there was no obvious alteration in the proportion of alpha and beta cells, and that the abnormally large cells were beta cells. The acinar tissue was healthy.

Discussion

Graham and Oakley (1950) have suggested that the clinical picture produced by a tumour of the islet tissue of the pancreas may also be produced by diffuse hyperplasia of the islet cells, but Skillern and Rynearson (1953) have thrown doubt on this hypothesis, and suggest that, in some of the cases reported as showing diffuse hyperplasia of islet cells, a more careful search might have revealed a small tumour. In the case reported here, Whipple's (1938) criteria for the diagnosis of functioning islet-cell tumours were fulfilled, yet no tumour was found after very careful examination of the portion of pancreas removed at operation. It may be that a minute adenoma, not noted during the operation, still exists in the portion of pancreas remaining *in situ*, but this seems unlikely, as, during the five years the patient has been followed up, there has been no further evidence of hypoglycaemia. The histological appearances of the pancreas strongly suggest that a diffuse hyperplasia of the islet tissue was, in fact, present.

While partial resection of the pancreas does seem to have controlled the hypoglycaemic state of this child, complete 'cure' cannot be claimed, for it is not possible to forecast what may happen to the remaining islet cells. The hyperplasia is presumably due to some stimulating factor, possibly a pituitary hormone, which may continue to act, producing

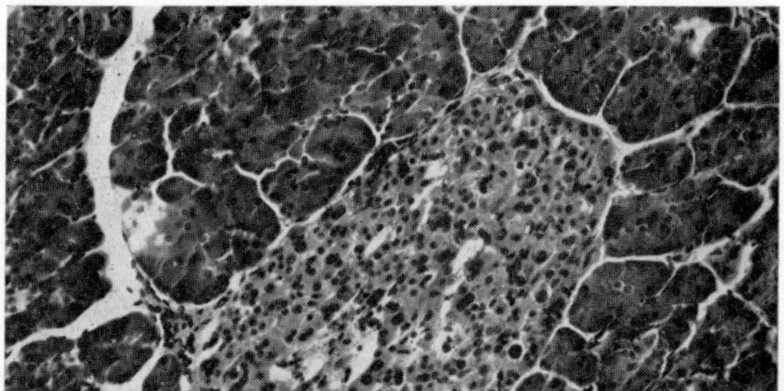

Fig. 1.—Photomicrograph of the pancreas showing an enlarged islet of Langerhans (× 120).

further hyperplasia or even exhaustion and death of the islet cells. Thus further attacks of hypoglycaemia may eventually occur or a state of diabetes mellitus be produced.

Nevertheless it seems likely that the mental defect of this patient may be related to the recurrent attacks of hypoglycaemia and, in retrospect, one wishes that the operation had been carried out earlier.

Summary

A baby started having convulsions at the age of 7 weeks. These fits generally occurred before the first feed of the day. He was investigated in hospital at the age of 8 months and was found to have a blood sugar level ranging from 32 to 42 mg. % at the onset of a fit. A diagnosis of islet cell tumour was made and two-thirds of the pancreas were removed. The blood sugar levels returned to normal and the fits were controlled. Histological examination of the resected portion of pancreas revealed a diffuse hyperplasia of islet cells, but no tumour was found.

No record of a similar case has been found in the British literature.

I would like to express my gratitude to Dr. Agnes MacGregor and Dr. R. F. Ogilvie for their help with the pathology of this case.

References

Agustsson, H., Tudor, R. B. and Chisholm, T. C. (1947). *J. Amer. med. Ass.*, **134**, 1202. (Abstract of *J. Lancet*, **67**, 190 (1947).)
Callaway, J. M. (1946). *J med. Ass. Ga*, **35**, 164.
Cushing, H. (1930). *Lancet*, **2**, 119.
Garland, H. (1957). *Brit. med. J.*, **2**, 969.
Graham, G. and Oakley, W. G. (1950). *Quart. J. Med.*, **19**, 21.
Howard, J. M., Moss, N. H. and Rhoads, J. E. (1950). *Int. Abstr. Surg.*, **90**, 417.
Skillern, P. G. and Rynearson, E. H. (1953). *J. clin. Endocr.*, **13**, 587.
Whipple, A. O. (1938). *J. int. Chir.*, **3**, 237

EXTENDED EXCHANGE TRANSFUSION IN PRE-HYDROPIC INFANTS

BY

EILEEN M. O'NEILL and RONALD R. GORDON

From the City General Hospital, Sheffield

(RECEIVED FOR PUBLICATION AUGUST 5, 1958)

Exchange transfusion in the immediate treatment of haemolytic disease of the newborn is now a fully established procedure with more or less agreed indications for its use (Allen and Diamond, 1957). Up till now the procedure has been mainly used to prevent kernikterus and in this it has been eminently successful both in the 'clinical' and the 'pathological' varieties of this condition. It can be said that in any unit in which facilities for proper exchange transfusion are available kernikterus should no longer be a problem in haemolytic disease due either to Rhesus, ABO or other incompatibility.

The deaths still encountered in haemolytic disease of the newborn are of two types: those which occur *in utero* resulting in stillbirth and those in which the babies are born alive but die within a few hours either before, during, or after the first exchange transfusion. The main cause of death in the first type is hydrops foetalis, which is essentially severe heart failure occurring *in utero*; in the second type the cause of death is probably also heart failure so that the term 'pre-hydrops' would be a fairly accurate description of this clinical condition. It is mainly with this group of pre-hydropic infants that we are concerned in this communication.

Before discussing this group further, however, we must explain that in our view these deaths are in quite a different category from those described by Campbell (1955). In his cases the babies were relatively mildly affected and it was only because of the fear of later jaundice that an exchange was undertaken. In them the babies were perfectly well until they suddenly collapsed and it was felt that there was probably a severe biochemical upset affecting perhaps the serum potassium (Campbell, 1955) or serum citrate (Kelsall and Vos, 1955). We have been fortunate in having no experience of this type of case and it seems that no satisfactory explanation for them is, as yet, forthcoming (Farquhar and Smith, 1958).

In contrast, the pre-hydropic babies are born with a low cord haemoglobin (under 10 g. %) and are clinically pale and either not jaundiced or only mildly so. The cord blood bilirubin is usually high and may be very high. In addition, the babies are usually ill with rapid respirations which often become grunting in character and there is often some oedema. The liver and spleen are both enlarged and there is sometimes a profuse purpura. The fact that haemolysis is proceeding rapidly is shown by the high reticulocyte count in the cord blood. These babies are on the verge of, or in, heart failure (Mollison and Cutbush, 1949), as is shown by the high venous pressure recorded when the catheter is passed up the umbilical vein. Even with the use of exchange transfusion the mortality in this group is still high.

The occurrence of pre-hydropic infants is well documented in the literature and they are usually shown as dying from heart failure. In the report of Mollison and Walker (1952), out of 79 deaths during the first week of life 17 were due to this cause: eight of these died in spite of treatment by simple or exchange transfusion. Walker and Neligan (1955) in their own series of 250 treated cases of haemolytic disease, reported deaths attributable to the disease and, of these, five were due to heart failure, comprising the largest single cause of death. Walker and Mollison (1957), recently reviewed the deaths from the disease in England and Wales and reported that in two years (1953 and 1955), there were 312 and 315 deaths respectively: of these, 58 and 55 were attributed to heart failure although all of them did not necessarily have 'proper' treatment. In fact, of these 113 infants, in only 75 was exchange transfusion attempted, 57 of them dying during the procedure. They reported a further group of 69 infants in the two years who were said to die of 'hydrops foetalis', this is probably the severest degree of the condition we are discussing and, in our view, it is not of necessity fatal. We feel that the name 'hydrops' should be kept only as a pathological term since it has, by usage, an implication of death or impending death; the name, 'pre-hydrops' could then be applied to all those born alive who show any of the signs of heart failure. If one includes the cases in Walker and Mollison's (1957) series which were classified as born alive 'with hydrops', out of a total of 627 deaths in two years, 182 (113+69) were attributed to heart failure; in the same period 187 were attributed to kernikterus. The deaths from kernikterus are likely to decrease further with the years so that heart failure as a cause of death will become relatively more important. The management of these infants is still a difficult problem (Walker and Neligan, 1955).

It is usually recommended that the cord be clamped early and that before starting exchange transfusion blood should be taken off so as to reduce the venous pressure. The amount varies between 20 ml. and 80 ml. It has also been suggested that instead of taking it off all at once a larger amount of blood should be removed than is transfused in the early stages of the exchange until a suitable 'venesection' has been achieved (Walker and Neligan, 1955). It is not often stressed, however, that it may be difficult and even dangerous to reduce the venous pressure and that even when reduced it may rise again during the subsequent exchange transfusion: yet most paediatricians know this and also that accurate measurements of the venous pressure are difficult to record especially at the start of the transfusion.

It has also been suggested (Murray and Norman, 1957) that digitalis should be given to reduce the venous pressure, but if this is followed by ordinary exchange transfusion it seems likely that quite a proportion of the drug will be removed before becoming effective (Wheeler and Ambuel, 1957). It could, however, be a useful adjuvant in the treatment: it was not used in either of the two recent severe cases we now report who died, nor in the third case which recovered.

Case Histories

Case 1. S.B. was the second affected child in the family, and the estimated maturity was 36 weeks. Delivery was normal, and the cord clamped immediately. Birth weight was 5 lb. 5 oz. The cord blood showed a positive Coombs test: Hb 42% (6·3 g. %); serum bilirubin 12 mg. %; reticulocyte count 50%. From the start the baby was ill, grunting and cyanosed, although there was no oedema and no purpura. Exchange transfusion by the umbilical route was started two hours after delivery and the venous pressure was found to be high, the blood gushing round the catheter making accurate measurement impossible. A further 20 ml. were removed after the catheter was in position and the venous pressure was then normal. The exchange consisted of 540 ml. in and 560 ml. out. The blood used was three days old. The time taken was 60 minutes. On completion the venous pressure had risen to 15 cm. of blood, and just afterwards the baby became suddenly more cyanosed, gasped a few times, and died. A post-transfusion specimen of the baby's blood showed a potassium level of only 21·1 mg. % (5·9 mEq/l.). Autopsy showed dilatation of the right ventricle but nothing else.

Case 2. K.T. was the second affected child in the family, the previous one having hydrops foetalis. The estimated maturity was 39 weeks. There was antepartum haemorrhage due to type 2 placenta praevia. A.R.M. was performed and the delivery was uneventful. Birth weight was 6 lb. The cord was clamped immediately. Cord blood results showed a positive Coombs test: Hb 30% (4·2 g. %); bilirubin 4·6 mg. %; reticulocytes 52%.

The child's general condition from the start was poor: there was extreme pallor and slight jaundice; the respirations were grunting; there were many petechiae but no oedema. Exchange transfusion was started one hour and 50 minutes after birth. Once again the venous pressure was high and was brought down to normal by the removal of 50 ml. of blood. An exchange of 350 ml. was then effected; at first the baby's general condition improved but the transfusion had to be stopped at the above level because of a sudden deterioration 36 minutes after starting. At this stage the venous pressure had risen to 20 cm. although it was normal before starting the exchange proper. Despite calcium gluconate and coramine the baby died and once again the cause of death at autopsy appeared to be heart failure. Two bottles of blood were involved in this exchange, the first being one day old and the second six days old.

These two babies were born exceedingly anaemic and very ill. They were both in heart failure and in both the high venous pressure was relieved before the exchange was started. Even so the failure was progressive, resulting in a further rise of venous pressure throughout the exchange and terminating in death. We felt, therefore, that this method was not entirely satisfactory although we realized that infants just as severely affected had been treated similarly with recovery (Watson, Crosse and Hatchuel, 1954; Walker and Neligan, 1955). We felt that, since in other forms of chronic anaemia, rapid transfusion may kill the patient (Sharpey-Schafer, 1945), too rapid exchange transfusion might also do so, especially as we had evidence of a rise in venous pressure during the exchange. It seemed possible, therefore, that if we removed a considerable amount of blood to relieve venous pressure we could replace it by means of a slow drip in the same way as for any other chronic anaemia; during the procedure also the pressure could be watched and if it increased further then another venesection could be performed. This involved being prepared to leave the catheter in position for a prolonged period but this, of course, has been done previously in the treatment of anuria without harm (Russell, Dewhurst and Brace, 1954). In such critically ill infants we felt that it was completely justified to do so, although we fully agree with Wheeler and Ambuel (1957) that a catheter should not be left in the umbilical vein for several days just because a repeat exchange might be necessary.

When Case 3 was seen we had the opportunity to try out this system of what might be called 'extended exchange transfusion'.

Case 3. P.P. was the first affected child in the family. There was slight A.P.H. at 30 weeks, but a normal full-term delivery. Birth weight was 8lb. 2oz. and the cord was clamped immediately. Cord blood showed a positive Coombs test: Hb 40% (5·9 g. %), bilirubin 14 mg. % and reticulocytes 40%. At birth the baby was very pale and slightly jaundiced; there was no oedema and no bleeding. Respirations were rapid and shallow and there was some cyanosis. Whilst waiting for the blood to be prepared the condition became even worse and the respirations became grunting in character. It was, therefore, decided to perform a slower form of exchange transfusion to try and avoid the disappointments of the previous two cases.

At the age of 2½ hours the transfusion was started via the umbilical route. Again the venous pressure was found to be exceedingly high and so, in spite of the severe anaemia, 100 ml. of blood were withdrawn with marked clinical improvement as well as improvement in the venous pressure, although even then it did not come down completely to normal. On this occasion, instead of proceeding to the complete exchange following the venesection, a transfusion of suitable blood was allowed to run into the umbilical vein very slowly over the next eight hours. During this time the baby received 200 ml. of blood which was a little more than we had anticipated. At this stage the baby was becoming dyspnoeic again so a further 60 ml. of blood were withdrawn with considerable improvement both clinically and in the venous pressure. From this point onwards further amounts of blood were removed at intervals whilst the slow drip was continued until the anaemia was fully corrected and the baby was out of failure. From then on small amounts of blood were removed and transfused at the same sitting and eventually it was felt safe to perform a complete exchange to remove the circulating bilirubin which had reached 16 mg. %. A summary of the treatment, which was certainly fully 'extended', is given in the accompanying appendix. It can be seen that the process lasted 63 hours.

In addition to the usual warmth, oxygen, calcium gluconate and vitamin K, intramuscular penicillin and streptomycin were given from the first day as a prophylactic. A final blood sample, taken at the end of the transfusion, grew only coagulase negative staphylococci in one bottle: the serum calcium at that time was 9·2 mg. % (4·6 mEq/l.), the potassium was 13·0 mg. % (3·3 mEq/l.) and the serum bilirubin 9·0 mg. %.

Progress was slow and the baby was feeble and moderately jaundiced for 15 days. The liver remained enlarged and the skin became 'sclerematous'. Slowly she improved, however, but it was three weeks after her birth before she was fit enough to go home. Since then progress has been perfectly satisfactory.

Discussion

We appreciate that this infant could have survived with ordinary exchange transfusion, as has been reported before (Watson *et al.*, 1954; Walker and Neligan, 1955). We do not think that the method used has not in some way been used previously since it may differ only slightly from the 'leisurely' exchange referred to by Farquhar and Smith (1958), and of course many people have probably left the catheter in position for lengthy periods.

On the other hand we believe that the idea of leaving the catheter in and performing the exchange gradually in the way described is a reasonable method to use in certain cases.

In retrospect, we think that in our Case 3 we probably removed and replaced too much blood in the first stage and in future would aim at 50 ml. amounts in and out unless the venous pressure was so high that clinical improvement could not be obtained except by greater venesection. We would probably make use of digitalis in further cases also since it might have time to become effective. The aim of treatment at this stage is to bring the patient out of heart failure as quickly as possible. Once immediate improvement has been obtained the anaemia should be corrected fairly slowly by means of a drip transfusion; removal and replacement, by slow drip, can then be continued until the baby is completely out of heart failure. Only then should any real attempt be made to remove the infant's red cells, and this, as well as the reduction in the serum bilirubin, can be effected by repeated exchange transfusions. In our case it took about 48 hours to correct the venous pressure and the anaemia and by that time the height of the serum bilirubin called for a full exchange. As a result a much greater volume of blood than usual was required to treat this infant and a total of 1,650 ml. was used.

It is possible that in the future some extended exchange technique, if found to be of value, may be more often required since it seems possible that more of these severely affected babies may be seen.

It was shown by Watson *et al.* (1954) that in families with a bad history better results might be obtained by early induction of labour with immediate exchange transfusion of the premature baby, than by leaving the pregnancy to continue and result in stillbirth. The idea of premature induction of labour in sensitized women has also recently been advocated by Kelsall, Vos and Kirk (1958). The main reason why premature induction was so strongly condemned by Mollison and Walker (1952) was because of the high incidence of kernikterus in the resulting premature babies. As Walker *et al.* (1957) indicate, it is unlikely that this high incidence of kernikterus would occur today owing to the much greater use of repeated exchange transfusion. For this reason early induction does not now hold the same terrors as it did and it seems likely that it will be more fully used in the future, especially if a means can be found to determine when the foetus is severely affected. The objective then will be to convert a hydropic baby which dies *in utero* into a pre-hydropic one with a chance of survival. We believe that in the management of these very ill infants extended exchange transfusion may be found to be of value.

Summary

The term 'pre-hydrops' as applied to some babies suffering from haemolytic disease of the newborn is described.

A method of treating such babies by means of an extended exchange transfusion is given, with details in a single case.

References

Allen, F. H. and Diamond, L. K. (1957). *New Engl. J. Med.*, **257**, 705.
Campbell, W. A. B. (1955). *Arch. Dis. Childh.*, **30**, 513.
Farquhar, J. W. and Smith, H. (1958). *Ibid.*, **33**, 142.
Kelsall, G. A. and Vos, G. H. (1955). *Ibid.*, **2**, 161.
——, —— and Kirk, R. L. (1958). *Brit. med. J.*, **2**, 468.
Mollison, P L. and Cutbush, M. (1949). *Brit. med. J.*, **1**, 123.
—— and Walker, W (1952). *Lancet*, **1**, 429.
Murray, J. and Norman, A. P. (1957). *Proc. roy Soc. Med.*, **50**, 711.
Russell, C. S., Dewhurst, C. J. and Brace, J. C. (1954). *Lancet*, **1**, 902.
Sharpey-Schafer, E. P. (1945). *Lancet*, **2**, 296.
Walker, W. and Mollison, P. L. (1957). *Ibid.*, **1**, 1309.
Walker, W., Murray, S. and Russell, J. K. (1957). *J. Obstet. Gynaec. Brit. Emp.*, **64**, 573.
—— and Neligan, G. A. (1955). *Brit. med. J.*, **1**, 681.
Watson, H. B., Crosse, V. M. and Hatchuel, W. L. F. (1954). *Ibid.*, **1**, 679.
Wheeler, W. E. and Ambuel, J. P. (1957). *Pediat. Clin. N. Amer.*, **4**, 383.

APPENDIX

Summary of Extended Exchange Transfusion

9.3.58. 11.5 p.m. Born. Hb 40%. Bilirubin 14·0 mg. %.

10.3.58. 1.30 a.m. Exchange transfusion started. Venous pressure very high. 100 ml. blood withdrawn followed by slow drip of partly packed red cells.

10.50 a.m. Venous pressure high. 60 ml. blood withdrawn and drip continued. Total blood in 200 ml. Total blood out 160 ml.

6.50 p.m. Venous pressure high. 50 ml. blood withdrawn. Total blood out 210 ml. Total blood in 259 ml. Drip continued.

11.50 p.m. Venous pressure normal. 50 ml. blood withdrawn followed by exchange of 30 ml. Total blood out 290 ml. Total blood in 339 ml. Drip continued.

11.3.58. 9.30 a.m. Hb 108%. Bilirubin 15 mg. %. Venous pressure normal. 50 ml. blood withdrawn followed by exchange of 50 ml. Total blood out 390 ml. Total blood in 576 ml. Drip continued.

5.38 p.m. Venous pressure normal. 60 ml. blood withdrawn followed by exchange of 210 ml. Total blood out 660 ml. Total blood in 895 ml. Drip continued.

11.30 p.m. 50 ml. blood withdrawn. Total blood out 710 ml. Total blood in 931 ml. Drip continued.

12.3.58. 10.15 a.m. Hb 104%. Bilirubin 16·0 mg. %. 10 ml. blood withdrawn. Total blood out 720 ml. Total blood in 978 ml. Drip continued.

2.15 p.m. 40 ml. blood withdrawn followed by exchange of 640 ml. Total blood out 1,400 ml. Total blood in 1,650 ml. Drip stopped.

13.3.58. Hb 110 %. Bilirubin 9·0 mg. %.

26.3.58. Hb 77%. Bilirubin 2·0 mg. %.

MASSIVE ADRENAL HAEMORRHAGE IN THE NEWBORN

BY

EILEEN E. HILL and JOHN A. WILLIAMS

From the Children's Hospital, Birmingham

(RECEIVED FOR PUBLICATION AUGUST 12, 1958)

Intra-abdominal haemorrhage in the newborn is a diagnostic and therapeutic challenge; the site of the haemorrhage is commonly the liver or adrenal, rarely the other organs. (Lundquist, 1930; Potter, 1940; Henderson, 1941). If the haemorrhage is profuse it may lead to rupture of the capsule of the organ and intraperitoneal haemorrhage. In the case of adrenal haemorrhage in the newborn most authors have concentrated on post-mortem findings, many of the infants being stillborn. The first reported case to be successfully treated was that of Corcoran and Strauss (1924). Since then eight other surviving infants in whom adrenal haemorrhage was diagnosed have been described and these cases are tabulated (Table 1).

The following case report describes an infant suffering from haemorrhage into the adrenal with rupture of the capsule and intraperitoneal extension of the haemorrhage. From a review of the literature this would appear to be the first newborn infant to survive this complication. Twenty-five similar cases which ended fatally are tabulated for comparison (Table 2).

Case Report

The mother, weighing 18 st. 10 lb., was admitted to the Birmingham Maternity Hospital at the twenty-seventh week of her eleventh pregnancy because of hypertension. Her blood was Group O Rhesus negative and contained blocking antibodies. Two previous infants had haemolytic anaemia due to Rhesus incompatibility. The father was heterozygous for the Rhesus factor. The mother was in hospital a month, her blood pressure being 160/90, she was then discharged and re-admitted at the thirty-fourth week. Labour was induced surgically by rupture of the membranes at the thirty-seventh week, the indications being hypertension, oedema and the previous history of Rhesus incompatibility. The liquor was clear.

TABLE 1

SUMMARY OF RECORDED RECOVERIES FROM INTRAPERITONEAL HAEMORRHAGE

Author	Delivery	Sex	Clinical Features and Day of Onset	Treatment
Corcoran and Strauss, 1924	Precipitate	M.	4 day. Fever, vomiting, pallor. Palpable mass left side obstructing colon	Laparotomy and removal of blood clot from left adrenal
Goldzieher and Greenwald, 1928	Prolonged labour. Forceps. Primipara	F.	2 d. Fever, pallor, cyanosis, convulsions, temperature 103° F. Palpable mass right side	Transfused and given adrenal extract 4 and 12 d. Mass slowly disappeared
Arnold, 1930	Normal	M.	4 d. Pallor, listlessness, palpable right-sided mass	Transfused 120 ml. blood
	Podalic version Breech extraction	F.	3 d. Pallor, anorexia, pyrexia, abdominal distension 7 d. Convulsions, palpable right-sided mass	Transfused 95 ml. blood
Goldzieher and Gordon, 1932	Normal		7 hr. rapid respirations, shrill cry, cyanosis. Small abdominal mass. Blood sugar normal. Haemoglobin 70%	Intramuscular blood
	Normal		2 d. cyanosis, rapid respirations, abdominal distension. 3 d. fever. Right-sided abdominal mass.	Transfused 100 ml. blood
	Asphyxiated		3 d. rapid respirations Temperature 105° F. Palpable left-sided mass	Intramuscular blood
Emery and Zachary, 1952	Forceps	M.	2 d. fever, pallor, listlessness. Palpable mass right side	Laparotomy and removal of blood clot from right adrenal capsule
Marin *et al.*, 1955	Difficult breech		3 d. pallor, cyanosis. Palpable mass left side	Laparotomy. Nephrectomy and adrenalectomy, both organs surrounded by blood

TABLE 2

SUMMARY OF RECORDED FATAL CASES WITH INTRAPERITONEAL HAEMORRHAGE

Author	Delivery	Sex	Clinical Features and Day of Onset	Death (day)	Site of Haemorrhage
Riesman: quoted Hamill, 1901		F.		9	L. adrenal. Intraperitoneal rupture
Norris, 1900			Congenital heart disease	10	R. adrenal and intraperitoneal
Mattei, 1863				4	L. adrenal and intraperitoneal
Spencer, 1891	Stillborn	F.			R. and L. adrenal and intraperitoneal haemorrhage from left
	Breech. Stillborn. Hydrocephalic	F.			R. adrenal and intraperitoneal Rupture R. lobe of liver
	Mild hydrocephalic. Forceps delivery failed, Breech extraction	M.	Child only just alive when born	1	R. adrenal and intraperitoneal
Prudden, 1899	Normal		Breathed and fed badly	4	R. adrenal and intraperitoneal
Hodenpyl, 1890	Normal		3 d. Sudden collapse	3	R. adrenal and intraperitoneal. Subcapsular hepatic haemorrhage
Hervey, 1870			10 d. Sudden collapse	10	R. adrenal and intraperitoneal
Fiedler, 1870	Normal		4 d. Sudden abdominal distension, dyspnoea	4	R. adrenal 4-5 oz. intraperitoneal blood
Milroy, 1884	Rapid	M.	Pale, cold. Dyspnoea	12 hr.	R. adrenal and intraperitoneal
Tuley, 1892	Very short	M.	3 d. pyrexia. 4 d. respiration 72 laboured. Weak pulse 200. Painful expression. Tense abdomen	4	R. adrenal and 8½ oz. in peritoneal cavity
Hamill, 1901	Normal primipara	M.	2 d. temperature 103° F. Pallor. Restless, cyanosis, rapid respiration	3	R. adrenal and 6 oz. in peritoneal cavity
Lundquist, 1930	Breech extraction	M.	Shocked at birth. 5 d. convulsions. 6 d. mass left side	7	L. adrenal and intraperitoneal
	Extraction. Difficulty with shoulders	M.	Schultze resuscitation. Convulsions 2 d.	2	L. adrenal and intraperitoneal
	Normal primipara	M.	Asphyxiated. 6 d. pallor off feed. Resistance left side abdomen	6	R. adrenal and intraperitoneal
	Normal primipara	M.	4 d. pallor. Abdominal distension	4	R. adrenal and intraperitoneal
	Normal primipara	M.	5 d. pallor. Refused feed	5	R. adrenal and intraperitoneal
	Uterine inertia. Forceps extraction	M.	5 d. Sudden collapse	5	R. adrenal and intraperitoneal
	Transverse lie. Breech extraction	M.	Found dead	2	L. adrenal and intraperitoneal
Arnold, 1930	Normal primipara	M.	4 d. Pallor, air hunger. Convulsions abdominal distension	5	R. adrenal and intraperitoneal
	Podalic version. Breech extraction		3 d. Sudden collapse with abdominal distension. Petechiae	3	R. adrenal and intraperitoneal 200 ml. of blood
Goldzieher and Gordon, 1932	Normal		3 d. Cyanosis. Pallor. Rapid respirations. Fever 101·8° F. Purpura. Blood sugar 10 mg. at 88 hr. Bilateral abdominal masses	4	Bilateral, with 3 oz. of blood in peritoneal cavity
Kohlbry and Wells, 1945	Forceps		Pallor. Cyanosis. Air hunger. Vomiting. Abdominal distension	4½ hr. (Transfused)	R. adrenal and intraperitoneal
Emery and Zachary, 1952	Normal		Pallor, rapid collapse	2	R. adrenal and intraperitoneal

Three days later as labour had not started pitocin was given and labour commenced. After four hours 20 minutes a male infant weighing 7 lb. 14 oz. was delivered through a cervix which was not fully dilated. The multiparity and the obesity of the mother made controlled delivery difficult. The infant was a little pale and shocked at birth but was quickly resuscitated following clearing of the air passages. He was not jaundiced, the liver and spleen were not enlarged, the cord blood was Group A Rhesus negative, Coombs test negative, with a bilirubin of 0·8 mg./100 ml. Unfortunately clotting of the blood prevented estimation of the haemoglobin level.

The infant's condition gave rise to no concern until the morning of the third day when he was noticed to be pale. The haemoglobin was 12·1 g./100 ml. An hour later he became fretful and resented examination. His respirations became shallow and rapid, and cyanosis developed. The rectal temperature was 96·6° F. The differential diagnosis at this stage lay between an overwhelming infection, or an intracranial or intra-abdominal haemorrhage. Penicillin and streptomycin were given. The child's condition further deteriorated, the pallor increased, the heart sounds became soft and a definite resistance to palpation was present on the right side of the abdomen. Within 15 minutes the infant's breathing ceased but the heart continued to beat. Meanwhile, a rapid transfusion of 80 ml. of blood was given through an umbilical catheter and cortisone 5 mg. and vitamin K 2·5 mg. were given intramuscularly; respirations recommenced and the colour improved. Two hours later breathing again became rapid and a further 5 mg. of cortisone was given intramuscularly. The child improved sufficiently to be transferred to the Children's Hospital. He was still pale, with peripheral cyanosis, though the haemoglobin was now 16·8 g./100 ml. The abdomen was tense, and again resistance was felt more over the right side. The respirations were rapid and shallow and during examination twitching of the face and arms was observed. An accurate diagnosis seemed essential for the carrying out of further treatment. Hepatic haemorrhage with rupture of the capsule was considered the most likely, but the convulsions pointed rather to an adrenal haemorrhage. It was therefore decided to do a laparotomy if abdominal paracentesis confirmed the presence of intraperitoneal blood. Blood was cross matched and an intravenous drip set up.

Abdominal paracentesis, one inch below the right costal margin in the anterior axillary line, produced 4 ml. of unclotted blood. The child was therefore anaesthetized and the peritoneal cavity opened by an incision parallel to the right costal margin. A large quantity of free blood and clots were removed from the peritoneal cavity. Inspection of the liver showed it to be intact. The right suprarenal capsule, however, was grossly distended by a blood clot and blood was present round the right kidney. The appearance of the kidney and adrenal closely resembled a tumour. The left suprarenal felt normal. After evacuation of the clot the adrenal capsule was packed with fibrin foam. No bleeding points were located and the abdomen was closed. The blood clot was later reported by Dr. A. H. Cameron to contain adrenal cortical tissue (Fig. 1).

The immediate post-operative condition was satisfactory. For two days the child remained on intravenous fluids to which hydrocortisone, 12·5 mg., was added each 24 hours. Thereafter oral feeds were tolerated. Cortisone in decreasing doses was given over a further five days. At no time did the child's condition or the serum electrolytes indicate adrenal insufficiency. The wound healed rather slowly but the infant's general condition remained excellent.

Discussion

Various factors seem to be concerned in the production of haemorrhage into the adrenal gland.

Trauma. Throughout the literature, trauma, at or soon after birth, is considered to be the main cause of intra-abdominal haemorrhage. In Lundquist's (1930) series of 18 adrenal haemorrhages only five deliveries were normal. Three of the infants had been delivered rapidly because of prolapse of the cord. Podalic version, forceps extraction and breech deliveries are all mentioned. Rogers (1934) in his paper on rupture of the liver describes three cases in which labour was induced medically with pitocin and it is interesting that this drug was used in our case. In 10 of the 25 fatal cases, labour was recorded as abnormal. In the reports of the infants who recovered details are fuller and seven of the 10 deliveries were abnormal. Birth weights are often above average (Henderson, 1941) and corresponding with this there is a preponderance of male infants.

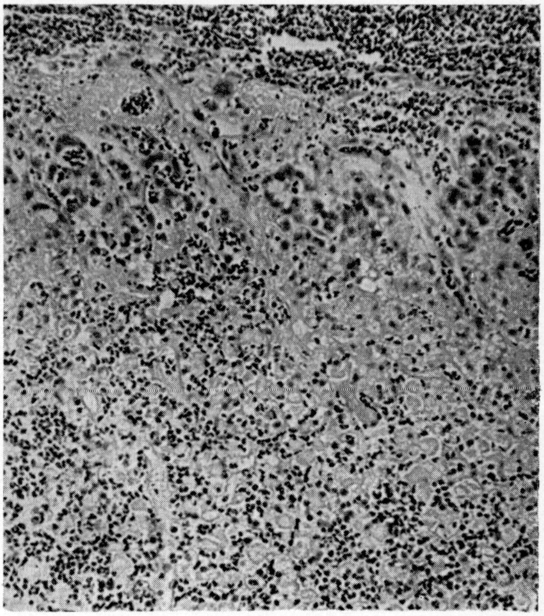

FIG. 1.—Adrenal haemorrhage showing 'permanent' cortical tissue between the external haematoma and the internal haemorrhagic 'foetal cortex'.

Asphyxia. Asphyxia probably plays a minor part in the causation of large haemorrhages though small bilateral adrenal haemorrhages, in themselves insufficient to cause death, are a common finding in asphyxiated infants. In such cases haemorrhages are usually found at other sites and these asphyxial haemorrhages are not a feature in the cases under discussion (Arnold, 1930; Henderson, 1941).

Coagulation Defect. A lowered prothrombin level would appear to be of considerable importance, for the time of onset of the symptoms of acute haemorrhage into the adrenals is the second to seventh day which coincides with the age at which haemorrhagic disease of the newborn occurs (Arnold, 1930; Marin, Graham and Kickham, 1955). In the earlier writings, before hypoprothrombinaemia was known to occur, haemophilia is mentioned as an aetiological factor (Townsend, 1894; Morison, 1908).

Infection. Infection, which is the commonest cause of adrenal haemorrhage in the older child, is not often found in this group of infants.

Adrenal Vascularity and Involution. At birth the adrenals are relatively large having an average combined weight of 6·5 g. which is reduced by the age of 2 to 3 months to 3·51 g. (Tähkä, 1951). Direct trauma, unlikely to cause damage to the relatively much smaller gland of the older child, may well affect the larger gland of the newborn. The change in size is entirely due to the involution of the foetal cortex (Kern, 1911; Baar, 1954). During this process extreme hyperaemia with congestion and dilatation of capillaries occurs chiefly in the inner zone which comprises 80% of the foetal cortex. There is also a breaking down of the structure of this zone which may lessen any support given to the capillaries and make them more liable to rupture from increased congestion or external pressure. Areas of the outer, more compact layer of cortex may, as in our case, be found in the clot of blood suggesting that haemorrhage does indeed start in the inner hyperaemic layer (Hamill, 1901; Marin *et al.*, 1955).

Anatomy. In 18 of the 25 fatal cases the right gland alone was affected; in two the haemorrhage was bilateral and in five left sided only. In the surviving infants haemorrhage was considered, clinically or proved at laparotomy, to be on the right side in six out of the 10 cases. The explanation of this right-sided preponderance is considered to be the different venous drainage of the adrenals. The vein from the right gland drains directly into the inferior vena cava and is therefore more liable to be affected by pressure on the inferior vena cava during delivery or during resuscitation. The vein from the left adrenal drains into the smaller renal vein (Mattei, 1865). Magnus (1911) believes that the right adrenal gland, having the liver anteriorly and ribs posteriorly, is also more liable to direct compression.

Clinical Findings. The clinical findings are discussed fully by Goldzieher and Gordon (1932) in their paper on suprarenal haemorrhage. They divide the signs into those due to acute adrenal insufficiency on the one hand and acute haemorrhage on the other. The former consist of rapid respirations, pyrexia, purpura, metabolic upsets, convulsions and cyanosis, abdominal pain, vomiting and diarrhoea. The general effects of the latter are shock, collapse, weak pulse, cold extremities, pallor and air hunger, whilst the local effects are a distended abdomen and a palpable mass. It is not known whether there is any change in serum electrolytes in the acute phase suggesting adrenal insufficiency. A low blood sugar of 10 mg./100 ml. was recorded by Goldzieher and Gordon (1932) in one infant six hours before death from bilateral adrenal haemorrhage with intraperitoneal rupture. In practice awareness of the condition and recognition of the clinical picture has far more bearing on the immediate prognosis. Pyrexia and convulsions may be present but the important signs are, as in the case described, the sudden onset of a pneumonia-like illness with the addition of abdominal distension or a palpable abdominal mass.

Minor haemorrhages into the adrenals insufficient to cause clinical signs in the neonatal period may later present as calcification of the adrenals with or without signs of adrenal insufficiency. The finding of bilateral adrenal calcification following adrenal haemorrhage at birth has been reported by Snelling and Erb (1935). Gardner (1957) describes an infant with bilateral calcification presumably following birth trauma due to a footling presentation, who showed signs of adrenal insufficiency. Classical Addison's disease in children may be the result of haemorrhage into the adrenals in the newborn (Williams and Robinson, 1956). Larger haemorrhages especially when bilateral would certainly be expected to cause death from adrenal insufficiency and no surviving case has been found though many fatal cases with large bilateral suprarenal haemorrhages are recorded.

Where the haemorrhage is large but unilateral the clinical picture may be far less dramatic without definite signs of adrenal insufficiency or acute blood loss. In this instance the abdominal mass is the main finding. In the case reported by Corcoran and Strauss (1924) the distended adrenal had, by pressure on the descending colon, caused signs of intestinal obstruction. Marin *et al.* (1955) report the case of an infant who had a normal kidney and a haemorrhagic adrenal removed in the belief that it was a Wilms' tumour. The adrenal capsule was distended with old blood clots in which calcium was found. Only the cortex of the adrenal was intact. We have found an exactly similar case to this in the records of the Children's Hospital.

Where haemorrhage is extensive blood loss may be so acute that even when the diagnosis is correctly made the infant dies before treatment can be instituted (Arnold, 1930).

Treatment. In infants with symptoms and signs suggestive of acute intra-abdominal haemorrhage replacement of the blood loss is the most urgent need. The umbilical vein is a convenient route for transfusion in the newborn. This is one of the few neonatal emergencies which call for rapid transfusion and amounts up to 100 or even 200 ml. of blood may be required. As much as 8½ oz. of blood have been recovered from the peritoneal cavity (Tuley, 1892). Vitamin K should be given.

Whether the child should be subjected to laparotomy is debatable. It should not be necessary when the infant's condition improves rapidly after transfusion and remains satisfactory. In the surviving infants not operated on, the palpable abdominal masses have been noted to disappear. In suspected intraperitoneal haemorrhage the method of abdominal paracentesis strongly advocated by Rogers (1934) can be used to confirm the diagnosis. In cases where haemorrhage appears to be continuing, especially in those, the majority, where the exact site of haemorrhage is in doubt, laparotomy is advisable and may be life saving.

Adrenal extract was first used by Goldzeiher and Greenwald (1928) in the treatment of adrenal haemorrhage in the newborn. They believed that it was an important factor in the infant's survival. However, Arnold (1930) did not consider that any of the infants he describes died from adrenal insufficiency. We have no proof that our case was helped by steroid therapy but in the initial collapsed state, when the infant's condition was critical, and certainly after the confirmation of adrenal haemorrhage, its use seemed advisable. Now that steroid therapy is so readily available it is hoped, that with the recording of further survivals, its use can be better assessed.

Summary

A case surviving extensive haemorrhage into the right adrenal with rupture into the peritoneal cavity is described. Twenty-five similar but fatal cases are tabulated with nine other surviving cases who did not show intra-peritoneal haemorrhage.

The aetiology, clinical picture and treatment is discussed.

The need for urgent diagnosis and treatment if the child is to survive is stressed.

We wish to thank Dr. B. Wood and Mr. M. I. D. Noble for permission to publish the case. We are very grateful to Mr. B. Wood for his advice and encouragement and to Dr. A. H. Cameron for the histological report. We would also like to thank Mr. J. Williamson for the photograph and Mrs. Harris for clerical assistance.

REFERENCES

Arnold, D. P. (1930). *Amer. J. Dis. Child.*, **40**, 1053.
Baar, H. S. (1954). *Lancet*, **1**, 670.
Corcoran, W. J. and Strauss, A. A. (1924). *J. Amer. med. Ass.*, **82**, 626.
Emery, J. L. and Zachary, R. B. (1952). *Brit. med. J.*, **2**, 857.
Fiedler (1870). *Arch. Heilk.*, XI, 301.
Gardner, L. I. (1957). *Pediat. Clin. N. Amer.*, **4**, Nov., p. 896.
Goldzieher, M. A. and Gordon, M. B. (1932). *Endocrinology*, **16**, 165.
—— and Greenwald, H. M. (1928). *Amer. J. Dis. Child.*, **36**, 324.
Hamill, S. McC. (1901). *Arch. Pediat.*, **18**, 81, 161.
Henderson, J. L. (1941). *J. Obstet. Gynaec. Brit. Emp.*, **48**, 377.
Hervey (1874). *Bull. Soc. anat. Paris*, 1870, 2 ser., **15**, 263.
Hodenpyl (1891). *Proc. N.Y. path. Soc.*, 1890, p. 67.
Kern, H. (1911). *Dtsch. med. Wschr.*, **37**, 971.
Kohlbry, C. O. and Wells, A. H. (1945). *Minn. Med.*, **28**, 1002.
Lundquist, B. (1930). *Acta obstet. gynec. scand.*, **9**, 331.
Magnus, G. (1911). *Berl. klin. Wschr.*, **48**, 1119.
Marin, H. M., Graham, J. H. and Kickham, C. J. E. (1955). *Arch. Surg. (Chicago)*, **71**, 941.
Mattei, R. (1863). *Sperimentale*, **11**, p. 28.
—— (1865). *J. méd. Chirurg. Pharmacol. (Bruxelles)*, **41**, 322.
Milroy, W. F. (1884). *Amer. J. Obstet. Dis. Women*, **17**, 772.
Morison, B. G. (1908). *Lancet*, **1**, 1620.
Norris, C. (1900). *Proc. N.Y. path. Soc.*, March.
Potter, E. L. (1940). *J. Amer. med. Ass.*, **115**, 996.
Prudden (1899). Quoted by Hamill, *Proc. N.Y. path. Soc.*, p. 92.
Riesman (1901). (Quoted by Hamill.) Post-mortem records. University Hospital, Philadelphia.
Rogers, G. (1934). *Amer. J. Obstet. Gynec.*, **27**, 841.
Snelling, C. E. and Erb, I. H. (1935). *J. Pediat.*, **6**, 22.
Spencer, H. R. (1892). *Trans. obstet. Soc. Lond.* (1891), **33**, 203.
Tähkä, H. (1951). *Acta pediat. (Uppsala)*, **40**, Suppl., 81.
Townsend (1894). (Quoted by Hamill.) *Amer.Pediat. Soc. Reports*, Vol. VI.
Tuley, H. E. (1892). *Arch. Pediat.*, **9**, 842.
Williams, A. and Robinson, M. J. (1956). *Arch. Dis. Childh.*, **31**, 265.

BOOK REVIEWS

Principal Infectious Diseases of Childhood. By NELLES SILVERTHORN. (Pp. ix+102. 28s.) Toronto: University Press; London: Oxford University Press. 1958.

The field of infectious diseases of children is such a rapidly changing one that frequent appraisal of the position is desirable. Occasionally with delay in publication techniques of treatment have changed or new diagnostic methods become available.

This compact book presents a reasoned summary of all the common infections of childhood from the standpoint of the clinician. The material is presented under five headings: infections in the newborn, infectious or communicable diseases, infections of the nervous system, virus diseases, and non-virus respiratory infections. It is not intended to replace the standard textbooks to which reference for detail of diagnosis and treatment is recommended.

Where diagnostic laboratory facilities are available, their aid in problems of childhood is at times invaluable. This book omits reference to the laboratory diagnosis of smallpox. In cases of purulent meningitis a firm diagnosis and guide to treatment is frequently available from blood culture when the cerebrospinal fluid has not provided an organism. This might have been commented upon in the diagnosis of these conditions.

The absence of diagrams and illustrations is commendable in a book of this nature in which the text is essentially concise. The book will prove of value to public health workers, family doctors and students.

Tuberculosis in White and Negro Children.

Vol. I. By JANET B. HARDY. The Roentgenologic Aspects of the Harriet Lane Study. (Pp. vii+122; illustrated. 60s.)

Vol. II. By MIRIAM E. BRAILEY. The Epidemiological Aspects of the Harriet Lane Study. (Pp. 103; 8 figures. 36s.) Massachusetts: Harvard University Press. London: Oxford University Press. 1958.)

This work comes from the Harriet Lane Tuberculosis Clinic of the Johns Hopkins Hospital and was initiated by Dr. Edwards Park in 1928. The first volume, by Dr. Janet Hardy, is a beautifully produced book; it begins with a succinct account of the anatomy of the thoracic lymphatic system and the tracheo-bronchial tree. This is followed by 240 illustrations, 230 of which are radiographs, describing the normal variations, non-tuberculous conditions which must be differentiated, and the serial x-ray stories of many of the patients. There is a final section on bronchoscopy and bronchography, their indications and contra-indications and the techniques available. Everything about this book is first class; all the illustrations are outstandingly good and as an atlas it is a mine of information for reference.

The second volume, by Dr. Miriam Brailey, deals with the prognosis and statistics of the patients studied. The author attempts to determine the prognosis of tuberculous infection in children in the form of a statistical analysis based on the records of 1,329 children, 437 white and 892 negro, investigated in the Harriet Lane Tuberculosis Clinic between 1928 and 1945. Follow-up was continued till 1950.

The story of the planning of the investigation and of the results obtained is clearly and interestingly unfolded. Details are given of the initial chest x-ray findings, the incidence of extrapulmonary lesions, the mortality according to age, sex, initial findings and intrafamilial exposure. There were 140 deaths from tuberculosis, 20 among the white children and 120 among the negroes and, in addition, 40 children, 15 white and 25 negro, died from conditions other than tuberculosis.

The mortality was 9% for white children and 22% for negroes in those cases where initial infection occurred before the age of 3 years. When infection was first discovered after the age of 3 years, the mortality was 0·8% for white children and 8% for negroes. In the first group 78% of the deaths were due to tuberculous meningitis with or without miliary involvement, 12% to post-primary tuberculous pneumonia and 5% to reinfection pulmonary tuberculosis. In the second group 39% of deaths were due to meningitis, 5% to tuberculous pneumonia and 50% to reinfection pulmonary tuberculosis.

In investigating the risk of developing reinfection pulmonary tuberculosis it was found that the annual reinfection rate in the white children was only 0·034%, whereas in the negroes it was 0·33%. Further, the mortality rate in these cases was much higher in negroes and the risk of reinfection in girls was five times greater than in boys. Where exposure was continued after primary infection the incidence of reinfection within a 10-year period was three times higher than in those who escaped subsequent exposure. It is clear, therefore, that although reinfection in white children presents no real problem this does not hold true for negroes (and other susceptible subjects) in whom reinfection increases the risk of the development of phthisis.

Despite the fact that the picture described here has been completely changed as a result of chemotherapy and B.C.G., it nevertheless merits study for it is full of valuable information, the story of a well planned co-operative effort, and of considerable historical interest.

It is to be warmly commended to all interested in the study of the many facets of childhood tuberculosis.

Roentgen Diagnosis of Abdominal Tumours in Childhood. By CHARLES M. NICE, Jr., ALEXANDER R. MARGULIS and LEO G. RIGLER. (Pp. viii+74; 52 figures. 30s.) Springfield, Illinois: Charles C. Thomas; Oxford: Blackwell Scientific. 1957.

This is a book which contains useful advice on the interpretation of radiographs of the abdomen in childhood, and for the most part the advice is based on straightforward radiography, either without a contrast medium or simply with a barium meal or enema or an intravenous pyelogram.

This is just the sort of help which the paediatrician or surgeon would welcome, but the book is poorly written in the sense that it is difficult to read, and also contains a lot of trite phrases which do nothing but produce irritation in the reader, e.g. 'There is much to be said for making an attempt to make a diagnosis before surgery'. As an example of obscurity or unhappy phraseology we have the following: 'As, with the exception of haemangiomas, other tumours of the liver do not show calcification, its presence is an important differential point'.

The book is a curious mixture of first class material well arranged in a very practical way, and the overstatement of the obvious. 'Many possible avenues of approach can be used: the division into solid and cystic, into neoplastic, congenital, traumatic and inflammatory. The neoplastic can further be subdivided into benign and malignant'. This sort of statement may be all right in a textbook for nurses, but to spend time and space on it in a book 'intended for radiologists, paediatricians and surgeons interested in the preoperative diagnosis of tumours of childhood' detracts from its other very obviously good points. To have 52 first-class radiographs illustrating the problems of diagnosis of tumours in childhood available in a compact book of this sort is fine. For this reason it is a good reference book to have in a hospital library, provided one does not expect much help from the written portion.

Recent Advances in Paediatrics, 2nd ed. Edited by DOUGLAS GAIRDNER. (Pp. viii+378; 82 figures. 48s.) London: J. and A. Churchill. 1958.

The appearance of the first edition of *Recent Advances in Paediatrics* in 1954 filled a notable gap in British paediatric literature providing, as it did, in a relatively small compass, a survey and a balanced appraisal of the current state of knowledge of many aspects of paediatrics in which notable advances had been made in the preceding decade. The second edition will undoubtedly be no less welcome, for its aim and general plan are the same and the standard of its predecessor is amply maintained.

The content of the present volume is, of course, entirely new and the subjects have been chosen 'to display the growing edge of paediatrics today, the theoretical interest as well as the practical importance of a subject entering into the choice'. The first chapter on changes in the circulation at birth and the effects of asphyxia ranges widely over the field of animal physiology, from which much light has been shed in recent years on the darkness which still clouds our vision of the rapidly changing physiological scene during the first hours and days of independent existence. This is in many ways the most interesting and stimulating chapter in the book and of peculiar value in that it summarizes recent work in a field which is of vital importance to us as paediatricians but which few of us can hope to cover successfully in the original literature.

The selection of subjects is again admirable for on all of them there is something new to say and in several the time is clearly ripe for stock taking. It has become clear in recent years that the aetiology of jaundice in the newborn is more diverse than we had suspected and the two chapters devoted to this subject present a clear picture of the present position. Spina bifida cystica and hydrocephalus remain among the more difficult problems of infancy but considerable technical advances have recently been made in their management and it is useful to have here a definitive statement based on a wide experience of both conditions. The chapter on hypothyroidism is a fine illustration of how careful study of a few cases of a rare disorder can add to our understanding of a basic physiological process. The editor himself is responsible for the chapter on the haematology of infancy, a subject to which he has made considerable contributions: a large part of this chapter is devoted to the details of iron metabolism and haemopoiesis which are not elsewhere readily available with reference to this particular age period.

Other chapters deal with physical growth, the nephrotic syndrome, tuberculosis, rheumatic fever, the deaf child and pyrogenic osteitis, and a remarkably high standard is maintained in all of them.

There is an ample selection of references at the end of each chapter and the index is both accurate and adequate. This can be thoroughly recommended as a well written and well produced book of wide interest and usefulness and the editor and his associates are to be congratulated on their valiant efforts to keep us up to date.

Étude des Carences Protidiques Observées Chez l'Enfant en Pays Tropical (Kwashiorkor). By HENRI DUPIN. (Pp. 169; 55 figures. No price given.) Paris: Librairie Arnette. 1958.

This is a doctorate thesis presented in the Faculty of Science of the University of Paris. The author works in Dakar and therefore his views can be taken to represent the French school of thought on kwashiorkor. He cites, however, nearly 300 references, has obviously read widely and he presents his own original observations against a sound background. One of his main interests seems to be in regard to the liver lesions of this widespread disorder with particular reference to the possible arrest of progress towards cirrhosis when an adequate protein intake is secured. The photographs of biopsy material are of varying quality.

Krankheiten der Neugeborenen. Edited by ALBRECHT PEIPER. (Pp. ix +131; illustrated. DM. 19.40.) Leipzig: Georg Thieme. 1958.

Neonatal Paediatrics. Edited by W. R. F. COLLIS. (Pp. xiii+301; 35 figures. 30s.). London: W. Heinemann. 1958.

Here are two books on the care of the newborn from abroad: the first in German from Leipzig, and the second in English from Dublin. And they serve to remind one that traditions and customs play a large part in life, and what may be taken for granted in one place may seem very odd from another; also that different conditions of life often account for big differences in outlook.

Professor Peiper's book with 12 contributors is a rather brief straightforward textbook addressed, one would say, to aspiring paediatricians and senior students taking higher examinations. The quality of the contribution varies from excellent to very moderate indeed, and in some chapters there is a strong impression that the author is writing from the literature rather than from personal experience. Indeed, reference, and deference, to authors and publications are freely dispersed throughout the text. There are, however, good chapters on the general care of the newborn and also on staphylococcal infections, both by Dr. Hans-Christoph Hempel, on respiratory physiology and disturbances by Dr. Harald Thomas, and a particularly interesting chapter by Dr. Anne Marie Stieve on the neonatal manifestations of Listeriosis, an acute and subacute widely disseminated septicaemic condition giving rise to widespread granuloma-like lesions. The condition is due to a diphtheria-like organism now named *listeria monocytogenes*, and only very occasional cases have been reported outside Germany, including a few in this country, though there appears to have been a comparatively widespread outbreak in Leipzig, Halle, and one or two other neighbouring towns. The organism is endemic in some animals and occurs in adults, and it might well be that cases are occurring in this country and passing unrecognized.

The Irish book, with 20 of the 27 contributors coming from Dublin, has a parochial outlook of which even the authors seem to be aware. The editor in his preface, for instance, says to his prospective readers that he is 'aware that some of the methods advocated here are not universally accepted . . . but we think this better than trying to reach an agreed mean', and in another chapter almost apologizes for the exceedingly original and excellent idea of establishing a centre for the treatment of pyloric stenosis in a maternity hospital. In yet another chapter Dr. Collis says 'We do not presume to teach or even advise our colleagues who no doubt have evolved their own drill'; or again, on a chapter devoted to the prevention of tuberculosis (Dr. Dunlevy), 'We would particularly not wish to give advice, say, to the Tuberculosis Medical Officers of a large English city . . .'. This deprecating tone might be becoming if this were a better book. But though a few of the chapters, on the care of the premature, for instance, by Dr. Collis and Dr. Moran, and on respiratory conditions by Dr. Brian McNicholl, and on vomiting, also by Dr. Collis, are good, the book, on the whole, is disappointing. It suffers from too many authors, many of them specialists in their own field but not apparently in neonatal practice, and in these chapters conditions are constantly being discussed which have little relevance to the neonatal situation. The chapter on the heart, for instance, contains Paul Wood's classification of congenital heart disease based on 900 cases, many of them adults, but only a few scrappy lines on cardiac failure, and nothing at all on how to manage an infant with severe cyanosis, anoxic attacks, impending or overt heart failure. Again, do molluscum contagiosum, urticaria pigmentosa (illustrated by the back view of a child well on in the toddler stage), or even infantile eczema, really occur in Dublin neonates? Chapter 14 gives adequate accounts of haemolytic disease and haemorrhagic disease of the newborn, but fails to discuss the basic considerations regarding red cell and haemoglobin formation in the foetus, about which so much of such interest has been published recently, and so is able to state that the anaemia of prematurity is caused by damage to blood forming organs consequent on infection, impaired liver function and 'the general state of immaturity of all blood forming tissue . . .'. The chapter on water-electrolyte metabolism does little to clarify a very difficult subject, defines milli-equivalent as 'the amount of acid or base which the ion is capable of neutralising', and prints a table (p. 54) of instructions in which '85 per cent. saline intravenously or subcutaneously' and '0·2 per cent. glucose in 0·45 per cent. saline' are advised for the treatment of salt loss; misprints, obviously, but not conducive to helping a puzzled student.

There is ample room for a good book on neonatal paediatrics, but what surely is needed is that each subject should be approached with the realization that most of the conditions will be specific for this age group, and all will need to be approached specifically from a strong, well informed, not only paediatric, but neonatal point of view.

In contrast, however, there is one gem in this collection of very semiprecious stones. Dr. McCance and Miss Widdowson have written a brief chapter on renal function in the newborn in lucid, simple and economical English. These two authors have illuminated an exceedingly difficult and still unclear subject and for this chapter only the book is perhaps worth the 30s. that it costs in this country.

Paediatrics for the Practitioner—Supplement, 1958. Edited by WILFRID GAISFORD and REGINALD LIGHTWOOD. (Pp. v+146; illustrated. 35s.). London: Butterworth. 1958.

The supplement for 1958 to this by now well-known textbook of children's diseases contains original articles on chemotherapy, behaviour disorders, urology, chromatography in clinical paediatrics and encephalography. There are also 33 pages of Noter-up, a section containing material which corrects, amplifies and expands the earlier volumes of text. The high standard set by previous contributors is well maintained and the small volume is delightfully produced.

Tetanie. By HANS JESSERER. (Pp. xii+191; 46 figures. DM 29.70.) Stuttgart: Georg Thieme. 1958.

This is another in the series of monographs published by Georg Thieme, Stuttgart, and it maintains the standard commonly expected of their publications. The study is based on experience gained from 680 cases of tetany seen in the first medical and paediatric clinics of the university over a period of 12 years in postwar Vienna. It suggests an extraordinarily high incidence of the disease, even for Vienna which had earned the epithet 'tetany city' many years ago.

Unfortunately the author omits a statistical analysis of his material which might have provided a great deal of interesting information, in particular for the paediatrician. The rachitogenic form still ranks high in his account of tetany in childhood although Dr. Jesserer admits that it has lost somewhat in numerical significance. This is surprising as rickets and this type of tetany have practically disappeared in this country.

The classification of the tetany syndrome of the adult is also applied to the child with only minor variations. In the hypocalcaemic group are included the rachitogenic, enterogenous and hypoparathyroid forms as well as tetany complicating renal disease and following the administration of cation exchange resins. In the normocalcaemic groups are listed idiopathic tetany, tetany resulting from organic brain lesions, hyperventilation, infections, poisonings and loss of chloride ions due to excessive vomiting.

A short chapter deals with tetany in the neonatal period.

Dr. Jesserer insists on limiting the term tetany to conditions presenting at one time or another the characteristic tetanic spasms as an expression of the increased neuromuscular irritability, and he separates an 'idiopathic' tetany from the symptomatic variations. Idiopathic tetany occurs in young adults or adolescents; the blood calcium is within normal range, and its pathogenesis is attributed to increased irritability of cerebral centres.

Reading of the book is made a little cumbersome through the interpolation of large numbers of case records, some of purely historical interest and taken from the earlier literature on the subject. Only a quarter of the book is devoted to tetany in the young—understandably, as the author is a physician with limited paediatric interests.

On the whole this is a good review of the subject and over 600 references provide the background.

Advances in Pediatrics, Vol. 10. Edited by S. Z. Levine and five Associated Editors. (Pp. 362; illustrated. 67s.) Chicago: Year Book Publishers. Distributed in Great Britain by Interscience Publishers, London. 1958.

The tenth volume of this series is perhaps topical in that two of the seven articles deal with psychological principles in paediatric practice and convulsive disorders in infants and children. Dr. Sabin's review of the prevention of poliomyelitis by vaccination epitomises the problems and progress made in this subject but contains little for the up-to-date paediatrician. Papers on the treatment of tuberculosis, staphylococcal infections in nurseries and muscular disorders of childhood follow the usual lines, and there is a short but valuable section on the transfer of antibodies from mother to child from Vahlquist.

This annual, or nearly annual, collection of review articles by leading authorities serves a useful purpose in ensuring that the children's doctor short of reading time can, with the minimum of study, keep himself aware of what and where the growing edge of paediatrics is, while the references following each paper enable him to look up in the original publications any points on which he needs further information.

Many of the juicier subjects have already been dealt with in earlier volumes, and perhaps the time is nearing when some form of 'Noter-up' such as is produced by Gaisford and Lightwood for *Paediatrics for the Practitioner* will be desirable for *Advances in Pediatrics*. A growing point in paediatrics does not cease growth merely because a topical review article has been written about it, and the editor of *Advances in Pediatrics* must certainly be wondering when, in the light of very recent advances, he will have to commission articles on subjects already discussed in earlier volumes of the series.

PAEDIATRIC PATHOLOGY CLUB

Proceedings of the Fourth Annual Meeting

The fourth meeting of the Paediatric Pathology Club was held in the Ciba Foundation, London, on November 14 and 15, 1958. Forty members and guests attended.

Dinner was taken at the Royal Society of Medicine, when a gift was presented to Dr. W. W. Payne on his retirement.

The general topic for discussion at the meeting was Neonatal Liver Disease, on which the principal speakers were Dr. W. W. Payne, Dr. G. R. Newns, Dr. M. Bodian, Dr. J. A. Dudgeon, and Sir Roy Cameron.

The following papers were presented:

Summaries of Original Papers

N. J. Brown (Bristol). 'Neonatal Hepatitis in Twins.' Identical twins were born at 37 weeks' gestation. The mother gave no history of illness during pregnancy; she had never been jaundiced or had a blood transfusion. Her blood group was A Rh positive and Kahn test was negative. There were two previous healthy children.

Twin 1 was well until the tenth day when he became deeply jaundiced with pale stools, slight diarrhoea and mild pyrexia. The jaundice cleared after four months but the liver and spleen gradually enlarged and there was, over the next six years, progressive increase of liver damage as judged by liver function tests. Spider naevi and oesophageal varices developed and he died aged 7. Necropsy showed death to be due to haemorrhage from oesophageal varices. The liver showed a severe cirrhosis with coarse irregular scarring. Microscopically there was marked fibrosis with an apparent increase in small bile ducts and round cell infiltration in the portal areas.

Twin 2 was born in white asphyxia and his condition was poor throughout. He died on the second day and was not jaundiced. Necropsy (performed by Dr. R. Aidin) revealed two small tentorial tears and extensive atelectasis. The liver was yellowish green in colour and the gall bladder contained clear mucoid fluid. The bile ducts were normal. Microscopically the liver cells showed marked vacuolation and some loss of outline. 'Bile thrombi' were present in the canaliculi but the bile ducts were not dilated. There was a moderate amount of erythropoietic activity. There was slight but definite fibrosis and some inflammatory exudate of round cells and occasional polymorphs in the portal tracts.

It is reasonable to suppose that these uniovular twins both suffered from some form of hepatitis in the neonatal period, and, by virtue of the fact that Twin 2 died from unrelated causes, we were afforded the opportunity of studying the same disease at two different stages.

H. B. Salt and O. H. Wolff (Birmingham). 'Serum Lipoprotein Electrophoresis Patterns in Neonatal Liver Disease.' Serum lipoproteins were separated electrophoretically into three fractions, designated omega, beta and alpha, and the bound lipids evaluated quantitatively. The lipoprotein lipid patterns and their graphical representations were shown for the normal infant and the various types of neonatal jaundice.

In haemolytic disease of the newborn the alpha-lipro-protein lipid tends to be low; this depletion is relieved immediately after exchange transfusion, but reappears. It has been observed even three weeks later, at which time the beta-lipoprotein was greatly increased. In severe physiological jaundice, alpha-lipoprotein was not depleted, though some diminution of beta-lipoprotein was evident.

In biliary atresia beta-lipoprotein was greatly increased and alpha-lipoprotein somewhat depleted. Later, when biliary cirrhosis had developed, beta-lipoprotein was lower and alpha-lipoprotein much depleted. The development of an 'omega-beta plateau' appeared to be further evidence of biliary cirrhosis (? presence of an abnormal lipoprotein component).

In neonatal hepatitis in the early stages, beta-lipoprotein was elevated (though typically not so greatly as in biliary atresia) and alpha-lipoprotein greatly diminished. With good progress the patterns became more normal, but if cirrhosis developed both beta- and alpha-lipoproteins became depleted, and the omega-fraction vanished.

In a case of haemolytic anaemia of unknown aetiology, uncomplicated by liver damage, alpha-lipoprotein was normal and beta-lipoprotein was depleted. Apart from physiological jaundice, this is the only type of jaundice in which alpha-lipoprotein was not decreased. Later, when the infant was no longer jaundiced the pattern was quite normal.

The significance of these findings was discussed in relation to lipid metabolism in neonatal liver disease. Electrophoretic lipoprotein-lipid patterns may be a useful guide in the differentiation of biliary atresia and neonatal hepatitis, but cannot be claimed to be sufficiently specific to provide results of diagnostic certainty.

R. H. Wilkinson (London). 'Liver Function Tests in the Newborn.' The examination of faeces and urine for pigments is helpful but the examination of serum for alkaline phosphatase, turbidities, and protein fractions is not so helpful in testing liver function in the newborn child. Enzymic studies on glucuronide conjugation show these are sensitive indicators of liver function. The work of Kove, Goldstein and Wroblewski (1958) on serum glutamic oxalacetic and serum glutamic pyruvic transaminases was described to show how enzymatic tests of liver function may be helpful.

Kove, S., Goldstein, S. and Wroblewski, F. (1958). *J. Amer. med. Ass.*, **168**, No. 7, 860.

T. E. PARRY (Cardiff). 'Amino-aciduria in Liver Disease.' Urines from five children suffering from severe liver disease were examined for amino acids by paper chromatography. The cases consisted of (*a*) a boy aged 7 years and two girls age 11 years and 12½ years who died from cirrhosis of the liver, (*b*) a girl, age 13 years who died in hepatic coma due to acute hepatic necrosis, and (*c*) a girl of 16 years who recovered from a severe attack of infective hepatitis.

All cases showed a generalised amino-aciduria which was slight when the urine was examined six months before death but heavy during the terminal illness. The heaviest amino-aciduria was encountered in two specimens, one from cirrhosis and one from acute hepatic necrosis, collected from the bladder at autopsy following death in hepatic coma. An amino-aciduria of considerable severity was encountered in the case of infective hepatitis at the height of the illness when mental symptoms (mainly drowsiness) predominated; this gradually diminished and the fourth specimen, collected three weeks later, yielded a normal chromatogram.

The amino acids encountered in diminishing order of concentration were: glycine, serine, threonine, alanine, glutamine, lysine, glutamic acid, cysteic acid, valine, ethanolaninc, tyrosine and aspartic acid. The hydroxy-amino acids threonine and serine produced particularly prominent spots during the terminal coma, whereas tyrosine produced only faint spots. The heavy amino-aciduria at the height of the hepatic coma in these cases supports the view that changes in the amino acid pattern of body fluids may be an important factor in the pathogenesis of hepatic coma.

J. A. DUDGEON (London). 'Virus Aspects of Hepatic Disease in Infancy.' Various methods for establishing the aetiology of viral disease were briefly discussed. Emphasis was laid on the need to establish a clear-cut causal relationship between viral agents isolated from body tissues or secretions and the underlying pathological process, in both natural and experimental infections. Some method of handling a virus in the laboratory, either in animals or in tissue culture, was an essential pre-requisite for all such work, in particular for immunological studies. Against this background, a number of viruses were considered that were capable of causing hepatic disease in infancy and early childhood: virus A (IH or infective hepatitis); virus B (SH or serum hepatitis); herpes simplex; cytomegalic inclusion disease or salivary gland viruses and Coxsackie virus B.

Hepatitis in adults could be caused by either virus A or B, which had similar but not identical properties. Less was known about the pathology of these two infections in infancy. Virus A was known to be responsible for mild hepatitis, usually non-icteric, in infancy and early childhood, but cases were uncommon before 6 to 9 months of age. Even less information was available as to the role they played in neonatal hepatitis. Both virus A and virus B could be regarded as potential aetiological agents after transplacental infection; virus B seemed to be the more likely, in view of the prolonged viraemia known to occur. However, causal relationship could only be established when these viruses could be handled in the laboratory. Some aspects of recent work on laboratory transmission in chimpanzees and in tissue culture were discussed.

Herpes simplex has recently been recognized as a cause of neonatal hepatitis. A review was made of cases of disseminated herpes with a fulminating infection and widespread visceral lesions, together with the pattern of herpes simplex infection at this age and its relation to prematurity. Laboratory studies pointed to a close causal relationship between virus and disease.

Interest in the relationship between cytomegalic inclusion disease and hepatitis has been aroused by recent studies on this virus (salivary gland virus) in tissue culture. In Boston, strains of virus have been isolated in human skin tissue culture from liver biopsy material in which multinucleate cells were present and also from one case of 'neonatal hepatitis' in which no cytomegalic cells could be found in the liver. More evidence is required before causal relationship can be established.

Evidence of hepatitis has been obtained in two recent series of cases of infantile myocarditis due to Coxsackie virus B. This virus should also be considered when investigating cases of viral hepatitis.

N. E. FRANCE (London). 'Lung Changes in Cystic Fibrosis of the Pancreas.' The lungs in six cases of cystic fibrosis of the pancreas aged between 15 months and 8 years were examined by serial sections of large slices of lung about 1·5 cm. thick in an attempt to correlate the pathological and radiological findings. In contrast to children under 3 months of age where mucus plugs in the bronchi were the only lesions suggestive of cystic fibrosis of the pancreas, these older children showed a number of characteristic changes.

The earliest lesion appeared to be a thickening of the bronchial and bronchiolar walls by a chronic inflammatory exudate into the peribronchial tissues, later involving the adjacent alveoli which became collapsed and showed an epithelial lining. Extensive longstanding segmental collapse was infrequent. Upon these slowly progressive lesions were superimposed a number of changes of infective nature, several of which were associated in individual cases. These included inflammation and destruction of the bronchial mucosa, the occurrence of numerous small abscesses in the peribronchial tissue frequently rupturing into bronchi, and multiple peripheral abscesses especially in the subpleural regions ultimately draining into bronchioles. These lesions were associated with progressive dilatation of bronchi and bronchioles and the formation of old abscess cavities containing air and lined by fibrous tissue with little evidence of inflammation; many of the latter were surrounded by small emphysematous bullae.

K. RHANEY (Dundee). 'Enterogenous Cysts and Congenital Diverticula of the Alimentary Canal.' Enterogenous cysts and congenital diverticula of the alimentary canal are known to be frequently associated with congenital defects of the vertebral bodies. The vertebral lesions are best studied radiologically and appear to be due to defective fusion of the sclerotomes around the notochord, giving rise to hemivertebrae and the various forms of anterior spina bifida. Not uncommonly there is also evidence of abnormal segmentation of the sclerotomes.

In Case 1* an enterogenous cyst in the posterior mediastinum traversed the diaphragm, having probably arisen from the duodenum. It was accompanied by defects of bony fusion and of segmentation in the bodies of the cervico-dorsal vertebrae.

In Case 2 a diverticulum extended from the distal end of a short oesophagus through a hole in the cartilaginous plate bridging an anterior spina bifida and was attached to an abnormal spinal cord in the cervical region.

In Case 3 a neurenteric connexion was found in an anencephalic foetus with rachischisis of the neuro-spinal axis and widely divergent hemivertebrae. A diverticulum extended from the distal end of a short oesophagus through a hole between the cervico-dorsal vertebrae and was apparently connected to the neural tissue in the cervical region.

In Case 4 an enterogenous cyst lay within the cervical spinal cord of a newborn infant. The cyst was lined with gastric mucosa and had perforated, causing an abscess and acute meningitis. This infant, like the other three, had an abnormally short neck, presumably caused by defective formation of the vertebral bodies. The development of an enterogenous cyst within the spinal cord is probably due to protrusion of endoderm into the neuro-ectoderm where it subsequently becomes detached from the developing gut when the vertebral bodies develop around the notochordal rod.

JAMES B. AREY and ANGELO DIGEORGE (Philadelphia). 'Gonadal Dysgenesis in Infants and Children.' The present report concerns the morphological alterations in the gonads of nine patients with gonadal dysgenesis. Their ages varied from 2 days to 7 years; only one was more than 12 months of age when the diagnosis was established.

Three infants in whom the diagnosis was established by biopsy of the gonads are still living. Although there was some doubt as to the phenotypic sex of each of these three infants, all of them were genotypic males. A small urogenital sinus, a uterus and a unilateral fallopian tube were present in each of these three infants, and an abnormal gonad was demonstrable on the side on which the fallopian tube was present; a relatively normal testis was present on the opposite side. Histological sections of the affected gonad in each instance revealed scattered cords of cells suggesting primitive testicular tubules. Sections of the opposite (unaffected) gonad revealed normal testis.

* Cases 1, 2 and 4 are reported in detail in *J. Path. Bact.* (in press)

In addition, six patients with gonadal dysgenesis died, four as a result of other congenital malformations. All six were phenotypic females and each had a normal-appearing uterus and fallopian tubes. Two of the six were genetic males, two were females, and in two the histologic preparations were unsatisfactory for the determination of the genetic sex. The small size of both gonads was obvious macroscopically in the infant aged 3 months and in the older child, but was not recognized in the younger infants. Histological sections revealed a similar pattern in both gonads of any single patient in this group. In three patients the structure was recognisable in at least some areas as ovarian in nature, although the number of primordial ova was greatly diminished as compared with normal ovaries from infants and children of comparable ages; in a girl 7 years old only nine ova were identified in over 200 sections of ovary. In the other three infants in this group the gonads consisted of small cords of cells suggesting primitive testicular tubules.

The morphological alterations obviously vary in different patients with gonadal dysgenesis. In the present series the changes consist of bilateral ovarian hypoplasia, bilateral testicular dysgenesis and unilateral testicular dysgenesis. The diagnosis of gonadal dysgenesis should be suspected in any phenotypic female with severe congenital malformations, but the alterations in the affected gonads may not be apparent macroscopically in young infants.

G. S. ANDERSON (Newcastle). 'Congenital Goitre due to Potassium Chlorate.' Amongst 31 women, all having a history of repeated abortion and then treated during a further pregnancy with potassium chlorate, seven produced infants with a congenital goitre. Five of the 31 pregnancies resulted in stillbirths of which two showed a goitre, whilst of 26 liveborn infants five showed a goitre. In the three goitrous infants who survived, the neck swelling subsided within a few weeks and the children have made normal progress. On one child radioactive iodine studies carried out shortly after birth revealed a hypothyroid state.

Satisfactory histology of the thyroid was obtained from the two liveborn goitrous infants. One died at 16 hours with a thyroid weighing 18 g. The other died at 4 days and the thyroid weighed 23·5 g. These thyroids showed different histological patterns: one had a relatively normal histological appearance whilst the other showed epithelial hyperplasia but of a type having little resemblance to that seen in adult thyroid disease.

The relatively large number of congenital goitres from a small group of women (who previously had not, apparently, produced a goitrous infant) coupled with the close chemical formula of potassium chlorate to potassium perchlorate (a known anti-thyroid drug) suggests that the chlorate ion has an anti-thyroid effect.

J. HART-MERCER (Newcastle). 'Sudden Death in an Asthmatic Boy on Prednisone Therapy, associated with a General Arteriolar Disease.' Attention was drawn to the unexpected histological finding of widespread arteriolar damage in a boy of 7 years whose uncomplicated but incapacitating bronchial asthma had responded satisfactorily to Prednisone therapy. The steroid had mostly been given at a maintenance dosage of 5 mg. daily but over rather long periods, totalling over 12 months. He had been very well; but he was taken ill suddenly with vomiting, headache and convulsions, and died in a few hours.

Autopsy showed few gross changes beyond pulmonary and cerebral oedema, moderate hepatomegaly and adrenal cortical atrophy, and death was attributed to acute adrenal insufficiency due to the indirectly suppressive action of Prednisone.

Many focal arteriolar lesions were found in liver and spleen. The affected arterioles were mostly of small calibre and showed nodular hyaline eosinophilic intimal thickenings with displacement and narrowing of the lumen. Frozen sections showed considerable sudanophil and doubly refractile lipid in these intimal plaques as well as in the Küpffer cells of the hepatic sinusoids. There was no fibrinoid necrosis or arteriolitis and no focal change in the related tissue parenchyma. Further scanty arteriolar lesions were found in the heart (210 g.) and periadrenal tissue.

SIR ROY CAMERON. 'Experimental Evidence of Reversibility of Liver Disease.'

G. R. OSBORN (Derby). 'Giant Cell Hepatitis in a Family of 16.'

M. BODIAN (London). 'Histopathology of Liver Disease in Infancy.'

F. A. LANGLEY (Manchester). 'Thymic Hyperplasia following B.C.G. Vaccination.'

The next meeting of the Club will be held at Bristol, on October 23 and 24, 1959.

EDITORIAL NOTE

The Editorial Board of the *Archives of Disease in Childhood* feel that the method of citing references without titles is uninformative.

Authors are, therefore, asked in future to include the title of the article cited when compiling a list of references.

BRONCHIECTASIS IN CHILDREN: ITS MULTIPLE CLINICAL AND PATHOLOGICAL ASPECTS

BY

HOWARD WILLIAMS and R. N. O'REILLY

From the Clinical Research Unit, Royal Children's Hospital, Melbourne

(RECEIVED FOR PUBLICATION DECEMBER 12, 1958)

There has been considerable controversy concerning the aetiology, pathology and pathogenesis of bronchiectasis ever since Laennec's original description in 1819. The two principal and most widely accepted theories of pathogenesis have been first, that the disease was primarily due to bronchial damage from infection, the weakened bronchi then dilating, and second, that pulmonary collapse was the primary cause, bronchial dilatation initially being due mainly to secondary mechanical factors. Pathological studies have revealed a wide variety of lesions. In some the essential structure of the bronchi and bronchioles was completely destroyed by infection, in others the component parts of the bronchial wall were normal. Collapse of the affected lobes or segments was a feature in some, but not in others. Interstitial inflammation of the adjacent lung could be either pronounced or absent. Clinical studies have also revealed great diversity of features in different patients. The mode of onset may vary from an insidious onset with bronchitis in infancy to an acute onset with either severe pneumonia or pulmonary collapse. Some patients have no symptoms and live a normal life, others have much cough and sputum and die early from pulmonary suppuration. Some have chronic sinus infection and wax keratosis, others never show these features.

What is the explanation of this diversity of clinical and pathological features, and theories of pathogenesis? Two explanations are possible: first, there are all grades of severity of a disease entity which may be caused by a variety of infections, and second, there are a number of separate diseases each with a different pathology and clinical pattern but all with the one common gross morphological feature of bronchial dilatation. This problem has been considerably elucidated in recent years by detailed clinical and pathological studies. It is now well known that primary pulmonary tuberculosis (Kent, 1942; Jones, Peck and Willis, 1946; Veeneklaas, 1952; and Williams and Anderson, 1953) and fibrocystic disease of the pancreas (Zuelzer and Newton, 1949; Bodian, 1952; Sant' Agnese, 1955) give rise to bronchiectasis, and that both diseases have distinctive pathological and clinical features. Whitwell (1952) in a morbid anatomical study of bronchiectatic lobes resected surgically described three separate pathological entities, atelectatic, saccular and follicular bronchiectasis and indicated that there were distinctive clinical features in each group. He was unable to classify a considerable proportion of his material.

In a study of the development of bronchiectatic lesions in a wide variety of patients, we have been able to classify them into a number of definite groups according to their primary pathology. In a series of 650 patients with bronchiectatic lesions we have studied 241 of them from the inception of the disease process and followed them for periods of four to 10 years. The following classification is submitted but it is proposed to give details of the first two groups only, those with subacute pyogenic collapse and those with non-specific infective bronchiolitis and interstitial pneumonia, as the pathology and clinical features of the other groups are better known and understood.

(1) Sub-acute pyogenic pulmonary collapse ..	37
(2) Non-specific infective bronchiolitis and/or interstitial pneumonia	57
(3) Fibrocystic disease of the pancreas ..	56
(4) Primary pulmonary tuberculosis	53
(5) Congenital malformations of the bronchial tree	16
(6) Miscellaneous lung infections	22
Total ..	241

Subacute Pyogenic Pulmonary Collapse

Permanent and Reversible Bronchiectatic Changes. The common association of bronchiectasis and collapse both clinically and pathologically in humans, and experimentally in animals led to the assumption that pulmonary collapse was the major factor causing bronchiectasis. Warner and Graham (1933), Anspach (1934). Lee Lander and Davidson (1938), Fleischner (1940), Brennemann (1943), Lee Lander (1946) and Coope (1948) have all expressed this view. It has been also demonstrated that bronchial dilatation in a collapsed lobe may disappear if the lobe re-expands, by Findlay (1935), Jennings (1937), Lee Lander (1946) and Field (1949).

Material and Methods. Subacute pyogenic pulmonary collapse has been arbitrarily defined as a pyogenically infected collapsed lobe or segment which has been collapsed between six weeks and one year. After one year it was considered to be chronic. Collapse associated with fibrocystic disease of the pancreas or tuberculous glands was excluded in these patients. Of the 37 children in the group, non-specific respiratory infection was the cause of collapse in 16, pertussis in 11, measles in two, allergic bronchitis in four, foreign body in two and post-operative causes in two. All the patients were studied clinically, special note being made of previous general health and respiratory disease. The follow-up period has varied from four to 10 years. Special methods of study were serial antero-posterior and lateral chest radiographs, bronchoscopy and bronchogram. The sputum was cultured for pathogenic organisms using standard 6% horse blood agar plates with a meat infusion broth base. Special techniques for culture of *Haemophilus influenzae* were not used routinely.

Age, Sex Incidence, Predisposing Factors. All different age groups were represented, four children being under 2 years, 20 between 2 and 6 years and 13 between 6 and 14 years. Eighteen of these were boys and 19 girls. All except five children had been in previous good health. Four of the five had previous manifestations of an allergic diathesis, while the fifth had suffered from recurrent respiratory infections. An uncle of one patient had bronchiectasis.

Onset and Symptoms. In all patients the onset of the illness was a clearly defined episode with either acute respiratory infection, pertussis, morbilli, an attack of allergic bronchitis, a post-operative complication or inhalation of a foreign body. The two outstanding clinical features were, first, persistent cough following the initial respiratory infection, and second, constitutional symptoms of ill health. There were no characteristic features about the cough, although some parents described it as 'chesty' or as if 'phlegm were present', but no child spontaneously expectorated sputum. The constitutional symptoms were those common to any low grade infection, namely pallor, languor, poor appetite, loss of weight and often continuous or intermittent low grade fever.

Clinical Signs. The patients did not look well, their muscle tone and posture was poor and all except three had lost weight. Three had upper respiratory tract infection. Physical signs in the chest were localized to the affected lobe or lobes and usually minimal. Diminished air entry and crepitations were characteristic of the majority, but tubular breathing was heard in four. Postural coughing over the examiner's knee (Fig. 1) and urging the child to 'cough and spit it up' was frequently successful in demonstrating the presence of mucopus in the bronchial tree.

Radiological signs of lobar collapse were un-

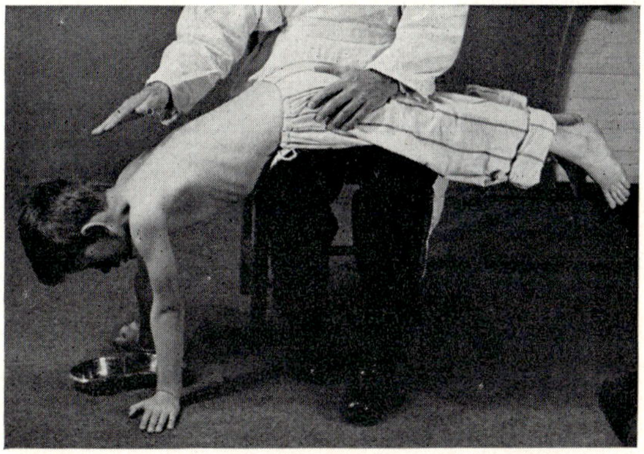

FIG. 1.—Showing method of posturing child to obtain sputum.

TABLE 1
LOBAR DISTRIBUTION

Unilateral					Bilateral				
RML	RLL	RML and RLL	LLL	LLL and Lingula	RML RLL LLL	RLL, LLL Lingula	RLL and Lingula	RUL LLL	RML and LLL
1	5	10	8	3	2	2	4	1	1

equivocally demonstrated in all patients, the lesion being unilateral in 27 and bilateral in 10. The right lung was involved alone in 16, the left alone in 11. Table 1 gives details of the lobar distribution.

Bacteriology. The sputum of 34 of the 37 patients was cultured. Table 2 gives the results.

TABLE 2

BACTERIOLOGY OF SPUTUM OF 34 PATIENTS WITH SUBACUTE PYOGENIC COLLAPSE

Staphylococcus aureus	6
Staphylococcus aureus and *Streptococcus pneumoniae*	2
Staphylococcus aureus and *β. haemolytic Streptococcus*	1
β. haemolytic Streptococcus	4
Streptococcus pneumoniae	2
Streptococcus pneumoniae and *β. haemolytic Streptococcus*	1
Haemophilus influenzae	2
No pathogens isolated	16
Total	34

Bronchoscopy and Bronchogram. At bronchoscopic examination all patients had mucopus in the affected lobar bronchus but the bronchial lumen was not occluded by either mucous plug, mucosal swelling or glandular pressure. In 28 patients the affected lobar branches showed mild inflammatory changes, in three a red granular appearance, and in six it was normal. After the mucopus was aspirated by sucker, more was expelled from the peripheral part of the bronchial tree when the patient was made to cough by lightening the anaesthesia.

Radio-opaque oil instilled into the bronchial tree demonstrated dilated crowded bronchi. The dilatation affected the middle divisions of the bronchial tree, and was saccular in seven and cylindrical in 30. The smaller bronchi and bronchioles were not demonstrated as oil failed to enter these structures (see Cases 1, 2, 3).

Treatment. Two principles of treatment were followed in these patients. The first was chemotherapy to promote resolution of the infection, the second postural coughing and physiotherapy to clear the bronchial tree of secretions and to aid re-expansion of the collapsed lung. Chemotherapy was limited in many patients in the early part of this study to courses of one to two weeks sulphonamide or penicillin therapy, but later one of the tetracycline group of drugs was used for periods of four to six weeks. Postural coughing and physiotherapy was carried out in most patients but in children under 3 years it is extremely difficult if not impossible to get them to cough voluntarily or carry out any breathing exercises.

Course of Disease. Fig. 2 illustrates the varied course that the disease followed. In 16 patients resolution was complete, while seven were left with permanent collapse and bronchiectasis. Partial resolution occurred in 14 patients leaving varying degrees of patchy bronchiectasis and collapse. Those patients in whom complete resolution occurred were usually diagnosed early, were usually of an age when they could co-operate with physiotherapy and were usually given adequate chemotherapy. In contrast those with failed or partially failed resolution were frequently diagnosed later, were younger and treatment was not so effectively administered.

All patients with complete resolution have remained well during the average follow-up period of six years. Of the seven patients with failed resolution, three had persistent cough and sputum and were cured by lobectomy, while the remaining four became symptom free one to two years after the initial infection and have dry bronchiectasis. Ten of the 14 patients with incomplete resolution have remained symptom free and in good health, while the remaining four temporarily developed some cough and sputum following a respiratory infection. Only one of the patients developed wax keratosis.

Case Reports

Case 1: Example of Complete Resolution. S.H. was a normal healthy girl until she attended school at the age of 5 years in February, 1951. Following a series of colds she was left with persistent cough and became pale and languid and refused to eat. When examined at the age of 5½ years she was thin, pale and looked ill. There was impaired percussion note, diminished air entry and crepitations over the left lower lobe and a chest radiograph showed collapse of the left lower lobe. Postural coughing produced five or six blobs of yellow mucopus, culture of which grew *β. haemolytic Streptococci.* Bronchoscopic examination showed mucopus in the left lower lobe bronchus, the mucosa of which was slightly inflamed but the lumen was patent. A bronchogram demonstrated collapse and cylindrical bronchial dilatation of the three basic segments of the left lower lobe (Fig. 3a).

Following treatment with penicillin, physiotherapy and postural coughing, she gradually lost her cough and sputum and in eight weeks had regained her normal health and weight. Clinically and radiologically the signs of collapse of the left lower lobe cleared. Bronchoscopy and bronchogram 12 weeks later confirmed re-expansion of the lobe and demonstrated a normal bronchial tree (Fig. 3b). The child has been observed for 6 years and has remained well and symptom free.

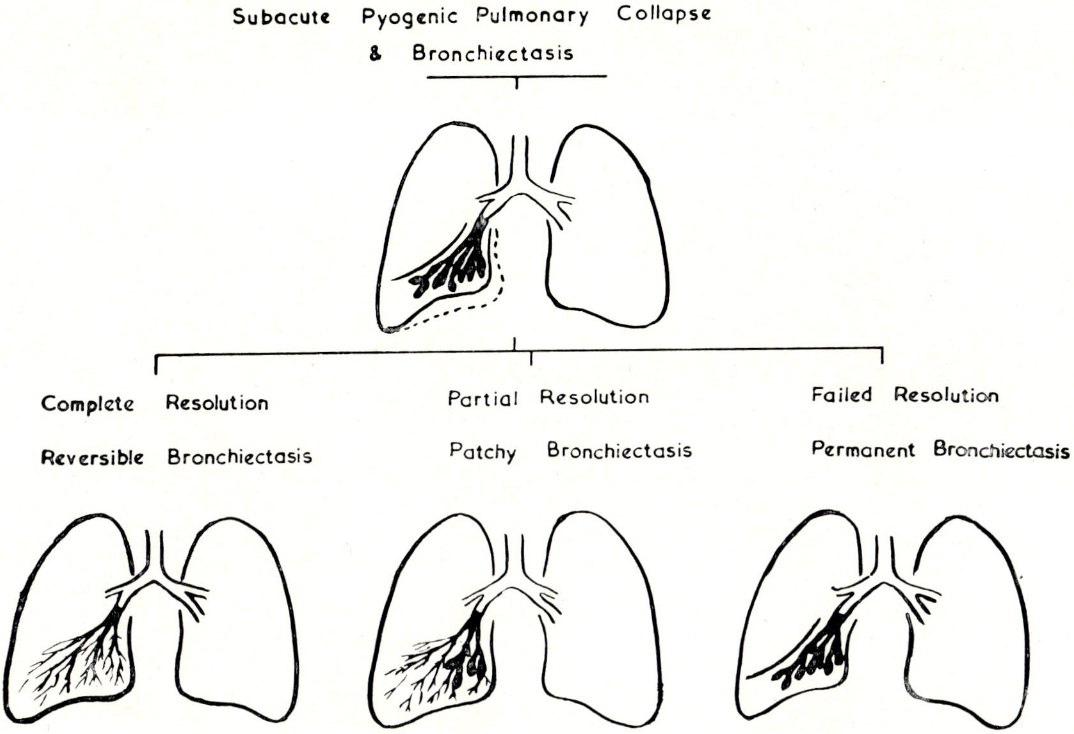

FIG. 2.—Diagrammatic representation of course of subacute pyogenic pulmonary collapse.

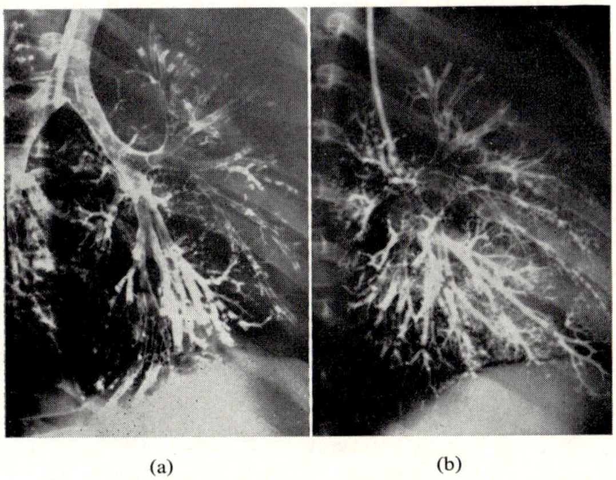

FIG. 3A.—Case 1, aged 5½ years. Showing collapse and cylindrical dilatation of three basic segments of left lower lobe following respiratory tract infection two months previously.

FIG. 3B.—Showing re-expansion of collapsed lobe and return of bronchial tree to normal. Bronchogram 12 weeks after Fig. 3A.

Case 2: Example of Incomplete Resolution. In February, 1950, M.P., a healthy boy of 6 years, developed an acute respiratory tract infection which was diagnosed as 'pneumonia' by his family doctor. Temporary improvement followed one week's sulphonamide therapy but his cough persisted and two weeks later the 'pneumonia' relapsed. Despite treatment with penicillin he remained sick and had a persistent cough. When admitted to hospital seven weeks after the original infection he appeared pale and listless and had clinical and radiological evidence of collapse of the right lower and middle lobes. Postural coughing produced blobs of yellow mucopus, culture of which failed to detect the presence of pathogenic organisms. At bronchoscopy mucopus was found in the right lower lobe bronchus but the bronchogram showed collapse, and saccular and cylindrical bronchiectasis of the right middle and lower lobes, except the axillary basic segment (Fig. 4a).

Following treatment with penicillin, physiotherapy and postural coughing, his general condition steadily improved and his cough and sputum cleared in two months. A bronchogram three months later was normal except for some slight fusiform dilatation of the more proximal bronchial divisions of the dorsal and posterior basic segments (Fig. 4b). He has been observed during the past seven years and has remained in excellent health with no cough.

Case 3: Example of Slow Incomplete Resolution. R.B., aged 2½ years, contracted a respiratory tract infection in November, 1949, for which he was given

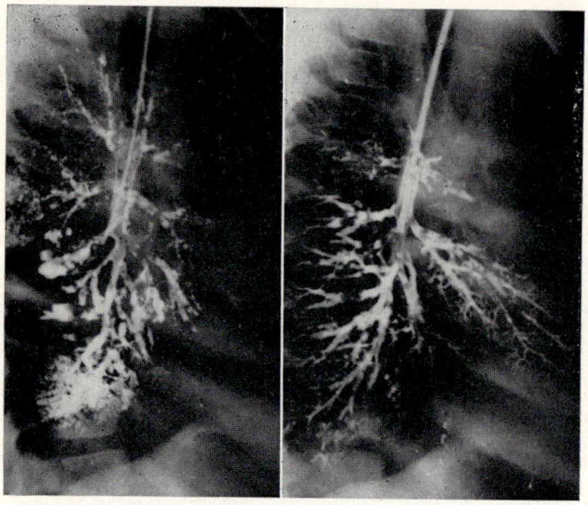

(a) (b)

FIG. 4A.—Case 2, aged 6 years. Pneumonia seven weeks previously. Showing collapse and cylindrical dilatation of right middle lobe and saccular and cylindrical dilatation of all segments of right lobe with exception of axillary basic segment.

FIG. 4B.—Bronchogram three months after Fig. 4A, showing expansion of right middle lower lobes and a little residual fusiform dilatation of bronchi of dorsal and posterior basic segments.

penicillin for six days. Following this illness the child remained listless and pale, with low grade fever and a cough. When admitted to hospital five weeks later he had both clinical and radiological evidence of collapse of the right lower and middle lobes. On postural coughing he produced blobs of sputum, culture of which failed to detect pathogenic organisms. Bronchoscopic examination showed the mucous membrane of the right bronchus to be reddened, swollen and granular in appearance and the lumen contained mucopus. A bronchogram (Fig. 5a) showed collapse with saccular and cylindrical bronchiectasis of the right lower and middle lobes.

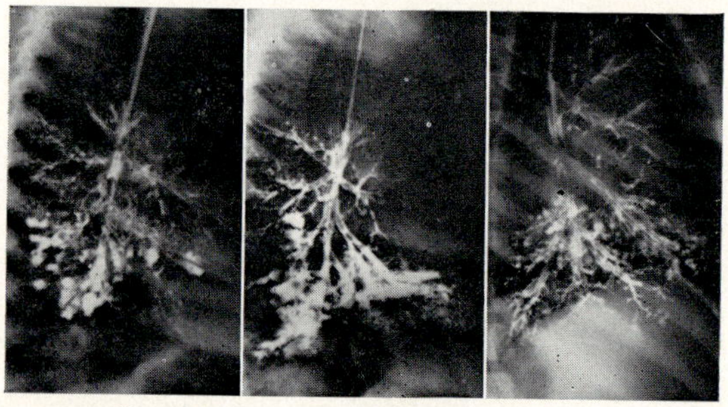

(a) (b) (c)

FIG. 5A.—Case 3, aged 2½ years. Respiratory tract infection, cough and malaise for 5½ weeks. Bronchogram showing collapse and cylindrical and saccular bronchial dilatation of right lower and middle lobes.

FIG. 5B.—Three months after Fig. 5A. Only change is slight re-expansion of right middle lobe with some alveolar filling.

FIG. 5C.—One year after Fig. 5B. Showing considerable re-expansion of right lower and middle lobes with residual fusiform dilatation of most of bronchi.

Treatment with penicillin and sulphonamide was given for only two weeks with slight improvement in his cough, but he was still not well and the right lower and middle lobes remained collapsed. He was too young to co-operate with physiotherapy and postural coughing. Bronchoscopic examination three months later showed a little mucopus in the right bronchus but the redness and oedema had cleared. A bronchogram (Fig. 5b) showed the right lobe was still collapsed and bronchiectatic but the right middle lobe had partially expanded, although bronchiectasis was still present.

The child slowly improved in general health and radiologically the opacity in the right lower and middle lobes gradually cleared. Another bronchogram one year later showed that the right lower and middle lobe had partially expanded and that patchy fusiform bronchiectasis involving the more proximal bronchial divisions was present in most segments (Fig. 5c).

During the following eight years he has gradually improved and over the past four years has been in excellent health. If he contracts a cold he may develop a little cough and sputum for one to two weeks.

Non-Specific Infective Bronchiolitis and/or Interstitial Pneumonia

Generalized, Patchy and Progressive Bronchiectatic Changes. Many workers among whom are McNeil, Macgregor and Alexander (1929), Robinson (1933), Ogilvie (1941), Churchill (1949), and Whitwell (1952) have shown that destructive mural bronchitis and bronchiolitis and interstitial pneumonia cause bronchiectasis and that pulmonary collapse is not an essential feature. In the following group of 57 patients it will be shown how chronic non-specific infective bronchiolitis and/or interstitial pneumonia may give rise to either generalized, patchy or progressive bronchiectatic changes and that pulmonary collapse, while it may occur, is not an essential pathological feature.

Material and Methods. Fifty-seven patients with bronchiectasis in whom the lesion commenced clinically as non-specific infective bronchiolitis and/or interstitial pneumonia were observed from the inception of the disease. All patients had negative Mantoux tests and none had fibrocystic disease of the pancreas. Methods of study were the same as in the patients with subacute pyogenic collapse.

Age, Sex Incidence, Predisposing Factors. Forty-nine of the 57 children were under the age of 2 years when the disease commenced; 31 were under 1 year, 18 between 1 and 2 years and five between 2 and 3 years, and only three were over the age of 3 years. Thirty-one of the patients were girls and 26 were boys.

These infants appeared to be in good health before the onset of respiratory infection. Eight of them exhibited manifestations of allergy either before or after the onset of the respiratory infection. A familial history of chronic sinus infection, chronic bronchitis and bronchiectasis was a feature of this group. Four siblings, one parent and three aunts had proven bronchiectasis of a similar pattern. A history of chronic cough with sputum suggestive of bronchiectasis or chronic bronchitis was obtained in 10 of the parents, in nine uncles or aunts, and three cousins.

Onset and Symptoms. In 42 of the 57 patients the disease commenced insidiously with a running nose and cough following either teething, a cold or bronchitis. In five it developed during pink disease. In the remaining 15 a definite illness, such as morbilli, pertussis or bronchopneumonia initiated the symptoms.

Persistent cough, continuous or intermittent nasal discharge, sudden attacks of fever, and general ill health were the dominant features in all patients. Ill health was manifested by lack of energy, fretfulness, irritability, poor appetite and slow weight gain. The cough often sounded as if secretion was present in the bronchial tree and in the more severely affected patients the breathing was often rattly and wheezy in character. Nasal discharge was often mucopurulent but at times mucoid in character. Febrile episodes, which were often mistaken for attacks of pneumonia, were very characteristic and occurred every few weeks or months. The onset was usually quite sudden and the attack would often rapidly abate after several days but in some persisted for longer.

Clinical Signs. Many of these children looked constitutionally ill, were often pale, undersized and had poor muscle tone and posture. Thoracic kyphosis, bilateral Harrison's sulcus and pot belly were frequently noted. Respiratory movement was poor and was mainly in the upper part of the thoracic cage. Mucopurulent or mucoid nasal discharge, with an obstructed nasal airway and oedematous red or pale mucous membrane was observed in most patients. Crepitations were the characteristic clinical sign, and in the severely affected patients were heard all over the chest, while in the others they were heard over a wider area than the lesions demonstrated both radiologically and bronchographically. Rhonchi were often heard in the severely affected patients. Thirty-six patients developed wax keratosis.

Bacteriology. It was difficult to obtain sputum from these infants and the only completely reliable way was by bronchoscopic aspiration. Irritation of the back of the throat by a spatula would result in coughing in some infants and if sputum was coughed into the pharynx it was aspirated. Sputum cultures were carried out in seven infants by pharyngeal aspiration and in 22 by bronchoscopic aspiration. In only one was a pathogenic organism, *Staphylococcus aureus*, cultured. However, it must be pointed out that the sputum obtained by bronchoscopic aspiration was contaminated by ether vapour and this could have been a reason for failure to culture gram negative organisms. Later these 57 children learned to expectorate mucopus and on culture the sputum in 51% grew a pathogenic organism, either β. *haemolytic Streptococcus*, *Streptococcus pneumoniae*, *haemophilus influenzae*, *Staphylococcus aureus* or *bacillus proteus*.

Radiological Signs. In many patients whose illness commenced insidiously plain radiographs were either normal or showed only a prominent broncho-vascular pattern. In some, particularly those in whom the disease followed bronchopneumonia, morbilli or pertussis, haziness or mottling was observed in either the lower lobes, right middle lobe or lingula. Lobar or segmental collapse was present in only 10 patients when first examined, but it developed in nine other patients later. The lingula and right middle lobe were the lobes most frequently affected.

Bronchoscopy and Bronchogram. Mucopus was aspirated from the affected lobar or segmental bronchi and only mild inflammatory changes were noted in the bronchi. In those severely affected the bronchiectatic lesions involved both upper and lower lobes. In those less severely affected, gravity seemed to play a part in determining the distribution of the lesions, for the dependent lobes namely the lower lobes, right middle lobes and lingula were affected. The lesions were commonly bilateral with the left side usually more affected than the right, and if the lesion was unilateral, it was usually the left side. The early bronchiectatic lesions usually affected the more peripheral part of the bronchial tree (Case 5)

Course of Disease. These patients were arbitrarily divided into three sub-groups according to the severity of the illness and the pattern of bronchiectatic changes. Fig. 6 illustrates these changes. The most severely affected had generalized bronchiectatic changes which were either fusiform, cylind-

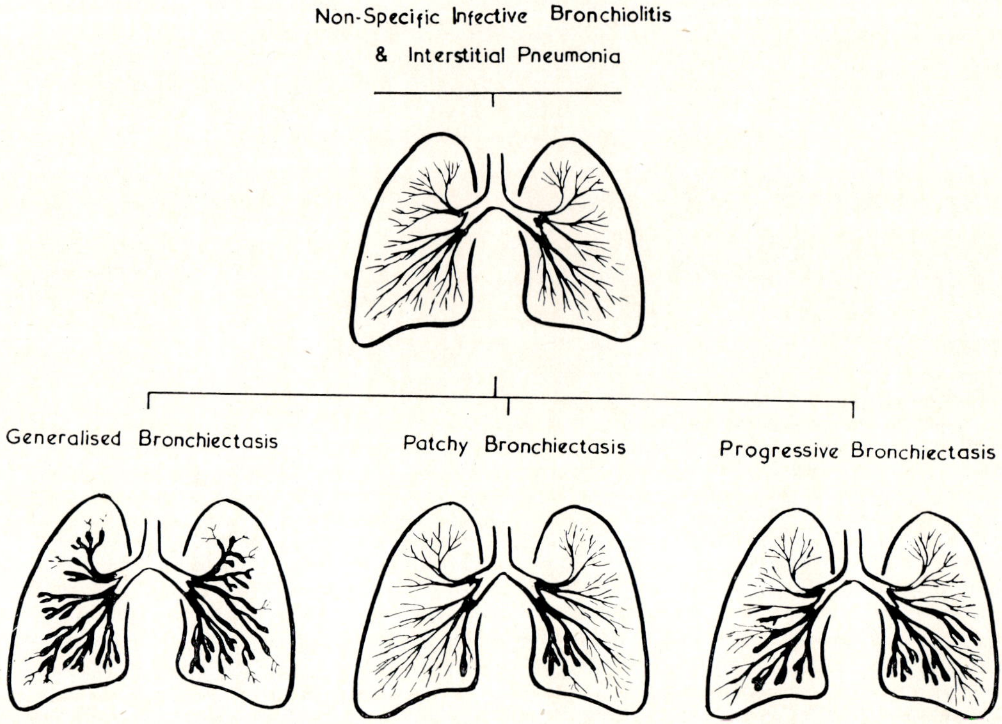

FIG. 6.—Diagrammatic representation of varied lesions that may occur in non-specific infective bronchiolitis and interstitial pneumonia.

rical or saccular in type. These children were constitutionally ill and their growth was stunted. As they grew older and could co-operate in clearing their bronchial tree of secretions, their general health improved and feverish attacks abated.

A group of 19 patients, in whom the symptoms were much less severe, had bronchiectatic changes which were either localized or patchy in distribution. In 12 the lesions were bilateral and in seven unilateral. As these patients grew older the symptoms of cough and nasal discharge ameliorated and two of them became symptomless apart from temporary cough and sputum following a respiratory infection.

In a group of 27 patients bronchiectatic changes were observed to develop in a lobe or segment previously demonstrated as normal bronchographically. Clinically this lung was affected early, as crepitations were constantly present long before bronchiectatic changes were demonstrated. It is emphasized that progression did not refer to extension of bronchiectatic changes in a segment already so affected. The most frequent pattern of development of the lesions was initial involvement of the left lower lobe and lingula and then the right middle and right lower lobes. All combinations of progressive changes have been observed in both lower lobes, lingula and right middle lobe. In 17 patients a new lobe was involved and in eight it was on the opposite side. In 10 patients a new segment was involved in an already affected lobe. Seven of the 27 patients underwent lobectomy of either one or two lobes in an attempt to remove all bronchiectatic areas. All seven patients developed bronchiectasis in another lobe, and in only two was it attributable to post-operative collapse.

Case 4: Example of Severe Generalized Type. G.L., was a normal baby of healthy parents but his maternal uncle had proven bronchiectasis. In 1954 his mother developed non-tuberculous pleurisy, and one week later at the age of 4 months he developed a cough, rattling breathing and nasal discharge, and was considered to have bronchitis. These symptoms persisted and at the age of 7 months he was found to have crepitations and inspiratory and expiratory rhonchi over the entire chest. Sputum, which was coughed into the mouth, was examined bacteriologically on two occasions but no pathogenic organisms were cultured. Prominent broncho-vascular markings with emphysema of the lung fields were seen in the plain radiographs. Bronchoscopy at the age of 10 months showed much mucopus in the bronchial tree and bronchograms showed extensive fusiform bronchiectatic changes in the entire right lung and the major part of the left lung (Fig. 7).

Empirical treatment with one of the tetracycline group of drugs in the dose of 15 mg. per kg. of body weight was given intermittently over the next four years. During the first two years his general health was not good and he had frequent feverish attacks and his breathing would often be rattly. However, for the past year his general health has been much better and he has not had more than two minor feverish attacks. This change has been due to his ability to cough and clear his bronchial tree of secretion.

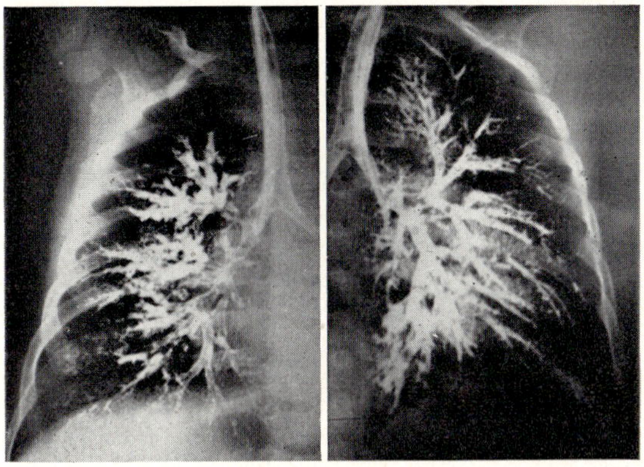

FIG. 7.—Case 4, aged 10 months. History of six months' cough, rattling breathing, feverish attacks and nasal discharge. Bronchogram showing extensive fusiform bronchiectatic changes in right lung and in left lower lobe, lingula and pectoral segments of left upper lobe.

Case 5: Example of Progressive Group. W.S. was the third child of healthy parents but a maternal uncle was considered to have bronchiectasis. When 15 months of age he developed a mild respiratory tract infection and was left with persistent cough and purulent nasal discharge. When examined in 1948, six weeks after the initial infection, he was a thin infant with purulent rhinorrhoea, slight inspiratory and expiratory wheeze and widespread fine crepitations over both lower lobes, right middle lobe and lingula. Radiological examination of his chest showed prominent hilar shadows and broncho-vascular markings in both lower lobes. The cough, nasal discharge and febrile episodes persisted. At the age of 3½ years a bronchogram revealed a normally filled bronchial tree, except for slight stumping of one small bronchus in the posterior basic segment of the left lower lobe (Fig. 8a). A further bronchogram at the age of 6½ years, however, showed patchy irregular cylindrical bronchiectasis of all segments of left lower lobe, lingula and right middle lobes and of the axillary basic segment of right lower lobe (Fig. 8b).

From the age of 6½ years to 11 years his general health slowly improved, he lost his attacks of fever and his cough and nasal discharge lessened. At this time only a few crepitations could be heard over both lower lobes after coughing and he was able to expectorate only an occasional piece of mucopus. A bronchogram at the age of 11 years showed more pronounced bronchiectatic changes in the affected areas and in addition the retro-cardiac and posterior basic segments of right lower lobe were affected.

Case 6: Example of Progressive Bronchiectasis following Surgery. M.W. was the first child of healthy parents. No familial history of bronchiectasis or other chronic respiratory illness was elicited. When aged 2 months she insidiously developed a running nose, rattling chesty cough and later suffered with frequent feverish attacks. When first seen at the age of 8 months in 1948, she was underweight, did not look well and crepitations were heard over both lower lobes and lingula. Radiological examination of the chest showed a little haziness over the left lower lobe and the broncho-vascular lung markings were rather accentuated. The symptoms, signs and radiological changes persisted and a bronchogram at 3 years of age showed patchy irregular cylindrical bronchiectasis of the three basic segments of the left lower lobe, but the lingula and entire right lung were normal. These bronchographic changes were the same at 5 years of age.

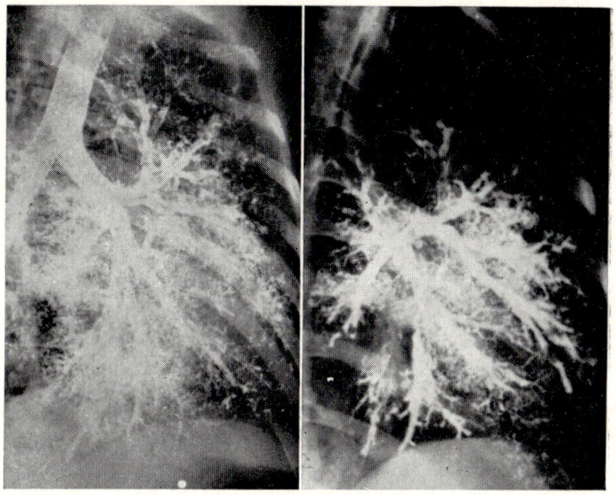

(a) (b)

FIG. 8A.—Case 5, aged 3½ years. Cough, nasal discharge and episodes of fever since age of 15 months. Bronchogram showing normal filling with exception of one small bronchus in posterior basal segment.

FIG. 8B. Aged 6½ years. Bronchogram three years after Fig. 8A. Showing patchy cylindrical lesions in all segments of left lower lobe and lingula. No collapse.

When aged 6 years a left lower lobe lobectomy was performed. No post-operative collapse occurred but the cough, nasal discharge and febrile episodes persisted unabated. One year later a further bronchogram showed well marked bronchiectatic changes in the lingula and pectoral segments of left upper lobe, the right lung being apparently normal. Owing to persistent symptoms and ill health a left upper lobectomy was carried out at the age of 7½ years. Again no benefit followed and her general health remained poor and her sputum became profuse and offensive. Steadily inflammatory changes progressed in the right lung and her general health deteriorated, death following two and a half years later at the age of 10 years. Autopsy revealed extensive bronchiectatic changes with interstitial pneumonia in all segments of the right lower lobe and right middle lobe and less marked changes in the right upper lobe.

Discussion

Comparison of the two groups of patients, those with subacute pyogenic collapse and those with non-specific infective bronchiolitis and/or interstitial pneumonia reveal considerable differences in the pathology, pathogenesis, clinical features and course of the illness. Pulmonary collapse was the constant initial basic pulmonary lesion in the former, while it was an infrequent and incidental finding in the latter group. In the collapse group, bronchial dilatation was always present initially, and as the lesions were often reversible it is improbable that the dilatation was due to bronchial damage in many patients. In the bronchiolitis and interstitial pneumonia group, bronchiectatic lesions were not always present initially but often developed as the lesion clinically progressed. Once the bronchiectatic lesions were present they remained and reversible changes were never observed. The pattern of many of these lesions was similar to that in fibrocystic disease of the pancreas, in which widespread bronchiectatic lesions often developed from an extensive suppurating bronchiolitis. In fibrocystic disease the viscid tenacious mucus is an important factor in determining the generalized nature of the lesions, whereas gravity with poorer drainage of the dependent lobes and a poor cough reflex were important factors in the latter group. The group of patients with bronchiolitis corresponds to the patients with follicular bronchiectasis reported by Whitwell (1952), who showed that destructive mural bronchitis and bronchiolitis and interstitial pneumonia was a common cause of bronchiectasis and that pulmonary collapse was not an essential feature.

Comparison of the clinical features and course of the disease in both groups is best set out in table form (Table 3). This clinical evidence strongly supports the view that these are two different respiratory tract diseases.

TABLE 3
CLINICAL FEATURES AND COURSE OF DISEASE IN TWO GROUPS

Clinical Feature	Subacute Pyogenic Collapse	Non-Specific Infective Bronchiolitis and Interstitial Pneumonia
Age incidence	Occurs at all ages but commonest between 2-6 yr.	Usually under 2 yr. Uncommon after 3 yr.
Type of onset	Acute with either pneumonia, non-specific respiratory infection, pertussis or morbilli	Insidious with bronchiolitis in approx. 75%. Acute with bronchopneumonia, pertussis or morbilli in approx. 25%
Chronic upper respiratory infection ..	Rarely present	Always present: usually persistent, otherwise recurrent
Wax keratosis	Rare	Common: present in two-thirds
Physical signs	Always localized to affected lobe or lobes, and often unilateral and unilobar. Usually crepitations and rales, and diminished breath sounds	Initially widespread bilateral crepitations especially in lower half of chest. Clinical signs more extensive than bronchographic evidence of the disease
Clinical course	Frequently become dry and symptomless 1-2 yr. after initial infection	Nasal discharge, cough, sputum and febrile episodes persist through childhood, but often between ages of 10-14 yr. symptoms become less severe
Radiological	Collapse always initially present	Early: frequently little or no evidence of parenchymatous disease, especially in those with insidious onset Later: mottling, haziness and collapse may occur
Bronchiectasis	Frequently unilateral, and right side more commonly involved than left. Dilated bronchi usually those of the more proximal divisions of the bronchial tree. Often reversible, never generalized or progressive	Commonly bilateral and left side more extensively involved than right. Initially dilated bronchi usually those of peripheral parts of bronchial tree. Lesions may be generalized, localized or progressive. Never reversible
Bacteriology	Pathogenic organisms isolated in early stages of over 50% cases	No specific pathogens isolated in early stages in in majority
Genetic	No familial history of bronchiectasis or chronic respiratory disease	Familial history of proven bronchiectasis in 14% and of chronic sinusitis, bronchitis and probable bronchiectasis in 38% of siblings, parents and immediate relatives

Treatment

Three principles were the basis of the treatment of the majority of these patients. The first principle was early diagnosis to forestall some of the destructive inflammatory changes, the second was chemotherapy to assist resolution of the infection, and the third was physiotherapy and postural coughing to restore lung function and clear the bronchial tree of secretions.

In the collapse group very satisfactory results occurred in those patients in whom an early diagnosis was made, and effective chemotherapy, physiotherapy and postural coughing instituted. In the bronchiolitis group, the results were not nearly as satisfactory for two reasons. First, chemotherapy had to be used empirically as a pathogenic organism could not be isolated in the majority of patients. One of the tetracyclines in doses of 15-20 mg. per kg. of body weight has seemed to be the most satisfactory drug. Second, difficulty was experienced with postural coughing and physiotherapy as the majority of children were under the age of 3 years. There is little doubt that inability to restore lung function was the factor of major importance in hindering the recovery of these children. It was very evident that when they were old enough to learn to clear their bronchial tree of secretions, there was very great clinical improvement and the course of the disease was in many cases arrested. Later active physiotherapy and games helped greatly to improve both general health and respiratory function.

Surgical treatment of those patients with collapse and bronchiectasis who had persistent symptoms gave excellent results. However, seven children of the bronchiolitis group who had a lobectomy subsequently developed bronchiectatic lesions in lobes previously demonstrated to be normal bronchographically. Ginsberg, Cooley, Olsen and Kirklin (1955) and others have reported similar unsatisfactory results in some children. The three premises on which the surgical treatment of bronchiectasis is based, namely that the disease is a focal one and not a general infection of the lung, second that it is not a progressive disease, and third, that a bronchogram will delineate diseased and healthy lung tissue, are not valid in this latter group. Firstly, there is good evidence to believe that the disease in some patients is a general infection of the upper and lower respiratory tract, secondly the lesions are progressive in some patients, and thirdly a lobe may be clinically infected long before there is bronchographic evidence of disease in that lobe. Moore, Kobernick and Wigglesworth (1949) showed that lung segments considered normal bronchographically showed evidence of inflammatory changes in the bronchioles. It is considered that the role of surgical resection in the bronchiolitis interstitial pneumonia group of patients should be limited to those patients who have a lobe completely destroyed by infection or by collapse and infection and who have much sputum and cough: removal of such a lobe is best deferred until the second decade when the child can co-operate with physiotherapy and when any infective lesions in other parts of the lung have been observed to be stable and not progressive.

Summary

Two groups of patients, one with subacute pyogenic pulmonary collapse, the other with non-specific infective bronchiolitis and/or interstitial pneumonia have been shown to develop bronchiectasis.

The pathology, pathogenesis, clinical features and course, bacteriology and familial history of the two groups are different.

Treatment by chemotherapy, postural coughing and physiotherapy resulted in complete or partial resolution of the collapse and bronchiectasis in the many patients with subacute collapse. Similar treatment was much less effective in the other group owing to inability to carry out effective postural coughing and physiotherapy as the majority were under 3 years of age. In addition, chemotherapy could not be used specifically as pathogenic organisms were not isolated in most patients.

Bronchiectasis should be regarded as the end stage of a number of distinct diseases. The clinician, by recognizing the early stages of those diseases which cause permanent pulmonary damage and bronchiectasis, may do much to prevent their more serious manifestations.

References

Anspach, W. E. (1934). *Amer. J. Dis. Child.*, **47**, 1011.
Bodian, M. (1952). *Fibrocystic Disease of the Pancreas*, p. 135. Heinemann, London.
Brennemann, J. (1943). *Dis. Chest*, **9**, 39.
Churchill, E. D. (1949). *J. thorac. Surg.*, **18**, 279.
Coope, R. (1948). *Diseases of the Chest*, 2nd ed. Livingstone, Edinburgh.
Field, C. E. (1949). *Pediatrics*, **4**, 21.
Findlay, L. (1935). *Arch. Dis. Childh.*, **10**, 61.
Fleischner, F. (1940). *Amer. Rev. Tuberc.*, **42**, 297.
Ginsberg, R. L., Cooley, J. C., Olsen, A. M. and Kirklin, J. W. (1955) *J. thorac. Surg.*, **30**, 331.
Jennings, G. H. (1937). *Brit. med. J.*, **2**, 963.
Jones, E. M., Peck, W. M. and Willis, H. S. (1946). *Amer. J. Dis. Child.*, **72**, 296.
Kent, E. M. (1942). *Amer. Rev. Tuberc.*, **46**, 524.
Laennec, R. T. H. (1819). *A Treatise on the Diseases of the Chest and on Mediate Auscultation*, 4th ed. Translation by J. Forbes Longman, London, 1834.
Lander, F. P. Lee (1946). *Thorax*, **1**, 198.
—— and Davidson, M. (1938). *Brit. J. Radiol.*, **11**, 65.
McNeil, C., Macgregor, A. R. and Alexander, W. A. (1929). *Arch. Dis. Childh.*, **4**, 170.
Moore, J. R., Kobernick, S. D. and Wiglesworth, F. W. (1949). *Surg. Gynec. Obstet.*, **89**, 145.
Ogilvie, A. G. (1941). *Arch. intern. Med.*, **68**, 395.
Robinson, W. L. (1933). *Brit. J. Surg.*, **21**, 302.
Sant'Agnese, P. A. di (1955). *Dis. Chest*, **27**, 654.
Veeneklaas, G. M. H. (1952). *Amer. J. Dis. Child.*, **83**, 271.
Warner, W. P. and Graham, D. (1933). *Arch. intern. Med.*, **52**, 888.
Whitwell, F. (1952). *Thorax*, **7**, 213.
Williams, H. and Anderson, C. (1953). *Quart. J. Med.*, **22**, 295.
Zuelzer, W. W and Newton, W. A. (1949). *Pediatrics*, **4**, 53.

RESPIRATORY STRIDOR PRODUCED BY AN ABERRANT PULMONARY ARTERY

BY

W. H. SCHUTT and P. M. ROBB

From the Royal Hospital for Sick Children, Edinburgh

(RECEIVED FOR PUBLICATION DECEMBER 10, 1958)

Of recent years increasing interest has been shown in congenital abnormalities of the heart and great vessels because of the possibility of successful surgical correction in certain types of defect. The following case presented as one of congenital stridor in which an anomalous vascular ring was diagnosed clinically and eventually confirmed at autopsy; its exact nature was unsuspected and would have perplexed the operating surgeon. It is for this reason that the case is being published.

Clinical History

The child, a male infant, was admitted to the hospital aged 1 month.

The pregnancy had been normal and at 36 weeks' gestation the mother was delivered of twins, one of which was quite normal. The other, our patient, was an obvious mongol. His birth weight was 5 lb. 9 oz.

While in the maternity hospital the child did well but soon after discharge he developed a slight nasal discharge and some difficulty with feeding.

One week prior to admission he began to have attacks during which he would choke and become blue and very limp. Gentle patting on the back would be followed by recovery. Usually these turns lasted for no longer than a minute and occurred two or three times a day.

On arrival at hospital the diagnosis of mongolism was confirmed. He was also found to have a marked inspiratory stridor with suprasternal and subcostal indrawing. Crying precipitated marked cyanosis. A soft systolic murmur was audible over the precordium but no other abnormality of the cardiovascular or respiratory systems was detected. Routine haematological investigations and a teleradiogram were within normal limits.

The child was placed in an oxygen tent and over the next 48 hours seemed to improve considerably. The stridor persisted, but no further cyanotic attacks occurred until the evening of the third day after admission. These then gradually became more frequent and it was at this stage that a vascular ring constricting the trachea was suspected. No confirmatory radiographic studies were undertaken, however, and the child died on the fifth day in hospital.

Findings at Autopsy. At autopsy it was confirmed that a vascular ring was compressing the trachea.

A persistent left superior vena cava was present, draining into a dilated coronary sinus (see Figs. 1 and 2).

The pulmonary trunk arose normally from the right ventricle. Just before it curved beneath the arch of the aorta, it gave off the ductus arteriosus, which was patent (see Fig. 2). When it reached the right border of the aortic arch, the pulmonary trunk divided into three; the two smaller divisions passed to the upper and lower lobes of the right lung respectively, while the larger division curved sharply to the left, running posterior to the trachea, between it and the oesophagus, to reach the hilum of the left lung (see Fig. 3). The trachea was thus enclosed in a vascular ring composed of the anomalous left pulmonary artery posteriorly and the left upper pulmonary vein anteriorly (Fig. 1). The pressure by the upper left pulmonary vein on the anterior surface of the trachea was reinforced by the arch of the aorta and the left superior vena cava. The lungs showed generalized emphysema.

A moderate quantity of clear fluid was found in the peritoneal cavity. The liver, spleen, and kidneys showed nothing of pathological interest beyond moderate venous congestion.

Discussion

Vascular rings produced by various anomalies of the aorta and its branches causing compression of the trachea have been recognized and successfully treated for some time, but stridor caused by an anomalous left pulmonary artery seems not to have been recorded until 1954 (Welsh and Munro, 1954). Since then, four further cases have been recorded (Potts, Holinger and Rosenblum, 1954; Morse and Gladding, 1955; Wittenborg, Tantiwongse and Rosenberg, 1956—two cases). Respiratory obstruction in these cases is usually fairly severe, but there may be slight differences in its manifestation depending on whether the obstruction involves the right main bronchus only or the distal portion of the trachea and consequently whether the child has unilateral or bilateral emphysema. Three infants

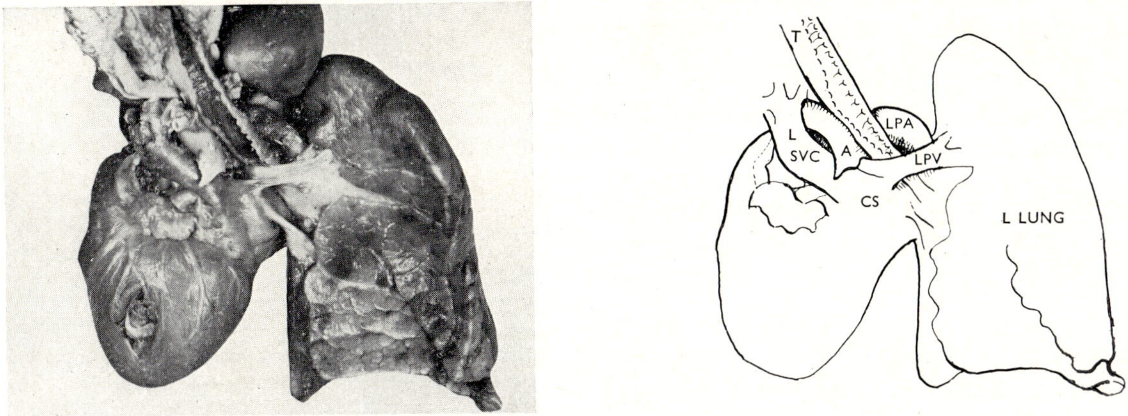

FIG. 1.—Left lung and heart seen from left. Trachea (T.) encircled by left pulmonary artery (L.P.A.) and left pulmonary vein (L.P.V.) reinforced anteriorly by aorta (A.) and left superior vena cava (L.S.V.C.) which drains into coronary sinus (C.S.).

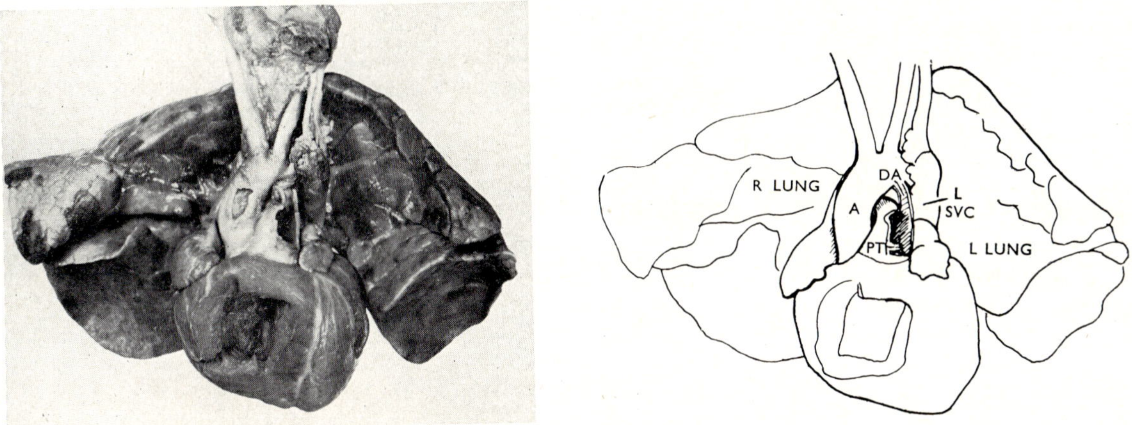

FIG. 2.—Heart and lungs seen from front, showing undivided pulmonary trunk (P.T.) curving beneath aorta after giving off ductus arteriosus (D.A.). A. Aorta.

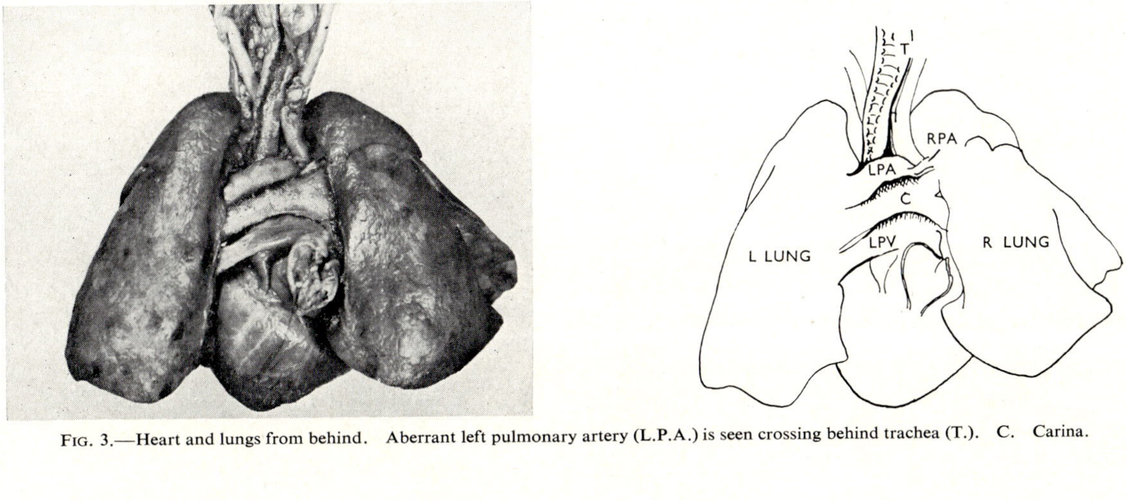

FIG. 3.—Heart and lungs from behind. Aberrant left pulmonary artery (L.P.A.) is seen crossing behind trachea (T.). C. Carina.

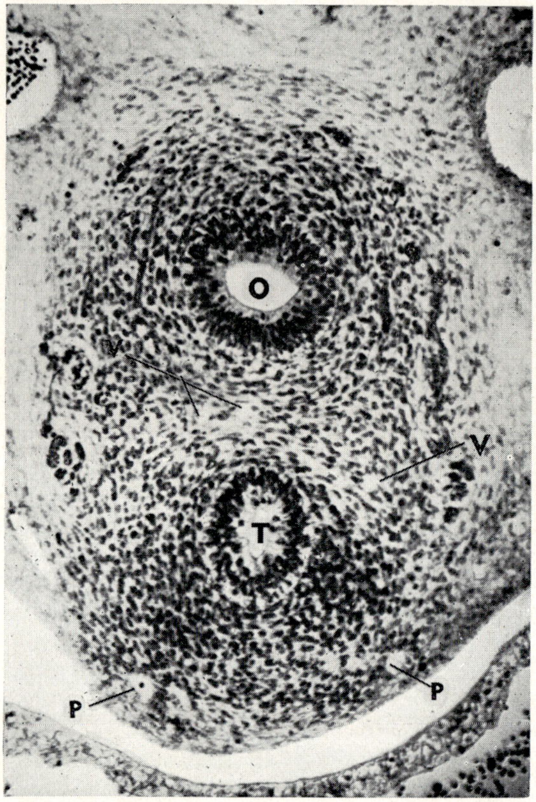

FIG. 4.—A transverse section of the trachea (T.) and oesophagus (O.) from a six-week, 9.0 mm., human embryo. The two pulmonary arteries (P.) are seen ventral to the trachea. Vessels (V.) of the foregut splanchic plexus are present within the mesenchyme which surrounds the trachea and which lies between the trachea and oesophagus. × 200.

with anomalous left pulmonary arteries have been submitted to surgery. One child died of cardiac arrest before any attempt could be made to correct the fault (Welsh and Munro, 1954); one died 11 days after operation (Morse and Gladding, 1955); and one survived and showed dramatic improvement (Potts *et al.*, 1954). In the case of the child who died during the operation the trachea was compressed by the anomalous artery; in the other two cases the right main bronchus was compressed and the method used was division and anterior transplantation of the left pulmonary artery. It is probable that the site of the compression is an important factor in determining whether or not the fault can be successfully corrected. A child with a compressed right main bronchus and one emphysematous lung might stand a better chance than a child with a compressed trachea and bilateral emphysema. Another important factor is the presence or absence of additional anomalies. Of the six patients with aberrant left pulmonary arteries (including ours), two had a persistent left superior vena cava which would add to the surgeon's difficulties (neither of these was operated on), and two were mongols.

Embryological Considerations. According to Jordan and Kindred (1948) rudiments of the pulmonary arteries appear in two places. One branch grows from the base of the sixth arch towards the lung primordium and the other from the mesenchyme surrounding the lung primordium towards the sixth arch. It is conceivable that the downgrowth from the sixth arch might fail to occur on the left side and that the vessels from the left lung primordium would then connect with the developing right pulmonary artery instead of the left. The connexion would take place by way of a channel formed from the vessels of the foregut splanchnic plexus surrounding the trachea and lying between trachea and oesophagus. This can be well visualized on looking at Fig. 4 (Muir, 1958).

Summary

A case of an aberrant left pulmonary artery producing stridor is described. The literature is briefly reviewed and the treatment of the condition discussed. The embryology is considered.

We would like to express our appreciation to Dr. D. M. Douglas for permission to publish this case and much encouragement. We would also thank Professor R. W. B. Ellis and Dr. A. R. Macgregor for much helpful criticism and advice.

REFERENCES

Jordan, H. E. and Kindred, J. E. (1948). *Textbook of Embryology*, 5th ed. D. Appleton-Century Company, London and New York.
Morse, H. R. and Gladding, S. (1955). *Amer. J. Dis. Child.*, **89**, 351.
Muir, A. (1958). Personal communication.
Potts, W. J., Holinger, P. H. and Rosenblum, A. H. (1954). *J. Amer. med. Ass.*, **155**, 1409.
Welsh, T. M. and Munro, I. B. (1954). *Arch. Dis. Childh.*, **29**, 101.
Wittenborg, M. H., Tantiwongse, T. and Rosenberg, B. F. (1956). *Radiology*, **67**, 339.

BONE LESIONS OF URTICARIA PIGMENTOSA IN CHILDHOOD

BY

MARTIN H. LEES and C. ERIC STROUD
From The Hospital for Sick Children, Great Ormond Street, London

(RECEIVED FOR PUBLICATION NOVEMBER 4, 1958)

Urticaria pigmentosa is a dermatosis characterized clinically by areas of pigmented skin which show marked urtication when a stimulus such as a scratch or a pinprick is applied. Initially they occur as pink urticarial lesions, but instead of fading they persist as oval or round, light or dark brown macules or, less commonly, papules or nodules.

Histologically, the skin lesions show an increased number of mast cells in the dermis, and probably it is their high histamine content which accounts for the facility with which urtication occurs. The mast cells contain not only an abnormally high content of histamine (Riley, 1953; Riley and West, 1953), but also a great excess of heparin (Oliver, Bloom and Mangieri, 1947).

In recent years the concept of a generalized disease due to mast cell proliferation has been gaining ground. Mast cell infiltration of parenchymatous organs has been reported (Ellis, 1949; Reilly, Shintani and Goodman, 1955; Berlin, 1955; Brodeur and Gardner, 1956; Loewenthal, Schen, Berlin and Wechsler, 1957; Rider, Stein and Abbuhl, 1957), and the appearance of mast cells in the peripheral blood has been called a mast cell leukaemia (Hissard, Moncourier and Jacquet, 1950; Waters and Lacson, 1957).

The discovery by Sagher, Cohen and Schorr (1952) that bone lesions could be associated with urticaria pigmentosa has led others to investigate the condition from this aspect (Clyman and Rein, 1952; Calnan, 1953; Asboe-Hansen, 1953; Grupper, 1954; Parmentier, 1954; Bluefarb and Salk, 1954; Cordero, 1954; Degos, 1955; Reilly *et al.*, 1955; Stark, Van Buskirk and Daly, 1956; Deutsch, Ellegast and Nosko, 1956; Schorr, Sagher and Liban, 1956; Sagher, Liban, Ungar and Schorr, 1956; Zak, Covey and Snodgrass, 1957).

These accounts show a striking variability in the incidence of osseous abnormalities and also in the form and characteristics of the lesions.

The admission of an 8-year-old girl with urticaria pigmentosa, paraplegia and bone changes in the spine (Case 1) led us to re-examine 31 other children, who had been patients at this hospital, with a diagnosis of urticaria pigmentosa.

Scope of the Survey

Questions were put to the parents of each child concerning the onset, course and behaviour of the skin disorder. A history suggestive of intermittent or continuous release of histamine or heparin was sought.

Physical examination of each child was made with particular reference to evidence of coagulation disorder, hepatomegaly, splenomegaly, or clinical evidence of bone involvement.

A skeletal survey consisted of a lateral radiograph of the skull, an anteroposterior view of the chest, and single radiographs of the dorsal and lumbar spine, and of the upper and lower limbs. Haematological evidence of a coagulation disorder was sought; in all patients, haemoglobin, bleeding-time and clotting-time were estimated. The serum cholesterol was also estimated in each case. In those with evidence of systemic or bony abnormality the urine was examined for excess 5-hydroxyindole-acetic acid, as this metabolite of serotonin has been found in excess in cases of systemic mast cell disease.

Thirty-two children were examined. Four showed unequivocal bony abnormalities (Cases 1-4), one of whom also had an enlarged spleen. Case 5 had associated coeliac disease together with generalized osteoporosis. Case 6 had gross hepatomegaly, thought to be the result of bacterial cholangitis. Case 7 had unexplained splenomegaly.

Case Histories

Case 1. P.W., an 8½-year-old white girl, was admitted to this hospital under the care of Dr. Wilfrid Sheldon on August 6, 1957. Most of her life had been spent in Mombasa, Kenya. She had three healthy siblings.

At the age of 1 week she developed blotchy patches

on the skin of her trunk, neck and limbs; these were at first red but subsequently became brown and now are seen to have all the characteristics of urticaria pigmentosa.

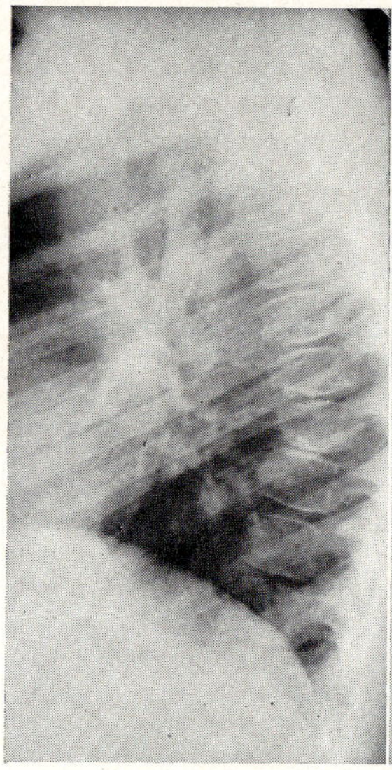

FIG. 1.

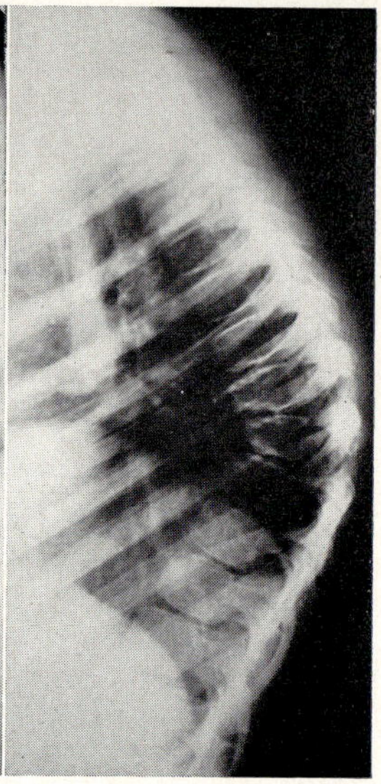

FIG. 2.

FIG. 1.—Case 1. Thoracic spine, showing appearances similar to Scheuermann's disease (August, 1957).
FIG. 2.—Case 1. Thoracic spine (January, 1958).

When 2 years old she had a febrile illness lasting eight weeks, during which she lost the use of both legs and partially of her right arm. She made a complete recovery except for slight weakness of her right leg, which caused a persistent limp.

She remained well until the age of 7 years 11 months, when her right leg became weaker and she started falling down. Four months later her left leg also became weak and she had progressive difficulty in walking; shortly afterwards there was difficulty in starting micturition. In the two weeks before admission to hospital she complained of pins and needles in both legs.

She was a cheerful, intelligent girl. Her skin showed unequivocal urticaria pigmentosa. In the central nervous system there were signs of spastic paraplegia more marked on the right than on the left, with sensory loss involving the posterior columns and spinothalamic tracts, but with no definite sensory level. Tendon reflexes were very brisk in both legs, the right side more so than the left; there were bilateral extensor plantar responses. She was just able to walk unaided and her gait was typically spastic; other systems were entirely normal.

Radiographs of the spine showed a mid-dorsal kyphosis with wedging of the bodies of T7 and T8 and narrowing of the adjacent disc spaces. The anterior parts of these two vertebral bodies were involved by an osteolytic process, similar in appearance to Scheuermann's disease. Skeletal survey was otherwise negative.

Haemoglobin was 100%, Mantoux negative to 1:100 and W.R. negative. Bone marrow was normal. No excess 5-hydroxyindoleacetic acid was discovered in the urine. Bleeding and clotting times were normal. Cerebrospinal fluid was under 200 mm. pressure, the child was rather upset by the procedure and Queckenstedt's test was not conclusive. A myelogram on August 15, 1957, showed that there was an arachnoid cyst situated posterior to the spinal cord, extending from T7 to T11. It communicated with the subarachnoid space below.

A skin biopsy was taken at the time of myelography and showed the typical appearances of urticaria pigmentosa.

A laminectomy was performed by Mr. Kenneth Till. It was possible to remove approximately nine-tenths of the cyst, leaving the subarachnoid space entirely free of obstruction.

Microscopy of the cyst wall showed that it was formed of collagenous tissue, containing scanty fibroblasts and a few polymorphs, but no mast cells. The bone fragments from laminectomy were also examined microscopically but showed no mast cell infiltration. The area of bone involved by the osteolytic process was on the anterior surfaces of the vertebrae and was not available for biopsy.

Post-operatively, her walking appeared to improve, though the physical signs were unchanged, apart from an increase in her dorsal kyphosis.

Five months post-operatively it was evident that her walking was deteriorating and a repeat myelogram showed that there was again a partial block at the level

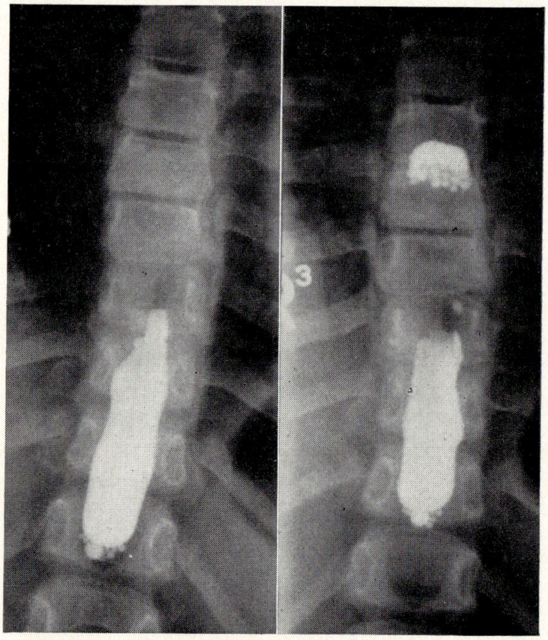

FIG. 3.—Case 1. Myelogram. August, 1957. Showing arachnoid cyst extending from T.7 to T.11.

of T9 and the contrast medium again filled the cyst which was previously demonstrated.

On January 29, 1958, Mr. Kenneth Till carried out a further laminectomy of T6, T7 and T11. The cyst was this time lined with a membrane much thicker and more opaque, and was also more extensive, reaching up to T7 and down to T12. It was possible to remove only a small portion of the cyst.

Post-operatively she was seen by Dr. I. G. Williams who thought that in view of the poor prognosis irradiation was justified, accepting the hazard of producing a radiation myelitis. Irradiation was therefore given.

Three months after the second operation she is definitely walking better, though there has still been little change in the physical signs.

Case 2. L.P., 10-year-old girl, developed urticaria pigmentosa at the age of 5 months. When aged 8 years she started to complain of abdominal pains, vaguely related to meals. A barium meal was normal, but the spine showed the appearances of Scheuermann's disease affecting the vertebral bodies T7, T8 and T9 (Fig. 4). Bone marrow was normal. Haemoglobin was 83% and bleeding and clotting times were normal. Serum cholesterol was 197 mg. %.

There was no kyphosis and the deformity of the vertebral bodies did not appear to cause any disability.

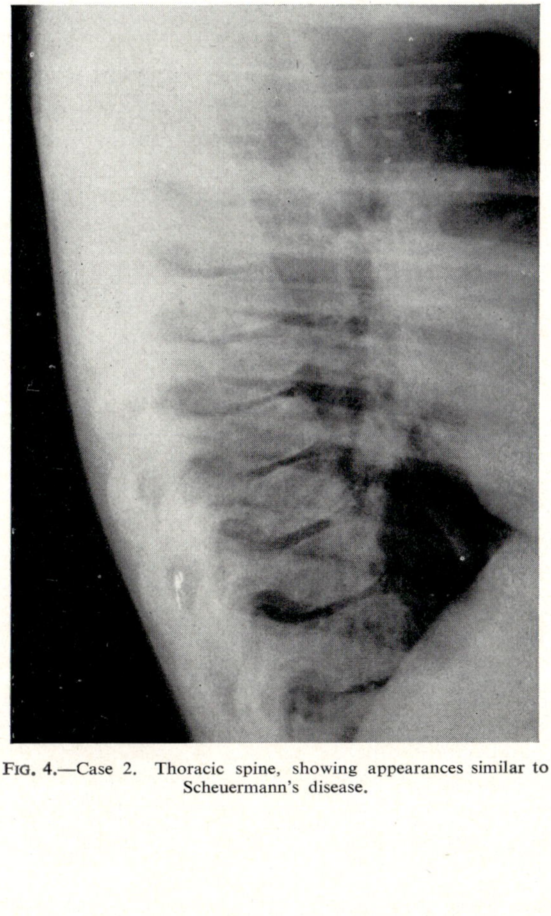

FIG. 4.—Case 2. Thoracic spine, showing appearances similar to Scheuermann's disease.

The abdominal pain of which she occasionally complained had none of the characteristics of root pain.

Case 3. S.B., a 3-year-old-girl, developed urticaria pigmentosa a few weeks after birth. Her general health

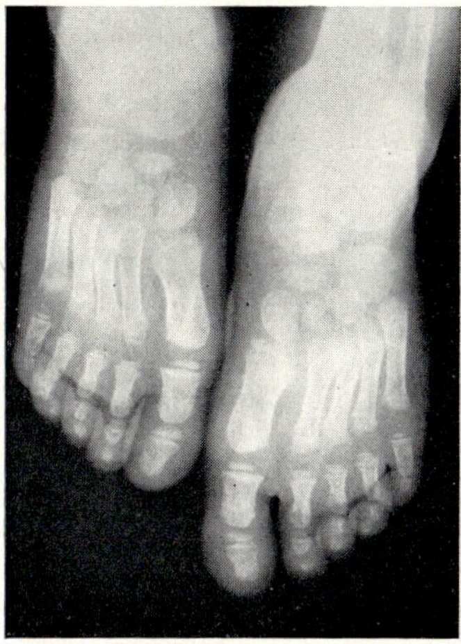

FIG. 5.

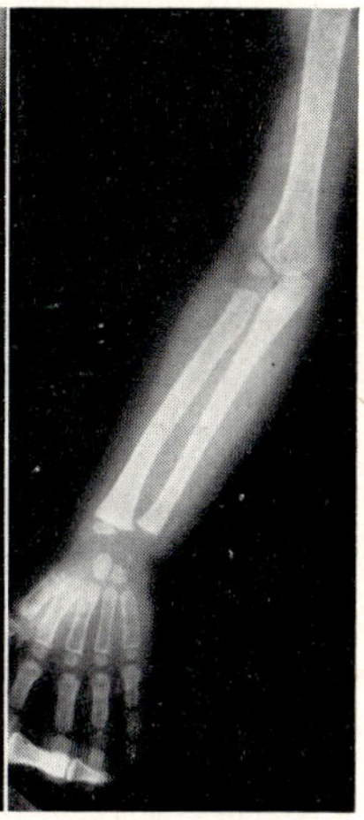

FIG. 6.

FIG. 5.—Case 3. Radiograph of feet, showing osteoporosis.
FIG. 6.—Case 3. Radiograph of arm, showing osteoporosis.

was excellent, except for occasional vomiting bouts. On physical examination her liver was found to be enlarged to 5 cm. below the right costal margin and the spleen palpable 3 cm. below the left costal margin.

Skeletal survey showed generalized osteoporosis (Figs. 5, 6). Serum cholesterol was 127 mg. % and the haemoglobin 82%. Bleeding and clotting times were normal.

Case 4. J.A., an 11-year-old boy, developed urticaria pigmentosa at the age of 3 months. No abnormality was found on physical examination, but radiographs of the knees showed increased tubulation at the ends of the femora, and on the medial aspects there were small exostoses.

Case 5. S.D., a 2-year-old girl, developed urticaria pigmentosa at the age of 3 months. Birth weight was 6 lb. 6 oz., and at the age of 8½ months she was admitted to this hospital under the care of Dr. B. E. Schlesinger for investigation of failure to thrive; she weighed only 10 lb. 13 oz.

A diagnosis of coeliac disease was made and she was put on a gluten-free diet. She gained 3 lb. in the next month and a further 4 lb. in the next four months. Skeletal survey showed generalized bone decalcification which has reverted to normal after treatment on a gluten-free diet.

Case 6. R.G., a 13-month-old boy, was admitted to this hospital under the care of Professor A. A. Moncrieff with an eight-week history of fever, anorexia and drowsiness. On admission his temperature was 103·4° F., his liver was enlarged 7 cm. below the right costal margin and urticaria pigmentosa was present.

Mr. H. H. Nixon performed a laparatomy; there were several ounces of free fluid in the peritoneal cavity, and the liver was uniformly enlarged and firm.

Dr. Martin Bodian reported that a skin biopsy confirmed the diagnosis of urticaria pigmentosa and that liver biopsy showed the appearances of a bacterial cholangitis with excessive numbers of histiocytic reticulum cells. No mast cells were seen.

Dr. I. A. B. Cathie reported on the bone marrow; the smear taken before treatment showed marked toxic granulation of myelocytes, giving appearances very similar to the mast cells described in cases of mast cell leukaemia (Hissard *et al.*, 1950; Waters and Lacson, 1957). However, the granules did not stain heavily with toluidine blue and the marrow reverted to normal following antibiotic therapy.

Treatment was begun with intramuscular penicillin and streptomycin, and continued with Gantrisin. The temperature returned to normal, the liver rapidly diminished in size, and so a diagnosis of bacterial cholangitis appeared to be substantiated.

The case shows a clinical similarity to that reported by Rider *et al.* (1957) where a 2½-year-old girl presented with urticaria pigmentosa, fever and hepatosplenomegaly. In their case, however, there were mast cells in the bone marrow and 25-30 mast cells per high power field in the liver: there was improvement without antibiotic therapy.

The clinical picture of Case 6 is unusual since, in spite of gross enlargement of the liver, there was no jaundice, neither was there any alteration in the liver function tests, as is usual with bacterial cholangitis associated with hepatomegaly of this degree. Final judgment on the relationship, if any, between this child's urticaria pigmentosa and his liver disease cannot yet be made.

Case 7. G.W., a 2-year-old boy, developed urticaria pigmentosa at the age of three days. The rash spared only the hands; on the buttocks it tended to be confluent, but elsewhere was in the form of macules ½-1 cm. in diameter. The spleen was palpable 1 cm. below the left costal margin, but otherwise there was no abnormality. Haemoglobin was 84%. Bone marrow showed a highly active but normal picture. Skeletal survey showed no abnormality.

Discussion

Urticaria pigmentosa is described in most text books of dermatology as a harmless but interesting dermatosis, occurring predominantly in children and usually undergoing spontaneous regression around the time of puberty.

In our series, 29 of the 32 gave a history of onset between the age of 3 weeks and 6 months; the other three arising at 10 months, 1 year and 6 years respectively.

Eight children were seen over the age of 10 years. In five of these the lesions had gone and in two the condition had much improved. In only one had the lesions persisted unchanged. This confirms the favourable prognosis usually given that the rash will clear up at, or before, puberty.

The form of the lesions seems to fall into three groups. They may be deeply pigmented, small, usually measuring less than ¼ in. in diameter, and situated mainly around the neck and shoulders (nine examples). Alternatively, the lesions are widespread, less pigmented, large, up to 2 in. in diameter, often confluent and involving chiefly the trunk and proximal parts of the limbs (22 examples). Rarely there is a solitary patch of urticaria pigmentosa; in one of our cases it was on the cheek. Our series included a pair of uniovular twins, both of whom showed urticaria pigmentosa. All the cases produced the characteristic urtication, following pinprick or scratch. No papular or nodular lesions were seen. Some of the cases had been verified by skin biopsy and nearly every case had been seen personally by Dr. R. T. Brain. Three had had wheezing attacks in the past, but antihistamine drugs had not been tried for their relief.

The striking variability of the bone lesions associated with urticaria pigmentosa has already been mentioned. Sagher and Schorr (1956) collected all the reported cases up to that time and found that they fell into two main groups. In one there was generalized cystic osteoporosis of the ribs with thickening of the bony trabeculae; stippling of the bony structure in the skull and thickening of the skull tables; generalized sclerosis of the pelvic bone and vertebrae. In the other, calcified deposits and decalcified areas of various sizes were seen in humerus, radius, femur, skull and shoulder.

The osteoporotic lesions found in Case 3 correspond well with the generalized type described by Sagher. The exostoses in Case 4 might well have nothing to do with the disease, but are nevertheless abnormal. The radiological changes similar to Scheuermann's disease in Cases 1 and 2 constitute a previously undescribed variant in the bone lesions of urticaria pigmentosa.

The presence of bone lesions in 12·5% of our cases of urticaria pigmentosa and in 36·5% of Sagher's series is strongly suggestive of a definite association and not of an incidental finding.

Unfortunately, none of the patients in our series has been suitable or willing to allow bone biopsy, but this has been carried out in three other reported cases. Stark *et al.* (1956) described a 55-year-old man in whom urticaria pigmentosa had been present since the age of 13 years: there were generalized radiological bone changes and a rib biopsy stained with toluidine blue and Giemsa-Wolbach showed many mast cells in the bone marrow. Zak *et al.* (1957) described a 58-year-old woman with urticaria pigmentosa and hepatosplenomegaly. Radiologically, the spine, thorax and pelvis were diffusely involved in a combined osteolytic-osteoblastic process, the appearances being highly suggestive of metastatic neoplasm. Bone from the right iliac crest stained with polychrome methylene blue (Unna) showed numerous mast cells.

Schorr *et al.* (1956) followed the case of a woman of 55. She had had a skin eruption diagnosed as urticaria pigmentosa for five years and on skeletal survey showed marked sclerosis of the whole of the bony structure of the vertebrae and pelvis. The radiographic bone changes were progressive and she died in July, 1955, after developing enlargement of liver, spleen and lymph nodes associated with monocytic leukaemia. Autopsy revealed osteosclerosis and myelosclerosis of bones and dense accumulations of mast cells in many of the marrow spaces. In addition there was monocytic infiltration of most of the internal organs and in the bone marrow.

Williams (1952) showed that tissue mast cells in small numbers are a normal constituent of human bone marrow and this is also the view of Johnstone (1956). They may be increased in numbers in a wide variety of pathological states, but the very great increase in the numbers of mast cells in the cases described by Stark *et al.*, Zak *et al.* and Schorr *et al.*, are surely indicative of an actual mast cell infiltration as the cause of the bony lesions.

Summary

A review of 32 children with urticaria pigmentosa disclosed four cases in which there were significant bone lesions. Two children showed changes similar to those seen in Scheuermann's disease, an association not previously described: in one of these there was an arachnoid cyst and paraplegia. A further three cases showed coincident abnormalities, coeliac disease in Case 5, bacterial cholangitis in Case 6 and unexplained splenomegaly in Case 7.

The incidence of osseous abnormalities is far greater than that to be expected from a random 32 children. The evidence for regarding these lesions as the result of mast cell infiltration is discussed.

For permission to report these cases and for helpful criticism, it is a pleasure to record our thanks to Dr. Wilfrid Sheldon, Professor A. A. Moncrieff, Dr. R. T. Brain and Dr. B. Schlesinger. We are also indebted to Dr. J. Sutcliffe, Dr. R. D. Hoare and Dr. G. N. Weber for their expert opinions in interpreting the radiographs, to Dr. Martin Bodian for the histological reports, and to Dr. I. A. B. Cathie for his opinion on the bone marrows. We thank also Mr. Derek Martin for the radiograph reproductions.

References

Asboe-Hansen G. (1953). *Acta derm.-venereol.* (*Stockh.*), **33**, 471.
Berlin, C. (1955). *A.M.A. Arch. Derm.*, **71**, 703.
Bluefarb, S. M. and Salk, M. R. (1954). *Ibid.*, **70**, 376.
Brodeur, P. and Gardner, L. I. (1956). *New Engl. J. Med.*, **254**, 1165.
Calnan, C. D. (1953). *Proc. roy. Soc. Med.*, **46**, 544.
Clyman, S. G. and Rein, C. R. (1952). *J. invest. Derm.*, **19**, 179.
Cordero, A. (1954 . *Minerva derm.* (*Torino*), **29**, 55. Abst. *Ann. Derm. Syph.* (*Paris*), **82**, 189. 1955.
Degos, R. (1955). *Act. dermo-sifiliogr.* (*Madr.*), **46**, 759.
Deutsch, E., Ellegast, H. and Nosko, L. (1956). *Hautarzt*, **7**, 257.
Ellis, J. M. (1949). *Arch. Path.* (*Chicago*), **48**, 426.
Grupper, C. (1954). *A.M.A. Arch. Derm. Syph.*, **69**, 109.
Hissard, R., Moncourier, L. and Jacquet, L. (1950). *C.R. Acad. Sci.* (*Paris*), **231**, 253.
Johnstone, J. M. (1956). *Amer. J. clin. Path.*, **26**, 60.
Loewenthal, M., Schen, R. J., Berlin, C. and Wechsler, L. (1957). *A.M.A. Arch. Derm.*, **75**, 512.
Oliver, J., Bloom, F. and Mangieri, C. (1947). *J. exp. Med.*, **86**, 107.
Parmentier, J. (1954). *Les lesions osseuses de l'urticaire pigmentaire.* Thèse, Paris.
Reilly, E. B., Shintani, J. and Goodman, J. (1955). *A.M.A. Arch. Derm.*, **71**, 561.
Rider. T. L., Stein, A. A. and Abbuhl, J. W. (1957). *Pediatrics*, **19**, 1023.
Riley, J. F. (1953). *Science*, **118**, 332.
—— and West, G. B. (1953). *J. Physiol.* (*Lond.*), **120**, 528.
Sagher, F., Cohen, C. and Schorr, S. (1952). *J. invest. Derm.*, **18** 425.
——, Liban, E., Ungar, H. and Schorr, S. (1956). *Ibid.*, **27**, 355.
—— and Schorr, S. (1956). *Ibid.*, **26**, 431.
Schorr, S., Sagher, F. and Liban, E. (1956). *Acta radiol.* (*Stockh.*), **46**, 575.
Stark, E., Van Buskirk, F. W. and Daly, J. F. (1956). *A.M.A. Arch. Path.*, **62**, 143.
Waters, W. J. and Lacson, P. S. (1957). *Pediatrics*, **19**, 1033.
Williams, G. T. (1952). *Amer. J. clin. Path.*, **22**, 1039.
Zak, F. G., Covey, J. A. and Snodgrass, J. J. (1957). *New Engl. J. Med.*, **256**, 56.

A LONGITUDINAL STUDY OF THE GROWTH AND DEVELOPMENT OF PREMATURELY AND MATURELY BORN CHILDREN

PART IV. MORBIDITY

BY

CECIL MARY DRILLIEN

From the Department of Child Life and Health, Edinburgh

(RECEIVED FOR PUBLICATION OCTOBER 31, 1958)

This paper, which is the fourth in a series presenting findings in a long term study of growth and development in a sample of nearly 600 prematurely and maturely born children, describes the health history of the group in the first 2 years of life. A description of the sample and methods of investigation is given elsewhere (Drillien, 1958).

The children were visited at six-monthly intervals, and a history taken of any illness necessitating medical attention or hospital admission. It is realized that what constitutes an 'illness' for the individual mother depends on her temperament, the type of home, and whether the child is first or later born. The middle class mother with a first baby tends to call in the doctor for minor ailments, while the poor working class mother with a large family may ignore quite obvious ill-health. For this reason an illness has only been included in the subsequent analysis if there appeared to have been some degree of definite constitutional disturbance or pathology. It was also obvious that the better type mothers remembered and recorded their children's illnesses accurately, whereas the mother from a lower social grade tended to under-estimate the number of disease incidents. If differences are found in incidence of illness in different types of home, it is likely that the recorded differences are smaller than those actually occurring.

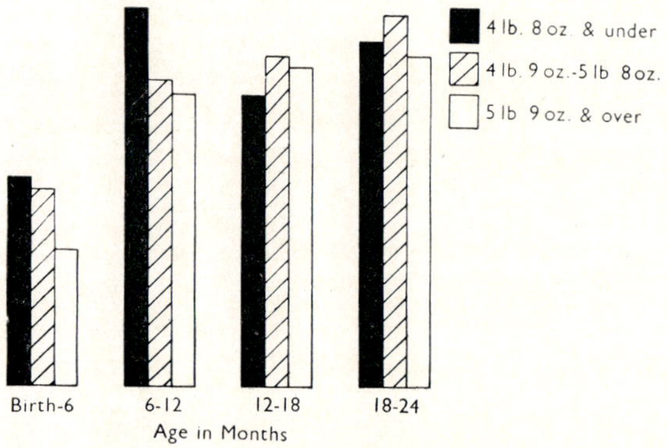

FIG. 1.—Total medical illness in the first two years of life by birth-weight and age.

Patterns of Morbidity in the First Two Years

Fig. 1 illustrates the relative amount of medical illness suffered by different birth weight groups during four six-monthly periods. Fig. 2 divides the total morbidity into five sections: respiratory disease, infections of ear, nose and throat, gastro-intestinal infections, specific fevers, and all other conditions. The prematurely born appear to suffer from more illness in the first year, especially from respiratory infections, in spite of the fact that there are more firstborn children in this group. In the second year there is little difference in the total amount of ill-health, the larger born children tending to have rather more illness, chiefly owing to an increase in incidence of specific fevers and also of tonsillar and middle-ear infections. This is probably due to the increased risk of acquiring infections from siblings, and the earlier age at which these children are allowed out to play. It is noteworthy that throughout the first two years, respiratory infections account for more than half of all illness necessitating medical attention.

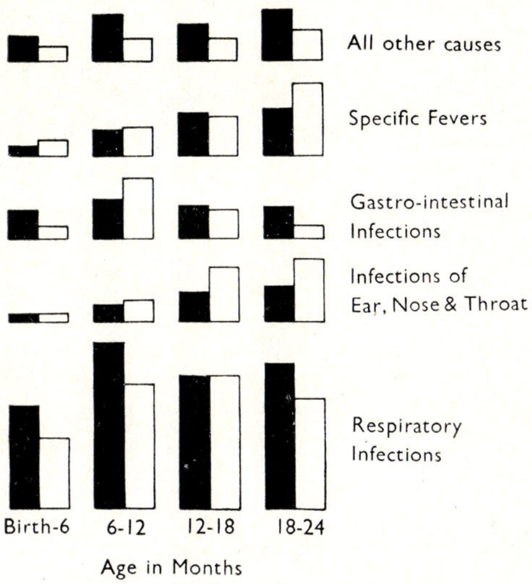

FIG. 2.—Relative morbidity by diagnostic category.
Black = premature
White = mature

Respiratory Infections. The incidence of respiratory disease and infections of the throat and middle ear has been analysed in more detail, an endeavour being made to group the illness according to the severity of the condition. The following scoring has been adopted for each six-monthly period:

(1) Frequent head colds, one or two chesty colds, influenza (defined as a febrile attack of uncertain origin), whooping cough described as being mild, laryngitis and pharyngitis.

(2) Frequent chesty colds, tonsillitis, whooping cough described as being severe.

(3) Bronchitis, croup, otitis media with discharge, measles or whooping cough complicated by bronchitis.

(4) Pneumonia, laryngo-tracheo-bronchitis, measles or whooping cough complicated by pneumonia.

It might be expected that the amount of respiratory illness would be affected by the number of older siblings, the efficiency of the mother and the standard of housing, as well as by birth weight. The child with several siblings was found to have a higher incidence of respiratory infection than the only child, as well as of all other infective conditions, but it does not necessarily follow that the presence of older children in the family is of major importance. It was found that the standard of maternal care was highly correlated with parity, as seen in Fig. 3. In families with five or more children, 70% were considered to be receiving poor or only fair maternal care, whereas when the survey child was first born, care was satisfactory in 83% of cases. It is difficult to differentiate the relative effect on the morbidity rate of maternal care and number of older siblings, as in only 10% of the cases receiving the best care were there more than two older children, and in only 3% of firstborn children was maternal efficiency considered poor. In the subsequent analysis the incidence and severity of respiratory infection is related to maternal efficiency only, but it should be remembered that in those cases where efficiency is fair or poor there will be the added risk to the child of infection carried by other members of the family.

Fig. 4 shows the amount of respiratory infection in the first two years, according to the scoring given above, by birth weight and maternal efficiency. A very striking difference is seen between children

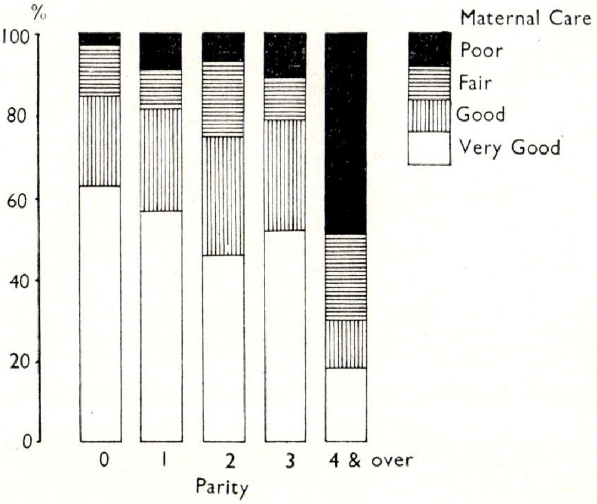

FIG. 3.—Standard of maternal care by parity of mother.

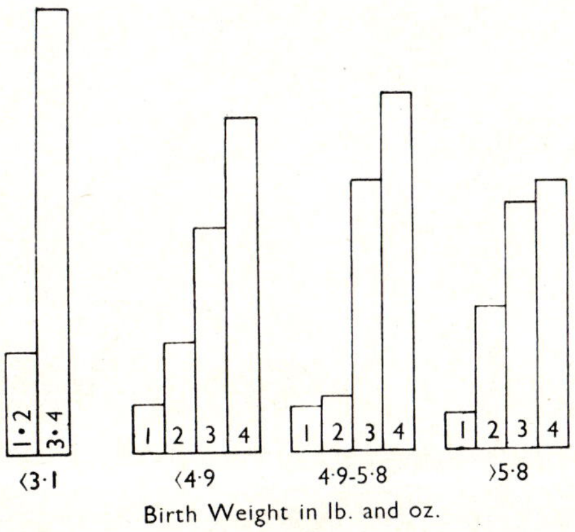

FIG. 4.—Amount of respiratory illness in first two years by maternal care and birthweight.
Care: 1 = very good. 2 = good. 3 = fair. 4 = poor.

receiving the best and worst care, this difference being most marked in the prematurely born, in spite of the fact that more of these children are first born. A smaller group of children who were 3 lb. or less at birth is also being studied, and the figure gives the comparative amount of respiratory illness in this group for two grades of maternal care, efficiency grades one and two, and three and four being combined to give larger numbers. Here the amount of illness in the best maternal efficiency group is only slightly higher than that for the larger birthweight groups, but children of this low birthweight receiving the poorest care show a very much higher infection rate than children from similar backgrounds who were bigger at birth.

In estimating the effect of housing on the amount of respiratory illness, the difficulty again arises that poor housing and low maternal care commonly go together. Fig. 5 demonstrates the amount of respiratory illness by birthweight in the best and worst housing accommodation in those cases where maternal care was satisfactory. In the prematurely born, there is a definite excess of respiratory illness associated with poor accommodation, though there is very little difference in those who were mature at birth. The other half of the figure shows the amount of respiratory illness by birthweight where maternal care was poor, for those accommodated in municipal housing compared with children in poorer housing. In the smallest born, and also those who were mature at birth, there was considerably more illness in those who might be considered adequately housed, these findings probably being due to the apparent increased susceptibility to respiratory infections in children of low birthweight, and to the fact that nearly all the maturely born children were members of large families. Adequate housing by itself does not diminish the amount of illness. There is no doubt that money available for food and clothing decreases considerably when a family with one wage earner moves into a municipal house at three or four times the previous rent, and with extra overhead expenses. During the age period studied, 32 children were removed from poor overcrowded accommodation into municipal houses. In only one case did the mother consider that the child's health had improved. It was striking how little illness was encountered in really poor accommodation, if maternal care was good, but most of these mothers restricted their families to one or two children until re-housing was possible. On the other hand, when a poor type family was re-housed, the pattern of living usually continued along the same lines, shared beds being the rule. Between the ages of 2 and 4 years the number of families

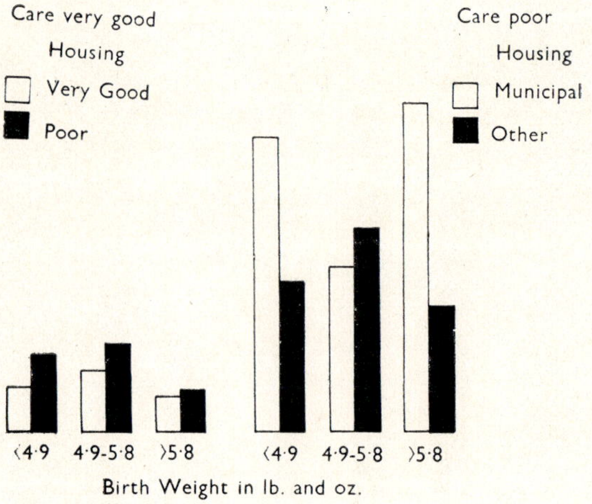

FIG. 5.—Amount of respiratory illness in certain types of housing by maternal care and birthweight.

rehoused has increased, and it may be possible at a later date to estimate more accurately the effect of re-housing on health. The incidence of respiratory illness was found to be considerably higher in prematurely born boys than in girls, but it also happens that in this sample there was an excess of poor maternal care in the male group. When the sexes were compared according to whether care was satisfactory or unsatisfactory it was found that prematurely born boys had between 20 and 30% more respiratory illness than girls for all grades of maternal care, but no difference was found between maturely born boys and girls from similar homes. The apparent increased susceptibility of boys to lower respiratory infections is confirmed by local and national figures. In the Report of the Department of Health for Scotland (1957) for 1956 the notifications for all forms of pneumonia in the under-5-year-old group are 35% higher for boys than girls. Deaths attributed to pneumonia and bronchitis in Edinburgh for the same year and age group were 19 per 1,000 for boys and two per 1,000 for girls.

Gastro-intestinal Infections. The incidence of gastro-intestinal infections reached a peak during the second half of the first year, when the child was being introduced to solid foods. No marked difference was found in incidence in different birthweight groups, although, as would be expected, the incidence increased with increasing size in family. Fig. 6 shows the relative amount of gastro-intestinal infection according to the standard of maternal care.

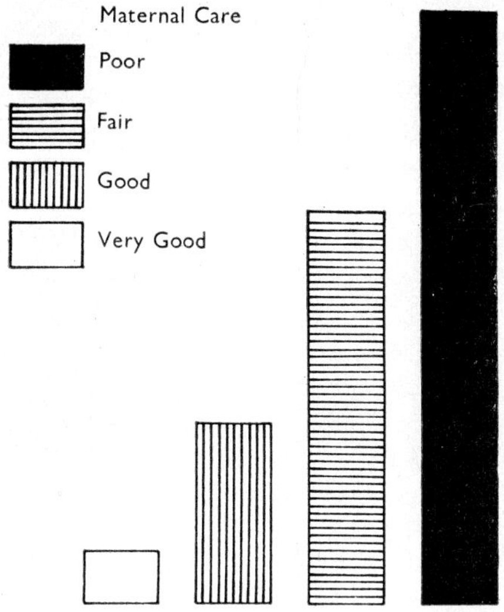

FIG. 6.—Gastro-intestinal infections by maternal care.

Mild digestive disorders with little constitutional disturbance, and parenteral diarrhoea and vomiting associated with another infection have not been included. Gastro-enteritis and dysentery of moderate severity have been scored 1, and more serious conditions necessitating admission to hospital have been scored 2. The risk of gastro-intestinal infection increases markedly as maternal care deteriorates. It is noteworthy that of a total of 327 children receiving the best care only two were admitted to hospital with gastro-intestinal infections during the first two years of life. In the worst maternal efficiency group there were 14 admissions for a total of 63 children.

Specific Fevers. Table 1 gives the numbers of children in the sample who contracted various specific fevers during the first 2 years of life, and also the incidence for firstborn children, and those with older siblings.

Measles and whooping cough were the commonest infectious diseases during this period, and these two conditions have been analysed in more detail. It was found that the incidence of measles and whooping cough was correlated both with size of family and maternal efficiency. There was no significant difference in susceptibility to infection between the prematurely and maturely born. The level of care in the premature group was lower, but the larger number of firstborn children cancelled out this effect.

TABLE 1

INCIDENCE OF CERTAIN SPECIFIC FEVERS

Specific Fever	Firstborn No.	Firstborn Per cent.	Later Born No.	Later Born Per cent.	Total No.	Total Per cent.
Measles	35	12·2	58	19·1	93	15·7
Whooping cough	21	7·3	30	9·9	51	8·6
Chicken pox ..	5	1·7	24	7·9	29	4·9
Rubella	6	2·1	3	1·0	9	1·5
Mumps	1	0·3	7	2·3	8	1·4
Others	2	0·7	—	—	2	0·3
	70		122		192	

TABLE 2

INCIDENCE OF MEASLES AND WHOOPING COUGH BY MATERNAL EFFICIENCY

Maternal Efficiency	Children Affected: First born (%)	Children Affected: Later born (%)	Children Affected: Total (%)	Severe Cases (%)
	Measles			
1 and 2 ..	10·7	16·4	13·4	9·7
3 and 4 ..	23·3	25·0	24·4	29·0
	Whooping Cough			
1 and 2 ..	6·6	7·3	6·9	9·4
3 and 4 ..	11·6	16·7	15·0	52·6

Table 2 gives the incidence of measles and whooping cough by maternal efficiency for firstborn children and those with older siblings, and also the percentage of total cases which were considered to be severe. The illness was called severe when there was considerable constitutional disturbance and a prolonged convalescence, and when there was a complicating bronchitis or pneumonia. The incidence of measles and whooping cough was twice as high for those children who were receiving poor or only fair maternal care, both for firstborn children and those with older siblings. In addition, the proportion of cases classified as being severe was three times as high for measles, and more than five times as high for whooping cough.

It seems likely that the efficient mother is more conscientious about protecting her child from infection, this being made easier by the better standard of housing, and that when infection does occur, the child who has been well nourished and whose general health has hitherto been good is less likely to suffer from a severe attack or lower respiratory complications. As would be expected, the proportion of children receiving protective immunization against whooping cough is higher for those receiving satisfactory care, 77·2% compared with 42·6% in those cases where care was unsatisfactory. No statistically significant differences were found in case incidence of protected and unprotected children after maternal care and number of older siblings had been taken into account. However, numbers are small. It may be possible at a later date to estimate more accurately the protection afforded by immunization.

Skin Diseases. Table 3 gives the number of skin diseases requiring medical attention by two grades of maternal efficiency. As would be expected, there was a much higher incidence of septic skin infection where maternal care was unsatisfactory. It is of interest that 18 out of a total of 19 cases of infantile eczema occurred in children receiving satisfactory care, whose mothers appeared to be rather above average in intelligence. The affected children also appeared to be above average intelligence. This, too, was the only skin condition which occurred predominantly in the prematurely born, only four of the 19 cases being seen in full term infants.

TABLE 3

INCIDENCE OF SKIN DISEASES BY MATERNAL EFFICIENCY

	Maternal Efficiency			
	1 and 2		3 and 4	
	No.	Per cent	No.	Per cent.
Impetigo and other septic skin conditions	13	2·8	22	17·3
Abscesses and recurrent boils	9	1·9	5	3·9
Infantile eczema	18	3·9	1	0·8
Other skin conditions	6	1·3	2	1·6

Other Infections. During the two-year period only eight cases of infectious illness were recorded other than those already considered. These were: meningococcal meningitis (3), pneumococcal meningitis (1), tuberculous meningitis (2), and pyelitis (2). All cases of meningitis occurred in the prematurely born.

Accidents. Thirty cases of accident or injury were treated in hospital during the two-year period. These are set out by cause in Table 4. There was no difference in incidence between children whose care was satisfactory (5% of total children at risk) and unsatisfactory (5·5%). As would be expected, the majority of accidents (83%) occurred in the second year of life. Twice as many accidents occurred in boys, and three times as many in the maturely born, due to the earlier age of walking. No accident was fatal.

TABLE 4

ACCIDENTS REQUIRING HOSPITAL TREATMENT

Burns and scalds	12
Fractures and dislocations	6
Cuts requiring stitches	6
Swallowed foreign bodies	3
Concussion	2
Poisoning	1
Total	30

Congenital Defects. Table 5 gives the number of congenital defects found in different birthweight groups, and also the incidence of minor and major defects, the latter involving risk to life or considerable handicap. Both minor and major handicaps increase strikingly with decreasing birthweight. This would be expected, as the child with a congenital abnormality is likely to be born before term. No social gradient could be demonstrated in the incidence of congenital defect.

TABLE 5

CONGENITAL ABNORMALITIES BY BIRTHWEIGHT

	Birthweight (lb. oz.)		
	4·8 and under	4·9 to 5·8	5·9 and over
No. of children at risk	165	214	213
Microcephaly	2	—	—
Cerebral palsy	6	1	1
Mongolism	—	—	1
Congenital deafness	4	—	—
Congenital cataract	—	2	—
Other congenital eye abnormalities	1	—	1
Cleft palate	—	1	—
Congenital stridor	—	—	1
Congenital heart lesions	1	1	—
Pyloric stenosis	3	2	1
Other abnormalities of digestive tract	1	2	—
Inguinal hernia	9	1	2
Umbilical hernia (requiring operative treatment)	—	—	3
Congenital dislocation of hip	1	—	—
Talipes	—	1	—
Absence of limb	—	1	—
Asymmetry of limbs	—	1	—
Haemangiomata	6	3	2
Total	34	16	12
Percentage	20·6	7·5	5·6
Major abnormalities	16	8	3
Percentage	9·7	3·7	1·4
Minor abnormalities	18	8	9
Percentage	10·9	3·7	4·2

All Other Conditions. Table 6 sets out all other conditions requiring medical treatment or hospital admission. Nearly all cases classified as 'failure to thrive' also had an obvious anaemia. As would be

TABLE 6

ALL OTHER CONDITIONS REQUIRING MEDICAL TREATMENT

	Premature	Mature
Failure to thrive and anaemia	26	2
Recurrent convulsions	4	—
Thrombocytopenic purpura	1	—
Pink disease	1	—
Recurrent acidosis	1	—
Squint	12	2
Flat foot, knock knees, bow legs	17	1
Sternomastoid tumour	3	—
Facial palsy	1	—
Rectal prolapse	1	—
Hydrocoele	1	1
Mesenteric adenitis	1	1
Venous thrombosis (foot)	1	—

expected, these cases occurred predominantly in the premature group, anaemia of prematurity being a well recognized condition. It is noteworthy, however, that three-quarters of these cases were receiving unsatisfactory maternal care. Of 18 cases of marked flat foot requiring treatment, 17 occurred in the premature group.

Hospital Admissions. Table 7 gives the number of children admitted to hospital for medical reasons in the first 2 years of life, and also the total number of admissions by birth weight. It will be seen that twice as many prematurely born children were admitted to hospital, and the total number of admissions was two and a half times as high as in the mature control group.

Table 8 gives total admissions for different diagnostic categories, and shows that nearly one-half of hospital admissions in the premature group were due to lower respiratory infections.

Deaths. Ten children out of the total of 595 died before reaching their second birthday. Details of their deaths are set out in Table 9. The numbers are too small to draw any general conclusions, but a few points seem to stand out. All deaths except one occurred in the premature group of 381 children (death rate, 23·6 per 1,000 children surviving for longer than 28 days after birth). In another investigation of the later development of children who were 3 lb. or less at birth, six deaths occurred in the first two years out of a total of 65 children (death rate, 92·3 per 1,000 surviving children). Seven of the ten children were males, although numbers of males and females in the sample are about equal. Six of the 10 children were twins, although only 38% of the total sample were twin births. Maternal efficiency was considered to be unsatisfactory (efficiency grade three or four) in one-half of the cases. Of the total sample of children. 20% were considered to be receiving unsatisfactory care.

TABLE 7

HOSPITAL ADMISSIONS BY BIRTHWEIGHT

Birthweight (lb. oz.)	No. of children admitted per 100 children at risk	No. of admissions per 100 children at risk
4·8 and under	18	25
4·9-5·8	19	26
5·9 and over	9	10

TABLE 8

HOSPITAL ADMISSIONS FOR MEDICAL ILLNESS BY CAUSE AND BIRTHWEIGHT

	Premature	Mature
Lower respiratory infections	42	3
Convulsions (? cause)	5	1
Dysentery, gastro-enteritis	22	6
Tonsillitis, laryngitis, otitis media	6	3
Specific fevers	8	5
Skin infections	3	1
Other infections	6	1
All other causes	7	2
Total	99	22
No. of children at risk	381	214

Discussion

In the report of the study of health and sickness experience in the first year of life in Newcastle (Spence, Walton, Miller and Court, 1954), the following sentence occurs: 'In the study of these

TABLE 9

DEATHS IN THE FIRST TWO YEARS OF LIFE IN 595 CHILDREN SURVIVING FOR LONGER THAN 28 DAYS

Birthweight (lb. oz.)	Sex	Twin or single birth	Age at death (months)	Cause of Death	Maternal Efficiency
2·7	F	T	6	? Found dead in cot	1
3·0	M	S	4	Pneumonia	4
3·12	M	T	5	Cerebral sinus thrombosis	1
3·13	M	T	24	T.B. meningitis	4
4·7	M	T	6	Whooping cough. Gastro-enteritis	1
4·13	F	S	3	Pneumonia	3
4·14	M	S	17	Pneumococcal meningitis	1
5·0	M	T	1	Pneumonia	4
5·6	F	S	15	T.B. meningitis	2
6·1	M	T	3	? Found dead in cot	4

families and in attempting to correlate their environments with the health of the children, there emerged one dominating factor, the capacity of the mother.' The current study of the health of prematurely and maturely born children in Edinburgh confirms this finding. For all birthweights, morbidity rates, and severity of infective disease were highly correlated with maternal efficiency, prematurely born children being affected to a greater extent by adverse environmental conditions than maturely born children from similar homes.

In the Newcastle study, 85% of total recorded illness was infective in origin, which compares closely with the Edinburgh findings of 85% for prematurely born and 90% for the mature control group. Nearly one-half of the total morbidity was due to respiratory infections, as was also found in a recent survey reported by Grundy and Lewis-Faning (1957).

For all types of infection, the prevalence and severity of the condition varied inversely with the standard of maternal care. The excess morbidity of prematurely born children in the first year of life is largely accounted for by the lower standard of maternal care in this group, but there does appear to be a small but definite excess of lower respiratory infections in those smallest at birth. This susceptibility to bronchitis and pneumonia of prematurely born children was noted by Douglas and Mogford (1953). Douglas reported that the excess in lower respiratory infections was found even when the premature infant was reared in an apparently favourable environment, which is contrary to the findings in the present investigation. In the Edinburgh sample very little difference was found between the incidence and severity of respiratory infections in children receiving the best maternal care, but there was a marked difference between the smallest and larger born where maternal efficiency was poor. It seems probable that the failure to note a social morbidity gradient is accounted for by the fact that the better type mother is more likely to remember and record her child's illnesses accurately, especially as the children studied by Douglas were seen at infrequent intervals: 2 months, 2 years, and 4½ years. Similarly, in an investigation of morbidity in the first 5 years of life in Luton (Dykes, Grundy and Lewis-Faning, 1953), no social morbidity gradient could be demonstrated after the exclusion of bronchitis and pneumonia in the first year. In this study, sickness was defined as a condition requiring treatment in bed for 48 hours, a visit from the doctor, or a condition leaving a recognizable disability. The mother from the higher social grades is more likely to treat minor illness seriously than the poor mother with a large family, as well as to remember her child's illnesses in retrospect.

Only small social group differences were found by Douglas and Blomfield (1958) in the incidence of measles and whooping cough, though children from poor families contracted these infections at an earlier age. The influence of housing and maternal care was considered to be negligible. Again, it is likely that there has been under-reporting on the part of the poorer mothers. In another paper, discussing the reliability of longitudinal surveys, Douglas and Blomfield (1956) report that of 1,296 mothers who stated at 2 years that their child had contracted whooping cough and/or measles, 96 failed to report this at 4½ years, failure to remember occurring predominantly amongst poor type mothers.

Summary

The health history has been studied of a group of nearly 600 prematurely and maturely born children in Edinburgh in the first two years of life.

The following conclusions were reached:

More than 85% of all illness requiring medical attention was infective in origin, nearly one-half of this being due to respiratory infections. Prematurely born children suffer from more medical illness in the first year of life, especially from respiratory infections.

The incidence and severity of respiratory infection is highly correlated with the standard of maternal care. Prematurely born children are affected to a greater extent by an adverse environment than maturely born children from similar homes. No great difference was found in the incidence of respiratory infections in different types of housing, for children receiving similar care. Prematurely born boys appeared to be more susceptible to respiratory infections than girls.

The incidence and severity of gastro-intestinal infections is highly correlated with the standard of maternal care.

The incidence and severity of measles and whooping cough is also highly correlated with standard of care both for firstborn and later born children. No statistically significant difference in case incidence was found between children who had or had not received protective immunization against whooping cough.

Infective skin conditions were associated with unsatisfactory care. Infantile eczema was found predominantly amongst intelligent children of good type mothers.

No social gradient was demonstrated in the incidence of accidents, most of which occurred in the second year of life. The incidence was highest amongst maturely born boys.

The incidence of congenital defects, both major and minor, increased with decreasing birth weight. No social gradient could be demonstrated.

Hospital admissions for medical illness were considerably higher in the prematurely born, especially for lower respiratory infections. Details are given of deaths.

The health experience of the Edinburgh group is compared with that of similar surveys, and some reasons put forward for certain discrepancies observed.

It is a pleasure to thank Professor R. W. B. Ellis for his assistance and encouragement throughout.

This research programme is being supported by a grant from the Scottish Hospital Endowments Research Trust.

REFERENCES

Department of Health for Scotland (1957). Report for 1956. H.M.S.O., Edinburgh.
Douglas, J. W. B. and Blomfield, J. M. (1956). *Milbank mem. Fd Quart.*, **34**, 227.
——, —— (1958). *Children Under Five.* Allen and Unwin, London.
—— and Mogford, C. (1953). *Brit. med. J.*, **1**, 748.
Drillien, C. M. (1958). *Arch. Dis. Childh.*, **33**, 417, 423.
Dykes, R. M., Grundy, F. and Lewis-Faning, E. (1953). *Brit. J. prev. soc. Med.*, **7**, 31.
Grundy, F. and Lewis-Faning, E. (1957). *Morbidity and Mortality in the First Year of Life.* Eugenics Society, London.
Seiler, H. E. (1957). Annual Report of the Public Health Department for 1956. Edinburgh.
Spence, J., Walton, W. S., Miller, F. J. W. and Court, S. D. M. (1954). *A Thousand Families in Newcastle upon Tyne.* Oxford University Press, London.

A CASE OF IDIOPATHIC PULMONARY HAEMOSIDEROSIS WITH MYOCARDITIS

BY

S. CAMPBELL and C. A. J. MACAFEE

From the Royal Belfast Hospital for Sick Children and the Department of Pathology, the Queen's University of Belfast

(RECEIVED FOR PUBLICATION DECEMBER 1, 1958)

Idiopathic pulmonary haemosiderosis is a not uncommon condition characterized clinically by anaemia, haemoptysis, and radiological changes in the lung fields. It was first described by Ceelen (1931), and the clinical and pathological findings of the disease have been fully reviewed by Wyllie, Sheldon, Bodian and Barlow (1948). This case is presented because of the association of myocarditis with the pulmonary lesions of idiopathic pulmonary haemosiderosis.

Case History

The black rectangles on the diagram indicate the hospital admissions of the patient (Fig. 1). He was first seen at the age of 7 in 1950 when he complained of increasing tiredness and shortness of breath of five months' duration. He was the eleventh child in a family of 12, the remainder of whom are quite healthy. On examination he was a thin, pale child with an enlarged liver, but there were no other abnormal clinical findings.

He was admitted for investigation and his blood picture showed an iron deficiency anaemia with a haemoglobin of 7·4 g./100 ml. (50%). Unfortunately at this time he had Sonne dysentery and was transferred to the Fever Hospital.

He was next seen in 1953 when again he had a history of pallor, and was now coughing and spitting up blood. On admission to hospital his blood picture showed an iron deficiency anaemia with a haemoglobin of 5·75 g./100 ml. (39%). His serum bilirubin was 0·2 mg. %. His liver function tests were normal but he had an increase of urobilinogen in his urine. A barium swallow and radiographs of the chest showed nothing of note. He was transfused with blood and discharged on oral iron.

He remained relatively well during 1954 but was readmitted in January, 1955, as his haemoglobin had again fallen to 5·05 g./100 ml. (34%). He was again transfused. In March, 1955, he had an oesophagoscopy and punch liver biopsy done by Professor H. W. Rodgers. Both these investigations gave normal findings.

In November, 1955, he had a phlyctenular conjunctivitis, and in view of this had a radiograph of the chest which showed widespread areas of consolidation. At this time the diagnosis of acute idiopathic pulmonary haemosiderosis was made by Dr. O. D. Fisher, on the basis of the history of haemoptysis, episodes of profound anaemia, and the radiographic pulmonary changes. This diagnosis was confirmed by a lung aspiration biopsy which showed haemosiderin-laden macrophages. There was a reticulocytosis of 33% in his peripheral blood at this time and his bone marrow showed a marked erythropoiesis. An E.C.G. was normal.

In February, 1956, he had a splenectomy done by Professor H. W. Rodgers, and following this he was well

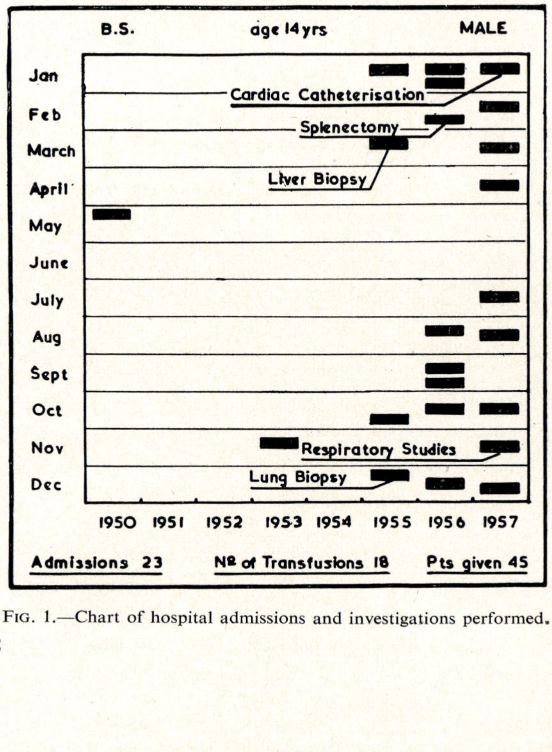

FIG. 1.—Chart of hospital admissions and investigations performed.

until August, 1956, when his haemoglobin had again fallen and he required transfusions.

In January, 1957, cardiac catheterisation was carried out by Dr. J. F. Pantridge and the findings excluded pulmonary hypertension.

In March, 1957, haemosiderin was demonstrated in his gastric washings. Treatment with cortisone was then commenced, but was without effect and the drug was discontinued in October when he was admitted with fever and sudden onset of severe pain in the left lumbar region. His urine showed evidence of a coliform infection which was treated with an eight-day course of chloramphenicol.

In November, 1957, he was admitted in cardiac failure. He had cyanosis, peripheral oedema, crepitations at both bases, and gross hepatomegaly. He responded well to digoxin and his haemoglobin rose spontaneously from 8·88 g./100 ml. (60%) to 13·3 g./100 ml. (90%). Following this respiratory studies were carried out by Professor O. L. Wade who reported that the findings were compatible with lung fibrosis.

He was readmitted in December, 1957, again in gross cardiac failure, and with a haemoglobin of 9·2 g./100 ml. (62%). He died within a few hours in cardiac failure and there were no symptoms of a pulmonary crisis. At no time was there any jaundice or finger clubbing.

He had a fever only on two occasions, when he had a urinary infection and when he was in cardiac failure.

Findings at Autopsy. The body was that of a 14-year-old boy of small stature and average nutrition. There were no palpable superficial lymph nodes or other external lesions of note. The main pathological lesions were in the lungs, heart, lymph nodes and left kidney.

The heart weighed 250 g. and was enlarged for a boy of this age. No congenital or other valvular lesions were present. The right ventricle was hypertrophied, measuring 9 mm. The left ventricle was dilated, its endocardium was rather opaque, and the myocardium mottled, with pale areas suggestive of fibrosis (Fig. 2). No mural thrombi were noted.

The lungs showed a striking picture. *In situ* they failed to collapse when the chest wall was opened and each had a blotchy red pleural surface. On section they were of a deep rusty colour with intense congestion and a poorly defined alveolar pattern at the bases, whereas at the apices the alveolar pattern was more distinct The cut surface gave a uniformly positive prussian blue reaction for iron (Fig. 3).

The hilar and paratracheal lymph nodes were markedly enlarged (the largest being 5×3×2 cm.) and gave a positive reaction for iron.

The liver was enlarged (1,100 g.) and showed only terminal congestion.

The right kidney (130 g.) was normal in appearance. The left kidney (60 g.) showed a healed infarct involving the upper two-thirds of the renal substance.

The brain, bone marrow, and all other organs were normal.

Histological Examination. Heart : many sections of the left ventricle were examined and all showed a marked degree of fibrosis, chiefly in the inner third of the myocardium. There were infiltrations of polymorphs, large mononuclears and lymphocytes between the patches of fibrosis, and eosinophils were noted in some areas. The picture was that of a myocarditis of some duration and probably progressive at the time of death. There were no deposits of iron in the myocardium (Fig. 4).

Lungs : many sections were studied and the following different features were noted. Many haemosiderin-filled macrophages were seen lying in foci in the alveoli, and also a few in the interstitial tissues. There was evidence of terminal haemorrhage with red blood cells in the air spaces. The alveolar walls showed extensive fibrosis with much thickening of the parenchyma. The walls of the small arteries showed a number of striking features. In haematoxylin and eosin sections the elastic tissue was often fragmented and stained dark blue. It gave a positive prussian blue reaction for iron. The fragmentation was associated with accumulations of giant cells sometimes forming ill-defined granulomata (Figs. 5 and 6). A few of the vessels showed an acute arteritis, with necrosis of their walls, and infiltrations of polymorphonuclear leucocytes and lymphocytes in all coats (Fig. 7). The elastic tissue of the alveolar septa showed a similar alteration with much iron impregnation and fragmentation.

Paratracheal lymph nodes : the sinuses were filled with large numbers of iron-containing macrophages. Vascular changes were also present, the elastica of the blood vessels within the lymph nodes showing iron impregnation, fragmentation and giant cell reaction, as found in the lung. There were also many plasma cells scattered throughout the lymph node.

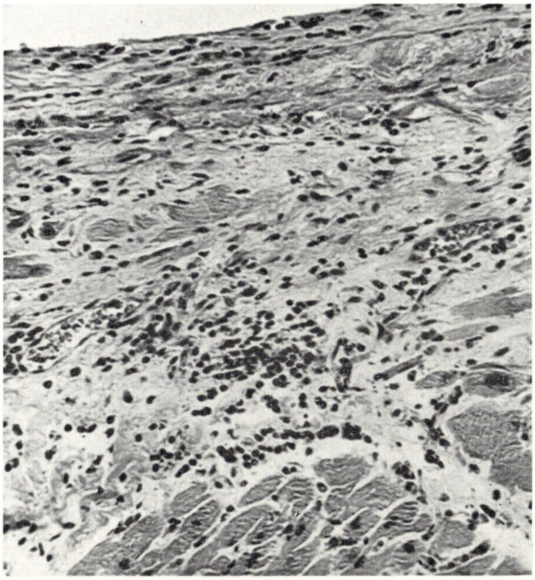

Fig. 4.—Section of the myocardium showing subendocardial fibrosis and inflammatory cell infiltration. H. and E. × 100.

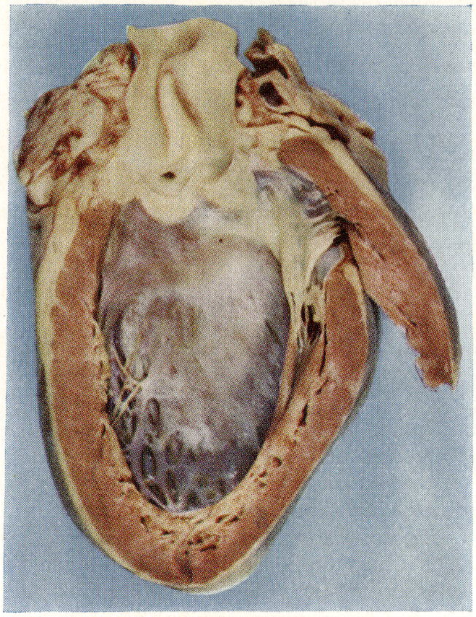

FIG. 2.—Heart showing left ventricular dilatation with patchy fibrosis of the myocardium.

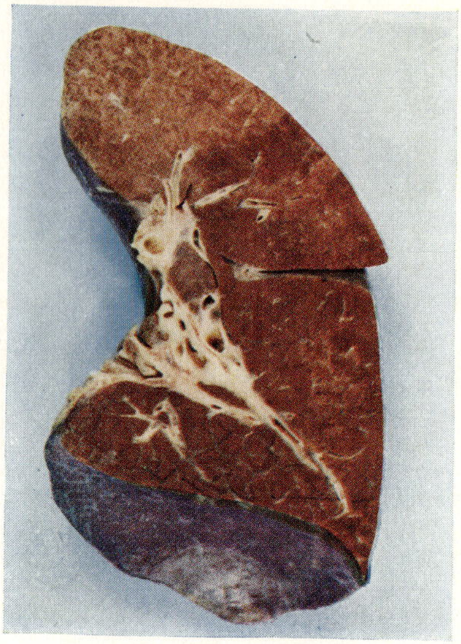

FIG. 3.—Right lung showing intense haemosiderin staining of the cut surface.

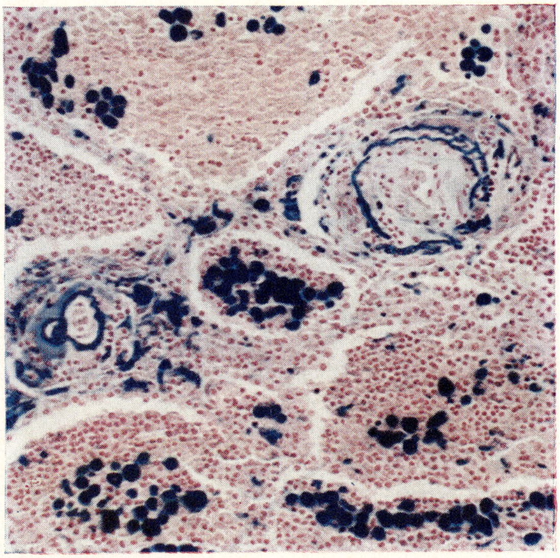

FIG. 5.—Section of the lung showing iron filled macrophages in air spaces and impregnation of elastic tissue of blood vessels with iron. Stained by Perls' method. × 100.

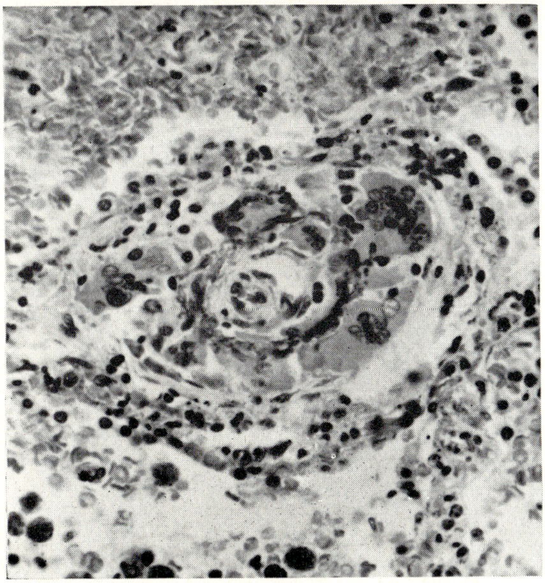

FIG. 6.—Section of small pulmonary artery showing iron impregnation and fragmentation of the elastic fibres with marked giant cell reaction. H. and E. × 350.

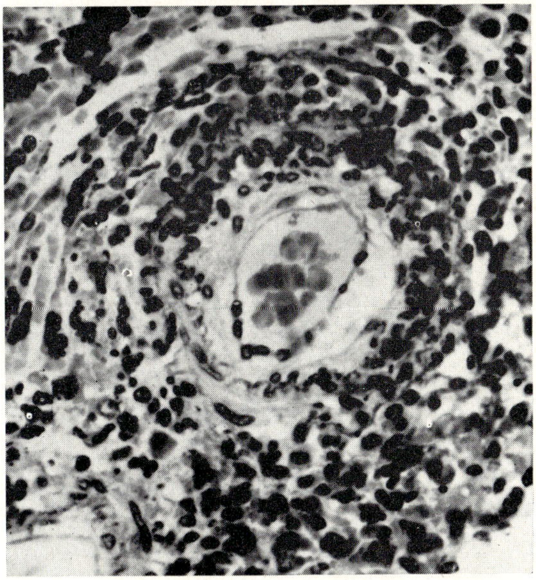

FIG. 7.—Section of pulmonary artery showing arteritis with inflammatory reaction in all coats. H. and E. × 350.

No iron was found in the sections of liver, spleen or bone marrow.

Discussion

The diagnosis of idiopathic pulmonary haemosiderosis was suspected clinically in this case by the presence of anaemia, recurring haemoptyses, and radiological changes in the lung fields, the diagnosis being confirmed by lung biopsy. The autopsy findings, while in keeping with this diagnosis, show one or two unusual features. The occurrence of a myocarditis, for example, is of some interest. It is well known that pulmonary haemosiderosis may develop secondary to advanced cardiac failure such as in mitral stenosis, occasionally hypertension, and other lesions of the left side of the heart. The possibility of a relationship of this myocarditis to the pulmonary lesions must therefore be considered. Review of the literature reveals that some form of myocarditis in association with idiopathic pulmonary haemosiderosis is not a rare occurrence.

At present about 70 cases of idiopathic pulmonary haemosiderosis have been reported. Out of 65 of these, 28 have been confirmed by autopsy; in five it was stated that a 'myocarditis' or 'myocardial change' was present (Gellerstedt, 1939; Glanzmann and Walthard, 1941; Waldenström, 1944; Scheidegger and Dreyfuss, 1945; Soergel, 1957). However, in only eight cases is a histological examination of the myocardium mentioned: Soergel, though he mentioned two cases with a subacute myocarditis, does not describe what histological changes were seen. Wigod (1955) reported a case in a child aged 15 months in which the heart weighed 85 g. (normal weight 47 g.). The right ventricle was 3 mm. thick and the left 8 mm. Histologically there was some vacuolation of the muscle fibres due to fat. Another case worth noting is that of Walton and Williams (1951) in a man aged 19 years, who died in heart failure. At autopsy the heart was enormously enlarged, weighing 1·1 kg. Unfortunately no histological examination of the myocardium is described. It is difficult to explain such gross cardiac enlargement merely as a result of the pulmonary lesions. It is evident therefore that pulmonary and cardiac changes may occur together in this disease.

As far as the lungs are concerned these showed all the characteristic features that have been described in idiopathic pulmonary haemosiderosis, namely, the iron-filled macrophages, the alveolar haemorrhages, the thickening of the alveolar walls, and changes in the elastic tissue in the vessels and the alveolar walls. The associated arteritis has previously been described by Anspach (1939). Similarly the hilar lymph nodes are typical in that they contain iron-filled macrophages. One feature that has not previously been reported, as far as we are aware, is the great number of plasma cells in the lymph nodes, but their significance is uncertain.

Ceelen (1931) originally suggested that the pulmonary lesions were due to a primary elastic tissue disorder. However, the pulmonary lesions are now believed to develop as a result of a local excess of iron from repeated haemorrhages. The iron becomes deposited in the parenchyma and particularly in the elastic tissue fibres. These fibres in turn undergo fragmentation which then stimulates a foreign body giant cell reaction. The same appearances occurred in the blood vessels in the lymph nodes where there was also a heavy local deposition of iron. Similar fragmentation of the elastica and foreign body granulomata may be seen in the metastatic calcification of the lung occurring in myelomatosis. This supports the idea that the elastic tissue changes are merely secondary but leaves unsolved the problem of what is the basic defect which allows haemorrhage to occur. The possibility of an allergic mechanism has been suggested by Steiner (1954).

A very similar picture can be found in the lungs in mitral stenosis of long duration (Lendrum, 1950). The main difference is that in mitral stenosis the iron-filled macrophages are arranged in foci and the hilar lymph nodes contain little or no iron. But this may be purely a difference of degree. What one must, in fact, consider, is whether the pulmonary lesion in this case is truly idiopathic, or secondary to the left ventricular failure from the myocarditis. One year before death it was found that pulmonary hypertension was not present on cardiac catheterisation. This tends to exclude a long period of heart failure though terminally there was gross heart failure. On the whole, however, the pulmonary changes were more advanced than is normally seen in pulmonary haemosiderosis of cardiac origin, and the case is therefore more likely to be of the idiopathic type. A further possibility exists, that the tissues of the heart and lungs are attacked simultaneously by the same aetiological agent, the nature of which is at present unknown.

Though it is impossible to reach any definite conclusion as to the relationship of the myocarditis to the pulmonary lesions, it is felt that closer clinico-pathological study including histological examination of the heart should be made in all cases of this nature. In the past most attention has been focused on the pulmonary lesions, and the myocardium has not always been investigated histologically.

The only other incidental finding was that of the renal infarct, which has been reported on one other occasion (Schoeniger, Tucker and Bolande, 1958). In this present case it was probably of embolic origin from the left ventricle.

Summary

A case of 'idiopathic' pulmonary haemosiderosis in a boy of 14 years is reported. The condition which was diagnosed clinically by gastric washings and lung biopsy, was confirmed at autopsy.

Therapy with splenectomy and cortisone was used without effect.

A severe myocarditis was found and its possible relationship to the pulmonary lesions is discussed.

We wish to thank Professor F. M. B. Allen for permission to publish the clinical details of this case. We are also indebted to Professor J. H. Biggart and Dr. E. F. McKeown for much helpful criticism and advice. The photography is the work of Mr. D. Mehaffey. We also thank the Northern Ireland Hospital Authority for a grant in aid of publication.

References

Anspach, W. E. (1939). *Amer. J. Roentgenol.*, **41**, 592.
Ceelen, W. (1931). In *Handbuch der speziellen pathologische Anatomie und Histologie*, ed. F. Henke and O. Lubarsch, band 3, teil 3, p. 20. Springer, Berlin.
Gellerstedt, N. (1939). *Acta path. microbiol. scand.*, **16**, 386.
Glanzmann, E. and Walthard, B. (1941). *Mschr. Kinderheilk.*, **88**, 1.
Lendrum, A. C. (1950). *J. Path. Bact.*, **62**, 555.
Scheidegger, S. and Dreyfus, A. (1945). *Ann. Paediat. (Basel)*, **165**, 2.
Schoeniger, E. L., Tucker, A. S. and Bolande, R. P. (1958). *Radiology*, **70**, 191.
Soergel, K. H. (1957) *Pediatrics*, **19**, 1101.
Steiner, B. (1954). *Arch. Dis. Childh.*, **29**, 391.
Waldenström, J. (1944). *Acta radiol. (Stockh.)*, **25**, 149.
Walton, M. and Williams, A. A. (1951). *Brit. med. J.*, **2**, 390.
Wigod, M. (1955). *New Engl. J. Med.*, **253**, 413.
Wyllie, W. G., Sheldon, W., Bodian, M. and Barlow, A. (1948). *Quart. J. Med.*, (n.s.) **17**, 25.

CONGENITAL HEART BLOCK

BY

R. W. SMITHELLS* and E. B. OUTON

From St. James' Hospital, Leeds

(RECEIVED FOR PUBLICATION NOVEMBER 28, 1958)

Congenital heart block is an uncommon condition. Before 1920 only seven acceptable cases had been recorded. With the widespread introduction of clinical electrocardiography further examples were reported from all parts of the world and when Yater, Lyon and McNabb (1933) reviewed the subject they were able to collect 44 cases which satisfied their diagnostic criteria.

Since then many more instances of congenital heart block have been recognized but, despite the increasing number of reports, few include anatomical and histological findings. In a recent survey of the subject Donoso, Braunwald, Jick and Grishman (1956) could find records of autopsies in only 17 instances, with adequate histological studies in seven.

These seven cases are summarized in the accompanying table together with an eighth case here reported. A further case (Wallgren and Winblad, 1937, Case 1) is also included although no E.C.G. is available and the criteria of Yater (1929) are therefore not fulfilled. However, there can be little doubt that the infant had congenital heart block (Table 1).

Case Report

Peter W. was born on May 8, 1957, weighing 6 lb. 1 oz. His mother had had one previous child and four miscarriages. She had rheumatic heart disease and a past history of pulmonary tuberculosis. She had been well throughout the pregnancy. One of her brothers had died at the age of 6 months with congenital heart disease.

The foetal heart rate was about 60 per minute before labour began. During labour the midwife recorded the same rate. The baby was born by breech delivery and showed blue asphyxia. He was given artificial respiration, oxygen and stimulants and recovered in about 20 minutes. Thereafter he became dyspnoeic and cyanosed during feeds. These symptoms became more marked and at the age of 2 days he was transferred to St. James' Hospital, Leeds, under the care of Dr. E. C. Allibone.

On admission his temperature was 97° F. (36° C.), pulse 48 per minute and respirations 60 per minute. When quiet he was a good colour but when crying or feeding he became cyanosed. The heart size could not be determined accurately. No thrill was felt. There was a loud, blowing systolic murmur audible over the entire praecordium. The femoral pulses were present. There was no oedema. The lungs were clear.

The clinical diagnosis was congenital heart disease with heart block. An E.C.G. showed complete atrio-ventricular dissociation with an atrial rate of 130 per minute and a ventricular rate of 47 per minute (Fig. 1).

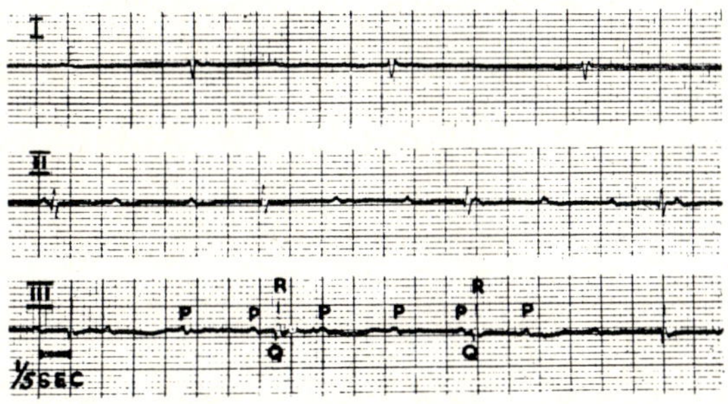

FIG. 1.—E.C.G. showing complete heart block.

He was nursed in oxygen and was taken out only for feeds which he took reasonably well from a bottle. Later his condition deteriorated and he was fed by oesophageal tube.

At the age of 4 days an apical diastolic murmur was clearly audible in addition to the systolic murmur. Two days later his temperature rose to 101° F. (38·4 °C.) and he remained febrile until he died at the age of 9 days. No change in the pulse rate was noted when the temperature rose.

Pathology. At autopsy the brain showed widespread subarachnoid haemorrhage, which was considered to be anoxic in origin. Many areas of haemorrhage and collapse were seen in the lungs, especially in the lower lobes.

The heart weighed 38 g. (after fixation in 10% formalin). Apart from slight dilatation of both ven-

* Present address: Department of Child Health, Alder Hey Hospital, Liverpool 12.

TABLE 1
HISTOLOGICAL STUDIES IN CONGENITAL HEART BLOCK

Author and Date	Clinical Features	Age at Death	Electrocardiogram			Autopsy Findings			Histological Findings
			Type of Block	Heart Rate A	Heart Rate V	VSD	ASD	Other Abnormalities	
Wilson and Grant (1926)	Cyanosis. Systolic thrill and murmur	15 m.	2:1		60–100	+	—	Big aorta, small pulmonary artery	Strands from normal AV node. Much fibrous tissue
Yater (1929)	Cyanosis. Systolic murmur	18 d.	Complete	116	47	+	+	Situs inversus except ventricles. Patent ductus arteriosus	AV node in two parts separated by fibrous tissue
Yater, Lyon and McNabb (1933)	Cyanosis. Dyspnoea. Systolic murmur	2 m.	Complete	150	50	+	+		Bundle separated from node by fibrous tissue
Yater, Leaman and Cornell (1934)	Cyanosis. Systolic murmur	17 h.	Complete	100	50	+	+		Node almost completely severed from bundle
Wallgren and Winblad (1937)	?	10 m.	No E.C.G.		40	—	—	? Fibro-elastosis	Node separated from bundle by fibrous tissue
	Cyanosis. Dyspnoea. Systolic murmur	3 m.	Complete	156	40	—	+		Node separated from bundle.
Wendkos and Study (1947)	Cyanosis. Dyspnoea. Systolic murmur	3 d.	Complete	135	50	—	—	Patent ductus arteriosus. Coarctation	No bundle found
Turpin, Lenègre and Chassagne (1947)	Terminal cyanosis. Systolic thrill and murmur	7 m.	Complete	150	75	+	—	Both atria entered R. ventricle. L. ventricle rudimentary	? agenesis of bundle
Smithells and Outon .. (1959) present case	Cyanosis. Dyspnoea. Systolic and diastolic murmurs	9 d.	Complete	130	47	—	—		Node separated from atrial muscle by collagenous tissue

A = atrial. V = ventricular. AV = atrioventricular   ASD = atrial septal defect. VSD = ventricular septal defect.

tricles it appeared normal with fully developed interatrial and interventricular septa. The foramen ovale and ductus arteriosus were probe patent. All other organs appeared normal.

Two blocks from the heart and two blocks from each lung were kept and embedded in paraffin for histological examination.

The first block from the heart was taken from the right atrium and included its junction with the superior vena cava and the upper half of the crista terminalis. It was sectioned transversely from above downwards. The second block included the lower two-thirds of the interatrial septum and the upper two-thirds of the interventricular septum. In it the septa were sectioned transversely, from behind downwards and forwards.

Each section was 10μ thick and every tenth section was mounted. Of these, the first and every succeeding tenth section were stained with haematoxylin and van Gieson. Section 54 of block 2 was later restained with phosphotungstic acid haematoxylin.

The lung blocks were cut transversely from the middle of each of the main lobes, sectioned at 6μ and stained with haematoxylin and eosin (Figs. 2, 3, 4).

HEART. In sections 3 to 48 of block 1 the sino-auricular node was seen as a wedge-shaped mass of interlacing muscle fibres and fine connective tissue surrounding the nodal artery and lying between the more clearly defined bundles of atrial muscle.

One hundred and thirty-eight sections from block 2 were examined in order to study the condition of the atrio-ventricular node and bundle. A small area of muscle appeared in the right side of the lower interatrial septum (section 52, Fig. 2). It was surrounded by collagenous connective tissue, continuous on the left with the aortic ring and above and anteriorly with the septum membranaceum. In section 54 the area had become a compact bundle of pale, striated muscle receiving a small artery (Figs. 3 and 4). This structure was regarded as the atrioventricular node. Its appearance agreed closely with the description of the full-term node given by Duckworth (1952). Its continuation as the bundle of His ran along the base of the septum membranaceum in succeeding sections. A branch passed down the left side of the interventricular septum, enclosed in a fine connective tissue sheath but the right branch was not clearly identified. No muscular connexion between the atrial myocardium and either the node or the ventricular myocardium was seen in the sections examined. No epithelial inclusions were seen in the septal tissues.

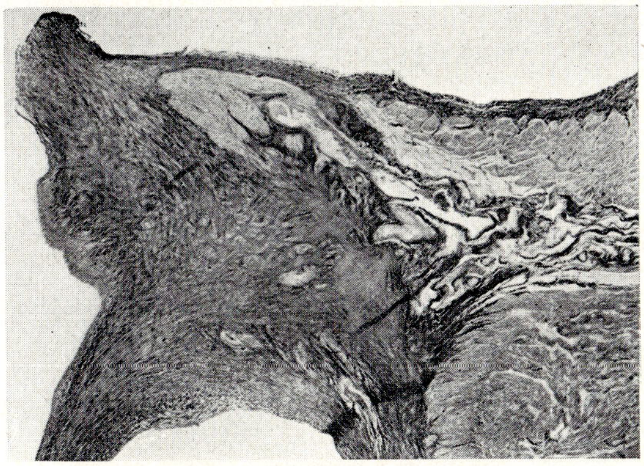

FIG. 3.—Atrioventricular node receiving small artery. Section 54. H. and van Gieson. × 16.

LUNGS. All sections showed patchy but widespread oedema and haemorrhage, usually associated with plugs of hyaline material in the alveolar ducts and terminal bronchioles.

The cause of the total heart block was considered to be a separation of the atrial myocardium from the atrio-ventricular node by collagenous connective tissue. The immediate cause of death was probably hyaline membrane disease. No infective cause of the pyrexia was found in the material examined.

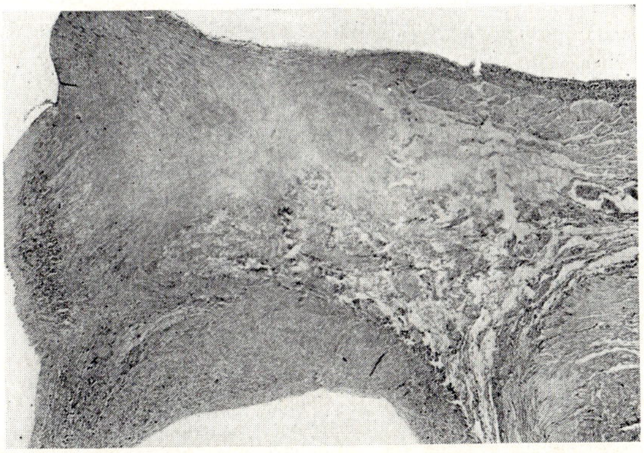

FIG. 2.—Centre above, connective tissue enclosing small area of muscle. Right above, atrial muscle. Right below, ventricular muscle. Left below, aortic ring. Section 52. H. and van Gieson × 22.

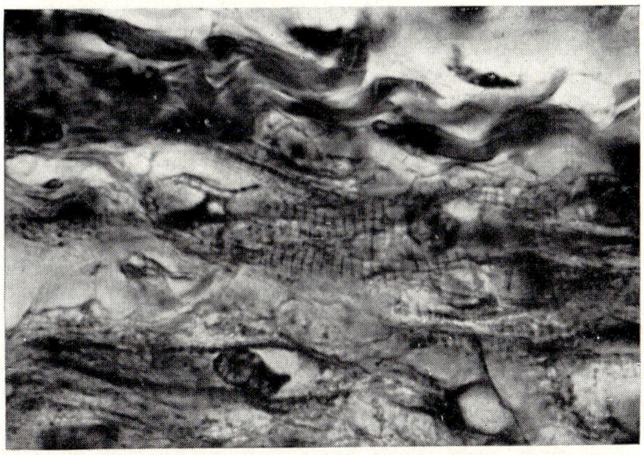

FIG. 4.—Part of atrioventricular node, showing striated muscle fibres. Section 54. Phosphotungstic acid-haematoxylin. × 650.

Discussion

Patients dying with congenital heart block are frequently found to have ventricular septal defects at autopsy. This has given rise to some misunderstandings. First, ventricular septal defect has in the past been regarded as capable of causing heart block by anatomical interruption of the AV bundle. Second, it has been assumed that a patient with congenital heart block is likely to have a ventricular septal defect and such a lesion has often been diagnosed on the basis of a systolic murmur only. The presence of a diastolic murmur or cyanosis in some of these patients has been regarded as confirmatory evidence of an underlying malformation.

Development of the Conducting System. The development of the conducting system in the human heart is still a subject for debate but it has been established in the sheep (Field, 1951). First the atrioventricular bundle appears by differentiation *in situ* in the posterior and inferior walls of the common ventricle. The ventricular cavities are subsequently excavated on either side of the bundle so that it comes to lie in the free margin of the interventricular septum. Later the atrioventricular node arises by differentiation of tissue close to the central fibrous body. The bundle subsequently achieves anatomical and physiological continuity with the node. The sino-atrial node appears much later after the heart has started beating.

To result in complete atrioventricular dissociation the conducting system must be interrupted either at the AV node, or in the bundle above its bifurcation. This localization is confirmed by the normal QRS complexes usually seen on the E.C.G. The usual histological finding in congenital heart block is separation of the bundle from the node by fibrous tissue (see Table 1). In the case described above the node lacked continuity with the atrial muscle. In two reported cases (Wendkos and Study, 1947; Turpin, Lenègre and Chassagne, 1947) little or no conducting tissue has been identified. Rarely, heterotopic epithelial inclusions are found (Willis, 1958).

Even in the presence of gross malformations in the region of the AV node, continuity of the conducting tissues is usually achieved. In patients with large defects of the membranous interventricular septum, ostium primum defects and persistent A.V. canal, disturbances of conduction are only exceptionally found. The anatomy of the conducting system in these conditions has been demonstrated by Reemtsma and Copenhaver (1958).

Congenital Heart Block with Cardiac Malformations. In spite of earlier beliefs, there is no association between heart block and isolated ventricular septal defect. When these two disorders co-exist additional anomalies are almost invariably present. Of particular interest is the association of heart block, ventricular septal defect and corrected transposition of the great vessels. Walker, Cooley, McNamara and Moser (1958) operated on 69 children for closure of V.S.D. Three of them had associated corrected transposition and these all showed heart block.

Congenital Heart Block without Malformations. It is important to emphasize that congenital heart block may occur without any associated malformation. Indeed, this is probably the usual situation in patients surviving early childhood since uncomplicated congenital AV block is a relatively benign condition. Keith, Rowe and Vlad (1958) reported 23 cases of heart block in children of whom only six had associated anomalies. The almost invariable presence of heart malformations in children who die with heart block indicates that it is the malformations, not the dysrhythmia, which cause death.

Symptoms and Signs in Isolated Congenital Heart Block. Congenital heart block is usually symptomless although exertional dyspnoea is not uncommon in early life and Stokes-Adams attacks may occur. A systolic murmur is audible in about 90% of cases and mitral diastolic flow murmurs are not uncommon. Minor degrees of cardiac enlargement are usual.

Congenital heart block may be associated with intermittent or permanent cyanosis in early life which later disappears. White, Eustis and Kerr (1921) reported a mongol with congenital heart disease. At birth cyanosis was present and became more marked on crying. Five weeks later cyanosis was less marked and at the age of 11 weeks it had disappeared. Systolic and, later, diastolic murmurs were present and the clinical diagnosis was ventricular septal defect with patent ductus arteriosus.

Romberg and White (1924) describe an infant with heart block who was cyanosed at birth. At 9 months of age cyanosis was only seen when the child cried. At 10 months old, cyanosis was no longer seen. Systolic and diastolic murmurs were heard.

Aylward (1928) reported two siblings with congenital heart block. His clinical diagnosis was later given electrocardiographic support by Aitken (1932). The first child showed cyanosis and exertional dyspnoea when first seen but these had disappeared by the age of 6 years. There is no mention of a heart murmur. The second child was cyanosed only for the first 2 weeks of life and no murmur was heard.

Walker *et al.* (1958) report three children with heart block, V.S.D. and corrected transposition of the great vessels. One showed cyanosis up to the age of 8 years, after which it gradually disappeared.

An infant with complete heart block usually has a ventricular rate about one-third of normal. It seems improbable that this could be entirely compensated for by an increased stroke volume until the heart has had time to enlarge. Cardiac output will therefore be small and tissue oxygenation defective. On exertion oxygen demands increase, but no appreciable increase in heart rate is possible. Peripheral cyanosis is then likely to appear or become more marked. As the child grows the ventricular rate approximates more closely to the normal and the capacity of the ventricles increases. Exertional dyspnoea and cyanosis may then disappear.

Summary

The case is reported of an infant with congenital heart block who died at the age of 9 days. During life intermittent cyanosis with systolic and diastolic murmurs suggested a cardiac malformation but at autopsy the heart was macroscopically normal. Histological studies showed a normal atrioventricular node and bundle but the node was separated from atrial muscle by connective tissue.

We wish to thank Dr. E. C. Allibone for permission to publish this report; Dr. W. Goldie for the autopsy findings and the heart and lung specimens; and Professor R. A. Willis, Dr. G. M. Bonser and Dr. P. R. Evans for their helpful comments. We are indebted to Mr. G. Stansfield for cutting the sections and to Mr. J. Hainsworth for the microphotographs.

References

Aitken, J. K. (1932). *Lancet*, **2**, 1375.
Aylward, R. D. (1928). *Brit. med. J.*, **1**, 943.
Donoso, E., Braunwald, E., Jick, S. and Grishman, A. (1956). *Amer. J. Med.*, **20**, 869.
Duckworth, J. W. A. (1952). M.D. Thesis. Edinburgh.
Field, E. J. (1951). *Brit. Heart J.*, **13**, 129.
Keith, J. D., Rowe, R. D. and Vlad, P. (1958). *Heart Disease in Infancy and Childhood*, 1st ed. Macmillan, New York.
Reemtsma, K. and Copenhaver, W. M. (1958). *Circulation*, **17**, 271.
Romberg, E. C. and White, P. D. (1924). *Boston med. surg. J.*, **190**, 591.
Turpin, R., Lenègre, J. and Chassagne, P. (1947). *Arch. franç. Pédiat.*, **4**, 617.
Walker, W. J., Cooley, D. A., McNamara, D. G. and Moser, R. H. (1958). *Circulation*, **17**, 249.
Wallgren, A. and Winblad, S. (1937). *Acta paediat. (Stockh.)*, **20**, 175.
Wendkos, M. H. and Study, R. S. (1947). *Amer. Heart J.*, **34**, 138.
White, P. D., Eustis, R. S. and Kerr, W. J. (1921). *Amer. J. Dis. Child.*, **22**, 299.
Willis, R. A. (1958). *The Borderland of Embryology and Pathology*, 1st ed. Butterworth, London.
Wilson, J. G. and Grant, R. T. (1926). *Heart*, **12**, 295.
Yater, W. M. (1929). *Amer. J. Dis. Child.*, **38**, 112.
——, Leaman, W. G. and Cornell, V. H. (1934). *J. Amer. med. Ass.*, **102**, 1660.
——, Lyon, J. A. and McNabb, P. E. (1933). *Ibid.*, **100**, 1831.

CONGENITAL ANOMALIES ASSOCIATED WITH CEREBRAL PALSY AND MENTAL RETARDATION

BY

RONALD S. ILLINGWORTH

From the Department of Child Health, the University of Sheffield and the Children's Hospital, Sheffield

(RECEIVED FOR PUBLICATION DECEMBER 15, 1958)

In the past 12 years 800 children with mental retardation or with cerebral palsy have been seen in the Children's Hospital, Sheffield, by the Department of Child Health. While looking through punch-card summaries of these cases, it became obvious that there was a much higher incidence of associated congenital anomalies in children with mental retardation without cerebral palsy than in those with cerebral palsy whether retarded or not. In view of the fact that in many ways there is a close similarity between the aetiological factors of the two conditions, it was felt that an analysis of the associated anomalies and their incidence in the two groups would be of interest. This paper analyses, therefore, the incidence and nature of associated congenital anomalies in the two groups of children.

Method of Study

The study is based on 300 children with cerebral palsy (excluding hydrocephalus), and 500 children with mental retardation without cerebral palsy. They are all consecutive cases, and constitute all the children seen with these conditions by the Department of Child Health in the past 12 years. They include all cases in which the diagnosis of mental retardation or of cerebral palsy was made and indexed, and therefore are not in any way selected. They include all degrees of severity, from the most trivial symptomless cerebral palsy and the most trivial degree of mental retardation, even including those children who are commonly considered to be in the normal range of intelligence (e.g. with an I.Q. of 90 or 95), to the most severely incapacitated idiots with a level of intelligence so low that it was unscorable. Many of those with a trivial degree of mental retardation formed part of another study on the predictive value of developmental tests in infancy (Illingworth, 1959). They may not necessarily be representative of mentally retarded children and those with cerebral palsy as a whole, but it is difficult to think of any reason why the series to be discussed should be significantly different from any larger series elsewhere.

For the purposes of the study, cases of pre-natal or natal origin have been separated from those of post-natal origin. Tables 1 and 2 show the aetiological factors in the two groups of children, as far as they could be ascertained. There were some children in whom the correct category was uncertain. The defect in the so-called acute infantile hemiplegia,

TABLE 1

AETIOLOGICAL TYPES OF CEREBRAL PALSY*

Pre-natal or Natal (278)	
Simple or non-specific (including spastic forms, athetosis, ataxia, tremor, rigidity and mixed forms)	266
Sturge-Weber syndrome	4
Cerebral angioma	1
Schilder's disease	4
Pelizaeus-Merzbacher syndrome	1
Friedreich's ataxia	1
Von Willebrand's syndrome with cerebral haemorrhage and hemiplegia	1
Post-natal Origin (22)	
Sequelae of pyogenic meningitis	4
Encephalitis or post-infectious encephalomyelitis	11
Trauma	2
Cerebral vein thrombosis	3
Malignant hypertension	1
Fallot's tetralogy with cerebral vein thrombosis	1

* Excluding hydrocephalus.

TABLE 2

AETIOLOGICAL TYPES OF MENTAL RETARDATION*

Pre-natal or Natal (465)	
Mongolism without congenital cardiac lesion (some with other defects)	63
Mongolism with congenital cardiac lesion (some with other defects)	16
Simple or non-specific	362
Phenylketonuria	5
Gargoylism	2
Tuberous sclerosis	3
Akinetic seizures with hypsarrhythmia developing in a previously clinically normal child	14
Post-natal Conditions (22)	
Sequelae of encephalitis	10
Post-infectious or post-immunization encephalomyelitis	8
Pyogenic meningitis	2
Trauma	1
Cerebral vein thrombosis	1
Uncertain Category (13)	
Degenerative conditions of the brain (including two of Von Bogaert's syndrome)	13

* Excluding cerebral palsy.

for instance, and in children who developed normally for five or six months and then suddenly deteriorated with a simultaneous development of akinetic seizures ('hypsarrhythmia') was thought likely to be of pre-natal origin. As it happens, none of these children in either group had any associated anomalies.

For the purposes of this study, I have included only those children in whom the defect was thought to be of pre-natal or natal origin. Mongolism being a separate entity, and the associated anomalies found in mongolism being well known, the 79 examples of this condition are not analysed separately, except only for the incidence of congenital heart lesions (16 in 79 children). This is, therefore, a study of 278 children with cerebral palsy and 386 children with mental retardation.

Results

The incidence of associated congenital anomalies in the 278 children with cerebral palsy is shown in Table 3. Defects of hearing and defects of vision, other than cataract, optic atrophy, choroidoretinitis and retrolental fibroplasia, have not been included. The list includes 19 children, one with a cleft palate, five with serious eye conditions, and one with congenital heart disease. Details of these children cannot be given here, because space will not permit.

In contrast to Table 3, Table 4 shows the incidence of associated anomalies in the 386 children

TABLE 3

CEREBRAL PALSY: ASSOCIATED CONDITIONS OR SYNDROMES IN PRE-NATAL OR NATAL FORMS (19)

Pièrre Robin syndrome with spina bifida, abnormal toes, congenital pyloric stenosis and spastic quadriplegia	1
Cataract, hepatosplenomegaly, spastic quadriplegia and convulsions	1
Congenital heart disease with transposition of the viscera, athetosis and convulsions	1
Optic atrophy with syndactyly, mental deficiency and athetosis	1
Optic atrophy (including two with convulsions)	6
Retinal changes with convulsions, hemiplegia and mental deficiency	2
Aplastic or hypoplastic anaemia	3
Lipoidosis with a mixed form of cerebral palsy and convulsions	1
Steatorrhoea with athetosis and mental deficiency	1
Precocious puberty with convulsions, mental deficiency and hemiplegia	1
Precocious puberty, spastic quadriplegia, retrolental fibroplasia and convulsions	1

TABLE 4

MENTAL RETARDATION WITHOUT CEREBRAL PALSY, ASSOCIATED CONDITIONS OR SYNDROMES IN PRE-NATAL OR NATAL FORMS, EXCLUDING MONGOLISM

Cardiovascular Anomalies (4)	
Congenital heart disease alone	4
Cranial Anomalies (13)	
Hypertelorism (includes one with megalencephaly)	4
Craniostenosis	2
Abnormal shape (excluding microcephaly, simple asymmetry, and flat occiput)	5
Frontal hyperostosis	1
Abnormal shape, with abnormally small interpupillary distance	1
Facial Anomaly (1)	
Beaked nose and peculiar facies	1
Ocular Anomalies (16)	
Optic atrophy (includes two with convulsions)	9
Retrolental fibroplasia	1
Choroidoretinitis with convulsions	1
Bilateral cataract	1
Congenital nystagmus	1
Buphthalmos	1
Cerebromacular degeneration with convulsions	1
Coloboma with convulsions	1
Skeletal Anomalies (7)	
Chondrodystrophy	1
Congenital stippled epiphyses	1
Gross dwarfism	1
Congenital fusion of radius and ulna	1
Congenital absence of radius	1
Congenital dislocation of hip	1
Syndactyly	1
Musculoskeletal and Neuromuscular (9)	
Congenital hypotonia (includes one with convulsions)	5
Congenital facial diplegia (Möbius syndrome)	1
Congenital bulbar palsy	1
Myasthenia gravis	1
Myopathy	1
Cleft Palate (7)	
Alone (includes two with convulsions)	6
With micrognathia (Pièrre Robin syndrome)	1
Deafness (severe)	5
Anaemia (3)	
Hypoplastic	2
Cyclic neutropenia	1
Congenital Laryngeal Stridor	2
Toxoplasmosis	2
Complete Aphasia (age 10)	1
Congenital Obliteration of Bile Ducts	1
Steatorrhoea (including one with convulsions)	3
Amino-aciduria with Convulsions	1
Ichthyosis	1
Miscellaneous Syndromes (27)	
Micrognathia, talipes, divarication of the recti, incurving little finger	
Micrognathia, optic atrophy, congenital heart disease, talipes, microcephaly, torticollis, congenital abnormality of cervical spine, branchial fistula, congenital dermal sinus, cranial abnormality, convulsions	
Micrognathia, permanent facial palsy, severe foot deformity	
Cleft palate, syndactyly, incurved little finger, epicanthus	
Linear naevi, choroidoretinitis, kyphoscoliosis, optic atrophy, craniostenosis, prolonged middle finger	
Linear and diffuse pigmented naevi, valgus deformity of foot, splenomegaly, optic atrophy, frontal hyperostosis, congenital dermal sinus, hypertrophied middle finger of each hand	
Optic atrophy with congenital dislocation of hip and convulsions	
Optic atrophy with scoliosis and convulsions	
Optic atrophy with deafness and convulsions	
Optic atrophy, enophthalmus, congenital heart disease, hypotonia and convulsions	
Optic atrophy, congenital heart disease, extensive naevoid formation, congenital defect of kidney	
Cataract, congenital heart disease and hypospadias	
Congenital paralysis of the right internal rectus muscle of the eye, with talipes	
Severe strabismus with high arched palate and convulsions	
Choroidal degeneration with deafness	
Spasmus nutans	
Rubella syndrome (cataract and congenital heart disease) with ichthyosis	
Arachnodactyly, hypertelorism, congenital intestinal obstruction	
Arachnodactyly and deafness	
Lobster hand	
Hypotonia, deafness and deformity of the ears	
Hypotonia, steatorrhoea, strabismus, hepatic dysfunction, peculiar facies	
Congenital heart disease with megalencephaly	
Congenital insensitivity to pain with anhydrosis and convulsions	
Klippel-Feil syndrome with meningocoele and kyphoscoliosis	
Mandibulo-facial dysostosis, optic atrophy, hairy mole of forehead, low hair line, accessory nipples, convulsions	
Congenital dislocation of hip and abnormal skull	

with mental retardation, giving details of those anomalies in 103 children. Minor defects, such as abnormalities of the ears, or minor degrees of strabismus, have been excluded. Deafness is only mentioned when it is severe. Cranial and facial anomalies have only been mentioned when they are very obvious. The list includes nine with congenital heart disease, 30 with serious eye lesions, and eight with cleft palate. The list concludes with 27 mixed syndromes of considerable interest which will not be further described here.

It will be seen that the incidence of associated congenital anomalies in children with cerebral palsy is 19 out of 278 children (6·8%), and that in children with mental retardation is 103 out of 386 children (26·4%).

Discussion

Studies of the ante-natal history of mothers who have given birth to children with mental deficiency or cerebral palsy have shown that there are many features in common in the antecedents of these conditions. In both groups of conditions there is a greater incidence of antepartum haemorrhage, toxaemia, and other conditions leading to anoxia in the foetus, than is found in pregnancies leading to the delivery of a normal foetus (Lilienfeld and Parkhurst, 1951; Pasamanick and Lilienfeld, 1955; Lilienfeld and Pasamanick, 1955). Hence the observation that the incidence of associated anomalies is 6·8% in a group of 278 unselected children with cerebral palsy, as compared with one of 26·4% in 386 children with mental retardation, indicates, as one would expect, that there are other contributory factors, possibly largely genetic, which operate differently in the two groups.

It may be argued that the two groups are not strictly comparable in that while all the children in one group are mentally retarded, some of the children in the cerebral palsy group are not. It has already been explained, however, that children with only trivial degrees of mental retardation have been included in the former group, while it is known that only a small number of children with cerebral palsy have an I.Q. of over 100 (the figure given by Dunsdon (1952) being 8%) while 50% have an I.Q. of less than 70 (Illingworth, 1958). Nevertheless, 16 of the 19 examples of associated anomalies occurred in children with cerebral palsy who had a low level of intelligence.

The high incidence of cleft palate and congenital heart disease in the mentally retarded group is of interest. It was shown elsewhere that the mean I.Q. of children with cleft palate is slightly lower than that of the normal population (Illingworth and Birch, 1956). Ireland, Witham and Harper (1955) found that the incidence of congenital heart disease in 723 mental defectives in institutions was 2·35%, while the incidence in the series of retarded children described above (excluding mongols) was 9 in 372 (2·41%). Ireland *et al.* remarked that this incidence is seven times higher than that in the general population, and that even when mongols were excluded, the incidence was still several times higher than that in the general population.

Summary

The incidence of associated congenital anomalies in an unselected group of 278 children with cerebral palsy of pre-natal or natal origin is compared with that in 386 children with mental retardation of pre-natal or natal origin, excluding mongols.

The incidence of associated anomalies was 6·8% in the children with cerebral palsy and 26·4% in the children with mental retardation alone.

The high incidence of cleft palate and congenital heart disease in the mentally retarded group is noted.

The implications of these findings are discussed.

References

Dunsdon, M. I. (1952). *The Educability of Cerebral Palsied Children.* Newnes Educational Publishing Co., London.
Illingworth, R. S. (1958). *Recent Advances in Cerebral Palsy.* Churchill, London.
—— (1959). *Arch. Dis. Childh.* In the press.
—— and Birch, L. B. (1956). *Arch. Dis. Childh.*, **31**, 300.
Ireland, C. R., Witham, A. C. and Harper, H. T. (1955). *New Engl. J. Med.*, **252**, 117.
Lilienfeld, A. M. and Parkhurst, E. (1951). *Amer. J. Hyg.*, **53**, 262.
—— and Pasamanick, B. (1955). *Amer. J. Obst. Gynec.*, **70**, 93.
Pasamanick, B. and Lilienfeld, A. M. (1955). *J. Amer. med. Ass.*, **159**, 155.

HYDRANENCEPHALY AND ALLIED DISORDERS

A STUDY OF CEREBRAL DEFECT IN CHINESE CHILDREN

BY

C. S. MUIR

From the Department of Pathology, University of Malaya

(RECEIVED FOR PUBLICATION DECEMBER 21, 1958)

It is proposed to present 11 cases of cerebral defect. Six of these can be classed as hydranencephaly, the others show varying degrees of cerebral mantle tissue loss. The diagnosis and aetiology of these defects will be discussed and pictorial evidence produced to show that hydranencephaly is probably the end result of a graduated series of cerebral cortical defects.

Hydranencephaly is defined by Potter (1952) as 'an abnormality consisting of a complete or almost complete absence of the cerebral hemispheres. The leptomeninges and dura are completely formed occupying their normal positions in the skull'. Although Bettinger (1940) attributes the name of the condition to Cruveilhier (1835), and although the latter describes the anomaly and illustrates his case with an excellent colour plate, he does not in fact use the word, remarking, 'Il y a deux espèces d'anencéphalies: l'anencéphalie hydrocéphalique et l'anencéphalie avec l'absence de la voûte craniènne, du plutôt avec dejettement et deformation des os de la voûte'. He continues, 'Dans l'un et l'autre cas l'absence du cerveau doit être produite par la mème cause'. It seems that Spielmeyer (1905) was the first to use the word in the title of his paper, 'Ein hydranencephales Zwillingspaar'.

The number of reported cases is probably about 70. Reliable figures are difficult to obtain as various authors have not hesitated to extend the definition to suit their own specimens. Others, e.g. Picaza, Cardelle and Martin Jimenez (1955) who would abolish the term altogether, hide within their term 'hydroencephalodysplasia' undoubted cases of the classical condition. Yet others, like Kåss (1951), erroneously describe their cases as being examples of gross hydrocephalus.

The classification of the condition, like many others whose aetiology is uncertain, is in dispute. Earlier authors were content to use the descriptive term 'hydranencephaly' and leave it at that. Yakovlev and Wadsworth (1946) after a detailed histological study of two cases suggest the name 'schizencephaly'. They considered the defect to be a true cerebral agenesia, with congenital clefts of the cerebral mantle, and hydrocephalus. Cohn and Neumann (1946) consider 'severe bilateral porencephalia'* to be the proper classification, while Picaza *et al.* (1955) coin the term 'hydroencephalodysplasia'. By this they connote any defect in the cerebral mantle associated with hydrocephalus. They describe 23 cases covering the range of specimens illustrated in this paper. Their series included three post-mortem examinations and 10 exploratory craniotomies. This classification has much to recommend it despite the clumsiness of name, as it links hydranencephaly with a wider range of similar disorders.

Crome and Sylvester (1958) suggest 'hydrencephaly' as being a more appropriate name, since, in fact, the lesion is quite unrelated to anencephaly.

Morbid Anatomy

Hydranencephaly. No two specimens of hydranencephaly are exactly alike. The average case shows at the base of the skull, sitting above the tentorium cerebelli, two prominent knuckles, representing the basal ganglia. From these, there sweeps forward into the anterior cranial fossa a thin membrane composed of immature nervous tissue elements and adherent pia-arachnoid (Bettinger, 1940): the membrana gliae limitans. This may peter out, or may continue closely applied to the pia-arachnoid

* Strictly porencephaly means a loss of cerebral substance resulting in a fistula between subarachnoid space and lateral ventricle. It is held that such fistulae are probably rare and most authors, including the writer, use the term largely to connote a loss of cerebral substance of such degree that the cavity of the lateral ventricle may be seen from the outside.

as a paper-thin sheet which passes posteriorly to join the posterior portion of the cerebral vestiges, thus enclosing the ventricular cerebrospinal fluid and separating it from the sub-arachnoid space. The cells in this membrane are immature and often contain a large connective tissue admixture. Moser (1952) suggests these few glial cells may survive by virtue of a better blood supply.

The lateral and third ventricles are absent, the choroid plexus lying free, posterior to the basal ganglia. Rarely the choroid plexus may be absent (Yakovlev and Wadsworth, 1946).

The olfactory nerves are usually present, although they may be represented by localized thickenings in the nervous tissue sheet mentioned above (Moser, 1952). Najman (1953) was unable to find a first nerve in his case.

The optic nerves are usually present; microphthalmia is common. Although the other cranial nerves are usually present, the fourth has been noted to be absent (Gerundo, 1955).

Detailed neuroanatomical and histological descriptions of the lesion are extant, those of Yakovlev and Wadsworth (1946) and of Moser (1952) being particularly valuable. The latter paper also contains an exhaustive review of the German language literature.

Porencephaly. The morbid anatomical picture of porencephaly varies with the extent of the cerebral defect. The range of defects commonly met with can be seen in the illustrations in this paper.

Causes

If one examines the literature one finds that hydranencephaly has been blamed on many agents, viral, chemical and vascular.

Kåss (1951) reports on a male infant who died at the age of 8 weeks with severe hydrocephalus and microphthalmia. The child had been delivered by caesarian section as the foetal skull had, on radiographic examination of the maternal pelvis, looked abnormally large. At birth it proved to be 46 cm. in circumference enlarging to 50 cm. just before death. Laboratory tests for toxoplasmosis and syphilis were negative. Necropsy revealed the typical picture of hydranencephaly: a normal cerebellum, pons and medulla, the cerebrum being represented by a mass of white tissue the size of a walnut. The mother of this child had suffered from epidemic hepatitis in the second and third months of pregnancy.

Ilberg (1901) found histological evidence of syphilis in the liver and spleen of his case.

Thelander, Shaw and Piel (1953) found the meninges of the right frontal region to be diffusely infiltrated with small calcified flecks and suggested that a toxoplasma infection may have been responsible.

Conte, McCammon and Christie (1945), reviewing proven cases of congenital abnormality in children whose mothers had rubella in the first three months of pregnancy, found that four of the five cases which they had themselves collected, showed cerebral aplasia. Unfortunately, they do not state what they mean by this term.

Olive and DuShane (1953) describe a child whose mother had attempted at the fourth month of pregnancy to induce abortion by the intra-uterine injection of formaldehyde. At necropsy shortly after birth her child showed bilateral absence of the anterior halves of the cerebral hemispheres.

The mother of Case 3 of Yakovlev and Wadsworth (1946) had made repeated attempts to induce abortion by the ingestion of unspecified drugs. At autopsy the child, aged 21 months, showed the classical intracranial features of hydranencephaly.

Johnson (1938) describes a 6½-month-old child who had always been weak, and whose weight gain since birth was but 420 g. Enlargement of the head and microphthalmia were the salient clinical features. The head showed the phenomenon of transillumination, air studies revealing an external hydrocephalus and a small brain. Necropsy confirmed the radiological picture, frontal lobes, fornix, mammillary bodies and the aqueduct of Sylvius being absent. The third ventricle was rudimentary. The mother, it transpired, had been given *x*-ray therapy 17, 24 and 32 days after the probable date of conception, receiving in all 1,150 r in air. The uterus, it was estimated, received 400 r.

Gerundo (1955) suggested, on histological grounds that the choroid plexus might be abnormally active, thus causing a severe internal hydrocephalus.

Marburg and Casamajor (1944) consider that venous thrombosis or stasis, especially of the deep cerebral veins is the most likely cause.

Spielmeyer (1905) found that the vessels on the surviving cortex, especially those of the cerebellum, were thin walled, dilated and showed a remarkable tendency to become confluent and form cavernous spaces.

It thus seems that either there may be a multiplicity of aetiological agents, or that all the maternal infections reported are fortuitous.

A major divergence of opinion exists as to whether the cortical tissue is laid down and then destroyed, or whether it is suppressed *ab initio*.

Crosby (1944) who examined Watson's (1944) Case 1 from an anatomical aspect, was of the opinion, after she had lightly packed the covering membranes which lay over the rudimentary cerebral vestiges, that the brain had developed for some five months and then regressed. Edinger and Fischer (1913) described in their case convolution-like indentations of the pia-arachnoid and deduced that the cortical tissue had developed normally and then regressed. Picaza *et al.* (1955) describe in one of their cases pseudo-convolution-like markings on the skull bones but felt that they were due to pressure from the underlying fluid rather than showing any relationship with the cortex. Not all cases of hydranencephaly show a covering membrane, let alone convolutional markings.

Spatz (1935) describes experiments to show that foetal brain tissue reacts differently from that of the adult if subjected to gradual deprivation of blood supply, stating that such tissue liquefies leaving lacunae of cysts, whereas the adult would respond by 'fibrosis'. Becker (1949) injected into the carotid artery of newborn puppies a paraffin-olive oil mixture with a melting point of 40° C. Necrosis and gradual resorption ensued, the end result in a year or so being a smooth walled cavity enclosed by a 'hydranencephalic' membrane. Vogel and McClenahan (1952) occluded the major cerebral arteries of day-old chicks by electrocautery. By this means they produced marked retardation of cortical development, the forebrain in survivors often remaining as a thin walled cyst. Thelander *et al.* (1953) found in the liver and spleen of their case large collections of pigment which they believed must represent destroyed brain tissue. Gerundo (1955) noted that in the cytoplasm of the cells of the choroid plexus there were many pigment granules which he stated were haematogenous. Moser (1952) describes the thin layer of brain tissue present as having abundant haemosiderin deposits. Others such as Najman (1953) have been unable to find any haemosiderin, or, at most, a very little (Hunziker, 1947).

Yakovlev and Wadsworth (1946) point out that if the brain develops and is then destroyed, it would be reasonable to assume that the dependent cell stations would show secondary destruction or atrophy, e.g. the nuclei of origin of the thalamo-cortical projection fibres. They demonstrated that this is so in adult cases of porencephaly following cerebral thrombosis, while in hydranencephaly there is rather hyperplasia of these basal nuclei. They feel that the anatomical lesions are consistent with a primary inhibition of differentiation of the neural tube before the second month of intra-uterine life. This contention is supported by the timing of the foetal injury in the cases of Johnson (1938) and Kåss (1951).

A similar condition has been reported in calves (Whittem, 1957).

Racial Incidence. The condition has hitherto been reported, in the main, in persons of Caucasian stock. Picaza *et al.* (1955) found several cases among mulattoes; Montagné and Du'ong Bá-Bành (1950) found one in a Vietnamese infant; Gerundo (1955) found one in a Chamorro child in Guam. This paper records, for the first time, to the best of the author's belief, its occurrence in Chinese. Search of the autopsy records of the Singapore General Hospital for the past 10 years (over 20,000 autopsies) failed to reveal the condition in either Indians, Pakistanis, Sikhs, or Malayans.

Clinical Features

Hamby, Krauss and Beswick (1950) suggest the following points as being of use in the systematic investigation of the condition.

(1) **Recognition of Characteristic Clinical Pattern.** Picaza *et al.* (1955) aptly described the condition as one of functional decortication. As this term could well be applied to any child under the age of 3 weeks it is not until this age is reached that suspicions that something is amiss may be aroused. The most constant feature is a hyper-irritability. Moro's, the startle, and grasp reflexes are usually present. The child may whine incessantly in a mechanical sort of way, presenting as it does so, an indifferent facies. The child usually suckles normally and feeding difficulties may not arise until shortly before death. The eyes are frequently affected showing inco-ordinate movement, marked strabismus and nystagmus. Microphthalmia is not uncommon. The pupils react to light (Yakovlev and Wadsworth, 1946), the optic discs are, as a rule, pale. Simple optic atrophy was noted in half of the cases reported by Picaza *et al.* (1955). Dissociated movements were noted by Olive and DuShane (1953).

The most constant physical finding is enlargement of the head which usually occurs in the first few weeks, although this feature may not become apparent until about the third month. Some show this cranial enlargement at birth; in only one, however, had the enlargement required craniotomy to effect delivery (Hurowitz, 1936).

Various authors have from time to time described assorted concomitant findings. Both of Watson's (1944) cases were severely jaundiced. Picaza *et al.* (1955) found five of his hydroencephalodysplasia cases to be very cyanosed at birth. Half of his series showed convulsions, either generalized or Jacksonian, a feature not noted by any other author. Thelander *et al.* (1953) noted difficulty in establishing respiration, while Edinger and Fischer (1913), Kåss (1951), and Moser (1952) noted that their cases had great difficulty in maintaining the body temperature. Such features, although they may assume importance in a particular child are of little consequence in diagnosis.

In short, the picture is one of little spontaneous activity, cranial enlargement and eye disturbances.

(2) **Transillumination of Head.** This simple test was first described by Strasburger (1910) who noted that in cases of severe hydrocephaly, i.e. those in which the residual brain tissue was less than 1·0 cm. thick, a light placed behind the child's head in a darkened room would cause it to glow red all over. Onsalo (1933) constructed a special box for this purpose. In recent years the test has been brought to the notice of paediatric workers by Hamby *et al.* (1950). They liken the colour obtained on transillumination to the orange-red light which emanates from an ornamental Japanese lantern. The mother of one of the cases of these latter authors noticed that her child's head glowed when it was brought near a table lamp.

Despite its simplicity this test can give a very accurate picture of the intracranial contents as any residual brain tissue shows up as a dark patch. When the head is transilluminated the pupils appear to glow red. Most authors seemed convinced of the value of the test (Beswick, 1948; Najman, 1953).

(3) **Fontanelle Puncture.** Fontanelle puncture seems to yield little information and in the days before antibiotics was a sure passport to a septic meningitis (Johnson, 1938). The cerebrospinal fluid protein may be raised (Thelander *et al.*, 1953), or normal (Picaza *et al.*, 1955). There may be xanthochromia at the first tap; the cell count varies from child to child. Injection of a dyestuff into the spinal theca may show communication with the remnants of the ventricular system. The degree of agenesis is not related to the presence or absence of spinal block. When the fluid is withdrawn it may be replaced by air. If sufficient is injected the state of the cranial cavity may be very accurately determined, especially if the head be inverted when taking skiagrams. Watson (1944) counsels against this procedure as one of his cases had severe convulsions after the fluid was removed. Picaza *et al.* (1955) concur, remarking that air studies are not well tolerated, as if the degree of agenesis is severe they are not infrequently followed by respiratory syncope and infection.

(4) **Electroencephalography.** E.E.G. shows a characteristic complete absence of electrical activity over those areas which lack subjacent brain tissue. Relatively minor defects can be detected in this way. All writers seem agreed that this is a constant finding.

(5) **Angiography.** Angiography presents a pathognomonic picture. As the internal carotid is usually hypoplastic the operative procedure is difficult (Picaza *et al.*, 1955). Care should be taken not to mistake superficial temporal and meningeal arteries for cerebral vessels. Thelander *et al.* (1953) showed the circle of Willis to be intact but very small. They felt this was an effect, rather than the cause, of the lack of brain tissue.

Diagnosis ante-mortem is of importance if only to obviate the adoption of children suffering from this defect, as in Case 1 of this series. Beswick (1948) reports on a child who had been adopted at the age of 1 week having been pronounced normal by a competent paediatrician. Parents should be warned of the poor prognosis. Edinger and Fischer (1913) describe a child who lived to the age of 3½ years, the oldest on record.

Case Histories

Case 1.—J.J.N., a 2-week-old female Chinese, was admitted to the General Hospital, Singapore, on April 12, 1957, for investigation of jaundice and cranial enlargement. The child had been adopted on the fourth day of life. At that time the foster-mother had noticed mild jaundice. The child had suckled poorly, slept fitfully and 'lay crying all night'. Since birth the child had had several twitching attacks each lasting a few seconds. The birth weight was 8 lb., the child being delivered in hospital at term. The officiating midwife noticed no abnormality.

On admission the child was mildly icteric, the skull circumference 38 cm. The temperature was subnormal and remained so for the rest of the child's life. The pupils reacted to light sluggishly, the eyes remaining turned downwards at all times. There was a rough systolic murmur near the cardiac apex, the muscle tone was hypertonic, the tendon reflexes present.

The haemoglobin was 83% (Haldane); the blood group B Rh positive. Coombs direct test was negative, as was the Kahn. A subdural tap was performed, the fluid withdrawn being moderately xanthochromic. The protein level was 100 mg. %, the cell count four lymphocytes per c.mm. Cerebrospinal fluid obtained from the spinal theca gave identical results. Shortly after this procedure all the limbs became spastic. On April 22, 1957, the left eye was noted to be purulent. Despite treatment the process advanced and the cornea became ulcerated. Evisceration was recommended and carried out by Dr. K. Y. Wong. The child died on May 2, 1957.

An autopsy was performed (861/57). Externally the child was mildly jaundiced; the skull circumference was 41 cm. A small high interventricular septal defect was noted in the heart. The pulmonary valve was bicuspid. Both cerebral hemispheres were absent. Two small knuckles of white matter, 2 cm. in diameter, represented the basal ganglia. There were no lateral or third ventricles. The choroid plexus was stained a light brown, and was seen to lie posterior to and between the twin eminences of the basal nuclei. A thin membrane about 2 mm. thick swept forward from the basal nuclei into the anterior cranial fossa which continued, closely applied to the pia-arachnoid, across the vault of the skull, to rejoin the cerebral vestiges posteriorly, thus enclosing the cerebrospinal fluid. The optic and other cranial nerves were present (Fig. 1).

Medulla, pons, cerebellum and tentorium cerebelli appeared normal. The carotid vessels, although smaller than usual, appeared otherwise normal. The circle of Willis was intact, although anterior and middle cerebral vessels were practically vestigial, petering out after a centimetre or so.

The superior sagittal sinus was present, but the lumen was much smaller than is usual. The inferior sagittal sinus appeared normal.

Histology. The membrane anterior to the basal nuclei varied considerably in thickness from place to place. Essentially it showed two fairly distinct layers: that in apposition to the subarachnoid space and its attendant vessels was composed principally of large polyhedral cells with an abundant cytoplasm and a rich fibrillary network: that exposed to the intracerebral C.S.F. showed much fewer glial cells, a corresponding decrease in fibrils, and many more microglial cells (Fig. 2). There was no ependymal lining. No neurones were seen.

One small ependymal inclusion was present 2 mm. below the surface of the right basal nuclei.

Haemosiderin was present in moderate amounts in that part of the membrane near the subarachnoid space, and a great deal more in the tissues of the subarachnoid space themselves. Occasional haemosiderin and lipid-laden macrophages were seen throughout the nerve tissue of the basal nuclei.

Morphologically the choroid plexus appeared normal. The H. and E. section showed the choroidal cells to be masked by a light brown pigment. This proved to be haemosiderin.

Comment. Classical hydranencephaly, moderate amounts of haemosiderin present in addition to ependymal inclusions in the basal nuclei. The membrana gliae limitans is similar in structure to that described by others (Crome and Sylvester, 1958).

Case 2. S.M.K., a 9-day-old Chinese female infant, was admitted to the General Hospital, Singapore, on July 3, 1958, with a history of progressive jaundice since birth, associated with difficulty in feeding.

Examination revealed a marked jaundice and a slight pyrexia. Heart and lungs appeared normal. Reflexes and muscle tone appeared normal. Haemoglobin 100% (Haldane), W.B.C. 19,600 per c.mm., the differential count being within normal limits. The child died 12 hours after admission.

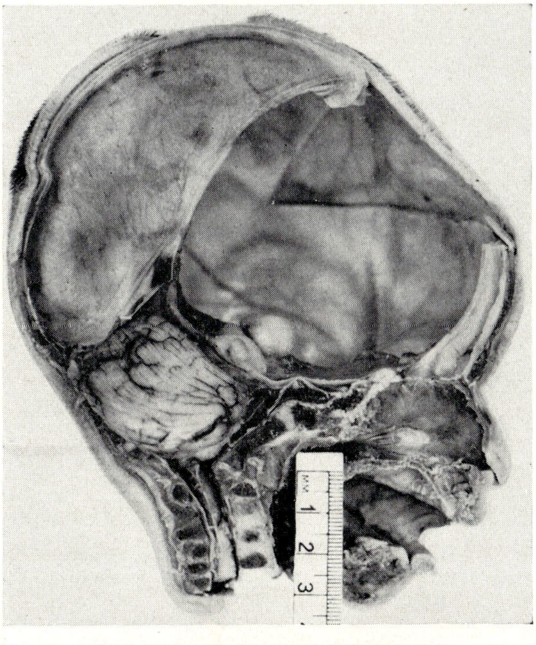

Fig. 1.—(P.M. 861/57). Skull hemisected in saggital plane. Normal cerebellum, intact falx, and basal nuclei are clearly seen.

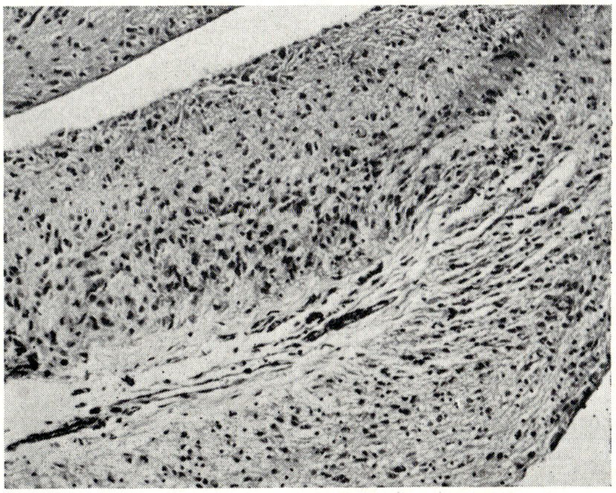

Fig. 2.—(P.M. 861/57.) The membrana gliae limitans, folded over on itself in this section, is composed of two fairly distinct layers: an outer cellular, in apposition to the subarachnoid space, and an inner, less cellular, in contact with the intracerebral C.S.F. H. and E. × 110.

At autopsy (1283/58) a few minor areas of collapse were noted in both lungs, principally at the free margins of the lower lobes. The skull was of normal external diameter (29·8 cm.). Removal of the calvarium revealed a classical case of hydranencephaly. There was complete absence of the cortex.

The dura was covered by a thin brownish, relatively tough layer of tissue which showed numerous dimples and lacunae (Fig. 3).

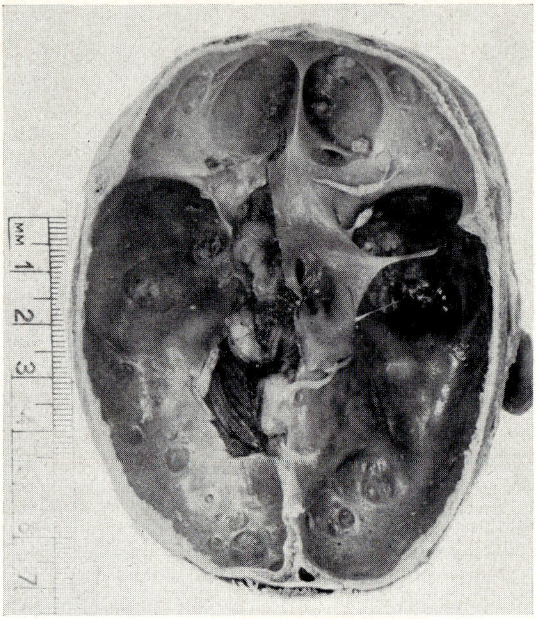

FIG. 3.—(P.M. 1283/58.) Absence of cerebral hemispheres, a distorting band of membrane in right middle cranial fossa, and numerous dimples, or ulcers, in dura.

In this membrane were numerous focal collections of mid-brown amorphous pigment, the largest measuring about 0·5 cm. across.

The basal nuclei were very small. Between them and attached medial to them was a prolongation of the brown layer of tissue mentioned above, which swept up over the basal nuclei to merge with that flooring the cranial fossae. At the right antero-lateral margin a strand of tissue distorted this funnel shaped opening to the right so that on casual inspection the basal nuclei were not visible. At the base of this opening lay the choroid plexus and the opening of the acqueduct of Sylvius. Beneath the membrane lay well formed optic and olfactory nerves. The remainder of the cranial nerves and the pituitary gland appeared normal. The circle of Willis was intact although the blood vessels were very small. The middle cerebral vessel passed just posterior to the chiasma to ramify on the inferolateral surfaces of the funnel mentioned previously.

HISTOLOGY. In the region of the basal nuclei the dura was lined on its inner surface by varying thicknesses of primitive nerve cells, heavily infiltrated with microglia. From place to place there were breaks in the dura, resulting in small undermined 'ulcers' corresponding to the dimples seen with the naked eye. The lumina of these hiatuses were filled with haemosiderin-laden foamy macrophages (Figs. 4, 5). In the floor of the lesion numerous other haemosiderin-laden cells were present, in addition to a few capillary vessels. An occasional calcified area was present. In the six sections taken from varying areas of the cranial fossae, the subarachnoid space was for the most part obliterated.

The choroid plexus appeared normal, showing light haemosiderin deposits in the choroidal cells.

No ependymal inclusions were seen in the sections taken.

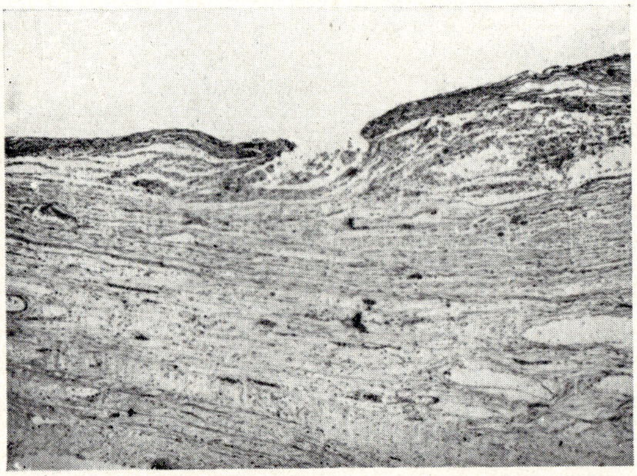

FIG. 4.—(P.M. 1283/58.) Cross-section of one of the ulcers seen in Fig. 3. Dense layer on surface represents membrana gliae limitans, below which subarachnoid space is obliterated, all being densely adherent to dura. H. and E. × 35.

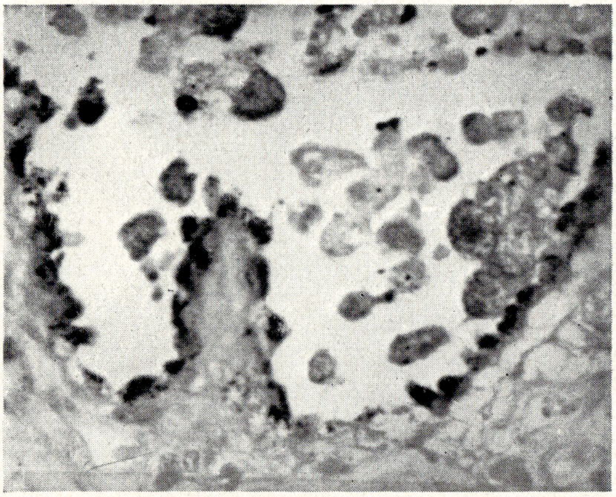

FIG. 5.—(P.M. 1283/58.) The floor of another such ulcer is lined, and lumen filled, by foamy haemosiderin laden macrophages. Perls' stain × 375.

Comment. Partial obliteration of the subarachnoid space has been noted by Crome and Sylvester (1958). This specimen shows classical hydranencephaly associated with massive haemosiderin deposits.

Case 3. L.K.E., a 6-day-old female Hylam child, was admitted to the General Hospital, Singapore, on February 11, 1958, with a history of refusal to take feeds since birth. Three days after birth the child was noticed to be jaundiced, the pigmentation deepening rapidly, till on the seventh day the serum bilirubin was 20 mg. %. Examination of the spinal cerebrospinal fluid revealed a yellowish fluid whose protein level was 200 mg. %, the other findings being within normal limits. The child declined rapidly, dying on March 1, 1958.

An autopsy was performed (396/58). Externally the child was deeply jaundiced. The liver was enlarged soft and greenish in colour. The spleen appeared normal.

The cranial cavity showed classical hydranencephaly (Fig. 6). The basal nuclei were rather small, the left being 15 mm. across, the right 10 mm. There was a vestigial hippocampus on the right side only, with a few rudimentary gyri on the under-surface. On the same side, adjacent to the right pituitary fossa, was a small pedunculated mass of nerve tissue 15 mm. in diameter. Between the basal nuclei lay the floor of the third ventricle and the choroid plexus.

A thin tenuous sheet of nerve tissue swept forward from the anterior aspect of the basal nuclei into the anterior cranial fossa. The olfactory nerves were represented by cord-like localized thickenings in the sheet. The optic and other nerves were present. The eyes appeared normal. The circle of Willis was present, but all vessels, including the posterior cerebral artery, were very small.

Histology. The choroid plexus showed brownish discolouration, but otherwise appeared normal. Stains for haemosiderin revealed heavy deposits within the choroidal cells.

Sections of basal nuclei and hippocampus showed haemosiderin to be present not only on the surface, but within the brain substance. The liver was congested, the sinusoids appearing wider than is usual. The portal tracts were normal, containing a few focal collections of nucleated cells. There were moderately large amounts of haemosiderin within all the liver cells. The spleen was congested and showed moderate amounts of haemosiderin.

Comment. Classical hydranencephaly with heavy intracranial, and moderate intrahepatic deposits of haemosiderin.

Case 4. N.M.K., a 2-year-old Chinese female infant was admitted to the General Hospital, Singapore, on May 9, 1958, complaining of difficulty in feeding. During the previous two days there had been episodes of epistaxis, associated with a mild fever.

The head was much enlarged, being 42 cm. in circumference. There was bleeding from the mouth and nose, deep cyanosis of the lips, and marked pallor of the mucous membranes. The child was flaccid and in coma. Crepitations were heard at the lung bases. Death occurred four hours after admission.

An autopsy was performed (891/58). A confluent bronchopneumonia was found in all lobes of both lungs. The spleen was multilobulate, being represented by nine spleniculi held together by delicate connective tissue strands.

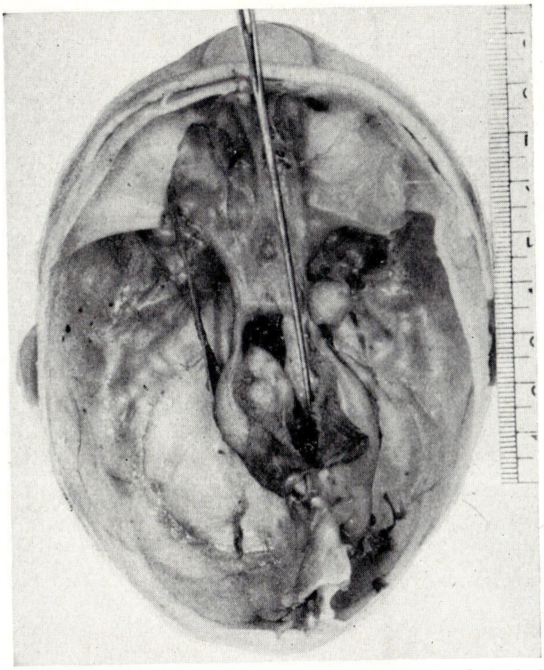

Fig. 6.—(P.M. 396/58). The intracranial appearances of classical hydranencephaly. Probe is in aqueduct of Sylvius, and is flanked on either side by choroid plexuses.

The brain showed a lesser degree of defect than the previous specimens. A fine membrane enclosed 580 ml. of cerebrospinal fluid and was attached to the lips of the defects. On the left there was a thin rudimentary hippocampus with normal appearing gyri on the under surface. The convolutions on the upper surface were broad, indistinct and flattened. On the right side was a lobe which was neither truly temporal nor occipital measuring 3×2 cm. Both lobes showed numerous areas of brownish deposit, both on the surface, and within their substance, measuring up to 5 mm. across. The cranial nerves were present. The eyes were very small. The choroid plexuses appeared normal. The cerebellum was represented by a large single cyst, which contained within its lumen the choroid plexus of the fourth ventricle.

The circle of Willis was present although the vessels were all very small. The vertebral, basilar and posterior cerebral vessels appeared normal. The sagittal sinuses appeared normal.

HISTOLOGY. The lateral margin of the superior surface of the hippocampus showed the point of attachment of the thin nervous tissue sheet. This contained a few nerve cells and moderate numbers of microglia. This sheet became closely applied to the substance of the occipital lobe, blending with the underlying tissue, yet it could be followed as a separate entity on account of linear deposits of calcium. These corresponded more or less, but not entirely, to the haemosiderin deposits. Multinucleate macrophages were seen in relation to these calcium deposits (Fig. 7). Elsewhere within the lobe haemosiderin lay in two forms, either loosely scattered or within foamy macrophages several of which were multinucleate.

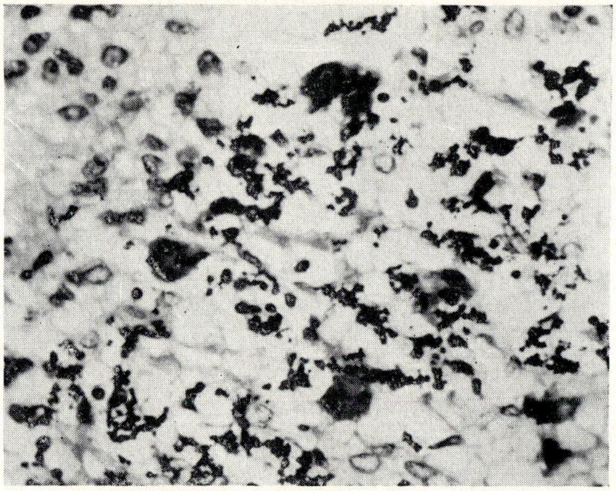

FIG. 7.—(P.M. 891/58). Several multinucleate giant cells surrounded by calcium deposits. H and E. × 375.

A similar appearance was seen in the temporal lobe and in the basal nuclei. Many foamy haemosiderin-laden macrophages were to be found in the Virchow-Robin spaces of small blood vessels (Fig. 8).

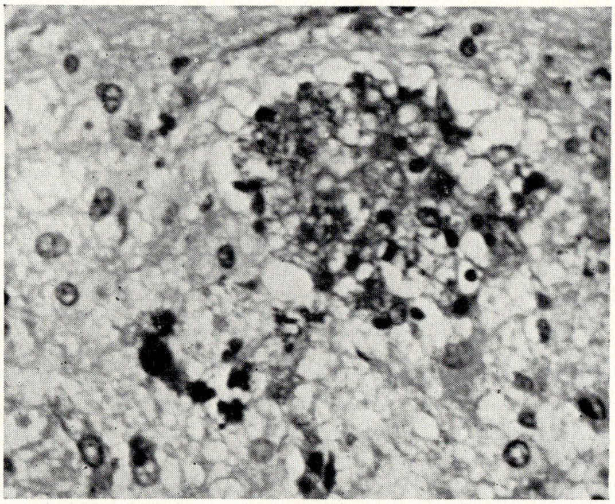

FIG. 8.—(P.M. 891/58.) Numerous foamy macrophages in a Virchow-Robin space. H. and E. × 375.

The wall of the cystic cerebellum was thin, and showed some post-mortem change. Within it there were numerous blood vessels, in whose Virchow-Robin spaces there were large aggregations of haemosiderin-laden foamy macrophages. In several of these areas cholesterol clefts were seen (Figs. 9, 10).

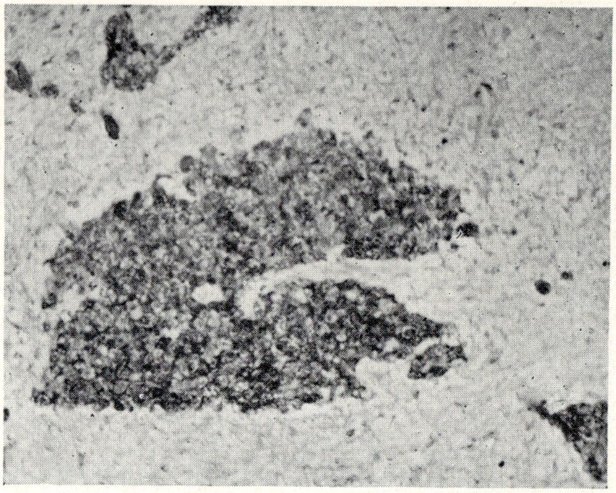

FIG. 9—(P.M. 891/58.) Haemosiderin-laden macrophages in cerebellum. Perls' stain × 35.

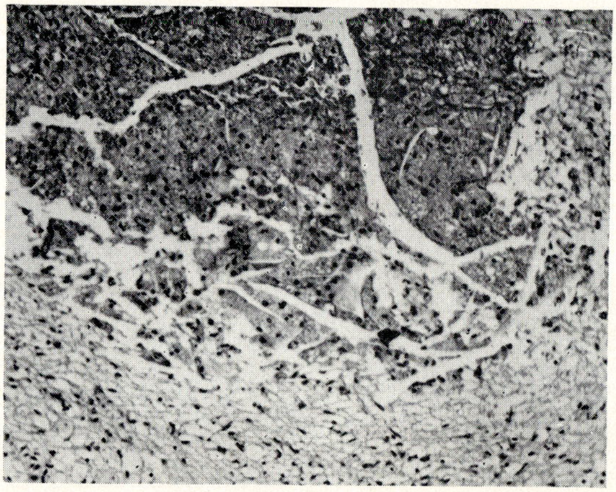

FIG. 10.—(P.M. 891/58.) Cholesterol clefts within aggregations of macrophages. H. and E. × 110.

The choroid plexuses appeared normal, although heavily laden with haemosiderin (Fig. 11).

In a few places the retina showed various degrees of focal atrophy, the ganglion cells being absent and the nuclear layers represented by one or two cells. Elsewhere, although the retina had stripped off the pigment epithelium, appearances were normal. No haemosiderin was seen.

Comment. Classical hydranencephaly showing massive intracranial deposits of haemosiderin. In addition, in this case, there is a cerebellar lesion and mutilobulation of the spleen.

Case 5. T.S.H., a 2-year-old female Teochew, was admitted to the General Hospital, Singapore, on March 12, 1958, with a complaint of inability to eat for the past four months. The child was very emaciated, and had multiple septic sores on the scalp. Crepitations were heard at the right lung base. The child died eight hours after admission.

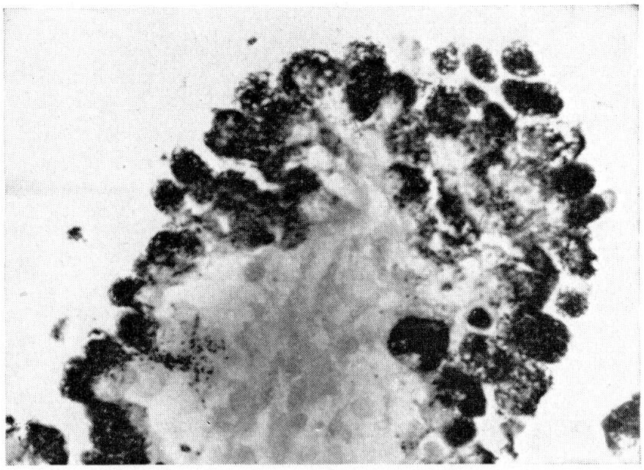

FIG. 11.—(P.M. 891/58.) Heavy deposits of haemosiderin within choroidal cells. Perls' stain × 375.

An autopsy was performed (475/58). The lungs showed early bronchopneumonic change. The brain showed the appearance of hydranencephaly (Fig. 12). The basal nuclei were very much enlarged measuring 3·5×2×2 cm. Towards the occiput were rudimentary hippocampi. From the anterior end of the basal nuclei a thin sheet of nerve tissue sprang forward to blend imperceptibly with the pia and enclose the cerebrospinal fluid. The circle of Willis was intact although anterior and middle cerebral vessels were very small. The eyes appeared normal.

HISTOLOGY. Sections taken at intervals of 2 mm. through the basal nuclei showed that the medial aspect was clothed by an incomplete flattened ependymal layer of cells. Beneath this lay a rather condensed layer of glial tissue at the under surface of which numerous blood vessels were seen. Within the substance of the grey matter at one place about 20 ependymal rosettes were present (Fig. 13).

Haemosiderin was present in very small amounts, not in the superficial layers but deeper down within the basal nuclei, principally in paravascular macrophages.

More posteriorly in the basal nuclei several larger vessels were found just beneath the surface and in this region haemosiderin was much more prominent, although by no means heavy.

Section of the hippocampus showed haemosiderin in moderate amounts deep within the remnant, more superficially, and within the walls of the attached membrana gliae limitans. A small ependymal inclusion was present.

Comment. Classical hydranencephaly occurring in an older infant, showing ependymal inclusions in the basal nuclei and hippocampus. Haemosiderin is present in small quantities.

Case 6. T.S.S., a 1-month-old female Teochew child, was admitted to the General Hospital, Singapore, on July 19, 1957, and was immediately placed on the dangerously ill list. The mother stated that the child's head had started to enlarge rapidly two weeks after birth. The child, a first baby, had been delivered in hospital, weighed 7 lb. 5 oz. at birth and had been regarded as quite normal. Feeding, as is common in Singapore, had been on condensed milk. Twenty-four

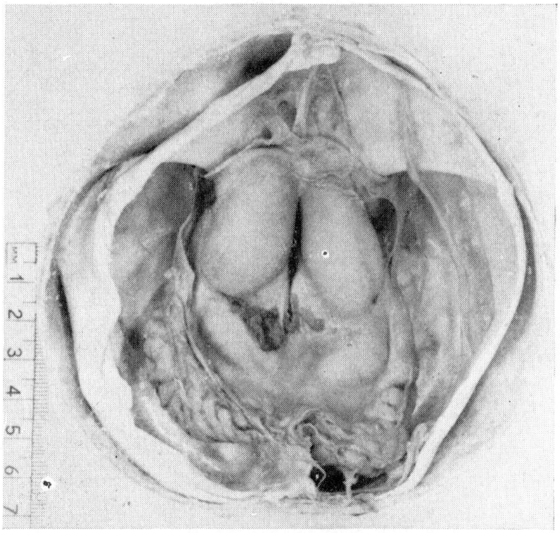

FIG. 12.—(P.M. 475/58.) Gross enlargement of basal nuclei and rudimentary hippocampi.

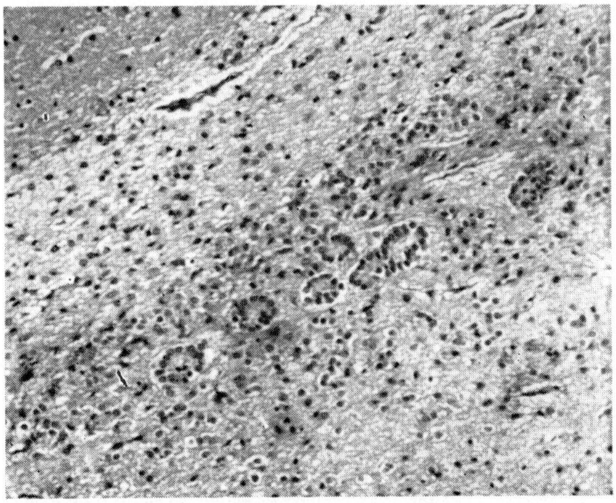

FIG. 13.—(P.M. 475/58). Ependymal rosettes within basal nuclei. H. and E. × 110.

hours before admission the child had become fevered, had vomited and then passed several loose stools.

The nutritional state of the child was poor, the pharynx inflamed; auscultation over the lung bases revealed many crepitations. The tendon reflexes were present although muscle tone and power were poor. Despite treatment with antibiotics the child died next day.

An autopsy (1543/57) was performed. The lungs showed patches of bronchopneumonic consolidation. The circumference of the skull was 42 cm. The cranial cavity contained about 500 ml. of clear cerebrospinal fluid. There was complete absence of the cerebral hemispheres (Fig. 14). The basal nuclei were much enlarged measuring on the right 2×1·5×1·5 cm., and on the left 3×1·5×1·5 cm. Posterior to the enlarged basal nuclei, partially filling the posterior cranial fossa,

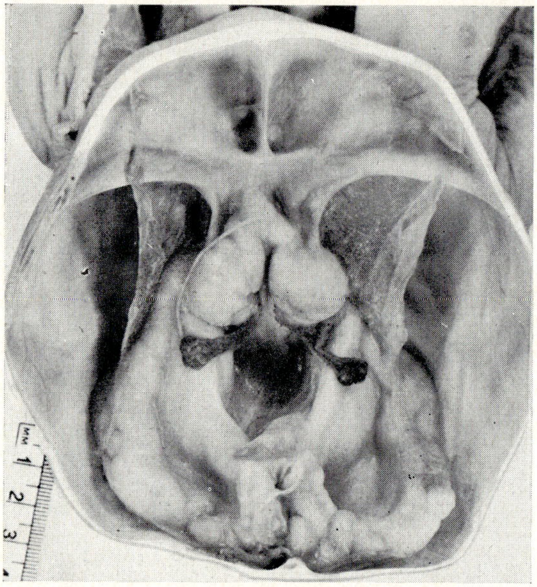

FIG. 14.—(P.M. 1543/57.) Appearances of hydranencephaly, the thin membrane being particularly well seen in this specimen.

were imperfectly formed hippocampi, attached to the margin of which was a thin tenuous membrane which enclosed the cerebrospinal fluid. The under-surface of the hippocampi showed a few incomplete gyri. Between the hippocampi there emerged from two foramina, separated by a thin antero-posterior band of nerve tissue, the choroid plexuses. Running from the anterior end of this band a cord of nerve tissue 2 mm. thick ran to find attachment to the crista galli. The blood vessels although small appeared normal. The cranial nerves appeared normal.

HISTOLOGY. The basal nuclei appeared normal. Covering them was a dense glial layer some 2 mm. thick which showed, from place to place, focal collections of round cells, mainly close to small ependymal inclusions (Fig. 15). The nuclei were not covered by ependyma. Haemosiderin was present in large amounts about 1 mm. beneath the surface, and deeper within the grey matter. A small amount of haemosiderin was seen beneath the surface of the hippocampi remnant.

The membrana gliae limitans contained large numbers

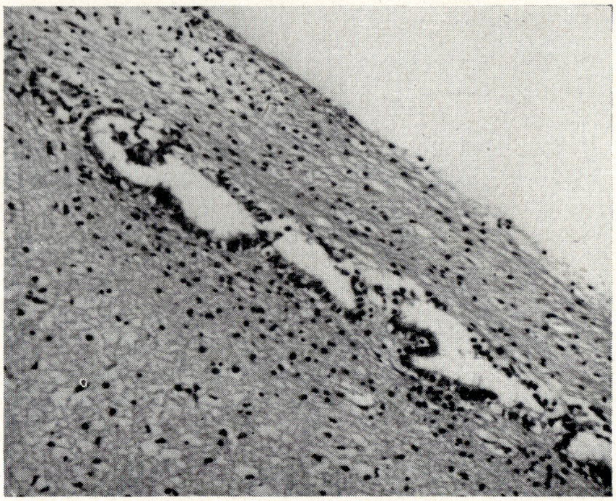

FIG. 15.—(P.M. 1543/57.) Ependymal inclusions just below surface of basal nuclei. H. and E. ×110.

of glial cells with an abundant cytoplasm and a rich fibrillary network. A small number of microglial cells were seen. The subarachnoid space, and the interstitial tissues around it, contained moderate numbers of haemosiderin laden macrophages.

The choroid plexus, which contained large amounts of haemosiderin, was otherwise normal.

Comment. Classical hydranencephaly. The basal nuclei show small ependymal inclusions. A moderate amount of haemosiderin is seen throughout.

Case 7. T.O.P., an 18-month-old female Chinese child, was admitted to the General Hospital, Singapore, on May 22, 1958, with a complaint of diarrhoea, cough and fever of two days' duration.

She was a small undersized child with a cleft palate. Temperature 99° F. Harsh rales were heard at the lung bases. The child died four days after admission.

An autopsy was performed (1002/58). There was a patent foramen ovale in the heart. Both lungs showed advanced bronchopneumonic change.

On opening the skull, a most bizarre abnormality was encountered (Fig. 16). There was complete absence of occipital, parietal and temporal lobes. In the region of the frontal lobes the anterior cranial fossa was partly filled by an oval plaque of cortical tissue. This showed no division into right and left lobes, gyri traversing the anterior surface from side to side without vestige of interruption. The superior and lateral edges of the brain tissue were rolled over, and attached to the margin of the defect posteriorly was a thin tenuous, often

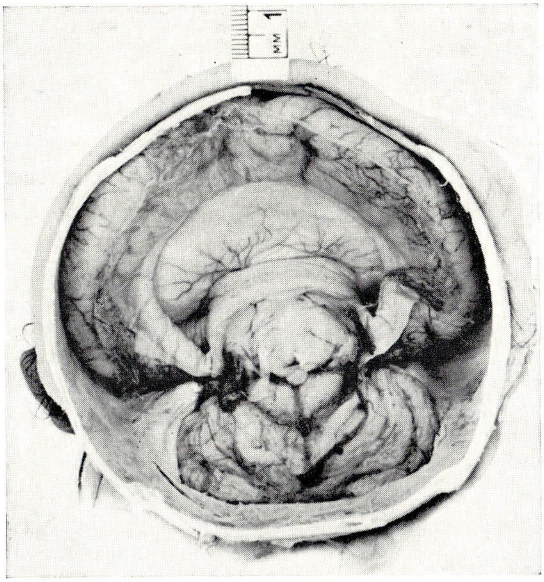

FIG. 16.—(P.M. 1002/58.) The peculiar frontal remnant with its folded-over posterior edge. The cerebellum and mid-brain are seen more posteriorly.

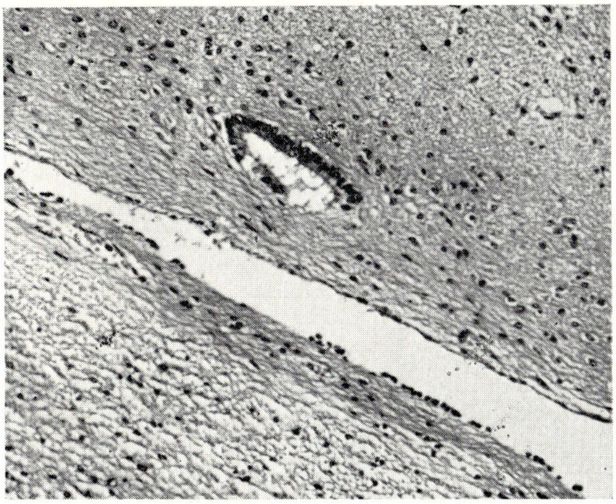

FIG. 17.—(P.M. 1002/58.) Ependymal inclusion within cortical tissue at folded-over edge seen in Fig, 16. H. and E. × 110.

incomplete membrane. Apart from this vestige there was no other brain tissue above the tentorium cerebelli. Through the hiatus in the anterior portion of the tentorium a small portion of pons was visible, in the middle of which was a small foramen, the opening of the aqueduct of Sylvius.

Rudimentary optic nerves were present, but no olfactory nerve was seen. The cerebellum and pons appeared normal. The choroid plexus of the fourth ventricle was present and appeared normal; that of the lateral ventricle was not seen. The crista galli was absent. The falx cerebri was absent. The lateral and sigmoid sinuses were in their correct places. The circle of Willis was intact. The middle cerebral vessels were vestigial. The anterior cerebral vessels ramified over the frontal remnant.

HISTOLOGY. Sections of the cervical cord and pons appeared normal.

A section taken from the left lateral edge of the remnant in the anterior cranial fossa showed relatively normal cortical tissue, the cells being of the size, shape and orientation of those normally seen in the cortical areas. The inner aspect of the folded over posterior edge was lined by ependyma. Immediately subjacent to this lining several small ependymal inclusions were present (Fig. 17). Stains for haemosiderin revealed a few scattered focal collections of the iron containing pigment scattered, apparently at random, throughout the cortical tissue. The haemosiderin was for the most part present within macrophages.

Section of the kidney showed within the cells of the collecting convoluted tubules a dark brown granular pigment which did not take up the iron stain.

Comment. Bizarre anomaly with preservation of an anomalous frontal lobe. Ependymal inclusions seen, and small amounts of haemosiderin present.

Case 8. O.G.S., a male Hokkien aged 4 years, was brought to the General Hospital, Singapore, by his father on April 5, 1953, and died on his way from admission room to the ward. He had had a fever for several days and had vomited several times on the day of admission. The referring general practitioner had noted the temperature to be 100·2° F., slight rigidity of the neck, enlarged inflamed tonsils, harsh breath sounds, and had made a diagnosis of bronchopneumonia.

An autopsy was performed (581/53). The lungs showed a patchy bronchopneumonia. The right cerebral hemisphere seemed to be slightly enlarged, with a dilated lateral ventricle. The left cerebral hemisphere was represented by a rudimentary occipital lobe and hippocampus (Figs. 18 and 19). Along the free margin of the defect there was a fine sheet of nerve tissue which spread laterally from the large basal nuclei (2·5 × 4 cm.) to peter out after some 2 cm. This nervous tissue sheet was supported by the pia arachnoid. The cerebellum appeared normal. The cerebral peduncles were present and appeared to be equal in size. The choroid plexus was normal. The circle of Willis was present, the vessels on the left being very small, the middle cerebral vessel running laterally as far as the edge of the nerve tissue sheet.

HISTOLOGY. The basal nuclei were covered by a thin layer of white matter, beneath which numerous small blood vessels ran parallel to the surface. There was no ependymal covering, or ependymal inclusions. Small focal collections of haemosiderin were present throughout, principally in relation to small blood vessels.

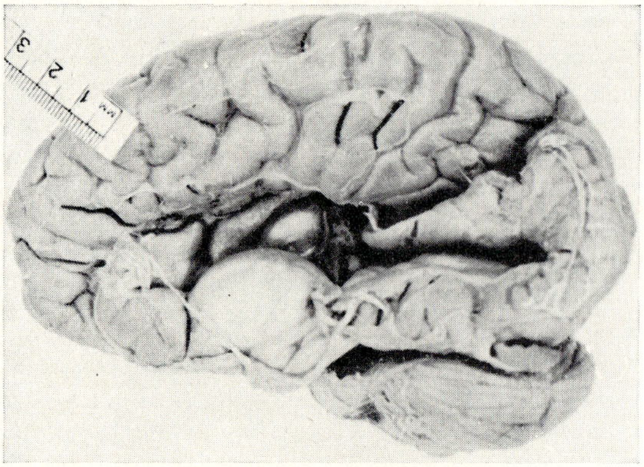

FIG. 18.—(P.M. 581/53.) Lateral view of brain showing absence of left frontal, temporal and parietal lobes.

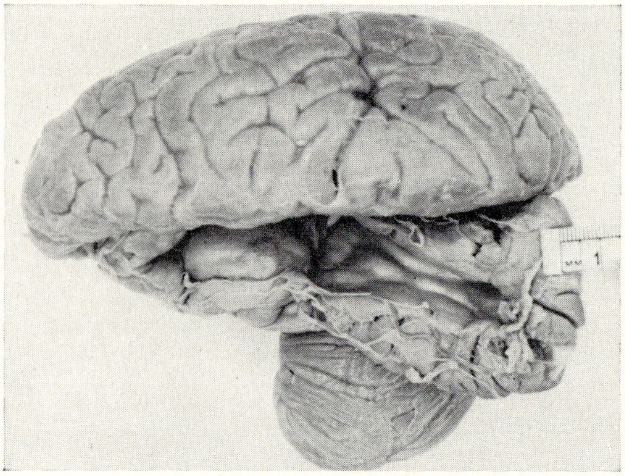

FIG. 19.—(P.M. 581/53.) Same brain as in Fig. 18, seen from above. Note the large basal nuclei.

The roof of the exposed posterior horn of the left lateral ventricle was not lined by ependyma. Very small amounts of haemosiderin were present.

The cells of the choroid plexus looked somewhat degenerate. Haemosiderin was present in moderate amounts.

Sections of the right and left middle cerebral arteries revealed no abnormality, that on the right being approximately double the size of the other.

Comment. In this specimen there is agenesis of the left cerebral hemisphere only. The portions remaining are those supplied by the posterior cerebral artery. Moderate amounts of haemosiderin are present in the brain tissue near the defect, there being no evidence of fibrosis.

Case 9. L.L.P., an 8-year-old Chinese girl, was admitted to the General Hospital, Singapore, on September 13, 1958, with a complaint of cough, fever, dyspnoea, and fits of one day's duration. The temperature was 103·6° F. Numerous coarse crepitations were heard at the lung bases. The child was noted to be a mental defective, and was the size of a 3-year-old. She died shortly after admission.

An autopsy was performed (1821/58). The principal lesion in the brain was the presence of two defects on the supero-lateral aspects of both frontal lobes. The defect on the right was the smaller, being 3 cm. long and approximately 1 cm. wide. Around the defect was an area of microgyria extending over the greater part of the hemisphere. A similar appearance obtained on the left. Here the defect was larger, measuring 3 cm. by 2 cm. and was again surrounded by microgyri (Fig. 20). Only the occipital lobe on this side showed gyri that approached normal.

Both defects communicated with enlarged lateral ventricles, the septum pellucidum being absent. The corpus callosum was present. The inner walls of the ventricles were irregular and showed several rests of grey matter, principally around the defects. This irregularity of the inner surface extended into the posterior horns. The circle of Willis was normal. The end branches of the left and right middle cerebral arteries ramified over the surface of the brain posterior to the defects.

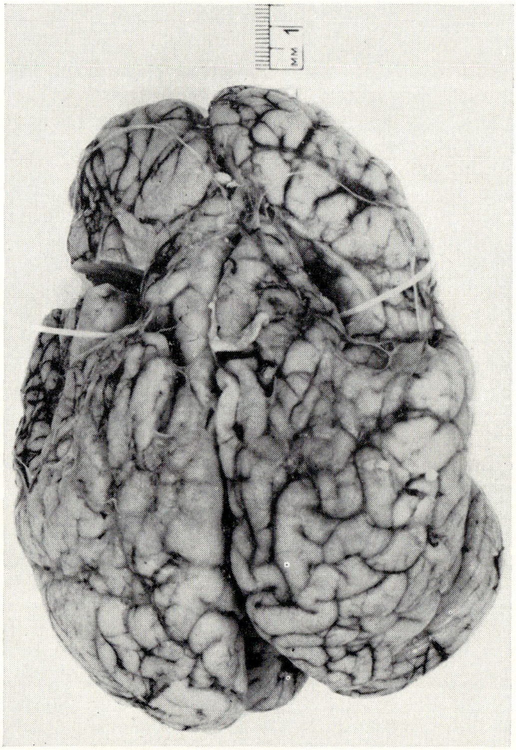

FIG. 20.—(P.M. 1821/58.) Brain viewed from above shows white plastic rod passing into one porencephalic defect and out of another on opposite side.

The choroid plexuses and the remainder of the brain appeared normal.

HISTOLOGY. At the edge of the lateral lip of the defect on the left side, on the superior aspect of the brain, was an area composed of glial fibres and blood vessels, No fibrous tissue was seen. This region was heavily infiltrated with microglia. Small amounts of haemosiderin were present, principally lying free in the subjacent brain. The walls of these blood vessels were heavily stained by a brownish pigment of uncertain nature.

Small petechial haemorrhages were seen in the basal nuclei. Within the left basal nucleus, running laterally, and well removed from the aqueduct of Sylvius were a series of small ependymal inclusions (Fig. 21). The choroid plexus was normal. No haemosiderin was present.

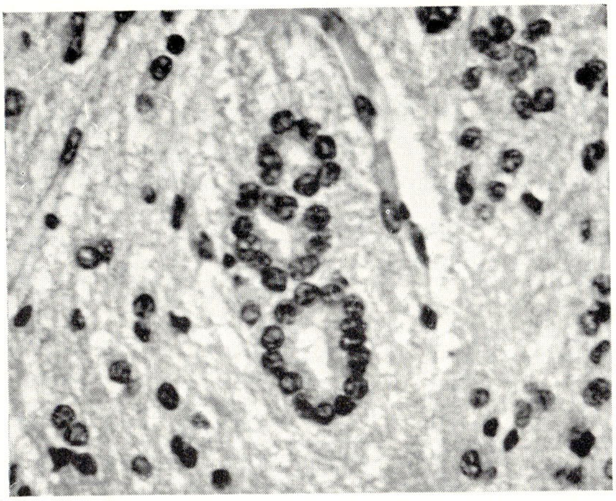

FIG. 21.—(P.M. 1821/58.) Ependymal cells deep within left basal nucleus. H. and E. × 375.

Comment. Bilateral porencephaly. The micropolygyria suggests pre-natal origin (Greenfield, Blackwood, McMenemey, Meyer and Norman, 1958). Very small amounts of haemosiderin present, also peculiar ependymal inclusions.

Case 10. N.P.K., a male Teochew, aged 7 years, was brought to the General Hospital, Singapore, on February 7, 1952. Investigation by H.M. Coroner revealed that the boy, who had been in apparent good health, had fallen when running about with his friends. He lost consciousness and died on his way to hospital.

An autopsy was performed (191/52). The contents of the thoracic and abdominal cavities appeared normal. Externally the head, which appeared larger than usual, showed a contusion 3 cm. in diameter over the right forehead. Under the scalp there was a haematoma corresponding in size to the surface contusion. The left lateral ventricle communicated with the subarachnoid space through an opening about 2 cm. in diameter in the region of the Rolandic fissure some 1·5 cm. from the vertex (Fig. 22). The subarachnoid space over the left cerebral hemisphere was distended with blood-stained cerebrospinal fluid. The sulci of the right hemisphere were less prominent than usual. The left middle cerebral vessel passed between the temporal and frontal lobes to gain the surface of the brain and then passed upwards in the sulcus below the defect. No thrombosis or other lesion was seen in the vessel. There was no septum lucidum but the corpus callosum was present.

HISTOLOGY. A section taken from the lip of the defect showed that at the under-surface of the lip within the brain substance there were large collections of macrophages containing haemosiderin. In this area the Virchow-Robin spaces of several of the small blood vessels showed a dense cellular infiltrate composed of round cells and larger macrophages (Fig. 23). No fibrous tissue was seen in the region.

The right middle cerebral artery showed no abnormality. The choroid plexus contained small amounts of haemosiderin.

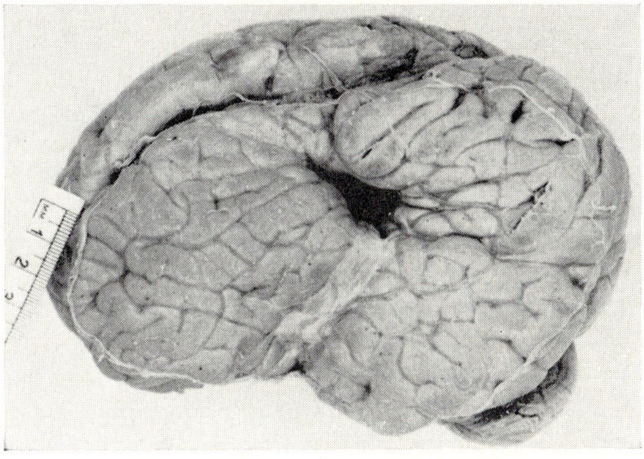

FIG. 22.—(P.M. 191/52.) Single left sided porencephalic defect. Note smooth edge. (Cf. Fig. 25.)

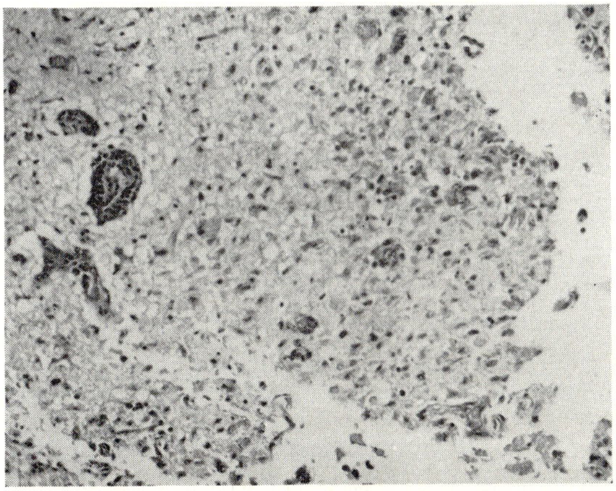

FIG. 23.—(P.M. 191/52.) The lip of the porencephalic defect contains many macrophages, a large number of which are within the Virchow-Robin spaces. H. and E. × 110.

Comment. Unilateral porencephaly with haemosiderin laden macrophages at the lip of the defect.

Case 11. G.H.W., a 3-year-old male Teochew child, was admitted to the General Hospital, Singapore, on November 7, 1957, with a complaint of cough and fever of five days' duration. The child appeared to be a mongol. Crepitations were heard over the lung bases. There was a rough systolic murmur maximal in intensity over the third left interspace. Despite treatment the child died three days later.

An autopsy was performed (2331/57). The lungs showed a well marked bronchopneumonia. There appeared to be early bronchiectatic change in the right upper lobe.

The heart was enlarged, weighing 85 g. There was marked hypertrophy of the right ventricle and a marked dilatation of the right auricle associated with a large atrial septal defect and a high ventricular septal defect. The ductus arteriosus was patent.

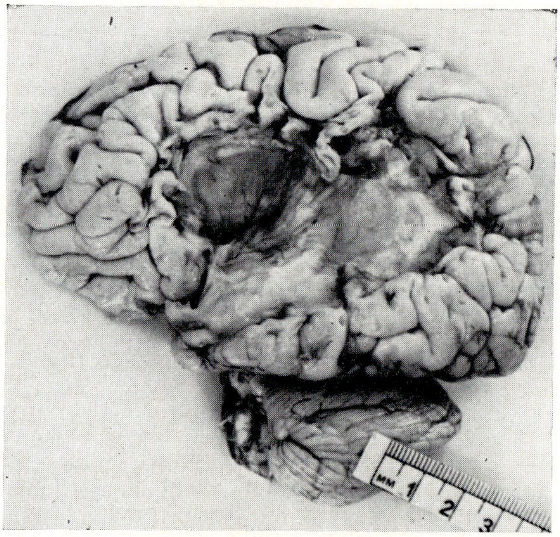

FIG. 24.—(P.M. 2331/57.) A well marked parietal lobe defect. The covering membranes have been largely removed to show sclerogyria at lip of defect, and tough dense membrane separating sub-arachnoid space from lateral ventricle.

The left cerebral hemisphere showed a large defect of the temporo-parietal region 8 × 5 cm. in size (Fig. 24). This defect had a well marked sclerosed rim to which a thickened, dense, highly vascular, pia arachnoid was firmly adherent. The fibrous tissue which bridged the defect was closely applied to a very thin layer of nerve tissue approximately 1 mm. thick, thus separating the membranes from the cavity of the lateral ventricle.

Search for a left middle cerebral artery failed to reveal even the vestiges of such a vessel, although the anterior and posterior cerebral vessels were present in their usual situations. The vessels on the right side of the circle of Willis were normal.

There was no other intracranial abnormality.

HISTOLOGY. A section taken through the middle of the defect in the coronal plane revealed a dense fibrovascular membrane firmly adherent to the lip. This blended imperceptibly with the subjacent white matter (Fig. 25) which in consquence contained many capillaries and much fibrous tissue. Large numbers of foamy macrophages were present in this area. The membrane was continued downwards closely applied to a thin nervous tissue septum which separated it from the cavity of the lateral ventricle. This septum was lined on the ventricular aspect by ependyma. Stains for haemosiderin showed the region of sclerogyria and the subjacent brain tissue and the membrane to contain much iron, both free and in macrophages, the latter being grouped round vessels and in the Virchow-Robin spaces. Elsewhere the membranes appeared normal.

Comment. Defect in temporoparietal region associated with apparent absence of middle cerebral artery. This lesion is probably post-natal in origin.

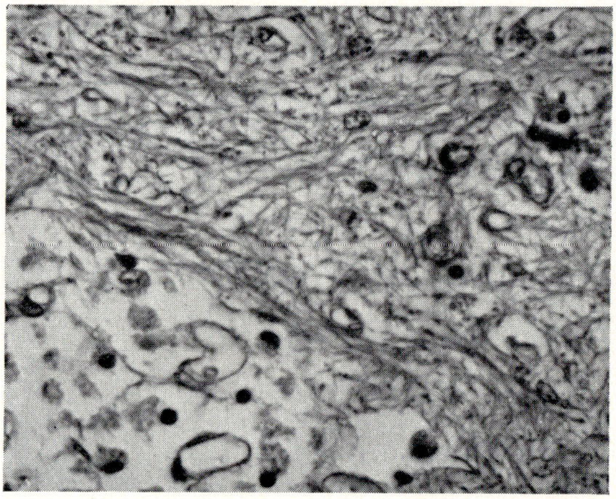

FIG. 25.—(P.M. 2331/57.) Interlacing fibrous tissue within brain substance at edge of defect. Note numerous capillaries. Picro-Mallory × 375.

Discussion

If one assumes that there is a primary inhibition of differentiation of the primitive nervous tube before the end of the second month of intra-uterine life, the mechanism of production of the subsequent defects is easily explained. This was realized as long ago as 1889 by Schattenberg who wrote, 'if one assumes that in the area of the cerebral mantle corresponding, for example, to the future central convolutions, there occurs in the cerebral wall an arrest of growth in thickness, then in the course of continual growth of the brain the surrounding parts will first overhang this area and then will eventually develop a pit formed by the rolled in surface of the brain'. The larger the area affected the more likely is it that pressure of the ventricular cerebrospinal fluid will force the cerebral remnants against the membranes. Thus the larger the area initially damaged, the more like classical hydranencephaly and the less like porencephaly will the end result be.

This theory assumes that some toxin or viral agent causes the initial lesion. It is true that many neurotropic viruses have a predilection for particular parts of the mature nervous system, and there seems no reason why a foetal brain should not similarly be affected. If this thesis be accepted, then one must perforce envisage a process with local death of a relatively small amount of developing nervous tissue, perhaps a cubic centimetre for a foetus up to the second month of intra-uterine life, and at most a small amount of local haemorrhage. One would not, if an adherent of this hypothesis, expect to see small, let alone large, amounts of haemosiderin in the cranial cavity, or elsewhere at autopsy. This theory does, however, neatly explain the presence of ependymal cells within the caudate nucleus or at the margin of a porencephalic defect as being a portion of the original pia-ependymal seam of a cleft in the cerebral mantle (Yakovlev and Wadsworth, 1946).

The contention that the damage occurs before the end of the second month is supported indirectly by the finding of a multilobulate spleen in Case 4.

Hitherto, this very rare malformation has been recorded only in association with gross anomalies of the heart and great vessels (Miller, 1925; Greenberg 1957). As the splenic primordium, an area of thickening in the dorsal mesogastrium, is first seen when fusion of the atrio-ventricular cushions is taking place about the thirty-sixth day after conception, it has been held that the factors interfering with the proper fusion of the cushions may also affect the developing spleen. If this be so, then it may be that such an agent acting about this time could also damage the developing brain.

If one accepts Yakovlev and Wadsworths' interpretation of the significance of ependymal inclusions (as in Cases 1, 5, 6, 7 and 9) and the supporting evidence of the multilobulate spleen, then it becomes clear that the defects in fact do have their origin at an early date. The presence of considerable amounts of haemosiderin in such cases is, however, very difficult to explain away.

As Kundrat (1882) has pointed out in his study of porencephaly, the distribution of most of these defects is within that of the Sylvian arteries. This fact, he felt, was in itself sufficient grounds for believing that all such defects were due to softenings, the end result of local circulatory disturbances.

This is an attractive theory. In substantiation one would expect to find either diseased blood vessels, or at least organized thrombi within their lumina, such as Yakovlev and Wadsworth (1946) were able to demonstrate in their Case 5. While it is true that complete recanalisation might occur after a thrombotic episode, that no trace should be found of such a lesion in any of the vessels in this series stretches credibility. The presence of haemosiderin could easily be explained as haemorrhage from damaged blood vessels in the area of softening might well be expected. The later in intra-uterine life the episode occurred, and the more extensive it proved to be, the larger the amount of haemosiderin one might expect to see. Similarly if death occurred a long time after birth much of the haemosiderin originally found might be metabolized.

In this series the presence of various amounts of haemosiderin in all of the specimens has been amply demonstrated; no arterial or venous lesions have been, however, found.

An intracranial haemorrhage, subsequent to softening, or as a primary event, would be associated with local destruction of nervous tissue. The liberated blood pigments, and lipids, would be taken up either by surviving microglia, or by blood-borne macrophages. Much of the free pigment in the ventricular space would percolate into the Virchow-Robin spaces with the cerebrospinal fluid to become fixed there in macrophages (Figs. 8, 9, 23) some of the remainder being fixed by the macrophages in the meninges. Much of the rest could pass into the blood stream via the Pacchionian bodies, after passing through the fourth ventricle and the aqueduct of Sylvius, and thence become trapped in liver and spleen.

The small amount of lipid seen in the sections may be accounted for by the imperfect myelination of the foetal brain.

Much stress has been laid on the survival of the basal ganglia. If it be remembered that the basal nuclei receive blood not only from the anterior cerebral artery, which supplies the anterior portion of the putamen, but also by the middle cerebral artery, via its medial striate branches, and by the postero-medial central branches of the posterior cerebral artery (Gray, 1954) it will be readily appreciated that this portion of the brain is in a much better position to withstand loss of a portion of its blood supply than most others. It will have been observed that, with the exception of Case 7, the portions of brain missing are, in the main, those supplied by the anterior and middle cerebral arteries. In Case 8 with unilateral absence of a portion of the left hemisphere, the parts remaining are the cuneus, lingual gyrus, uncus, hippocampal gyrus, and the interior temporal gyrus, a textbook description of the distribution of the posterior cerebral artery.

This predilection for those areas of the brain which do not receive blood from the vertebral system, might suggest some anomaly of the carotid system. Although hypoplastic, no anomaly was found in these vessels in this series. Granted many of the carotid vessels were small in calibre, but with the exception of Case 11 (which is discussed separately below), all were present, patent and appeared normal on histological examination. The hypoplasia is almost certainly secondary to the loss of cerebral substance.

The choroid plexus was in all cases normal. Apart from a superficial deposition of haemosiderin nothing could be found that would in any way support the contentions of Gerundo (1955) that there might be an excessive production of cerebrospinal fluid.

Case 11 shows many features not found in other specimens: an absent blood vessel, and a defect in the cerebral substance covered by a dense vascular fibrous tissue sheet firmly welded to a rim of distorted nerve tissue. This sclerogyria is very suggestive of repair following some vascular disturbance. Although Yakovlev and Wadsworth (1946) maintain that such a disturbance occurring either before or after birth may give rise to the same end result, it is felt that in the light of descriptions by others, such as that of Raskin (1958), a picture such as is seen in Case 11 is much more likely to be the result of birth trauma to a vessel.

Rabson (1952) describes a case of porencephaly in a newborn baby in which abnormally large blood vessels were present in the brain tissue at the margin of the defect. Numerous haemosiderin-laden macrophages were present in the ventricular cavity and in the overlying meninges. He does not state whether there was any lesion of the blood vessels supplying the area affected. The absence of fibrous tissue around this defect which must have been there before birth, suggests that it is only in the post-natal lesion of vascular origin that fibrous tissue will be formed at the edge of such a defect.

While Yakovlev and Wadsworth (1946) considered that both hydranencephaly and porencephaly might have two origins, some in which there was a primary agenesis, and others caused by some encephaloclastic process, ante-natal or post-natal, the author feels that such a division is not entirely satisfactory having demonstrated features of both haemorrhage and agenesis in several of his specimens.

Summary

Six cases of hydranencephaly, and five of lesser degrees of cerebral defect, occurring in Chinese children, principally female, are presented.

The clinical diagnosis of hydranencephaly is discussed.

Various aetiological theories are discussed in the light of the gross and microscopic appearances of the specimens.

It is concluded that (*a*) hydranencephaly and the porencephalies represent varying degrees of the same pathological process, and (*b*) the evidence available does not support any one cause for the lesions to the exclusion of another.

I wish to thank Professor R. Kirk for kind help and criticism, Dr. C. Elaine Field for permission to quote briefly from case histories, and Dr. T. Balasingham (Cases 2, 3, 4, 5), Dr. E. B. La'Brooy (Cases 6, 8, 10) and Dr. W. K. Gin Lee (Case 7) of this Department for access to their autopsy notes and material. Thanks are also due to Mrs. Mary Low who cut the sections, Mr. V. Nalpon who took the photographs, Messrs. Liu, Rai and Seerangan who assisted with the specimens, and Mr. P. A. Samuel who typed the script.

References

Becker, H. (1949). *Dtsch. Z. Nervenheilk.*, **161**, 407 and 446.
Beswick, W. F. (1948). *N.Y. St. J. Med.*, **48**, 2364.
Bettinger, H. F. (1940). *Med. J. Aust.*, **2**, 375.
Cohn, R. and Neumann, M. A. (1946). *J. Neuropath. exp. Neurol.* **5**, 257.
Conte, W. R., McCammon, C. S. and Christie, A. (1945). *Amer. J. Dis. Child.*, **70**, 301.
Crome, L. and Sylvester, P. E. (1958). *Arch. Dis. Childh.*, **33**, 235.
Crosby, E. C. (1944). Quoted by Watson (1944), *loc. cit.*
Cruveilhier, J. (1835). *Anatomie Pathologique du Corps Humain*, Vol. I, Livraison 15, plate 4. J. B. Baillière, Paris.
Edinger, L. and Fischer, B. (1913). *Pflüg. Arch. ges. Physiol.*, **152**, 535.
Gerundo, M. (1955). *J. Phillipp. med. Ass.*, **31**, 546.
Gray, H. (1954). In Gray's *Anatomy*, edited by Johnston, T. B. and Whillis, J. 31st ed., p. 747. Longmans Green, London.
Greenberg, S. D. (1957). *A.M.A. Arch. Path.*, **63**, 333.
Greenfield, J. G., Blackwood, W., McMenemey, W. H., Meyer, A. and Norman, R. M. (1958). *Neuropathology*, p. 328. Edward Arnold. London.
Hamby, W. B., Krauss, R. F. and Beswick, W. F. (1950). *Pediatrics*, **6**, 371.
Hunziker, K. (1947). *Mschr. Psychiat. Neurol.*, **114**, 129.
Hurowitz, J. (1936). *Schweiz. Arch. Neurol. Psychiat.*, **38**, 207.
Ilberg, G. (1901). *Arch. Psychiat. Nervenkr.*, **34**, 140.
Johnson, F. E. (1938). *J. Pediat.*, **13**, 894.
Kåss, A. (1951). *Acta. paediat. (Uppsala)*, **40**, 239.
Kundrat, H. (1882). *Die Porencephalie: Eine anatomische Studie.* Leuschner and Lubensky, Graz.
Marburg, O. and Casamajor, L. (1944). *Arch. Neurol. Psychiat. (Chicago)*, **52**, 170.
Miller, A. J. (1925). *Amer. J. Path.*, **1**, 467.
Montagné and Du'ong Bá-Bành (1950). Extrême-Or. méd., No. 3, p. 54.
Moser, E. (1952). *Ann. paediat. (Basel)*, **179**, 193.
Najman, E. (1953). *Ibid.*, **181**, 249.
Olive, J. T. and DuShane, J. W. (1953). *Amer. J. Dis. Child.*, **85**, 43.
Onsalo, E. (1933). *Arch. esp. Pediat.*, **17**, 410.
Picaza, J. A., Cardelle, G. and Martin Jimenez, R. (1955). *J. Neurosurg.*, **12**, 535.
Potter, E. L. (1952). *Pathology of the Fetus and the Newborn*, p. 431. Year Book Publishers, Chicago.
Rabson, S. M. (1952). Cited by Potter, E. L., p. 409, *loc. cit.*
Raskin, N. (1958). *Arch. Pediat.*, **75**, 332.
Schattenberg, R. (1889). *Beitr. path. Anat.*, **5**, 119.
Spatz (1935). Quoted by Watson (1944), *loc. cit.*
Spielmeyer, W. (1905). *Arch. Psychiat. Nervenkr.*, **39**, 807.
Strasburger (1910). *Dtsch. med. Wschr.*, **36**, 294.
Thelander, H. E., Shaw, E. B. and Piel, J. J. (1953). *J. Pediat.*, **42**, 680.
Vogel, F. S. and McClenahan, J. L. (1952). *Amer. J. Path.*, **28**, 701.
Watson, E. H. (1944). *Amer. J. Dis. Child.*, **67**, 282.
Whittem, J. H. (1957). *J. Path. Bact.*, **73**, 375.
Yakovlev, P. I. and Wadsworth, R. C. (1946). *J. Neuropath. exp. Neurol.*, **5**, 169.

INCIDENCE OF RHEUMATIC FEVER IN CEYLON

BY

STANLEY DE SILVA

From the Lady Ridgeway Hospital for Children and the Maternity Hospitals of Colombo, Ceylon

(RECEIVED FOR PUBLICATION NOVEMBER 19, 1958)

Conflicting views have been expressed about the incidence of rheumatic fever in the tropics. Fernando (1939) concluded that 'rheumatic infection is an important cause of heart disease among the hospital class of the population of Ceylon and accounts for from anything between one-fourth to one-fifth of the total cardiovascular diseases among them. The incidence, manifestations, virulence and progressiveness of rheumatic carditis scarcely differ in any important respects from what is seen in non-tropical countries'.

While this is probably quite true of rheumatic infection in the adult, it was thought fit to investigate its incidence and manifestations in the children in this country.

Incidence

In studying the incidence of the disease as it occurs in children in Ceylon, I have contrasted the incidence as seen in the Children's Hospital, Colombo, the General Hospital, Colombo, and The Hospital for Sick Children, Great Ormond Street, London. The Lady Ridgeway Hospital for Children (400 beds) is the only hospital for children in Ceylon and admits about 18,000 children up to the age of 12 years annually, with a daily out-patient attendance of about 1,200. It draws its patients mainly from Colombo but also from all parts of the island. The General Hospital (1,500 beds) is for adults only. I have chosen The Hospital for Sick Children, Great Ormond Street, for comparison as it is the largest children's hospital in England and also has about 400 beds.

I shall deal with the incidence of rheumatic fever in the Children's Hospital, Colombo, in the period 1953-57. During this five-year period 70,292 children were admitted to the hospital, and, of these, 560 were admitted for some form of rheumatic disease, an incidence of 0·7% of the total admissions. Two hundred and two of this group had signs of carditis, i.e. nearly 35% of those admitted for rheumatic disease and 0·2% of the total admissions (Table 1).

A more detailed study was made of the incidence in my unit of 75 beds during this period. It was found that out of a total of 13,656 children admitted there were 107 patients (0·78%) with rheumatic manifestation, and 34 of these children (i.e. 0·2% of the total admissions) showed cardiac manifestations. It will be seen again that in this unit 31% of the rheumatic children showed evidence of cardiac involvement. The pattern of the disease, in my unit, therefore, is very similar to that seen in the hospital as a whole.

There were 12 deaths due to rheumatic disease during this period, almost every death being due to cardiac disease, a death rate of 2% amongst those admitted with infection.

When this picture is compared with that seen at the General Hospital, Colombo, during the period 1952-57, out of a total of 355,401 admissions there were 3,538 admissions for rheumatic infection (i.e. 0·7% of admissions), amongst whom were 2,848 patients with carditis (0·8% of the total admissions).

TABLE 1

ADMISSIONS TO THE LADY RIDGEWAY HOSPITAL FOR CHILDREN: 1953-57

Admissions	1953	1954	1955	1956	1957	Five-year Total
Total per year	10,884	12,174	14,154	16,551	18,529	70,292
For rheumatic disease	99 (0·9%)	88 (0·5%)	81 0·5%)	128 (0·8%)	164 (0·8%)	560 (0·7%)
For carditis	33 (0·3%)	67 (0·4%)	28 (0·3%)	41 (0·2%)	33 (0·1%)	202 (0·2%)
Percentage of carditis among cases admitted for rheumatic infection	33%	76%	31%	44%	51%	35%

So, although the incidence of rheumatic infection is nearly the same in the child and in the adult, the incidence of carditis is four times greater in the latter. Further, while 202 children, or only 35% of the children with rheumatic infection, showed evidence of established cardiac involvement on admission, 2,848 adults, 80% of the rheumatic patients, showed cardiac involvement (Table 2).

It can therefore be concluded that in the tropics cardiac manifestations are more common in adults or occur at a much later age than in temperate zones.

I have compared these findings with those of Cox and Schlesinger (1955) who analysed the incidence of the disease as seen at The Hospital for Sick Children, Great Ormond Street. In showing a steady decline in the severity of the disease and its incidence in relation to hospital admissions during the last 30 years, they found that in the period 1919-20, out of 2,519 admissions to the hospital, there were 262 patients with rheumatic infection (10·8% of total admissions) of whom 148 showed evidence of cardiac involvement (56·5%). There were 22 deaths, a mortality of 8%. During the period 1946-50, out of 59 patients admitted with rheumatic infection, 35 showed evidence of cardiac involvement (59%). The incidence was much less during 1949-50, when, out of 4,917 admissions, only 31 (0·6%) showed evidence of rheumatic disease. In 1957, out of 19 patients admitted with rheumatic infection, 10 (52%) had evidence of cardiac involvement (Cox and Schlesinger, 1956).

While taking into consideration the marked decline in incidence of rheumatic infection as seen from the admissions to that hospital in recent years, one is struck with the very high incidence of carditis amongst those admitted with rheumatic infection: 56%, 59% and 52%, for the respective periods quoted.

It must be conceded that the pattern of the disease as seen in The Hospital for Sick Children, Great Ormond Street, may not be a true reflection of that seen in England as a whole. Nevertheless, although the incidence of the disease in this hospital has fallen from 10·8% to 0·7% to 0·2% in the three periods 1919-20, 1946-50, and 1957, the incidence of carditis in each period is 56%, 59%, and 52%, as compared with Ceylon where only 35% of children with rheumatic manifestations showed evidence of cardiac disease.

Clinical and Other Factors

The clinical manifestations in children are similar to those in adults in Ceylon though there are certain differences. For instance, children do not appear to have repeated attacks of swelling in the joints or pain flitting from joint to joint. Those we see in hospital have perhaps two or three attacks of joint pain, and the knee, ankle and, though rarely, the elbow, appear to be the only joints affected. The episode is usually trivial and almost forgotten by the time the cardiac symptoms and signs manifest themselves. Moreover, the attacks subside rapidly in a few days. This contrasts with the picture seen in young adults: if they do give a history of joint pains they emphasize the severe nature of the attacks and their frequent recurrence over a period of years.

Cutaneous Manifestations. These are extremely rare in this country. During the last five years we can recall only three cases in this hospital in which subcutaneous nodules were present. It is amusing to see students searching for skin manifestations in the dark skinned children in this country. They are not seen even in the lighter skinned children of Ceylon. One of the rare examples of subcutaneous nodules is shown in Fig. 1.

TABLE 2

INCIDENCE OF RHEUMATIC DISEASE IN FOUR UNITS

	Lady Ridgeway Hospital for Children	My Unit (L.R.H.C.)	General Hospital Colombo	Great Ormond Street			
Period	1953-57	1952-57	1952-57	1919-20	1946-50	1949-56	1957
Admissions: Total per year	70,292	13,656	355,401	2,519		4,917	7,968
For rheumatic diseases	560 (0·7%)	107 (0·7%)	3,538 (0·1%)	262 (10·8%)	59	31 (0·6%)	19 (0·2%)
For carditis	202 (0·2%)	34 (0·2%)	2,848 (0·8%)	148 (0·6%)			10 (0·1%)
Percentage of carditis among cases admitted for rheumatic diseases	36%	31%	80%	56·5%	59%		52%
Total deaths and mortality	12 (2%)			22 (8%)			

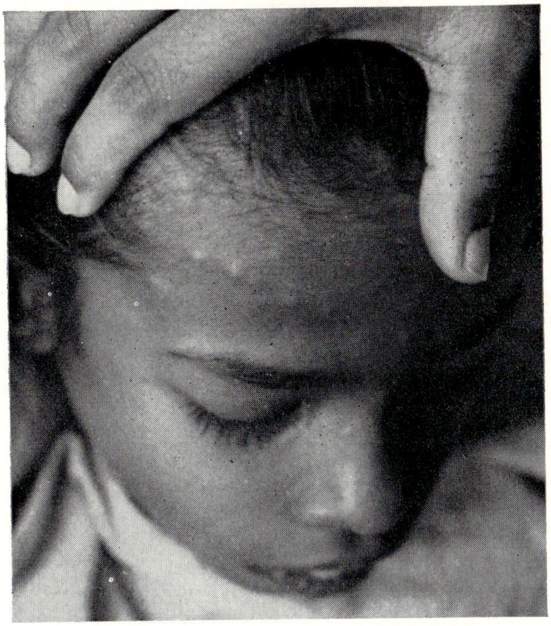

FIG. 1.—Subcutaneous nodules in a coloured child.

Cardiac Manifestations. Although only 0·2% of the total admissions to the Children's Hospital during the five-year period showed cardiac manifestations, it is interesting that only about 30% of those with rheumatic infection showed some cardiac lesions in contrast to the incidence of 80% seen in adults. The commonest lesion is mitral stenosis, which accounts for about 80% of the lesions seen in children. Aortic lesions by themselves are very rare in children, only one child with such lesions being seen in five years in my unit. A combined lesion is sometimes seen, and, extremely rarely, an isolated pericardial effusion.

Chorea. Chorea is a very uncommon manifestation of rheumatism in Ceylon. Out of 560 children there were only 13 (0·2%) cases of chorea during the five-year period. This is a very striking contrast to the incidence seen in the temperate climate. For instance, in The Hospital for Sick Children, Great Ormond Street, in 1919-20 the incidence was 62% among 262 children and in 1946-50 39% among 59 children. Chorea is also very rarely seen in the adult in Ceylon and equally rarely does the adult give a history of chorea in childhood.

Age Incidence. Only children under 12 years of age are admitted to the Children's Hospital. The disease is seldom or never seen in the toddler or in the child under 8 years of age, and most of the cases seen in the hospital are nearer 12.

Economic Considerations. Rheumatic infection appears to be common in children of the poorer classes in the towns: labourers, artisans and traders. It is seldom seen in the village population. It is perhaps true that the village population is not so readily attracted to the hospitals as the town dweller, but with easier facilities for travel in recent years the hospital does draw a very large number of children from the rural areas. The impression gained is that the incidence is low in the rural areas and higher among the poorer people in the towns, while among the upper and middle classes in the towns it is distinctly uncommon. I have seen only four cases among 3,000 patients in private practice during the last 10 years. I believe that this is so even among the adult population.

Effect of Malnutrition. In a country like Ceylon where malnutrition is rife, and seen particularly in hospital practice, one would expect a serious infection like rheumatic infection to take a heavy toll. However, manifestations of rheumatic infection are conspicuous by their absence in the large numbers of malnourished children we come across daily.

Conclusions

Rheumatic fever appears to run a mild course in childhood in Ceylon.

The most common age of occurrence is in late childhood, from about 9 to 12 years.

Cardiac complications in childhood are much less common than in temperate climates and appear in a later age group, in early adult life.

The mortality in childhood is less than in England.

Cutaneous signs are very rarely seen.

Chorea is extremely rare in children in Ceylon.

REFERENCES

Cox, P. J. N. and Schlesinger, B. E. (1955). Paper read at Royal Society of Medicine on May 25, 1955. *Gt Ormond Str. J.*, No. 11, p. 38.

——, —— (1958). Personal communication.

Fernando, P. B. (1939). *Quart. J. Med.*, **8**, 261.

HERPES SIMPLEX VIRUS INFECTION: DISSEMINATION IN ASSOCIATION WITH MALNUTRITION

BY

D. McKENZIE, J. D. L. HANSEN and W. BECKER

From the Red Cross Children's Hospital and Departments of Pathology and Child Health, University of Cape Town, and the C.S.I.R. and U.C.T. Virus Research Unit, Department of Pathology, University of Cape Town

(RECEIVED FOR PUBLICATION NOVEMBER 11, 1958)

Eight cases of disseminated herpes simplex infection unassociated with infantile eczema have been found at autopsy during the period September, 1957, to April, 1958. All but two of these were grossly malnourished.

Herpetic stomatitis is very much more common than is generally appreciated. Routine studies carried out in our virus laboratory have revealed that many of the more severe and atypical forms of stomatitis are due to the herpes simplex virus, and in the past must have been diagnosed as stomatitis due to Vincent's angina or moniliasis.

While herpes simplex infection usually manifests itself as a lesion localized to the epithelial surfaces of the lips, face and mouth, widespread systemic involvement does from time to time occur. Dissemination in association with infantile eczema (eczema herpeticum or Kaposi's varicelliform eruption) is well known, but in recent years a fulminating illness due to widespread dissemination of the herpes simplex virus, quite unassociated with eczema, has been reported by several investigators.

On histopathological grounds, Hass (1935) suggested that the necrotic liver and adrenal lesions found in a premature infant at autopsy were due to systemic dissemination of the herpes simplex virus. Encephalitis in the newborn due to herpes simplex virus has been recorded by several authors (Smith, Lennette and Reames, 1941; Wildi, 1951; Florman and Mindlin, 1952; France and Wilmers, 1953), hepatic necroses due to the same agent have been described (Quilligan and Wilson, 1951; Zuelzer and Stulberg, 1952; France and Wilmers, 1953; Pugh, Newns and Dudgeon, 1954; Brain, Pugh and Dudgeon, 1957) while necrotic adrenal lesions have been noted in association with eczema herpeticum (Zuelzer and Stulberg, 1952; Brain *et al.*, 1957). With the exception of two cases in Group II of Zuelzer and Stulberg (1952) and one case of Brain *et al.* (1957), all cases recorded have occurred in the neonatal period. Of interest in our series is that all the children were between 9 and 16 months of age.

Clinical Features

The clinical features of the eight cases are summarized in Table I. In all save one convulsions occurred before admission, and in all but one there was clinical evidence of gross malnutrition. The one case with proved pneumococcal meningitis falls into a rather different category.

The cerebrospinal fluid in five of the remaining seven cases was examined on admission and was normal. A further specimen of the C.S.F. from Case 5 was examined four days after admission and proved to be abnormal with a protein of 170 mg. %, positive globulin test and 25 lymphocytes but normal sugar content. Autopsy revealed an encephalitis in this instance.

The occurrence of a bleeding tendency in half our cases confirms the similar observation made previously (Zuelzer and Stulberg, 1952).

Virus Studies. Virus studies were undertaken on tissues removed at autopsy from Cases 4, 7 and 8.

Tissue slices were taken from the liver and other organs and stored in separate containers. A suitable portion of each tissue was weighed and ground up to make a 10% emulsion in Hank's lactalbumen hydrolysate medium (Melnick, 1956), containing penicillin in a concentration of 100 units/ml., streptomycin 100 μg/ml., neomycin 100 μg/ml., and mycostatin 25 units/ml. After centrifugation of the emulsion at 10,000 r.p.m. for 10 minutes, 0·1 ml. amounts of the supernatant fluid were inoculated into HeLa tissue and/or monkey kidney tissue roller-tube cultures. The supernatant fluid was tested for bacteriological sterility and the remainder was ampouled and stored in dry ice.

TABLE 1

SUMMARY OF CASES

Case No.	Race and Sex	Age (months)	Weight (lb. oz.)	Symptoms	Stomatitis	Hepatomegaly	Signs of Malnutrition	Convulsions	Other Findings	Death after Admission (days)
1	Col. F.	16	—	Arrived O.P.D. *in extremis* with severe stomatitis: died before admission	Yes	—	Kwashiorkor	—	—	On admission
2	Col. F.	12	9 13	Diarrhoea and vomiting for 5 d. Convulsions, 1 d.	N.R.	Yes	Gross marasmus	Yes	Raised serum sodium and chloride. Apyrexial	2
3	Col. F.	12	11 14	Diarrhoea and vomiting for 4 w.	Yes	Yes	Kwashiorkor	Yes	Purpura	8
4	Native M.	15	14	Diarrhoea and vomiting for 3 w.	Yes	Yes	Kwashiorkor	Yes	Purpura	7
5	Col. M.	9	9 7	Diarrhoea, vomiting, cough for 3 w. Sore mouth for 1 w.	Yes	Yes	Malnourished	Yes	Pyrexia bleeding tendency	4
6	Col. M.	15	20 13½	Stomatitis for 3 d. Convulsions for 1 d.	Yes	No	None	Yes	Pyrexia	1
7	Col. F.	12	13 5	Sore mouth for 2 w. Convulsions for 1 d.	Yes	Yes	Kwashiorkor	Yes	Pyrexia bleeding tendency	4
8	Native M.	14	N.R.	Sordes. Pneumococcal meningitis	N.R.	N.R.	Malnourished	Yes	—	17

The tubes were incubated at 37° C. in a revolving drum and examined each day for cytopathogenic effect. Two serial subcultures were made, using larger inocula of 0·2-0·3 ml. before a specimen was assumed to have no virus present.

Virus titrations were carried out on the stored supernatant fluids from those specimens in which virus had been detected. Tenfold dilutions of the fluids were made in Hank's lactalbumen hydrolysate medium containing 5% rabbit serum (freed of inhibitor and heat-inactivated), and these were inoculated in 0·1 ml. amounts into tissue culture tubes, using three or four tubes per dilution. The results are indicated in Table 2.

Cytopathogenic effect produced by the herpes simplex virus in these cases was striking and distinctive. The virus was identified by a standard neutralization technique using herpes simplex immune serum prepared in mice, and controls set up under the same conditions with normal mouse serum. In the case of each isolation these virus observations were checked by the production of encephalitis in mice and typical pocks on the chorioallantoic membrane of the developing chick embryo.

TABLE 2

VIRUS ISOLATIONS

Case No.	Specimens Examined	Virus Isolation	Titre $TCID_{50}$/ml.
4	Liver	Positive	Not done
7	Liver	Positive	$10^{8 \cdot 0}$
	Spleen	Positive	$10^{3 \cdot 0}$
	Lung	Positive	Less than $10^{1 \cdot 0}$
	Heart, tongue, kidney, adrenal, brain, blood	Negative	
8	Liver	Positive	$10^{8 \cdot 25}$
	Spleen	Positive	$10^{6 \cdot 75}$

Two commercial preparations of gamma globulin were titrated for inhibition of cytopathogenic effect by the herpes simplex virus isolated from Case 7. The one preparation neutralized 50 TCD_{50} when diluted 1/1200, the other when diluted 1/1400. Case 7 received 3 ml. of the latter preparation of gamma globulin on the third day before death, and the serum (heat-inactivated) from the autopsy was found to neutralize 50 TCD_{50} only at a dilution of less than 1/2.

Morbid Anatomy and Histology. The autopsy findings are summarized in Table 3. In six of the eight cases macroscopic lesions were found in the liver. These are so characteristic that in Case 8, who died of pneumococcal meningitis, the pathologist performing the autopsy was able without hesitation to identify the liver lesion as being due to herpes simplex infection. Where the lesion was not visible macroscopically the histological appearances were such that there was no doubt as to the aetiology.

Tongue. In the majority no resemblance to the

TABLE 3

SUMMARY OF AUTOPSY FINDINGS

Case No.	Hepatic Necrosis	Adrenal Necrosis	Comment
1	Microscopic	Microscopic	—
2	Macroscopic	No	Bronchopneumonia
3	Macroscopic	Microscopic	—
4	Macroscopic	Microscopic	Bronchiolitis. Virus isolated from liver
5	Microscopic	Microscopic	Encephalitis
6	Microscopic	Microscopic	Round worms ++
7	Macroscopic	No	Infarct of spleen. Virus isolated from liver, spleen, lungs
8	Macroscopic	Microscopic	Pneumococcal meningitis. Splenic lesions possibly attributable to herpes simplex virus. Virus isolated from liver, spleen

The first detectable abnormality appeared to be swelling of the epithelial cell nuclei with fragmentation of the chromatin network and loss of basophilic staining, the central portion of the nucleus remaining unstained save for basophilic stippling caused by chromatin fragmentation. The nucleus continued to increase in size and the chromatin and nucleolus became marginated, resulting in an apparent increase in thickness of the basophilic nuclear membrane; at the same time eosinophilic intranuclear inclusion bodies became apparent as rounded globules, some occurring singly and occasionally several in one nucleus. These eosinophilic bodies increased in size and, where multiple, appeared to coalesce so that large eosinophilic bodies almost filled the swollen nucleus with a clear unstained halo between them and the nuclear membrane. At this stage the nucleolus was no longer recognizable and some nuclei were extremely irregular in outline, with the indentations of the nuclear membrane imparting a bizarre appearance to the nucleus (Fig. 3).

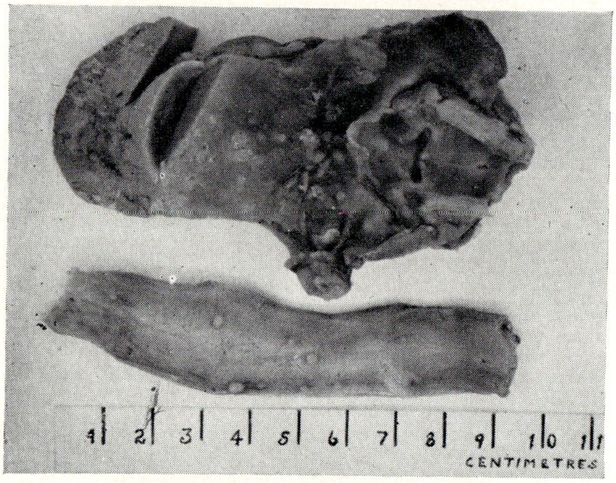

FIG. 1.—Tongue and oesophagus showing hypertrophic lesions caused by herpes simplex virus.

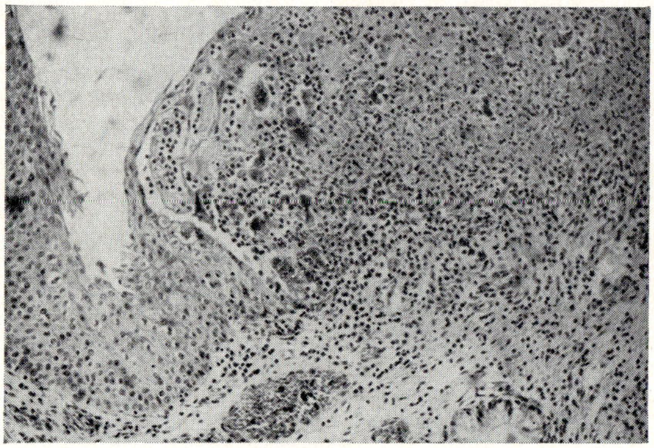

FIG. 2.—Margin of herpetic ulcer in tongue showing epithelial giant cells. H. and E. × 90.

vesicular nature of the original lesion was recognizable. The vesicles had become confluent, and large areas of the surface of the tongue had been replaced by superficial serpiginous ulcers. Occasionally the lesions were more hypertrophic, yellow in colour and slightly raised above the surface (Fig. 1).

Microscopically there was superficial ulceration without penetration into the underlying muscle. The surface epithelium had sloughed away leaving an area of necrosis covered by a fibrinous exudate in which only occasional polymorphonuclear cells were present. At the margin of the lesion characteristic epithelial giant cells were seen mainly lying free in the area of ulceration, and in these and in nuclei of the adjoining epithelial cells nuclear inclusions were visible (Fig. 2).

In the epithelial cells at the margin of the ulcer a cytoplasmic change also became apparent. There was ballooning of the cell and the cytoplasm lost its eosinophilic staining and became clear. No inclusion bodies were seen in adjacent superficial glands. The earliest stage of the inclusions were seen in the cells next to but outside the ulcer, the final stages prior to destruction of the nucleus being at the very edge of the ulcer.

Oesophagus. The oesophagus was affected in four of the eight cases. In three of these there were punched out ulcers up to 2 mm. in size over the lower third to half of the oesophagus. In the

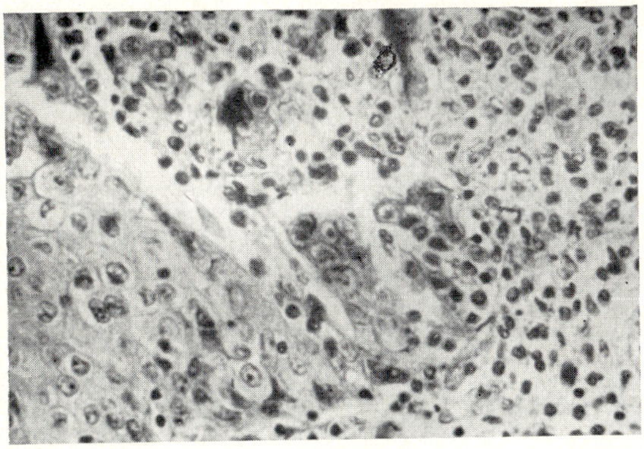

FIG. 3.—Nuclear inclusions in epithelial cells of tongue. H. and E. × 160.

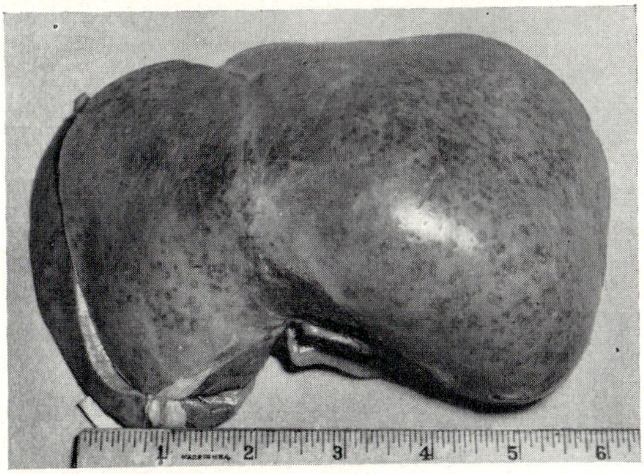

FIG. 4.—Liver showing the characteristic circular areas of necrosis.

remaining case there was a mixed picture of yellow nodules up to 3 mm. in diameter and raised approximately 1 mm. above the surface and small punched-out superficial ulcers up to 1 mm. in size. A small zone of congestion surrounded the nodular lesions and similar lesions were present in the pyriform fossae (Fig. 1).

Microscopically the appearances were very similar to those seen in the tongue, apart from the nodular lesions, which consisted of heaped-up fibrinous exudate with some epithelial cells. No giant cells were seen in our sections but nuclear changes in the epithelium at the ulcer margin paralleled those described in the tongue.

Liver. In six of the eight cases there was a macroscopic lesion of the liver, associated with a gross degree of fatty infiltration. The lesions were so striking that they may be regarded as pathognomonic of herpes simplex infection. Their size varied, presumably with duration, from pin head foci of necrosis just visible with the naked eye to areas up to 3 mm. in size. Unless these had become confluent each was a perfect circle, dead white in colour, with a surrounding zone of hyperaemia or haemorrhage giving a target-like appearance to the whole and sharply demarcating the affected tissue from the surrounding liver parenchyma (Fig. 4). There did not appear to be any regularity of distribution of these lesions in the liver substance, and they were scattered in haphazard fashion both under the capsule and on section. There were no obvious differences between the two lobes in frequency of the lesions. In some cases the lesions were strikingly uniform in size while in others the widely varying size suggested different ages in dissemination and development.

Microscopically the extent of parenchymal involvement varied from 10% in the least involved to 75% in the most severely affected (Fig. 5). In most the lesions were multilobular though in the smaller and presumably earlier lesions they were lobular and situated more in the mid- and peripheral zones than centrally.

Whether large or small the necrotic focus was infarct-like to the extent that both parenchyma and stroma were equally destroyed. In the centre usually only nuclear remnants were apparent, but in the early lesions in addition haemorrhages were evident with red cells lying free in the area of necrosis. The necrotic area merged abruptly into surviving liver parenchyma in which the only detectable abnormalities were in cell nuclei. There was no evidence of inflammatory reaction or of proliferation of liver cells, but there was dilatation of sinusoids over a narrow zone surrounding the lesion.

In more extensive and presumably older lesions the area of necrosis was far more extensive, and red cells were not recognizable as such in the centre,

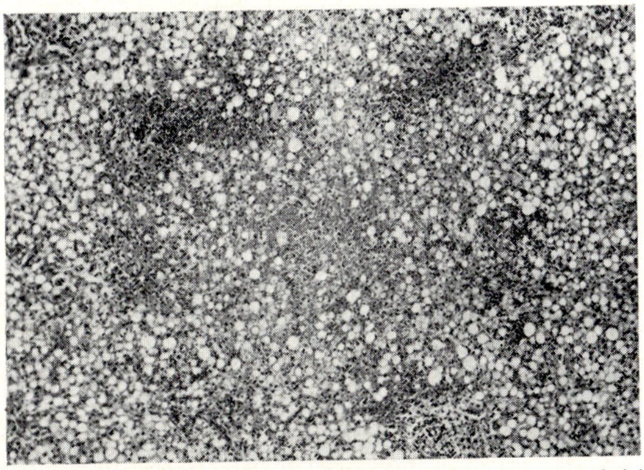

FIG. 5.—Liver: the large central area of necrosis is surrounded by haemorrhage. H. and E. × 150.

but formed a homogeneous pool of laked blood merging with the necrotic background.

The feature of greatest histopathological interest was the presence of intranuclear inclusion bodies (Fig. 6). There appeared to be two patterns of development of these structures. Whether the different forms of nuclear change seen were all intermediate between normal nuclei and nuclei with fully mature inclusion bodies or whether varied pathways of development took place was impossible to say. However not all stages, nor even similar stages, were recognizable in all sections. It is reasonable to believe that the more mature inclusions are likely to be in the centre and the earlier stages at the periphery. For this reason the peripheral cells are taken as the starting point for the purpose of describing the nuclear changes.

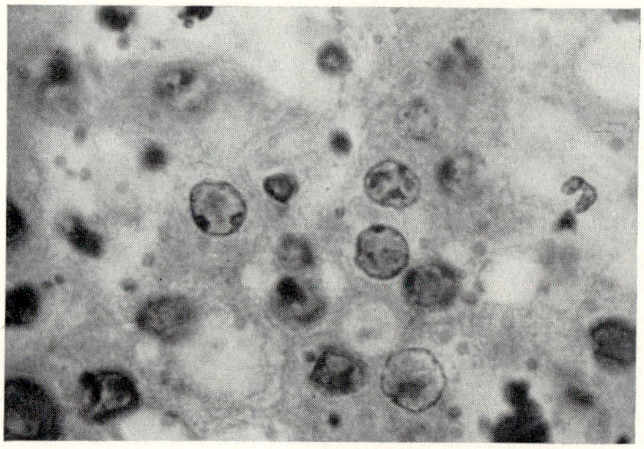

FIG. 6.—Intra-nuclear inclusions in liver cells. H. and E. × 800.

What was regarded as the earliest indication of infection was a swelling of the nucleus and loss of staining density. The chromatin was fragmented and appeared as basophilic stippling of the nucleoplasm which was otherwise unstained; the nucleolus was present and was at this stage near the nuclear membrane. Nearer to the necrotic focus the nuclei seemed to have lost their nucleoli, and the chromatin was marginated and presented as an irregularly staining basophilic lining to the nuclear membrane resembling a string of pearls. The remainder of the nucleus was generally uniformly eosinophilic and homogeneous, and no individual inclusions could be identified though the nucleus as a whole had increased in size. Occasional nuclei, however, instead of the uniform eosinophilic background appeared to contain small eosinophilic bodies scattered throughout. Towards the centre of the lesion the nuclei while still larger than normal were somewhat smaller than in the previous stage. The whole nucleus was filled with a more compact, denser homogeneous eosinophilic material and only the nuclear membrane took up the basophilic dye. At this stage the outline of the nucleus was irregular and crenated and some of the inclusions under high power objective showed a more purplish than eosinophilic character. Examination under oil immersion showed that what appeared to be a homogeneous inclusion was really a honeycomb of small round eosinophilic bodies set in a bluish coloured matrix, the whole filling the entire nucleus.

The apparent alternative pathway of development did not appear as clear-cut as that just described. Here again the earliest stage was enlargement of the nucleus, fragmentation of chromatin and loss of basophilic staining, margination of chromatin and

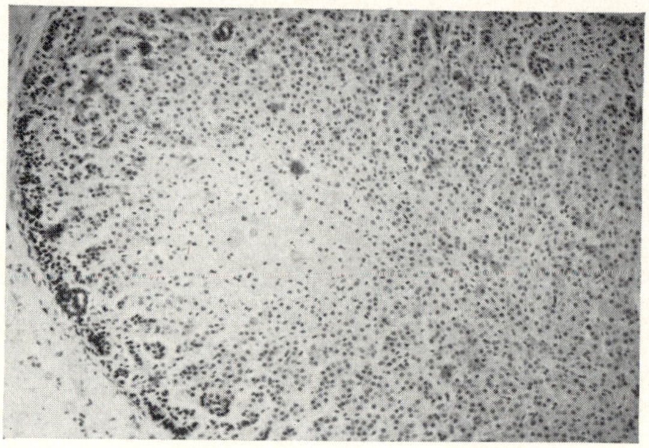

FIG. 7.—Area of necrosis in adrenal cortex. H. and E. × 80.

nucleolus and eventual loss of the latter. The inclusions, however, were slightly different. The first forms seen were cells containing a single, or several, large globular eosinophilic bodies in the nucleus. In some nuclei these were uniform in size, in others larger forms suggesting coalescence were also found. Towards the centre of the lesion inclusions were again single and eosinophilic, but did not fill the enlarged nucleus, and a distinct unstained halo lay between the eosinophilic inclusion body and the basophilic nuclear membrane. Subsequent stages seemed to parallel those already described above.

Hass (1935) described two types of inclusion body, one eosinophilic and one basophilic and traced their development. While two types of inclusions seem to occur in our cases, basophilia of these was not prominent save in the later stages. Whether there are in fact two separate lines of development or whether the nuclear changes described are in reality manifestations of various stages in a single pathway of development of virus within the infected nucleus is a matter for conjecture.

Adrenals. No macroscopic lesions were seen in any of these cases, though they have been described in association with disseminated herpes simplex infection and infantile eczema (Brain *et al.*, 1957). Microscopic lesions were seen in five cases (Fig. 7).

Microscopically areas of necrosis were seen in both medulla and cortex. In the cortex there was always a thin rim of normal tissue between the capsule and the necrotic area. The lesion was essentially similar to that in the liver allowing for the differences in the tissue structure. Nuclear inclusions were present, but not with the frequency or variation of those in the liver. The earliest change in the nucleus was increase in size and clearing of the nucleoplasm which showed basophilic stippling due to fragmentation of chromatin. The chromatin became marginated and inclusion bodies appeared in the nucleus showing either as eosinophilic stippling or a homogeneous eosinophilic mass filling the nucleus. Occasionally an unstained halo separated the eosinophilic inclusion from the nuclear membrane.

Spleen. In Cases 7 and 8, though not visible macroscopically, there were small necrotic infarct-like lesions in the spleen.

Although the virus was isolated from these spleens in high titre and not from the blood, the absence of inclusions make it difficult to be certain that the lesions were the result of the herpes simplex virus.

Brain. In all cases with the exception of Case 8, the brains were tense and oedematous and in some congested. Oedema and congestion are not uncommon findings in association with malnutrition. In Case 5 in addition to the oedema and congestion the meninges appeared thickened and gelatinous though no inflammatory exudate was visible.

Microscopically the leptomeninges showed oedema and scattered infiltration by lymphocytic cells. The brain was congested and oedematous but in addition there was minimal lymphocytic perivascular cuffing, suggesting a true meningo-encephalitis.

Other Organs. Other organs examined macroscopically and microscopically included pancreas, lungs, kidneys and myocardium. In none of these were lesions ascribable to the herpes simplex virus found. The trachea and large bronchi showed no macroscopic lesions, but were not examined microscopically. This is an unfortunate omission, as in a subsequent case, not included in this series, typical and extensive lesions have been seen in the trachea and bronchi. The smaller bronchi and bronchioles encountered in sections of the lung showed no nuclear changes in the lining epithelium. The lung parenchyma in all instances was normal.

In the pancreas there was some duct and acinar dilatation with accumulation in the lumina of eosinophilic material; and in some a minor degree of acinar atrophy: these appearances are not infrequently seen in association with kwashiorkor and malnutrition, and a relationship to the herpes simplex infection is unlikely.

Vascular lesions as described by other authors in the liver (Zuelzer and Stulberg, 1952; Williams and Jack, 1955) and in the spleen (Williams and Jack, 1955) were not seen in our cases.

Discussion

Widespread dissemination of the herpes simplex virus with lesions in internal organs is no new entity (Smith *et al.*, 1941; Wildi, 1951; Quilligan and Wilson, 1951; Florman and Mindlin, 1952; Zuelzer and Stulberg, 1952; France and Wilmers, 1953; Pugh *et al.*, 1954; Williams and Jack, 1955; Brain *et al.*, 1957), and the unusual features of our cases are the older age group in which they occurred and the frequent association with malnutrition.

As far as we are aware similar observations have not been previously recorded in South Africa, although in clinical experience herpetic gingivo-stomatitis is relatively common in the Union in the 1 to 5-year age group. Whether the number of cases of systemic herpes simplex infection seen in this relatively short period implies a sudden increase of virulence in the local strain of virus, or whether the incidence of overt infection reached epidemic proportions it is impossible to say.

Several authors have noted that the incidence of primary local herpetic infections is higher in the lower socio-economic group (Andrewes and Carmichael, 1930; Burnet and Lush, 1939; Scott, Coriell, Bland and Burgoon, 1952) and that the greatest number of those susceptible to infection are between 6 and 24 months of age (Burnet and Williams, 1939; Scott *et al.*, 1952). The general pattern of infection seen locally substantiates this, and we would suggest that where malnutrition is an accompaniment of poor socio-economic conditions the chances of dissemination of herpes simplex gingivo-stomatitis to internal organs may be increased.

Though no figures are available in South Africa to indicate the ratio of subclinical to clinical infection, Coetzee (1955) has shown that 100% of the sera of adult Bantu in the Pretoria area had antibodies to the herpes simplex virus. Anderson and Hamilton

(1949) showed that 100% of susceptibles in an orphanage in Australia became infected by 22 months of age, whereas McNair Scott *et al.* (1952), investigating lower income groups attending the out-patients clinic of the Children's Hospital of Philadelphia, found 64% had antibodies, and Burnet and Lush (1939) reported antibodies in 93% of persons attending a general hospital. From Coetzee's (1955) figures it would appear that the incidence of infection in the low socio-economic groups in South Africa is maximal.

We wish to stress the high specificity of the naked eye appearances of the liver when the necrotic foci are abundant, and indeed now regard it as diagnostic of disseminated herpes. In retrospect in five out of the eight cases the diagnosis could have been made with the naked eye. The microscopical appearances are also characteristic both in extent and type but focal necroses are not rare in the liver and the diagnosis might well be missed if one did not know of the herpetic lesion and no macroscopic specimens were available. Virus was isolated in high titre from the liver and spleen but not from the blood, and though the splenic lesions are not histologically specific, it is felt that they may well be due to localization of the virus at this site.

Treatment of these cases by other than symptomatic methods presents a difficult problem. Supportive measures and antibiotics are essential and there may be justification for steroid therapy where there is no question of infantile eczema and where dissemination of the virus is suspected. A case may however be advanced for massive gamma-globulin therapy in malnourished children with primary herpes simplex infection as a protective measure against dissemination.

Summary

Eight cases of disseminated herpes simplex virus infection in children 9 to 16 months of age are reported.

An association between malnutrition and dissemination of the virus is mooted.

Attention is drawn to the highly characteristic liver lesions and the histo-pathology of various organs is described.

Virus isolation was carried out in three cases with titration of virus in several organs in two of these.

The high incidence of infection in the lower socio-economic groups is briefly discussed.

We wish to thank Professor J. G. Thomson, Professor A. Kipps and Dr. C. J. Uys for advice and criticism; Dr. L. Anstey and Dr. C. J. Watson for the autopsies on Cases 5 and 8; Professor F. Ford for permission to use cases from his wards and Dr. J. F. W. Mostert, Superintendent of the Red Cross Children's Hospital, for permission to publish. Thanks are also due to Mr. B. Todt and Mr. W. Taylor for photographs.

REFERENCES

Anderson, S. G. and Hamilton, J. (1949). *Med. J. Aust.* **1**, 308.
Andrewes, C. H. and Carmichael, E. A. (1930). *Lancet*, **1**, 857.
Brain, R. T., Pugh, R. C. B. and Dudgeon, J. A. (1957). *Arch. Dis. Childh.*, **32**, 120.
Burnet, F. M. and Lush, D. (1939). *Lancet*, **1**, 629.
—— and Williams, S. W. (1939). *Med. J. Aust.*, **1**, 637.
Coetzee, J, N, (1955). *S. Afr. J. Lab. clin. Med.*, **1**, 52.
Florman, A. L. and Mindlin, R. L. (1952). *A.M.A. Amer J. Dis. Child.*, **83**, 481.
France, N. E. and Wilmers, M. J. (1953). *Lancet*, **1**, 1181.
Hass, G. M. (1935). *Amer. J. Path.*, **11**, 127.
Melnick, J. L. (1956). In *Diagnostic Procedures for Virus and Rickettsial Diseases*, 2nd ed. American Public Health Association, New York.
Pugh, R. C. B., Newns, G. H. and Dudgeon J. A. (1954). *Arch. Dis. Childh.*, **29**, 60.
Quilligan, J. J. and Wilson, J. L. (1951). *J. Lab. clin. Med.*, **38**, 742.
Scott, T. F. McN., Coriell, L., Bland, H. and Burgoon, C. F. (1952). *J. Pediat.*, **41**, 835.
Smith, M. G., Lennette, E. H. and Reames, H. R. (1941). *Amer. J. Path.*, **17**, 55.
Wildi, E. (1951). *Rev. neurol.*, **84**, 201.
Williams, A. and Jack, I. (1955). *Med. J. Aust.*, **1**, 392.
Zuelzer, W. W. and Stulberg, C. S. (1952). *A.M.A. Amer. J. Dis. Child.*, **83**, 421.

CHRONIC ULCERATIVE COLITIS IN CHILDHOOD

A FOLLOW-UP STUDY

BY

RONALD C. KING,* ARTHUR E. LINDNER and H. MARVIN POLLARD

From the Department of Internal Medicine, Gastroenterology Unit, University of Michigan Medical School, Ann Arbor, Michigan

(RECEIVED FOR PUBLICATION OCTOBER 28, 1958)

Although chronic ulcerative colitis may well have been known to Sydenham (1848), it was only comparatively recently that Helmholz (1923) first recorded the occurrence of the condition in children with an account of five cases. Since that time the disease has become increasingly recognized as a condition of childhood and larger series have been reported from America (Jackman, Bargen and Helmholz, 1940; Bargen and Kennedy, 1955; Holowach and Thurston, 1956; Meeker and Goff, 1956), from Australia (Covernton, 1949), from Sweden (Lagercrantz, 1955), and more recently from England (Schlesinger and Platt, 1958). Jackman *et al.* (1940) found, as a result of follow-up studies, that over half of their 95 children had either become worse or had died, whereas a more recent investigation concerning 126 children (Bargen and Kennedy, 1955) revealed a much more optimistic prognosis.

Between July 1, 1947, and June 30, 1956, a total of 391 patients attended the University Hospital with chronic ulcerative colitis. Of these 52 (13·3%) were aged 15 years or less when the disease first appeared. In an attempt to assess the prognosis of the condition as seen in childhood at this large medical centre, a follow-up study was initiated, the results of which form the basis for this communication.

The medical records of the 52 patients were studied and cases were included only if the clinical story of chronic diarrhoea was supported by negative bacteriological findings and positive radiological or sigmoidoscopic evidence. Six of the patients had been seen as out-patients but the remainder had all been investigated or treated in hospital. Simple questionnaires were then prepared and despatched and satisfactory information was obtained in 51 instances, a follow-up rate of 98·1%. When surgery had been performed or death had occurred in other hospitals these were written to and the relevant surgical or autopsy details obtained.

Clinical Details. Thirty-one (59·6%) of the patients were male and 21 (40·4%) female. Details of age distribution and duration of the disease are shown in Tables 1 and 2. The period of follow-up ranged from one to 26 years, with an average of nine years. The extent of radiological involvement and the sigmoidoscopic appearances are summarized in Table 3. The most constant radiographic finding was loss of the normal haustral markings, and this involved the entire colon in 30 (57·7%) of the cases. Terminal ileal involvement

TABLE 1

DETAILS OF AGE AT ONSET, AGE AT WHICH FIRST SEEN AT UNIVERSITY HOSPITAL, AND AGE AT TERMINATION OF FOLLOW-UP

Age at Onset of Disease (yr.)	Patients (No.)	Age when First Seen at University Hospital (yr.)	Patients (No.)	Age at End of Follow-up* (yr.)	Patients (No.)
1	—	10	2	15	5
2	—	11	1	16	2
3	—	12	4	17	2
4	—	13	12	18	4
5	1	14	8	19	3
6	—	15	8	20	5
7	1	16	2	21	1
8	1	17	2	22	2
9	4	18	2	23	2
10	2	19	3	24	3
11	3	20	1	25	2
12	13	22	1	26	1
13	8	23	1	27	3
14	11	24	2	30	1
15	8	25	1	31	2
		28	1	34	2
		33	1	39	2
	52		52		42

* Excluding nine deaths and one untraced patient.

* In receipt of a Clinical Fellowship of the American Cancer Society.
Present address: St. Bartholomew's Hospital, London.

TABLE 2

DURATION (IN YEARS) OF DISEASE WHEN FIRST SEEN AND TOTAL DURATION TO DEATH, SURGERY, OR TERMINATION OF FOLLOW-UP

Duration when First Seen (yr.)	Patients (no.)	Total Duration (yr.)	Patients (no.)
Less than 1	15	1	1
1	10	2	4
2	8	3	5
3	3	4	4
4	5	5	3
5	2	6	3
7	1	7	4
9	1	8	3
10	3	9	3
14	1	10	2
15	1	11	3
17	2	12	4
		13	2
		15	1
		16	3
		17	1
		19	2
		21	1
		23	1
		26	1
	52		51

TABLE 3

EXTENT OF RADIOLOGICAL INVOLVEMENT AND SIGMOIDOSCOPIC APPEARANCES

Barium Enema	Patients (no.)	Sigmoidoscopy	Patients (no.)
Not done (N.D.) ..	3	N.D.	2
Normal (N.) ..	7	Grade 1	1
Distal (D.) ..	6	Grade 2	3
Left side (L.) ..	5	Grade 3	36
Right side (R.) ..	1	Grade 4	10
Total (T.) ..	18		
Total + terminal ileum (T.I.) ..	12		
	52		52

(Grade 1: oedema. Grade 2: granularity. Grade 3: granularity + bleeding. Grade 4: Grade 3 + ulceration.)

was evident in 12 (23%). Patients in whom barium enema was normal or in whom this investigation had not been performed all had diagnostic appearances on sigmoidoscopy, while 46 (88·5%) of the children had incontrovertible sigmoidoscopic evidence of chronic ulcerative colitis. Seven (13·5%) showed pseudo polyp formation and a stricture was found in one case. Forty-one (79%) of the children had haemoglobin levels below 13 g. % (Haldane) while 11 (21%) had levels below 10 g. %.

Results of Follow-up. Fifty-one of the 52 patients (98·1%) were satisfactorily followed up and of these nine (17·6%) were dead. Eight of the deaths (15·7%) occurred directly or indirectly as a result of the ulcerative colitis (Table 4), while the ninth was due to portal cirrhosis, probably unrelated to mild ulcerative colitis. Carcinoma of the colon developed in four cases (7·8%) all of whom had had the disease for nine years or more (Table 4). Twelve of the patients (23·5%) underwent excisional surgery with one post-operative death. This youth had severe colitis of four years' standing and in addition to a colectomy had also had duodeno-colic and jejuno-colic fistulae excised. In the remainder operations were performed as follows: ileostomy and total colectomy (5); ileostomy, total colectomy and abdomino-perineal resection of the rectum (4); sub-total colectomy with ileo-sigmoid anastomosis (2). Two patients underwent surgery for isolated fistulae (one ileal, one rectal) while six others were operated on for unrelated conditions. The surviving group of 42 patients was therefore divided into 11 who had undergone excisional surgery and 31 who had not.

Perusal of the completed questionnaires enabled a

TABLE 4

DETAILS OF FATAL AND NEOPLASTIC CASES

Patient	Sex	Age of Onset (yr.)	Duration	Age of Death (yr.)	Sigmoidoscopy	Barium Enema*	Cause of Death	Surgery
35	M.	9	2	11	3	L.	Exacerbation	Nil
44	M.	12	2	14	2	D.	,,	,,
46	F.	11	1	12	3	N.D.	,,	,,
51	M.	9	4	13	3	T.	Post-operative	Excision of colon, and entero-colic fistulae
52	F.	14	5	19	3	N.D.	Exacerbation	Nil
29	M.	12	14	26	3	T.I.	Carcinoma	Laparotomy
42	M.	10	21	31	3	T.I.	,,	,,
50	F.	9	15	23	4	T.I.	,,	,,
33	M.	13	9	Alive and well 3 years post-operatively	3	T.I.		Colectomy, and excision of carcinoma

* Abbreviations as in Table 3.

detailed assessment to be made of the patients' condition at the end of the follow-up. Five (45·5%) of the surgical group were underweight for their height as compared with nine (29%) of the medically treated patients. Nine (82%) of the surgical group were working or attending school or college regularly, while 30 (97%) of the medical group were similarly employed. Eight of the surgical group were aged 19 years or more at the termination of the follow-up. Of these, three (37·5%) were married with children, four (50%) were unmarried, while the status of one was not known. Twenty-two of the medical group were aged 19 or more at the termination of the follow-up and of these 12 (54·5%) were married, seven (32%) with children. Nine (82%) of the surgical group stated that their condition was excellent, one (9%) with an ileo-sigmoidostomy lacked energy, while in one case insufficient time had elapsed since operation for an opinion to be given. By contrast only 17 (55%) of the medical group described their condition as excellent and could be considered inactive, while 14 (45%) were having persistent symptoms with more than four motions a day and the intermittent passage of blood and/or mucus. Only 2 (18%) of the surgical group had required further admission to hospital (revision of ileostomy, drainage of perineal abscess) but 14 (45%) of the medical group had been subsequently admitted to hospital on account of the colitis. Three (27%) of the surgical group had suffered episodes of ill health not necessitating admission but 14 (45%) of the medical group had been inconvenienced in this way.

Discussion

The clinical features of the cases considered here do not differ in any important respects from recently described series. The present status of chronic ulcerative colitis in childhood has been well summarized by Lyons (1956), and in our patients no new pathological or aetiological factors were discovered, neither were any new diagnostic methods employed. Treatment was along orthodox lines, with rest, diet, antispasmodics, antibiotics and steroids, with blood transfusion and psychiatric or surgical intervention when necessary.

The unpredictable and at times fulminant course of ulcerative colitis in childhood makes it difficult to relate the condition at the time of examination with the ultimate outcome. Complete involvement of the colon will usually imply a more serious state and although this has been shown to affect the prognosis adversely in adults (Cullinan and MacDougall, 1957) such is not the case in childhood (Lyons, 1956). It is true that nine (75%) of the patients who came to surgery had total involvement when seen at the University Hospital as against 16 (52%) of the medical group, and similarly the four patients who developed colonic neoplasms had the entire colon and also the terminal ileum affected. However, of the five patients who died during acute exacerbations of the colitis, three had radiographic examination of the colon and of these only one had total involvement. In the remaining two the distal colon only was affected. Rapid progression and spread of the condition must have occurred as both died within a few months of being seen. A symptomatic appraisal of the patients treated medically reveals a similar lack of correlation between the extent of involvement and ultimate condition. Twenty-four of the 31 patients in the medical group had abnormal colon radiographs, 16 with total and eight with distal or segmental involvement. Reference to Table 5 reveals that patients with localized

TABLE 5

RELATION OF SUBSEQUENT SYMPTOMS TO DEGREE OF INVOLVEMENT ON BARIUM ENEMA WHEN SEEN AT UNIVERSITY OF MICHIGAN HOSPITAL

X-ray	Total involvement (16) (%)	Segmental (8) (%)	Normal (7) (%)
More than four motions daily	31	37·5	0
Blood in stools	31	25	29
Mucus in stools	31	50	14
Periodic ill health	56	75	43
Further hospitalization	31	37·5	43

involvement in fact suffered more subsequent inconvenience from their colitis than those in whom the entire colon was affected, while those in whom only the sigmoidoscopy was abnormal suffered less. Of the 28 patients in the medical group with Grade 3 or 4 sigmoidoscopic changes, seven (25%) continued to pass four or more motions a day, 10 (35·7%) persistently passed blood or mucus, 17 (60·7%) experienced periods of ill health, while in 11 cases (39·3%) this had necessitated further admission to hospital.

The incidence of malignant degeneration is high (7·8%). Even more striking is the early age at which the neoplasms occurred, the average age at the time of death from or diagnosis of the neoplasm being 25·25 years. There is now little doubt that chronic ulcerative colitis is a pre-malignant condition in both adults and children. The recorded incidence of carcinoma varies, in adults, depending on whether the material is derived from medical or surgical sources. Thus in medical series Sloan, Bargen and Gage (1950) reported 109 instances of neoplasm in 2,000 cases, Kiefer, Eytinge and Johnson (1951), nine in 458, Weckesser and Chinn (1953), four in 118, Banks, Korelitz and Zetzel (1957), nine in 245, and Cullinan and MacDougall (1957) six in 346, whereas from surgical sources Kiefer *et al.* (1951) recorded 10 in 226, Lyons and Garlock (1951) nine in 226, Hurt (1954) two in 18, Bacon, Yang, Carroll, Cates, Villalba and McGregor (1956) 12 in 84, and Thorlakson (1956) 12 in 182. The tendency for malignant change to occur increases, not unexpectedly, with the duration of the colitis, and in the series reported by Lyons and Garlock (1951) 36% of those who had had the disease longer than 12 years developed carcinomata. This susceptibility to carcinoma of the large bowel has been variously estimated as from five times (MacDougall, 1954) to 66 times (Kiefer *et al.*, 1951) that of the normal population. The growths may have multifocal origins (Gelber, Hawthorne and Gelb, 1955) and usually progress rapidly. Fewer reports are available concerning colitis and malignancy in children, but Tidrick and Hickey (1956) recorded six cases, all of whom developed their colitis in childhood, while Meeker and Goff (1956) described one similar case. In larger series Lagercrantz (1955) reported six instances of malignant degeneration in 150 children, Bargen and Kennedy (1955) six in 139, and Schlesinger and Platt (1958) two in 60. To date only five authentic cases of neoplasm complicating ulcerative colitis during childhood have been described (Wilcox and Beattie, 1956). Four (16·7%) of our 24 patients who had had the disease longer than nine years developed carcinomata, a figure which should weigh very heavily in favour of excisional surgery when the management of the long standing chronic disease is being considered. The case for surgery becomes even stronger when one compares the operative mortality with the risk of malignant degeneration (Hagan and Hagan, 1957).

Six (75%) of the eight patients who died from their colitis were male. Excluding deaths from neoplasm the remainder all occurred within five years of onset, three being within two years of the first appearance of the disease. It is interesting to note that only one of these five patients underwent surgery and he only when his condition was desperately complicated by duodeno-colic and jejuno-colic fistulae, and it is reasonable to suppose that some of these lives might have been saved had surgical treatment been more readily undertaken. Lyons (1956) has recently summarized the two main indications for surgery in chronic ulcerative colitis of childhood as (1) danger to life, and (2) invalidism. Under the first heading come such situations as acute fulminating toxaemia, haemorrhage, and perforation, impending or actual, while invalidism may be the result of intractability, stricture, pericolic abscess, fistulae or polyposis.

The risk of malignant degeneration in the long standing case is so real that we consider this also constitutes a very definite danger to life and provides another indication for elective surgery. The tendency now is to perform ileostomy with colectomy and rectal resection in one or two stages, although in some cases ileo-rectal anastomosis may be possible. The age at which surgery is performed will depend very much on the patient's condition, but it is interesting to note that of the six patients who underwent surgery after the age of 18 only one was underweight at the time of the termination of the follow-up, while of the five patients who were operated on before the age of 18, four were subsequently underweight. The results of surgery in this small series were excellent in 82% and compare very favourably with the 45% of medically treated patients who were enduring chronic ill health and, of course, the risk of later malignant degeneration.

Some interesting facts relating to mortality and surgical treatment emerge when comparisons are made between the 26 cases first seen before and the 25 cases first seen after July, 1951. As regards age of onset and extent of radiological and sigmoidoscopic involvement the two groups are comparable, although those in the first group had a much longer duration of the disease. The same principles of medical treatment were applied to all patients (six in the first group and eight in the second receiving steroids) while excisional surgery was employed in seven and five cases respectively. The two striking differences are in mortality and time at which surgery was performed. Excluding deaths from carcinoma, the mortality in the first group (15·4%) is nearly four times that of the second (4%). Although improvements in medical treatment may be partly responsible one cannot escape the conclusion that earlier surgery also played a part in lowering the mortality. In the first group surgical treatment was employed, on average, eight years after the onset and within three years of first being seen at the University Hospital, while in the second group operation was performed, on an average, within four years of the onset and within seven months of first being seen.

Table 6 summarizes the overall results of the follow-up. A childhood condition in which 27·4% of the sufferers continue with chronic ill health and from which 15·7% die, constitutes a serious challenge to medical science. In the absence of any more effective conservative remedy the results of this

TABLE 6

OVERALL RESULTS IN 51 CASES FOLLOWED UP

		Number	Percentage
Treatment: Medical	Asymptomatic	17	33·3
	Recurrent symptoms	14	27·4
Surgical	Asymptomatic	9	17·6
	Lacking in energy	1	2·0
	Too early to assess	1	2·0
Death	Acute exacerbation	4	7·8
	Post-operative	1	2·0
	Carcinoma of colon	3	5·9
	Unrelated	1	2·0
		51	100·0

investigation suggest that these figures might be improved by the more frequent use of surgery in the early acute condition and by its ultimate employment in the long standing chronic case.

Summary

Fifty-one of 52 children (98·1%) with chronic ulcerative colitis were successfully followed up for from one to 26 years after the onset of the disease.

Eight (15·7%) had died as a result of the colitis, four (7·8%) had developed carcinoma of the colon, and 12 (23·5%) had undergone excisional surgery, with one (2%) post-operative death.

Of the patients who had had the disease longer than nine years 16·7% developed colonic neoplasms.

Of 31 patients managed medically 14 (45%) continued with active disease, and 17 (55%) appeared to be inactive, whereas nine (82%) of the patients who survived surgery described their condition as excellent.

Analysis of the results suggests that both the morbidity and the mortality rates would be improved by the more frequent employment of surgical measures both in the early acute, and in the long standing chronic case.

We would like to express our appreciation to Mrs. Jean Waters and her staff of the University Hospital Follow-up Unit for their splendid co-operation in this study, to Dr. Robert J. Bolt for his helpful suggestions and review of this material, and to Mrs. A. Milne for secretarial assistance.

REFERENCES

Bacon, H. E., Yang, L. M. O., Carroll, P. T., Cates, B. A., Villalba, G. and McGregor, R. A. (1956). *Amer. J. Surg.*, **92**, 688.
Banks, B. M., Korelitz, B. I. and Zetzel, L. (1957). *Gastroenterology*, **32**, 983.
Bargen, J. A. and Kennedy, R. L. J. (1955) *Postgrad. Med.*, **17**, 127.
Covernton, J. (1949). *Clin. Rep. Adelaide Child. Hosp.*, **1**, 230.
Cullinan, E. R. and MacDougall, I. P. (1957). *Lancet*, **1**, 487.
Gelber, I., Hawthorne, H. R. and Gelb, A. (1955). *Gastroenterology*, **28**, 836.
Hagan, W. H. and Hagan, H. (1957). *Sth med. J. (Bgham, Ala.)*, **50**, 99.
Helmholz, H. F. (1923). *Amer. J. Dis. Child.*, **26**, 418.
Holowach, J. and Thurston, D. L. (1956). *J. Pediat.*, **48**, 279.
Hurt, L. E. (1954). *Ann. Surg.*, **139**, 838.
Jackman, R. J., Bargen, J. A. and Helmholz, H. F. (1940). *Amer. J. Dis. Child.*, **59**, 459.
Kiefer, E. D., Eytinge, E. J. and Johnson, A. C. (1951). *Gastroenterology*, **19**, 51.
Lagercrantz, R. (1955). *Acta paediat. (Uppsala)*, **44**, 302.
Lyons, A. S. (1956). *Pediat. Clin. N. Amer.*, Feb. 1956, p. 153.
—— and Garlock, J. H. (1951). *Gastroenterology*, **18**, 170.
MacDougall, I. P. M. (1954). *Brit. med. J.*, **1**, 852.
Meeker, I. A. and Goff, P. (1956). *West. J. Surg.*, **64**, 545.
Schlesinger, B. and Platt, J. (1958). *Proc. roy. Soc. Med.*, **51**, 733.
Sloan, W. P., Bargen, J. A. and Gage, R. P. (1950). *Gastroenterology*, **16**, 25.
Sydenham, T. (1848). *The Works of Thomas Sydenham*, Vol. 1, p. 166. Sydenham Society, London.
Thorlakson, R. H. (1956). *Surg. Gynec. Obstet.*, **103**, 41.
Tidrick, R. T. and Hickey, R. C. (1956). *J. Iowa St. med. Soc.*, **46**, 485.
Weckesser, E. C. and Chinn, A. B. (1953). *J. Amer. med. Ass.*, **152**, 905.
Wilcox, H. R. and Beattie, J. L. (1956). *Amer. J. clin. Path.*, **26**, 778.

PHYSIOLOGICAL JAUNDICE

BY

A. A. CUNNINGHAM

From the Kingston Hospital

(RECEIVED FOR PUBLICATION NOVEMBER 19, 1958)

Davidson, Merritt and Weech (1941), using the 'micro' method where blood was obtained from the heel, the usual amount collected being 0·5 ml., carried out a detailed study of bilirubin levels of 132 infants during the neonatal period. Correlated levels revealed that, at a concentration of 4-5 mg. % per 100 ml. serum, approximately half of the infants had jaundice. They also found that there was a highly significant association between the level of bilirubin in serum from the umbilical cord and the subsequent intensity and duration of jaundice in the infant. Billing, Cole and Lathe (1954) studied normal newborn babies selected to provide a wide range of birth weights. Heel prick blood was collected with heparin or oxalate and 0·05 to 0·2 ml. of plasma was used in quantitative estimation by Van den Bergh diazo technique. It was found that the influence of birth weight on the amount of pigment extended through the range of birth weights from 3-9 lb. and was most fully extended among small infants where plasma concentration often rose to 12 mg. % or above. They estimated that in certain circumstances the liver capacity to excrete pigment was reduced to 1-2% of normal. Meyer (1956) using venous samples of blood investigated serum bilirubin levels in 93 babies, of whom 46 were premature, who did not develop kernikterus. Babies under 2,000 g. (4 lb. 6 oz.) had levels rising on the sixth day, babies of 2,000-2,500 g. levelling out, and babies over 2,500 g. with falling levels on the sixth day.

The first stage in our research project was to find methods of bilirubin assay which could easily be applied to babies in the maternity unit. With the co-operation of Dr. D. Stark Murray, Kingston group pathologist, this was accomplished by Mr. J. M. Daly, chief biochemical laboratory technician. The tests were primarily designed to meet our needs in the treatment of haemolytic disease.

* This report is part of a wider investigation covering the field of neonatal jaundice which was a prizewinning entry in the 1958 competition for research work sponsored by the South-West Metropolitan Regional Hospital Board.

Details of the Daly 'Macro' and 'Micro' Methods of Bilirubin Assay

The 'Macro' Method. This method was prompted by the need for quick and reliable estimations of serum bilirubin levels in cord blood from infants of rhesus negative mothers with antibodies. The method had to satisfy the following conditions: (*a*) the colour had to be of sufficient intensity to give accurate absorptiometric readings over the range of 0·5-5·0 mg. % which meant that a serum dilution factor greater than 1 in 10 was undesirable; (*b*) the solution had to be free from turbidity; (*c*) sufficient solution had to be available for satisfactory readings; (*d*) the method had to combine speed with simplicity and reliability.

PRINCIPLE. Diazo reagent is added to the serum; simultaneous colour production and protein precipitation takes place with the addition of the alcohol/ether mixture. The proteins are then removed by centrifugation and the colour intensity of the clear supernatant fluid is measured photometrically (see Note 3).

REAGENTS. Absolute industrial spirit: ether: a mixture of equal volumes of each.

Van den Bergh diazo reagent: Solution A. Dissolve 1 g. of sulphanilic acid in 15 ml. of concentrated HCl. and make up to 1 l. with water. Solution B. Dissolve 0·5 g. of sodium nitrite in water and make up to 100 ml.

Mix 10 ml. of Solution A with 0·3 ml. of Solution B.

(*a*) DIRECT REACTION. In a centrifuge tube place: (1) 0·5 ml. diazo reagent plus 0·5 ml. serum; (2) add 4 ml. of distilled water and mix; (3) transfer to a 1 cm. cuvette and read at one minute and again at 15 minutes.

(*b*) INDIRECT REACTION. (Total bilirubin.) In a centrifuge tube place: (1) 0·5 ml. serum plus 0·5 ml. diazo reagent; (2) add 4 ml. of the alcohol/ether (50% v/v) mixture. Stopper with a rubber bung and mix well; (3) centrifuge for three minutes; (4) read in the colorimeter 10 minutes after the addition of the alcohol/ether reagent, using a wavelength of 540 millimicrons (Ilford filters 404 or 625); (5) read the result on a calibration curve.

CALIBRATION CURVE. Weigh out 20 mg. of dry bilirubin (B.D.H.) and dissolve in about 4 ml. of N/10 sodium hydroxide. Wash this into a 200 ml. volumetric flask with several flushes of water and make up to the mark. From this stock solution make up a series o standards containing 0·5, 1·0, 1·5, 2·0, 2·5, 3, 4, 5, 6, 7, 8, 9, 10 mg. % bilirubin by suitable dilution with saline. Each one of these standards is then put through Stages 1 and 2 for total bilirubin and the extinction values read after maximum colour has developed. This usually takes about half an hour. A calibration curve is then prepared from these data.

NOTES. (1) The bilirubin standard must be made up fresh and the calibration curve prepared immediately. (2) After the addition of the alcohol/ether mixture the contents of the tube should be well mixed or a clear supernatant will not be obtained after centrifuging. (3) Ensure that the centrifuge used is of a type suitable for spinning inflammable mixtures of the alcohol/ether type. (4) If the bilirubin level exceeds 10 mg. % dilute the serum with saline to bring it into this range. (See comparison chart, Fig. 1.)

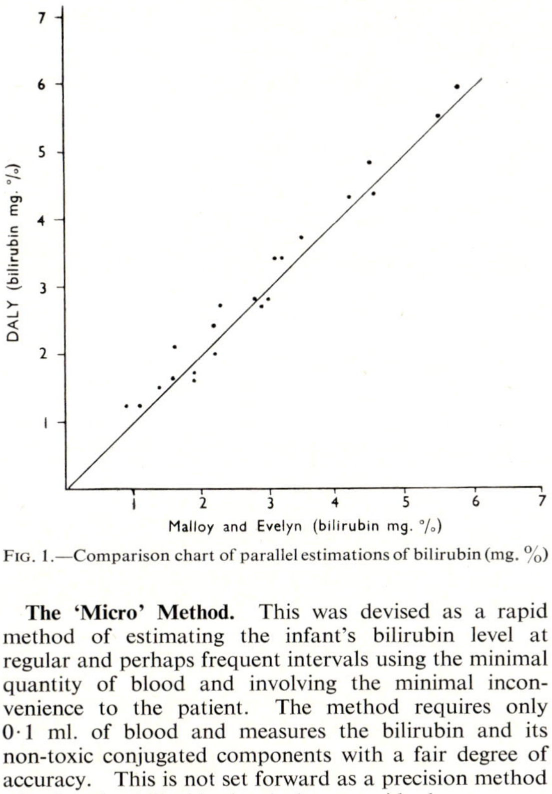

FIG. 1.—Comparison chart of parallel estimations of bilirubin (mg. %)

The 'Micro' Method. This was devised as a rapid method of estimating the infant's bilirubin level at regular and perhaps frequent intervals using the minimal quantity of blood and involving the minimal inconvenience to the patient. The method requires only 0·1 ml. of blood and measures the bilirubin and its non-toxic conjugated components with a fair degree of accuracy. This is not set forward as a precision method of estimating bilirubin, but it does provide the necessary information quickly and gives reasonably accurate results in the range of 3-20 mg. % of serum bilirubin.

PRINCIPLE. A micro-quantity of blood is added to a tube containing 0·85% sodium chloride solution. The tube is then centrifuged and the icterus of the serum measured photometrically.

METHOD: (*a*) TOTAL BILIRUBIN. (1) 0·1 ml. of blood is obtained from a heel stab and washed into a tube containing 2·9 ml. of 0·85% saline. Care must be taken to avoid haemolysis. (In this laboratory a 1 cm. diameter E.E.L. tube is used and has been found perfectly satisfactory in practice.) (2) Mix well by inversion and centrifuge for five minutes; (3) read in the colorimeter using a blue (Ilford 303) filter or, if a spectrophotometer is preferred, transfer the clear supernatant to a 1 cm. cuvette and read at 480 millimicrons using saline as blank; (4) read result against the calibration curve.

(*b*) DIRECT BILIRUBIN. (1) Take 2 ml. of the above supernatant fluid and pipette it into another 1 cm. E.E.L. tube or cuvette; (2) add 1 ml. of diazo reagent; (3) mix and stand at room temperature for 15 minutes; (4) read in colorimeter using a green filter (Ilford 404) or if a spectrophotometer is preferred at 540 millimicrons; (5) read result against calibration curve.

NOTES. (1) The blood must be collected with care as any trace of haemolysis affects the readings. Ether and not alcohol should be used to sterilize the skin. (2) If a spectrophotometer is available, the transmission at 578 millimicrons should be measured. This should not be lower than 90%. (3) Lipochromes do not appear to interfere at the dilution used. (4) A haemoglobin estimation is always done at the same time.

CALIBRATION CURVE FOR TOTAL BILIRUBIN. A sample of heparinised blood is obtained from a patient with obstructive jaundice (i.e. with a high direct component). Mix thoroughly and pour off a fraction of the sample into a centrifuge tube. Spin and estimate the bilirubin content according to the 'macro' method described. Place another fraction in a P.C.V. tube and estimate its value. This should be in the region of 50%±2%.

The curve is then prepared by taking 0·1, 0·09, 0·08 ml. etc. down to 0·01 ml. of the heparinised whole blood sample and making up the volume in each case to 0·1 ml. with a well mixed heparinised blood sample from an unjaundiced patient. These samples are washed into 2·9 ml. of saline and treated according to the Stages 1, 2, 3 and 4 as for total bilirubin. Plot a graph.

In this laboratory the original calibration curve was prepared from a sample of blood containing a serum bilirubin of 20 mg. %, a haemoglobin of 102% and P.C.V. of 49%. This curve has been repeatedly checked throughout the recorded series and found to be quite constant so that slight variations in haemoglobin and P.C.V. content do not appear to influence the result very greatly.

CALIBRATION CURVE FOR DIRECT BILIRUBIN. After reading the total bilirubin samples above, transfer 2 ml. of the supernatant fluids to 1 cm. E.E.L. tubes or cuvettes and treat the samples according to Stages 2, 3, 4 and 5 as for direct bilirubin. Plot a graph.

Present Investigation

It was decided to investigate a sequence of 1,000 babies born in the maternity unit of Kingston Hospital from April 1, 1957, onwards, over a period of seven months. We eliminated from the investigation all babies of 2½ lb. and under, those suffering from haemolytic disease of the newborn and a few who did not live long enough to develop jaundice. The babies were visited daily and an estimate of the jaundice made clinically in daylight as far as possible. Bilirubin estimations were carried out at various stages in an effort to find the day of maximal staining. Table 1 gives a résumé of the results.

For control purposes, estimations were carried out on 50 babies of various weights on various days of life at a time when no clinical jaundice was detectable, even after pressing the skin in a good light. In 45 out of 50 cases, the total bilirubin was less than 3 mg. %. In each of three cases the total was 3 mg. %, in one case it was 3·5 mg. % and in another 4·5 mg. %. This shows that there is a small error in clinical judgment. Lighting, texture of the skin and the high red cell count are factors which cause this difficulty of assessment.

In our series it was quite possible that cases of jaundice of a few hours' duration were missed, so it was decided that it would be more accurate to analyse only those cases of jaundice with a total bilirubin content of over 5 mg. %. The results are shown graphically on the accompanying charts (Figs. 2 and 3) where bilirubin total and direct estimations are plotted against weight in pounds, with standard deviations in each group. Table 2 gives the percentage in each weight group in relation to the total number of babies in the survey.

It will be seen that there were 140 babies with a maximal total bilirubin over 5 mg. %=14% of total and of these there were 34 with maximal bilirubin over 10 mg. %=3·4% of total. Furthermore, it would appear that about 70% of babies weighing 4½ lb. or less at birth will develop maximal jaundice to a level of over 5 mg. % and about 30% to over 10 mg. %. In addition, seven out of 63, i.e. approximately 11% of all premature babies will produce a maximal bilirubin percentage of 15 mg. % or more and it is in this group that the danger of kernikterus arises.

Exchange transfusion is the only treatment we have to control the rise of bilirubin concentration, but this is a procedure fraught with considerable danger to small babies and it is difficult to decide at what level the procedure should be carried out or repeated.

Exchange transfusions were carried out in three cases in this series.

Case Notes

Case 1. J.A., a male twin (1), was born following antepartum haemorrhage with first loss six days prior to admission and quite heavy loss during the day of admission. The mother, aged 19, had had three children (two miscarriages in two previous years at two to three months). J.A. cried in one minute and respirations were feebly established in two minutes. The baby weighed 3 lb. 11½ oz. when admitted to the Premature Baby Unit, and oxygen was given throughout the day. The mother's blood group was A Rh.+ve, baby's A Rh.+ve. On the second day at 5 a.m., the baby had a severe cyanotic attack. Intragastric oxygen was given with coramine and lobeline about half an hour later as respirations were intermittent and the heart beat extremely weak. Penicillin and streptomycin were given intramuscularly. On the third day, the baby's general condition was still poor and tent oxygen was continued. Bilirubin total 13·5 mg. %, direct 3·5 mg. %. On the fourth day his condition had improved slightly. Bilirubin total of 12 mg. %, direct 4·0 mg. %. On the fifth day his general condition was fair, but jaundice was very marked. Total bilirubin 18·0 mg. %, direct 7·0 mg. %.

TABLE 2

CASES WITH MAXIMAL TOTAL BILIRUBIN

Weight (lb.)	Total Cases	Over 5 mg. % (No.)	Over 5 mg. % (%)	Over 10 mg. % (No.)	Over 10 mg. % (%)
2½ –3½ } premature babies	11	9	= 82	6	= 55
3½+–4½ } premature babies	15	9	= 60	2	= 13
4½+–5½ } premature babies	37	13	= 35	7	= 19
5½+–6½	150	22	= 15	5	= 3
6½+–7½	333	40	= 12	6	= 2
7½+–8½	304	30	= 10	7	= 2
8½+–9½	130	15	= 12	1	= 0·8
9½+–10½	16	2	= 12	—	—
Over 10½	4	—	—	—	—
	1,000	140	= 14	34	= 3·4

TABLE 1

JAUNDICED BABIES : MAXIMAL TOTAL BILIRUBIN (MG. %)

Weight (lb.)	All Babies	5—3	10—5	15—10	20—15	Over 20	Total
2½+– 3½ ..	11	1	3	4	1	1	10
3½+– 4½ ..	15	2	7	1	1	—	11
4½+– 5½ ..	37	5	6	7	—	—	18
5½+– 6½ ..	150	23	17	5	—	—	45
6½+– 7½ ..	333	63	34	6	—	—	103
7½+– 8½ ..	304	54	23	7	—	—	84
8½+– 9½ ..	130	8	14	1	—	—	23
9½+–10½ ..	16	1	2	—	—	—	3
10½+–11½ ..	4	—	—	—	—	—	—
	1,000	157	106	31	2	1	297

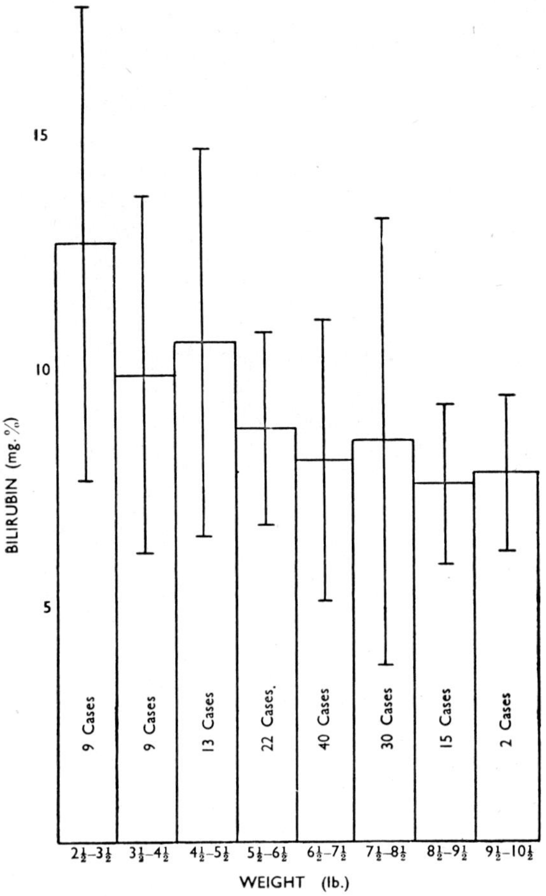

Total bilirubin:
in babies with total bilirubin over 5 mg. %.

lb.	Average	S.D.
2½- 3½	12·7	5·1
3½- 4½	9·8	3·8
4½- 5½	10·6	4·0
5½- 6½	8·7	2·0
6½- 7½	8·0	2·9
7½- 8½	8·4	4·6
8½- 9½	7·6	1·7
9½-10½	7·8	1·7

* The limits of one standard deviation are shown as a vertical line.

FIG. 2.—Total bilirubin estimation plotted against weight in pounds, with standard deviation in each group.

On the evening of the fifth day when the jaundice appeared to be very severe and the baby became listless and ill, it was decided to carry out an exchange transfusion. After 90 ml. the child's condition was so poor that transfusion was discontinued. The child's shocked condition did not, however, respond to resuscitative measures, and the child died about 40 minutes after the transfusion was stopped; at autopsy there was marked cerebral oedema, but no evidence of kernikterus.

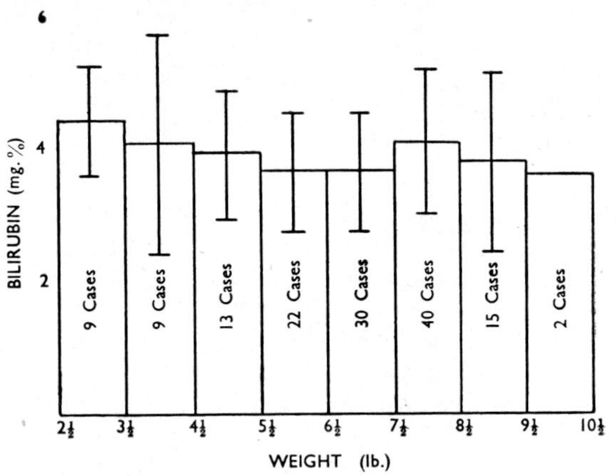

F,G. 3.—Relationship between birthweight and maximal-direct bilirubin (linked with maximal total). The limits of one standard deviation are shown as a vertical line.

Direct bilirubin (conjugated):
in babies with total bilirubin over 5·0 mg. %.

lb.	Cases	Mean	One S.D.
2½- 3½	9	4·5	0·8
3½- 4½	9	4·1	1·6
4½- 5½	13	4·0	1·0
5½- 6½	22	3·7	0·9
6½- 7½	40	3·7	0·9
7½- 8½	30	4·1	1·1
8½- 9½	15	3·8	1·3
9½-10½	2	3·6	—
	140		

FIG. 3.—Direct bilirubin estimation plotted against weight in pounds with standard deviation in each group.

Case 2. D.A., a male twin (2), brother of the above twin, was born by breech delivery. He cried in one minute, and respiration was established in two. Birth weight was 3 lb. 3 oz. Both legs were discoloured and oedematous. His blood group was A Rh.+ve. On the first day the child passed a melaena stool on two occasions. Vitamin K 2·5 mg. was given intramuscularly. On the second day there were several melaena stools. Jaundice at 24 hours. On the third day the baby was deeply jaundiced. Total bilirubin 13·5 mg. %, direct 3·5 mg. %. Exchange transfusions was carried out in the evening of the third day. Intramuscular digoxin 0·0625 mg. was given before transfusion. The bilirubin total fell from 15 mg. % at the onset to 9 mg. % towards the end of the transfusion. The total exchange was 240 ml. in and 243 ml. out. The child's condition was very poor throughout the night following the transfusion and there were grunting respirations all the time. He had improved slightly on the fourth day. Bilirubin total 12·0 mg. %, direct 4·0 mg. %. On the fifth day jaundice again was deep. Bilirubin total 22·0 mg. %, direct 8·0 mg. %. A second exchange transfusion was started, but after 20 ml. great difficulty was experienced with clotting in the catheter and it was decided to discontinue the operation. Dextrose saline, 50 ml., was given intravenously.

Jaundice was still very deep on the sixth day. There were no signs of kernikterus in the central nervous system. Bilirubin total 26·0 mg. %, direct 6·0 mg. %. On the seventh day jaundice was still deep. Again there were no signs of kernikterus. Bilirubin total 24·0 mg. %, direct 8·0 mg. %. On the ninth day bilirubin total 16·0 mg. %, direct 4·0 mg. %, and on the fifteenth day bilirubin total 4·5 mg. %, direct 2·0 mg. %.

This baby made good progress in the neonatal period, developed anaemia on the thirty-third day of life and was given 75 ml. of fresh blood. He continued to make good progress, gained weight, and since then has developed into a normal healthy baby.

Case 3. J.D., male. The mother was admitted with severe antepartum haemorrhage. There was a normal vertex delivery, and the birth weight was 3 lb. 3 oz. He cried weakly in one minute, and then respiration became grunting in character. His condition improved after intragastric oxygen for half an hour. The child was placed in an oxygen tent. There was a melaena stool on the first day, and again on the second with fresh blood. Synkavit, 1 mg., was given intramuscularly. Jaundice was noticed at 30 hours. On the third day jaundice increased. Bilirubin total (a.m.) 9·0 mg. %, direct 4·0 mg. %. Stools contained a large amount of fresh blood. By evening the bilirubin total was 11·5 mg. %, direct 4·0 mg. %. In spite of the considerable amount of fresh blood in the stools, the haemoglobin remained high. It was decided to carry out a small exchange transfusion using very fresh blood, primarily with the object of treating the haemorrhagic disease yet also to control the bilirubin concentration. The transfusion was completed in 1 hour (110 ml. in and 110 ml. out) by which time the baby's condition showed signs of deterioration. The respirations were shallow and grunting and there were some twitching jerking movements which responded quickly to chloral hydrate sedation. On the fourth day a dark melaena stool was passed on two occasions. Bilirubin total 10 mg. %, direct 3·5 mg. %. On the fifth day his general condition was much improved. Bilirubin total 10·0 mg. %, direct 4·0 mg. %. The improvement continued on the sixth day. Melaena stool. Bilirubin total 16·5 mg. %, direct 4·0 mg. %. On the seventh day bilirubin total 15·0 mg. %, direct 7·0 mg. %.

The jaundice lasted in all about 13 days. The lowest weight was 2 lb. 9¼ oz. on the fourteenth day, and from then onwards progress was steady and uneventful, apart from the development of anaemia in the sixth week of life. This case emphasizes the value of a small exchange transfusion, using fresh blood, in the treatment of haemorrhagic disease where the haemoglobin is high and the baby very small.

The quick methods of bilirubin assay were of particular value in following up the jaundice in these three cases. It is interesting to speculate on the danger of bilirubin, but one feels that in the development of kernikterus in premature babies there are probably other factors as well as the increased level of bilirubin.

It is also to be noted that a small percentage of babies weighing over 5½ lb. will develop comparatively high levels of jaundice. The percentage appears to vary very little with birth weight in this group or with period of gestation and it is rather remarkable that the figures for, say, 8½-lb. babies are little different from those of, say, 6-lb. babies.

The incidence of jaundice, especially as it appeared to be similar in the various weight groups over 5½ lb., suggested that there might be some cause which operated at all weights in non-premature babies. Rhesus incompatibility was excluded in all cases as routine, but ABO or other blood group incompatibility was much more difficult to recognize. Severe cases of ABO haemolytic disease can generally be diagnosed clinically even without the help of laboratory aids, but mild cases present a problem. Unlike rhesus disease, ABO incompatibility cannot be anticipated by antenatal testing. However, since the work of Boorman, Dodd and Trinick (1949) more cases of ABO haemolytic disease have been recognized. Valentine (1958) selected from 1,000 unselected live births all babies showing jaundice in the first 24 hours of life. Of 21 so investigated, seven were cases of rhesus haemolytic disease. The jaundice of the remaining 14 he considered to be due to ABO haemolytic disease. He concluded that ABO haemolytic disease can occur in a clinically recognized form as often as once in 71 births and may arise in 7% of AB incompatible mother/child pairs, i.e. three times as commonly as rhesus haemolytic disease.

In this series, we had 24 cases where jaundice was detected about 24 hours after birth or less. The mother and baby blood groups are shown in Tables 3 and 4.

TABLE 3

BABIES WITH JAUNDICE 24 HR. OR LESS AFTER BIRTH: 24 PAIRS

Blood Group:										
Mother's ..	O	O	O	A	A	A	B	A	B	O
Baby's ..	A	B	O	A	O	AB	O	B	?	?
Totals ..	4	1	7	6	1	1	1	1	1	1

TABLE 4

ABO INCOMPATIBLE PAIRS WITH MOTHER'S BLOOD GROUP O JAUNDICE 24 HR. OR LESS AFTER BIRTH: 5 PAIRS

Blood Group:					
Mother's	O	O	O	O	O
Baby's	B	A	A	A	A
Baby's weight (lb. oz.) ..	4·13	6·3½	7·3	7·13	8·13
Maximal bilirubin (mg. %) ..	15·0	7·5	7·5	5·5	12·0

We then surveyed those cases of physiological jaundice where the maximal bilirubin was over 10 mg. % (34 in all) (Tables 5 and 6).

TABLE 5

ABO MOTHER/CHILD GROUPS
BABIES WITH MAXIMAL BILIRUBIN OVER 10 MG. %: 34 PAIRS

Blood Group :								
Mother's	O	O	O	A	A	B	A	A
Baby's	A	B	O	A	O	O	?	?
Total	7	1	10	12	1	1	1	1

TABLE 6

ABO INCOMPATIBLE MOTHER/CHILD PAIRS WITH MOTHER'S GROUP O: 8 PAIRS

Blood Group :								
Mother's	O	O	O	O	O	O	O	O
Baby's	A	A	A	A	A	A	B	A
Baby's weight (lb. oz.) ..	5·4	7·13	7·9	5·5	6·15½	3·3	4·13	8·13
Maximal bilirubin (mg. %)	12·0	10·5	12·5	15·0	13·5	16·5	15·0	12·0

In this short series, the babies of three of the OA pairs and that of the OB pair were premature. We did not have the facilities for carrying out extensive blood type grouping such as that which Valentine used, but if one excludes prematurity the number of cases of ABO haemolytic disease in our series must have been very limited, if indeed any cases existed at all. The babies from the ABO incompatible mother/child pairs were clinically no different from those where there was ABO compatibility.

The incidence of group A persons in the general population in this part of southern England is slightly higher than that for the British Isles as a whole, so if ABO haemolytic disease is as common as Valentine suggests there should be more evidence of it in a series of this kind. Our experience, therefore, does not support Valentine's work.

Apart from prematurity, we have not been able to separate any other cause for so-called 'physiological jaundice'. Vitamin K was given sparingly in doses of 1-2·5 mg., one dose only in each case, to premature babies and to a trivial number of other babies after complicated obstetric procedures. We did not consider vitamin K in this dosage to be a factor. There was no evidence of syphilis or sepsis, or blood disease in any of our cases.

Cord Blood Estimations

In a further series of babies, an effort was made to correlate the level of cord bilirubin with subsequent jaundice, but in practice this was most difficult and quite unrewarding. It was quite impossible to get a succession of cases, for complicated obstetric procedures, quick removal of the placenta, concentrated obstetric work, etc., made the collection of samples extremely difficult, and at times impossible. It was also disturbing to find that certain samples taken by skilled operators soon after birth were unsatisfactory because of slight haemolysis. This haemolysis, presumably due to enzyme action, occurred between one and 10 minutes after birth. The result of the investigation, therefore, applied to random samples taken as and when convenient.

Table 7 shows the correlation between weight and cord blood bilirubin estimations in 80 babies who did not subsequently develop clinical jaundice:

TABLE 7

CORD BLOOD TOTAL BILIRUBIN ESTIMATION IN 80 BABIES WITHOUT SUBSEQUENT CLINICAL JAUNDICE

Weight (lb.)	Up to and including 1·5 mg. %	Over 1·5 to 2·0 mg. %	Over 2·0 to 2·5 mg. %
	(no.)	(no.)	(no.)
Over 5½ to 6½ ..	6	1	1
Over 6½ to 7½ ..	16	10	3
Over 7½ to 8½ ..	10	8	6
Over 8½ to 9½ ..	11	3	2
Over 9½ to 10½ ..	3	—	—
Total (80) ..	46=57·5%	22=27·5%	12 =15%

Table 8 shows the cord blood total bilirubin estimation in 39 babies who subsequently developed clinical jaundice:

Of the babies without clinical jaundice all had a total bilirubin in the cord blood of 2·5 mg. % or less and of this total, 57·5% had a total cord blood bilirubin of 1·5 mg. % or less. Of those with clinical jaundice, 38·4% had a cord bilirubin over

TABLE 8

CORD BLOOD TOTAL BILIRUBIN ESTIMATION IN 39 BABIES WHO LATER DEVELOPED CLINICAL JAUNDICE

Weight (lb.)	Up to and including 1·5 mg. %	Over 1·5–2·0 mg. %	Over 2·0–2·5 mg. %	Over 2·5 –3·0 mg. %	Over 3·0 mg. %
Over 5½ to 6½	2	2	3	4	1
Over 6½ to 7½	—	3	4	3	1
Over 7½ to 8½	—	3	3	3	1
Over 8½ to 9½	—	2	2	1	—
Over 9½ to 10½ ..	—	—	—	1	—
Total (39) ..	2=5·1%	10=25·6%	12=30·8%	12=30·8%	3=7·6%

TABLE 9

Sex	Weight	Blood	Group*	Cord Bilirubin (mg. %)		Day of Maximal Total Bilirubin (mg. %)†								
	lb. oz.	Mother	Baby	Total	Direct	2	3	4	5	6	7	8	9	10
M	7 9	A+ve	A+ve	1·6	0·3	—	—	7·5	7·5	—	9·0	—	11·0	8·0
						—	—	(3·0)	(3·0)	—	(4·0)	—	(4·0)	(3·0)
F	5 13	O+ve	O+ve	2·5	0·6	—	7·5	10·5	9·0	—	—	7·5	—	—
						—	(3·0)	(4·5)	(3·5)	—	—	(4·0)	—	—
F	5 14	A+ve	A+ve	1·3	0·6	6·5	—	3·0	3·0	—	—	7·5	—	—
						(2·5)	—	(1·5)	(1·5)	—	—	(4·0)	—	—
M	7 9	O−ve	A−ve	3·4	0·0	4·5	—	4·5	—	—	—	—	—	—
						(2·0)	—	(2·0)	—	—	—	—	—	—
M	8 2	B+ve	O+ve	1·6	0·0	3·0	7·5	—	—	—	—	—	—	—
						(0·0)	(2·5)	—	—	—	—	—	—	—
M	7 13	A+ve	A+ve	3·0	0·5	—	—	—	4·5	—	—	—	—	—
						—	—	—	(1·5)	—	—	—	—	—
M	7 12	A+ve	A+ve	3·0	0·75	—	3·0	—	—	6·0	5·0	—	—	—
						—	—	—	—	(2·5)	(2·0)	—	—	—
M	7 8	A+ve	B+ve	2·7	0·75	—	7·5	7·5	7·5	—	—	—	—	—
						—	(2·5)	(2·5)	(2·5)	—	—	—	—	—
M	6 10	O+ve	A−ve	3·6	1·0	3·5	—	4·5	—	—	—	—	—	—
						(0·5)	—	(1·5)	—	—	—	—	—	—

* Positive and negative signs refer to Rh+ve and Rh−ve
† (Direct component in parenthesis)

2·5 mg. % and only a small percentage had a cord bilirubin over 3 mg. %. The highest figure in the series was a cord blood bilirubin of 3·6 mg. % (direct 1·0 mg. %)—a male child weighing 6 lb. 10 oz. who subsequently developed a mild degree of jaundice only, reaching a maximal total bilirubin of 4·5 mg. % (direct 1·5 mg. %) on the fifth day. The other babies with a cord blood bilirubin of over 3 mg. % all developed a comparatively mild degree of jaundice around 5 mg. % at the maximum. The great variety in results is shown in Table 9 by some examples.

This short investigation, carried out under great difficulty (and not very popular in the obstetric department) showed that estimations of cord bilirubin were of very little value in forecasting the subsequent development of jaundice. We could not find the correlation which other workers have reported.

Summary

A series of 1,000 consecutive babies born in the maternity unit of Kingston Hospital was studied with particular reference to the incidence of so-called 'physiological jaundice'. The series did not include cases of diagnosable haemolytic disease, premature babies under 2½ lb. in weight and those babies who died before jaundice could be determined; 14% of the babies developed a maximal bilirubin over 5 mg. % and of the total 3·4% developed a maximal total bilirubin over 10 mg. %.

Of the premature babies, 63 in all, 11 developed a maximal bilirubin concentration of 15 mg. % or more; three of these had exchange transfusion, one of whom died, but the other two made a good recovery and are normal healthy children.

The incidence and severity of so-called physiological jaundice is most marked in premature babies and is presumably associated with immaturity of liver function; in about 10% of these babies there is some risk of the development of kernikterus. In babies over 5½ lb. in weight at birth, about 2% developed jaundice with a maximal bilirubin level over 10 mg. %, but there did not appear to be any danger of kernikterus in these cases. Contrary to the work of Valentine (1958), we did not find any evidence to justify a diagnosis of ABO haemolytic disease as a causative factor, even in those babies who developed jaundice within 24 hours of birth.

In a second series of 119 babies, taken at random (80 without clinical jaundice and 39 with clinical jaundice) no correlation of value could be found when cord blood estimations were linked with the development of subsequent jaundice.

I should like to acknowledge the help and co-operation received from Dr. D. Stark Murray, group pathologist, and Dr. B. Meade, consultant biochemist, of the Kingston Group Laboratory, and Dr. A. F. Huston, assistant paediatrician. I must particularly thank Mr. G. Gray and Mr. J. M. Daly, senior laboratory technicians, who collected and tested most of the blood samples, also Miss J. MacIntyre, Matron, Miss C. M. Bowen, superintendent midwife, and many sisters and nurses from the Maternity Unit, without whose devoted care, nursing skill and goodwill, an investigation of this type would be of no avail.

REFERENCES

Billing, B. H., Cole, P. G. and Lathe, G. (1954). *Brit. med. J.*, **2**, 1263.
Boorman, K. E., Dodd, B. E. and Trinick, R. H. (1949). *Lancet*, 1, 1088.
Davidson, L. T., Merritt, K. K. and Weech, A. A. (1941). *Amer. J. Dis. Child.*, **61**, 958.
Meyer, T. C. (1956). *Arch. Dis. Childh.*, **31**, 75.
Valentine, G. H. (1958). *Ibid.*, **33**, 185.

THE DIAGNOSIS OF MENTAL RETARDATION IN INFANCY

A FOLLOW-UP STUDY

BY

R. S. ILLINGWORTH and L. B. BIRCH

From the University of Sheffield and the Children's Hospital, Sheffield, and the Institute of Education, University of Sheffield

(RECEIVED FOR PUBLICATION DECEMBER 22, 1958)

There seems to be an increasingly firm conviction among psychiatrists and psychologists that developmental tests in infancy have little or no predictive value. For instance, Bowlby (1951) wrote in his famous monograph that 'mental tests have no predictive value in the first 18 months of life'. Kirman (1953) wrote that 'few people are so bold as to claim to be able to measure intelligence in babies or to predict the future course of their mental development'. Eysenck (1953) wrote that 'intelligence testing before the age of 6, or 5 at the earliest, should be discouraged', because, he said, 'testing before the age of 2 has no predictive accuracy at all for adult intelligence'. Apgar, Girdany, McIntosh and Taylor (1955) wrote of the meagre value of Gesell rating of adaptive behaviour at 2 years as compared with the Stanford Binet test at 5 years. Wittenborn (1957) concluded that developmental tests were of very little value in determining the intelligence of babies for the purposes of adoption. Sontag, Baker and Nelson (1958) wrote that levels of I.Q. at pre-school age have hardly any predictive value. Karelitz (1958) wrote that ' it is now recognized that psychological tests of infants cannot be used to predict the child's future development'. Kirman (1958) wrote 'in regard to mental deficiency it is possible to recognize only severe mental defect at an early stage', and 'the predictive value of tests under the age of 5 years is very low'.

Many of these statements are incontrovertible. Correlation coefficients calculated between the results of assessments of ability made first in infancy and later in childhood are known to be very low. When the first assessment is made before the age of 2 years they commonly approximate to zero and may even be negative (Bayley, 1940).

Until a correlation coefficient rises to the order of 0·9 prediction of one variable from another is very little superior to a prediction based upon chance. It is frequently forgotten, however, that a low correlation between two sets of scores may not be incompatible with reasonably accurate prediction within certain narrow limits within the total range of the two measures. If the two measures follow an approximately Gaussian distribution and if the particular narrow limits, within which accurate prediction is possible, lie at either extreme of the distributions, then the contribution of the relatively few scores involved may be negligible in the calculation of a product moment correlation coefficient. It seems that such is the case in the prognosis of mental retardation, for it has long been known that the I.Q. of dull children is much more constant than it is in normal or super-normal children (Terman and Merrill, 1937). For this reason psychologists (e.g. Valentine, 1950), who would not subscribe to the general usefulness of early testing, have advocated procedures, including tests, for early diagnosis of mental defect, and Goodenough (1949) commented, 'in as much as radical changes in the treatment of backward and feeble minded children are more likely to depend upon the results of mental tests than is the case with children of normal or superior intelligence, the greater dependability of the intelligence quotient at the lower levels is a matter of considerable importance for those actively concerned with the welfare of children'. Vernon did not rule out early testing for the detection of mentally defective children when he wrote 'indeed the various tests of developmental level sometimes applied to babies from 0 to 2½ years provide practically no indication of later intelligence, except perhaps in cases of severe mental defect' (Vernon, 1957).

We imagine that any paediatrician would agree that in the majority of cases the diagnosis of severe mental retardation can readily be made in

TABLE 1

AGE OF DIAGNOSIS OF MENTAL RETARDATION WITH OR WITHOUT CEREBRAL PALSY*

Age of Diagnosis (months)	Mental Retardation Alone		Mental Retardation with Cerebral Palsy		Total	
	Total	Percentage of whole	Total	Percentage of whole	Total	Percentage of whole
0-3	27	6·4	11	6·0	38	6·3
Second 3	39	9·3	8	4·4	47	7·8
6-12	52	12·4	28	15·4	80	13·3
12-24	60	14·3	36	19·8	96	16·0
Later than 24	240	57·4	99	54·4	339	56·5
Total	418		182		600	

* Cases of mongolism, cretinism, hydrocephalus and anencephaly excluded.

infancy, though no one would deny that there are some cases which present great difficulty.

In the last 11½ years in the Department of Child Health, at the Children's Hospital, Sheffield, of 600 consecutive children thought to be mentally retarded, other than cases of mongolism, cretinism, hydrocephalus or anencephaly, the diagnosis was made in 261 (43·9%) before the second birthday (Table 1).

The report which follows concerns the first part of a follow-up study of children who were thought to show retardation of mental development in infancy, however slight and uncertain.

Method of Study

The study is based on 135 children who were considered by members of the Department of Child Health to be mentally retarded when first examined. All were under the age of 2 and all were born in 1953 or before. Cases of mongolism, cretinism, hydrocephalus and anencephaly were excluded. Children with cerebral palsy have been included, provided that a diagnosis of mental retardation was made. Subsequent reports will deal with children born in 1954 and later, when they reach the age of 5 years. In five children the mental retardation followed tuberculous meningitis, in three it followed pyogenic meningitis, and in two it followed encephalitis. The others were of pre-natal or natal origin. Three cases were complicated by congenital hypotonia, and three by blindness.

Every possible effort has been made to ensure that all cases thought to be retarded have been included. A triple check on the indexing of diagnoses is in use, and we do not think that any cases have been missed from our list. We can certainly say that every case indexed as mental retardation has been included in the study. There is therefore no question of the cases being in any way 'selected'.

The original diagnosis was made on the basis of simple developmental tests culled from the Gesell schedules, including as many different fields of development as possible. We did not, in other words, make the mistake of relying on motor tests alone for our opinions. We paid great attention to the developmental history, and followed that by the physical and developmental examination, interpreting our findings in the light of the history, as was done in the Yale Clinic of Child Development under Gesell. The method of developmental study has been summarized elsewhere (Illingworth, 1957). The diagnoses were made in the ward or in the out-patient department in the course of ordinary out-patient work, but not in a special clinic. About 95% were seen by the senior author of this paper (R.S.I.) but in some the initial diagnosis was made by other members of the Department of Child Health.

The age of the initial diagnosis of retardation is shown in Table 2.

TABLE 2

AGE OF INITIAL DIAGNOSIS OF MENTAL RETARDATION

Age (months)	Number	Percentage of Whole
0 to 3	19	14
3¼ to 6	17	13
6 to 12	41	30
12 to 24 ..	59	43

It will be seen that the diagnosis was made in the first three months in 19 children; in the first six months in 36 children, and in the first year in 77.

The majority of the children have been under continual observation in the out-patient department. Once a diagnosis of retardation was made, however, the child was included in the study even though subsequent observation indicated that the initial opinion was incorrect.

The follow-up study was based on intelligence

tests carried out by school medical officers, educational psychologists and by the Institute of Education. The usual test employed was that of Terman and Merrill. The patients came from a wide area, mostly within a radius of about 80 miles, and further uniformity in testing was impossible.

The oldest child at the time of follow-up was 10 years of age.

Children not Traced. Two children could not be traced: (1) the son of an itinerant gipsy. The boy was seen at the age of 18 months, when a diagnosis of spastic quadriplegia with amentia was made. He was not seen again; (2) a girl of 3 months was admitted to the hospital on account of vomiting. There was some retardation of motor development and it was thought that the knee jerks were exaggerated. She was thought to be slightly retarded. The following note was included in the letter to the family doctor: 'A definite prognosis as to the mental retardation cannot yet be given, and the baby will obviously need further observation to determine the progress of development.' By the age of 6 months it was decided that she was normal. The opinion was confirmed at 11 months, and she was not seen again. She subsequently emigrated.

Results

The results are summarized in Table 3. Of the 77 children in whom the diagnosis of mental retardation was made in the first year, 26 had died, and one was not traced. Of the 59 children diagnosed in the second year, six had died and one could not be traced. Most of the deaths occurred at home, so that autopsy findings were available in only 10, all of whom had gross brain anomalies obvious to the naked eye. Of the remaining 22 who died, the diagnosis of severe mental deficiency had been confirmed by intelligence tests after the age of 5 in one, but we cannot provide evidence of the correctness of the diagnosis in the remainder, who died before the fifth birthday. Most of them, however, had been under continued observation in the out-patient department, and the diagnosis was not altered in any.

Of the remaining 101 children, 59 on follow-up examination were ineducable, 24 had an I.Q. of 50 to 75, 13 had an I.Q. of 76 to 94, and five had an I.Q. of 100 or more. Table 3 shows an attempt to correlate the grading in infancy with that at school age. It must be emphasized that the grading in infancy was a rough one only in most cases. It will be seen that of 67 children who were thought to have severe mental retardation in infancy, 55 were subsequently proved to be ineducable: while of 20 children who were thought in infancy to be slightly retarded, only two proved to be ineducable.

The five children who were thought in infancy to be retarded, but who were later shown to have an I.Q. of 100 or more, are of special interest. Below are summaries of their case histories:

TABLE 4

CORRELATION BETWEEN ROUGH GRADING IN INFANCY AND SUBSEQUENT I.Q. SCORE

Degree of Retardation	Rough Grading in Infancy	Grading at School Age: Ineducable	Grading at School Age: I.Q. over 50
Severe	66	55	12
Moderate	16	6	10
Slight	20	2	18
Total	102*	63	40

* One died.

TABLE 3

FINAL ASSESSMENT OF RESULTS

Age of Initial Diagnosis (months)	Mental Retardation Alone (MR) or Mental Retardation with Cerebral Palsy (CP)	Intelligence Test Results (I.Q.): 100+	76–94	50–75	−50	Died: Autopsy evidence of gross cerebral anomaly	Died after 5th birthday proved mental defective	No autopsy	Not Traced
0–3 . .	MR	1	3	1	2	3	1	1	1
	CP	—	1	1	1	1	—	2	—
3–6 . .	MR	—	—	3	6	2	—	2	—
	CP	—	—	—	1	1	—	2	—
6–12 . .	MR	—	3	2	12	1	—	4	—
	CP	3	—	3	6	1	—	5	—
12–24 . .	MR	—	4	7	21	1	—	2	—
	CP	1	2	7	10	—	—	3	1
Total . .		5	13	24	59	10	1	21	2

Case 1. This boy was admitted at the age of 2 months with a history of frequent convulsions for the previous three weeks. He was found to be backward in development. He had begun to smile in response to his mother at 2 months and to vocalize at 3 months. There was complete head lag in ventral suspension and when he was pulled to the sitting position. At 4½ months the head control was that of an 8 to 10-week-old baby. A subdural tap was negative, but an air encephalogram was thought to show some cortical atrophy. At 10 months he was thought to be average in development.

On follow-up examination at the age of 9 years he was found to be a normal child with an I.Q. of 122.

Comment. There was good reason for considering that the prognosis here was poor. It is well recognized that air-studies often correlate badly with developmental potential, but in this case there was the combination of retarded development with a history of frequent convulsions.

Case 2. This boy was found at the age of 7 months to have a spastic hemiplegia. An assistant, without stating his reasons, wrote that the boy had a low level of intelligence, but added that it was difficult to be sure. He was still thought to be mentally retarded at the age of 3. The diagnosis of hemiplegia was confirmed, but at the age of 7 his I.Q. was 100.

Comment. The difficulty of assessing the intelligence in cases of cerebral palsy is well known. Perhaps this boy could be termed a 'slow starter'.

Case 3. This interesting girl was seen just before her first birthday. She had been slightly retarded in her developmental history. She had been born at term. She had begun to smile at the age of 11 weeks, to grasp an object voluntarily at 6 months, and to imitate her parents at 8 months. She was not able to sit, the motor development being that of a 5-month-old child. The opinion expressed was 'minimal birth injury, almost normal mentally'. At the age of 9 she had virtually no physical disability, and the I.Q. was 118.

Comment. In retrospect the diagnosis was correct. At the age of 9 the girl was not as nimble on her legs as other children, but there was no definite disability. There was unquestionably a mild generalized retardation when she was first seen a few days before her first birthday.

Case 4. This boy caused great difficulty in diagnosis. He was seen just before the first birthday, on account of backwardness in development. He was unable to sit without support, or to chew, but had begun to say single words with meaning. The comment written was 'There is a striking dissociation in his development. I think that he shows a combination of mental retardation with physical defect. Further observation is essential'.

At the age of 3 years athetoid movements became obvious. At the age of 4 he was a typical athetoid child with an I.Q. of 100.

Comment. In retrospect one feels that one would make the same mistake again.

Case 5. This boy with kernikterus was seen at the age of 1 year, 11 months. The comment made was, 'I think that his I.Q. is 80 to 90, but that may turn out to be an underestimate'. At the age of 5 it was 100.

Comment. This underestimate of his ability was so trivial that it was of no significance.

The intellectual potential of 11 other children was considerably underestimated. Four of them were seen in the first year, and the remainder in the second year. Only two had cerebral palsy. Of the nine thought to be severely retarded, five were later found to have an I.Q. of 50 to 75, and the others had an I.Q. of 86, 87, 88 and 94 respectively. Of the other two, one was thought to have a developmental quotient of 50 to 60, while the I.Q. proved to be 80: and the other was thought at 9 months to have a D.Q. of 60, while the subsequent I.Q. was 80.

Four children fared less well than was expected. Three of these had cerebral palsy. Two were seen in the first year. Two were thought to be slightly retarded in infancy: one was given a D.Q. of 60, and another was thought to be moderately retarded. All were later found to be ineducable.

It is interesting that while 16 fared better than we expected, only four fared materially worse than expected. This fact alone should emphasize the need for caution in giving a developmental prognosis.

Discussion

It is clearly incorrect to assert without qualification that developmental tests in infancy have no predictive value. There are obvious difficulties, in that there are so many variable factors which may affect development. There are children who appear to be backward at first, and who subsequently catch up to the average, or at least reach a much higher level than was expected. There are children who are average at first and subsequently deteriorate, as a result of a degenerative disease of the brain, encephalitis, lead poisoning, hypoglycaemia, or other causes. There are great difficulties in making a correct estimate of the capability of an infant with cerebral palsy. The fact remains, however, that mental retardation can be diagnosed in infancy, at least in a high proportion of cases.

For practical purposes the diagnosis of mental retardation is probably the most important single function of developmental tests in infancy. It is particularly important for the assessment of suitability for adoption. Though it may be of academic interest, it is not of much practical importance to be able to predict whether an infant is going to have an I.Q. of 110 or 140: but it may well be important to know whether he will have an average I.Q. or one of about 70: and it may certainly be important to know whether he is likely to have an I.Q. of about 50. For practical purposes, therefore, developmental tests in infancy are of great value, and we disagree entirely with those who assert the opposite.

We are particularly anxious to emphasize that the estimates made in children discussed in this paper were made in the ordinary busy out-patient clinic or in the ward. They were not made in a special clinic. They were made by the paediatrician in the ordinary course of his work, in the presence of students and postgraduates, and not by a psychologist. That, we feel, is as it should be. Rough developmental assessment must be part of the routine daily work of any paediatrician.

We have deliberately not discussed all the difficulties of developmental assessment. We have set out merely to present a factual statement of our findings. We do not propose to discuss the difficulties of predicting mental superiority in an infant. We aimed at proving that in one aspect, and that the most important from the practical point of view, developmental tests in infancy are of the utmost value.

No one should think that the art of developmental prognosis is easy. It is beset with innumerable hazards. This must be emphasized, for it would be a tragedy to tell a mother that a child is going to be an idiot when in fact he will be normal or a genius. The wise paediatrician does not give a prognosis to the mother until he is certain, and in very many cases that can only be after repeated examinations have clearly demonstrated a retarded rate of developmental progress.

Summary

It has been shown that developmental tests in the first two years of life have an invaluable predictive value with regard to the early diagnosis of mental retardation.

The study was based on 135 children in whom mental retardation was diagnosed in the first two years, even though subsequent observation showed that development had become normal. In 77 of these the diagnosis was made in the first year. Cases of mongolism, cretinism, hydrocephalus or anencephaly were excluded. Intelligence quotients were estimated at the age of 5 to 10. Two children could not be traced. Thirty-two died, and in the 10 in whom an autopsy was carried out, a gross cerebral anomaly was found.

Of the remaining 101 children, 59 on follow-up examination were found to be ineducable (I.Q. below 50), 24 had an I.Q. of 50 to 75, and five had an I.Q. of 100 or more.

It was noted that while only four children fared worse than was expected, some 16 children fared better than the original developmental level had led us to expect.

We wish to thank the following doctors for their great help and co-operation, without which this study would have been impossible: S. Childs, C. D. Cormac, R. Barnes, H. M. Cohen, D. G. Davies, H. B. Davies, R. J. Donaldson, J. L. Emery, F. Ferguson, J. Fielding, R. Glenn, T. S. Hall, C. C. Harvey, E. G. Herzog, G. Higgins, H. Everley Jones, J. B. S. Morgan, G. A. W. Neill, E. G. M. Oates, J. W. Pickup, J. A. W. Reid, Llywelyn Roberts, T. E. Roberts, J. Main Russell, H. L. Settle, J. A. Stirling, M. C. Taylor, J. B. Tilley, H. G. Watson and J. M. Watt.

References

Apgar, V., Girdany, B. R., McIntosh, R. and Taylor, H. C. (1955). *Pediatrics*, **15**, 653.
Bayley, N. (1940). "Mental Growth in Young Children." In *Intelligence: Its Nature and Nurture*. Thirty-ninth Year Book of the National Society for the Study of Education. Part II: *Original Studies and Experiments*, p. 11. Public School Publishing Co., Bloomington, Illinois.
Bowlby, J. (1951). *Bull. Wld Hlth Org.*, **3**, 355.
Eysenck, H. J. (1953). *Uses and Abuses of Psychology*. Pelican Books, Harmondsworth.
Goodenough, F. L. (1949). *Mental Testing*. Rinehart, New York.
Illingworth, R. S. (1957). *The Normal Child*, 2nd ed. Churchill, London.
Karelitz, S. (1958). *Ann. Paediat. Fenn.*, **4**, 1.
Kirman, B. H. (1953). *J. ment. Sci.*, **99**, 531.
——— (1958). *Brit. med. J.*, **2**, 1215.
Sontag, L. W., Baker, C. T. and Nelson, V. L. (1958). *Monogr. Soc. Res. Child Development*, **23**, No. 2.
Terman, L. M. and Merrill, M. A. (1937). *Measuring Intelligence*. Houghton Mifflin, Boston.
Valentine, C. W. (1950). *Psychology and Its Bearing on Education*. Methuen, London.
Vernon, P. E. (1957). *Secondary School Selection: A British Psychological Society Inquiry*. Methuen, London.
Wittenborn, J. R. (1957). *The Placement of Adoptive Children*. Charles C. Thomas, Springfield, Illinois.

CONGENITAL HYDROCEPHALUS IN MONOVULAR TWINS

BY

V. GELLMAN

From the Department of Pediatrics, University of Illinois, Chicago, U.S.A.

(RECEIVED FOR PUBLICATION JANUARY 2, 1959)

Congenital hydrocephalus in monovular twins is very rare. Borle (1953) published an extensive review of the cases reported since 1899 which purported to demonstrate the familial character of hydrocephalus. Her work covered the English, American and European publications and included seven pairs of monovular twins with hydrocephalus occurring in each twin (Booth, 1911; Siemens, 1924; Weise, 1935, de Lange, 1936; Fischer, 1942, Polman, 1950; Klein, Bersot and Borle, 1953). However, the presence of hydrocephalus was not definitely proven in some of these cases.

For example, in Booth's case the evidence for hydrocephalus is scant. His twins were 2½-year-old female pyopages united in the sacrococcygeal region. They were bright and intelligent, but the shape of their heads was 'peculiar'. They had bulging foreheads and flat vertices. Booth suggested that the children had almost a hydrocephalic appearance but he gave no further evidence to support his impression.

Siemens described identical twin brothers aged 4 months. Their head circumferences were 45·5 cm. and 45 cm. respectively. Both had cerebral atrophy and severe external hydrocephalus of unknown aetiology. The author postulated a hereditary aetiological factor.

The twins described by Weise survived until adult life. Their head circumferences were 58 cm. and 57 cm. respectively. Each had a mild degree of hydrocephalus. Both were retarded and in addition one had syringomyelia.

De Lange (1936) described twins aged 8 months with head circumferences of 46 cm. and 45 cm. Their skulls were natiform from birth and they both had a mild degree of rickets. Their anterior fontanelles were bulging and in one the cerebral spinal fluid pressure was increased. The author believed that hydrocephalus was the cause of the skull deformity.

The cases reported by Fischer (1942) were probably not congenital hydrocephalics. Their head circumferences at birth were 32 cm. and 33 cm. Enlargement of the head was first noticed in early childhood. The twins both died and at autopsy definite signs of meningitis were seen.

Polman (1950) made only a brief reference to a pair of hydrocephalic twins who were 'presumably monozygotic'. No further details were given.

The patients reported by Borle (1953) herself were a pair of male monovular twins. Head enlargement became apparent in each twin sometime between 2 and 6 months. There was no accompanying illness, but convulsions began at about 8 months. At 2 years their head circumferences were 53 and 54 cm. respectively. The anterior fontanelles were still open and radiographs of the skull showed changes typical of hydrocephalus. Both boys were mentally retarded. They began to walk at 2 years and to talk at 4 years. There was in addition another hydrocephalic sibling.

In 1956 Cohn, Weinburg and Rockaway published a report on the birth of achondroplastic monovular twins with hydrocephalus, who died soon after birth. The mother was subsequently delivered of a third hydrocephalic achondroplastic infant. In the case of the twins, the hydrocephalus was caused by bony hypertrophy in the region of the foramen magnum obliterating the subdural and epidural space. One can assume, therefore, that the hydrocephalus was not primarily of genetic origin but secondary to the changes in the skull due to achondroplasia.

Of the eight cases mentioned above, the hydrocephalus in two pairs of twins was secondary to some other aetiological factor (Fischer, 1942; Cohn *et al.*, 1956). This leaves six cases which may support the theory that some cases of congenital hydrocephalus are genetically determined. A seventh case is presented.

Case Report. S. and N. were 5-year-old identical twin boys who were delivered at term after a normal pregnancy by caesarian section because of interlocking heads. The boys weighed between 8 and 9 lb. at birth. They presented no feeding problems, sat at 4 months, walked at 18 months, and had no serious illnesses. However, at

5 years they both developed stomatitis and were taken to their physician. He was impressed by the large size of their heads and their obvious mental retardation, and referred them to hospital.

The parents were Palestinian Arabs. The father was 60 and the mother 33. They were both healthy and of average intelligence, although their knowledge of English was limited. The sister and brother, aged 4 and 3 years respectively, were normal. A sibling born before the twins had died at 3 days of unknown cause. According to the mother this infant had had a normal head size.

S. and N. were physically well-developed boys. S. was 129 cm. tall and weighed 64 lb., and N. was 129 cm. tall and weighed 63½ lb. Their head circumferences were 55 and 56 cm. respectively. Apart from their obviously large heads, vacant, open-mouthed expression (see Fig. 1), and slowness of affect, there were no abnormal physical findings on examination. They were quiet, bashful boys who seemed to lack animation and who were extremely dependent on their parents. During one week in the ward they neither talked to each other nor played with the other children, but cried constantly for their mother.

Relevant laboratory investigations are listed in Table 1.

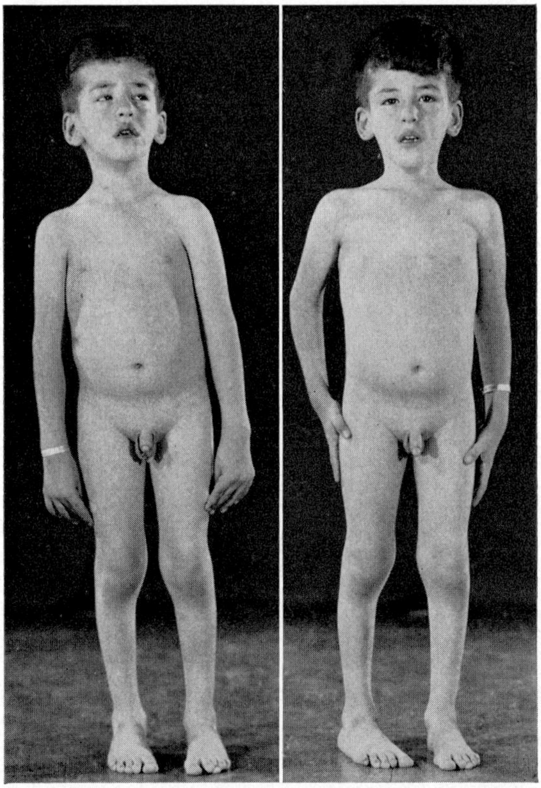

FIG. 1.—N.J. and S.J., aged 5 years. Both children have large heads and vacant expressions.

TABLE 1

LABORATORY INVESTIGATIONS

Test	S	N.
Hb.	12 g./100 ml.	10·7 g./100 ml.
W.B.C.	6,000/c.mm	6,000/c.mm.
Blood group	O Rh+ (/cDE/Rh_2)	O Rh+ (/cDE/Rh_2)
Serum W.R.	N.*	N
Serum Kahn	N	N
Serum cholesterol	459 mg./100 ml.	388 mg./100 ml.
P.B.I.†	5·8 mg./100 ml.	11·6 mg./100 ml.
I_{131} uptake	28·6% (patient spilled some of dose)	23%
Urine:		
Albumin	N	N
Sugar	N	N
Sediment	No casts	No casts
C.S.F.:		
Protein	29 mg./100 ml.	16 mg./100 ml.
Cells	Few RBC/c.mm.	2 RBC/c.mm.
W.R.	N	N
Kahn	N	N
Colloidal gold	0000000000	0000000000
Toxoplasma dye test	N	N
Bone age	Compatible with that of a 2-3-year-old male	Compatible with that of a 2-3-year-old male

* N=negative.
† Blood samples were taken soon after iodine mouth washes.

Electroencephalograms in both patients showed 14 and 6 per second positive spike seizure activity in both hemispheres.

Pneumoencephalography in both patients showed an increase in the size of the skull. In the case of S., the occipito-frontal diameter was 20·5 cm., the biparietal diameter was 17·5 cm., and the height 16·5 cm. In the case of N., the occipito-frontal diameter was 21·5 cm., the biparietal diameter was 17·5 cm., and the height 18 cm. There was moderate symmetrical distension of the ventricular system in both patients. These findings are compatible with hydrocephalus. The dorsum sellae and sutures were normal.

Psychological testing was attempted in both children but was difficult because of lack of co-operation. N. was described as 'untestable' but it was the examiner's impression that he was retarded. The test on S. revealed intellectual limitation of a degree which could not be accurately determined.

Comment

Occasionally it is possible to find an exogenous factor such as syphilis, meningitis, toxoplasmosis, or obstetrical trauma as the underlying cause of congenital hydrocephalus. Frequently, however, no organic cause can be detected. In such cases the question of a genetic factor arises, particularly when the condition occurs in monovular twins. The fact that there is a strong familial tendency to congenital hydrocephalus would also support the genetic theory.

In the case of the twins presented above, toxic factors and obstetrical trauma were eliminated. The history and investigations suggested that this was an authentic case of congenital hydrocephalus in monovular twins. It is postulated that the hydrocephalus was of genetic aetiology. In the presence of mental retardation the high cholesterol values and the retarded bone age are suggestive of hypothyroidism. However, the patients were of normal stature and other tests of thyroid function did not confirm this diagnosis.

Summary

The case histories are reported of identical twins with congenital hydrocephalus and mental retardation. The rarity of such cases is demonstrated by a brief review of the publications on this subject. The cases are presented in support of the theory that some examples of congenital hydrocephalus may be genetically determined.

I wish to express my thanks to Dr. Heyworth N. Sanford for permission to publish the cases, and to Dr. Ira M. Rosenthal for helpful criticism of the paper.

REFERENCES

Booth, J. A. (1911). *Brit. med. J.*, **2**, 653.
Borle, A. (1953). *J. Génét. hum.*, **2**, 157.
Cohn, S., Weinberg, A. and Rockaway, F. (1956). *Amer. J. Obstet. Gynec.*, **72**, 1346.
De Lange, C. (1936). *Arch. Dis. Childh.*, **11**, 39.
Fischer, H. (1942). *Z. ges. Neurol. Psychiat.*, **174**, 264.
Klein, D., Bersot, H. and Borle, A. (1953). *Confin. neurol.*, **13**, 158
Polman, A. (1950). *Genetica* **25**, 29.
Siemens, H. W. (1924). *Die Zwillings pathologie*, p. 82. J. Springer Berlin.
Weise, G. (1935). *Arch. Psychiat. Nervenkr.*, **103**, 191.

A CASE OF RUPTURE OF THE HEPATIC DUCT IN A NEWBORN INFANT

BY

JOAN P. WRIGHT and HELEN E. WORSLEY
From the Duchess of York Hospital for Babies, Manchester

(RECEIVED FOR PUBLICATION NOVEMBER 19, 1958)

A successfully treated case of a perforation in the biliary system of a newborn infant is presented. Cases have been reported in which bile peritonitis has occurred in association with rupture of a congenital cyst of the common bile duct (Byrne and Bottomley, 1953). Only six cases of perforation in the biliary tract have been found in which symptoms began in the neonatal period and in which the biliary system at laparotomy appeared otherwise normal (Caulfield, 1936; Mason, Sidbury and Guiang, 1954; Pettersson, 1955).

Case History

E.A.W. was the first child of healthy parents and was born in a maternity home on April 14, 1958, weighing 7 lb. 14 oz. Delivery was normal and she was perfectly well until the fifth day. It was then reported that the stools were pale and that she was reluctant to take feeds. On the ninth day she vomited after every feed, was pale and unwell and was transferred to the Duchess of York Hospital under the care of Dr. S. K. Guthrie. On examination the child was apyrexial and was in good general condition. She was very slightly icteric and there was minimal abdominal distension with general tenderness. No signs of free fluid in the abdominal cavity were elicited. The stools were pale and the urine a normal colour.

Investigations. Haemoglobin was 15·7 g., E.S.R. was 3 mm. in one hour, and W.B.C. was 3,000 (polymorphs 45%, eosinophils 1%, plasma cells 1%, lymphocytes 51%, monocytes 2%). Serum bilirubin (micro.) 2·4 mg. %. There was a trace of bile pigments in the urine, but no urobilinogen. A straight radiograph of the abdomen was normal.

Progress Report. After admission the child continued to pass clay-coloured stools and to vomit after every feed. By the following day her general condition had deteriorated; she had become slightly dehydrated and there was increasing abdominal distension. At this stage she was noticed to have a yellow stain extending from the right hypochondrium to the right iliac fossa. Within a few hours this staining had spread to the hypogastrium and the left iliac fossa. A surgical opinion was sought and the child was seen on the day after admission by Mr. N. F. Kirkman, who decided to carry out an immediate laparatomy.

Operative Details. A transverse epigastric incision was made. There was bile staining of all deep tissues and a moderate amount of free bile in the peritoneal cavity. A small irregular hole about ½ cm. in length was found in the hepatic duct near the hilum of the liver. There was a small area of necrosis surrounding the perforation and a little inspissated bile in the lumen of the duct. The gall-bladder was empty. A probe was passed without difficulty into the lumen of the duct and apart from the perforation the biliary tract appeared normal. The bile duct was drained externally by a rubber catheter with side holes which was passed through the perforation and along the duct towards the duodenum. Separate drains were placed in the peritoneal cavity through stab wounds to drain the right and left paracolic gutters, and the abdominal wall was closed.

Post-operative Progress. An intravenous infusion had been started pre-operatively and was continued for 48 hours. She was given initially 250 ml. N/5 saline in 4·3% dextrose followed by 5% dextrose in water. On the second post-operative day she was given 100 ml. of whole blood. Throughout this period small feeds were given and were retained and the child's general condition was good. On the second day she passed a small stool containing bile. On the eighth day a choledochogram was performed using 1 ml. of lipiodol; this showed normal hepatic and common bile ducts, the dye passing freely into the duodenum. The catheter draining the bile duct was removed and the child made an uneventful recovery. When seen at 3 months of age she was in all respects a normal child.

Comment

The cause of the rupture was not obvious at operation and the following aetiological factors have been considered.

Infection. Although the child had a mild infection of the umbilicus there was no evidence of infection in the hilum of the liver and the possibility of necrosis of the duct following infection is therefore discounted.

Birth Trauma. There are many cases in which rupture of the liver was caused by birth trauma (Genell, 1930; Potter, 1940; Arden, 1946 and 1951). In none of these cases was there any damage to the biliary tract. It is difficult to postulate a strain to the biliary tract leaving the liver intact.

Congenital Abnormality. In the case reported here a plug of inspissated bile was found in the duct distal to the site of perforation. This caused obstruction of the duct, pale stools having been noticed from the fifth day. On the ninth day the patient started to vomit after every feed and was obviously not as well. We suggest that the perforation occurred at this stage, giving rise to the later signs of abdominal distension and bile staining of the skin. Byrne and Bottomley (1953) reported a case of congenital cyst at the junction of the cystic and hepatic ducts, this being the site of rupture. Pettersson (1955) reported four cases, in three of which he found no obstruction in the ducts, but in one of which he found a plug of mucus at the ampulla of Vater. These four cases had all ruptured at the junction of the cystic and hepatic ducts, and, quoting Byrne and Bottomley, Pettersson suggested that this site may be subject from an embryological point of view to structural weakness or diverticulae. He suggested that a stenosis of the duct or a plug in the duct or ampulla of Vater would be a contributory factor. The case reported here had many similarities to those described by Pettersson. The initial symptoms of vomiting and pale stools, and the later signs of peritonitis being present in all cases. At operation the appearance of the perforation was similar, but in this case occurred in the hepatic duct just above its junction with the cystic duct. We suggest that a congenital weakness was present at this unusual site and that the theory of Pettersson as to the causation of the rupture is applicable to this case.

Summary

A successfully treated case of rupture of the hepatic duct with symptoms presenting at the fifth day of life is reported. Possible causes are considered with special reference to the theory postulated by Pettersson (1955).

We wish to thank Dr. S. K. Guthrie and Mr. N. F. Kirkman for permission to publish this case and for their helpful advice.

References

Arden, F. (1946). *Med. J. Aust.*, **1**, 187.
Byrne, J. J. and Bottomley, G. T. (1953). *A.M.A. Amer. J. Dis. Child.*, **85**, 694.
Caulfield, E. (1936). *Ibid.*, **52**, 1348.
Genell, S. (1930). *Acta obstet. gynec. scand.*, **9**, 180.
Mason, L. B., Sidbury, J. B. and Guiang, S. (1954). *Ann. Surg.*, **140**, 234.
Pettersson, G. (1955). *Acta chir. scand.*, **110**, 192.
Potter, E. L. (1940). *J. Amer. med. Ass.*, **115**, 996.

BOOK REVIEWS

Management of the Newborn, 2nd ed. By ARTHUR H. PARMELEE. (Pp. 368; 47 figures. 64s., $8.50.) London: Interscience Publishers. Chicago: Year Book Publishers. 1959.

The second edition of Professor Parmelee's charming book on what he himself calls the ' Story of the Newborn' retains much of its original form with newly written chapters on retrolental fibroplasia, oxygen therapy and staphylococcal infections, fairly extensive revision on material relating to hyaline membrane syndrome, resuscitation, and infants of diabetic mothers as well as considerable bringing up to date here and there throughout the book. Though not a textbook in the ordinary sense, and though a spate of books on the neonate have appeared since the first edition in 1952, this slim volume remains the most readable and perhaps the best book on its subject. It is not encyclopaedic but contains all and more that the student and the practitioner needs. Each subject is made to sound interesting because Professor Parmelee has chosen to write on subjects that have aroused his own interest and because he writes in English prose which is simple and lucid and in a very direct way reflects his own feelings and even his own senses. For instance, when describing local cyanosis he says 'light friction with the finger will often cause a normal pink colour to return to the cyanotic area but in a few minutes cyanosis again appears'; and in subcutaneous fat necrosis the areas 'feel not unlike buttons when grasped by their firm edges'; again, of a newly born infant 'the skin has a velvety softness more delicate than anything else I have ever felt'. This sort of personal writing, which might easily become embarrassing, is woven into the substance of the text in such a way as both to lighten its reading and illuminate his meaning.

As always in American books, the paper and printing and general get up is of a high standard.

L'Hérédité en Ophtalmologie. By JULES FRANÇOIS. (Pp. vii+876; 629 figures. Fr. fr. 8,000.) Paris, Masson et Cie. 1958.

This is a most useful book. It is in four parts. The first gives a general account of mendelian genetics, and includes a chapter on elementary statistics. The second describes the general applications of genetics in ophthalmology: the recognition of discrete clinical entities from their genetic behaviour; the detection of carriers; the value of a knowledge of genetic risks in the early treatment of genetic disorder; genetic counselling and eugenic considerations. The third gives a full account of the disorders of the eye known to be genetically determined. The fourth describes the genetically determined syndromes in which the eye is also involved. It is the last which would be of most interest to paediatricians.

Each section is well illustrated, and the accounts of conditions where genetics are difficult, for example the errors of refraction, are well balanced. English-speaking medical practitioners already have a good text-book covering much the same ground to consult, Professor Sorsby's *Genetics in Ophthalmology*. This French book is more detailed, and contains a fuller list of references to the continental literature, so it will form a useful supplement.

Le Mongolisme. By ROBERT LÉCUYER. (Pp. 152. Fr. fr. 1,500.) Paris: G. Doin. 1958.

The study of mongolism has for some time reached a dead end and almost no new material factors have been added to our knowledge for over 30 or more years, while the only important change in the state of these curious children has been that for the most part they now survive into adult life. This painstaking monograph surveys the subject in a general way, and presents the principal problems of diagnosis, aetiology and treatment with considerable detail. The author brings with him 39 cases which help to enliven the rather dry, arid survey of the literature of which the monograph is almost entirely composed.

All the known factors are presented, and many of the better known fantasies about aetiology are also discussed. In the chapter on aetiology all theories break down against the irreducibly meagre, well established and ever verifiable factors of maternal age and the occurrence in both of monozygotic, but not of dizygotic, twins. The chapter on treatment is perhaps the most successful in this monograph and the author points out that since development in these children is in general slow and various phases are passed through slowly, and in particular the mongols' dependence on maternal care and affection and a happy family life is unduly prolonged so that he can suffer from deprivation, hospitalization, and the like for just so long as he remains a mental toddler; and that this may be well on into the seventh and eighth year or later. He claims that many of the difficulties, aggressiveness, uncouthness and lapses into imbecility, have their roots in unhappy childhood, and might have been avoided by greater sympathy and love.

Working in an institution the author nevertheless realizes the conditions there for mongols fall very far short of the optimum, and would like to see established some kind of organization for more home care and boarding out for them when they have the misfortune to be rejected by their parents. This is an important point to have made and one that should be appreciated by all those coming into contact with these unfortunate children. There is an extensive and useful bibliography.

Le Nouveau-né Thérapeutique Médicale. Prevention et Soins. By MARCEL LELONG, FRANÇOIS LEPAGE and ALFRED ROSSIER. (Pp. 238; 6 figures. Fr. fr. 2,500.) Paris: G. Doin. 1958.

The Bibliothèque de Therapeutique Médicale adds another manual of treatment to its already long and on the whole distinguished list. This library sets out to present scientifically based therapeutic practice related closely to clinical medicine, and is aimed at the practising physician and specialist. The volume under review, on the care and treatment of the newborn, is edited by Marcel Lelong who contributes two chapters. Apart from a chapter on infections it confines itself to the physiological hazards that face the foetus during the perinatal period. Eight chapters cover respectively obstetrical trauma, foetal anoxia, white asphyxia—*mort apparante*, haemorrhagic disease, haemolytic disease, neonatal feeding, infection and prematurity. The approach is in the main didactic, the literature being drawn on chiefly to illustrate the theme, and the book is in the main the expression of neonatal paediatrics as practised at the Clinique de Puériculture of the Hospital of Saint Vincent de Paul and the Centre de Prematurés de L'Ecole de Puériculture. Each chapter introduces its subject with a careful discussion of physiological and pathological considerations upon which is based the prevention and treatment that follow. This rational framework sets a serious tone and a high level is maintained throughout, with perhaps the best contributions from Lelong in his account of foeto-neonatal anoxia, its amelioration and treatment, and the review by Dr. Alagille of the mechanisms giving rise to haemorrhage in the newborn.

With some notable exceptions the care of infants is, as might be expected, much the same in Paris and London. However, adrenaline, camphor and cognac (which sounds more effective than humble brandy) are more used and indeed perhaps more useful than other medullary and cardiac stimulants. After all, as Marcel Lelong reminds us, Goethe was rescued from profound asphyxia by the midwife: 'elle plongea le bébé dans une bassine pleine de vin chaud, après quoi il se reanima et commença à vivre . . .'. Vitamin K is reckoned ineffectual, administered to the infant, for the prevention of hypoprothrombinaemia or of haemorrhagic incidences, at least in premature infants; Largactil is freely used to combat various kinds of 'shock', and a kind of moderate cooling to 34 to 35°C is administered for three to five days to premature infants suffering from *cyanose, le tonus, l'agitation et sur toutes les manifestations de choc en general*, using Largactil, phenergan and gardenal. Both the early, isochromic, and the later, iron deficient, anaemias of prematurity claim to be avoided by repeated weekly transfusion of 10 to 15 ml. of citrated blood. These, and some other practices, may sound strange to English ears, but are given logical justification in the text, and may stimulate some of us to look into cherished beliefs.

The printing and paper are excellent; the binding paper backed. There are but six rather oddly chosen illustrations, and the text contains several misprints, mistakes and slipped decimal points, most of which have been corrected in *errata*. The French is easy.

SOME RESPIRATORY AND CARDIOVASCULAR PROBLEMS AFTER BIRTH*

BY

G. S. DAWES

From the Nuffield Institute for Medical Research, University of Oxford

It is a privilege to speak in memory of Sir George Frederic Still. Still was born in 1868. He took a classical degree at Cambridge and studied medicine at Guy's Hospital. In 1897, at the age of 29, when medical registrar and pathologist to The Hospital for Sick Children, Great Ormond Street, he published a paper 'on a form of chronic joint disease in children', an original and accurate description of what became widely known as 'Still's disease'. In 1906, at the age of 38, he became the first Professor of the Diseases of Children in the United Kingdom, at King's College. He spent the rest of his life looking after children, and in the advancement of knowledge of their diseases.

Thirty years ago, in 1928, Still became the first President of the British Paediatric Association. He must already have seen great changes in the practice of medicine, and it would have been hard to believe that there were even more revolutionary advances just ahead. But the years that followed, years of unemployment, of international crisis, and of war, were accompanied by an astonishing tide of medical discoveries. These came partly from the observations of practising physicians, from a better understanding of the natural history of disease. They came partly from fundamental investigations, from the development of chemotherapeutic agents and antibiotics, from advances in anaesthesia and surgical technique, from a host of different investigators all over the world. These discoveries have had a great influence on the expectation of life of children in this country. In Fig. 1 is plotted the total number of deaths, in England and Wales, by age up to 12 years, for 1928 and 1957. The total number of live births registered were 660,267 in 1928, and 723,381 in 1957. There are several interesting points about these figures. Firstly, there has been a great general improvement in the last 30 years; no elaborate statistics are needed to make this apparent. Secondly, during the first week of life the improvement is very much less than that at subsequent periods. Thus deaths during the first week were 2·16/1,000 live births in 1928; they were still 1·39/1,000 in 1957. The result is that, in 1957, 10,177 children died from natural causes in the first seven days of life, and only 9,994 during the next seven years. These figures are startling; very similar ones are reported from other countries. The stillbirth rate, which was 22·5/1,000 live births in 1957, has remained about the same for the last ten years. There were therefore more than 16,000 stillbirths, as compared with a loss of 10,177 during the first week after birth in 1957.

At or after birth there are, therefore three types of problem which demand attention: (1) Stillbirth;

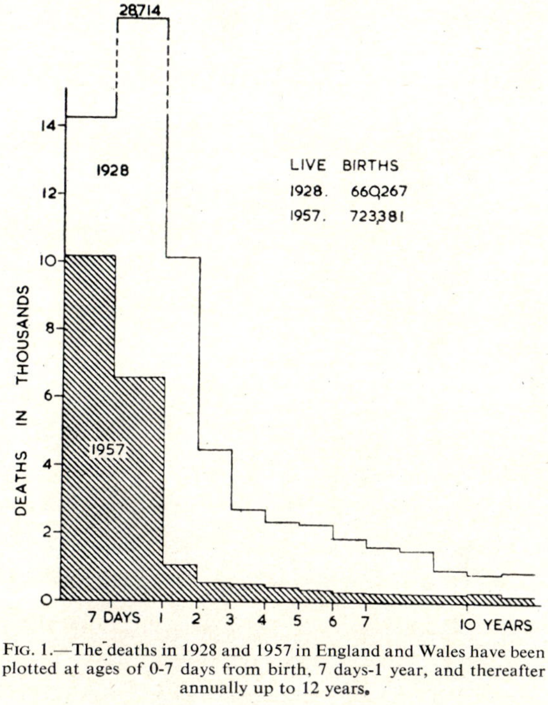

FIG. 1.—The deaths in 1928 and 1957 in England and Wales have been plotted at ages of 0-7 days from birth, 7 days-1 year, and thereafter annually up to 12 years.

* The Still Memorial Lecture presented to the meeting of the British Paediatric Association in Scarborough in April, 1959.

this is an obstetric rather than a paediatric problem. (2) Immaturity, atelectasis and postnatal asphyxia, which together account for more than half neonatal deaths, according to the Registrar-General's tables. We may add hyaline membrane disease to this group. (3) Spastic paralysis, since it is widely believed that asphyxia at birth may be one cause of this condition.

I propose to talk about experiments upon animals in relation to these problems. Animal experiments can be useful in two ways. Firstly it may prove possible to reproduce a disease in experimental animals. For example Ashton and his colleagues were able to cause retrolental fibroplasia by exposing young animals to high O_2 concentrations, and hence to incriminate this as an important factor in causing the disease. Sometimes a naturally occurring disease in animals appears very similar to that in man. Thus toxaemia of pregnancy occurs in sheep, and a report has appeared which suggests that hyaline membrane disease may occur in the thoroughbred foal. These provide direct lines of attack upon the diseases in question.

The second way in which animal experiments can help is in providing background knowledge of biological mechanisms. It is about this aspect of research upon the newborn that I propose to talk, and to illustrate by examples. Although a great deal of work has been done over the last 50 years on such fundamental problems as the control of the circulation and breathing, and the effect of changes in the environment of the adult animal and man, very little attention has been paid to the newborn. We therefore have several general biological problems to tackle. Is the small newborn animal in these respects an exact miniature replica of the adult? Or are there features of its physiological behaviour which are peculiar to its size and youth? Some babies are born before the normal period of gestation is ended. They are immature, but what do we mean by immature in quantitative terms? Are their blood pressure and cardiac output less? Can we measure their cardiovascular and respiratory reflexes, and their ability to withstand asphyxia? Perhaps their physiological behaviour is different, not only in degree, but also in kind, from that of adults? We also have to consider species differences. When a physiological mechanism has been shown to exist in animals, it may be possible to show that it also exists in the baby, and I hope to give examples of this. But I do not mean thereby to suggest that the intellectual traffic is all one way. There are many examples where observations upon the human infant have stimulated research upon animals, often with unexpected results. There are therefore good reasons why paediatricians, physiologists and biochemists should work together in order to tackle the many problems which are of mutual interest.

Changes in the Circulation after Birth

The changes which take place after birth can be divided into two categories, the anatomical and the functional. I think we are now coming towards the end of a period when the anatomical changes were of predominant interest, and turning towards the functional. This can be illustrated by reference to the change in the circulation from the foetal to the neonatal condition. The work of Barcroft and his colleagues (Barclay, Franklin and Prichard, 1944; Barcroft, 1946) had suggested that the ductus arteriosus and foramen ovale were both closed within a few minutes after the establishment of normal breathing. We now have reason to believe that neither of these changes are normally complete for several days from birth. The most striking evidence with regard to the ductus arteriosus is the presence of a loud murmur in newborn lambs, calves and foals (Dawes, Mott and Widdicombe, 1955; Amoroso, Dawes and Mott, 1957), audible on the left side of the chest and radiating medially from the mid-axillary line. This murmur is undoubtedly due to turbulent flow of blood at high pressure from the aorta to the pulmonary trunk, as has been shown by cineangiograms and by measurements of the pressure and oxygen content of blood withdrawn from the great vessels. The murmur is abolished by ligation of the ductus arteriosus. The murmur normally appears within 10-15 minutes of birth and persists for as long as two days. It is only heard when the ductus is partly constricted, though even then as much as half the pulmonary blood flow may be passing through the ductus. There is now ample evidence that in human babies, also, the ductus arteriosus does not close completely and at once after birth. Thus Rowe and James (1957) and Adams and Lind (1957) have taken cineangiograms and catheterized newborn infants; they have calculated that a large proportion of pulmonary flow comes from the ductus arteriosus for several days after birth. The cardiac murmur from a patent ductus arteriosus, which is so easily and so regularly heard in lambs, was not so readily identified in children. It was not until last year that Burnard (1958) in a painstaking and fascinating piece of work, established its presence in more than one-third of human births. It was fascinating because he made the unexpected observation that the murmur in human infants was heard more frequently in association with a history of asphyxia and with a raised respiratory rate. We do not yet know what are the full implications of this association, for we still have so little factual information about the cardiovascular and respiratory systems in such infants.

Closure of the valve of the foramen ovale is effected by a change in the pressure relations between the left atrium and the inferior vena cava. In the foetus, blood normally passes from the inferior vena cava to the left atrium, but when ventilation is begun and the cord is tied, pulmonary blood flow increases and umbilical flow ceases. There is therefore a relative rise in left atrial pressure and a fall in inferior vena caval pressure, so that the valve becomes apposed to the foramen ovale during the greater part of the cardiac cycle. Barcroft (1946) concluded that since the blood of a newborn lamb became relatively well saturated with oxygen within a few hours of birth, it was unlikely that much blood passed as a right-to-left shunt through the foramen ovale. Yet the arterial blood of a newborn lamb is not wholly saturated with oxygen, and there was still the possibility of a small right-to-left shunt during a short period of the cardiac cycle only. Lind and Wegelius (1954) reported the passage of small quantities of contrast medium from the inferior vena cava to the left side of the heart in some human babies, but this might have been due to rapid injections of large quantities of contrast medium, which raises the pressure in the great veins. Recently Condorelli, Dagianti, Polosa and Giuliano (1957) have produced evidence of a very small right-to-left shunt in unanaesthetized lambs up to the fifth day from birth, using a dye-dilution method which involved an injection of only 0·2 ml. at a time. Weisbrot, James, Prince, Holaday and Apgar (1958) found a mean left atrial O_2 saturation of $93{\cdot}8 \pm 2{\cdot}6$ (S.D.) % (by passing a catheter from the umbilical vein) in 10 normal babies during the first hour of life. Therefore in the normal baby any such shunt must also be very small.

Nevertheless for some days after birth the anatomical pathways which are usually thought of as peculiar to the foetus are still not firmly shut. The reactions of the cardiovascular system after birth are therefore different from those of the adult. Firstly so long as there is a left-to-right shunt through the ductus, from aorta to pulmonary trunk, pulmonary blood flow is increased; this may be of some transient advantage, but the load on the left ventricle is also greater. Heart failure may occur for this reason. Secondly if the baby becomes asphyxiated the direction of blood flow through the ductus may reverse (James and Rowe, 1957) and venous pressure may rise, giving a large right-to-left shunt through the foramen ovale. It is abundantly clear that the neonatal circulation, though only a transitional form between the foetal and adult, requires careful study. It is also interesting that the same general conclusions have been reached from studies on both animals and babies.

Changes in Oxygen Consumption at Birth

So much for the anatomical side. We now have to consider function, and this is not a matter which can be discussed in isolation. It brings us straightaway to a consideration of size. Small animals have a large surface area relative to their body weight. Since heat loss is proportionate to surface area, the energy production of small mammals must be high, in order to keep their body temperature constant at 37-38° C. If metabolic rate is relatively high, then the consumption of oxygen, the production of carbon dioxide, respiratory movements and cardiac output are likely to be increased in proportion. These are matters which are almost self-evident; the consequences for the changes which occur after birth are considerable.

The oxygen consumption of a foetal lamb has been estimated by measuring umbilical blood flow and multiplying this by the umbilical arteriovenous oxygen difference. This gives a figure of some 4·5 ml./kg./min. in foetal lambs which have a reasonably high arterial O_2 saturation, say 50% or more. This figure falls within the normal range for the oxygen consumption of adult sheep; that is to say, the normal rate of O_2 consumption of the foetus, per unit body weight, is much the same as that of the ewe. But within a day after birth the lamb's resting oxygen consumption, measured directly, increases nearly threefold to a mean of about 12 ml./kg./min. (Dawes and Mott, 1959b, Fig. 2). This change is just about what might be anticipated from theoretical considerations, for the surface area of a newborn lamb is, weight for weight, approximately three times that of an adult sheep. Presumably this increase in oxygen consumption after birth may also occur in species other than the sheep. Some postnatal observations by Mount (1958) suggest that it may take place in piglets, but this is hardly direct evidence. So far there are no reliable estimates of the rate of oxygen consumption of human babies *in utero*; the newborn baby has an oxygen consumption of only 5-7 ml./kg./min. (Cross, Tizard and Trythall, 1957), but is usually better clothed and kept in a warmer environment than a newborn lamb.

We may here pause to consider the implications of some of these observations. They suggest that before birth the mechanisms are present and ready

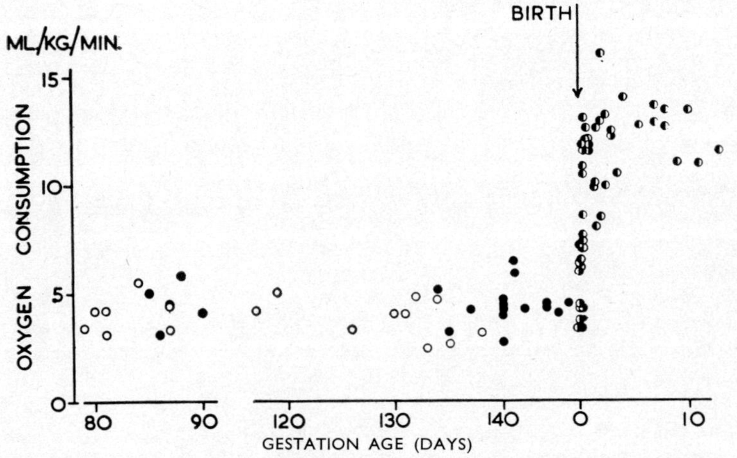

FIG. 2.—The rate of O_2 consumption/unit body weight has been plotted against gestation age in days for foetal lambs anaesthetized with pentobarbitone (O) or chloralose (●), and in days from birth in newborn lambs ventilated artificially (◑) or breathing spontaneously (◐). O_2 consumption increases about three-fold after birth (Dawes and Mott, 1959b).

to serve a radical change in metabolism and function. Such subtle matters as the regulation of appetite and of shivering in response to cold, which can hardly have been practised *in utero* are prepared and ready for use. After a day or two a lamb can maintain its body temperature in a laboratory at 20° C. without shivering; how this is achieved so rapidly we do not yet know.

Oxygen Consumption and Partial Oxygen Lack in the Newborn

I now propose to turn to a general consideration of the response to oxygen lack in the newborn. It is important to bear in mind the general opinion of physiologists about this matter, i.e. that in adult mammals, oxygen consumption is independent of the oxygen content of the inspired air, until this is lowered to such an extent that life is seriously endangered. This view was based on the fact that observations on man at high altitude did not suggest that metabolic rate was reduced. It was also supported by acute experiments on adult dogs. Oxygen consumption was not reduced until the arterial O_2 saturation fell below 40%, corresponding to 6% O_2 or less in the inspired air. At this point there was evidence of impending cardiovascular failure (Harrison and Blalock, 1927; Cordier and Mayer, 1935; Gorlin and Lewis, 1954). Finally many experiments on isolated enzyme systems have shown that they are able to accept oxygen at very low partial pressures, down to 5 mm. Hg or less, as compared with a normal partial pressure of 95 mm. Hg in the arterial blood of adult man.

In some species, and under certain conditions, O_2 consumption is indeed largely independent of the arterial O_2 partial pressure, and Fig. 3 shows such an experiment upon an adult sheep. However, when we turn to small animals, and in particular newborn animals, the results are different. One of the most important contributions in this field was the demonstration by Cross *et al.* (1955, 1957) that when the oxygen content of the inspired air is

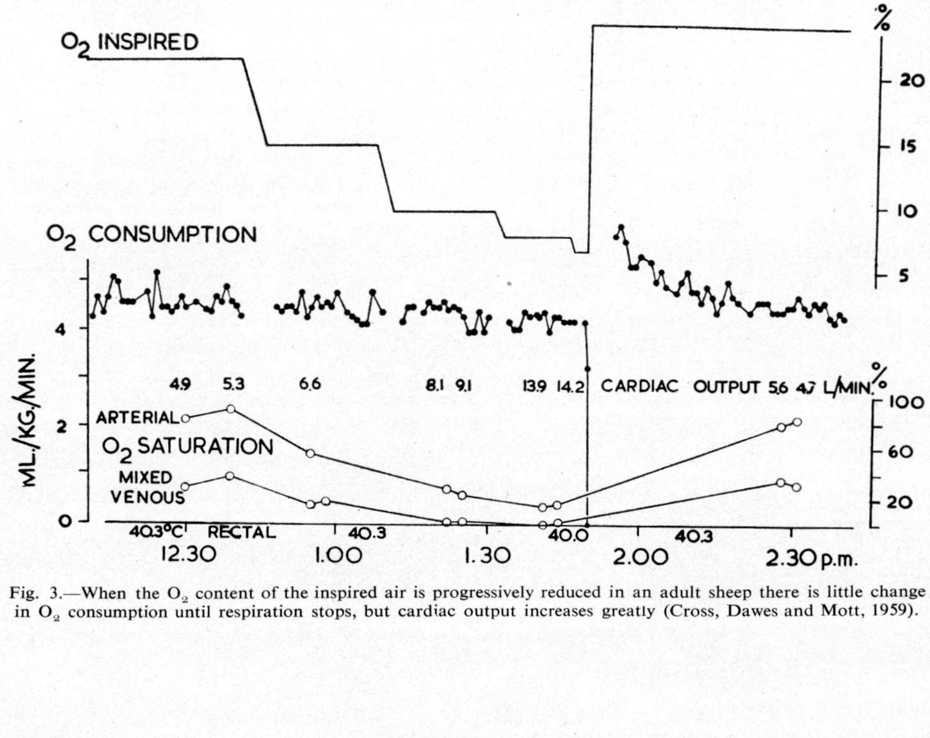

Fig. 3.—When the O_2 content of the inspired air is progressively reduced in an adult sheep there is little change in O_2 consumption until respiration stops, but cardiac output increases greatly (Cross, Dawes and Mott, 1959).

reduced, only from 20·9% to 15%, the rate of oxygen consumption falls in newborn babies. Since that time a similar phenomenon has been demonstrated in the newborn of a number of other species (Fig. 4).

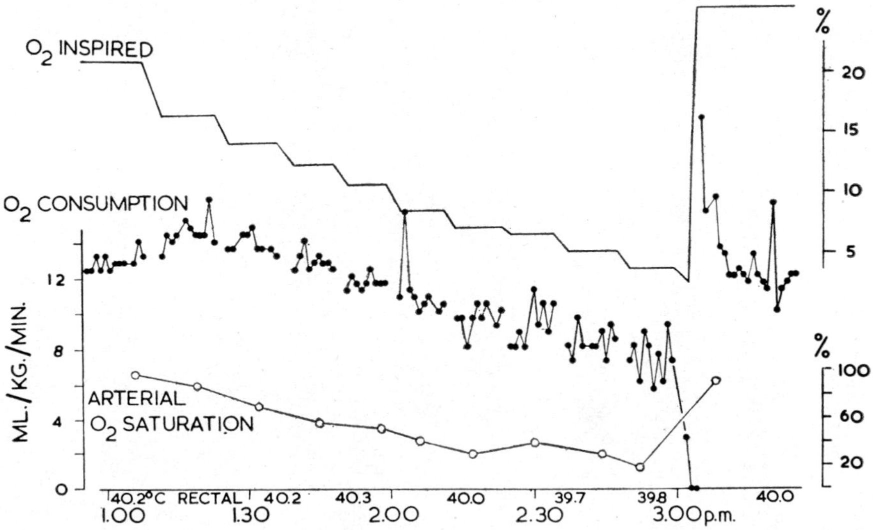

FIG. 4.—When the O_2 content of the inspired air is progressively reduced in a newborn lamb maintained at the neutral temperature, there is a considerable fall in O_2 consumption (Cross, Dawes and Mott, 1959).

The causes of the failure to maintain O_2 consumption during anoxia are not simple. The first factor to be considered is the environmental temperature. When a man or an animal is exposed to a cold environment his rate of oxygen consumption increases. He not only attempts to reduce heat loss by vasoconstriction in the skin, but he also spends more energy in an attempt to maintain his body temperature. On the other hand if he is exposed to a very warm environment he begins to pant, becomes restless, and once again his rate of oxygen consumption increases. There is therefore an intermediate range of environmental temperature at which oxygen consumption, at rest, is minimal. This is known as the neutral temperature. Small animals, such as mice and rats, when kept at their neutral temperature, show only a small fall in O_2 consumption during anoxia, but at lower environmental temperatures the fall is considerable (Lintzel, 1931; Chevillard and Mayer, 1935; Blood, Glover, Henderson and d'Amour, 1949; Flückiger, 1956). Hill (1958) has done a particularly thorough analysis of this phenomenon on newborn kittens and adult guinea-pigs, and has shown in both that the extra O_2 consumption which occurs on exposure to a less warm environment is particularly susceptible to oxygen lack. Fig. 5 demonstrates this phenomenon in a 60-day-old lamb. The O_2 consumption at the start of the experiment, breathing air at an environmental temperature of 19° C., was 120 ml./min. The environmental temperature was then lowered and O_2 consumption increased to 190 ml./min. When the lamb was given 10% O_2 to breathe, instead of air, O_2 consumption rapidly fell to 110 ml./min., i.e. just below what it had been before exposure to cold. When the oxygen content of the inspired air was raised, shivering began again and O_2 consumption increased. The fall in O_2 consumption during anoxia was just about equal to the increase on exposure to cold. This phenomenon is particularly easy to demonstrate in young animals or small animals, and one suspects that it is size, as much as youth, which is of importance.

There are other factors concerned with the inability of newborn animals to maintain their O_2 consumption during anoxia. Firstly, O_2 consumption falls if body temperature falls, and here small animals are particularly at a disadvantage because their heat capacity is low and their surface area relatively large. Secondly, in newborn lambs there is also a large fall in O_2 consumption during anoxia, even when the lamb is at its neutral temperature and when the deep body temperature is well maintained (Fig. 4). This fall is easy to demonstrate in a lamb a few days after birth, when O_2 consumption has increased from the foetal to the neonatal level (Fig. 6). But lambs which are 3 weeks old or more behave more like adults (Cross, Dawes and Mott, 1959). It would appear therefore that this is another phenomenon peculiar to the transition from foetal to neonatal life.

In summary then, O_2 consumption falls in anoxic newborn animals for a variety of reasons. Some of these are related to body size; it is by no means certain that immaturity of the physiological mechanisms can be blamed. And now, you may well ask, is the newborn animal the worse or the better off for its ability to dispense with part of its normal O_2 requirement? In so far as its body

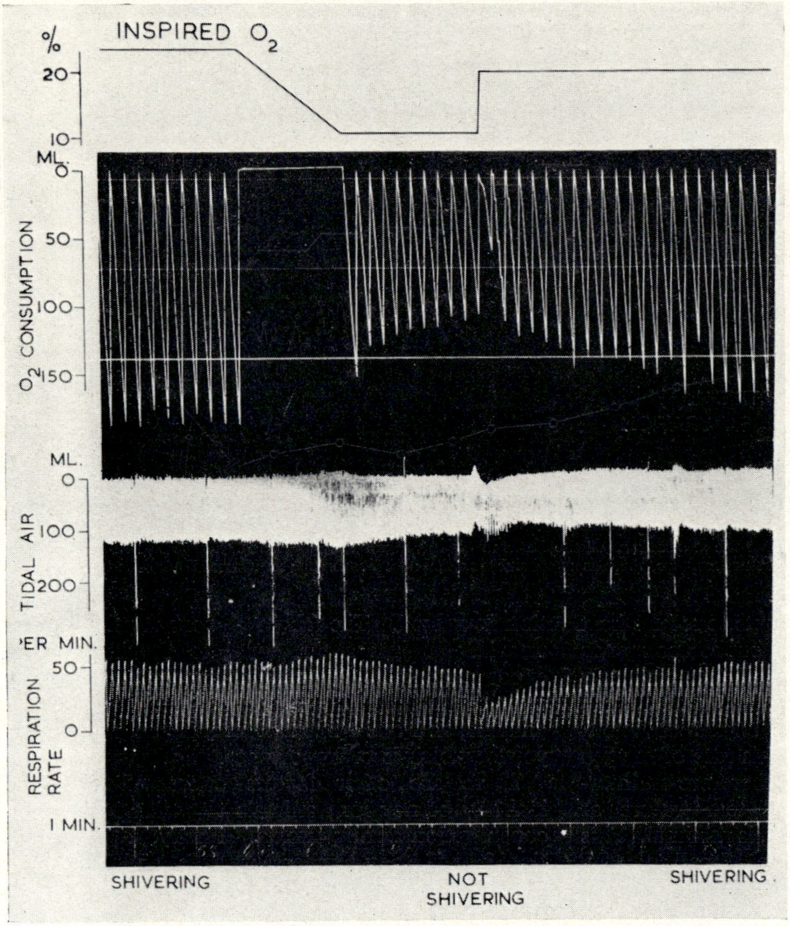

FIG. 5.—A lamb was placed in a low environmental temperature, in which it shivered. When the O_2 content of the inspired air was lowered, shivering ceased and O_2 consumption fell; when it was raised, O_2 consumption increased and shivering reappeared (Cross, Dawes and Mott, 1959).

in adults the hyperpnoea is maintained. Cross and Oppé (1952) concluded that the hyperpnoea was due to stimulation of the chemoreceptors and that the failure to maintain hyperpnoea was due to depression of the respiratory centre by oxygen lack. That seemed the only possible interpretation, but it was rather surprising that such a relatively small degree of anoxia should cause respiratory depression. Another group of workers in the U.S.A. failed to observe hyperpnoea on giving low oxygen mixtures to newborn babies at all (Miller and Smull, 1955), a result which led them to believe that the chemoreceptor mechanisms were not functional after birth. This is, on the face of it, an even more surprising conclusion. One would have expected that anoxic stimulation of respiration would be well-developed in the newborn, above all else. Was it possible, then, that there were some other circumstances about the experiments which led to these unexpected observations?

One possible approach was to try and see under what circumstances the same responses could be obtained in experimental animals. The newborn rabbit was chosen for this purpose. A preliminary investigation showed that the Hering-Breuer respiratory reflexes, the carotid chemoreceptor reflex and the pulmonary deflation reflex were all present and active in the rabbit at birth. This conclusion was verified by section of the appropriate nervous pathways, for the reflexes then disappeared. I do not propose to go into the experimental details, but would emphasize that it is important to have reached the conclusion in one species at least (and the rabbit is born in a relatively immature state, with its eyes closed and unable to fend for itself) that the crucial respiratory reflexes are well established at birth.

When newborn rabbits were exposed to low

temperature falls, I would surmise that it is worse off, but we still really do not know for sure. It is dangerous to assume that such mechanisms have a purpose. I think we should be satisfied for the moment to understand the mechanisms.

Respiration and Partial Oxygen Lack in the Newborn

We now come to a consideration of respiratory behaviour in the newborn, and the response to partial oxygen lack. During the past decade there have been several investigations of the control of respiration in the newborn infant. Dr. Kenneth Cross showed that when a baby was given 15% O_2 to breathe, it reacted by hyperpnoea which lasted only a few minutes. This was unexpected, because

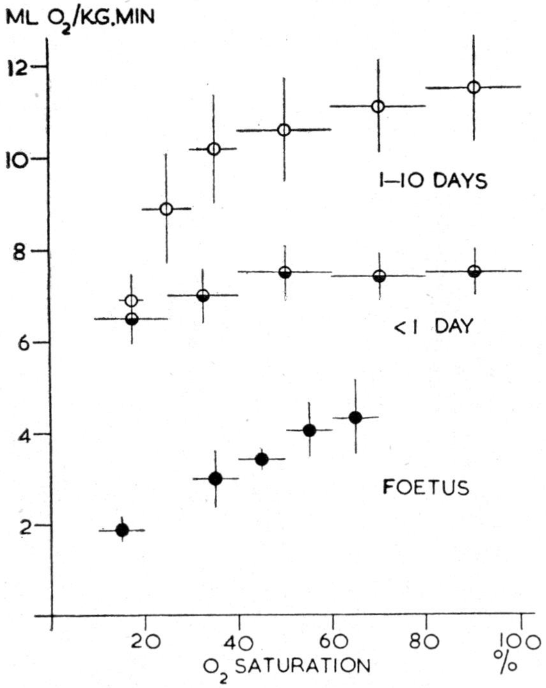

FIG. 6.—Diagram to show the behaviour of foetal and newborn lambs in response to anoxia. Ordinate, O_2 consumption/unit body weight; abscissa, arterial O_2 saturation. The vertical lines through each circle indicate the 95% confidence limits of the means, and the horizontal lines the range of the observations, all of which were made at the neutral temperature (Cross, Dawes and Mott, 1959).

oxygen mixtures at an environmental temperature above 30° C. the rate and depth of breathing was increased, and this increase was well-maintained (Fig. 7). But at lower ambient temperatures there was only a transient increase, or even a decrease in the minute volume of breathing (Dawes and Mott, 1959a). Subsequent experiments suggest that this phenomenon occurs in both newborn rabbits and lambs when exposed to a temperature rather below the neutral range, that is to say, in conditions in which the rate of oxygen consumption has already increased in response to cold, but with only a trivial fall of deep body temperature. We do not know if these observations provide an explanation for the respiratory findings on human babies; they may do so, but only experiment will determine this. Meanwhile we may note that, in newborn animals: (1) There is evidence of a full range of respiratory reflexes at birth, at the neutral temperature. (2) If the environmental temperature is lowered below the neutral range, oxygen consumption normally increases, but then (*a*) slight anoxia causes a considerable fall of oxygen consumption; and (*b*) the hyperpnoea in response to anoxia is poorly maintained, or even absent altogether.

I am not sure whether we should be justified in concluding that it would be wise to maintain a newborn infant, who was suffering from respiratory difficulties, at the neutral temperature (i.e. a high environmental temperature), but I should not be at all surprised if this does not prove to be the safest procedure in the long run. Only observations on newborn infants will tell us this.

The Task of the Circulation

Next there is the question of autonomic control of the circulation after birth. In the past a number of observations have been widely quoted, which purport to show that the autonomic nervous system is, in one respect or another, either not functional, or barely functional at birth. Thus it has been concluded that the vasomotor reflexes were not developed in the newborn rabbit, kitten or puppy until some days or weeks after birth. However,

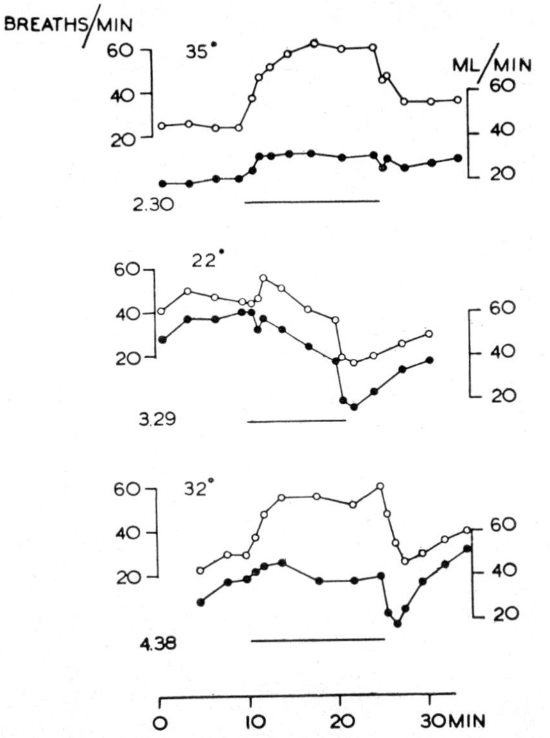

FIG. 7.—Rabbit 4 days old. Open circles respiratory rate; closed circles minute volume. During the periods indicated by the solid lines the rabbit breathed 11% O_2 instead of air. At an environmental temperature of 32-35° C. the rabbit showed a maintained hyperpnoea in response to anoxia, but at 22° C. the hyperpnoea was not maintained (Dawes and Mott, 1959a).

closer and more critical examination of the experiments on which these conclusions are based show them to be inadequate, in many respects, by present day standards. To take a very simple example, Soltmann (1877) reported that stimulation of the peripheral end of the vagus did not slow the heart in a newborn rabbit; Kellogg (1927) found that it did sometimes, but not always. Admittedly newborn rabbits are rather small, and weigh only about 50 g., but nevertheless with better instruments than were formerly available it is possible to show that vagal stimulation always slows the heart, and other evidence suggests that the vasomotor reflexes are present and functional. This may be regarded as a corollary of the evidence already quoted, that the respiratory reflexes are well established at birth in the rabbit.

What is equally important is the growing realization that the task with which the cardiovascular system of a newborn creature is faced is not the same, quantitatively, as that in an adult. Even after the foetal cardiovascular channels are completely closed, by a week or 10 days after birth, there are differences. The quantity of oxygen to be carried from the lungs to the tissues in each minute is greater, per unit body weight, than in the adult. Fig. 8 shows that cardiac output, per unit body weight, is greater in the newborn lamb than in the adult ewe. Thus a lamb weighing 10 kg. may have a cardiac output of 3 l./min. while a ewe of 50 kg. has a cardiac output of only 5 l./min. This is not wholly surprising, and it may be pertinent to recall that the heart rate of small animals is in general greater than that of large ones. The few measurements of foetal cardiac output so far available suggest that cardiac output increases after birth. And whereas the cardiac output of an adult sheep increases three to five fold during anoxia, that of lambs up to 60 days old shows little change. This is one of the most striking differences between the behaviour of young and adult sheep subjected to oxygen lack. It would have been tempting to conclude that autonomic control of the circulation was inadequately developed in the young lamb, were it not for the fact that cardiac output is already relatively so high (Fig. 8). There is little doubt that we have a great deal more to learn in this field, and there is a danger to be avoided of generalizing from one species. Unfortunately it is by no means easy to measure cardiac output on small animals.

The Ability to Survive in the Total Absence of Oxygen

There is another fascinating physiological attribute of very young animals which demands attention. This is their ability to survive periods of total oxygen lack which far exceed those which kill adults of the same species. To my mind this is one of the most important aspects of neonatal physiology, in relation to the clinical problems which are in the forefront of our minds. It is a matter which is of crucial importance if it is believed that some, perhaps many, cases of cerebral palsy result from asphyxia at birth. It may also serve to explain some of the bizarre pathological appearances in the lungs of infants which have died from respiratory difficulties after

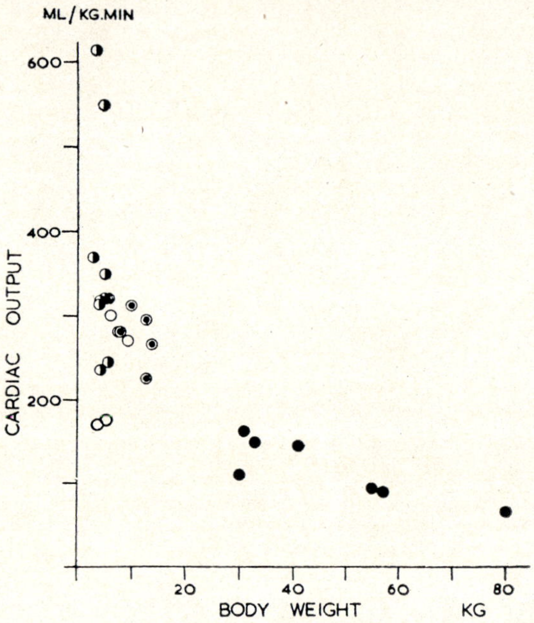

FIG. 8.—Cardiac output (Fick method) has been plotted against body weight for lambs less than 1 day old (◑), 2-12 days old (○), 20-60 days old (⊙) and for adult sheep (●), all while breathing air (Cross, Dawes and Mott, 1959).

birth, in that the heart can go on beating, and the lungs be expanded, in the presence of anoxia from which any adult would rapidly succumb.

It is strange that so little experimental work has been undertaken on this problem. The essential facts are well authenticated. Human babies have been delivered by caesarean section after the death of their mother and have survived. They have also survived prolonged periods of suffocation from various causes. When given 100% nitrogen to breathe, newborn rats live for as long as 50 minutes and kittens and puppies more than 20 minutes, while newborn guinea-pigs and lambs, which are more mature at birth, live for only seven to 10 minutes. Himwich, Bernstein, Herrlich, Chesler and Fazekas

(1942) have shown that administration of iodoacetate, which blocks the enzyme systems responsible for glycolysis, reduces the survival time of young animals in anoxia to that of adults. It is evident that in such young animals energy is obtained during anoxia by breakdown of carbohydrate to lactic and pyruvic acids, and that it is by deriving this energy that the animal can survive. One of the difficulties about such studies is that newborn animals are either very small, or if they are larger do not survive anoxia for long. It is therefore not easy to obtain serial blood samples and hence to study the biochemical changes during anoxia. However, foetal lambs, just over half-way through gestation, weighing 350-600 g., are suitable subjects for this purpose. The umbilical cord may be tied for as long as 40 minutes, with apparently complete recovery when it is then untied (Fig. 9). During the period of anoxia carbohydrate appears and lactic acid accumulates in the blood, rising first rapidly and then more slowly. The pH of the blood begins to fall within one minute of tying the cord, and reaches 7·0 which is very low indeed, on the average by 10 minutes. The most remarkable feature of these experiments was that most of the carbohydrate loss appeared to be from the heart, which at this period of life has very large reserves. More mature foetal lambs had less carbohydrate in their ventricular muscle, and were able to withstand total anoxia for a shorter period of time. In newborn animals also there was a linear relationship between the carbohydrate concentration in the ventricles of the heart before asphyxia, and the duration of survival as timed to the last respiratory effort. This holds not only for rats at different ages from birth, but also for rabbits and guinea-pigs (Fig. 10).

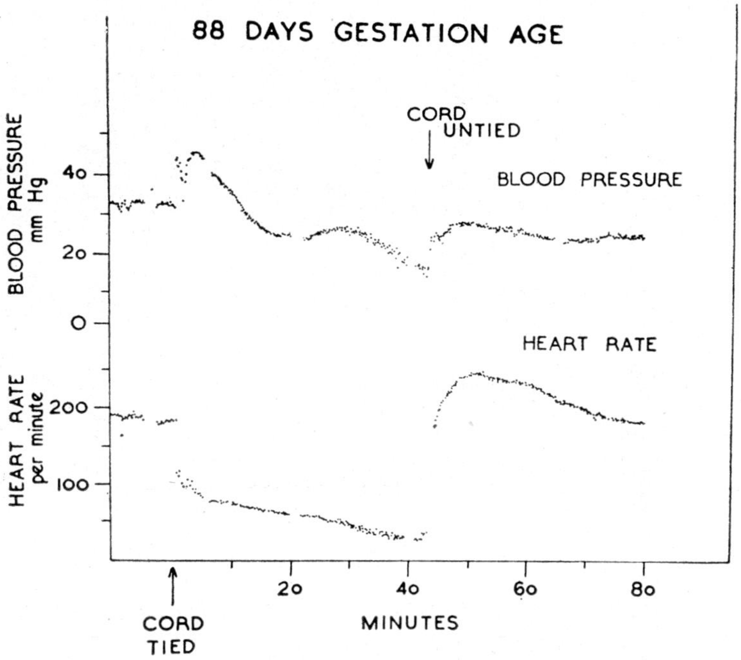

FIG. 9.—Foetal lamb of 88 days gestation age (term is 147 days). The umbilical cord was tied for 40 minutes and then untied, when blood pressure and heart rate recovered (Dawes, Mott and Shelley, 1959).

There is certainly more to the problem than the cardiac carbohydrate, since it is well known that the decapitated head of a newborn rat will continue to make gasping movements for as long as 20 minutes. Yet these results are interesting for several reasons. Firstly, they lead to a broader understanding of the means whereby whole animals survive total anoxia, and of the limitations thereto. It may be coincidence that there is a direct relation between the initial concentration of carbohydrate in the heart, and the duration of respiratory efforts; it may on the other hand be a causal relationship. As it is, these results make us consider once more whether it is the heart or the brain which usually succumbs first. There are a few tragic instances, in both children and adults, where the vegetative system has recovered from anoxia, but consciousness has never been regained. But if the cardiovascular system fails first then recovery is quite impossible. However effective ventilation is, oxygen cannot reach the brain if the output of the heart is inadequate, even though it may still be beating. It is therefore possible that the circulation may usually fail before there is irreversible damage to the brain. Secondly, these experiments must make us consider whether there are any means which can be employed to increase the duration of survival during total anoxia. Preliminary experiments have suggested that this is feasible; in some lambs the duration of survival has been doubled. But the optimal conditions have not yet been discovered, and at the present moment the method of treatment is hazardous. I do not want to indicate more than that the possibility exists. Thirdly, we must recognize that almost all babies are to some extent asphyxiated by the process of delivery, whatever the method and however expert the care. You have only to examine the published figures to recognize this. The mean figures for the arterial oxygen saturation in the umbilical cord are almost all less than 30%, with an O_2 partial pressure of only 8-16 mm. Hg. This is miserably low by any reasonable physiological standard, far less than the average for healthy foetal lambs. James, Weisbrot, Prince, Holaday and Apgar (1958) have recently published an interesting analysis of the biochemical changes in the blood of normal babies after birth. There was a systematic rise in *p*H and in the 'buffer base', indicating a recovery from metabolic acidosis, consequent on asphyxia at or before birth. The conclusion is inescapable that almost every baby at birth has had its carbohydrate reserves somewhat depleted by glycolysis, and begins an independent life with a blood *p*H considerably below the optimal. It is not at all surprising that some of these infants breathe poorly after birth; it is just as well that most of them can still make respiratory efforts when there is no measurable oxygen in the arterial blood at all.

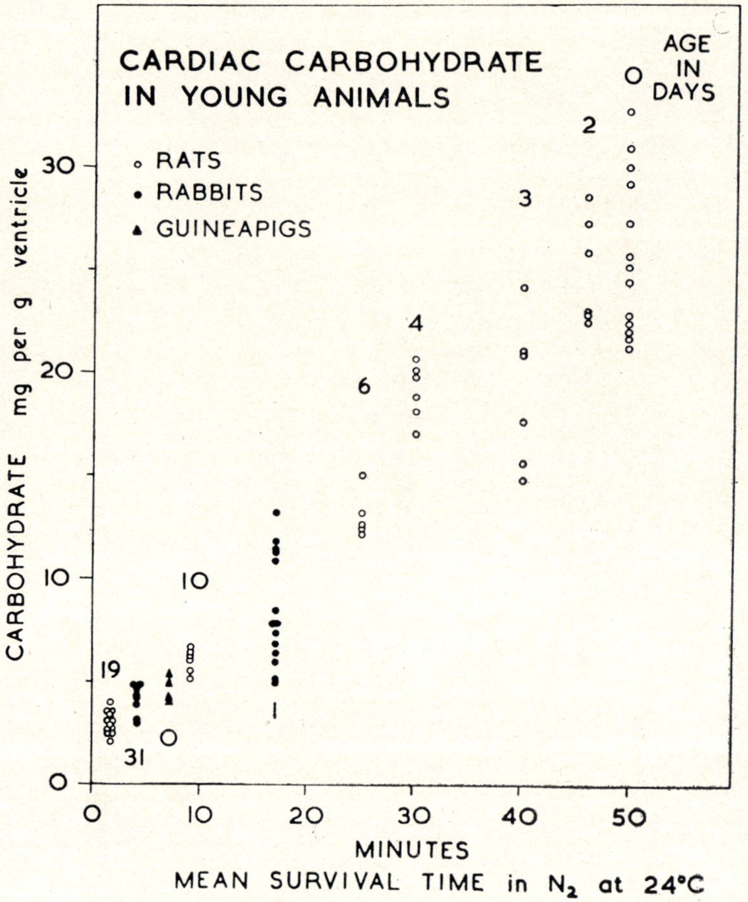

FIG. 10.—There is a roughly linear relationship between the mean survival time in nitrogen of young animals and the cardiac carbohydrate concentration before anoxia (Dawes, Mott and Shelley, 1959).

Conclusion

These animal experiments suggest that there is more to the newborn than at first appeared. He is neither a miniature replica of the adult, nor is he entirely helpless. He is not a weak creature, poorly endowed with the mechanisms which are required to maintain a constant internal environment.

A newborn animal is not only young, it is also small, compared with an adult of the same species, and it is growing rapidly. It is now evident that there is still something to be learnt about the way in which small animals, irrespective of youth, react to changes in their environment. Some of the reactions which were first thought of as characteristic of newborn creatures have been observed in adults (of other species) which are small in size. We should therefore be chary of concluding that any physiological mechanism in a newborn baby is immature, or underdeveloped, unless there are compelling reasons for doing so. McCance and Widdowson (1956) have provided an interesting example of this principle by showing that, because of their rapid growth, newborn piglets convert 90% of the nitrogen they ingest in a full diet into body protein. Hence the kidney does not need to be able to secrete more than a limited amount of urea. The kidney may be 'immature' by adult standards, but it is fully capable of doing the job it normally needs to do. Hence rapid growth rate, as well as size and environment, are most important factors to consider when assessing the physiological capabilities of a baby. We have seen that the course of the circulation in the newborn is in some respects different from that in the adult and that the responses to oxygen lack and to changes in environment temperature are also different. Yet the newborn creature is not passive; it is a complicated and highly integrated organism, and its behaviour deserves study for its own sake.

The biological mechanisms which I have endeavoured to describe have all presented problems in classical physiology. They could have been tackled with the methods which were available in 1928, when this Association was first founded, and when Still became its first President. There are several reasons why they have not been studied intensively. Some of these are of a technical nature; it is often tedious and sometimes difficult to perform experiments on small animals. But much more important has been the failure to realize that the problems even existed. With the realization that they do exist, and that nowadays more children die in the first seven days of life than during the next seven years, there is a challenge to further research that cannot be ignored.

I am grateful to the *Journal of Physiology* for permission to reproduce Figs. 3-10.

REFERENCES

Adams, F. H. and Lind, J. (1957). *Pediatrics*, **19**, 431.
Amoroso E. C., Dawes, G. S. and Mott, J. C. (1958). *Brit. Heart J.*, **20**, 92.
Barclay, A. E., Franklin, K. J. and Prichard, M. M. L. (1944). *The Foetal Circulation and Cardiovascular System, and the Changes that they Undergo at Birth.* Blackwell, Oxford.
Barcroft, J. (1946). *Researches on Pre-natal Life.* Blackwell, Oxford.
Blood, F. R., Glover, R. M., Henderson, J. B. and d'Amour, F. E. (1949). *Amer. J. Physiol.*, **156**, 62.
Burnard, E. D. (1958). *Brit. med. J.*, **1**, 806.
Chevillard, L. and Mayer, A. (1935). *Ann. Physiol. Physicochim. biol.*, **11**, 225.
Condorelli, M., Dagianti, A., Polosa, C. and Giuliano, G. (1957). *Atti del XIX Congresso della Società Italiana di Cardiologia*, p. 165.
Cordier D. and Mayer, A. (1935). *Ann. Physiol. Physicochim. biol.*, **11**, 199.
Cross, K. W., Dawes, G. S. and Mott, J. C. (1959). *J. Physiol. (Lond.)*, **146**, 516.
—— and Oppé, T. E. (1952). *Ibid.*, **117**, 38.
——, Tizard, J. P. M. and Trythall, D. A. H. (1955). *Ibid.*, **129**, 69P.
——, ——, —— (1957). *Acta paediat. (Uppsala)*, **46**, 265.
Dawes, G. S. and Mott, J. C. (1959a). *J. Physiol. (Lond.)*, **145**, 85.
——, —— (1959b). *Ibid.*, **146**, 295.
——, —— and Widdicombe, J. G. (1955). *Ibid.*, **128**, 344.
Flückiger, E. (1956). *Helv. physiol. pharmacol. Acta*, **14**, 369.
Gorlin, R. and Lewis, B. M. (1954). *J. appl. Physiol.*, **7**, 180.
Harrison, T. R. and Blalock, A. (1927). *Amer. J. Physiol.*, **80**, 169.
Hill, J. R. (1958). *J. Physiol. (Lond.)*, **143**, 64P.
Himwich, H. E., Bernstein, A. O., Herrlich, H., Chesler, A. and Fazekas, J. F. (1942). *Amer. J. Physiol.*, **135**, 387.
James, L. S. and Rowe, R. D. (1957). *J. Pediat.*, **51**, 5.
——, Weisbrot, I. M., Prince, C. E., Holaday, D. A. and Apgar, V (1958). *Ibid.*, **52**, 379.
Kellogg, H. B. (1927). *Proc. Soc. exp. Biol. (N.Y.)*, **24**, 839.
Lind, J. and Wegelius, C. (1954). *Cold Spr. Harb. Symp. quant. Biol.*, **19**, 109.
Lintzel, W. (1931). *Pflüg. Arch. ges. Physiol.*, **227**, 693.
McCance, R. A. and Widdowson, E. M. (1956). *J. Physiol. (Lond.)*, **133**, 373.
Miller, H. C. and Smull, N. W. (1955). *Pediatrics*, **16**, 93.
Mount, L. E. (1958). *J. Physiol. (Lond.)*, **142**, 57P.
Rowe, R. D. and James, L. S. (1957). *J. Pediat.*, **51**, 1.
Soltmann, O. (1877). *Jb. Kinderheilk.*, **11**, 101.
Weisbrot, I. M., James, L. S., Prince, C. E., Holaday, M. D. and Apgar, V. (1958). *J. Pediat.*, **52**, 395.

THE PUPILLARY MEMBRANE IN PREMATURE INFANTS

BY

BRUNO GANS

From the Premature Baby Unit, Lewisham Hospital, London

(RECEIVED FOR PUBLICATION JANUARY 5, 1959)

The presence or absence of a pupillary membrane is a valuable sign of immaturity in infants born before term. This fact has been noted by Continental authors. As no reference to it could be found in British medical publications since the war the following brief account may be of use.

In the 13 mm. embryo the annular vessel, a branch of the ophthalmic artery, forms an anastomotic ring round the rim of the developing optic cup. At the 17 mm. stage buds arise from this annular vessel. These ultimately form a series of loops which lie on the anterior surface of the lens. In the 40 to 60 mm. embryo there is an elaborate vascular network arranged in three tiers of arcades. After the fifth month of foetal life this network, the pupillary membrane, begins to atrophy. First the central tiers of arcades become progressively more attenuated and then disappear. As vascular involution proceeds the second arcade disappears behind the growing border of the iris. At term most of the loops have disappeared and only the first arcade remains. This forms a series of anastomotic vessels, the lesser circle of the iris (Duke-Elder, 1938). Minor remnants of the pupillary membrane are, of course, extremely common in full term infants (Seissiger, 1929) and indeed in the general population, particularly if their eyes are examined by means of a slit lamp.

The well-known difficulty of obtaining a good view of a premature infant's fundus oculi is due, in part, to the vessels of the pupillary membrane. On naked eye examination this structure is seen as a delicate blue-grey veil behind the pupillary aperture. After homatropin mydriasis the vessels constituting the membrane can be observed through the +20 lens of an ophthalmoscope. They form a spider's web which stands out black against the red retinal light reflex. To obtain a good view the examiner should hold the ophthalmoscope in his right hand and the infant's head in his left, using his left index finger to retract the upper lid. A nurse holds the baby's body and retracts the lower lid with her free index finger. Care must be taken not to let the cornea become dry by prolonged examination.

Fig. 1 shows the pupillary membrane of a 3-day-old infant weighing 2 lb. 2 oz. Figs. 2 and 3 represent the membrane of a baby weighing 2 lb. 12 oz. on the second and fourth day after birth. The marked reduction in the number and calibre of the vessels is noticeable. Figs. 4 to 8 illustrate the progressive changes taking place in the pupillary membrane of an infant observed from the third to the forty-first day of life, during which time her weight rose from 3 lb. 8 oz. to 5 lb. 1 oz.

During the last three years some 270 premature infants have been examined in the unit at Lewisham Hospital. From these observations it appears that the presence of a pupillary membrane, particularly if it is extensive, is a good though non-specific sign of immaturity. Schmöger (1955) found a clear-cut inverse relationship between the extent of the membrane and the length and weight of 302 premature infants whom he examined. It proved impossible to demonstrate such a simple relationship in the Lewisham material. Some small, though relatively mature, infants had no membrane or only one or two delicate threads. A similar finding is recorded by Huggert (1952) who found the membrane to be absent in two infants weighing less than 1,500 g. and in five infants weighing between 1,600 and 1,700 g. in a series of 66 premature infants, 11 of whom did have a pupillary membrane. In my experience, an easily seen membrane is present in the majority of immature babies, and almost always in those weighing less than 1,500 g. The number and size of the vessels closely parallels the degree of immaturity, and an extensive network appears to be a more reliable prognostic index than the baby's gestation period, its weight or the degree of its hypothermia. It closely agrees with one's clinical impression of the infant's viability.

The rate of vascular obliteration and disappearance of the membrane also follows closely the infant's general progress. Schmöger (1955) states that the membrane disappears within a few days of birth, almost always at the end of the first week, and at the latest in the second week. In my experience

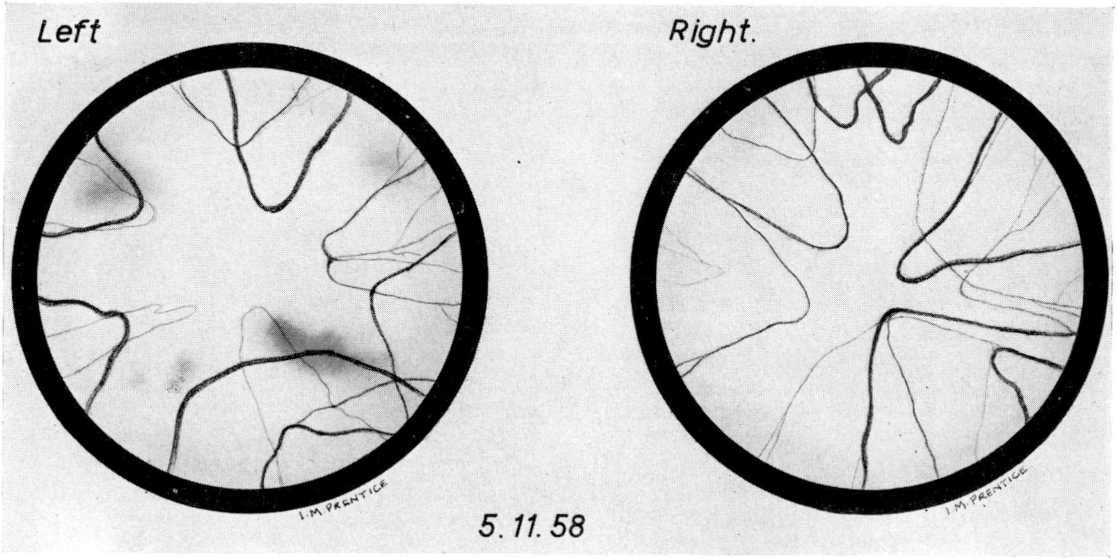

FIG. 1.—Pupillary membrane of 3-day-old infant weighing 2 lb. 2 oz

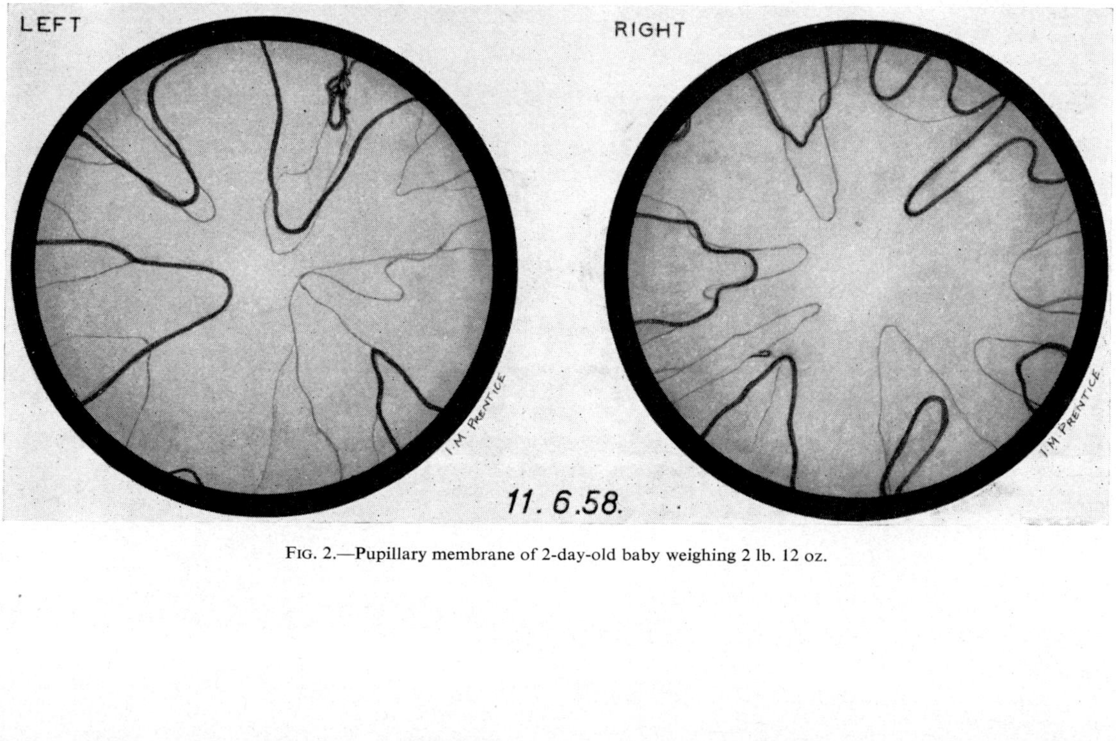

FIG. 2.—Pupillary membrane of 2-day-old baby weighing 2 lb. 12 oz.

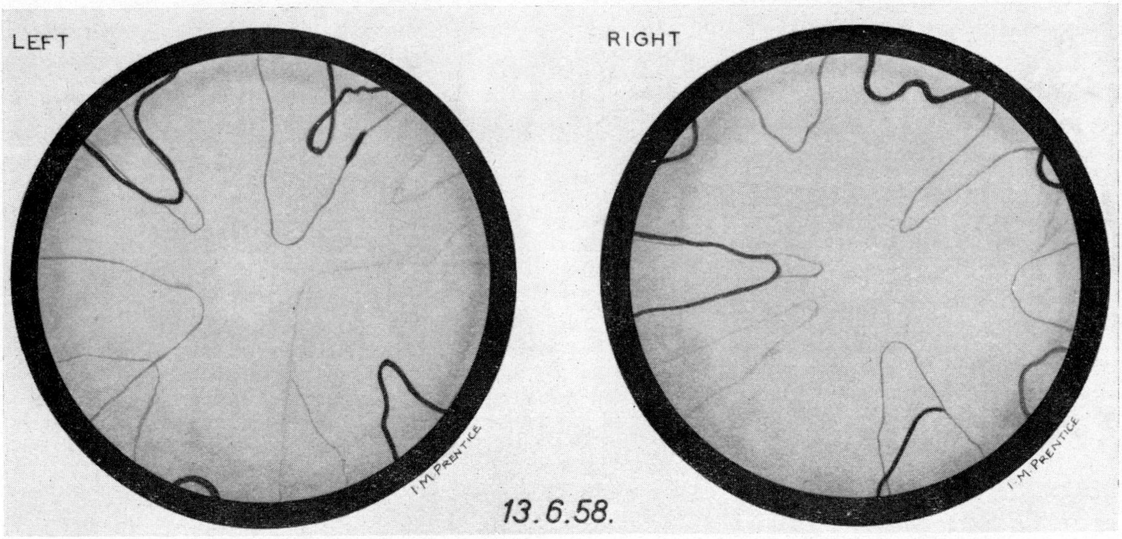

FIG. 3.—The same child as in Fig. 2 on fourth day after birth

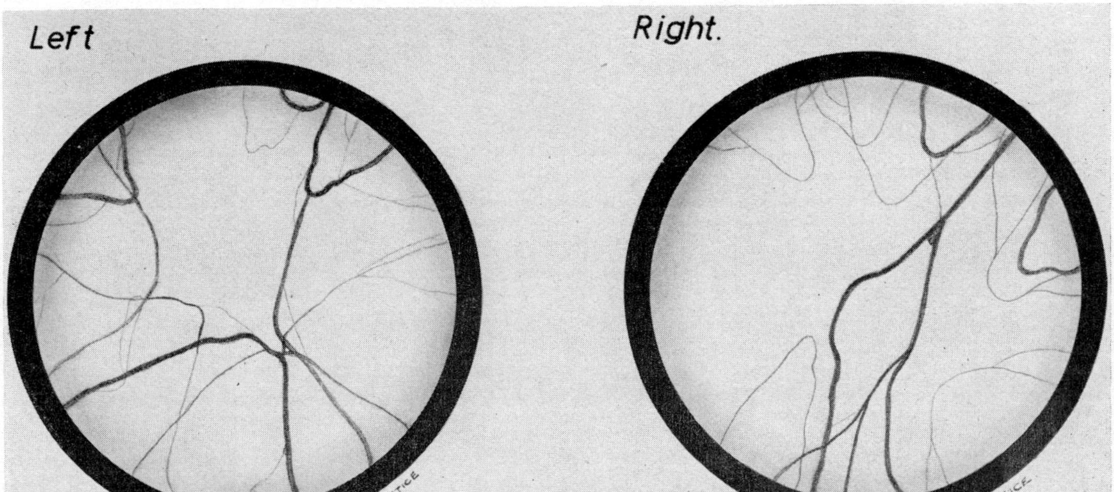

FIGS. 4-8.—Progressive changes in pupillary membrane of infant observed from 3 to 41 days old, during which time her weight increased from 3 lb. 8 oz. to 5 lb. 1 oz.

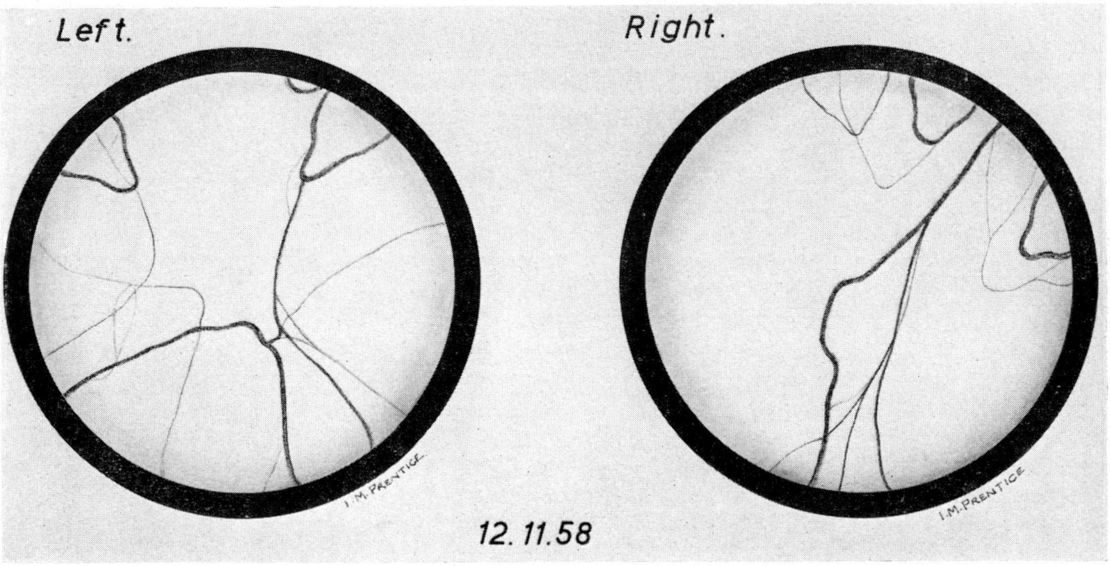
Left.
Right.
I.M. PRENTICE
I.M. PRENTICE
12. 11. 58

FIG. 5.

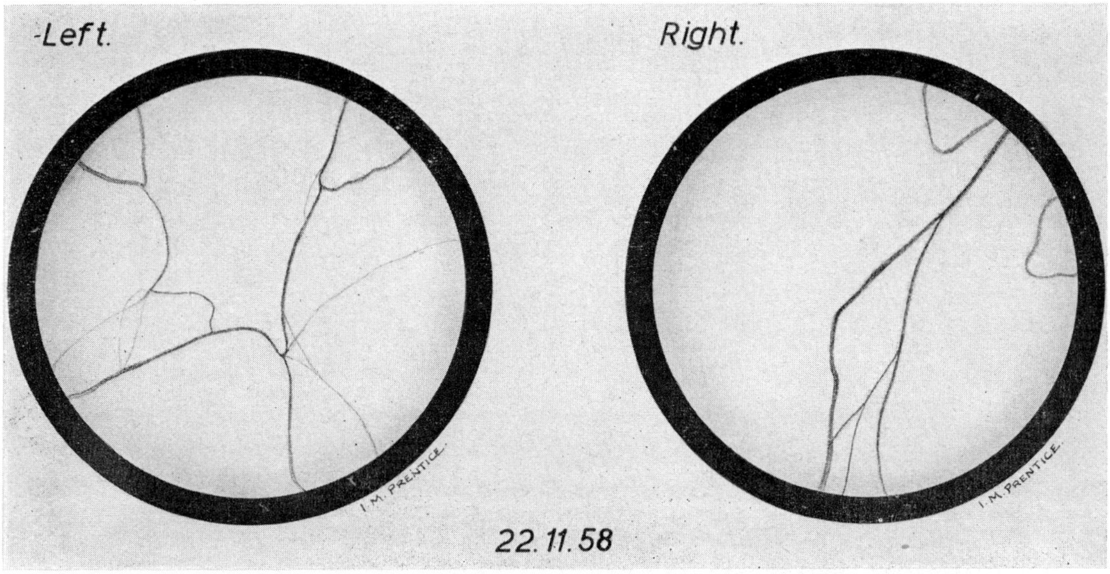
Left.
Right.
I.M. PRENTICE
I.M. PRENTICE
22. 11. 58

FIG. 6

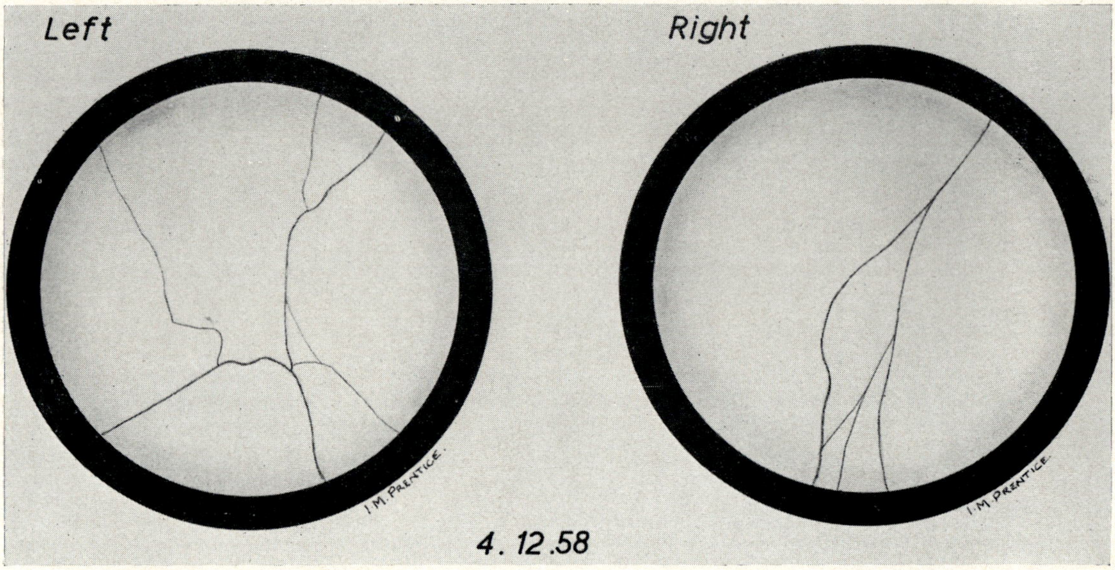
Left
Right
I.M. PRENTICE.
I.M. PRENTICE.
4. 12.58

FIG. 7.

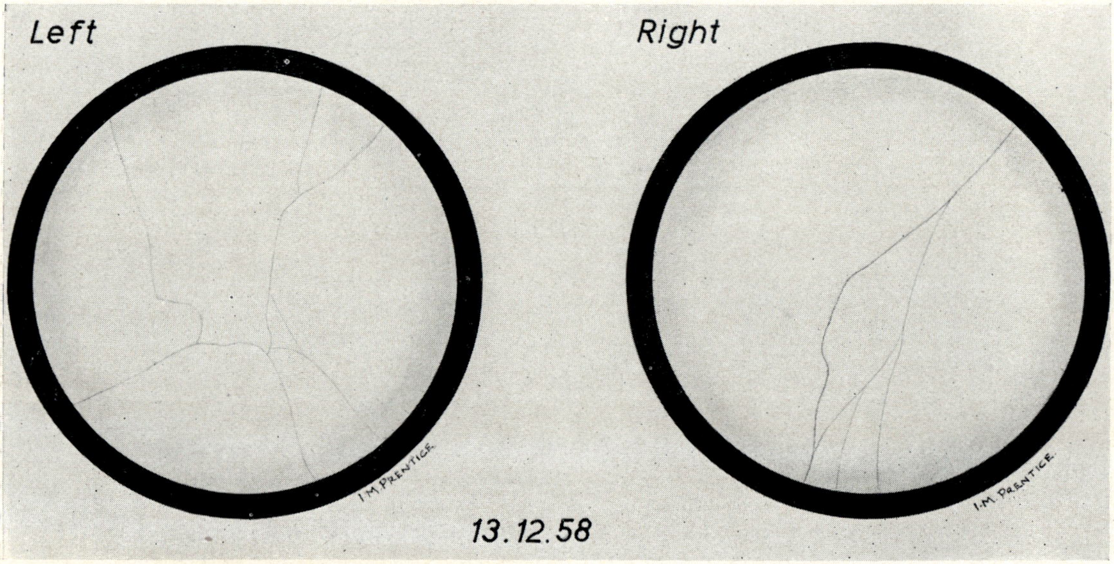
Left
Right
I.M. PRENTICE.
I.M. PRENTICE.
13.12.58

FIG. 8.

no hard and fast rule can be made about the time taken for the vessels to disappear. This finding would be expected if the assumption is correct that the pupillary membrane disappears *pari passu* with the infant's progressive maturation. Most infants are discharged from the unit when they weigh 6 lb. and in none of those discharged was a persistent pupillary membrane found. No doubt slit lamp examination would have revealed remnants, invisible through a simple lens, in the majority. In 104 children of originally low birth weight (1,020 to 2,500 g.), Wagner (1957) found no case of persistent membrane when these children were examined at the ages of 3 to 5 years.

Summary

The presence and extent of the pupillary membrane is a valuable index of immaturity in premature infants.

REFERENCES

Duke-Elder, W. S. (1938). *Textbook of Ophthalmology*, Vol. 1 (2nd impression). Kimpton, London.
Huggert, A. (1952). *Acta paediat. (Uppsala)*, **41**, 463.
Schmöger, R. (1955). *Kinderärztl. Prax.*, **23**, 433.
Seissiger, J. (1929). *Arch. Augenheilk.*, **100-101**, 302.
Wagner, G. (1957). *Klin. Mbl. Augenheilk.*, **131**, 326.

GLYCOGEN DISEASE

BY

S. VAN CREVELD

From the Paediatric Clinic of the University of Amsterdam

(RECEIVED FOR PUBLICATION JANUARY 13, 1959)

Since our first description of the hepatomegalic type of glycogen disease (van Creveld, 1928; Snapper and van Creveld, 1928) we have repeatedly reported on the condition of the patient described in that year and on a second patient described for the first time in 1932 (van Creveld, 1934, 1952, 1953). We have recently re-examined both patients and this paper reports our present findings which add a good deal to former findings.

Methods Used

(*a*) Intravenous glucose test: in Case 2 this was done in the usual way by giving a single intravenous injection of $\frac{1}{3}$ g. of glucose per kg. body weight in a 20% solution. In Case 1 the dose of intravenous glucose was determined according to the method of Jokipii and Turpeinen (1954). Here glucose is injected intravenously and slowly over a long period, thus imitating the normal process of absorption. This method might give information not easily obtainable by a single rapid injection. This could be of particular importance in this patient. The objection has been made against this method that individual blood glucose-time curves frequently show irregularities, and we therefore give the results obtained in our patient with reservation. He was given an injection of 5% glucose in distilled water over a period of 60 minutes at the rate of 340 mg. of glucose per minute.

(*b*) Epinephrine tolerance test: a blood sugar curve following the subcutaneous administration of 0·5 ml. of 1:1,000 solution of epinephrine.

(*c*) Glucagon tolerance test: a blood sugar curve following the intramuscular administration of 2·4 mg. of glucagon.*

(*d*) Repeated fasting blood sugar determinations. (*e*) Uric acid in blood under fasting conditions. (*f*) Cholesterol in plasma under fasting conditions. (*g*) Glycogen content of blood. (*h*) Serum proteins by method of Majoor (1947). (*i*) Sedimentation rate of erythrocytes. (*j*) Urine examination. (*k*) 17-hydroxycorticosteroids of blood.

* Glucagon (Lilly) was provided by Professor Rossi (Bern) and by Eli Lilly and Company, Indianapolis, (U.S.A.).

Case 1. Male, at present 38 years old. No complaints. Height 1·78 m., weight 87 kg. A physical examination disclosed no abnormalities; the liver was just palpable. He is married, and has two healthy sons, 7 and 8 years old respectively.

Case 2. Female, at present 32 years old. No complaints. Height 1·68 m., weight 66 kg. A physical examination disclosed no abnormalities; the liver was just palpable. She is married, and has a healthy son of 4 years.

Results and Comment

The results of the tests (*a*), (*b*) and (*c*) in both patients are summarized in Figs. 1 and 2, and those of the tests (*d*)-(*k*) in Table 1.

TABLE 1
TEST RESULTS

	Case 1	Case 2
Fasting blood sugar (mg./100 ml.)	75, 73, 70	83, 72, 79
Blood glycogen (mg./100 ml.)	27·5	8·2
Serum alkaline phosphatase (Bodansky units)	4·2	2
Cholesterol (mg./100 ml.)	340·5	173
Serum proteins (total) (g./100 ml.)	7·56	8·15
albumin	3·96	3·60
pseudoglobulin	2·34	2·87
euglobulin	1·26	1·68
Erythrocyte sedimentation rate (mm first hour)	8	7
Blood uric acid (mg./100 ml.)	5	6·2
Blood 17-hydroxycorticosteroids (mg./100 ml.)	8·1	

Case 1. Urine. (1) During glucose tolerance test: urine in fasting condition and during first hour of test free of acetone and reducing substance.

(2) During epinephrine tolerance test: urine at the end of the test: acetone positive, diacetic acid negative, reduction negative.

(3) During glucagon tolerance test: urine in fasting condition: acetone weakly positive, reducing substance negative. At 1, 2 and 3 hours after injection of glucagon, acetone present in all specimens of urine but reducing substances absent.

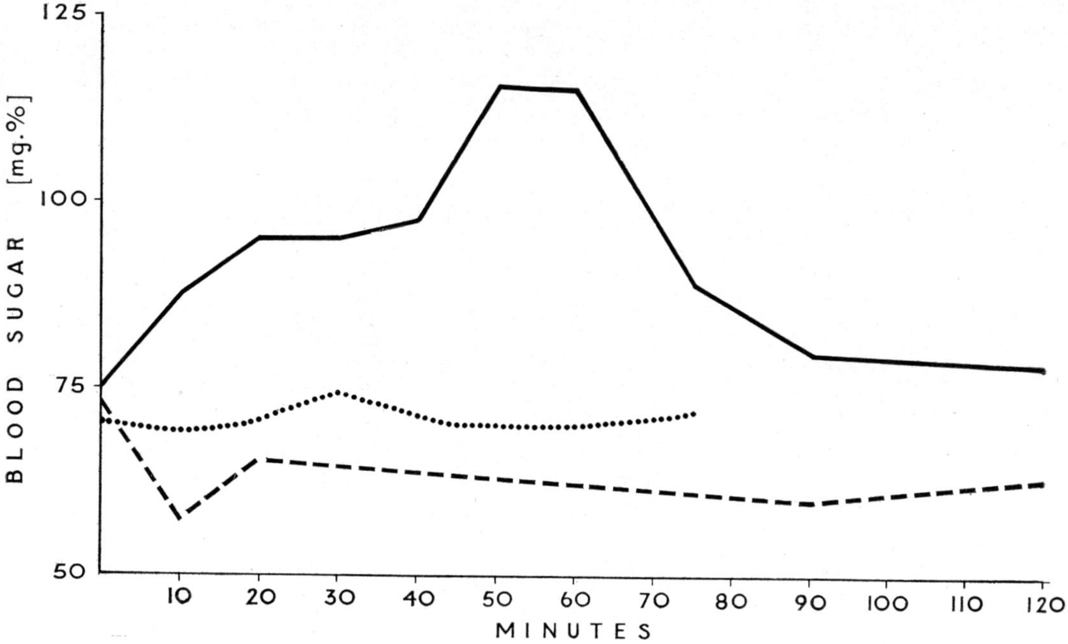

FIG. 1.—Patient 1: ——— Continuous intravenous glucose tolerance test for 60 minutes, - - - - Epinephrine tolerance test, ... Glucagon tolerance test.

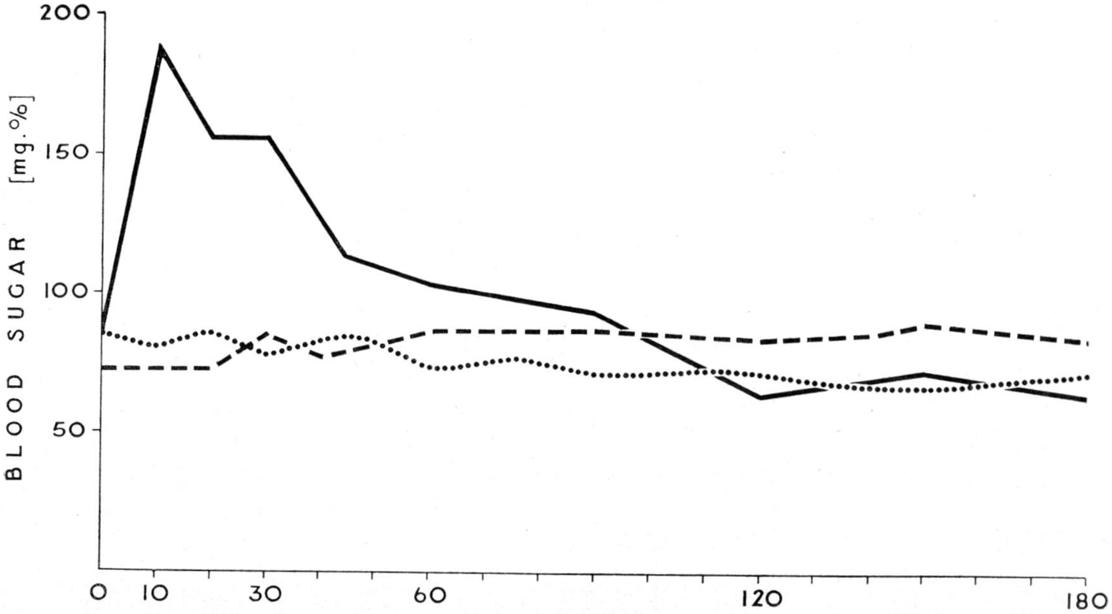

FIG. 2.—Patient 2: ———-Intravenous glucose tolerance test, - - -- - Epinephrine tolerance test, ... Glucagon tolerance test.

Case 2. Urine. (1) During glucose tolerance test: acetone and reducing substances absent from all specimens.

(2) During epinephrine tolerance test: under fasting conditions no acetone or reducing substances in the urine; 75 minutes and three hours after injection acetone present, reducing substances absent.

(3) During glucagon tolerance test: reducing substances absent from all urine specimens; one and a half hours and three hours after injection test for acetone weakly positive.

After the injection of glucagon both patients had temporary slight complaints, consisting of slight congestive complaints in Case 1 and slight nausea and chilliness in Case 2. These symptoms appeared in Case 1 between two and a half and three hours after the glucagon injection and disappeared in a few minutes. In Case 2 the symptoms appeared about one hour after the glucagon injection and lasted for about 20 minutes.

Results

The fasting blood sugar values in both patients are now, as in 1952, on the low side of normal. In the male patient (Case 1) cholesterol and glycogen in the blood are still increased. Blood uric acid, found to be increased by Jeune, Charrat and Bertrand (1957), was normal in both our cases. Acetone is absent from the urine in the fasting condition or is only weakly positive (before the glucagon tolerance test in Case 1). From the blood sugar curve after the continuous intravenous glucose test in Case 1, we can only say that at the end of the infusion the curve showed a distinct plateau. This could point to a difficulty in the fixation of glucose. After the end of the infusion a rapid decrease of the glucose to the fasting value occurred. In Case 2 the intravenous glucose tolerance curve was practically normal.

Following epinephrine administration the blood sugar level in Case 1 dropped immediately and remained depressed during the two hours of observation. In Case 2 this decrease was not observed, but an initial increase failed and half an hour after the injection a very slight increase followed which remained for the duration of observation. In both patients acetone appeared in the urine after epinephrine injection.

Glucagon in amounts which in normal adults cause a pronounced elevation in blood sugar concentration, produced no increase of blood sugar in either of our patients. As already noted both patients complained of slight transient symptoms following the glucagon injection.

17-Hydroxycorticosteroids in blood in Case 1 corresponded to the mean of six determinations (by F. Kuipers) in a normal adult.

Comment

As a result of this study it can be said that our two patients still show abnormalities of metabolism, especially as regards the absence of a hyperglycaemic effect following the injection of epinephrine and glucagon.

The effect of the injection of epinephrine is also abnormal as regards the appearance of acetone in the urine.

The lack of or an inadequate hyperglycaemic response to the administration of glucagon in children with this type of glycogen disease has already been noted by several authors (Ulström, Ziegler, Doeden and McQuarrie, 1952; Schulman and Saturen, 1954; Carson and Koch, 1955; Koulischer and Pickering, 1956; Gitzelmann, 1957). Here we may remark that even many years ago, long before glucagon was available, the absence of the so-called initial insulin-hyperglycaemia was noted in Case 2, when using an insulin which produced such a hyperglycaemia in normal individuals (van Creveld, 1934).

In a discussion at the Société de Pédiatrie de Paris in 1957 Clément (1957) remarked, without giving details, that in an adult with liver glycogen disease whom he had followed since early childhood the enlargement of the liver had disappeared and the blood sugar became normal, but that epinephrine and glucagon tests were still abnormal.

Esselborn, Davis and Hamblen (1950) described a female patient of 22 years in whom hepatomegaly disappeared with the onset of menstruation. However at the age of 22 hypoglycaemia, acetonuria and failure to respond to epinephrine still existed.

Gitzelmann (1957) in his studies on the glucagon problem in glycogen disease comes to the conclusion that the cases of glycogen liver could be divided into two groups. The first group should show a normal glycogenolysis after administration of glucagon, and in these cases acetonuria and hypoglycaemia should usually be absent. The second group should show decreased or only slight glycogenolysis after administration of glucagon.

In our cases hypoglycaemia and acetonuria were present for years and both cases still show a tendency to ketosis but no signs of glycogenolysis after administration of glucagon. In this respect there is therefore no agreement with the conclusions of Gitzelmann.

Both the absence of a hyperglycaemic effect after injection of epinephrine and the absence of such an effect after administration of glucagon in cases of glycogen liver is regarded as an expression of an existing enzymatic defect in liver glycogenolysis. Both hormones exert their effect by increasing the concentration of active phosphorylase which results in increased glycogenolysis and marked hyperglycaemia. The work of Cori and Cori (1952) and Cori and Schulman (1954) and of de Duve (1953) must also be mentioned in this respect. Starting from this effect of administration of glucagon some authors (Koulischer and Pickering, 1956; Gitzelmann, 1957) have already tried in cases of the hepatomegalic type of glycogen disease to influence the underlying defect in the enzyme glucose-6-phosphatase (Cori and Cori, 1952; Cori and Schulman, 1954) by long term glucagon administration either alone or combined with administration of thyroxine or a thyroid preparation. Here we must remark that the investigations of G. T. Cori have shown that the enzymatic deficiency is not always the same (Illingworth, Cori and Cori, 1956; Cori, 1957). Moreover, recent researches (Costa, Galansino and Foà, 1956; Galansino, Pozza, Costa and Foà, 1957) show that long term treatment with small doses of glucagon does not affect liver glycogen, whereas repeated large doses produce an increase in glycogen content.

The absence of response to the injection of epinephrine and glucagon in both our patients indicates that the enzymatic defect in glycogenolysis, whatever it may be (Cori and Cori, 1952; Cori and Schulman, 1954; Illingworth *et al.*, 1956; Cori, 1957), still exists. When notwithstanding this, the enlargement of the liver had already disappeared many years ago and both patients have grown normally, we must accept that the carbohydrate-metabolism has taken other ways than normal. Several possibilities can be considered here. Hubble (1954), taking advantage of the recommendation to give additional protein to children with glycogen disease (Bridge and Holt, 1945), noted an important increase in height over five years in a boy aged 6 years. In his opinion the requirement of protein for growth should decrease as age advances, so that more protein is available for gluconeogenesis. At the same time anabolic factors would be increasingly counterbalanced by the catabolic. Further studies may reveal more about the metabolism in adult cases of glycogen liver.

Summary

The results of some recent metabolic studies in two cases of the liver type of glycogen disease are reported. The patients are now 38 and 32 years old, and were described in detail for the first time respectively in 1928 and 1932.

In both cases a marked unresponsiveness to administration of both epinephrine and glucagon could still be demonstrated. The fasting blood sugar in both patients was repeatedly found to be normal or nearly normal, whereas the tendency to ketosis had decreased. Glycogen and cholesterol were still increased in the blood of one patient.

References

Bridge, E. M. and Holt, L. E. (1945). *J. Pediat.*, **27**, 299.
Carson, M. J. and Koch, R. (1955). *Ibid.*, **47**, 161.
Clément, R. (1957). *Arch. franç. Pédiat.*, **14**, 909.
Cori. G. T. (1957). *Mod. Probl. Pädiat.*, **3**, 344.
—— and Cori, C. F. (1952). *J. biol. Chem*, **199**, 661.
—— and Schulman, J. L. (1954). *Pediatrics*, **14**, 646.
Costa, E., Galansino, G. and Foà, P. P. (1956). *Proc. Soc. exp Biol. (N.Y.)*, **91**, 308.
Creveld, S. van (1928). *Ned. Maandschr. Geneesk.*, **76**, 304.
—— (1934). *Arch. Dis. Childh.*, **9**, 9.
—— (1952). *Ibid.*, **27**, 113.
—— (1953). *Postgrad. Med.*, **14**, 342.
Duve, C. de (1953). *Lancet*, **2**, 99.
Esselborn, V. M., Davis, C. D. and Hamblen, E. C. (1950). *J. clin. Endocr.*, **10**, 339.
Galansino, G., Pozza, G., Costa, E. and Foà, P. P. (1957). *Proc. Soc. exp Biol. (N.Y.)*, **94**, 417.
Gitzelmann, R. (1957). *Helv. paediat. Acta*, **12**, 425.
Hubble, D. (1954). *Lancet*, **1**, 235.
Illingworth, B., Cori, G. T. and Cori, C. F. (1956). *J. biol. Chem.*, **218**, 123.
Jeune, M., Charrat, A. and Bertrand, J. (1957). *Arch. franç. Pédiat.*, **14**, 897.
Jokipii, S. G. and Turpeinen, O. (1954) *J. clin. Invest.*, **33**, 452.
Koulischer, N. and Pickering, D. E. (1956). *A.M.A. Amer. J. Dis. Child.*, **91**, 103.
Majoor, C. L. H. (1947). *J. biol. Chem.*, **169**, 583.
Schulman, J. L. and Saturen, P. (1954). *Pediatrics*, **14**, 632.
Snapper, I. and Creveld, S. van (1928). *Bull. Soc. méd. Hôp. Paris* **52**, 1315.
Ulström, R. A., Ziegler, M. R., Doeden, D. and McQuarrie, I. (1952). *Metabolism*, **1**, 291.

Addendum

Since this article was written, together with Dr. H. G. Hers of the Laboratory of Physiological Chemistry, Louvain (Prof. C. de Duve), we have studied in both our patients the results of an intravenous galactose tolerance test, as was recommended in glycogen disease by Schwarz *et al.* (1957, *Paediatrics*, **19**, 585) for the evaluation of glycolytic pathways in the liver. In both cases the observed conversion of galactose to glucose pointed to the presence of an active glucose-6-phosphatase in the liver. A more precise diagnosis could not be made from this result.

THE SYNDROME OF HYPOPARATHYROIDISM AND STEATORRHOEA

BY

EIRIAN WILLIAMS and COLIN WOOD*

From The London Hospital

(RECEIVED FOR PUBLICATION JANUARY 29, 1959)

It is unusual for hypoparathyroidism and steatorrhoea to occur together. In steatorrhoea the plasma phosphorus is often low and the serum calcium either low or normal (Salvesen and Böe, 1953). Rarely there is marked elevation of the plasma phosphorus, denoting failure of parathyroid function, and symptoms of severe hypocalcaemia dominate the clinical picture.

The cases illustrating this association were reviewed by Jackson (1957). Some of these showed additional abnormalities such as hepatitis and adrenal failure, but hypoparathyroidism and steatorrhoea were the only constant features and interest has largely centred on the aetiological relationship of the one to the other.

Case History

First Hospital Admission. A girl aged 6 years was admitted to the Manchester Royal Infirmary on October 27, 1953, with acute meningo-encephalitis. For three weeks she had complained of increasing frontal headache and on the day before admission had had repeated epileptic convulsions, at least 50 during the course of the day. At the beginning of her illness she had also complained of cough and was prescribed sulphadiazine, but the drug had to be discontinued because of urticaria.

In June, 1953, urticaria had followed the use of penicillin and chlortetracycline for pneumonia, and on other occasions she had been found to be sensitive to phenobarbitone. Previous illnesses included measles, mumps, German measles and chickenpox, all before the age of 5 years.

At birth she was a month premature, weighing 5 lb., but her early development had been normal. Her parents and both her sisters, aged 11 and 4 years, were healthy.

On examination she was drowsy, temperature 99·2° F. with, at first, slight neck stiffness. There were no other abnormal findings.

The following investigations were carried out:

27.10.53. Serum calcium 10 mg. %. Inorganic phosphate 5 mg. %. Lumbar puncture: C.S.F. leucocytes 107 per c.mm. (polymorphs 27 per c.mm., lymphocytes 71 per c.mm., mononuclears 9 per c.mm.); protein 35 mg. %; sugar 53 mg. %; chloride 720 mg. %; Z.N. film, no tubercle bacilli seen. Culture sterile. Complement fixation tests for influenza A and B, Q fever, psittacosis and lymphocytic choriomeningitis were negative. Tests for cold agglutinins and agglutination with streptococcus M.G. were also negative.

She improved rapidly, during her stay in hospital had no more convulsions, and was discharged home after three weeks.

Second Hospital Admission. Four months later on March 6, 1954, she was admitted to the Royal Liverpool Children's Hospital. For six weeks her stools had been frequent, bulky, loose and pale, and for four weeks she had complained of cramps with carpopedal spasms due to tetany. The serum calcium on February 2 was 5·9 mg. % and inorganic phosphate 5·8 mg. %. Until admission she had been treated with parathormone and calcium intravenously, with some relief of symptoms.

On examination she was pale and thin; height 3 ft. 9 in., weight 2 st. 11 lb. Her tongue was clean and she was afebrile. There was moderate abdominal distension, liver and spleen being impalpable. Chvostek's sign was weakly positive.

Investigations showed: Haemoglobin 82%. W.B.C. 10,000 per c.mm. Serum calcium 7·2 mg. %. Inorganic phosphorus 6·0 mg. %. Radiographs of chest and bones were normal. Barium meal and follow-through examination showed slight segmentation of barium in the small intestine, with colon stasis and a redundant looped descending colon. The stools were large, pale, offensive and unformed. They contained no pathogenic organisms on culture. Trypsin was present to a dilution of 1/10.

She was treated with a low residue gluten-free diet containing 25 g. fat daily, and with vitamin D 2,000 units daily. Tetany improved, her weight increased 7 lb., but the stools were unaltered. She returned home on April 16.

Third Hospital Admission. The carpopedal spasms recurred, however, with attacks especially in the early mornings, and on June 3, 1954, she was re-admitted, having had parathyroid 20 U.S.P. units intramuscularly daily for 26 days and Collosol Calcium 2 ml. intramuscularly on alternate days.

* Present address: University of Maryland Department of Pathology, 31 S. Greene Street, Baltimore 1, Md, U.S.A.

It was now noted that her skin was dry and her nails longitudinally ridged. Serum calcium on June 4 was 9·7 mg. %, inorganic phosphorus 6·0 mg. % and plasma proteins 7·5 g. %.

Treatment was at first withheld and on June 21 the serum calcium was 7·7 mg. %, and the inorganic phosphate 6·0 mg. %. A week later calciferol 50,000 units daily by mouth was commenced. She was discharged on July 13.

Fourth Hospital Admission. At home tetany persisted despite treatment with a gluten-free diet, calciferol and calcium and on January 12, 1955, she entered the Royal Liverpool Children's Hospital for the third time. For four weeks, following a cold, attacks of tetany had been severe and prolonged, being partially relieved by intramuscular calcium gluconate and injections of parathyroid 25 U.S.P. units two or three times daily. Her appetite had been poor for a week and she had become slightly jaundiced. An epidemic of infective hepatitis was prevalent at the time.

The serum calcium was now 11·6 mg. %, inorganic phosphorus 6 mg. %. Plasma proteins 7 g. %, serum bilirubin 3 mg. % and alkaline phosphatase 23 King-Armstrong units. Chromatography of the urine revealed a normal amino acid output.

She was treated with calciferol 20,000 units daily and a gluten-free diet. Jaundice at first deepened and then gradually cleared. Tetany, however, persisted and bilateral lens opacities appeared leading to impairment of vision. On March 14 the serum calcium was 7 mg. %, inorganic phosphorus 4·3 mg. % and plasma proteins 5·5 g. %. On March 29 she was transferred to The London Hospital. During the journey, owing to her increased auditory acuity, she found the noise of the trains intensely distressing.

On examination at The London Hospital (at the age of 7 years 10 months, and 14 months after the onset of steatorrhoea and tetany) she was an intelligent, poorly nourished child, with moderate pallor and no jaundice. Height 3 ft. 11½ in. Weight 3 st. 3 lb. Her skin and hair were normal and nails soft and ridged. Her hands and feet were of normal proportions. A few teeth were carious, with hypoplasia of the enamel of the lower central incisors and lower permanent molars. Chvostek's and Trousseau's signs were strongly positive, but the limb reflexes were sluggish. The abdomen was distended. The liver and spleen were impalpable and there was no ascites. Bilateral lens opacities were obvious to the naked eye and visual acuity was reduced, R. 6/36 and L. 6/60.

Investigations showed the following results: 30.3.55. Serum calcium 4·8 mg. per 100 ml. Plasma phosphorus 8 mg. per 100 ml. Serum bilirubin 1·5 mg. per 100 ml. Alkaline phosphatase 26 King-Armstrong units. Thymol turbidity 4·1 units. Plasma proteins 8·1 g. per 100 ml. (albumin 4·4 g., globulin 3·7 g.).

3.4.55. Serum calcium 4·7 mg. per 100 ml. Plasma phosphorus 10·5 mg. per 100 ml.

20.4.55. Serum bilirubin 14·5 mg. per 100 ml. Alkaline phosphatase 26·0 units. Thymol turbidity 12·0 units. Plasma proteins 6·7 g. per 100 ml. (albumin 4·0 g., globulin 2·7 g.). Fat balance test (six days) 79% absorption on a diet containing 50 g. fat per day. Blood urea 36 mg. per 100 ml.

Radiological Studies. The bones showed slight generalized osteoporosis when compared with a normal control. Transverse growth lines were present in the metaphyses but there was no evidence of active rickets. The metacarpals were of normal length and no abnormal calcification was seen in the skull or elsewhere.

After two mouthfuls of a non-flocculating barium suspension the head of the barium column reached the ascending colon in three hours. Nothing was seen to suggest gross disease of the small intestine.

She was treated at first with calciferol 2,000 units daily by mouth and a gluten-free diet. From April 25 calciferol was given by intramuscular injection 100,000 units on alternate days, the dose being increased to 200,000 units on May 4 and to 500,000 units on May 11. Oral calcium lactate 8 g. daily increasing to 24 g. daily, pancreatin, folic acid and vitamins were also prescribed.

The serum calcium and inorganic phosphate levels returned towards normal, 8·2 mg. and 4·7 mg. per 100 ml. on June 1, 1955, and tetany disappeared. But in April jaundice returned with ascites, a flapping tremor and foetor hepaticus, and after repeated episodes of coma the patient died on June 8, 1955.

Summary of Autopsy (P.M. 229/55). A diagnosis was made of subacute hepatitis, idiopathic steatorrhoea and atrophy of parathyroid and adrenal glands. The parathyroids were not identified macroscopically. Lipid was absent and there was great focal atrophy in the cortex of both adrenals (together 5·5 g.). The pituitary (0·4 g.), thyroid (5·5 g.), pancreas (36·5 g.) and ovaries (together 3·2 g.) were normal. There was no glandular tissue at the site of the thymus. Skin and sclerae were jaundiced. There was serous ascites (800 ml.). The liver was grossly atrophied with several large areas of soft bile-stained and coarsely lobular regeneration nodules bordered by firmer, pale reddish-grey atrophied parenchyma (326 g.) (Fig. 1). The biliary system, hepatic and portal veins were normal as was the alimentary tract except for slight oedema of the mucosa of the terminal ileum. There was advanced fatty degeneration of the kidneys (together 163 g.); the remainder of the urinary tract was normal. The genital organs were infantile.

Serous effusion (114 ml.) was found in the right pleural cavity, and delicate fibrous adhesions throughout the right pleura. There was partial collapse and congestion of the lower lobes of the lungs. The larynx, trachea and bronchi were normal. There was enlargement of congested cervical and paratracheal lymph nodes (up to 2 cm. in diameter), and obsolete tuberculosis of one mesenteric gland. The brain was normal and there were no skeletal deformities, nor visible change in texture of right femur, vertebral bodies and ribs on section. Mixed haemopoietic and adipose marrow was found in the upper fifth of the femur. The calvaria was heavy without bossing. There was slight translucent mottling

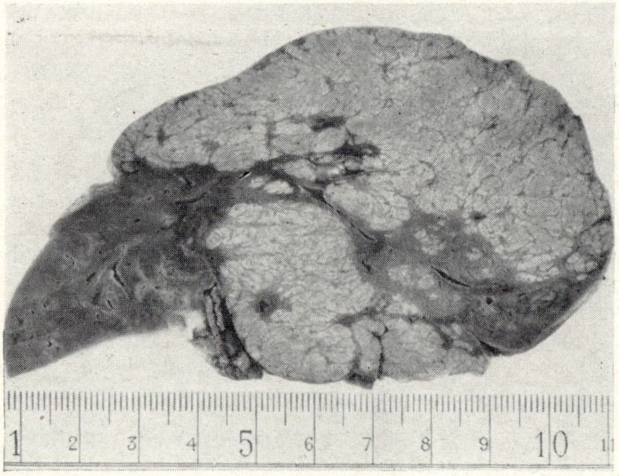

FIG. 1.—Gross atrophy of liver. Pale, coarsely lobular regeneration nodules. Coronal section.

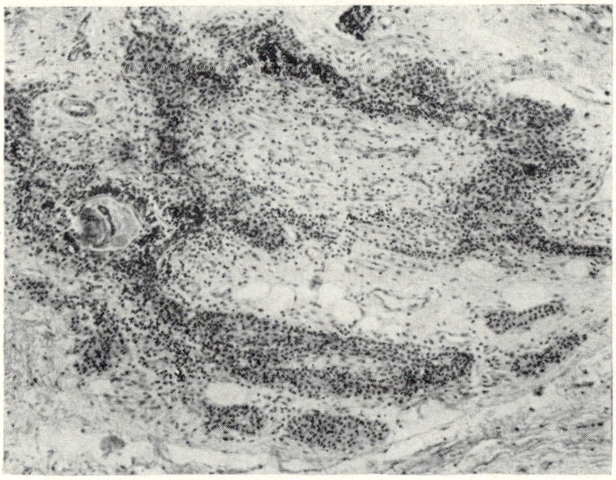

FIG. 2.—Parathyroid gland. Bands of two or more layers of epithelial cells, centrally replaced on one side of the field by lymphocytes, enclosing a Hassal's corpuscle. H. and E. ×75.

of teeth. She was a moderately nourished girl (weight 23 kg., length 122 cm.). Mean for 8 years: 26·35 kg. (Stuart and Stevenson, 1950) and 128 cm.

MICROSCOPIC EXAMINATION. PARATHYROIDS. Two glands were found in sections of paraffin-embedded tissue posterior to the right lobe of thyroid; they measured 0·7×0·5 cm., and 0·5×0·5 cm. The greater part of these glands consisted of vascular fibrous tissue surrounding solid islands and bands of well defined, somewhat vacuolated epithelial cells resembling parathyroid chief cells (Figs. 2 and 3) and centrally replaced by lymphocytes. There were occasional small separate acini lined by cuboidal cells (Fig. 4). In addition both glands contained several concentrically laminated bodies of eosinophilic material ringed by nucleated flattened squamous cells, resembling Hassal's corpuscles (Fig. 2). These lay in the centre of mainly peripheral islands and bands of parathyroid-like tissue, and were separated by lymphocytes from the epithelial cells of parathyroid type. There were also a few small cysts lined by low cuboidal epithelium, the larger of which contained cellular debris and structureless eosinophil material. Corresponding pieces of left cervical tissue included lobules of brown fat and small lymph glands but no parathyroid tissue.

THYMUS. No thymic or parathyroid glandular tissue was identified in the anterior superior mediastinal adipose tissue. A few lymph nodes were seen.

ADRENAL. There was diffuse uneven infiltration of the cortex with small lymphocytes, associated with disruption of the normal cellular pattern, congestion, and marked but uneven atrophy (Fig. 5). The medullary cells were widely separated; their cytoplasm was stringy and vacuolated.

THYROID. In sections of the right and left lobes the vesicles were packed with well-stained colloid and lined by low cuboidal cells. There was no lymphocytic infiltration, and no included parathyroid tissue.

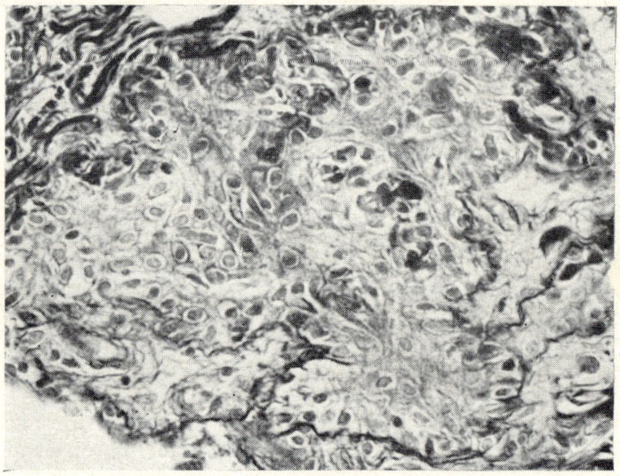

FIG. 3.—Parathyroid gland. Island of well defined epithelial cells, resembling chief cells. Masson's trichrome ×290.

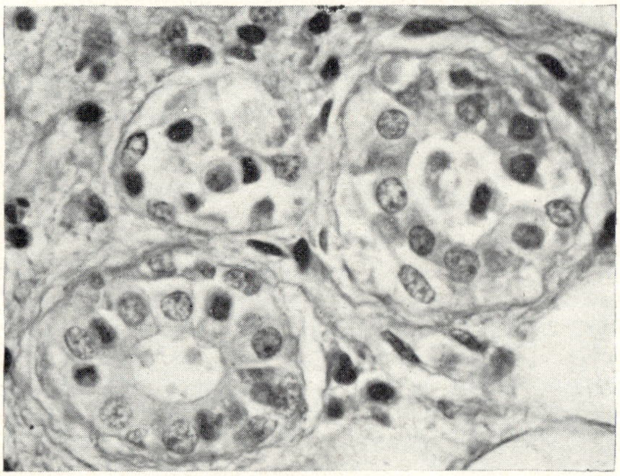

FIG. 4.—Parathyroid gland. Acini lined by cuboidal cells. Van Gieson ×650.

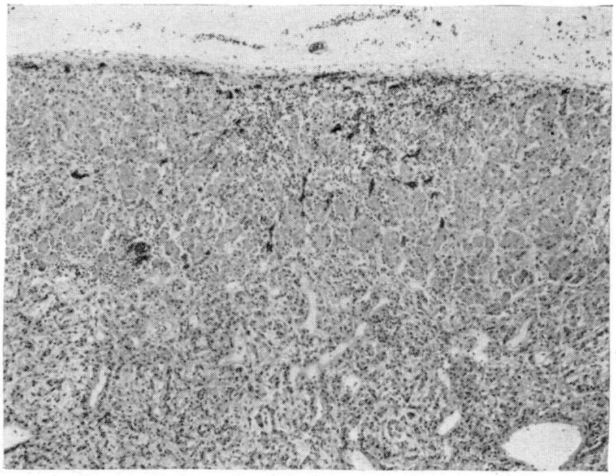

FIG. 5.—Adrenal cortical atrophy. The full thickness of cortex, and part of the medulla is showm. H. and E. ×48.

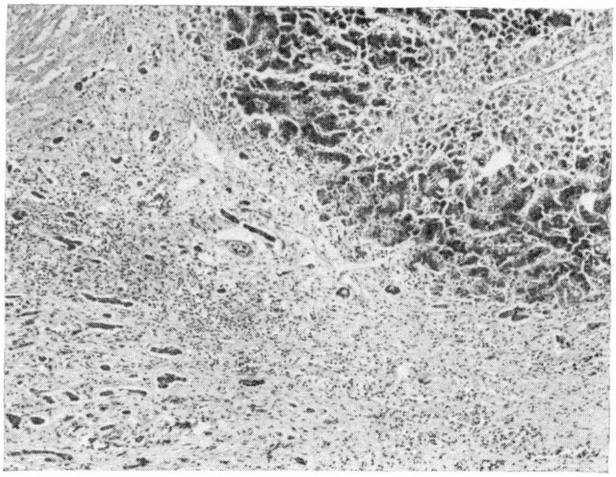

FIG. 6.—Hepatic regeneration nodule bordered by granulation tissue containing small bile ducts. H. and E. ×52.

PANCREAS. Abundant islets were seen in the moderately autolysed pancreas. There was no evidence of inflammation, fibrosis, or cysts.

PITUITARY. No abnormality seen. The basophil cells were numerically within normal limits.

OVARY. This contained several cystic primordial and atretic follicles.

LIVER. Coarse nodules of autolysed, regenerated liver cells, including areas of fatty change, were separated by granulation tissue. Here the lobules were collapsed, with a condensed reticulin framework, and showed marked lymphocytic infiltration, proliferation of surviving bile ducts, and periportal fibrosis (Fig. 6).

No abnormality was found in sections of small intestine, colon, mesenteric lymph node and submandibular salivary gland.

KIDNEY. There was conspicuous fatty degeneration of the tubular epithelium. The lipid was devoid of cholesterol esters.

BONES. Sections of the femoral head and greater trochanter, vertebra and costochondral junction were compared with control sections from a child of the same age (sudden accidental death). The epiphyseal cartilage of conjugation in the femoral head was narrower than in the control, and the zones of provisional calcification here and in the other epiphyses were very defective. There was little evidence of either osteogenesis or absorption of bone judging by the paucity of osteoblasts and osteoclasts.

Discussion

The main features in the seven previously reported examples of this syndrome have been summarized by Jackson (1957). The sexes have been equally affected and the age of onset has ranged from early infancy (Lowe, Ellinger, Wright and Stauffer, 1950) to 32 years. Salvesen (1957) attributes the hypocalcaemia in these cases to pre-existing hypoparathyroidism, the later development of steatorrhoea with faecal loss of calcium acting as an aggravating factor. But in none has hypoparathyroidism been evident clinically before the onset of steatorrhoea, and indeed in our patient the serum calcium was shown to be normal four months before the onset of this feature. On the other hand hypoparathyroidism complicating prolonged steatorrhoea might be due to secondary or 'exhaustion' parathyroid atrophy. In the patient described by Collins-Williams (1950) diarrhoea preceded tetany by 19 months, in Leifer and Hollander's (1953) by six months and in Jackson, Hoffenberg, Linder and Irwin's (1956) by two months. In our patient, however, this explanation cannot apply, for steatorrhoea and tetany appeared almost simultaneously.

The autopsy findings in two cases have failed to throw light on the pathogenesis of the hypoparathyroidism. In the case described by Castleman (1954) no parathyroid tissue was recognized. Similarly in ours no normal parathyroid glands or thymus were found in the sections of all the retrothyroid and anterior superior mediastinal connective tissue. Two epithelial glands were, however, identified in these sections. They were thought to contain parathyroid tissue, and if this interpretation is correct the glands were either hypoplastic, or extensively destroyed by necrosis, with inflammatory lymphocytic infiltration. The squamous corpuscles which each contained were regarded as inclusions of ectopic thymic tissue. This finding, however, does not provide evidence of congenital hypoplasia, for the combination of parathyroid and thymic tissues in the normal was carefully documented by Gilmour (1937, 1938) and is explained by their common embryogenesis.

In seeking the cause of steatorrhoea in these cases it would have been of interest to observe the effect of gluten withdrawal. But this was done only in ours, the patient's negative response tending to rule out the usual form of coeliac disease. Histopathological changes at autopsy in idiopathic steatorrhoea are few (Bockus, 1944) and it need only be said that in the present case there was no pancreatic disease, intestinal mucosal atrophy or intestinal lipodystrophy. The associated findings of hepatitis and adrenal disease in some of the others suggest that in these too the cause of the steatorrhoea was unusual. The hepatitis is unlikely to be nutritional due to malabsorption, because it rarely complicates other forms of steatorrhoea, and in the same way although in steatorrhoea the adrenals have sometimes been implicated in explaining some of its clinical manifestations, frank adrenal failure with corresponding histological changes do not occur. Furthermore, though parathyroidectomy in dogs has led to necrosis of liver cells (Larson and Elkourie, 1928) there can in this syndrome be no causal relationship between the hypoparathyroidism and hepatitis, because the one does not invariably follow the other.

It can reasonably be postulated that the agent causing the steatorrhoea is also directly injurious to the parathyroid glands and other organs. But whether it is a virus or the syndrome can be explained on the basis of hypersensitivity is conjectural. The case report by Leifer and Hollander (1953) can perhaps be quoted in favour of allergy. The patient had had asthma since the age of 2 years and there was a strong family history of childhood eczema. Our patient was sensitive to barbiturates, sulphonamides and certain antibiotics and the 'meningo-encephalitis' which preceded steatorrhoea in her case may also have been allergic. More significant perhaps were the autopsy findings of parenchymatous atrophy and lymphocytic infiltration in the parathyroid and adrenal glands. Similar changes are found in the thyroid in Hashimoto's disease and in the adrenals in idiopathic Addison's disease, both of which have been ascribed to auto-immunization (Roitt, Doniach, Campbell and Hudson, 1956; Anderson, Goudie, Gray and Timbury, 1957).

Indications of virus infection are equally scanty. Though our patient presented with atypical pneumonia and encephalitis, the only evidence of virus infection at autopsy was found in the liver. Here the appearances were those of post-necrotic cirrhosis following infective hepatitis, an infection which in the present case may even have been coincidental. Idiopathic hypoparathyroidism has been attributed to virus infection (Drake, Albright, Bauer and Castleman, 1939) and in one case (Leonard, 1946) the histological appearances of meningo-encephalitis were found in the hypothalamus at autopsy. In three cases (Cantarow, Stewart and Morgan, 1939; Leonard, 1946; Perlmutter, Ellison, Norsa and Kantrowitz, 1956) there were inflammatory changes in the liver, in the last two of these Addison's disease being a later development.

There is indeed closer affinity between so-called idiopathic hypoparathyroidism and the syndrome of steatorrhoea complicated by hypoparathyroidism, than between this syndrome and gluten-induced coeliac disease, and it can at least be concluded that in the syndrome steatorrhoea is aetiologically not the primary disorder.

Summary

A child aged 6 years 8 months developed steatorrhoea and hypoparathyroidism four months after an acute illness diagnosed as meningo-encephalitis.

She died of liver failure and autopsy revealed subacute hepatitis with atrophy of the parathyroid and adrenal glands. The alimentary tract was normal.

Previous examples of this syndrome are reviewed and its possible aetiology considered.

We are grateful to Dr. F. R. Ferguson, Professor N. B. Capon and Dr. Donald Hunter for permission to publish this case and to Dr. Hunter and Professor Dorothy Russell for their helpful advice and criticism.

REFERENCES

Anderson, J. R. Goudie, R. B., Gray, K. G. and Timbury, G. C. (1957). *Lancet*, **1**, 1123.
Bockus, H. L. (1944). *Gastroenterology*. Saunders, Philadelphia and London.
Cantarow, A., Stewart, H. L. and Morgan, D. R. (1939). *Endocrinology*, **24**, 556.
Castleman, B. (1954). In the case records of the Massachusetts General Hospital, *New Engl. J. Med.*, **251**, 442.
Collins-Williams, C. (1950). *Pediatrics*, **5**, 998.
Drake, T. G., Albright, F., Bauer, W. and Castleman, B. (1939). *Ann. intern. Med.*, **12**, 1751.
Gilmour, J. R. (1937). *J. Path. Bact.*, **45**, 507.
—— (1938). *Ibid.*, **46**, 133.
Jackson, W. P. U. (1957). *Lancet*, **1**, 1086.
——, Hoffenberg, R., Linder, G. C. and Irwin, L. (1956). *J. clin. Endocr.*, **16**, 1043.
Larson, E. and Elkourie, L. A. (1928). *Amer. J. Physiol.*, **85**, 387.
Leonard, M. F. (1946). *J. clin. Endocr.*, **6**, 493.
Leifer, E. and Hollander, W. (1953). *Ibid.*, **13**, 1264.
Lowe, C. U., Ellinger, A. J., Wright, W. S. and Stauffer, H. M. (1950). *J. Pediat.*, **36**, 1.
Perlmutter, M., Ellison, R. R., Norsa, L. and Kantrowitz, A. R. (1956). *Amer. J. Med.*, **21**, 634.
Roitt, I. M., Doniach, D., Campbell, P. N. and Hudson, R. V. (1956). *Lancet*, **2**, 820.
Salvesen, H. A. (1957). *Ibid.*, **1**, 1246.
—— and Böe, J. (1953). *Acta med. scand.*, **146**, 290.
Stuart, H. C. and Stevenson, S. S. (1950). In *Mitchell-Nelson Textbook of Pediatrics*, ed. W. E. Nelson, 5th ed. Saunders, Philadelphia.

THE TREATMENT OF CONGENITAL GALACTOSAEMIA

BY

NORMAN L. JONES and DAVID LEAK

From the British Military Hospital, Rinteln, Germany

(RECEIVED FOR PUBLICATION JANUARY 23, 1959)

Congenital galactosaemia is now a well recognized inborn error of metabolism and over 45 cases have been recorded (Andersen, 1957; Bennett, 1958). The underlying defect is the absence of the enzyme phospho-galactose uridyl transferase (Isselbacher, 1957), which catalyses the first stage of the conversion of galactose-l-phosphate to glucose; this results in an inability to metabolize galactose, and causes the intolerance to milk which characterizes the condition.

The clinical features of galactosaemia are of varying severity: for example, previously unsuspected cases have been recently discovered in mental defectives (Bergren, Donnell and Kalckar, 1958), while relatives of established cases may have an abnormal galactose tolerance test as the only manifestation of the disease (Holzel and Komrower, 1955). There is a marked contrast between these subjects and the acute form of the disease presenting with jaundice, hepatomegaly, galactosuria and amino-aciduria in the newborn, which, despite improved methods of diagnosis, still carries an appreciable mortality (Cox and Pugh, 1954; Clay and Potter, 1955; Holzel, Komrower and Schwarz 1957; Isselbacher, 1957).

Mason and Turner (1935) first described the successful use of a milk free diet in the treatment of an 11-month-old baby with galactosaemia; at the age of 24 years (though mentally retarded) he was able to tolerate small amounts of galactose (National Institutes of Health, 1957). In view of the recent increase of interest in this condition and the likelihood of its more frequent diagnosis, the purpose of this report is to evaluate the various diets which may be used, and to re-emphasize the necessity of the complete exclusion of lactose from the diet.

Case Report

C.S., a girl of 8 lb. 8 oz., was born after an uneventful pregnancy on February 18, 1958. Three days later she became slightly jaundiced and lethargic and during the following week became increasingly disinterested in feeding at the breast; half cream National Dried Milk was substituted. On March 1, 1958 (twelfth day) she weighed 7 lb. 1 oz., and was deeply jaundiced, the liver edge was palpable one inch below the costal margin and the abdomen was distended. She was apyrexial. Haemoglobin was 117% (17·4 g.), Coombs' test negative. Bilirubin was present in the urine, urobilinogen absent; there was a trace of albumin. Bile pigment was present in the stools. Over the next few days she developed a temperature of 100-101° F., which responded to empirical treatment with chloramphenicol and streptomycin. The liver increased in size and the serum bilirubin was 20 mg./100 ml.; thymol turbidity 2 units and alkaline phosphatase 40 King Armstrong units. On March 10 (twenty-first day) examination of the urine showed a reducing substance from which phenyl-lactosazone was formed with phenyl-hydrazine. Paper chromatography later confirmed that this specimen contained galactose and also cystine, l-tyrosine and l-leucine among other unidentified amino acids. On this day the half cream milk was replaced by a mixture containing Casilan (Glaxo), dextrose and water. There was a prompt response and after three days the serum bilirubin had fallen to 8 mg./100 ml. and the alkaline phosphatase to 25 K.A. units. The urine no longer contained a reducing substance though a trace of protein was still present. The weight had increased to 7 lb. 10 oz., the abdomen was less distended, and the liver smaller, but the spleen was now palpable. As this mixture was known to contain a small amount of lactose, a diet consisting of malt and soya (Soya Baby Food, Wander) was commenced on March 13 (twenty-fourth day). This was well tolerated at first but increasingly frequent loose stools prevented weight gain, and finally the diet was abandoned because of severe diarrhoea. The Casilan mixture was reintroduced but the diarrhoea continued and treatment with oral crystalloids was necessary to control the dehydration. A recurrence of fever on March 23 (thirty-fourth day) was due to a gluteal abscess which required incision and surgical drainage. On the same day feeding with half-strength L.L. Milk Food (Cow and Gate) was commenced. The food was taken well, but on the first day the infant had two generalized convulsions. The haemoglobin had now fallen to 57% (8·4 g.) and a small blood transfusion was given. Over the next six weeks, the L.L. Milk Food was well tolerated. However, the liver remained enlarged (two inches below costal margin) and the spleen became more prominent. The serum bilirubin was 1 mg./100 ml. and the alkaline phosphatase

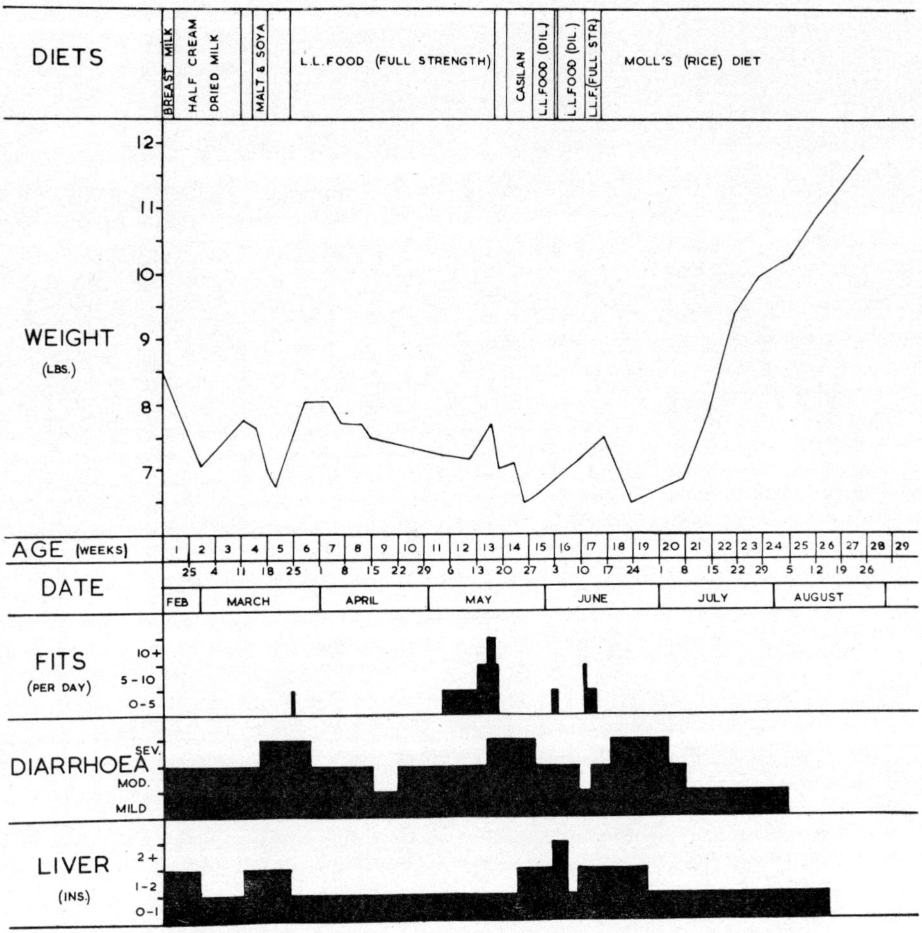

FIG. 1.—Chart illustrating the response to the various diets used. The periods in which no diet is indicated are those when simple dextrose-electrolyte solutions were used, except for the very short period in June, when a diet was used having Robinson's Patent Groats as its basis.

35 K.A. units. Urine chromatography revealed several unidentified amino acids but galactose was absent. During this period weight gain was only 10 oz. and attempts to increase this by adding arachis oil to the full strength food were unsuccessful.

On May 3 (aged 11 weeks) generalized convulsions recurred, and became increasingly frequent. They were unaffected by phenobarbitone gr. $\frac{1}{8}$ (8 mg.) b.d., but their frequency was decreased by giving 2 oz. of isotonic glucose-saline solution between the four-hourly feeds of L.L. Milk Food. Unfortunately on this regime the baby gradually lost weight, despite adequate fluid and calorie intake, and weighed only 7 lb. 2 oz. at the age of 12 weeks. To try and increase weight larger quantities of L.L. Milk Food were given more frequently; although there was an immediate weight gain, fits became increasingly frequent over the next four days, occurring about 30 minutes after starting each feed. Estimations of the blood electrolytes and serum calcium were within normal limits, but the non-fermentable blood sugar was high. The fits were thought to be due to galactose-induced hypoglycaemia and to prevent this one drachm of sugar was added to each feed. The incidence of fits was reduced but diarrhoea again became troublesome, and on the third day of this regime she lost 10½ oz. in 24 hours. Gram negative organisms and streptococci were present in the stools and treatment with intravenous fluids, including blood, and oral chloramphenicol, was given. Feeding with oral crystalloids and Casilan was slowly re-introduced. To prevent hypoglycaemia feeding with Casilan in 5% dextrose was tried, but a further severe attack of diarrhoea and dehydration required treatment with intravenous fluids. Feeding with Casilan and 5% dextrose was again slowly re-introduced, but on this regime she slowly lost weight and at the age of 14 weeks weighed only 6 lb. 10 oz. At this stage she refused her Casilan feeds, but it is significant that during the whole period of critical illness since L.L. Milk Food was discontinued no fits occurred. However, it was reluctantly decided to try again with L.L. Milk Food mixed in 5% dextrose, but the fits again recurred, although she maintained her weight. On June 3 (age 15 weeks), a one-third strength modified Moll's diet (using Robinson's Patent Groats) was tried. She took the food well for 12 hours but after a total of only 12 oz. of the mixture she became completely comatose, with a general flaccid paralysis, and loss of all reflexes. Her liver had increased in size to three inches below the right costal margin. The level of non-fermentable blood sugar was over 300 mg./100 ml. Intragastric tube feeding with a glucose solution of 1·75 g./kg. body weight was given, and the corneal and cough reflexes returned. Intragastric feeding with a solution containing 3·5 g. glucose/kg. body weight, 3 oz. three-hourly, was given for 18 hours by which time spontaneous movements had returned, and feeding with oral crystalloids could be commenced. It is quite remarkable that within 24 hours of stopping this modified form of Moll's diet the liver was enlarged to only half an inch below the right costal margin.

Feeding with L.L. Milk Food and glucose solution (3·5 g./kg.) was recommenced and although she gained 7 oz. in weight over the next two weeks the liver steadily increased in size, and the fits, always related to feeds, became more troublesome. A period of twitching lasting 60 minutes was finally terminated by intragastric tube feeding with the glucose solution.

On June 15 (age 17 weeks) a further modification of Moll's diet using a proprietary rice flour (Robinson's Baby Rice) in a 1 in 4 dilution, alternating with oral crystalloids, was commenced. A further attack of diarrhoea occurred after two days and the diet was temporarily replaced by oral electrolyte solutions. The Moll's diet was recommenced and over the next few days there was a marked improvement in her well-being: spontaneous activity increased, the monilia infection of the mouth healed, and she had less frequent bowel movements. During the next two weeks concentration of the Moll's diet was slowly increased to full strength, by which time (age 20 weeks) she weighed 6 lb. 10 oz. She was lively and took her feeds well. She cried lustily for the first time; the liver was palpable half an inch below the costal margin and the spleen was just tipped. In the first month of the full strength regime, she gained 3 lb., her mental and physical development showing similar improvement.

Weaning on to a lactose free selection of proprietary strained foods was commenced without incident at the age of 7 months.

An aqueous multivitamin solution (Abidec) 0·3 ml. daily was given throughout the illness, and the use of ferric ammonium citrate mixture for infants B.P.C. (30 minims t.d.s.) produced satisfactory increase in the haemoglobin.

Now at the age of 9 months she weighs 17 lb. 14 oz., and mental development corresponds approximately to that of a 7-month-old normal infant. The spleen is still palpable, but the liver is not enlarged and there are no cataracts. There are no urinary abnormalities, and the haemoglobin is 85% (12·7 g.).

The patient's brother (aged 3 years) excreted small amounts of galactose in the urine during a galactose tolerance test, but did not otherwise show any features of the disease. Normal results were obtained in the parents.

Discussion

This case illustrates the harmful effect of even small amounts of lactose in the diet of infants with galactosaemia. This may be due to the accumulation of galactose-1-phosphate in cells (Schwarz, Golberg, Komrower and Holzel, 1956), and indirectly to the production of hypoglycaemia.

Depression of blood glucose was found by Mason and Turner (1935) during galactose tolerance tests, and irreversible hypoglycaemia may follow them (Townsend, Mason and Strong, 1951). Several authors (Goldbloom and Brickman, 1946; Komrower, Schwarz, Holzel and Golberg, 1956) have also drawn attention to the depression of blood glucose in patients taking milk-containing foods, and, although unable to relate this to any specific symptoms, considered that it contributed to the impairment of cell metabolism. Cox and Pugh (1954) recorded convulsions in a child taking a half-cream dried milk whilst Clay and Potter (1955) in an infant receiving a diet containing Casilan found that the fits stopped when mixed feeding was introduced and suggested that a metabolic cause was responsible for them.

That the metabolic disorder underlying convulsions is the recurrent depression of blood glucose is suggested in the present case by the relationship of convulsions to feeding times, their increasing frequency as lactose containing foods were continued and their cessation following the complete exclusion of lactose. The failure of phenobarbitone to control the convulsions, whilst dextrose in high concentration reduced their incidence, together with the associated high level of non-fermentable blood sugar at the time of fits, also tend to support this. Hypoglycaemia may follow the ingestion of galactose because it is more rapidly absorbed than glucose and also tends to inhibit glucose absorption (Goldbloom and Brickman, 1946) and this may account for the occurrence of fits at meal times in the present case.

It follows that the complete exclusion of lactose from the diet in infancy should be the aim in all cases of galactosaemia; in the severer forms it is life saving, and it is suggested that it is no less important in milder cases. Mental deficiency and cataracts may follow an initial improvement with diets containing small amounts of lactose (Cox and Pugh, 1954), and these complications may be preventable.

Several diets have been recommended for the treatment of galactosaemia but some of them proved unsatisfactory for a variety of reasons. Malt and soya mixtures are lactose free and there have been several reports of their use (Townsend *et al.*, 1951; Bennett, 1958). Unfortunately, they may produce diarrhoea, as in this case. It has been suggested that this is caused by the high dextrose content and that half strength mixtures may not have this effect (Wokes, 1958). The preparation Nutramigen has been widely used in the United States with good results (Bruck and Rapoport, 1945; Isselbacher, 1957); it does, however, contain small amounts of lactose (Holzel *et al.*, 1957).

Mixtures containing Casilan have been frequently used, but are known to contain 1% lactose (Cox and Pugh, 1954; Clay and Potter, 1955). In this case improvement in jaundice followed its use, but there was little change in the weight or hepatomegaly.

L.L. Milk Food (Cow and Gate) has been recommended (The Hospital for Sick Children, 1958) and is said by the makers to contain less than 0·1% of lactose. In addition to the occurrence of convulsions in our patient, weight gain did not occur and there was again no change in liver size.

A diet was introduced by Moll and Stransky in 1922 for the treatment of chronic feeding disorders in children, permitting the exclusion of milk without restriction of calories. The basis of this diet is a milk free cereal, Moll and Stransky used biscuit flour, and egg. Holzel (1954) was first to use a modified form of this diet in cases of galactosaemia, using the cereal Farex (Glaxo) as the base (Holzel, 1954; Komrower *et al.*, 1956; Schwarz, Holzel and Komrower, 1958). This cereal now contains approximately 2·5% of lactose (Furnivall, 1958). Robinson's Patent Groats (J. and S. Coleman, Ltd.) have also been used (Holzel, Komrower and Schwarz, 1955); a mixture containing this cereal was used for only a short time in this case and was followed by a comatose state. Although there was strong evidence in favour of this being caused by its lactose content, none was found on testing the cereal using the phenylhydrazine reaction. The use of rice flour, which is lactose free, as the main ingredient for Moll's diet was recommended by Holzel *et al.* (1957), and this was the only diet found to be completely satisfactory in this case. Rapid improvement in general health, freedom from infection and reduction in liver size were followed by gain in weight. It is significant that no more fits have occurred, and although it is at present early to assess mental development satisfactorily, this appears to be progressing well. The use of this diet at an early age would probably avoid the necessity of intravenous therapy and blood transfusions which were essential in this case. A recipe for the diet used is given in the appendix below. Once mixed feeding is begun, the exclusion of lactose becomes somewhat simpler; tinned strained foods are widely used in weaning and a short list of suitable lactose free varieties is given in the appendix.

Some antibiotic suspensions commonly used in infants were tested for lactose by the phenylhydrazine method: suspensions of penicillin 'V' (Distaquaine 'V', The Distillers Company) and tetracycline (Achromycin, Lederle) were found to contain lactose, but chloramphenicol (Chloromycetin, Parke Davis) did not. It is suggested that where an oral antibiotic is indicated, this is the most suitable in cases of galactosaemia.

Summary

A case of severe galactosaemia in a newborn baby is described, with especial reference to the treatment. The various diets which have been recommended are reviewed; from their use in this case it is concluded that a completely lactose free diet is essential. A suitable form of treatment is described.

We express our thanks to Major S. M. Jarvis, R.A.M.C., for his constant advice and help, and to Mrs. K. Parnaby for help with the diet. It is a pleasure to record the never failing co-operation of the nursing and laboratory staff of this Hospital.

References

Andersen, D. H. (1957). In *Biochemical Disorders in Human Disease*, ed. R. H. S. Thompson and E. J King, p. 695. Churchill, London.
Bennett, C. E. (1958). *U.S. armed Forces med. J.*, **9**, 112.
Bergren, W. R., Donnell, G. and Kalckar, H. M. (1958). *Lancet*, **1**, 267.
Bruck, E. and Rapoport, J. (1945). *Amer. J. Dis. Child.*, **70**, 267.
Clay, P. R. and Potter, C. T. (1955). *Arch. Dis. Childh.*, **30**, 147.
Cox, P. J. N. and Pugh, R. J. P. (1954). *Brit. med. J.*, **1**, 613.
Furnivall, M. (1958). *Lancet*, **1**, 163.
Goldbloom, A. and Brickman, H. F. (1946). *J. Pediat.*, **28**, 674.
Holzel, A. (1954). *Med. Ill.*, **8**, 44.
—— and Komrower, G. M. (1955). *Arch. Dis. Childh.*, **30**, 155.
——, —— and Schwarz, V. (1955). *Lancet*, **2**, 92.
——, ——, —— (1957). *Amer. J. Med.*, **22**, 703.
Isselbacher, K. J. (1957). *Amer. J. clin. Nutr.*, **5**, 527.
Komrower, G. M., Schwarz, V, Holzel, A. and Golberg, L. (1956). *Arch. Dis. Childh.*, **31**, 254.
Mason, H. H. and Turner, M. E. (1935). *Amer. J. Dis. Child.*, **50**, 359.
Moll, L. and Stransky, E (1922). *Jb. Kinderheilk.*, **100**, 3.
National Institutes of Health (1957). Clinical Staff Conference on Galactosaemia. *Ann. intern. Med.*, **46**, 773.
Schwarz, V., Golberg, L., Komrower, G. M. and Holzel, A. (1956). *Biochem. J.*, **62**, 34.
——, Holzel, A. and Komrower, G. M. (1958). *Lancet*, **1**, 24.
Tattersall, G. (1958). Personal communication.
The Hospital for Sick Children (1958). *Diets for Sick Children*, 3rd ed., p. 16. London.
Townsend, E. H., Mason, H. H. and Strong, P. S. (1951). *Pediatrics*, **7**, 760.
Wokes, F. (1958). Personal communication.

APPENDIX

Suitable Foods Used in this Case

Modified Form of Moll's Diet. 6 oz. of Robinson's Baby Rice are mixed with 14 oz. of water. Two egg yolks are beaten with 3 oz. of glucose and added to this mixture.

Two egg whites, a pinch of salt and a pinch of bicarbonate of soda are finally added and the mixture is put in a dish greased with margarine and heated for half an hour in a saucepan of boiling water. The resulting pudding is diluted with equal parts of boiled water to make up the feeds. A more dilute form should be used initially.

List of Tinned Strained Goods (Heinz). Carrots, green beans, beef and liver soup, beef broth with beef and barley, bone and vegetable broth, apples and apricots with rice. Although peas are lactose free, they contain stachyose and paragalacto-araban which are metabolized to galactose (Tattersall, 1958).

PREGNANCY COMPLICATED BY DIABETES MELLITUS

A STUDY IN COMBINED OBSTETRIC AND PAEDIATRIC MANAGEMENT

BY

ANDREW M. CLAYE and W. S. CRAIG

From the Department of Obstetrics and Gynaecology and the Department of Paediatrics and Child Health, University of Leeds

(RECEIVED FOR PUBLICATION FEBRUARY 27, 1959)

Diabetes mellitus in association with pregnancy is an infrequent finding. The present paper gives the results of a series of 94 cases delivered in the Leeds Maternity Hospital during the period January 1, 1947, to August 31, 1958, inclusive. These results are the collective responsibility of a team consisting of an obstetrician, a physician experienced in diabetes mellitus, a paediatrician and their assistants. The results reflect also the value of highly skilled nursing care of the newly born baby.

Clinical Material

In the period during which the 94 women with diabetes mellitus were admitted there were 22,574 deliveries in the hospital. A large proportion of the mothers with diabetes mellitus were referred from the diabetic clinic at the Leeds General Infirmary.

Management

Obstetric. The obstetricians concerned do not hold identical views about management but in general apply the principles advocated by Peel (1955). Pregnancy is usually terminated at 36 or 37 weeks because of the liability of foetal death *in utero* to occur in the last weeks of pregnancy and because of the higher incidence of pre-eclampsia when pregnancy is allowed to continue to term. Only 24 patients were delivered at or after 38 weeks. Occasionally section or induction is performed earlier than the thirty-sixth week, the usual indication being pre-eclampsia. When premature labour begins spontaneously before 36 weeks vaginal delivery is awaited.

It would be incorrect to say that primigravidae have always been delivered by section. During the last three years however, section was performed on all primigravidae not delivered before 36 weeks. In multiparae with a satisfactory obstetric history, trial is given to vaginal delivery after induction usually not later than 37 weeks. A subsequent decision to perform section may be determined by the occurrence after induction of delay in going into labour, of slow labour or of foetal distress.

Paediatric. Importance is attached to postural drainage at the time of delivery but the stomach is not aspirated as a routine. During the early years of the study infants were nursed in open cots and use of an incubator was limited to babies with evidence of respiratory embarrassment, hypothermia or pronounced frailty. This policy was abandoned in 1953. Since then all newly born babies of diabetic mothers have been nursed for an initial period varying from 24 hours to one week in an incubator with the objects of providing optimum conditions for clinical observation and of favouring constancy of body temperature. Increased humidification of the air is employed only when there are signs of severe, persistent or progressively worsening respiratory distress suggestive of 'hyaline membrane disease'. Oxygen therapy is reserved for infants with sustained or intermittent attacks of cyanosis and infants with persistent respiratory distress. Intragastric administration has not been employed on any occasion. Premature infants are given ½ mg. Synkavit i.m. soon after birth.

Feeding is commenced as a routine on the second day of life, use being made of a bottle, a Belcroy or oesophageal tube according to the strength and capabilities of the infant. Human milk obtained from the mother or hospital banked breast milk is given for a minimum period of two weeks. The amounts of milk offered the infant are calculated on a basis of weight and estimated gestation. In general an infant receives each day 1½ oz. of milk per lb. (0·45 kg.) of body weight by the end of the first week and 2½ oz. per lb. body weight at the end of the second week of life. Reluctance to feed is not regarded as an adequate reason for reducing the amount of milk offered. In these circumstances oesophageal feeds are given by skilled nursing staff.

Antibiotics are employed in the presence of established infection but not as a prophylactic measure.

Results

(1) Maternal Mortality. There was one maternal death in the series. The patient was sent by her family doctor to book at 19 weeks, and the presence of maternal diabetes was first discovered at the ante-natal clinic. Referred back to her doctor for ante-natal care she was next seen when admitted to hospital in diabetic coma at 27 weeks. At the time of admission the blood sugar was 0·55 % and the urine contained a considerable amount of acetone and albumin. Despite treatment anuria developed and death occurred on the day following admission without the mother having been delivered. At post-mortem examination cortical necrosis of the kidneys was found.

(2) Foetal Loss According to Treatment. The results are summarized in Table 1. There was no example of multiple pregnancy. Sixty-nine infants survived the neonatal period. Eleven babies were stillborn and six died post-natally. There were seven abortions including three induced surgically, and the undelivered foetus of the mother who died.

TABLE 1

MATERNAL DIABETES MELLITUS: FOETAL LOSS ACCORDING TO OBSTETRICAL TREATMENT

Obstetrical Treatment	Total	Living*	Still-born†	Died	Abor-tion
Spontaneous labour ..	24	13	8	3	—
Spontaneous abortion ..	4	—	—	—	4
Died undelivered	1	—	—	—	1
Induced abortion (hysterectomy)	3	—	—	—	3
Induced labour	29	26	3	—	—
Caesarean section ..	35	32	—	3‡	—
Total ..	96	71	11	6	8
Less§ ..	2	2			
	94	69			

* A child is regarded as liveborn if he breathes or shows other signs of life after complete expulsion from his mother at any stage of pregnancy.

† A child who has issued from his mother after the twenty-eighth week of pregnancy but has not at any time after being completely expelled from his mother breathed or shown any other signs of life is considered to be stillborn.

‡ A fourth child died aged 6½ weeks from congenital heart disease.

§ Two patients, both of whose babies survived, are included against both 'Induced labour' and 'Caesarean section'. Both patients required section because the response to puncture of the membranes was unsatisfactory: abnormal uterine action developed in one, and ketosis in the other.

The total foetal loss was 25 in the series of 94 pregnancies. Seven of the 27 infants of patients who had pre-eclampsia did not survive, the rate of foetal loss among these mothers approximating closely to that for the whole series.

The highest foetal mortality occurs in the spontaneous labour group. There were eight stillbirths. Of these two occurred at or before 32 weeks and another was born at 36 weeks but had been dead for several weeks. These were probably unpreventable. Four babies died *in utero* at or after 36 weeks, their weights being 4 lb. 13 oz., 6 lb. 9 oz., 7 lb. 8 oz. and 8 lb. 2 oz. Earlier termination of pregnancy might have saved some and possibly all of these four babies. Caesarean section had been decided upon for the smallest of these babies but was delayed to allow the infant to increase in size. Unfortunately the foetal heart sounds disappeared two days before the date fixed for section. Trauma accounted for the eighth stillbirth. The baby presented by the brow, the outlet being described as contracted. Delivery was by mid-forceps after conversion to an occipito-posterior position.

Intra-uterine death had occurred before induction of labour was carried out in all the three stillbirths associated with this procedure. One died at 32 weeks. Another was born at 38 weeks, death having occurred at some unrecorded time previously. The third was to have had caesarean section but this was delayed because the patient had multiple abscesses and there was difficulty in controlling the diabetes. Meanwhile the foetal heart disappeared at 37½ weeks. Unfortunately none of the stillborn babies was submitted to post-mortem examination.

Three neonatal deaths occurred among infants in the spontaneous labour group. Autopsies were carried out on all three. The cause of death was shown to be due in one to severe haemolytic anaemia recognized during life and not attributable to rhesus incompatibility, and in another to gross developmental anomalies involving the heart and great vessels. Death of the third baby resulted from extensive intracranial haemorrhage secondary to bilateral tentorial tears, after delivery at 35 weeks, episiotomy having been omitted.

Thirty-five patients in the total series were delivered by caesarean section. There were three neonatal deaths in this group. Death in one infant was due to massive bilateral suprarenal haemorrhage, and in the other two babies was associated with the presence of hyaline membrane widely distributed throughout the lung structures.

(3) Neonatal Mortality. As already indicated there were six neonatal deaths in a total of 75 live births. Death took place within 18 hours of birth in all except the baby with haemolytic anaemia, who died aged 38 hours. Of the six infants the estimated gestation period was 36 weeks in the case of two and between 33 and 35 weeks in the case of the remaining four. One baby was not weighed. Birth weights of the remaining five infants averaged 5 lb. 13 oz., the smallest being 3 lb. 12 oz. and the largest 7 lb. 15 oz.

(4) Neonatal Morbidity. Congenital anomalies were noted in 10 liveborn babies. They consisted of developmental errors involving the heart (five), the facial appendages (one), microphthalmia (one), the urinary tract (one), the feet (one) and the skin (one). Congenital heart disease was associated in one case with hydrocephalus and absence of the right tibia and fibula. The urinary tract anomaly consisted of a recto-vesical fistula in a baby with gross talipes and extensive hirsuties. The skin anomaly consisted of a strawberry naevus. There was no apparent connexion between the duration or severity of the maternal diabetes and the occurrence of foetal anomalies. In all 10 mothers of babies with developmental errors, the diabetes had been effectively controlled before and during pregnancy. Control had been dietetic in four, and dietetic combined with insulin in six mothers. The duration of the maternal diabetes ranged from two months to 17 years and the age at onset from 13 to 33 years.

Localized bruising or petechiae were noted in 24 infants. In the majority the bruising was evident within 24 hours of birth but in a few it appeared at any time during the first three or four days of life. There were a few instances of bruising in situations known to have been subjected to slight but not abnormal pressure, but there was no history of local pressure in the majority of cases.

Superficial infection was noted in 31 babies. The eye and/or skin was involved in 28, the secretory glands in two, and the mouth in one. Ophthalmia in one infant was due to *Esch. coli* and the single example of buccal infection was monilial. *Staphylococcus aureus* was isolated in the remaining 29 babies. There was no example of deep or generalized infection.

Neuromuscular hyperexcitability commencing within 36 hours of birth was a feature of the clinical picture in 35 infants in the series. In its severest form the hyperexcitability presented as clinical tetany and was associated with a serum calcium level of less than 8 mg. per 100 ml. in 10 cases investigated biochemically. Convulsions occurred in two of these cases. In no baby were there symptoms due to hypoglycaemia.

Enlargement of the liver was a common finding. It was present in 48 infants. The degree of enlargement was considerable, the lower border of the organ being at or almost at the level of the umbilicus with the infant in the recumbent position. Precise measurement was not possible but, in assessing enlargement, the upper level of liver dullness was determined as a routine and account was taken of the extent to which the lungs had expanded. The consistence of the enlarged organ was invariably firm. Liver enlargement was found in the majority of the babies with superficial bruising and/or superficial infection and the infants showing marked reluctance to feed.

Enlargement of the liver was a feature of the majority of infants with a 'Cushing appearance'. The term 'Cushing appearance' refers to associated large size (macrosomia) having regard to the estimated gestation period; pendulous cheeks and heavy 'moon facies'; unusual coloration, consisting of a mulberry tinge giving place to what has been described as a 'sunset glow'; and generalized hypotonicity. This picture was present at birth in different degrees in 61 babies. In four cases the picture became increasingly obvious during the three or four days following birth. Disappearance of the Cushing characteristics was gradual and preceded by reduction in the size of the liver. The time taken for complete disappearance of the high coloured 'moon facies' varied from 10 days to four weeks. Cushing features were present in all the infants with evidence of neuromuscular excitability.

Fourteen infants (seven females and seven males) lacked the Cushing appearance. There was no abnormal clinical sign in 11 of these babies. Superficial infection was present in two infants, and acute respiratory embarrassment together with enlargement of the liver in one.

(5) Birth Weights of Liveborn Babies. Seventy-four of the 75 liveborn babies were weighed at birth. Birth weights varied from 2 lb. 13 oz. to 10 lb. 9 oz. and averaged 7 lb. 2 oz.

(6) Post-natal Weight Loss. Maximum weight loss in the first week of life ranged from 2 to 17% of the birth weight, averaging 7·8% for the 72 babies for whom adequate weight records were made. The day on which weight loss reached its maximum differed, varying from the second to the fifth day of life.

(7) Follow-up of Infants Surviving the Neonatal Period. Fifteen infants were followed up for a maximum period of six months, 25 for one year,

20 for three years and eight for five years. Follow-up took the form of clinical examination in 55 cases and of written enquiries sent to family doctors in 13 cases. Three children with congenital heart disease were alive at the age of 3 years. One infant died in hospital aged 6½ weeks from congenital heart disease first detected a few days after birth. Another child was found to be suffering from diabetes mellitus at the age of four years. A child suspected at the age of 8 months of being mentally defective was found to be deaf. Impaired hearing was suspected in another infant early in the second year of life. Deafness was confirmed and found to be severe by otologists in both these cases. Naevi not present at birth were found within six months of birth in four babies.

Otherwise the development of infants followed up in the series was found to be normal. The health histories of these babies were in no way unusual. Four infants in whom a clearly defined cardiac murmur of doubtful significance had been detected repeatedly in the first two weeks of life were found in the course of follow-up examination to be healthy and without any evidence of cardiac disease.

Discussion

The results of the management of pregnancy complicated by maternal diabetes mellitus are a measure of the effectiveness of teamwork by the obstetrician, physician, paediatrician and nursing staff. Control of the diabetes in the mothers in this study was undertaken by physicians with long experience of the condition. Pedersen, Bojsen-Møller and Poulsen (1954) have emphasized the particular importance of long term antenatal care. Our results serve to underline Miller's (1956) statement that the most meticulous regulation of carbohydrate metabolism and the best of pre-natal care are unable to reduce perinatal mortality to a level comparable to that in the non-diabetic population. Different opinions have been expressed concerning the relative merits of spontaneous delivery following induction and delivery by caesarean section. In our series there was no significant difference in mortality between the two methods, but no conclusion can be drawn from this observation as treatment was selected on the principles already described.

The highest mortality occurred among babies born following spontaneous delivery. Of the eight stillbirths it is possible at least that four might have been prevented had pregnancy been terminated earlier; and of the three neonatal deaths, one might have been avoided had episiotomy not been omitted.

Congenital anomalies were present in 10 babies. Miller (1956) comments upon the inadequacy of recorded findings and on the absence of statistics for purposes of comparison in a contemporary group of infants born to non-diabetic mothers. He recommends that the frequency and nature of anomalies found in the infants of diabetic mothers should be compared with the findings 'in concurrent non-diabetic populations preferably treated at the same institution as the diabetic group'. Table 2 summarizes the developmental errors found in other babies liveborn in the Leeds Maternity Hospital during the period January, 1947, to August, 1958. Livebirths excluding babies of diabetic mothers during this period numbered 22,196. Of these babies 716 (3%) had congenital anomalies. A comparison of these figures with the finding of abnormalities in 10 infants of the present series is not inconsistent with the view held by some authorities that anomalies occur with more than usual frequency in the babies of diabetic mothers.

TABLE 2

INCIDENCE OF ANOMALIES OF ALL DEGREES IN LIVE-BIRTHS OF ALL DEGREES OF MATURITY

Anatomical Location	Liveborn Children of	
	Non-diabetics (22,196)	Diabetics (75)
Skin and related structures	131 (0·6%)	1
Mouth and jaw	61(0·3%)	1
Limbs	198 (0·9%)	1
Spine and skull	97 (0·4%)	
Cardio-vascular	74 (0·3%)	5
Alimentary	41 (0·2%)	
Genito-urinary	72 (0·3%)	1
Mongol	29 (0·1%)	
Achondroplasia	1	
Fibrocystic disease	2	
Eye	3	1
Lungs	2	
Reticulo-endothelial	2	
C.N.S. (intracranial)	3	
Total	716 (3·0%)	10

Among livebirths in the present series congenital anomalies contributed directly to a fatal outcome in only two babies. In each case the anomaly was cardiac. One of the deaths occurred in the second month of life. Anomalies considered to be primary causes of death among the 22,196 liveborn babies delivered between January, 1947, and August, 1958, are summarized in Table 3. They total 106 of which less than one-third were related to the cardiovascular system. There was only one example among the babies of diabetic mothers of anomalous development of the central nervous system; this is the more striking considering the predominance of meningomyelocele in Table 3. Contrary to the experience of Peel and Oakley (1950) and, despite the fact that all babies were examined within a few hours of birth and again within the 36 hours preceding discharge from hospital, a strawberry naevus was found in only one infant.

TABLE 3

NUMBER OF ANOMALIES CONSIDERED TO BE THE PRIMARY CAUSE OF DEATH WITHIN TWO WEEKS OF BIRTH IN BABIES OF ALL DEGREES OF MATURITY BUT EXCLUDING BABIES OF DIABETIC MOTHERS

Cardio-vascular	30
Renal	9
Alimentary	8
Spine and skull	51
C.N.S. (intracranial)	3
Ichthyosis	1
Pulmonary	2
Diaphragm	2
Total	106

Prospects of neonatal survival are necessarily subject to the influence of premature birth. There were 75 liveborn infants. The estimated gestation period was less than 34 weeks in three, between 34 and 38 weeks in 53, and 38 weeks or more in 18 babies. The corresponding figure for one baby was uncertain. Of the six infants who died within 38 hours of birth (and representing all the neonatal deaths in the total series) the estimated gestation period was 36 weeks in the case of two, and between 33 and 35 weeks in the case of the remaining four. During the period January, 1950, to August, 1958,* approximately 1,610 infants with a birth weight of 5½ lb. or less and with an estimated gestation period of between 30 and 38 weeks were delivered in the Leeds Maternity Hospital. Of these infants 185 (11·6%) died in the hospital. In so far as these figures warrant tentative conclusions and recognizing that they apply only to the work of one particular hospital it seems that in the present series the risks of death due to premature birth were not increased as a result of maternal diabetes. This tentative conclusion is of special significance in that it provides suggestive evidence in support of the view already expressed that pregnancy might have been terminated earlier in some of the cases delivered spontaneously.

On balance we feel that in our series there has been a tendency to delay interference with pregnancy too long. It is probable that had pregnancy always been terminated at 35 weeks more babies might have been born alive and, in the absence of serious congenital anomalies, would have had good prospects of healthy survival. This view is in accord with those of Bachman (1952) and Peel (1955). The latter states that 'delivery at or before the thirty-sixth week reduces greatly the incidence of intra-uterine death without producing a corresponding rise in the neonatal death rate'.

Nevertheless the need remains for caution in early management by those responsible for the care of the infant of a diabetic mother. Experience in the present series agrees with that of Peel that the majority of deaths occur within a few days of birth. Indeed features of our series are that there was only one late fatality and that other deaths occurred not merely early but very early. Cardiac anomalies, vascular crises and hyaline membrane disease accounted for all the deaths. Both examples of fatal hyaline membrane disease occurred in infants delivered by caesarean section. No death was attributable or contributed to by infection. This is the more striking in view of the high incidence of infection in the series. The occurrence of 31 cases of superficial infection in 75 newly born babies of diabetic mothers compared very unfavourably with the incidence of approximately 8·5% of similar infections among all newly born infants in the hospital over the period January, 1947, to August, 1958.

Another feature of infants with infection in the series was enlargement of the liver. Clinical enlargement of the liver was present in 48 of the 75 liveborn babies. The enlargement might be evidence of the extramedullary haemopoiesis known to affect particularly the liver in babies of diabetic mothers (Miller and Wilson, 1943) although recorded postmortem findings do not suggest that the weight of the liver is significantly increased (Cardell, 1953; Warren and LeCompte, 1952). Alternatively the liver enlargement may reflect the abnormal glucose metabolism suggested by the asymptomatic hypoglycaemia detectable in the early days of life in many infants of diabetic mothers. There seems to be justification for suspecting that the offspring of diabetic mothers are liable to hepatic dysfunction. If this is accepted the tendency to bruising could be related to the disturbed function of the liver. The

* Reliable figures are not available for the years 1947, 1948 and 1949.

occurrence of clinical tetany in a proportion of these babies might be explained by the presence in the newly born infant's circulation of corticosteroids in abnormal amounts as a result of hormonal imbalance in the diabetic mother (Craig, 1958). Excess of circulating cortisone could explain the liability to infection, the Cushing appearance and the enlarged liver.

Initial progress following birth is likely to be slower in babies in whom macrosomia, the Cushing appearance and liver enlargement are pronounced. To judge by the present series progress is not characterized by abnormal weight loss. This observation is in keeping with the recorded findings of Farquhar and Sklaroff (1958) in connexion with the infants of diabetic women who, as in our series, were not subject to delayed feeding. The disappearance of the pseudo-oedema is to be explained not by abnormal fluid loss but by redistribution of body fluids between the intra- and extra-cellular spaces. Cortisone and thyroid have been suggested as adjuvants to treatment (Peel, 1958). We deprecate their use and attach emphasis to simplicity in medical and nursing care.

The results of the follow-up survey are reassuring. They suggest that congenital anomalies with a serious long term prognosis are unlikely to escape initial detection in the early weeks of life. While this is probably correct as a generalization an exception should be made of urinary abnormalities which are notoriously perplexing in early infancy. One child developed diabetes mellitus at the age of 4 years. In other respects the results of the follow-up survey provide no basis for thinking that the subsequent development and health of the babies of diabetic mothers surviving the neonatal period are in any way prejudiced.

Summary

A series of 94 cases in which pregnancy was complicated by diabetes mellitus is presented.

Obstetrical and paediatric management are outlined.

Foetal loss is discussed in relation to management.

Neonatal morbidity is described with special reference to congenital anomalies, infection, bruising and enlargement of the liver.

The results of a clinical follow-up of infants surviving the neonatal period are summarized.

We are greatly indebted to our senior colleagues on the obstetrical staff of the Leeds Maternity Hospital for permission to include mothers and babies under their care in this series. Dr. R. G. Paley was responsible for the medical supervision of most of the mothers. Assistance in studying maternal records was given by Dr. W. P. Black, and in following-up babies by Dr. A. Bogdan. We wish to pay tribute to the skill of the nursing staff undertaking care of the babies.

References

Bachman, C. (1952). *Amer. J. med. Sci.*, **223**, 681.
Cardell, B. S. (1953). *J. Obstet. Gynaec. Brit. Emp.*, **60**, 834.
Craig, W. S. (1958). *Pediatrics*, **22**, 297.
Farquhar, J. W. and Sklaroff, S. A. (1958). *Arch. Dis. Childh.*, **33**, 323.
Miller, H. C. (1956). *Advan. Pediat.*, **8**, 137.
—— and Wilson, H. M. (1943). *J. Pediat.*, **23**, 251.
Pedersen, J., Bojsen-Møller, B. and Poulsen, H. (1954). *Acta endocr. (Kbh.)*, **15**, 33.
Peel, J. H. (1955). *Brit. med. J.*, **2**, 870.
—— (1958). In *Neo-natal Paediatrics*, ed. W. R. F. Collis, p. 168. Heinemann, London.
—— and Oakley, W. (1950). Trans. 12th Brit. Congr. Obstet. Gynaec., London, 1949, p. 161.
Warren, S. and LeCompte, P. M. (1952). *The Pathology of Diabetes Mellitus*, 3rd ed. Lea and Febiger, Philadelphia.

VARICELLA ENCEPHALITIS

BY

J. D. HEPPLESTON, K. M. PEARCE and P. O. YATES

From Hope Hospital, Salford and the Department of Pathology, University of Manchester

(RECEIVED FOR PUBLICATION FEBRUARY 12, 1959)

The encephalitis which may complicate exanthematous fevers usually shows considerable perivascular demyelination of the white matter and for this reason is often thought of as primarily a disorder of the myelin. There is still some doubt as to whether the encephalitis of chickenpox is of this general type since although the disease is clinically not uncommon, in only seven cases have morbid-anatomical details been reported. Six of these reviewed by Waring, Neubuerger and Geever (1942) showed such histological variety that they felt unable to define a specific picture. Nevertheless several of the cases had shown perivascular demyelination. A very different picture was reported by Lander (1955) when he described a case of haemorrhagic encephalitis following varicella in a man of 36 years. Even in this case, however, the white matter was principally involved and there were some areas of demyelination. In the case reported below the cerebral grey matter was the site of maximal attack, illustrating yet another facet and supporting the view (Lumsden, 1958) that the essential lesion of post-exanthematous encephalitis is a vascular one.

Case Report

The patient, a girl aged 4 years and 9 months, was admitted to hospital on May 20, 1954. She was a well nourished child whose only previous notable illnesses had been measles and whooping cough.

Two weeks before admission she had developed a papulo-vesicular rash on the trunk with a few lesions also on the limbs, face and scalp. At the time she had been off colour and a diagnosis of chicken pox was made. She was not kept in bed. During the second week after the appearance of the rash she had been a little unsteady, falling forwards on a number of occasions. Four days before admission she awoke with a headache, but, despite this played outside with other children. Next day she became anorexic and lethargic. Her condition deteriorated and she was admitted to hospital in a stuporose state.

On examination after admission her trunk was covered with a rash, the lesions being in various stages of healing; many of those which had resolved had left small scars. From the appearance of the rash and the mother's description of its development there was no doubt that it was a healing chickenpox exanthem. Her heart, lungs, abdomen, ears and throat were clinically normal. She was a semi-comatose child who responded only slightly to requests made during examination. Her pupils were equal and reacted to light but her eye movements were irregular and unco-ordinated. As far as examination was possible no other signs of cranial nerve lesions were detected. At this time she appeared to be able to swallow normally. The retinae were normal and the optic disc margins well defined. She had some degree of right-sided hemiparesis, the arm being more affected than the leg. Her right knee and ankle jerks were increased and both plantar responses were extensor. There was no neck stiffness but Kernig's sign was positive, more so with the left leg than with the right. A provisional diagnosis of varicella encephalitis was made and lumbar puncture performed. This yielded clear cerebrospinal fluid under increased pressure. It contained 10 lymphocytes per c.mm.; 25 mg. of protein, 70 mg. of glucose, and 700 mg. of chlorides per 100 ml. A white blood count at this time showed a total of 14,200 per c.mm. (polymorphs 88%, lymphocytes 10%, monocytes 2%).

During the evening of her first day in hospital she developed convulsions, and for an hour there were periods, when she exhibited clonic movements of the right arm, leg and abdominal muscles. Her head and eyes jerked to the right; these movements occurred about once every second. At 10.20 p.m. the convulsive movements ceased spontaneously but she then appeared more deeply comatose and unable to swallow. During the night she developed further convulsions which were controlled with intramuscular phenobarbitone. To combat dehydration and maintain nutrition an intravenous drip was set up; through it 150 mg. of aureomycin were given. Her condition continued to deteriorate and further convulsions necessitated the use of intramuscular paraldehyde.

During the day of May 21 her condition remained much the same though she had no further convulsions. A further 200 mg. of aureomycin were given at 7.0 p.m., at which time she made hardly any response to external stimuli. Her pupils remained fully dilated and she appeared to have a rapidly progressive bulbar paralysis. At 5.20 a.m. the following day she died.

Necropsy. There were a few pock scars on the skin of the trunk. Apart from these and some pulmonary congestion, the only significant changes visible to the naked eye were in the brain. Here the grey matter of cerebral cortex and basal ganglia was pink and patchily swollen. The white matter appeared normal.

HISTOLOGY. The most striking feature was the localization of the inflammatory reaction to the grey matter (Fig. 1). Here there was swelling of capillary

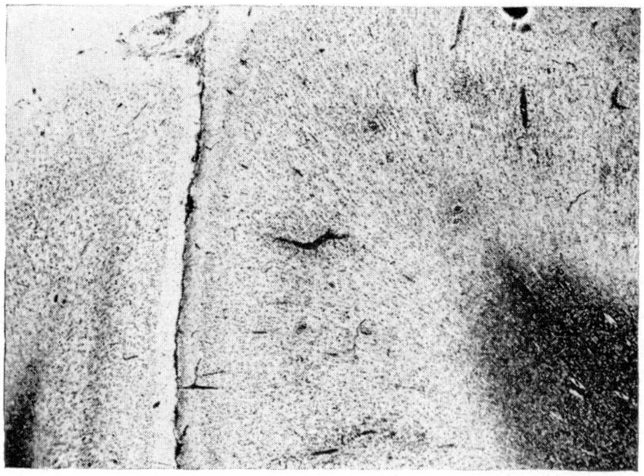

FIG. 1.—Cerebral cortex showing dilated venules and capillaries surrounded by zones of cellular reaction. The gyral white matter is free from demyelinating lesions. ×6

and venular endothelium (Fig. 2). The larger vessels were surrounded by a cuff of inflammatory cells, some of which were lymphocytes and plasma cells, but most were microglia. These latter cells showed mitotic activity. In contrast, the astrocytes were not prominent having only a little more cytoplasm than normal. Within the affected areas neurones were damaged showing a loss of Nissl substance and some cytoplasmic vacuolation. There were none of the changes of specific neuronal disease and no actual destruction or phagocytosis of nerve cells.

The vascular and inflammatory lesions were most common in the deeper layers of the cortex, often ending

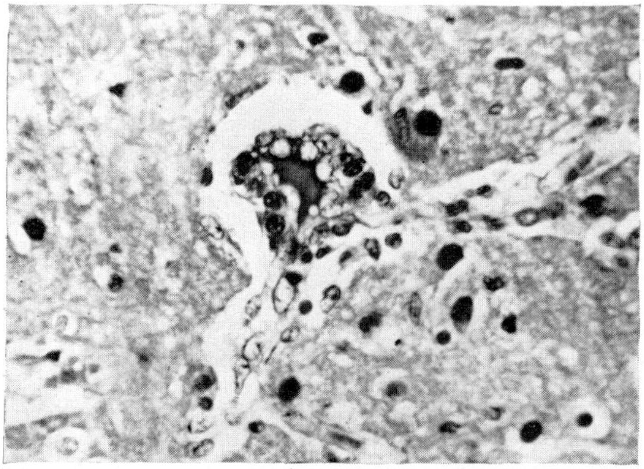

FIG. 2.—Small vessel from cortex with swollen endothelial cells and narrowed lumen ×440.

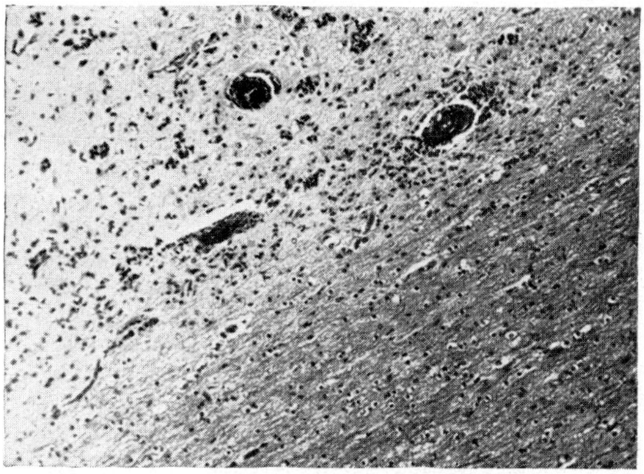

FIG. 3.—Blood vessels in deepest parts of the cortex 'cuffed' by inflammatory cells. Numerous reactive microglial cells confined to the grey matter. ×100.

sharply at the edge of the white matter (Fig. 3). They were present to approximately the same degree in all lobes of both cerebral hemispheres. Over large areas the lesions were confluent and no gyrus examined was without changes. In severely affected areas there was oedema of the cortex.

Elsewhere the grey matter was less severely involved than the cerebral cortex. Vascular endothelial lesions and microglial proliferation were present in the corpus striatum, thalamus, and the head of the caudate nucleus of both hemispheres. The hypothalamic nuclei, geniculate bodies, corpora quadrigemina, corpora mamillaria, substantia nigra, and red nuclei showed only a few changes. The mid-brain, pons and medulla were also slightly affected; no lesions were found in the cerebellar cortex or nuclei.

The white matter was involved in a few places only, usually beneath severely affected cortex. Here a few vessels had swollen endothelium with a cellular infiltration of their walls and a surrounding zone of reactive microglia. Rarely there was perivascular demyelination (Fig. 4).

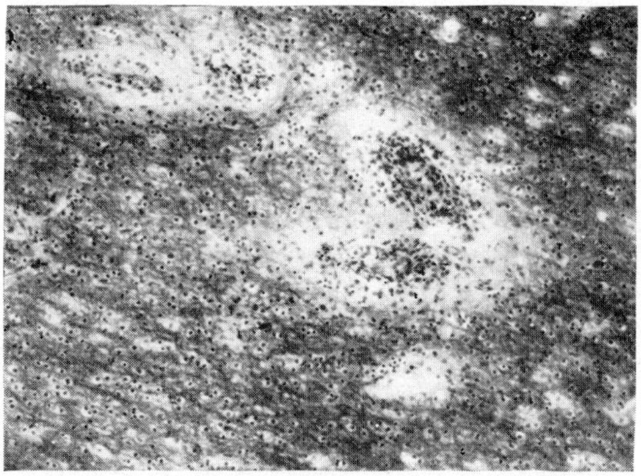

FIG. 4.—White matter of occipital lobe showing small blood vessels surrounded by lymphocytes and microglia which lie within pale perivascular zones of demyelination. Loyez ×100.

In mixed grey and white areas such as the corpus striatum the vascular lesions were more prominent in the grey matter—this predominance was greater than would be accounted for by the relative proportions of capillary bed in the two types of tissue. The cerebellar white matter, the optic tracts and cranial nerves were normal.

The upper cervical part of the spinal cord, which was the only part available for examination, showed none of the typical vascular or glial changes and the neurones were unaffected. There was, however, a striking degeneration of the myelin sheaths of most of both dorsal and ventral spinocerebellar tracts and to a lesser extent of the posterior and lateral parts of the dorsal columns (Fig. 5). The bundles running from the upper end of

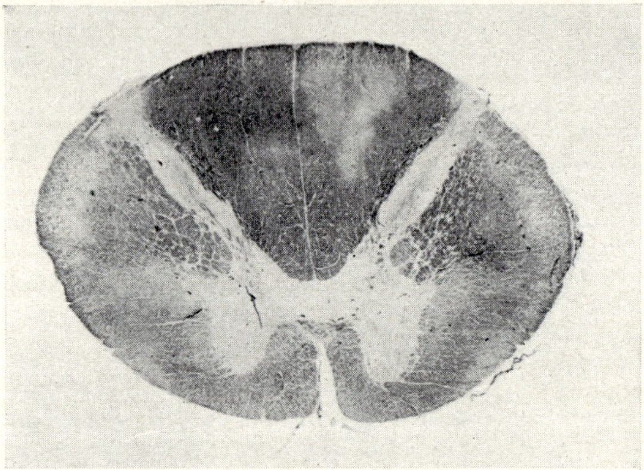

FIG 5.—Cervical cord showing ascending tract degeneration of dorsal and lateral columns. Loyez ×7.

Clarke's column to the dorsal spino-cerebellar tracts were degenerated with swollen myelin sheaths and fragmented axons. The spino-thalamic tracts were involved to a much lesser degree. Unfortunately no posterior root ganglia and no peripheral nerves were available for examination.

The meninges were infiltrated by lymphocytes, plasma cells and macrophages especially in regions where there was considerable underlying cerebral disease.

None of the viscera of the body showed any significant histological changes. A careful search did not reveal any vascular lesions comparable with those in the brain or any focal necrosis of tissue. No definite inclusion bodies could be demonstrated. An attempt to grow virus from the cerebral tissue was not successful; tissue culture techniques were not available at the time.

Discussion

Clinically neurological involvement in varicella is most commonly of a 'cerebellar' type in which ataxia, vomiting, nystagmus and occasionally speech changes are present (Underwood, 1935). However, recovery is usual and in the few pathological reports available appropriate lesions of the cerebellum or spinal cord were not recorded. The changes in the spinal cord in this case would undoubtedly account for the ataxia which preceded the encephalitis by several days. It is unfortunate that the origins of these ascending tract degenerations could not be examined. The cerebellum itself was not primarily affected. There are three notable features of the encephalitic process; the swelling of vascular endothelium, the intense proliferation of microglia and the occasional perivenular zones of demyelination. Each of these features is present in varying degrees in the encephalitis which follows not only chickenpox but also measles and vaccination against smallpox. Appelbaum, Dolgopol and Dolgin (1949) discussing the histological changes in measles encephalitis noted that vascular changes were common and in acute cases, where death occurred early, were widely distributed irrespective of the presence or absence of demyelination. In the cases dying later in the disease perivascular demyelination was usual and often extensive. Microglial activity was always marked though only at a late stage did these cells apparently begin to function as phagocytes. This intense cellular proliferation cannot be considered a direct response to necrosis of neurones or of myelin sheaths, since in many lesions it precedes the slightest evidence of such damage.

Six earlier pathological reports of varicella encephalitis were reviewed by Appelbaum, Rachelson, and Dolgopol (1953). They observed that though perivascular demyelination was the most prominent feature, changes in the grey matter occurred in almost all.

If the encephalitis is the result of direct viral attack then some evidence should be seen in cases dying of severe generalized chickenpox. Waring *et al.* (1942) reported such a case; a man aged 40 years died on the eighth day of illness. There was evidence of vascular damage in organs of the body and in the brain with focal necroses and petechial haemorrhages. Capillary endothelium was swollen in the cortex and white matter and the vessels, some of which were surrounded by haemorrhage, appeared to have undergone necrosis. Elsewhere the changes in the brain were a perivascular demyelination and microglial proliferation. On the other hand two cases described by Cheatham, Weller, Dolan and Dower (1956) showed vascular endothelial damage in many organs but the brains and spinal cords were normal. In both these latter cases the damaged endothelial cells contained intranuclear viral inclusion bodies. The evidence for direct viral attack on the vessels of the central nervous system is therefore somewhat contradictory. Moreover, encephalitis may follow chickenpox when the disease has apparently been extremely mild as in our case or indeed may appear during the period of regression of a more severe attack. Such factors suggest that the encephalitis is the result of some secondary phenomenon probably an abnormal antigen-antibody reaction. Support for this comes from the otherwise inexplicable changes of the microglia, which, unlike other glial cells, are closely related to the reticulo-endothelial system, and may be expected to react to the same stimuli as the vascular endothelium.

This concept of a non-specific aetiology is supported by Russell (1955) who emphasized the nosological unity of acute haemorrhagic leuco-encephalitis and acute disseminated encephalomyelitis of post-exanthematous type. She presented three cases in which encephalitis had followed an upper respiratory infection and in which lesions of two types were found. The one consisted of necrosis of arteriolar walls with a fibrinous, haemorrhagic and polymorphonuclear leucocytic exudation into the surrounding brain and the other a perivascular demyelination with intense microglial activity. She was able to find these two lesions characteristic of the two types of encephalitis, side by side in the same case. All her cases were adults and followed respiratory infections; none showed any evidence of an exanthematous disease. However, Lander (1955) described a case of undoubted acute haemorrhagic leuco-encephalitis of Hurst type complicating varicella. His patient was a man of 36 who developed encephalitis five days after the appearance of a typical but severe rash of varicella. Other members of his family including three children had had typical attacks. Lander described in addition to the haemorrhagic lesions, areas of perivascular demyelination; this was clearly a case of encephalitis of mixed type similar to those reported by Russell. There is, therefore, a broad group of cerebral lesions which may follow respiratory or gastro-intestinal infection in adults and the exanthematous illnesses in childhood. The interval between the onset of the primary illness and of the encephalitis varies from a few days to two or three weeks and it seems probable that the encephalitis is the result of an acquired sensitivity of the cerebral blood vessels to circulating antibody. In adults the lesion is more likely to take the form of an acute haemorrhagic leuco-encephalitis whether it follows the more common upper respiratory infection or the exanthemata as in Lander's case. In children it is most likely to be a non-haemorrhagic disseminated encephalomyelitis with perivascular demyelination as a prominent feature.

Summary

The clinical and pathological findings are reported in a case of post-varicella encephalitis in a girl of 4 years. There was little of the perivenular demyelination usually associated with post-exanthematous encephalitis, the predominant lesions being in the grey matter of cerebral cortex and basal nuclei. The conclusion reached is that the essential abnormality is damage to blood vessels possibly of an allergic nature.

We would like to thank Dr. R. I. Mackay under whose care the patient was admitted. The photomicrographs are the work of Mr. N. Mowat.

References

Appelbaum, E., Dolgopol, V. B. and Dolgin, J. (1949). *Amer. J. Dis. Child.*, **77**, 25.
——, Rachelson, M. H. and Dolgopol, V. B. (1953). *Amer. J. Med.*, **15**, 223.
Cheatham, W. J., Weller, T. H., Dolan, T. F. and Dower, J. C. (1956). *Amer. J. Path.*, **32**, 1015.
Lander, H. (1955). *J. Path. Bact.*, **70**, 157.
Lumsden, C. E. (1958). *Proc. roy. Soc. Med.*, **51**, 752.
Russell, D. S. (1955). *Brain*, **78**, 369.
Underwood, E. A. (1935). *Brit. J. Child. Dis.*, **32**, 83.
Waring, J. I., Neubuerger, K. T. and Geever, E. F. (1942). *Arch. intern. Med.*, **69**, 384.

NEUROLOGICAL SEQUELAE OF PERTUSSIS WITH PARTICULAR REFERENCE TO MENTAL DEFECT

BY

J. M. BERG

From the Fountain Hospital, London

(RECEIVED FOR PUBLICATION FEBRUARY 25, 1959)

Neurological complications associated with pertussis have long been known. Sears (1929) recorded that Sydenham (1624-1689) noticed that children with whooping cough might have difficulty in walking; cases of paralysis were described by Barrier (1842), Rilliet and Barthez (1843) and Trousseau (1866); and, according to Annell (1953), convulsions in pertussis were first described during epidemics in Copenhagen in 1775 and in Dillingen in 1811.

Many of those with neurological complications die during the acute illness, particularly if affected in the first two years of life, the mortality ranging from 33% to over 50% (Miller, 1956). Mortality rates up to 90% have been reported (Norberg, 1952). Perhaps about half the survivors recover completely, the remainder being left with physical and/or mental sequelae (Litvak, Gibel, Rosenthal and Rosenblatt, 1948; Miller, 1956). Of physical sequelae, epilepsy and paralyses are most frequent. In relation to mental sequelae, figures for complete recovery merit critical appraisal, as there is evidence that various personality and behaviour disturbances later in life are not infrequently related to pertussis in early infancy (Lurie and Levy, 1942; Byers and Rizzo, 1950; Annell, 1953). Without careful psychiatric follow-up, such cases may easily be classed as 'completely recovered' at the end of their acute illness. Frank severe mental retardation following pertussis is less likely to be missed, but has received little attention in the literature, particularly in this country. Such a case is here reported.

Case Report

No history of mental illness or defect, convulsions or other neurological ailments was elicited from a frank, co-operative mother in any of the following (relationships are to the patient):

Each of the four grandparents died between 69 and 75 years of age. The mother was 34 and the father 40 years old at the child's birth. There is a brother 12½ years older and a sister two and a half years younger. The mother has had no miscarriages or stillbirths. On the maternal side, two aunts and four uncles have between them eight children and seven grandchildren; on the paternal side, three aunts and three uncles have 13 children and five grandchildren.

The mother regularly attended an ante-natal clinic during her uneventful pregnancy. The child, a female, was born at full term on November 6, 1955, following an uncomplicated five-hour labour. Birth weight was 6 lb. 14 oz. (3·118 kg.). No abnormalities were noted neonatally, and the child thrived from the outset to the complete satisfaction of the parents and a welfare clinic she attended.

Progress was normal, without illness, till 10 months of age. By then, she could combine syllables like 'ma-ma', feed herself with small pieces of food, sit steadily without support, wave goodbye and understand several simple words. She had not been immunized against whooping cough.

Early in September, 1956 (aged 10 months) she developed a 'cold' associated with coughing which soon became paroxysmal and was accompanied by vomiting and an occasional whoop. On September 11 she was admitted to hospital with the diagnosis of whooping cough. On admission her temperature was 100° F., pulse rate 126 and respiratory rate 26 per minute. She was well-developed, well-nourished and in no acute distress. Apart from this, no abnormal physical signs were found. A post-nasal swab was negative for *H. pertussis*. The white blood count was 19,700 per cubic mm., with 81% lymphocytes. She was given chloramphenicol, mg. 150 six-hourly for five days.

No untoward developments occurred till September 16, when coughing spasms became more frequent and apnoeic periods replaced the whoop. An hour after the first of these apnoeic periods, the child was staring vacantly into space with all her limbs twitching. This lasted for some 15 minutes. She was not cyanosed and no abnormalities were noted on physical examination. She was sedated with chloral hydrate and put in an oxygen tent for two hours. The child was now placed on achromycin mg. 125 six-hourly for 11 days and phenobarbitone gr. ¼ thrice daily.

During the next week at least six such attacks occurred, now associated with cyanosis. On September 25 a particularly severe attack was accompanied by apnoea lasting several minutes. She became deeply cyanosed and stuporose, and normal breathing was only restored after 20 minutes of artificial respiration. No further apnoea or cyanosis was observed, though spasmodic coughing continued for 10 more days.

On September 28 she was noted to be drowsy, with twitching of all her limbs. The next day a lumbar puncture yielded a clear cerebrospinal fluid with 60 red cells per cubic mm., no white cells, 40 mg. protein per 100 ml., globulin not increased and a negative Wassermann reaction. Drowsiness persisted for some days with periodic screaming attacks and convulsive stiffening of the limbs. From October 1 she was given penicillin V mg. 60 six-hourly for 10 days, and, from October 2, intramuscular paraldehyde ml. 1 eight-hourly for four days. Gradually she became less drowsy but continued to be indifferent to her environment. It was then thought that she might be blind, though her fundi were normal. Apart from generalized hypertonicity, there were no other neurological signs.

During the rest of her stay in hospital restlessness, indifference and hypertonic limbs with brisk reflexes were the most notable findings. She had a transient internal strabismus. Clinically, the lungs were normal throughout. Intermittent pyrexia persisted from admission till October 12. No particular pyrexial pattern was associated with the attacks of apnoea, cyanosis and twitching.

The child was discharged on November 16 (aged $12\frac{1}{2}$ months) in good physical health, but restless and grossly demented. Apart from brisk reflexes, no neurological signs were present. Phenobarbitone, gr. $\frac{1}{4}$ twice daily, was prescribed. The mother described her child on discharge from hospital as 'like a broken doll. She stared all the time, but took no notice of anything'.

In this state she remained at home on phenobarbitone, and without fits, till January, 1957 (aged 14 months), when she was admitted to The Hospital for Sick Children, Great Ormond Street, for further assessment. It was noted that she could not sit unaided and that her behaviour was appropriate to a child of about 6 months. She could see and hear, and no abnormal physical signs, neurological or other, were found. An E.E.G. showed 'generalized abnormality compatible with a diffuse brain disorder'. She was discharged within a week, but readmitted a month later following a series of generalized convulsions associated with cyanosis and frothing at the mouth. Fits continued in hospital for a few days and were eventually controlled by phenobarbitone gr. $\frac{1}{2}$ thrice daily. Again no physical signs were noted and she was discharged.

Till now, December, 1958 (aged $3\frac{1}{12}$ years), she has remained at home without significant mental progress. She is given phenobarbitone, up to gr. 3 daily, as a prophylactic measure against convulsions which seldom occur unassociated with pyrexial illness. Febrile bouts of upper respiratory infection at $2\frac{1}{4}$ and $2\frac{1}{2}$ years of age were associated with convulsions without other neurological signs.

At present (aged $3\frac{1}{12}$ years) she is a well-developed, pretty child with no neurological or other physical signs.

The following psychological report was prepared by Dr. Mary Woodward: at the age of $3\frac{1}{12}$ years, on the Gesell Developmental Schedules, her developmental age was assessed as follows: locomotor scale (12-18 months), prehensory scale (40 weeks), adaptive scale (36-40 weeks), language scale (40 weeks), personal-social scale (44-52 weeks).

She was interested in most of the play material offered to her, though she preferred toys that made a noise.

She shows some unevenness in development. Her method of locomotion (crawling and walking with the aid of furniture) is that of an average year-old baby, whereas her climbing on to a large chair is more advanced behaviour. This is not usually developed until after the child has begun to walk alone. She is reported to take a few steps on her own occasionally, and it is possible that her walking has not developed further because she is timid.

Her language development also has some unusual features. She speaks the names of five people, correctly identifying each, but does not yet use other words denoting objects. She appears as yet to have no verbal comprehension. Personal-social development is also uneven in that she co-operates in dressing, but does not help to hold a cup; the latter response usually occurs much earlier.

Apart from locomotor development, her activities are in general those of the average child of 40 weeks, though her solution of simple problems and her awareness of unperceived objects are slightly in advance of this. She appears at present to be an imbecile.

Discussion

No example of mental deficiency as a sequel to pertussis has been established in the Fountain Hospital in the last 12 years. This hospital, with an average annual intake of 90 patients, admits children under 6 years, nearly all with I.Q.s below 50. As an attempt is made to elucidate the cause of the mental retardation in each case, it is unlikely that any substantial number of the total of over 1,000 children who have passed through the hospital in these 12 years owed their defect to whooping cough. However, several authors have indicated that mental defect may follow pertussis more often than is generally thought.

Lurie and Levy (1942) studied a successive group of 500 problem children seen at a child guidance home, 58 of whom had pertussis at or under 2 years of age. Of these 58, six showed progressive intellectual deterioration. Levy and Perry (1948) reported that, among 1,000 successive admissions to a Washington State Institution for children with I.Q.s of 70 or less, there were no fewer than 20 (2·0%) in whom 'there appeared to be a definite causal relationship between whooping cough and the intellectual retardation which followed'. Of these 20, eight were classified as idiots, eight as imbeciles and four as low-grade morons. Byers and Rizzo (1950) followed up for several years 35 children admitted to the Boston Children's Hospital with whooping cough contracted between 3 weeks old and 2 years. Six of these had intellectual or emotional difficulties which 'seemed sufficiently severe and persistent to compromise their competitive status'. One of the six was a microcephalic idiot and another a mental defective with an I.Q. of 37, both 'probably due to pertussis'. In view of such reports, it is worth bearing in mind the possible aetiological significance of pertussis in the many cases of mental defect where the causes are obscure.

A variety of neuropathological findings have been reported in cases of pertussis with neurological complications coming to autopsy. Haemorrhagic, inflammatory and degenerative lesions have been described, and many agents and mechanisms postulated to explain them. These include angiospasm, vascular stasis and mechanical damage to cerebral vessels; the action of toxins, viruses or other biological agents; and such factors as air emboli and spasmophilia. These theories were critically reviewed by Ellison (1934) and more recently by Litvak *et al.* (1948). In view of the varied pathological findings, it seems likely that all cases are not due to the same cause. With the report of cases in which there was no evidence of cerebral haemorrhage, this formerly much-favoured view of the aetiology lost ground. In recent years, cerebral anoxia, of whatever origin, has been widely regarded as the cause of neurological complications in some cases.

In the present case the association of apnoea with the neurological sequelae is striking. It is tentatively suggested that cerebral anoxia secondary to the apnoea was the basis for the subsequent clinical picture. It is noteworthy that, whatever the cause, it could produce cerebral damage sufficient to lead to imbecility and convulsions, but without paralysis or other persistent focal signs.

Summary

A case is reported of a normal girl who developed whooping cough at 10 months. During the paroxysmal stage there were frequent periods of apnoea and neurological complications developed, including drowsiness, twitchings of the limbs, hypertonic extremities with brisk reflexes and transient internal strabismus. Screaming attacks and restlessness were also noted. Therapy included chloramphenicol and achromycin. The child survived the acute illness in a grossly demented state and suffering from fits, but without neurological localizing signs. At $3\frac{1}{12}$ years she was assessed to be of imbecile level. The condition is tentatively attributed to cerebral anoxia consequent on severe apnoea occurring during the paroxysmal stage of pertussis.

Neurological sequelae of pertussis, with particular reference to mental defect, are briefly considered.

My thanks are due to Miss M. F. Craib for drawing my attention to the case and arranging various interviews; to Dr. W. H. Kelleher and Professor A. A. Moncrieff for access to clinical records; to Dr. G. Pampiglione for permission to quote from his E.E.G. report; to Dr. Mary Woodward for her psychological report; to Dr. J. C. McEntee and my colleagues at the Fountain Hospital for helpful suggestions.

REFERENCES

Annell, A.-L. (1953). Pertussis in Infancy as a Cause of Behaviour Disorders in Children. *Acta Soc. Med. upsalien.*, **58**, Supplement I.
Barrier (1842). Cited by Sears (1929).
Byers, R. K. and Rizzo, N. D. (1950). *New Engl. J. Med.*, **242**, 887.
Ellison, J. B. (1934). *Lancet*, **1**, 227.
Levy, S. and Perry, H. A. (1948). *Amer J. ment. Defic.*, **52**, 217.
Litvak, A. M., Gibel, H., Rosenthal, S. E. and Rosenblatt, P. (1948). *J. Pediat.*, **32**, 357.
Lurie, L. A. and Levy, S. (1942). *J. Amer. med. Ass.*, **120**, 890.
Miller, H. (1956). *Proc. roy. Soc. Med.*, **49**, 139.
Norberg, A. (1952). *Nord. Med.*, **47**, 776.
Rilliet, F. and Barthez, A. (1843). Traité clinique et pratique des Maladies des Enfants, Vol. 2, p. 215. Baillière, Paris.
Sears, W. G. (1929). *Brit. J. Child. Dis.*, **26**, 178.
Sydenham, T. (1624-1689). Cited by Sears (1929).
Trousseau (1866). Cited by Sears (1929).

CEREBRAL ATROPHY IN MICROCEPHALIC COUSINS

BY

PETER E. SYLVESTER

From the Fountain Hospital, London

(RECEIVED FOR PUBLICATION MARCH 4, 1959)

'There are secrets in all families.'
GEORGE FARQUHAR

Microcephaly is one of the commonest findings in low-grade mental defectives (idiots and imbeciles). It is associated with different forms of encephalopathy. Rarely, it occurs in families; Brandon, Kirman and Williams (pending) found that 114 unselected cases of microcephaly had 166 siblings of whom nine were also microcephalic. However, its occurrence in siblings or other relatives does not necessarily imply the same cause, though, when the nature of the lesions is similar, the possibility of a single disease being involved becomes likely. This was so in the following two children, who presented at necropsy granular and cortical atrophy (ulegyria) of a pattern often thought to follow cerebral birth trauma. However, this could be excluded in one child and was not definitely established in the other. The findings are reported since similar cases with familial association have not been recorded in the literature.

Family History

The two children, both boys, were first cousins, and gentiles. The father of one (Case 1) and the mother of the other (Case 2) were twins. Enquiry into the family tree (Fig. 1) failed to reveal evidence of similar illnesses in other members.

Nine years after the birth of Case 1, a healthy sister was born, who at 1 year of age was found to be developing normally. There had been no other pregnancies.

The three surviving siblings of Case 2 were all healthy and intelligent at the ages of 13, 10 and 2 years.

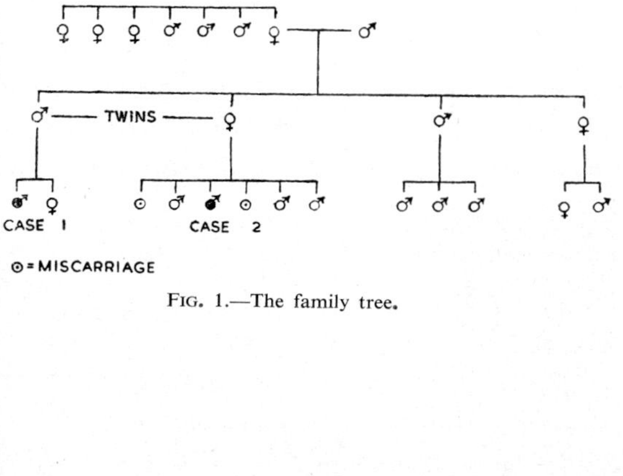

FIG. 1.—The family tree.

Case 1. He was the first child of a healthy mother, aged 24, and an unrelated, healthy father, aged 28. After a normal pregnancy, the infant was born at home. Presenting in the right occipito-posterior position and following a first stage lasting $36\frac{1}{2}$ hours, the second stage was uneventful and he was delivered with ease, the umbilical cord being wound loosely round his neck. However, he suffered from white asphyxia for which he received several injections of nikethamide over three days. The birth weight was 6·0 lb. (2·73 kg.). Jaundice did not develop. He had convulsions on the third day of life. The skull circumference was not recorded.

At 8 months of age, it became obvious that the child was not developing normally. He could neither hold up his head nor sit. There were doubts about his vision. Convulsions, consisting of sudden momentary jerks of the whole body and sometimes accompanied by vomiting, occurred frequently by day and night. He was taken for medical advice, and found to have severe mental retardation. There were bilateral diffuse lenticular opacities of a non-specific type, and the lenses were partially subluxated upwards and outwards. The palate was high-arched. A radiograph of the skull was normal.

He made no progress. Other milestones, crawling, standing, walking and talking, were not passed. During his second year, tonic spasms of his whole body followed by twitchings of the face, eyes, limbs and circumoral cyanosis occurred, these episodes lasting about a minute. Following convulsions, he often had bouts of crying which were impossible to soothe and continued day and night for several weeks.

The lenticular opacities were needled on several occasions and he was thought to be partially sighted.

At one time he seemed to know his parents' voices, but this was the only suggestion that he could ever hear.

Bronchitis, tonsillitis, pneumonia and several bouts of pyrexia intervened up to the time of admission to the Fountain Hospital at 5 years 10 months, when he had another attack of pneumonia. He was then a helpless, emaciated, barely conscious idiot, without any sort of rapport. A number of vague, restless and purposeless movements were noted; occasionally he stretched himself and brushed his right hand across his face. He had contractures of the right hand and foot.

There was a marked strabismus and nystagmoid movements to the right. The pupils, the right smaller than the left, were central and reacted to light but not convergence. There were peripheral lenticular opacities.

Lacking a blink reflex and ability to fix objects, he appeared to be completely blind. He did not react to a squeaky toy and, although the external and middle ears seemed normal, it was impossible to assess his auditory ability.

He was markedly hypotonic, and the tendon and abdominal reflexes could not be elicited. His I.Q. was 14 on the Vineland Scale.

His height was 40 in. (1·02 m.) and weight 28 lb. (12·7 kg.). The head circumference was 18½ in. (47·0 cm.) average normal for age and sex being 51·8 cm. (Westropp and Barber, 1956). The cranial index was 0·73 cm.

Radiography of the skull showed no bony abnormality. There was no albumen, sugar or phenylpyruvic acid in the urine.

He died suddenly at 5 years 11 months following a major fit during a meal.

Pathological Findings. The necropsy on the second day after death was performed by the coroner's pathologist. Death was due to severe subacute bilateral panpetrositis. Bronchopneumonia, with gross compensatory emphysema, was present at both bases, and terminal inhalation of stomach contents had occurred. The stomach was greatly distended and somewhat hypertrophic. A rather large liver showed numerous areas of focal necrosis. Apart from some congestion of the spleen and kidneys, and a small brain, other organs seemed normal.

The fixed brain, symmetrical in shape, with the cerebellum and brain stem, weighed 912 g. (average normal for age: 1,243 g.). Radiographically, the posterior horns of the lateral ventricles were slightly distended; there was no evidence of calcification. The superior temporal gyri were narrower than usual. At the right occipital pole occupying the tip, the medial aspect for 3 cm., and extending on to the medio-inferior margin for 1 cm., there was macroscopic ulegyria with 'cobblestone' appearance (Fig. 2). The left occipital pole looked normal. The ependyma was smooth and the meninges looked clear and could be stripped easily from the underlying cortex.

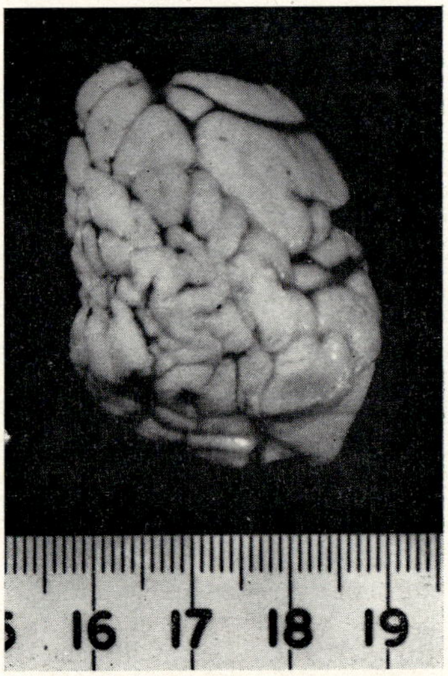

Fig. 2.—Case 1. Cortical atrophy at the tip of the right occipital lobe.

Histological Findings. Coronal sections of the frontal, temporal and occipital lobes, the basal ganglia, mid-brain, pons, medulla and cerebellum were embedded in celloidin, and sections stained by the usual neuropathological procedures—Nissl, Heidenhain, H.V.G., Mallory's P.T.A.H., Holzer, P.A.S., Greenfield's thionin, Nile blue sulphate and mucicarmine techniques. Frozen sections were used for Scarlet R, thionin, Holzer, von Kossa, Turnbull and Kultschitsky-Pal methods.

The most striking changes were in the occipital lobes where ulegyria affected several gyri above and below the post-calcarine sulcus (Fig. 3).

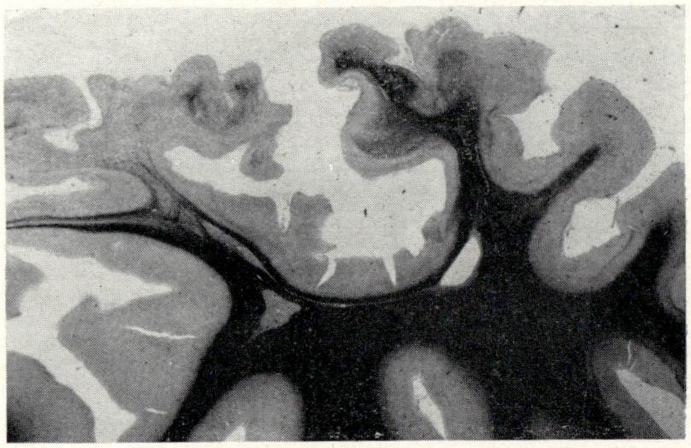

Fig. 3.—Case 1. Ulegyria with demyelination around the post-calcarine sulcus. Kultschitsky-Pal ×3.

Some of the gyri had been destroyed completely and the grey and white matter replaced by dense shrivelled glial scars, composed of three layers. The outermost layer was a rim of dense parallel glial fibres. The innermost layer consisted of a whorled knotty core of glial tissue with a network of collagen fibres—the remnants of blood vessels (Fig. 4). Between these two layers, glial strands ran, palisade fashion, at right-angles to the surface. Neither nerve cells nor myelin fibres had survived.

Less severely affected gyri showed incomplete destruction with many surviving nerve cells and myelin fibres. The profile of such a gyrus had a narrow stem surmounted by a large crown of apparently intact cortex with a normal cyto-architectonic structure. The stem was composed of a central core of glial tissue, which had replaced destroyed myelin tracts. Around this region some of the arcuate fibres remained, thus outlining an area of gliosed white matter. The surrounding grey matter was considerably thinned, nerve cells were reduced in number, and fibrous astrocytes were increased. In some areas of the stem, nerve cell loss was complete, notably in small laminar scars (Fig. 5) affecting layers 3

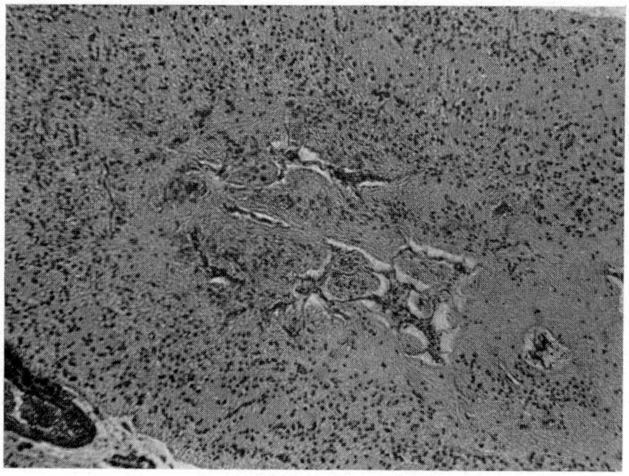

FIG. 4.—Case 1. Collagen tissue, the remnants of blood vessels, in the case of a destroyed gyrus. H.V.G. ×110.

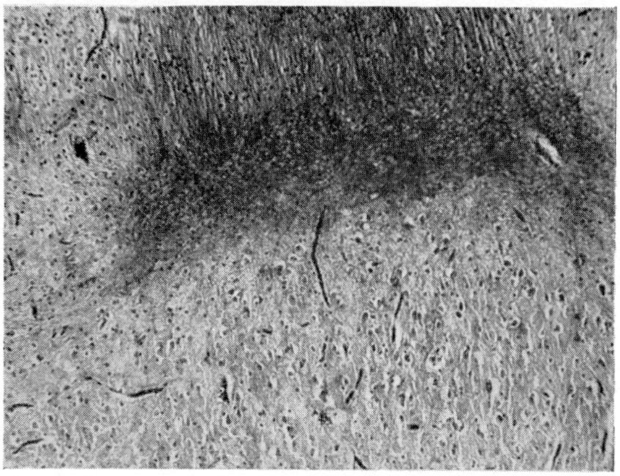

FIG. 5.—Case 1. A glial laminar scar in the grey matter. Holzer ×110

and 4. These small scars, semilunar in shape, were composed of a dense network of glial fibres from which glial strands radiated towards the surface, where they merged with a thick carpet of superficial glial fibres. Myelin fibres were absent from these scars, but those in adjacent areas were distorted. The cortical surface over these small scars was dimpled, thus accounting for the macroscopic appearance of granular atrophy.

Numerous metachromatic bodies were easily demonstrable in the white substance. They were small discrete globules much more numerous than the glial nuclei and varying in size from that of the nuclei to two or three times their size. They stained pink-violet by Greenfield's thionin method in celloidin sections and they were strongly P.A.S. positive. They stained with mucicarmine but not with Nile blue sulphate or Scarlet R.

The cyto-architectonic structure of the basal ganglia was normal. The white matter, containing a number of 'mucocytes', was well myelinated.

There was evidence of damage in other areas of the brain, notably demyelination with glial replacement in the corona radiata, the adjacent grey matter being markedly gliosed.

Astrocytes were increased in the molecular layer of the cerebellar cortex and Bergmann's cells were also present, especially towards the apices of the leaflets. There was no alteration in size and number of the Purkinje cells. There was neither demyelination, loss of granular cells, nor abnormality of the dentate nuclei.

The frontal and temporal lobes appeared normal. The optic nerves were well myelinated. Abnormality was not noted either in the Ammon's horn or in the brain stem.

The meninges and the blood vessels outside the scarred areas were normal. The ependyma overlying the calcar avis in the dilated posterior horn was partly denuded of cells, and there was periventricular gliosis.

Calcium could not be demonstrated. Compound granular corpuscles containing neutral fat were scattered in the atrophic cortex and collected around neighbouring blood vessels. Examination by polarized light failed to reveal doubly refractile material.

Case 2. He was the second child of a healthy mother, aged 26, and an unrelated healthy father, aged 27. The mother attended an antenatal clinic; her pregnancy was normal and her pelvis was considered adequate. Labour commenced at term and proceeded to a normal vertex delivery. The total duration of labour was 14 hours and 40 minutes and there was a post-partum loss of 5 oz. (135 ml.). The infant weighed 5 lb. 11 oz. (2·5 kg.); his umbilical cord measured 20 in. (50·8 cm.); his length was 19½ in. (48·6 cm.) and the head circumference 14 in. (35·6 cm.). Head moulding was thought to be absent. He was considered normal at birth and required minimal resuscitation. Complications were absent during the lying-in period and breast-feeding was satisfactorily established. Mother and child were discharged fit and well on the tenth day.

At 3 weeks of age he developed projectile vomiting after every feed. A diagnosis of congenital pyloric stenosis was made. A laparotomy was performed under 5% procaine local anaesthesia and open ether, but there was no evidence of pyloric 'tumour'. The post-operative period was stormy and vomiting continued. Slow improvement was achieved with atropine methonitrate and adjustment of feeds; nevertheless, vomiting was frequent. On the twenty-first day after operation he became cyanosed, tachypnoeic, and vomited copiously, and was placed in an oxygen tent. Ten days after this he developed a staphylococcal abscess of the thigh. Eventually his symptoms abated and he was discharged after 54 days in hospital.

Mental retardation was first suspected at nine months when he could not sit. Subsequently, he failed to pass other developmental milestones and never recognized his mother. Projectile vomiting continued. Epileptic fits developed, but there is no record of their character. He could not eat solid foods and, because of lack of progress, was again admitted to hospital at 23 months, when he was considered to be a blind, microcephalic mental defective. His head circumference was then 16½ in. (41·9 cm., average normal for age: 49·1 cm.). The back of his head was flattened. His reflexes and optic fundi were normal.

He was admitted to the Fountain Hospital at 4 years and 4 months, and classified as a microcephalic epileptic idiot with spastic diplegia. Feeble and helpless, he lay inertly in his cot with his legs partly drawn up and his right arm, flexed at the elbow and held rigidly against his body; occasionally he raised his left arm and stretched it. He drooled, resented being touched, and could neither sit nor hold up his head, flopping back when raised. He made no sounds other than a whimper.

His height was 34 in. (0·89 m.) and weight 20 lb. (9·1 kg.). The occipito-frontal circumference was 16¾ in. (42·5 cm., average normal for age and sex being 52·7 cm.). The cranial index was 0·78 cm. There was neither strabismus nor nystagmus. The lenses were clear. Pupils were central and circular, reacting equally to light. It was difficult to determine whether he had any vision. The external and middle ears were normal and he seemed to hear, showing excitement such as struggling and threshing his arms about when a tambourine was sounded. The legs were hypotonic with unequal knee jerks, that on the right being exaggerated. The plantar responses were equivocal.

Radiography of the skull revealed no bony abnormalities other than microcephaly. The W.R. was negative. Phenylpyruvic acid was absent from the urine. His blood group was O, M S M S, P+, cde/cde, Lu (a−), K−, Le (a−, b+), Fy (a−), Jk (a−). The cerebro-

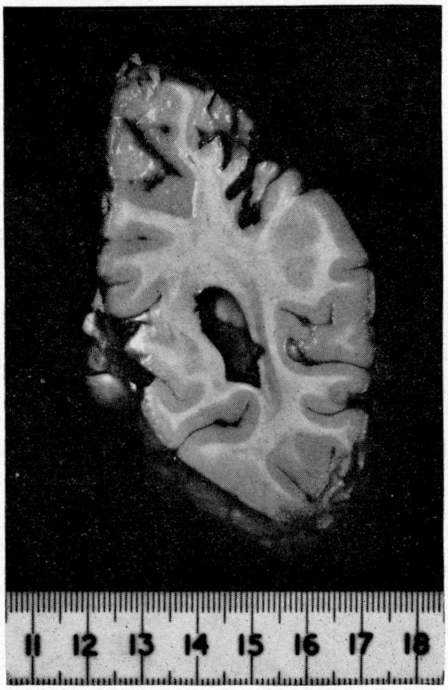

FIG. 6.—Case 2. Cortical atrophy affecting the superior occipital gyrus.

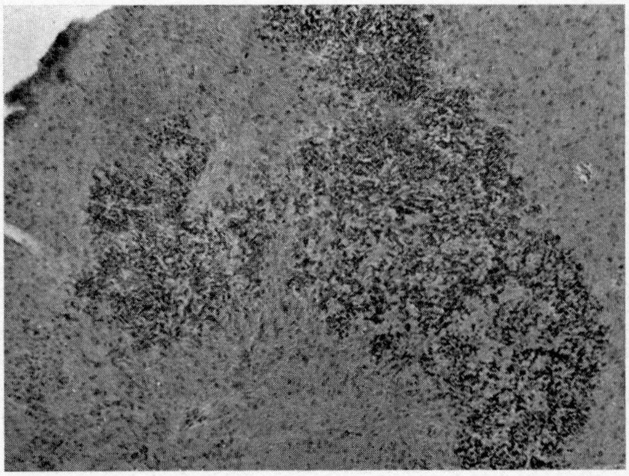

FIG. 7.—Case 2. Pseudo-calcium within the scar. Haematoxylin and carmine. ×110.

spinal fluid was normal. An E.E.G., taken at 6 years 4 months, showed a right posterior focus of sharp waves, but the left side showed so little rhythmic activity that a large destructive lesion on that side was considered possible. The dominant regular activity was in the theta range and had a rather sharp form. No alpha rhythm was present.

During his stay in hospital he made no mental progress and seven to 11 fits occurred each year. He had several respiratory infections, succumbing finally to bronchopneumonia at 6 years 5 months. Three days before death, a succession of fits began, with vomiting of food, during which the face twitched especially round the mouth. At first the arms were spastic and stimulation caused clonic spasms; meanwhile the legs remained hypotonic. Within 24 hours the spasticity and irritability spread to the legs until, 12 hours before death, he became comatose.

PATHOLOGICAL FINDINGS. At necropsy, on the day after death, the only significant findings, apart from those in the nervous system, were in the lungs and heart. Thick purulent sputum was present in the trachea and bronchi and in both lower lobes there were areas of lobular collapse, emphysema and bronchopneumonia. The foramen ovale was patent to a probe. Histologically, bronchopneumonia was confirmed. There were areas of alveolar collapse, inhalation and inflammatory pneumonia, alternating with areas of emphysema.

The fixed brain, rounded and symmetrical in shape, with the cerebellum and brain-stem weighed 826 g. (average normal for age: 1,235 g.). It was firm to touch, especially in the occipital poles, which did not completely overlap the cerebellum. Over the lateral aspect of both occipital lobes there was ulegyria, more marked on the left side. The corpus callosum was thinned in its posterior third. The basal ganglia seemed normal. Radiographically, there was dilatation of the posterior horns of the lateral ventricles; calcification was not seen. The ependyma was smooth and there was no naked-eye abnormality of the meninges.

HISTOLOGICAL FINDINGS. Representative sections were treated as in the previous case. In addition, sections from the parietal lobe and the spinal cord at the cervical, thoracic and lumbar levels were available.

As in Case 1, the most striking changes were in the occipital lobes where sclerosis affected several gyri in the external aspect of the lobes (Fig. 6). All layers of the sclerosed cortex were diseased. Nerve cells and white matter were destroyed and replaced by dense glial scars containing streaks of collagen, which were all that remained of obliterated blood vessels. Unlike Case 1, there were several deposits of pseudo-calcium within the scars (Fig. 7).

Several cysts, lined by dense glial tissue, were present in the sclerotic areas.

Demyelination, accompanied by fine gliosis, was present in the white matter adjacent to the cortical sclerosis.

Granular atrophy affected the cortex of the occipital lobe (Figs. 8 and 9), especially the depths of the sulci. It was more pronounced than in Case 1. Nerve cells and myelin fibres were absent from the glial scars, the more discrete of which extended toothlike from the surface into the grey matter; the intervening grey matter contained both nerve cells and myelin fibres.

There was a universal focal loss of nerve cells, with astrocytic replacement, in layers 3 and 4 throughout the occipital cortex. The visual cortex around the post-calcarine sulcus was affected by this nerve cell loss.

The meninges overlying the cortical scars were not thickened and contained normal-looking vessels. Haemorrhage was present in one area over the cortical scars. The normal-looking pia over the ulegyric scars was separated from the cortex by a thin layer of structureless picrophilic material.

Unlike Case 1, there was a widespread focal loss of nerve cells in layers 3 and 4 in the frontal lobe and also in the parietal cortex and the grey matter of the insula. 'Plaques fibromyéliniques' and marginal gliosis were noted in the parietal cortex.

The cyto-architectonic pattern of the basal ganglia was normal and there was no demyelination. Numerous metachromatic bodies were demonstrated in the white matter and, although they varied in size, many were large, about ten times the size of those in Case 1.

The cerebellum was well formed, and microscopically the organ looked normal.

The optic tracts were well myelinated and the cellular components of the external geniculate bodies were normal.

The Ammon's horn, brain stem and the spinal cord were normal.

Discussion

The type of lesions described are commonly thought to follow cerebral birth injury but this was absent in Case 2. Despite certain minor differences, the great measure of clinical and pathological similarity in the two cases makes a common disease likely.

Van Bogaert (1950) reported marbling in the thalamo-striate region of a brother and sister in whose family there were epileptic and mentally retarded members. Marbling of the basal ganglia and cortical atrophy are variants of scarring which is often thought to follow cerebral birth injury, and in van Bogaert's cases laminar necrosis and 'plaques fibromyéliniques' were demonstrated in the cortices. However, scarring may be produced in different ways and, in fact, there was no suggestion of a cause of cerebral birth injury other than the prolonged first stage of labour in Case 1.

In considering possible genetic factors, the opacities of the lenses and their subluxation in Case 1 may be important. According to Sorsby (1953), these lesions are usually due to dominant genes, but occasionally recessive inheritance occurs and this may have been the explanation for the present cases.

The head circumference of a microcephalic child may be within normal limits at birth. This was so in Case 2, whose head circumference at birth was 14 in. (35·6 cm.), but at 23 months it was 41·9 cm.;

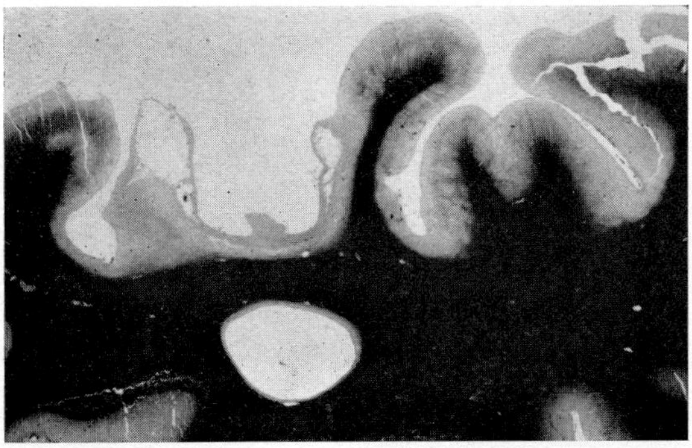

FIG. 8.—Case 2 Cortical atrophy of the occipital lobe with cyst formation. Kultschitsky-Pal ×3.

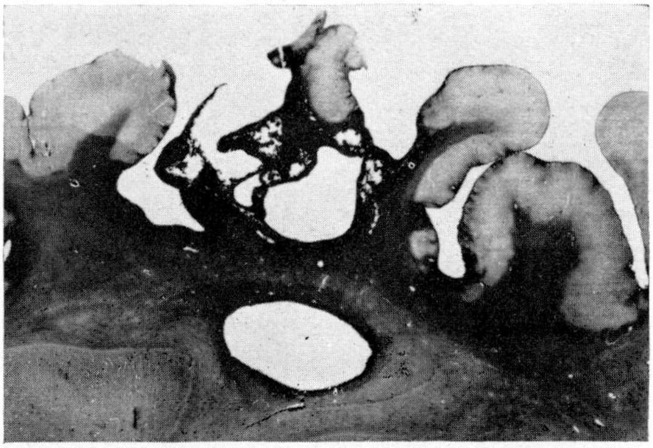

FIG. 9 —Case 2. Dense gliosis in a section at a similar level to Fig 8. Holzer ×3.

at 4 years and 4 months it was 42·5 cm.; and at 6 years and 5 months it was 44·0 cm. These last three figures are below three standard deviations from the mean for the age and sex.

Summary

The clinical and pathological aspects of microcephaly in two first cousins are described. Both children were blind, epileptic idiots. After death it was found that their brains were micrencephalic and showed cortical atrophy (ulegyria). Bilateral scarring affected the occipital lobes more than other parts of the hemispheres. In one child there was also widespread focal loss of cells throughout both hemispheres. Both brains showed laminar scars in the grey matter. One child had lenticular subluxation and opacities. It is suggested that the pathological changes in the brains might have been due to recessive inheritance.

Dr. B. H. Kirman gave me advice and Dr. L. Crome encouraged and guided me; Miss M. F. Craib gave valuable help with the family and social studies and members of other hospitals were most helpful in giving information. To all these I owe my thanks.

References

Bogaert, L. van (1950). *Mschr. Psychiat. Neurol.*, **120**, 169.
Kirman, B. H., Williams, C. E. and Brandon, M. W. G. (1959). *J. ment. Sci.* In the press.
Sorsby, A. (1953). *Clinical Genetics.* Butterworth. London.
Westropp, C. K. and Barber, C. R. (1956). *J. Neurol. Neurosurg. Psychiat.*, **19**. 52.

THE SIZE OF MENTAL DEFECTIVE BOYS*

BY

GORDON DUTTON

From Botleys Park Hospital, Chertsey

(RECEIVED FOR PUBLICATION FEBRUARY 2, 1959)

It is often stated that mental defectives are physiologically inferior to the rest of the population (Penrose, 1949), and Tredgold (1952) states that the life history of many of them shows a defective vitality of both body and mind. Goddard (1912) showed that stature and weight could be positively correlated with intelligence. These impressions are borne out by a casual glance at the inmates of any mental defective hospital but it seems worth while to take a closer look at the physical size of mental defective children for not all of them show this depression of growth. Mongols are a group of defectives who are obviously inferior physically to their normal brethren as far as height is concerned. The group of children suffering from organic lesions of the brain, having hemiplegia or some other motor deficit, are not always smaller than normal and when one comes to consider the undifferentiated type of defect one meets with those who are normal in size and those who are smaller than normal for their life age.

The physical size and development of mongols have been dealt with elsewhere (Dutton, 1959). This paper is concerned with the heights, weights and skeletal development of other groups of mental defective children, those suffering from an undifferentiated type of defect or from an organic brain lesion.

The undifferentiated group comprises those cases showing mental defect without evidence of a neurological lesion, epilepsy, psychosis or any other symptom complex allowing of a more precise classification. This group divides into two further sub-groups, those who are normal in height for their age and those who are markedly shorter than they should be. These two groups have been termed: (1) Non-pathological, those whose physical size is normal for their age. (2) 'Metabolic', those whose height is depressed by more than a year of height age (Dutton, 1958).

There are therefore for consideration four groups of mentally defective children. (The group of psychotic children was too small to make possible any valid conclusions and has therefore been omitted. Similarly cases of known metabolic error have been excluded.)

The four groups are:

(*a*) Organic	.. .. ..	31 cases
(*b*) Non-pathological	..	16 cases.
(*c*) 'Metabolic'	.. ..	22 cases
(*d*) Mongols	.. .. ..	50 cases

Material and Methods

All cases are considered to be mentally defective and are in the wards of a hospital specializing in the care of mental defectives.

The survey is confined to boys between the ages of 5 and 18 years. The bed allocation would not allow of sufficient girls for a worthwhile study.

Height. This was measured to the nearest 1/8 inch using a conventional stadiometer in the Standard Erect Position of Krogman (1950).

Weight. This was measured to the nearest ½ lb. nude apart from a pair of thin underpants, on a beam type of balance.

Skeletal Development. After considerable deliberation the inspectional method of Greulich and Pyle (1950) was selected since this is a well documented method that is economical and as only a single radiograph of the left wrist and hand is required it subjects the patient to the minimum amount of radiation. Each film was assessed on three separate occasions blind, and only after the mean of the three readings had been worked out was the name disclosed to the examiner.

Since skeletal development is expressed in years it was convenient to convert heights and weights into the same scale of measurement and this was done by reference to the tables of Sutcliffe and Canham (1950) which have been compiled from a

* This paper has been abstracted from a thesis entitled 'The physical approach to amentia' accepted by London University for the M.D. degree.

cross-sectional survey of a sufficiently large number of English children in recent years to allow a satisfactory comparison.

It is also possible to use the developmental ages in the same way as the mental age and obtain a developmental quotient (Talbot, Sobel, Burke, Lindemann and Kaufman, 1947). These workers found that the following formulae gave satisfactory results:

$$\frac{\text{Height age}}{\text{Life age}} \times 100; \quad \frac{\text{Weight age}}{\text{Life age}} \times 100;$$

$$\frac{\text{Skeletal age}}{\text{Life age}} \times 100.$$

The normal range for these methods is given as 80-120.

By using these formulae to obtain a developmental quotient it is possible to compare different age groups which would not be so easy if the raw figures alone were employed.

Results

Table 1 shows the means of the developmental quotients for height, weight and skeletal development in the four groups. This demonstrates that the mongols and the 'metabolic' group are similar as regards the depression of height and weight, whilst the other groups fall within the normal range. However here the similarity ends for it is only the 'metabolic' group that shows a significant depression in skeletal development.

TABLE 1

DEVELOPMENTAL QUOTIENTS FOR HEIGHT, WEIGHT AND SKELETAL DEVELOPMENT IN FOUR GROUPS OF MENTALLY DEFECTIVE BOYS

Group	$\frac{\text{Height Age}}{\text{Life Age}} \times 100$	$\frac{\text{Weight Age}}{\text{Life Age}} \times 100$	$\frac{\text{Skeletal Age}}{\text{Life Age}} \times 100$
Organic ..	86	92	95
Non-pathological ..	97	94	100
'Metabolic'	72	73	79
Mongols ..	68	77	95

The uniqueness of the 'metabolic' group is further shown by the fact that only 27·3% of them have a skeletal development within plus or minus 2 S.D. from the mean and the rest of them, 72·7%, have a skeletal development depressed more than 2 S.D. below the mean. These figures are practically the reverse of those obtained when one considers all the other groups together for then 74·2% have normal skeletal development and only 25·8% have their skeletal development depressed more than 2 S.D. below the mean.

Discussion

Growth and development are inherent biological attributes and it is surprising how easily normal growth is taken for granted, so that it is only when it fails to come up to our expectations that we think about it.

In the present series, the mentally defective boys comprising two of the four groups failed to grow normally, and one of these proved unique in showing developmental failure as well. It is important to make this distinction between development and linear growth because the two are under different hormonal control.

In the mongol group it is a striking fact that whereas height and weight are retarded skeletal development is normal. In sharp contrast to this, the group termed 'metabolic' shows pronounced retardation in skeletal development. This group also shows height and weight reduction but it must be borne in mind that these patients were segregated from the non-pathological group on the grounds that height was depressed by more than one year of height age; that is to say, the distribution curve of height of the original undifferentiated group was divided into two. The patients forming the tail of this curve were separated off as the 'metabolic' group and the remainder formed the non-pathological group. Hence, the 'metabolic' group, by definition, consists of patients of retarded height age and similarly those of the non-pathological group are of normal height age. Moreover, in so far as weight is positively correlated with stature, it is to be expected that the method of classification determines the normal weight age of the non-pathological group and the reduced weight age of the 'metabolic' group.

The growth disorder of mongols has already been described in detail (Benda, 1949; Dutton, 1959). The 'metabolic' group, in addition to the features already described, shows characteristic biochemical anomalies. The members of it are immature as regards steroid excretion, urinary non-protein nitrogen excretion and the level of alkaline phosphatase, whereas patients comprising the non-pathological group are normal in these respects. The details of these biochemical investigations have been described elsewhere (Dutton, 1958).

It thus appears that the patients of the 'metabolic' group, originally segregated from the remaining patients investigated by the absence of any evidence of an organic pathology and by showing the common feature of depressed height age, are also characterized by retarded development and by biochemical anomalies. From the standpoint of chemical anthropology (Macy and Kelly, 1957) it may be said that the 'metabolic' group displays widespread biological inferiority involving physical, mental and biochemical immaturity.

It might be argued that the developmental anomalies are directly related to the reduced stature of whatever cause and must therefore characterize anyone selected on the criterion of reduced stature. If this is so, then any patients belonging to the organic group who happen also to be of reduced height age should show the same biochemical and skeletal peculiarities. This has not been found to be so, for patients of reduced stature belonging to the organic group are normal in these respects. It therefore seems justifiable to assume the existence of a distinct 'metabolic' group of patients characterized by retarded skeletal development, depressed height age and biochemical immaturity. A basic biochemical abnormality seems most likely to underlie such a widespread disturbance of growth and maturation.

The non-pathological group now appears as the residue of patients after separation of all those in the series distinguishable by specific and detectable abnormalities. They are not mongols or epileptics, have no clinically demonstrable organic symptoms and are normal in respect of growth and physical development.

Many of the non-pathological group may be normal variants of the lower end of the distribution curve of intelligence. Possibly some of them are cases of protophrenia (Bourne, 1955), a suggestion that receives some support from the investigations of Hermelin and Kirwan (1958), who concluded after a study of the case histories that the incidence of pathological homes was greater in the non-pathological type than in patients from the other groups.

Summary

The results of an investigation into the heights and weights of mental defective boys are given, with the results of an assessment of their skeletal maturity.

Cases of undifferentiated mental defect can be further subdivided on a basis of physical size and skeletal maturity.

My thanks are due to Dr. J. M. Crawford, Physician Superintendent at Botleys Park Hospital, for permission to undertake this study on his patients, to the nursing staff for their help, to Mr. P. Purkiss, the laboratory technician at Botleys Park and Mr. E. Comer of the same hospital who took the radiographs, and above all to the patients who have good naturedly submitted to the various examinations.

References

Benda, C. E. (1949). *Mongolism and Cretinism*, 2nd ed. Grune and Stratton, New York.
Bourne, H. (1955). *Lancet*, **2**, 1156.
Dutton, G. (1958). M.D. Thesis. University of London.
—— (1959). *Arch. Dis. Childh.*, **34**, 46.
Goddard, H. H. (1912). *J. nerv. ment. Dis.*, **39**, 217.
Greulich, W. W. and Pyle, S. I. (1950). *Radiographic Atlas of Skeletal Development of the Hand and Wrist.* Stanford University Press, Stanford, California.
Hermelin, B. and Kirwan, E. (1958). *Lancet*, **2**, 1013.
Krogman, W. M. (1950). A Handbook of the Measurement and Interpretation of Height and Weight in the Growing Child. *Monogr. Soc. Res. Child. Develop.*, **13**, No. 3.
Macy, I. G. and Kelly, H. J. (1957). *Chemical Anthropology.* University of Chicago Press.
Penrose, L. S. (1949). *The Biology of Mental Defect.* Sidgwick and Jackson, London.
Sutcliffe, A. and Canham, J. W. (1950). *The Heights and Weights of Boys and Girls.* Murray, London.
Talbot, N. B., Sobel, E. H., Burke, B. S., Lindemann, E. and Kaufman, S. B. (1947). *New Engl. J. Med.*, **236**, 783.
Tredgold, A. F. (1952). *A Textbook of Mental Deficiency*, 8th ed. Baillière, Tindal and Cox, London.

TREATMENT OF TUBERCULOUS MENINGITIS

BY

W. MORTON FYFE

From the Department of Child Health, University of Glasgow and the Royal Hospital for Sick Children, Glasgow

(RECEIVED FOR PUBLICATION JANUARY 27, 1959)

When isoniazid is used for the chemotherapy of tuberculous meningitis the need for intrathecal therapy is controversial. A Scottish Joint Committee (1957) concluded from a comparative trial, including both adults and children, that intrathecal streptomycin is not now an essential part of the treatment. But, in fact, all the patients reported did receive intrathecal streptomycin for at least one week. Lincoln (1958) and Gaisford (1958) have abandoned intrathecal therapy but Smith, Vollum, Taylor and Taylor (1956) and Lorber (1956) maintain that some, not necessarily prolonged, treatment by the intrathecal route should be given and Miller (1958) concurs with this opinion. Since February, 1954, routine intrathecal therapy has been abandoned by one medical unit in the Royal Hospital for Sick Children, Glasgow, but retained by the other. In both units, however, the alternative method of treatment has occasionally been used when the clinician in charge judged this advisable. The purpose of the present paper is to compare the results obtained with these two methods of treatment.

Case Material

The material comprises 41 cases of tuberculous meningitis admitted to the Royal Hospital for Sick Children, Glasgow, between February 1, 1954, and December 31, 1957. In one case no treatment was given as the child died shortly after admission to hospital and the diagnosis was only established in the post-mortem room. Twenty cases received intrathecal streptomycin (Group 1) and 20 had no intrathecal therapy (Group 2). The age distribution of these patients and the stage of their disease at the start of treatment is shown in Table 1. The stage of the disease has been assessed on the patient's clinical condition as early, medium and advanced in the way described by the Medical Research Council (1948).

Three patients in Group 1 and five patients in Group 2 had a snowstorm appearance of the lungs on radiography and in five there were choroidal tubercles. One patient in each group had active spinal caries.

TABLE 1
AGE DISTRIBUTION AND STAGE OF DISEASE OF THE 40 TREATED CASES OF TUBERCULOUS MENINGITIS

Age (yr.)	Group 1			Group 2		
	E	M	A	E	M	A
0– 2 ..	3	6	0	1	5	2
3– 4 ..	0	5	1	4	1	0
5–10 ..	1	4	0	1	5	1
Total ..	4	15	1	6	11	3

E=early; M=medium; A=advanced

Bacteriological confirmation of the clinical diagnosis by smear, culture or guinea-pig inoculation of the cerebrospinal fluid was obtained in 17 cases in Group 1 and 15 cases in Group 2. Post-mortem examination confirmed the diagnosis in a further two cases in Group 2. One of the remaining three cases in each group had 'snowstorm lungs'.

Methods of Treatment

Group 1 (with Intrathecal Therapy)

Intrathecal Streptomycin. Dosage ranged from 25 to 50 mg. per injection according to age. Injections were given daily for a week, except in two cases where intrathecal therapy was stopped on the fifth and sixth days respectively. After the first week, injections were given on alternate days, twice weekly or weekly according to the physician's appraisal of the patient's progress. The number of intrathecal injections in the patients of this group ranged from five to 36.

Intramuscular Streptomycin. The daily dose was 20 mg. per lb. body weight (40 mg. per kg. body weight), given either as two divided doses (17 cases) or as a single injection (three cases). This was continued for five to seven months in 14 cases and for three to four months in five cases. One patient died in the fifth week of treatment.

Oral Isoniazid. The daily dose varied from 10 to 20 mg. per kg. body weight (5 to 10 mg. per lb. body weight). This was continued for between five and 10 months in 15 cases and for three to four months in four cases. The remaining patient was the one who died in the fifth week of treatment.

Additional Drug Therapy. Three patients were given para-aminosalicylic acid (P.A.S.). This was continued for one week in one, four weeks in another and 20 weeks in the third. One patient was given cortisone for four weeks and another prednisolone for 20 weeks.

Group 2 (without Intrathecal Therapy)

Intramuscular Streptomycin. The daily dose was 20 mg. per lb. body weight (40 mg. per kg. body weight), given either as two divided doses (one case) or as a single injection (19 cases). This was continued for five to six months in 14 cases and for three months in one case. Five patients died during their course of treatment. The duration of illness after the start of treatment in these cases was five days, three weeks, three months (two cases) and five months respectively.

Oral Isoniazid. The daily dose varied from 10 to 20 mg. per kg. body weight (5 to 10 mg. per lb. body weight). Except in the five cases where death intervened this was continued for six months to one year.

Additional Drug Therapy. P.A.S. was given to one patient for six weeks and to another for six months. Four patients received prednisolone. One patient was given intramuscular A.C.T.H. and intrathecal streptomycin (10 injections) during the last 17 days of his life. This patient is included in Group 2 as the intrathecal streptomycin did not alter the course of the illness.

Results

Recoveries. Seventeen patients in Group 1 and fifteen patients in Group 2 survived. Fourteen of the survivors in each group are well and have no detectable sequelae.

Relapses. Five patients in Group 1 had a relapse of the disease. In three, anti-tuberculous drugs were given initially for less than six months. One of these cases ended fatally. No patient in Group 2 has relapsed.

As a relapse can be regarded as a complication of the treated disease, the outcome of the relapse has been taken as the result of treatment in these cases. This has been done although one of the relapses was treated without intrathecal therapy.

Deaths. Three patients in Group 1 and five patients in Group 2 died. Of the five deaths in Group 2, one occurred from status epilepticus on the fifth day of treatment, one was in the case of a low-grade primary ament, while in the third case the tuberculous meningitis was the termination of advanced spinal caries and resulted from the rupture into the spinal subarachnoid space of a large paravertebral cold abscess.

Disabilities. Four survivors, three in Group 1 and one in Group 2, are disabled. All show mental retardation and various types of spastic palsy. One in Group 1, a girl, also has frequent convulsions and premature hypertrophy of the breasts.

One other child in Group 2, aged 2 years and admitted in the medium stage of the disease, had a right hemiplegia at the time drug treatment was completed. Eighteen months later he had made a complete recovery.

Factors Influencing Results

Stage of Disease. It is generally accepted that, apart from the nature of the therapy used, the most important factor governing the prognosis in tuberculous meningitis is the stage of the disease at the start of treatment. In both groups of the present study (Table 2) patients with advanced disease either died or had residual disabilities, whereas the majority (74% in Group 1 and 82% in Group 2) of patients in the early and medium stages made a complete recovery. The death of a boy in the early stage of the disease treated without intrathecal therapy (Group 2) was unexpected. However, he was a known low-grade mental defective which may have contributed to the fatal outcome. Comparison of the two groups shows that the preponderance of deaths in the group treated without intrathecal therapy was due to the death of two children who were in the advanced stage of the disease when

TABLE 2

EFFECT OF STAGE OF DISEASE ON RESULTS OF TREATMENT

Stage of Disease	Group 1			Group 2		
	Healthy	Disabled	Dead	Healthy	Disabled	Dead
Early ..	3	1	0	5	0	1
Medium ..	11	1	3	9	0	2
Advanced	0	1	0	0	1	2

treatment was started. One of these was the case associated with advanced spinal caries.

Age. When the results of treatment are related to the age of the patients at the onset of their illness it is seen that with one exception the deaths and disabilities were confined to children under 5 years of age (Table 3). The exception is again the case of the boy with advanced spinal caries. The less favourable prognosis of children under 3 years of age is recognized and has been shown to be due, at least in part, to delay in diagnosis (Medical Research Council, 1948; Lorber, 1954). In the present series the children under 5 years of age did tend to be in a later stage of the disease at the start of treatment than the older children. This is not apparent from Table 1 because of the wide range in the clinical condition of the patients included in the medium stage of the Medical Research Council classification.

TABLE 3

EFFECT OF AGE ON RESULTS OF TREATMENT

Age Group (yr.)	Group 1			Group 2		
	Healthy	Disabled	Dead	Healthy	Disabled	Dead
0– 2 ..	6	1	2	4	1	3
3– 4 ..	3	2	1	4	0	1
5–10 ..	5	0	0	6	0	1

Associated Miliary Tuberculosis. In neither group did an associated miliary tuberculosis of the lungs adversely affect the prognosis (Table 4). Indeed all the children with this association survived. This contrasts with the disproportionately high fatality rate in tuberculous meningitis associated with miliary tuberculosis when streptomycin was the only effective drug available (Russell and MacArthur, 1950).

TABLE 4

EFFECT OF ASSOCIATED MILIARY TUBERCULOSIS ON RESULTS OF TREATMENT

	Group 1			Group 2		
	Healthy	Disabled	Dead	Healthy	Disabled	Dead
With 'snowstorm' lungs	2	1	0	4	1	0
Without 'snowstorm' lungs ..	12	2	3	10	0	5

Spinal Block. Two children in Group 2 had a spinal block and both had prednisolone added to their therapy when the block was recognized. One had a spinal block on admission and recovered completely. The other, whose spinal block appeared during treatment, developed a progressive hydrocephalus and died. During prednisolone therapy, however, both showed clinical improvement and a fall in the protein content of the cerebrospinal fluid obtained by lumbar puncture.

Duration of Therapy. Five patients in Group 1 were treated with anti-tuberculous drugs for less than six months. Three of these had a relapse which was confirmed bacteriologically and one died. The fourth was given a further course of chemotherapy 15 months after the completion of his initial treatment because the radiological appearances in the chest showed deterioration. The fifth patient died. He was deeply unconscious with a progressive hydrocephalus after three months' treatment and, as the prognosis was regarded as hopeless, chemotherapy was stopped.

The short period of chemotherapy in these cases was probably responsible for the high relapse rate. Continuing daily intramuscular streptomycin for six months and daily oral isoniazid for a similar or an even longer period seems to be advisable if relapses are to be reduced to a minimum.

One patient in Group 2 was treated with intramuscular streptomycin for three months only but isoniazid was continued for nine months and this patient has remained well.

Method of Treatment. As complete recovery is the rule in the early stage of the disease and the exception in the advanced stage, Smith *et al.* (1956) consider that the results obtained in the medium stage are the most valuable for comparing the effectiveness of different methods of treatment. In the present series the recovery rate in the medium stage was 80% in the group receiving intrathecal therapy and 82% in the group treated without intrathecal therapy. By this criterion, therefore, the results of treatment were as good without intrathecal therapy as with it.

Discussion

There were 15 survivors from a group of 33 cases treated in this hospital with streptomycin alone (Russell and MacArthur, 1950). This is a survival rate of 45% and contrasts with 80% in the present series. As the proportion of early, medium and advanced cases is similar in the two series the higher survival rate in the present series is not due to earlier diagnosis and must be attributed to the inclusion of isoniazid in the therapeutic regime. It is disappointing that a decade has seen no progress in establishing the diagnosis at an earlier stage. In the present series the deaths and residual disabilities were almost entirely confined to children under 5 years of age, so that if improved results in the future are to be achieved by earlier diagnosis this disease must be constantly included in the differential diagnosis of unexplained illness in early childhood. The falling incidence of primary tuberculosis throughout the country may, in fact, tend towards delay in the diagnosis of tuberculous meningitis if doctors should fail to keep the possibility in mind in the case of young children with ' minor ' symptoms of only a few days' duration.

Comparison of the two groups in the present study suggests that the results to be obtained without intrathecal therapy are as good as those obtained when a small number of intrathecal injections are included in the treatment. The Scottish Joint Committee (1957) has pointed out that if a schedule of chemotherapy was ineffective an excessive mortality in the first 28 days of treatment and a high relapse rate would be expected. In the group treated without intrathecal therapy there have been no relapses and only one child died during the first 28 days of treatment. As this child became unconscious the day after treatment was started and died in status epilepticus on the fifth day of treatment it is unlikely that his death would have been prevented by intrathecal streptomycin. By these criteria therefore a combination of intramuscular streptomycin and oral isoniazid has proved in the present study to be effective treatment for tuberculous meningitis.

Conclusion

These findings are considered to indicate that daily intramuscular streptomycin for six months and daily oral isoniazid for a similar or an even longer period is the treatment of choice in the routine treatment of tuberculous meningitis in childhood at the present time. Adoption of this policy would avoid the hazards and discomforts of intrathecal streptomycin therapy in many cases of this disease. However, as superior results have not been shown to follow the withholding of intrathecal streptomycin, a limited number of intrathecal injections of streptomycin may still be advisable in children who are in the late stages of the disease when the diagnosis is established, and possibly in children whose disease does not show an early response to intramuscular and oral treatment.

Summary

Forty cases of tuberculous meningitis are reviewed. All of them were treated with intramuscular streptomycin and oral isoniazid. Twenty were also given intrathecal streptomycin in a minimum of five and a maximum of 36 injections. The results of treatment were as good without intrathecal therapy as with it. None of the children treated without intrathecal therapy had a relapse of the disease.

I wish to thank Professor Stanley Graham and Dr. J. H. Hutchison for helpful advice and criticism and for permission to publish this study of patients treated in their wards.

References

Gaisford, W. F. (1958). Quoted by Miller, F. J. W.
Lincoln, E. M. (1958). *Advanc. Pediat.*, **10**, 90.
Lorber, J. (1954). *Amer. Rev. Tuberc.*, **69**, 13.
—— (1956). *Brit. med. J.*, **1**, 1009.
Miller, F. J. W. (1958). In *Recent Advances in Paediatrics*, 2nd ed. p. 260., ed. D. Gairdner, Churchill, London.
Medical Research Council (1948). *Lancet*, **1**, 582.
Russell, S. J. M. and MacArthur, P. (1950). *Ibid.*, **1**, 59.
Scottish Joint Committee (1957). *Ibid.*, **2**, 756.
Smith, H. V., Vollum, R. L., Taylor, L. M. and Taylor, K. B. (1956). *Tubercle (London)*, **37**, 301.

PNEUMOCYSTIS PNEUMONIA ASSOCIATED WITH AGAMMAGLOBULINAEMIA

BY

J. G. B. RUSSELL

From the Royal Manchester Children's Hospital, Pendlebury

(RECEIVED FOR PUBLICATION JANUARY 27, 1959)

Infection with *Pneumocystis carinii* causes an interstitial cell pneumonia. It has been rarely reported in this country since Baar recorded a case in 1955.

The case reported here is of interest in that such an infection was associated with agammaglobulinaemia in a female infant.

Case Report

C.O., a female infant, had a birth weight of 6 lb. (2,720 g.). The parents were English and had one other normal child.

She was admitted to hospital at the age of 3 days because of abdominal distension and vomiting. This settled without specific treatment. She went home but was readmitted two weeks later with similar symptoms together with loose stools. Intravenous fluids were required and *E. coli* 0 26 was isolated from the stool. She was treated with neomycin, recovered and went home for two weeks before being readmitted again, dehydrated with diarrhoea and vomiting, and with abdominal distension. Following a course of tetracycline, she made satisfactory progress, gaining 2½ lb. (1,100 g.) in a month, reaching 9½ lb. (4,100 g.), but then had another attack of loose stools with gross abdominal distension. She was now aged 3 months and respiratory distress was noticed for the first time and was thought to be caused by the abdominal distension. A radiographic examination using a barium meal showed a distended colon, a rectum of normal calibre and coning in the rectosigmoid area. A diagnosis was made of Hirschsprung's disease, associated with enteritis. She failed to thrive.

She was transferred to the Royal Manchester Children's Hospital at the age of 5½ months. She then still weighed 9½ lb. There was gross abdominal distension with an empty rectum and she had a respiratory rate of 90 per minute associated with a bronchopneumonia. She was having loose offensive stools and vomiting. *E. coli* 0 26 was again isolated from the stool.

Tetracycline was given and she slowly improved. The *E. coli* 0 26 disappeared and 10 days after admission a laparotomy was carried out. The colon was dilated and appeared to cone to normal size at the pelvi-rectal junction. Biopsies were taken above and below this site and a colostomy carried out proximal to it. However, post-operatively the distension persisted; and as normal nerve plexuses were found in the biopsies, the diagnosis of Hirschsprung's disease was not confirmed.

She had continuous loose stools and vomiting, and required frequent intravenous fluids, including blood and plasma. An antibiotic resistant *Proteus morgani* was continually found in the faeces. From this time until her death the respiratory rate was rarely below 50 per minute and for several periods when she had signs of a bronchopneumonia was around 70 per minute. In between these exacerbations in the lungs there were persistent scattered crepitations, mainly at the bases. Radiographs taken at this time between attacks of bronchopneumonia were reported as normal. In retrospect, however, the lung fields do appear a little hazy. Because of the diarrhoea, large doses of potassium were given to maintain blood levels at a satisfactory value. She developed a bilateral otitis media, which did not respond to courses of erythromycin, novobiocin or streptomycin. The white cell count reached 12,000 per c.mm. with a polymorphic preponderance. The eosinophils were often absent and never rose above 130 per c.mm.

At this time, at the age of 7 months, the plasma proteins were examined by paper electrophoresis. It was found that the gamma globulin was only just detectable, although she had received blood and plasma before the estimation. The isohaemagglutinins were also reduced. The parents had a normal plasma electrophoretic pattern.

In view of her critical condition, it was decided to institute gamma globulin therapy without delay. She was given 0·5 g. of gamma globulin i.m. and 0·25 g. bi-weekly together with further blood transfusions. It was calculated that this would produce a level near the normal. This therapy had no apparent effect on her continuing diarrhoea and otitis media. Two weeks later a course of cortisone 5 mg. t.d.s. was given for three weeks, with novobiocin and streptomycin. Again the response was disappointing. She was given a short course of A.C.T.H. A week later she died at the age of 8 months. The immediate cause of death was a recrudescence of bronchopneumonia.

Autopsy (Dr. H. B. Marsden). Weight at death was 9 lb. 12 oz. (4,200 g.), and length $16\frac{1}{2}$ in. (41·5 cm.). She was a wasted child with marked abdominal distension. There was a left-sided colostomy.

The main findings were in the lungs. Weights: left lung 96 g. (normal 45 g.), right lung 118 g. (52 g.). The lungs were red-brown, solid throughout, with dilated bronchi containing pus. Microscopically there was extensive pneumonitis with acute and chronic inflammatory cells and plugs of exudate in the bronchial channels. The alveolar septa were thickened. Oedema, fibrin and haemorrhage with, in addition, foamy vacuolated material with swollen macrophages were seen in the alveoli (Fig. 1). Some of the vacuolated material could have been due to aspiration, but in parts there was a resemblance to *Pneumocystis* infection. There was a possible preponderance of reticulum cells. No plasma cells were seen. Silver impregnation (Le Tan Vinh, 1954) showed the presence of *Pneumocystis carinii*.

The large intestine was distended up to 4 cm. in diameter. It contained yellow liquid material and had a pale mucosa. Microscopically, the nerve supply was normal thus finally disproving the diagnosis of Hirschsprung's disease.

The reproductive organs were normal, confirming the female sex.

The only other relevant findings were in the lymph nodes. There were moderately sized nodes in the mesentery, and rather large red-black nodes in the thoracic and cervical regions. Microscopically, they showed an absence of plasma cells.

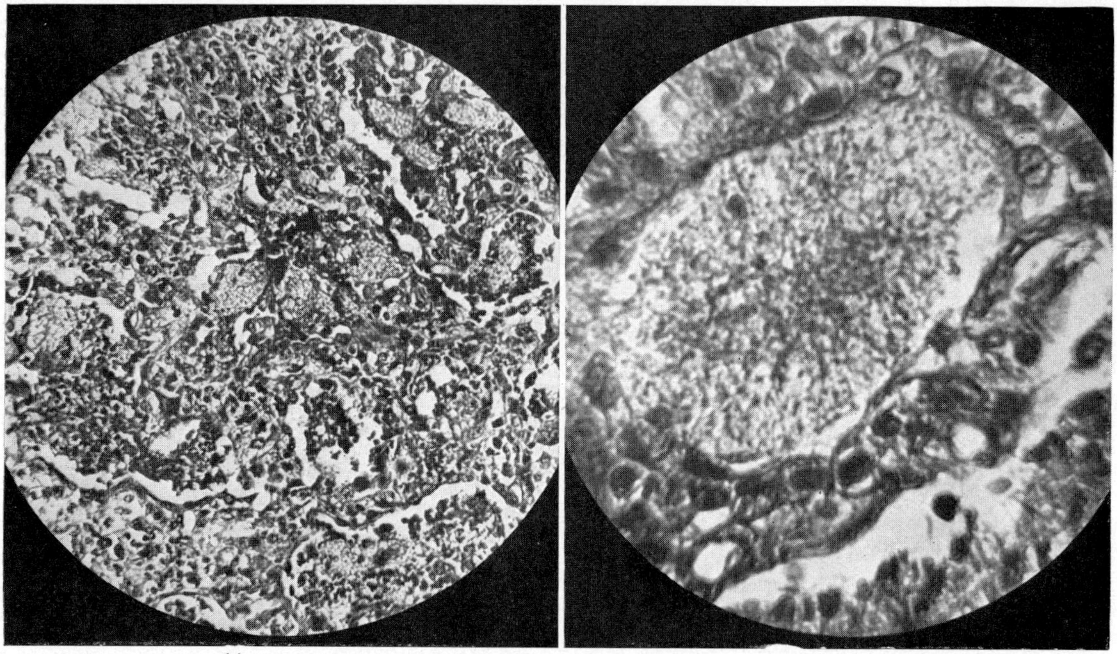

(*a*) (*b*)

FIG. 1.—Sections of lung, showing the foamy material lying in the alveoli, which was found to contain the *Pneumocystis* on silver staining (*a*) ×75. (*b*) ×650. Stain H. and E.

Comment

The diagnosis of agammaglobulinaemia was not finally confirmed before death in this case as it was felt that withholding treatment would seriously prejudice the baby's chances of survival. However, the diagnosis appeared to be confirmed by the absence of plasma cells in the necropsy material, which is the picture found in agammaglobulinaemia. This seems to be a true case of congenital agammaglobulinaemia because of the early onset of symptoms. In fact, the first attacks of enteritis occurred whilst the gamma globulin level in the child must have been near to that of the mother. The newborn's gamma globulin is maternally and perhaps placentally derived, and is as high as or higher than that of the mother. Yeivin, Salzberger and Olitzki (1956) have, however, shown that the antibodies of the enteric group, including *E. coli*, are present in much lower concentration in the newborn than in the mother's serum. Thus the newborn child is liable to attacks of enteritis, but the recurrent attacks in our patient due to the same organism are perhaps significant.

It is difficult to distinguish a true case of congenital primary agammaglobulinaemia from those cases in which there is an exaggeration of the physiological fall which occurs in the gamma globulin in infancy. Even in true agammaglobulinaemia, traces of gamma globulin can usually be detected. The true congenital form does not appear to have been previously reported in females. Harris and Schick (1954) gave unstated amounts of gamma globulin to female infants with antibiotic-resistant infections with good results, but made no measurement of the gamma globulin level. Pearce and Perinpanayagam (1957) reported the case of a female found to have agammaglobulinaemia from the age of 3 years. It was thought to be congenital because she had had recurrent infections from the age of 8 months. She had also an enlarged spleen and lymph nodes, which are common in the acquired form, and it seems likely that this was the acquired form starting at an unusually early age (*Lancet*, 1958). The diagnosis of agammaglobulinaemia was delayed in our case because it was thought not to occur in female infants.

Pneumocystis carinii is an aetiological agent of interstitial cell pneumonia. Infection with it has been reported in England only by Baar in 1955. Four cases have been reported from Scotland (Hutchinson, 1955; Bird and Thomson, 1957). Gerrard and Moore (1957) reported two similar cases from Canada. In each of these two latter reports agammaglobulinaemia in two boys was found to be associated with pulmonary *Pneumocystis* infection, and in each case a brother had also died of *Pneumocystis* infection. It seems reasonable to suppose that these siblings had also agammaglobulinaemia.

There are many cases reported from the Continent not associated with agammaglobulinaemia. Von Harnack (1954) was able to report 191 cases seen in Hamburg in four years, and there were over 700 cases in Switzerland in 1941-8 (Freudenberg and Tobler, 1950). It occurs in the first year of life, usually in infants who are premature, but less commonly also in debilitated older children. Rarely cases are reported in adults, generally with diseases of the reticulo-endothelial system. The incubation period is one to two months. There is an insidious onset of increasing dyspnoea. Physical signs are strikingly few in comparison with the marked respiratory distress, perhaps a few small patches of bronchial breathing, and a few coarse crepitations in some areas. Fever is absent or low grade. The mortality of diagnosed cases is about 20%, but probably many mild cases are not diagnosed. Radiographically, a diffuse ground glass appearance is generally found (Gajdusek, 1957). The hilar nodes are not enlarged. However, the picture appears to vary widely. In our patient, in between attacks of bronchopneumonia, the chest film showed little or no abnormality. Bird and Thomson (1957) noted fluffy opacities which became widespread and confluent. It may have been that the infection in our case was a terminal event as it apparently was in Hutchinson's first case, where the disease only lasted three days, but it seems more likely that it was responsible for the continuous dyspnoea which continued over the last four and a half months of her life.

The pulmonary infection was probably responsible for the continuous diarrhoea and abdominal distension, on which clinical attention was focused during the last months of her life. Whilst usually the presenting feature of *Pneumocystis* infection is dyspnoea, Hutchinson's second case also presented with vomiting, diarrhoea and loss of weight.

Histologically, in the lung there is extensive mononuclear infiltration of the septa. The alveoli are filled with exudate which, on high magnification, can be seen to be composed of masses of the parasite. If there is an associated agammaglobulinaemia the picture is modified in the absence of plasma cells. The organism, *Pneumocystis carinii*, has been classed as a protozoon, although some believe it to be a yeast.

Treatment has, until recently, been symptomatic, humid oxygen being the most effective agent. Tube feeding may be needed if the dyspnoea is severe. Antibiotics should be given as the diagnosis cannot be finally made on clinical examination, and in many cases there is an associated bacterial pneumonia. Antibiotics have no effect on the *Pneumocystis*. Gamma globulin has no effect even when there is an agammaglobulinaemia. It did not help our case, neither did it in Bird and Thomson's second one. Large doses of gamma globulin in this latter case did not affect the electrophoretic pattern of the serum proteins. Cortisone and corticotrophins are without effect. Recently success has been reported (Ivády and Páldy, 1958) using quinquivalent antimony compounds and aromatic diamidines.

The diagnosis of *Pneumocystis* infection is thus no longer of academic interest. Antibodies are formed and a complement fixation test has been developed (Haneke and Roser, 1958). There have been no reports of the organism being found in the sputum, but it seems reasonable to look. The white cell count shows an increase, with a polymorphic response, and an eosinophilia is often present. Gellis (1958) advocates lung puncture to confirm the diagnosis. The disease should always be suspected in a patient with an antibiotic-resistant pneumonia, or in one who has dyspnoea, especially if the physical signs are few. It may, however, present through the gastro-intestinal system.

Summary

A patient with *Pneumocystis carinii* pneumonia is described in whom there was associated agammaglobulinaemia. This latter seemed to be congenital in origin, and is unusual in that it occurred in a female infant.

My thanks are due to Mr. A. Jolleys, under whose care the patient was, for permission to publish, and to Dr. H. B. Marsden for the necropsy report, and to both for their criticism.

References

Baar, H. S. (1955). *J. clin. Path.*, **8**, 19.
Bird, T. and Thomson, J. (1957). *Lancet*, **1**, 59.
Freudenberg, E. and Tobler, W. (1950). *Ann. paediat.* (*Basel*), **175**, 185.
Gajdusek, D. C. (1957). *Pediatrics*, **19**, 543.
Gellis, S. S. (1958). *Year Book of Pediatrics*, 1958-59 series, p. 243. Chicago.
Gerrard, J. W. and Moore, D. F. (1957). *Canad. med. Ass. J.*, **76**, 299.
Haneke, K. and Roser, F. (1958). *Kinderärztl. Prax.*, **26**, 63.
Harnack, G. A. von (1954) *Ann. paediat.* (*Basel*), **183**, 224.
Harris, J. R. and Schick, B. (1954). *J. Mt Sinai Hosp.*, **21**, 148.
Hutchinson, J. H. (1955). *Lancet*, **2**, 844, 1196.
Ivády, G. and Páldy, L. (1958). *Mschr. Kinderheilk.*, **106**, 10.
Leading article (1958). *Lancet*, **1**, 1317.
Le Tan Vinh (1954). *Arch. franç. Pediat.*, **11**, 1035.
Pearce, K. M. and Perinpanayagam, M. S. (1957). *Arch. Dis. Childh.*, **32**, 422.
Yeivin, R., Salzberger, M. and Olitzki, A. L. (1956). *Pediatrics*, **18**, 19.

PERFORATION OF THE BOWEL IN HENOCH-SCHÖNLEIN PURPURA

BY

R. BASU

From the Alder Hey Children's Hospital, Liverpool

(RECEIVED FOR PUBLICATION FEBRUARY 20, 1959)

Perforation of the bowel in Henoch-Schönlein purpura has rarely been recorded in the literature. Two instances of this catastrophe are recorded here.

Case Reports

Case 1. D.J.S., a 4½-year-old boy, was admitted to the medical wards of Alder Hey Children's Hospital with a diagnosis of Henoch-Schönlein purpura. On the tenth day the child showed signs of intestinal obstruction and a mass was palpable in the right iliac fossa. He was transferred to the surgical wards with a diagnosis of intussusception.

At operation an ileo-ileal intussusception was reduced with some difficulty. The bowel was viable but there was some subserosal haemorrhage. The immediate post-operative period was very satisfactory, but, on the fifth post-operative day, the patient suddenly collapsed and on examination had signs of generalized peritonitis. After adequate intravenous therapy he was taken to the theatre.

At the second operation, on opening the peritoneal cavity, gas and faecal material were encountered. Two inches of the ileum were gangrenous and numerous large perforations were found in the healthy segment of gut, one foot proximal to the intussuscepted area. Resection of the gangrenous segment was carried out and the two ends of the bowel were exteriorized, as the condition of the patient did not permit an anastomosis. Post-operatively he was critically ill and died four days later.

AUTOPSY. Oesophagus: The mucosa of the lower third showed extensive ulceration but the muscle coat was intact.

Stomach: There was a rupture along the greater curve and posterior surface with escape of stomach contents into the peritoneal cavity. The edges of the rupture were soft and in parts congested. The rupture had certainly not been present for long before death.

Intestine: The intestine, above and below the ileostomy, was congested on the serosal surface and was oedematous throughout. There were small areas with petechial haemorrhages scattered throughout the whole length but no gross lesions were detected.

Spleen and kidney: These showed intense capillary congestion.

Lungs: They were moderately collapsed. Haemorrhagic areas were seen on the surface of all lobes and ante-mortem thrombi found in the radicles of the pulmonary arteries on both sides. There were multiple areas of infarction.

HISTOLOGY. The specimen of resected ileum consisted of approximately 30 cm. of ileum. The whole length of the gut was intensely injected with a patchy purulent exudate over the surface. There were numerous ragged perforations at various sites.

Microscopical examination of a section of the ileum, away from the perforations, showed an inflammatory serosal and subserosal reaction with congestion. At the edge of a perforation, the wall of the intestine showed haemorrhagic necrosis only.

The diagnosis was Henoch-Schönlein purpura perforation of the gut.

Case 2. T.R., a boy aged 8½ years, was admitted to the medical wards of an outlying hospital, with a diagnosis of Henoch-Schönlein purpura. He was treated with prednisolone 5 mg. twice a day. On the tenth day the abdomen started to distend and two days later signs of peritonitis developed. A straight radiograph of the abdomen revealed fluid levels. He was transferred to the surgical wards of Alder Hey Children's Hospital and at laparotomy a curious state of affairs was seen.

The peritoneal cavity could not be entered as the 'bowel' was adherent to the peritoneum. After careful dissection, the bowel was found to have three large perforations and was bound together, by adhesions, in one inextricable mass. I say 'bowel' because it was not possible to differentiate large from small gut. The three perforations were closed. A catheter was inserted into what one thought to be the proximal segment of gut and brought out through a separate incision.

After the operation the child was kept on continuous intravenous therapy and gastric suction for 15 days. His general condition remained fair but his state o nutrition suffered considerably. Ileus persisted and from the fifteenth post-operative day onwards Aminosol was administered through a polythene catheter which had been advanced into the inferior vena cava through the femoral vein. In spite of all care the patient died on the thirtieth post-operative day.

AUTOPSY. Heart and blood vessels: The right auricle and ventricle were distended. The mitral valve cusp had large adherent vegetations which appeared to be of recent origin. The inferior vena cava, below the renal veins, contained infected thrombi and so did the femoral and iliac veins.

Alimentary passages and peritoneum: The small bowel was matted together by adhesions. About 2 ft. away from the termination of the ileum, at the site of two sutured perforations, the adhesions were very dense and a further perforation was present. The gut appeared to be obstructed being grossly dilated proximal to this point and collapsed distally.

Brain: There was an early abscess in the substance, with an early pyogenic meningitis, of embolic origin probably.

Lungs: Some branches of the vessels contained ante-mortem clot, probably embolic in origin.

Kidney: There was gross pyaemic infarction with large abscesses in many areas. These grew Gram +ve cocci.

Discussion

Wolfsohn (1947) quotes Willan as having described visceral crises in purpura as early as 1808, thus ante-dating by 66 years Henoch's classical paper.

Henoch-Schönlein purpura, also known as allergic purpura, is characterized by: (1) Cutaneous manifestations, pleomorphic in character, involving mainly the extensor aspects of the limbs. (2) Colicky abdominal pain, vomiting, intestinal bleeding and intussusception. (3) Pain in the joints, haemarthrosis.

Other complications listed (Ackroyd, 1953) are (4) Bleeding from the gums and epistaxis. (5) Intracranial haemorrhages producing convulsions. (6) Nephritis, indistinguishable from Ellis' Type I nephritis, causing haematuria.

In this paper only the question of perforation of the bowel will be discussed. This complication has been seen only very occasionally. Ballin and Morse (1930) reported a case, an adult male with Henoch's purpura, in which perforation of the bowel occurred a few months after reduction of an intussusception. Unfortunately this case also died. Goldstein (1928) refers to haemorrhagic ulcers in the wall of the gut of patients with Henoch's purpura and considers that these perforate on very rare occasions.

Pathology

Kreidberg, Dameshek and Latorraca (1955) describe the lesions of Henoch-Schönlein purpura as acute perivasculitis in the walls of the small vessels occurring as a result of an immunologic mechanism. This was also observed in the two reported cases.

It is suggested that an acute vascular reaction, of this nature, in the small vessels could devitalize the wall of the bowel at several points and thus predispose to perforation. Nevertheless it is surprising, though fortunate, that this complication is so rarely seen. It must be presumed then that the reaction is not sufficiently severe to cause devitalization of the bowel wall.

Intussusception is the commonest surgical complication of this 'syndrome'. It requires prompt diagnosis and operation. Such an intussusception, if left untreated, may perforate and cause peritonitis due to the presence of non-viable gut. This also holds true to gangrenous bowel of any origin. But perforation of the bowel, as we have seen in these two cases, without any such cause is quite a separate entity. In Case 1 perforation of the bowel occurred in a healthy segment. Unfortunately Case 2 was complicated by bacterial endocarditis, due to infected emboli, and in addition had received prednisolone preoperatively. As perforation is not very common with this drug and as the endocarditis was post-operative, we can safely assume that this was another case of perforation *per se*.

Summary

Two cases of intestinal perforation, complicating Henoch-Schönlein purpura, are described.

I am grateful to Miss Isabella Forshall and to Mr. P. P. Rickham for permission to publish their cases and also for their help in the preparation of this paper. My thanks are also due to Dr. E. G. Hall for the post-mortem and pathological findings.

REFERENCES

Ackroyd, J. F. (1953). *Amer. J. Med.*, **14**, 605.
Ballin, M. and Morse, P. F. (1930). *Ann. Surg.*, **91**, 711.
Goldstein, E. (1928). *Med. Clin. N. Amer.*, **12**, No. 3 (New York Number), 869.
Kreidberg, M. B., Dameshek, W. and Latorraca, R. (1955). *New Engl. J. Med.*, **253**, 1014.
Wolfsohn, H. (1947). *Arch. Dis. Childh.*, **22**, 242.

THE NATURAL HISTORY OF THE PARTIAL THORACIC STOMACH (HIATUS HERNIA) IN CHILDREN*

BY

I. J. CARRÉ

From the Department of Child Health, Queen's University, Belfast

(RECEIVED FOR PUBLICATION FEBRUARY 9, 1959)

'It appears to me a most excellent thing for the physician to cultivate prognosis . . . he will manage the cure best who has foreseen what is to happen from the present state of matters.'

Notwithstanding the enormous medical achievements of the past half century this Hippocratic counsel remains today as fundamental a truth as when first propounded some 2,000 years ago. Regrettably, however, this aspect of medical knowledge is all too frequently ignored. There is no doubt that in the case of children with a partial thoracic stomach ('hiatus hernia', 'congenital short oesophagus') the divergent views expressed on prognosis and on the need for and value of particular forms of treatment emanate from a lack of a clear understanding of the natural history. The present review is aimed at remedying this deficiency and constitutes an attempt to outline the clinical progress of children affected with a partial thoracic stomach in the absence of either surgical or postural therapy.

Definition of Abnormality and Terminology

The following diagnostic criteria have been adopted. Only those children have been considered in whom a loculus of stomach could be demonstrated above the diaphragm either on radiological examination or at operation or necropsy. In all instances the protrusion of stomach has been through the oesophageal hiatus and the gastro-oesophageal junction has been situated within the chest at the upper aspect of the intrathoracic gastric loculus. The stomach has been the sole abdominal viscus demonstrated as protruding into the thorax (Fig. 1). Children with gastro-oesophageal incompetence but with no definite intrathoracic gastric loculus have not been considered.

The gastro-oesophageal abnormality, as defined, is referred to throughout as a 'partial thoracic stomach'. On the evidence available the use of a descriptive term has been preferred to one signifying a specific pathogenesis.

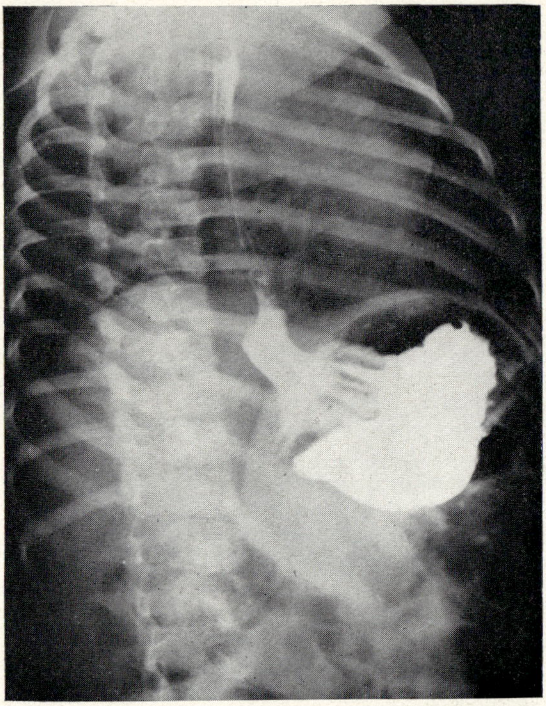

FIG. 1.—Example of a partial thoracic stomach in a 12-month-old child.

Material

The following review forms part of a study originally undertaken in 1951 at the Children's Hospital, Birmingham, and later continued at the Royal Children's Hospital, Melbourne, and the Royal Belfast Hospital for Sick Children. During

* This paper is based on part of a thesis accepted for the degree of M.D., University of Cambridge.

this period, 235 children with a proven partial thoracic stomach have been seen.

At the outset it is necessary to emphasize two major difficulties encountered in effecting this survey. The almost universal use of either surgical or postural methods of treatment since 1951 has meant that of patients diagnosed during subsequent years few could be considered in this review which is aimed primarily at outlining the clinical progress in the absence of either form of therapy. It follows that assessment of the clinical progress has had to be based on evidence relating chiefly to patients who attended hospital before 1951. As a result, though recognized as undesirable, it has none the less been necessary in carrying out this review to rely largely on retrospective evidence. The measures adopted to obviate errors inherent in such a retrospective study will be outlined in the appropriate sections.

Before 1951, a partial thoracic stomach was infrequently recognized in children. References to fewer than 100 children with an abnormality corresponding to a partial thoracic stomach were found in the medical literature published before 1951 (Carré, 1957). Thus, a second major problem was to collect a sufficiently large number of untreated patients to permit of analysis and conclusions. It appeared logical to assume that the greater number of children recognized as having a partial thoracic stomach subsequent to 1951 represented not a true absolute increase in incidence but merely reflected improved diagnosis and a greater awareness of the condition. This being so, it was argued that provided the abnormality persisted, even despite cessation of symptoms, it should be possible to recognize such cases in retrospect. To test this hypothesis, a separate retrospective follow-up study was undertaken (Carré and Astley, in preparation). Selected patients who had attended the Children's Hospital, Birmingham, between 1930 and 1950 with either an oesophageal abnormality or vomiting of undetermined cause were clinically and radiologically reassessed. As a result, over 40 previously unrecognized examples of the condition were discovered. The discovery of these cases resolved the shortage of untreated patients available for consideration.

Observations

Classification of Patients into Clinical Groups

For convenience of presentation the clinical progress of untreated children affected with a partial thoracic stomach is considered for each of three types of case: A. Survivors (i) Patients with no oesophageal stricture. (ii) Patients with a partial thoracic stomach complicated by a stricture of the oesophagus. B. Deaths.

A. Survivors. (i) Patients with no Oesophageal Stricture. In assessing the clinical progress of children considered in this section it has been necessary, for reasons already stated, to rely largely on parental retrospective information. It is, therefore, pertinent to consider the precautions taken to obtain as reliable a clinical history as possible.

All patients reviewed in this section were seen personally and one or both parents interviewed. A thorough and unhurried evaluation of the clinical progress was made at the time of interview. To provide for uniformity of information a case history sheet was drawn up listing specific points for enquiry. Questions to which answers appeared doubtful were listed with the parents' replies, if any, attached. These were then given to the parents for reconsideration at home. This provided them with an opportunity to reconsider the child's early history and to consult with other members of the family. If, on subsequent reflection, they considered their replies to have been inaccurate they were asked to return the list with their amended answers, or alternatively, such inaccuracies were corrected at the time of a subsequent interview.

In every instance it has been possible to augment and check the clinical history with case notes kept at the time of the child's original hospital attendance during infancy or early childhood. Whenever possible, information has been additionally checked by reference to maternity, health visitor and welfare clinic records and in a few instances by enquiry from the family doctor.

To ensure as much impartiality as possible in assessing the severity of symptoms, the following objective method has been used. Symptoms have been classified into the following categories of severity:

(i) Frequent: If vomiting and/or difficulty in swallowing solid food was noted to occur daily or at least on alternate days in children taking a normal diet for age. The routine use of a mashed diet occasioned by a child's inability to swallow solids has been interpreted as implying the existence of frequent symptoms despite the fact that the child on its mashed diet might have been having little or no vomiting or dysphagia.

(ii) Moderate: If vomiting and/or difficulty in swallowing solid food was noted to occur on an average of less than three times weekly but at least monthly in a child taking a normal diet for age.

(iii) Minimal: If vomiting and/or difficulty in swallowing solid food were absent or occurred on average less than once a month in a child taking a normal diet for age.

Selection of Patients. In addition to patients with an oesophageal stricture all children who had received either postural or surgical treatment previous to their last review have been excluded from this particular survey. Patients have also been excluded who had an associated unrelated chronic disorder which could have conceivably influenced their clinical progress.

Only children aged 4 years or more at the time of their last review have been considered. This age limit has been arbitrarily adopted so as to allow for as long a follow-up as possible while concurrently providing a sufficiently large group of patients to permit of conclusions.

Patients whose gastro-oesophageal abnormality was first diagnosed during life before three months of age have not been included. The progress of these infants has been considered separately in a 'prospective' review.

There were 53 patients available for study. At 4 years of age 26 had 'minimal' symptoms, 18 had improved but still suffered from 'moderate' symptoms while nine were vomiting daily or on alternate days. Further study of the symptomatic progress made by these children suggested that the clinical response to weaning on to solid food might serve as a useful prognostic guide. Of the 26 who were relatively free of symptoms at 4 years of age, 19 had shown improvement either before or at the time of weaning on to solids: of the 27 with 'frequent' or 'moderate' symptoms at 4 years, only two had improved with the introduction of mixed feeding (Table 1). On this basis, these children have been re-classified into two groups: Group I: Patients whose vomiting had improved either before or coincident with weaning on to solids. Group II: Patients whose symptoms either commenced, persisted unchanged or increased with the introduction of mixed feeding.

TABLE 1

CLINICAL PROGRESS OF 53 UNTREATED PATIENTS RELATED TO THE SYMPTOMATIC EFFECT OF WEANING ON TO SOLID FOOD

Classification of Symptoms at 4 Years	Number of Patients	Clinical Condition on Weaning: Improved	No change or worse
Minimal	26	19	7
Moderate	18	2	16
Frequent	9	0	9

The progress of patients in each group is illustrated in Figs. 2 and 3. The different clinical course followed by the majority of children in each group is evident. In Group I, only five of 21 children continued to have 'moderate' or 'frequent' symptoms after the age of 2 years and only two were not either completely or relatively free of symptoms by 4 years of age. By contrast, 30 of 32 children in Group II had 'moderate' or 'frequent' symptoms persisting after 2 years of age and 25 of these were still classified as having symptoms of at least 'moderate' severity when 4 years old. Moreover, a number of the older children in this latter group did not enjoy relative freedom of symptoms until many years later; of 15 aged 7 years or more when last reviewed, three had had symptoms of 'moderate' and four of 'frequent' severity up to 7 years.

A. Survivors. (ii) Patients with an Associated Oesophageal Stricture. The aim of this section of the review is to establish a clinical relationship between patients with an oesophageal stricture and those discussed in the previous section who were free of this complication. Clinical progress subsequent to the recognition of a stricture is not considered.

Thirty-six patients have been seen with both a partial thoracic stomach and an oesophageal stricture. In only one child was the onset of symptoms delayed until after 12 months of age. This patient had had no symptoms until the age

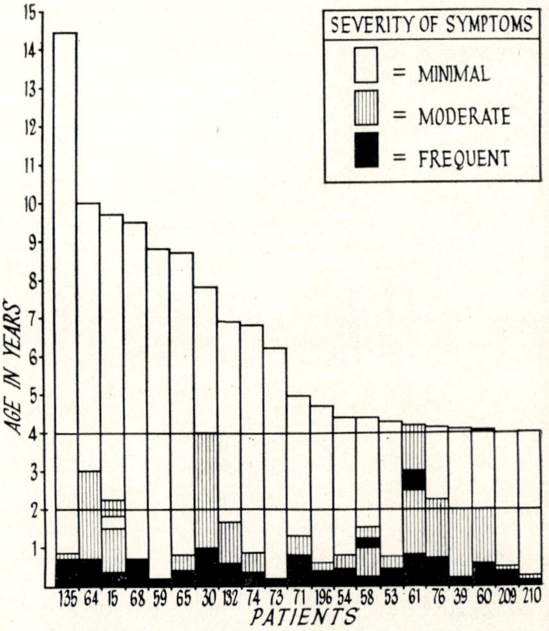

FIG. 2.—Clinical progress of 21 untreated Group I patients. Each column represents the clinical progress of a single patient.

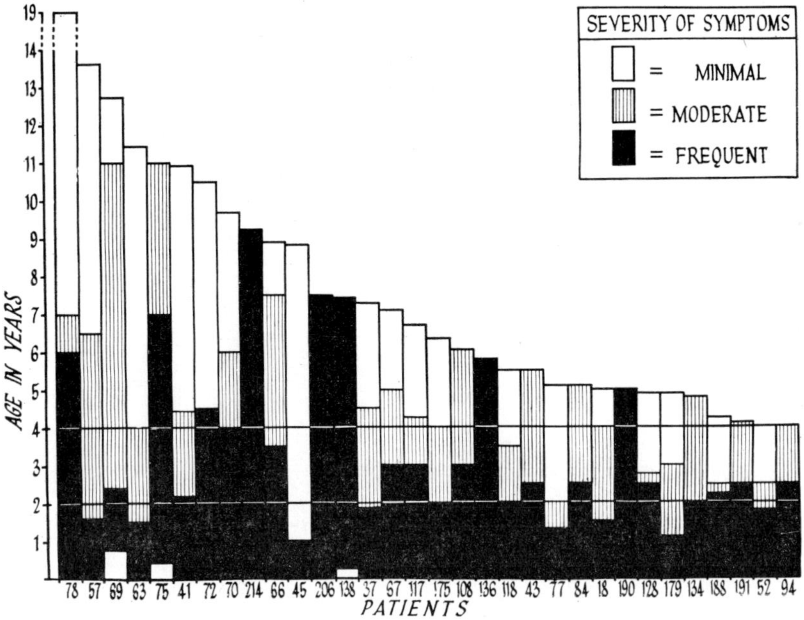

FIG. 3.—Clinical progress of 32 untreated Group II patients. Each column represents the clinical progress of a single patient.

of 5 years and 9 months. At this time she became critically ill with meningococcal septicaemia. During her illness she vomited repeatedly and this continued following her recovery. Radiological examination and oesophagoscopy confirmed the presence of an oesophageal stricture. The recognition of a partial thoracic stomach was made on review when she was aged 16 years and 4 months. Whether the partial thoracic stomach was present previous to her illness or developed subsequently as a result of cicatricial changes is conjectural.

It was not possible to determine accurately the age at which symptoms commenced in two other children. Of the remaining 33 patients, 30 had commenced vomiting within the first 4 weeks of life; the onset of symptoms in three patients had coincided with attempts to wean on to solid food.

In four instances the clinical response to weaning was uncertain. Of the remaining 31 patients whose symptoms had commenced in infancy, one child only was stated to have improved with weaning. Symptoms were recorded in three patients as starting with weaning, in eight as showing no improvement and in 19 as being definitely aggravated when weaning on to a solid diet was attempted. Nothing in the early clinical progress of these latter 30 patients distinguished them from the Group II children discussed in the previous section.

B. Deaths. In order to complete the assessment of the natural history a brief account is presented of the available data relating to the cause of death in children with a partial thoracic stomach.

The case records of 13 children who died with a proven partial thoracic stomach were available for study. None of these children had been treated by sustained posture; four had had surgical treatment. A necropsy was performed on 12 of these patients; the radiologically diagnosed partial thoracic stomach in the remaining child was confirmed at operation.

One child died of miliary tuberculosis when 3½ months old; the partial thoracic stomach was an incidental necropsy finding. The cause of death in two patients was unrelated to their gastro-oesophageal abnormality. The cause of death in a fourth child could not be accurately determined as a full autopsy report was not available.

Four children died following operative procedures. Three died within 48 hours of operation. In one, aged 3 weeks, a repair of a 'hiatus hernia' had been performed; two others, aged 2 years 3 months and 2 years 10 months, had had an oesophageal stricture resected and an oesophago-gastrostomy performed. The fourth patient was 13 years old. He died 23 days after having had an oesophageal stricture resected and an oesophago-jejunostomy performed. Death was due to a generalized peritonitis following on a break down of the anastomosis.

The fatal outcome in three children was attributed to inanition secondary to intractable vomiting. It is probable that biochemical disturbances contributed to the death of these infants. Unfortunately, biochemical data were not available. These infants were 10 weeks, 11 weeks and 4½ months old at the time of their death. One infant died when 5 months old from bronchopneumonia; additional contributory factors were prematurity, persistent vomiting from birth and marasmus. The remaining child died when 2 years 2 months old from bronchopneumonia and pneumococcal peritonitis. A gastrostomy had been performed four months previously. None of these latter five children had an oesophageal stricture.

The evidence though scanty suggests that in the absence of a complicating oesophageal stricture death in non-surgically treated patients is likely to occur during infancy from a combination of inanition, biochemical disturbances and infection.

Clinical Groups. On the basis of the evidence presented it is possible to define the following relatively distinct clinical groups:

Group		Change in Symptomatology on Weaning	Prognosis
Survivors	I	No symptoms or improved	Benign course. Majority free of symptoms by 2 years.
	II	No improvement or worse	(*a*) Prolonged clinical course with 'moderate' or 'frequent' vomiting and/or dysphagia commonly persisting to at least 4 years of age. No oesophageal stricture. (*b*) Symptomatology and progress dependent on presence of an oesophageal stricture.
Deaths			In the absence of an oesophageal stricture death likely to occur in early infancy from a combination of inanition, biochemical disturbances and infection.

Incidence of Clinical Groups

What percentage of all untreated clinically affected patients progress in a manner corresponding with each of the clinical groups outlined? A survey aimed at answering this question was undertaken at the Children's Hospital, Birmingham, during 1951-3. The following review is based on the results of that survey. Only information relating to patients attending the Children's Hospital, Birmingham, is therefore considered in this section.

In analysing the available data some degree of case selection has been necessary. Uncommon or difficult clinical problems tend to be referred to the Children's Hospital, Birmingham, from areas far removed from those routinely served by the hospital. As a result, in any paediatric problem an unduly large number of difficult and complicated cases are seen. For example, of patients with a partial thoracic stomach complicated by an oesophageal stricture, 16 of 25 (64%) came from homes outside the Birmingham City boundary. The comparable figures for patients with an uncomplicated partial thoracic stomach were 52 of 143 (36·4%). To obviate discrepancies which would arise from such irregular regional distribution, only patients living within the city have been considered.

Secondly, as the object of this survey is to evaluate the natural history in the absence of either surgical or postural treatment it has been necessary to rely almost exclusively on information relating to patients who attended hospital before 1951.

Despite this case selection, a true picture of the natural history cannot be obtained by merely comparing the number of patients corresponding with any one group with the total number available for study. This is mainly due to the fact that many of the patients were recognized following a clinical and radiological re-assessment of previously undiagnosed patients. These patients, who first attended hospital between 1930-50, were selected for review on evidence which suggested that they might have a partial thoracic stomach. Features which prompted selection were continued unexplained vomiting in early childhood and the presence of an oesophageal stricture, thereby automatically providing for preferential selection of severely affected children, i.e. Group II (*a*) and (*b*).

For this reason an alternative and more complex method of determining the relative incidence of each clinical group has had to be used. This has been done by estimating the number of children of each clinical group who could be expected to attend the Children's Hospital, Birmingham, within a period of four years. For convenience, these groups are considered in the reverse order to the previous section.

Deaths. Five children with a partial thoracic stomach were known to have died during the 10 years, 1940-50 inclusive. It is universally acknowledged that minor protrusions of the stomach through the oesophageal hiatus may be readily overlooked unless careful attention is paid to that area during the post-mortem examination. On the assumption that children with a partial thoracic stomach dying secondarily to the adverse effects of vomiting are likely to show autopsy evidence of oesophagitis, it would be expected that the pathological changes in the lower oesophagus would prompt a careful examination of that region. It is arguable that despite a typical clinical history and pathological changes in the lower oesophagus a minor degree of a partial thoracic stomach could still remain unrecognized. However, no record was found following a search of the autopsy records, for the four-year period 1947-50 inclusive, of a child with clinical features during life compatible with those of a partial thoracic stomach and who on necropsy had oesophagitis and ulceration of the lower oesophagus without a specifically mentioned intrathoracic cardia. During this same four-year period a minor degree of partial thoracic stomach was recorded as an incidental finding in one infant. Such an observation had not been made previously.

The probable authenticity of post-mortem evidence suggesting that death occurs infrequently in children with a partial thoracic stomach uncomplicated by an oesophageal stricture is supported by hospital records for the period during which this particular survey was in progress, i.e. 1951-3. No child with a partial thoracic stomach treated conservatively died during this period. Despite a careful routine examination of the oesophageal hiatus at autopsy no example of a partial thoracic stomach was detected during these years. I am grateful to Dr. H. S. Baar for this latter observation.

For these reasons it is considered that the post-mortem records for the four years 1947-50 inclusive reflect a reasonably reliable estimate of the number of untreated children dying as a result of clinical disturbances occurring in association with a partial thoracic stomach uncomplicated by an oesophageal stricture. During this time, two infants died from the effects of intractable vomiting; neither had been treated by posture or surgery. As almost half the total number of patients attending the Children's Hospital come from homes outside the city the mortality rate among infants of Birmingham residents may thus be approximately computed as one in four years.

Survivors. Group II (*b*). **Patients with an Associated Stricture of the Oesophagus.** During the 10 years, 1940-50, 14 children attending hospital were diagnosed as having a stricture of the lower oesophagus. Thirteen of these were traced and clinically reviewed. All were found to have an associated partial thoracic stomach on fluoroscopy. The untraced child lived outside the city boundary and the failure to review this patient is therefore immaterial to the present assessment. Only four of these children came from homes within the city, an incidence of one or two new cases every four years. By reason of the persistent and unpleasant symptoms associated with oesophageal obstruction it is certain that few, if any, children with an oesophageal stricture would fail to attend hospital. It is also extremely unlikely that an oesophageal stricture would remain undiagnosed. These results have therefore been accepted as providing a true indication of the occurrence of an oesophageal stricture among untreated children with a partial thoracic stomach living within the city of Birmingham.

Survivors. Group II (*a*). **Patients with no Oesophageal Stricture but with Symptoms Commonly Persisting to 4 years of Age and Later.** In an endeavour to obtain a reliable estimate of the incidence of this type of child, children who attended hospital during the four years 1947-50 inclusive, with unexplained vomiting persisting over the age of 6 months, were both clinically and radiologically reviewed. These years were chosen for the following reasons:

Patients would be at least 3 years old at the time of review. It was considered that this provided a reasonably long follow-up period for assessing the clinical progress, particularly with regard to the development of an oesophageal stricture.

An accurate list of all children with vomiting persisting over the age of 6 months was available for these years. This list was partly compiled from information kindly supplied by Dr. B. S. B. Wood.

Very few of the patients attending hospital during this period would have been treated by either posture or surgery.

As a result of this review it can be stated that of all patients attending hospital for the first time during 1947-50 and who were shown either then or later to have a partial thoracic stomach, 17 are known to have progressed in a manner comparable to that of Group II (*a*) patients; 11 lived within the City of Birmingham.

Survivors. Group I Patients Mostly Free of Symptoms by 2 Years of Age. The majority of children corresponding to this group show considerable symptomatic improvement during infancy. As a result, few are likely to attend hospital after the age of 12 months. It follows that unless diagnosed during infancy these particular children are likely to remain unrecognized.

In view of the greatly increased numbers diagnosed during infancy since 1951 it is certain that records before this date are unreliable with respect to this type of child. Since 1951, almost all infants have been treated by posture and are not therefore suitable for analysis. However, the years since 1951 provide an indication of the total hospital attendance of all groups. During the two and a half years period covered by this particular study, 41 infants under 12 months of age were diagnosed as having a partial thoracic stomach; 24 came from homes within the city. As these infants represent only those with sufficiently worrying symptoms to necessitate their attendance at hospital, these figures must be regarded as a conservative estimate of the true incidence.

It may thus be concluded that within a period of four years at least 38 infants from homes within the city will be brought to the Children's Hospital, Birmingham, because of symptoms associated with a partial thoracic stomach. Evidence has been presented indicating that of these patients one would probably die in infancy, two would have an associated oesophageal stricture (Group II (*b*)) and 11 others would suffer from vomiting or dysphagia for many years (Group II (*a*)) in the absence of postural or surgical treatment. It may be inferred, therefore, that 24 infants with a partial thoracic stomach attending hospital during a similar period would make an early spontaneous symptomatic recovery.

It is now possible to complete the assessment of he natural history by including the approximate proportion of all affected infants likely to correspond with each of the previously defined clinical groups. affected children progress in an identical manner during the early weeks of life irrespective of the eventual clinical outcome. No bias, therefore, should exist in favour of a particular clinical group in a series consisting of patients first diagnosed before 3 months of age. It is obvious that this would not apply to a series which included, for example, children originally diagnosed as having a partial thoracic stomach when between 12 and 18 months of age. For these latter children would represent mostly patients with persistent symptoms, i.e. Group II cases, as the mildly affected Group I type of child would be at this age either symptom-free or considerably improved and therefore unlikely to be brought to hospital for investigation. For this reason the recognition of a partial thoracic stomach during life before the age of 3 months has been adopted as an essential condition for consideration of patients in this analysis. As with the retrospective analysis, so allowance has had to be made for possible influences resulting from therapeutic procedures; children given postural treatment or who were operated on before the age of 12 months have been excluded.

Group		Change in Symptomatology on Weaning to Solid Food	Prognosis	Approx. % of all Clinically Affected Patients
Survivors	I	No symptoms or improved ..	Benign course. Majority free of symptoms by 2 years	60-65
	II	No improvement or worse ..	(*a*) Prolonged clinical course with moderate or frequent vomiting and/or dysphagia commonly persisting to at least 4 years of age. No oesophageal stricture.	30
			(*b*) Symptomatology and progress dependent on presence of an oesophageal stricture.	5
Deaths			No oesophageal stricture. Death likely to occur in infancy from combination of marasmus, biochemical disturbances and infection.	<5

'Prospective' Survey of Natural History

For reasons stated the preceding assessment of the natural history has, of necessity, been based largely on retrospective information. The following 'prospective' survey has been undertaken in an attempt to obtain confirmation of these deductions.

Evidence has been presented elsewhere (Carré, 1957) showing that with few exceptions clinically

Only nine of the 235 patients who have been seen qualify for consideration. The clinical progress of these children has been objectively assessed using the classification of symptoms previously described (Table 2). It will be seen that in five children

TABLE 2

PROGRESS OF NINE UNTREATED PATIENTS DIAGNOSED BEFORE 3 MONTHS OF AGE

Patient (Serial No.)	Clinical Progress (Severity of symptoms and age) Frequent	Moderate	Minimal	Age at last Review (yr.	m.)	Group
12	B* –4 y. 6 m.	4 y. 6 m.–6 y.	6 y. –LR	6	7	II*a*
14	B –LR			8	10	II*b*
19	3 d.–3 w.	3 w. –5 w.	5 w. –LR	7	9	I
20	B –3 m.	3 m. –4 m.	4 m. –LR	8	2	I
23	2 d.–3 w.	3 w. –5 w.	5 w. –LR	9	6	I
35	B –2 y. 6 m.	2 y. 6 m.–4 y. 6 m.	4 y. 6 m.–LR	6	10	II*a*
104	B –2 w.		2 w. –LR	6	8	I
183	8 d. –11 w.			11 w. (died)		—
203	B –5 m.	5 m. –11 m.	11 m. –LR	2	4	I

* Abbreviations: B=birth, d=days, w=weeks m=months, y=years, LR=last review.

symptoms improved spontaneously either before or coincident with weaning on to solid food (Group I patients). This improvement was subsequently maintained and from 12 months of age all five patients had remained free of troublesome symptoms up to their last review; four of these children were over 6½ years old. On the other hand, the three children whose vomiting had not improved with weaning (Group II patients) suffered from troublesome symptoms beyond 4 years of age. One (Case 35) had symptoms of 'moderate' severity until about 4½ years. Another (Case 12) had symptoms of similar severity until 6 years of age; this latter child when 17 months old had had a surgical repair of the 'hiatus hernia'. The third child (Case 14) developed an oesophageal stricture when about 2½ years old. The remaining patient (Case 183) died when 11 weeks old.

Allowing for the few patients studied these observations conform with the natural history deduced from the retrospective analysis. They also confirm that changes in symptomatology on weaning to solid food afford a useful guide to the patient's future progress.

Discussion

References to only 93 children with a gastro-oesophageal abnormality conforming to that of a partial thoracic stomach have been found in the literature published before 1951; only three publications referred to more than five patients (Carré, 1957). The frequently reported association of a partial thoracic stomach and an oesophageal stricture among these patients is striking. In the three series published by Findlay and Kelly (1931), Olsen and Harrington (1948) and Allison (1948), 21 of the 22 children mentioned had a stricture of the oesophagus. Of the remaining 71 children reported, 17 had an associated oesophageal stricture; in 24 insufficient information was provided for an accurate assessment to be made. Therefore, 38 of the 69 children, of whom sufficient information was available, were listed as having an associated oesophageal stricture. Judged by the high recorded incidence of concomitant oesophageal strictures the prognosis of children with a partial thoracic stomach appeared grave. At variance with this view were the conclusions of Lelong, Aimé, Aubin and Bernard (1939), Lelong, Lamy and Aimé (1940), Lelong, Aimé and Aubin (1941), Schmit (1940) and Bertoye, Bernheim and Moron (1946) who maintained that the disorder commonly underwent spontaneous cure. Supporting evidence was provided by isolated observations recorded by Christiansen (1941), Nadaud (1942), Kohler and Papillon (1946) and Nicod (1948). Each of these authors reported a single patient who had become symptom-free by 12 months of age. None of these children had an oesophageal stricture.

Despite the publication since 1951 of observations on larger series of affected children no clear picture of the natural history has evolved and similar differing opinions continue to be expressed. Belsey (1954) and Forshall (1955), for example, both regard the development of complications as constituting a major problem, while Carré (1952), Fox and Hunter (1954) and Swyer (1955) view the future of children with a partial thoracic stomach with comparative optimism. The knowledge of the natural history gained from this study provides both an explanation for such differing opinions and a rational basis for reviewing published information.

Excluding reports based on children considered in the present study (Carré, Astley and Smellie, 1952; Astley and Carré, 1954; Carré, 1957) all but one of the larger series published since 1951 have emanated from surgical clinics (Roviralta, 1952; Duhamel, Sauvegrain and Masse, 1953; Belsey, 1954; Waterston, 1954; Forshall, 1955). This raises two main considerations when interpreting these authors' observations. Firstly, many patients were treated surgically; the progress of such patients cannot be regarded therefore as indicating the natural outcome of the disorder. Secondly, because of the tendency for more severely affected patients to gravitate to surgical departments series published from these units will inevitably include a disproportionately large number of patients with complications. It is probable that most of the patients reported by these workers were of a type similar to those classified in this study as showing no improvement with weaning on to a solid diet (Group II). Such patients would be likely either to develop an oesophageal stricture or to suffer from persistent troublesome symptoms for many years. Unfortunately, the published information is inadequate for this contention to be conclusively substantiated but confirmatory support is provided by the number of reported patients who had an associated stricture of the oeosophagus: namely, five of 24 (Roviralta, 1952), nine of 49 (Duhamel *et al.*, 1953), 20 of 50 (Belsey, 1954), 20 of 132 (Waterston, 1954) and eight of 39 (Forshall, 1955). Addition of these figures shows that 62 of 294 children with a gastro-oesophageal abnormality corresponding to a partial thoracic stomach had an oesophageal stricture as well, an incidence of slightly over one in five. This compares closely with the frequency of one in six among Group II patients computed from this study. The somewhat higher incidence of oesophageal strictures among patients in the published series is probably due to the fact that whereas very few patients, if any, with an oesophageal stricture would fail to be referred for surgical treatment only a proportion of those without this complication would be likely to attend surgical departments. Moreover, as illustrated by the present study, patients with an associated stricture of the oesophagus are likely to include many referred from outlying areas not usually served by that hospital.

Before 1951, a partial thoracic stomach was uncommonly recognized in the absence of complications and hence any series which includes patients diagnosed before this date must inevitably include an excessively large number of severely affected patients. This fact is illustrated by Thomsen's (1955) publication, the only large series reported in addition to those considered. This author's series consists of 53 patients whose first hospital attendance was during the previous 30 years; of 28 who attended hospital before 1950, 14 had an associated stricture of the oesophagus, while of 25 who attended after that date only four had this complication. An interpretation of the prognosis based on an analysis of such a series without regard to this fact would obviously provide a completely misleading conclusion.

It is evident that the foregoing publications relate to selected material including a preponderance of severely affected patients. It can be appreciated how an uncritical evaluation of these reports could lead to a totally unrealistic and pessimistic attitude were such observations to be applied to all children affected with a partial thoracic stomach.

Symptoms attributable to a partial thoracic stomach commence within the first six weeks of life in over 90% of all clinically affected patients (Carré, 1957). As demonstrated in this study, symptoms in about two of every three of these children can be expected, in the absence of either postural or surgical treatment, to improve spontaneously during infancy. These observations afford an explanation for the more optimistic views on prognosis expressed by Roviralta (1952), Fox and Hunter (1954), Swyer (1955) and Plarre (1956) as these investigators have for the most part based their conclusions on a prospective review of patients diagnosed during early infancy. Moreover, the patients reported were, with few exceptions, treated by posture, a therapeutically beneficial procedure when instituted in early infancy (Carré, 1957). These authors' observations, therefore, do not truly reflect the natural history of the disorder but rather the outcome to be expected from treating infant patients by posture.

In 1953 Kelly published the results of a review of six of the nine patients previously reported by Findlay and Kelly in 1931. All had originally both a partial thoracic stomach and an oesophageal stricture. On review, these patients were between 23 and 30 years of age. All six were stated to be leading 'a normal active life' though not one was entirely free of symptoms.

Twenty-six of the patients reported by Thomsen (1955) were 5 years old or more at the time of their last review. Twenty-three suffered from troublesome symptoms beyond 4 years of age; 13 had an oesophageal stricture.

The literature contains reports of 19 other patients who had received neither postural nor surgical treatment other than dilatations for an oesophageal stricture during the first five years of life (LeWald, 1924; Wright, 1933; Christiansen, 1941; Nadaud, 1942; Huizinga, 1947; Schondel, 1947; Putney, 1948; Barrett, 1950; Pettersson, 1951; Nelson, 1953; Robb, 1954; Franklin and Henderson, 1955; Plarre, 1956). Two patients only were free of symptoms when last seen (Nadaud, 1942; Robb, 1954); 12 had an associated stricture of the oesophagus.

Thus, all reported long term retrospective reviews refer to patients with either an associated oesophageal stricture or symptoms persisting beyond 4 or 5 years of age. It is important that such reviews should be viewed in their correct perspective for although informative with regard to the progress of severely affected patients it is obvious that they do not in themselves provide a representative picture of the natural history.

It is apparent therefore that the published information does not provide a balanced and impartial picture of the natural history. However, it should theoretically be possible to obtain an indication of the overall prognosis by affecting a 'prospective' review of published cases similar to that described in this study. Reasons have been given for confining such a review to patients whose gastro-oesophageal abnormality was recognized during life and in early infancy. For only six of the reported patients given neither postural nor surgical treatment during the first 12 months of life can it be certain that the diagnosis was established in early infancy. Kohler and Papillon (1946) reported a child diagnosed at 12 days who was symptom-free when last seen at 12 months of age. Nicod (1948) and Humeau (1954) each reported a similar patient diagnosed at 3 months and 5 weeks and followed-up to 10 months and 15½ months respectively. The latter author also referred to an infant recognized as having a partial thoracic stomach at 2 weeks of age who died at 19 days from bronchopneumonia. One child reported by Robb (1954) was diagnosed at 4 months. This patient developed an oesophageal stricture. This worker also recorded a child diagnosed at 5 months of age as having an 'hiatus hernia'. This patient improved spontaneously, became symptom-free and had remained so to the time of her last review at 10 years. Thus, of these six reported patients, four made an uninterrupted symptomatic recovery, one developed a stricture of the oesophagus and one died. These observations are comparable to those recorded in this study.

In 1952 it was suggested that the clinical response to weaning to solid food might serve as a useful guide to the patient's future progress (Carré, 1952). The more extended observations recorded in this study have confirmed this view.

Summary

A review is described from which has been determined the natural history of the partial thoracic stomach in children. Evidence is also presented indicating that changes in symptomatology on weaning to solid food provide a useful guide to a patient's future progress.

It is concluded that about 60-65% of all clinically affected and untreated children pursue a relatively benign clinical course, the majority being free of symptoms by 2 years of age. With but few exceptions, these children show improvement either before or coincident with weaning on to solid food. Symptoms in a further 35% are not improved by weaning on to a mixed diet. Most of these patients suffer from troublesome symptoms up to 4 years of age and longer. A few of these latter children, representing about 5% of all patients, develop an oesophageal stricture. It has been estimated that in the absence of an oesophageal stricture less than 5% of all untreated patients would die.

It is suggested that neglect of the study of the natural history has been largely responsible for the differing views expressed on prognosis and on the need for and value of particular forms of treatment. By critically evaluating published information in relation to the knowledge gained from this study it has been possible to explain how the divergent opinions expressed have come to be formulated.

I am considerably indebted to Dr. R. Astley of the Radiology Department, Children's Hospital, Birmingham, not only for many radiological observations during the early part of this study but also for much valuable advice and ever-willing co-operation. I wish in addition to record my appreciation and gratitude to the following: Professor J. M. Smellie of the University of Birmingham to whom I am especially grateful for much support and encouragement; all members of the medical and surgical consultant staff of the Children's Hospital, Birmingham, the Royal Children's Hospital, Melbourne, and the Royal Belfast Hospital for Sick Children who have permitted me to examine and follow-up their patients; Dr. F. Plarre for the fluoroscopic examination of patients attending the Royal Children's Hospital, Melbourne, Dr. D. Boyd of the Royal Belfast Hospital for Sick Children for permission to undertake the fluoroscopic examination of patients in his department, and Dr. H. S. Baar of the Children's Hospital, Birmingham, for access to autopsy records.

References

Allison, P. R. (1948). *Thorax*, **3**, 20.
Astley, R. and Carré, I. J. (1954). *Radiology*, **62**, 351.
Barrett, N. R. (1950). *Brit. J. Surg.*, **38**, 175.
Belsey, R. (1954). *Ann. roy. coll. Surg. Engl.*, **14**, 303.
Bertoye, P., Bernheim, M. and Moron, M. (1946). *Arch. franç. Pédiat.*, **3**, 485.
Carré, I. J. (1952). *Arch. Dis. Childh.*, **27**, 300.
—— (1957). M.D. Thesis. Cambridge.
——, Astley, R. and Smellie, J. M. (1952). *Lancet*, **2**, 1150.
Christiansen, H. (1941). *Acta radiol. (Stockh.)*, **22**, 360.
Duhamel, B., Sauvegrain, J. and Masse, N. P. (1953). *Poumon*, **9**, 33.
Findlay, L. and Kelly, A. Brown (1931). *J. Laryng.*, **46**, 797.
Forshall, I. (1955). *Arch. Dis. Childh.*, **30**, 46.
Fox, E. G. and Hunter, J. L. P. (1954). *J. Irish med. Ass.*, **34**, 136.
Franklin, R. H. and Henderson, I. D. (1955). *Arch. Dis. Childh.*, **30**, 55.
Huizinga, E. (1947). *Ned. T. Geneesk.*, **91**, 1132.
Humeau, A. (1954). M.D. Thesis. Univ. Bordeaux.
Kelly, H. D. Brown (1953). *Proc. roy. Soc. Med.*, **46**, 943.
Kohler, C. and Papillon, J. (1946). *Arch. franç. Pédiat.*, **3**, 485.
Lelong, M., Aimé, P., Aubin, A. and Bernard, J. (1939). *Bull. Soc. méd. Hôp. Paris*, **55**, 145.
——, Aimé, P. and Aubin, A. (1941). *Presse méd.*, **49**, 106.
——, Lamy, M. and Aimé, P. (1940). *Bull. Soc. méd. Hôp. Paris*, **56**, 681.
LeWald, L. T. (1924). *Radiology*, **3**, 91.
Nadaud, P. (1942). *J. Radiol. Électrol.*, **25**, 139.
Nelson, T. Y. (1953). *Aust. N.Z. J. Surg.*, **22**, 192.
Nicod, M. (1948). *Praxis*, **37**, 745.
Olsen, A. M. and Harrington, S. W. (1948). *J. thorac. Surg.*, **17**, 189.
Pettersson, G. (1951). *Acta paediat. (Uppsala)*, **40**, Suppl. 83, p. 73.
Plarre, F. E. (1956). *Med. J. Aust.*, **2**, 241.
Putney, F. J. (1948). *Ann. intern. Med.*, **28**, 1094.
Robb, D. (1954). *Aust. N.Z. J. Surg.*, **24**, 18.
Roviralta, E. (1952). *Les Vomissements du Nourrisson*. Flammarion, Paris.
Schmit, L. (1940). M.D. Thesis. Paris.
Schondel, A. (1947). *Nord. Med.*, **33**, 419.
Swyer, P. R. (1955). *A.M.A. Amer. J. Dis. Child.*, **90**, 421.
Thomsen, G. (1955). *Acta radiol. (Stockh.)*, Suppl. 129.
Waterston, D. (1954). *Proc. roy. Soc. Med.*, **47**, 536.
Wooler, G. H. (1948). *Thorax*, **3**, 53.
Wright, A. J. (1933). *J. Laryng.*, **48**, 773.

BRITISH PAEDIATRIC ASSOCIATION

Proceedings of the Thirtieth Annual General Meeting

The Annual Meeting of the British Paediatric Association was held at the Royal Hotel, Scarborough, from April 22 to 25, 1959.

BUSINESS PROCEEDINGS. Dr. John Forest Smith took the Chair as President, and the following members were present:

> I. McA. Anderson, E. C. Allibone, J. Apley, G. C. Arneil, Cécile Asher, A. D. Barlow, J. Bowlby, Frances Braid, P. T. Bray, E. G. Brewis, F. S. W. Brimblecombe, D. Browne, R. W. Brookfield, T. A. Brand, W. A. B. Campbell, W. H. P. Cant, I. A. B. Cathie, T. Colver, Beryl D. Corner, E. C. R. Couper, S. D. M. Court, Christine Cooper, J. Crooks, V. Mary Crosse, J. Craig, W. S. Craig, G. Davison, M. E. Disney, D. M. Douglas, A. C. Doyne Bell, S. P. Dundon, H. L. Ellis, R. W. B. Ellis, J. L. Emery, P. R. Evans, H. G. Farquhar, H. V. L. Finlay, J. O. Forfar, Isabella Forshall, W. F. Gaisford, W. H. Galloway, Sylvia K. Guthrie, E. W. Hart, J. L. Henderson, W. Henderson, J. B. Heycock, C. J. Hodson, A. Holzel, D. V. Hubble, F. P. Hudson, J. H. Hutchison, R. S. Illingworth, N. M. Jacoby, Ursula James, R. T. Jenkins, H. Jolly, H. Everley Jones, J. J. Kempton, C. W. Kesson, G. M. Komrower, J. Lorber, P. MacArthur, R. A. McCance, D. MacCarthy, A. M. MacDonald, Agnes MacGregor, M. MacGregor, Helen M. M. Mackay, R. C. Mac Keith, T. P. Mann, J. H. Moseley, G. H. Newns, D. N. Nicholson, A. P. Norman, J. N. O'Reilly, A. P. M. Page, W. H. Patterson, W. W. Payne, C. P. Pinckney, L. J. Prosser, T. S. Rodgers, K. B. Rogers, B. E. Schlesinger, L. G. Scott, C. C. de Silva, R. A. Shanks, W. Sheldon, J. M. Smellie, R. E. Smith, T. Stapleton, R. E. Steen, W. P. Sweetnam, P. N. Swift, K. H. Tallerman, Dorothy Taylor, John Thomson, J. P. M. Tizard, D. H. Wallace, H. R. E. Wallis, C. Warren, A. G. Watkins, I. G. Wickes, H. P. Williams, D. A. J. Williamson, B. D. R. Wilson, D. W. Winnicott, B. S. B. Wood, Barbara Woodhead, S. Yudkin.

Professor A. M. Claye, President of the Royal College of Obstetricians and Gynaecologists, Dr. Geoffrey Dawes (George Frederic Still Memorial Lecturer) and Mr. G. J. Piller were the guests of the Association.

The following were present as guests of members of the Association:

> J. Alpert (U.S.A.), H. Angelman, M. W. Arthurton, Margaret Baber, J. Bate, A. C. Blandy, B. D. Bower, A. H. Cameron, K. Cameron, A. Clark, J. D. Crawford (U.S.A.), R. D. G. Creery, Pamela Davies, E. E. Doyle, O. D. Fisher, G. Gearty, H. Van Gelderen (Holland), Marcia Hall, E. E. Hill, T. S. Ingram, R. J. Isaac, P. M. Jeavons, J. Jones, O. Kauste (Finland), A. C. Kendall, B. M. Laurence, D. N. Lawson, D. Macaulay, J. C. Macaulay, Anne McCandless, Margaret Middleton, J. N. Montgomery, A. Moore, B. O'Donnell, Eileen M. O'Neill, M. W. Partington, J. H. Peel, M. G. Philpott, J. D. Pickup, Jackson Rees, K. Rhaney, J. R. Robert, E. G. G. Roberts, J. Rubie, J. Sakula, M. J. Simpkiss, A. H. Snaith, A. L. Speirs, J. M. Stansfeld, D. G. H. Stone, L. B. Strang, James Thomson, D. G. Vulliamy, H. J. Weston (New Zealand), R. H. R. White, R. H. White-Jones, R. Wigglesworth, H. Williams (Australia), O. H. Woolf, T. Wright.

The Annual General Meeting was held on April 23, 1959.

The Minutes of the last meeting, which had been published in the *Archives of Disease in Childhood*, were received and approved.

ELECTION OF OFFICERS. The following were elected:

> PRESIDENT: Dr. R. C. Lightwood
> PRESIDENT-ELECT: Professor A. V. Neale
> TREASURER: Professor A. G. Watkins
> SECRETARY: Dr. E. W. Hart

EXECUTIVE COMMITTEE, 1959-62:

> Dr. P. R. Evans, Dr. A. White Franklin, Dr. Victoria Smallpeice, Dr J. P. M. Tizard.

ELECTION OF MEMBERS. The following were elected:

HONORARY MEMBERS

Dr. J. Forest Smith, Dr. J. A. Fraser Roberts, Dr. Helen M. M. Mackay, Dr. W. W. Payne, Professor L. S. Penrose.

CORRESPONDING MEMBERS

Dr. C. Elaine Field (Singapore), Professor C. A. Janeway (Boston), Professor J. H. P. Jonxis (Groningen), Professor M. Lelong (Paris), Dr. A. Thomas (Paris).

ORDINARY MEMBERS

H. Angelman, M. W. Arthurton, Margaret D.

Baber, J. A. Black, A. C. Blandy, N. Butler, R. D. G. Creery, S. B. Dimson, E. E. Doyle, O. D. Fisher, T. N. Fisher, J. L. Garvie, R. J. Isaac, A. C. Kendall, A. C. Kirby, B. M. Laurence, D. N. Lawson, D. Macaulay, J. C. Macaulay, Anne E. McCandless, W. J. Matheson, Margaret Middleton, D. Morris, T. C. Noble, M. G. Philpott, J. D. Pickup, R. H. Pugh, E. G. G. Roberts, J. Rubie, J. Sakula, A. L. Speirs, D. G. H. Stone, James Thomson, D. G. Vulliamy, R. H. White-Jones, R. Wigglesworth, O. H. Woolf, T. Wright.

The Treasurer's report and statement of accounts for the year 1958-59 were received and adopted and the auditors were re-appointed for the coming year.

The report of the Executive Committee was received and approved and is printed below.

The proposal to increase the subscription to the Association to five pounds a year to include the subscription to the *Archives of Disease in Childhood* was carried by a large majority.

The warm thanks of the Association were expressed to Dr. P. R. Evans at the expiry of his five years' work as Honorary Secretary.

Report of the Executive Committee 1958-59

OBITUARY. The Association has suffered the loss of two honorary members, Dr. D. N. Nabarro and Dr. T. Pearse Williams, and of a corresponding member, Dr. H. Helmholz.

EXECUTIVE COMMITTEE

The Committee's members are: J. Forest Smith, K. H. Tallerman, R. Lightwood, A. G. Watkins, P. R. Evans, A. C. Doyne Bell, D. MacCarthy, R. C. Mac Keith, E. W. Hart, I. A. B. Cathie, Isabella Forshall, F. F. Kane, M. MacGregor, J. Apley, D. V. Hubble, P. MacArthur, L. G. Scott.

The following are invited to attend as observers: Cécile Asher (Ministry of Education), Dorothy Taylor (Ministry of Health), W. P. Sheldon—from April 1959 (Ministry of Health), J. C. R. Buchanan (Colonial Office).

The Committee met in November, 1958, and February and April, 1959. In addition to receiving reports from sub-committees (see below) the following matters were among the more important considered:

1. LIAISON WITH BRITISH MEDICAL ASSOCIATION. The two Associations are often asked to give evidence to committees and so on but have no ready mechanism for finding out when this is occurring or for comparing points of view. Attempts are being made to remedy the deficiency but so far nothing has been achieved except an agreement in principle. It should however be added that the Public Health Committee of the B.M.A. has for years sent its agenda and minutes to the secretary of the B.P.A.

2. ARCHIVES OF DISEASE IN CHILDHOOD. At the last Annual General Meeting the Executive was asked to consider and recommend whether subscription to the *Archives* at £3 0s. 0d. a year should be compulsory for all ordinary members, or whether to continue, as at present, the payment of £4 4s. 0d. a year if one wishes to subscribe. The Executive recommends the block subscription, *i.e.* £2 0s. 0d. annually as subscription to the Association and in addition £3 0s. 0d. annually for the *Archives*.

3. CHILDREN IN ADULT WARDS. Discussion and investigation (the latter conducted by M. MacGregor) of the number of children in adult wards have continued. It seems that about 16% of children are in adult wards but there are wide local variations. It was pointed out that the Faculty of Ophthalmology recommended in 1958 that children having eye operations should be cared for in ophthalmic departments; subsequently the report of the Platt Committee on the Welfare of Children in Hospital appeared, in which this special point is adequately dealt with.

4. QUEEN MARY'S HOSPITAL, CARSHALTON. After considering a letter and documents submitted by the Physician-Superintendent of this hospital, the Executive affirmed the Association's support of the policy advocated in the 1957 report of the Paediatric Committee of the Royal College of Physicians of London and asked to be kept informed of developments.

5. INVITATION FROM SWEDISH PAEDIATRIC SOCIETY. An invitation for 20 members to visit Sweden in September, 1960, was accepted.

6. POLIOMYELITIS CONGRESS. It was agreed that the Association should do what it could to further the success of the International Poliomyelitis Congress to be held in London in 1960.

7. CANADIAN JOINT MEETING. It was agreed that the joint meeting of the Canadian and British Associations should be held in Britain during July, 1961.

8. GENERAL PHYSICIANS. It was decided to enquire how many paediatric sessions were being conducted by general physicians. Most regions have supplied the information requested.

9. COMMONWEALTH VISITOR. Following a suggestion made by D. Gairdner, it was decided to try to raise money to assist a paediatrician from the

Commonwealth to visit Britain each year at a time which would allow him to attend the annual meeting.

10. THE COUNCIL. It was agreed to propose in 1960 alterations of the Rules so that the Executive Committee should change its name to The Council. Membership of the Executive Committee is almost always initiated by the proposal of the name of a candidate by one of the members of the Committee at its February meeting. Rule 4 permits any member of the Association to propose candidates and it is hoped that in future proposals will be sent in, in the same way as proposals for membership of the Association.

11. MEMBERSHIP. In view of the unprecedented increase in membership occurring from 1958 to 1960 it was decided to nominate for election only consultant paediatricians, and to take an early opportunity to debate future membership policy with regard to other specialists, such as paediatric surgeons and children's psychiatrists.

12. PAEDIATRIC EDUCATION. Some years ago a W.H.O. questionnaire on paediatric education in Europe was circulated. We were asked this year to follow it up by sending a representative to Zürich to discuss 'some selective measure which will increase definitely the standard of paediatric education', but declined, as we thought the initial enquiry did not provide a reliable basis for the discussion.

13. OTHER TOPICS. Other matters discussed were: arrangements for the annual meeting; nomination of members of the Association and its committees; preventive aspects of child health; accidents in childhood; formation of the Paediatric Research Society and the Paediatric Visiting Club; Niehans' treatment for mongolism; and the Report to the Government of Northern Ireland on Child Guidance and Speech Therapy.

STANDING COMMITTEES

CHILD PSYCHOLOGY: J. Apley, R. C. Mac Keith, Mildred Creak, D. V. Hubble, R. Mayon-White, A. A. Moncrieff, C. T. Potter, D. MacCarthy.

Report on psychiatric services for children sent to all paediatricians; report of proceedings submitted November, 1958, and April, 1959.

NURSING: A. G. Watkins, Mildred Creak, W. P. H. Sheldon, D. J. Waterston, R. S. Illingworth.

No report.

TROPICAL MEDICINE: R. Lightwood, R. W. B. Ellis, Cicely Williams, M. MacGregor, A. A. Moncrieff, A. G. Watkins.

Reported October, 1958: post-graduate education in this country to be fostered; secondment to overseas territories should be facilitated.

JAMES SPENCE MEDAL: The Secretary, N. B. Capon, C. G. Parsons, R. A. McCance, F. J. W. Miller.

No recommendation yet made.

JOINT COMMITTEE WITH R.C.O.G.: P. R. Evans, F. J. W. Miller, J. H. Hutchison, R. Lightwood, A. A. Moncrieff.

No report.

REPRESENTATIVES:

- National Association for Mental Health: R. C. Mac Keith
- U.K. Committee for Poliomyelitis: E. W. Hart
- Maternity and Midwifery Committee of Ministry of Health: J. Forest Smith
- Standing Tuberculosis Committee of Ministry of Health: W. S. Gaisford
- Joint Tuberculosis Council: W. S. Gaisford
- Standing Maternity Hospital Report Committee of R.C.O.G.: A. A. Moncrieff
- Medical Advisory Committee of Nursery Schools Association: L. G. Scott
- Leonard Parsons Memorial Committee: S. Graham
- Editorial Committee, *Archives of Disease in Childhood:* see list in *Archives*

AD HOC COMMITTEES

SCHOOL CLINICS: Cécile Asher, A. C. Doyne Bell, R. C. Mac Keith.

Recommendations about referring children for second opinions and about medical treatment at school clinics sent to South-East Metropolitan Regional Paediatric Society and to Ministry of Education.

SOFT DRINKS: P. R. Evans, W. W. Payne.

Report sent to Ministry of Agriculture, Fisheries and Food.

COMPOSITION OF MILK (COOK COMMITTEE): E. W. Hart, W. A. B. Campbell, I. A. B. Cathie, J. Thomson.

Written evidence sent; the Committee has now asked for oral evidence as well.

MEDICAL CARE OF ADOLESCENTS: D. V. Hubble, R. Gordon, R. C. Mac Keith, Victoria Smallpeice, R. E. Smith.

Report sent to Royal College of Physicians Paediatric Committee and to British Medical Association; published in *The Lancet*.

HALF CREAM CONDENSED MILK: Helen Mackay, P. MacArthur, Winifred Young.

Comments sent to Ministry of Agriculture, Fisheries and Food.

SKIMMED MILK WITH ADDED FAT: Helen Mackay, P. MacArthur, Winifred Young.

Letter approving labelling sent to Ministry of Agriculture, Fisheries and Food.

ADOPTION: MEDICAL EXAMINATION: R. C. Mac Keith, D. MacCarthy, A. White Franklin.

Report on examination before adoption sent to Standing Conference of Adoption Societies.

ADOPTION: LORD CHANCELLOR'S MEDICAL REPORT: P. R. Evans, R. C. Mac Keith, D. MacCarthy, A. White Franklin.

Comments sent to the Ministry of Health.

ARTIFICIAL INSEMINATION: W. S. Craig, E. W. Hart, A. P. Norman, C. O. Carter.

Report sent to Home Office Departmental Committee.

INFECTIOUS DISEASES HOSPITALS: R. H. Dobbs, F. F. Kane, M. MacGregor, Dorothy Taylor.

No report.

QUESTIONNAIRES

One of the admirable features of the Association is the facility it offers for quick surveys which may answer questions which are being asked urgently, e.g. do we see ariboflavinosis? It is the good response which makes these exercises so valuable. In the recent enquiry about parents in hospital, carried out for the Nuffield Foundation, 96% of those in clinical paediatric practice replied, a truly remarkable figure. The results have not yet been analysed, but I hope they will be available to us before long.

SCIENTIFIC SESSIONS

G. C. ARNEIL (Glasgow). 'Nephrosis in the Early Months of Life.' During the past few years 168 cases of the nephrotic syndrome were followed up at the Royal Hospital for Sick Children, Glasgow. Sixty-four (38%) were aged less than 2 years at the time of onset of the disease. This finding differs from the incidence in other areas. The various factors which may have contributed to the high incidence in these young patients were discussed. Four cases of congenital nephrosis were seen and all died. The prognosis of these young patients was found to differ significantly according to sex, and to the duration of oedema. The results of long-term follow-up are included.

W. W. PAYNE (London). 'A Comparison of Different Forms of Therapy in Nephrosis.' Three periods of treatment were reviewed, pre-antibiotics, antibiotics and antibiotics plus steroids. In the first group approximately 50% recovered and 50% died. In the second group 53% recovered and 32% died, and in the third group 40% recovered and 45% died.

The causes of death in the first group were mainly of infective origin, only 17% being from uraemia. In the second group 50% were from uraemia and in the third group 55%. In the second group individual treatments, diuretics (urea, water, mersalyl), resins and thyroid showed that time is the main factor causing healing since no treatment at all other than diet and antibiotics gave the best result. Steroids gave no better results until long-term treatment (six months or more) was given, when a remission rate, higher than the expected 50%, was obtained.

B. D. BOWER and P. M. JEAVONS (Birmingham). 'The Prognosis of Infantile Spasms.' Thirty patients with infantile spasms starting before the age of 12 months were followed by clinical and E.E.G. examinations for periods varying from 18 months to four years. The authors' scoring system was used to assess the severity of E.E.G. abnormality. All the first E.E.G.s were abnormal, 11 being hypsarrhythmic. At 2½ years of age half the patients were free of spasms and over one-third had normal E.E.G.s; only two had hypsarrhythmic E.E.G.s. There was no general mental improvement, but two were mentally normal at 2½ years. The E.E.G.s of patients in the perinatal injury group were on average more abnormal than those of the cryptogenic group but up to 2½ years the incidence of spasms in the two groups was the same.

Corticotrophin was given to seven other patients. Spasms were controlled and E.E.G. improvement occurred in five, but mental retardation was unchanged.

M. J. SIMPKISS (London). 'Anaemia and Kwashiorkor.' Children with kwashiorkor were more anaemic than controls. Both groups had reticulocytosis, a low serum iron and the same incidence of malaria and kwashiorkor. Anaemic kwashiorkor children had broad thin red cells and a cellular marrow, often macronormoblastic.

All kwashiorkor children were given skimmed milk. Some were given folic acid, intramuscular iron or both. In all groups there was a big unexplained fall in haemoglobin and later a rise. Reticulocytosis occurred at the beginning of treatment with an eventual rise in haemoglobin. The fall was not due to increased plasma volume. The final haemoglobin was higher in cases given iron and folic acid.

T. T. S. INGRAM (Edinburgh). 'The Fertility of Mothers of Diplegic Children and the Fate of Their Conceptions.' The reproductive performance of 76 mothers of diplegic children was compared with that of mothers of children suffering from other forms of cerebral palsy and of mothers from the general population. The mothers of diplegic children had had fewer pregnancies than those in the other groups though their average age was slightly greater. There were fewer conceptions in the years immediately preceding and following the birth of the diplegic child than at earlier or later periods.

Excluding from consideration the pregnancies which resulted in the birth of the patients, only 62% of other conceptions had produced healthy siblings who survived at the time of the study. In a high proportion there had been abnormalities of pregnancy, labour or delivery.

There appears to be an aetiological relationship between diplegia and impaired reproductive performance of the mother.

J. H. PEEL (London). 'The Baby of the Diabetic Mother.' The causation of the unavoidable, high perinatal mortality in pregnant diabetics remains uncertain. Foetal loss may be due to intra-uterine foetal death or to early neonatal death associated with the pulmonary syndrome of the newborn.

The evidence suggests that antenatal environmental factors play a part in the early neonatal mortality as well as in causing intra-uterine death. King's College Hospital has work in progress in an attempt to assess the extent and significance of foetal anoxia as follows:

1. Determination of uterine blood flow by means of radioactive sodium clearance tests.
2. Determination of oxygen saturation of foetal cord blood.
3. Cord haemoglobin levels at birth.

The importance of bed rest in the last weeks of pregnancy was emphasized. Attempts to determine hormonal placental function in the mother were described and the results of cortisone administration to the newborn in a series of babies presented.

G. GEARTY (Liverpool). 'A Review of 25 Cases of Patent Ductus Arteriosus Diagnosed and Treated Surgically during the First Year of Life.' The value of clinical, E.C.G. and radiological findings and of other ancillary investigations was discussed and illustrated.

Reference was made to the very large ductus and its additional problem of diagnosis.

The differentiation of a patent ductus from other lesions in infancy was considered and the difficulties of diagnosis when a patent ductus arteriosus is associated with other malformations, such as coarctation of the aorta, tricuspid atresia and pulmonary stenosis, were discussed.

H. J. WESTON (London). 'Analysis of the Results of Surgical Treatment of Congenital Heart Disease.' An analysis of the results of, and difficulties with, surgery on children up to 12 months of age who suffer from congenital heart disease was presented. This surgery has been performed mainly by Mr. David Waterston at The Hospital for Sick Children, Great Ormond Street, London. The series totalled about 120 cases during the years 1955-1957 inclusive.

A. H. SNAITH (London). 'Oestrogen Excretion in Childhood, in Health and Disease.' No adequate figures for oestrogen excretion by children in health or disease are available. The recently developed method of Brown has made this possible and figures were given for normal boys and normal girls up to the age of 15. Figures for oestrogen excretion in precocious puberty in girls, in cases of adrenal and ovarian tumours and in gynaecomastia were given. The origin of the urinary oestrogens in children and the interpretation of the figures obtained in pathological conditions were discussed.

JACKSON REES (Liverpool). 'Anaesthetic Methods Applied to the Treatment of Respiratory Disease in Infancy.' The communication defined respiratory insufficiency as a disproportion between cellular respiration and gaseous exchange, and suggested that such a disproportion is the proximal cause of death in cases of acute respiratory disease in infancy.

The way in which modern anaesthetic methods may be applied therapeutically to restore the equilibrium between metabolic requirements and gaseous exchange in cases of respiratory insufficiency was described, and examples were given of the successful application of each of these methods.

R. C. MAC KEITH (London). 'Micturition Induced by Giggling: ? Cataplexy.' A boy aged 9 and a girl aged 10 wetted themselves when they giggled but not when they coughed. Once started the micturition continued till the bladder was empty, even if the child stopped giggling earlier. The girl's mother had had similar trouble until she was 14 years old. In each case the problem was discussed and rapid improvement followed and persisted.

The symptom might be a variant of cataplexy or of epilepsy. In cataplexy muscular inhibition on laughter is seen; local forms are known. Micturition occurs with some minor epileptic seizures, which themselves may follow specific stimuli. The children reported probably had originally an abnormality of bladder control, but, when seen, their symptom was being perpetuated by anxiety.

GEORGE FREDERIC STILL MEMORIAL LECTURE. Dr. Geoffrey Dawes (Oxford) delivered the George Frederic Still Memorial Lecture entitled 'Respiratory and Cardiovascular Problems after Birth'.

A discussion on 'The Problems of the Regional Paediatrician' was held on the evening of April 23, 1959.

The President opened the discussion by outlining problems of which he had been notified and 25 members spoke subsequently. The problems discussed were: co-operation with infectious fever units; filling junior staff appointments; difficulties of deputies to cover leave periods; the sense of isolation of regional paediatricians and the desirability of close liaison with regional teaching centres and how this could be achieved; the need of some regions for more paediatric cover which was not sufficient to justify another full appointment.

The meeting felt that more knowledge on these points was required and the President decided that this should be referred to the Executive for further enquiry.

A. M. MacDonald won the Ulster Cup golf competition.

BOOK REVIEWS

Collected Papers: Through Paediatrics to Psycho-Analysis. By D. W. WINNICOTT. (Pp. ix+350; 20 figures. 35s.) London: Tavistock Publications. 1958.

Many paediatricians on both sides of the Atlantic are concerning themselves more and more with the child's view of the world, and in particular with the ways in which the developing human organism adapts with varying success to his crises and anxieties. When this experiential aspect of child development is studied there are apt to be consequences for the observer of a rather unique and personal kind: the realization that some of the child's problems are still active in ourselves. This is among the most significant of the problems facing contemporary paediatrics. What are the repercussions on training of the need for an awareness of the factors underlying the behaviour of children and the paediatrician's work on himself which this entails? This is one of the major themes of Dr. Winnicott's book.

Together with his three other recent publications (Winnicott, 1957a; 1957b; 1958) this book should be available wherever paediatrics and the training of paediatricians are seriously discussed. Barbara Korsch's admirable summary of the relevant American literature should also be added to this list (Korsch, 1958).

The lucidity and freshness of approach with which Dr. Winnicott writes need no emphasis here. Many of the articles are among the rather rare British contributions to the classics of paediatric psychiatry, e.g. Transitional Objects and Transitional Phenomena.

REFERENCES

Korsch, B. (1958). In *Advances in Pediatrics*, Vol. 10. Edited by S. Z. Levine, Year Book Publishers, Chicago.

Winnicott, D. W. (1957a). *The Child and the Family*. Tavistock Publications, London.

—— (1957b). *The Child and the Outside World*. Tavistock Publications, London.

—— (1958). In *Modern Trends in Paediatrics*, 2nd series. Edited by A. Holzel and J. P. N. Tizard. Butterworth, London, p. 250.

Growth and Development of Children, 3rd ed. By E. H. WATSON and G. H. LOWREY. (Pp. 334; 74 figures. 58s.; \$7·75.) London: Interscience Publishers. Chicago: Year Book Publishers. 1958.

This useful manual on the growth and development of children is now appearing in its third edition. There have been numerous alterations and almost every chapter has been extensively revised, whilst that on the role of endocrines has been rewritten. The book is aimed at the student wanting to learn and the practitioner, general and paediatric, needing a handy reference book, and as such it is adequate for its purpose. Its range is comprehensive, namely from the newly fertilized gamete to adolescence. Growth is described organ by organ and amply illustrated by figures, charts and graphs; heredity and environment and their inter-relationships are mentioned, and so are energy metabolism and the nutritional needs from all stages of foetal life onwards; endocrine factors, emotional, psychological and behavioural development, each have a chapter, and finally there is a not very useful chapter on abnormal growth. All this in 300 pages ! Indeed perhaps too much has been attempted, and some chapters have suffered as a result. Material and many of the graphs, charts and figures have been taken from the literature or borrowed from units throughout the countries on both sides of the Atlantic so that the book makes no pretence of contributing original work. It remains, however, a useful quick book of reference on many aspects of the main themes of growth and development in children.

Ergebnisse der Bluttransfusionsforschung, Vol. 4. Bericht der 7 Tagung der Deutschen Gesellschaft für Bluttransfusion in Berlin vom 20-21 Juni, 1958. (Pp. iv+280; 52 figs.; Sw.Fr. 32.25.) Basel/New York: S. Karger. 1959.

The topics chosen for the meeting of which this volume represents the proceedings were: blood and plasma fractions; blood and plasma transfusion in paediatrics; and the medico-legal aspects of transfusion. A series of papers and a short discussion on each of these subjects are followed by a miscellaneous collection of papers on other aspects of blood transfusion.

The subjects of the six papers in the paediatric section range from the purely social aspect of erythroblastosis to details of laboratory technique. Had they been more closely linked, a composite picture of German views on exchange transfusion or some other aspect of transfusion in childhood might have emerged; individually, these disparate contributions add little to our knowledge of their subjects, which are already well covered in various standard monographs.

The other sections will be of interest chiefly to those who have to deal with the laboratory aspects of blood transfusion; amongst those papers which are also of clinical interest may be mentioned that of van Loghem and his associates on leucocyte antibodies as a cause of transfusion reactions and a short review (in French) of the problems of platelet transfusion by Eyquem and Maupin.

Neurological and Psychological Deficits of Asphyxia Neonatorum. Edited by WILLIAM F. WINDLE. (Pp. xiv+336. 83 figures; £3.) Oxford: Blackwell Scientific Publications. Springfield, Illinois: Charles C. Thomas. 1958.

This work is the edited report of a conference held at the University of Puerto Rico in 1956 and attended by

28 American research workers in the fields of anatomy, physiology, psychology, paediatrics, obstetrics and neurology.

There are 13 chapters concerned with the physiology, pathology, and effects of anoxia at or before birth in producing cerebral palsy and mental deficiency, two chapters devoted to the behaviour of infant monkeys and their breeding and care, and four to the recorded proceedings of round table conferences.

Of the greatest interest are those chapters concerned with experimental neonatal asphyxia in animals, mainly guinea-pigs. But species differences are such that more will be learned in relation to human problems by experimental studies on other primates, and Dr. Windle and his colleagues are now undertaking such investigations with Macaca monkeys established as a free living colony on the island of Santiago off Puerto Rico. To assess the effects of neonatal asphyxia, special tests have had to be devised to measure intelligence and learning abilities in animals and these are described in relation to both guinea-pigs and monkeys.

This is an important book and could be read with profit by all concerned with problems of the newborn infant. Over 500 references are listed.

One minor protest must be entered. In his foreword Dr. E. Harold Hinman deplores the fact that 3% of the population of the United States (that is, nearly 5 millions) are considered as mentally retarded. But, for as long as a mentally retarded person is defined as one whose intelligence is less than two standard deviations from the mean for the population, there will always be 3% of any population who are 'mentally retarded'. It would be as true to say, and as absurd to deplore, that 50% of the population was below average intelligence.

Le Syndrome de Guillain-Barré et les Polyradiculo-névrites Aigues avec Dissociation Albumino-cytologique dans le Liquide Céphalo-Rachidien. By R. COIRAULT, A. LARCAN and P. DAVIDOU. (Pp. viii+200. 32s. 6d.; Fr. fr. 2,000.) Paris: Masson. 1958.

This is a monograph covering all aspects of the Guillain-Barré polyradiculitis, its history, clinical manifestations and complications, differential diagnosis, its multiple aetiology, its pathology and treatment. The work is well arranged and plentifully illustrated by case histories, and some 800 references are listed. Even in a monograph of this size some aspects of the subject receive scant attention. For instance, the important complication of raised intracranial pressure is discussed in one short paragraph, corticosteroid therapy is described by reference to the literature, but not apparently from personal experience, and the life-saving treatment of respiratory paralysis is allotted seven lines.

The original description of polyradiculitis with 'dissociation albumino-cytologique' in the cerebrospinal fluid was by G. Guillain, J. Barré and A. Strohl in 1916. Why has Dr. Strohl not received eponymous fame? There must be a story behind this.

Convulsive Disorders of Children. By D. H.-C. CHAO, R. DRUCKMAN and P. KELLAWAY. (Pp. vi+151; 25 figures. 42s.) London and Philadelphia: W. B. Saunders & Co. 1958.

This book or monograph is addressed, the preface tells us, to residents in the Blue Bird Circle Children's Clinic, Houston, Texas, and is based primarily on the collected experiences of the Clinic since its inception in 1949. It is in fact a simple and concise account of childhood convulsions and is admirably suited, as a vademecum, to final year students, house physicians and candidates for general medical and paediatric examinations. It is well written, beautifully produced, and incorporates excellent short illustrative case reports. At the end there is a table relating to the indications, dosage, toxicity, etc. of 15 drugs in common use. The authors seem curiously uninterested in prognosis, about which nothing is said, or in the social implications of epilepsy in relation, for instance, to parents and family or to schooling. The chapter on electro-encephalography describes clearly the common abnormal patterns but omits a description of the normal tracings. On the whole it is a useful little book to have at hand, but is perhaps rather expensive at 42s.

Untersuchungen zur klinischen Problematik der progressiven Muskeldystrophie. By JOACHIM BRUGSCH and KATHARINA BROCKMANN-ROHNE. (Pp. 54; 27 figures; D.M. 9.80.) Leipzig: Georg Thieme. 1958.

This monograph is based on the clinical experience of 214 cases of muscular dystrophy seen since 1948. The authors divide the condition into three clinically and prognostically distinct groups: (1) ascending infantile progressive muscular dystrophy; (2) the more benign scapulo-humeral and facio-scapulo-humeral forms; and (3) atypical forms including the 'para musculodystrophics', myotonia dystrophia, etc.

Much stress is laid throughout on the necessity for close collaboration between the paediatrician, the neurologist, the orthopaedic surgeon and the dietician, and they emphasize that a positive approach is essential in this condition.

Drug therapy with prostigmine, vitamin E, choline, glutamic acid, etc., and special diets are regarded as merely supportive though of some importance, but early diagnosis and early physiotherapeutic and orthopaedic treatment are essential.

The illustrations are clear. Some details of the biochemical disturbances and the genetic basis of some of the cases are given. A useful reference list is appended.

This is a useful monograph setting out the experiences of one team of workers but one which does not really add anything very new to our understanding of this group of conditions.

THE MAINTENANCE OF STABILITY IN THE NEWLY BORN*

1. CHEMICAL EXCHANGE

BY

R. A. McCANCE

From the Medical Research Council Department of Experimental Medicine, Cambridge

Sir Leonard Parsons was a very good friend to me. I met him first in the uneasy days just before the last world war, through an old colleague of mine who had gone to work in his department. He welcomed the idea that we should begin some joint work there and fostered my newly born interest in infant physiology till it was old enough to look after itself. I remember many stimulating visits to the Children's Hospital to discuss our results and Sir Leonard's leisured kindness on every occasion, in spite of all the administrative tasks which were pressing upon him at that time. We met again in very much happier circumstances at the British/Swiss Medical Congress which was held in Basel in 1946, and there his presence of mind may have been the means of saving my life. We had been talking about undernourished children in Germany, where my colleagues and I had been working, and I was so absorbed by listening to what he had to say about the clinical aspects of undernutrition in children one lovely September day outside 'Les Trois Rois' that I should certainly have been run over had he not pulled me back in time.

It was therefore a great privilege and also a pleasure to be invited to give these lectures, for it allows me an opportunity of helping to commemorate the man we all admire and to whom I owe so much.

The composition of the body, as revealed by chemical analysis, remains remarkably constant from hour to hour and from day to day. The efficiency of adults depends upon this, or in other words upon the maintenance of stability outside and inside the cells. This does not imply stasis, as the word homoeostasis might suggest, or indeed any constancy among the individual molecules, for each and every component of the body is in a state of intensely rapid flux. Few of the molecules in my plasma, for instance, were there a few minutes ago, yet its volume and temperature have altered very little in the last four or five hours, and the concentrations of glucose, sodium and potassium in it were much the same this morning as they were the day before yesterday. There is no need to multiply examples of this overall stability in adult life, for it has been implicit in the whole of physiology since the time of Claude Bernard (1865). Various aspects of it have been presented recently and very readably from different points of view by Hubble (1957), McIntosh (1957) and Pickering (1958). It is enough for the moment to emphasize that this overall stability is the result of a great number of the physical and chemical characteristics of the body being maintained in so-called 'steady states'. The internal temperature, the blood pressure, the volume of the plasma, its *p*H, the concentration of sugar, sodium and potassium in it, and in the cells, are all good examples. There are almost no limits to the number of these 'steady states' within the body.

When an adult is living in the physiological environment for which he was evolved, the stresses and strains of its daily life are rarely enough to break down the mechanisms which maintain the steady states, but a high altitude will do it and so will a very hot climate or too little drinking water, and so will disease. Most of the infections, for instance, alter the setting of some of the thermal regulating mechanisms, which then allow the temperature of the body to rise and maintain it in an abnormal steady state (Pickering, 1958). Nephrosis again raises the volume of extracellular fluid in the body by altering the setting of the controls and, so long as the nephrosis persists, the abnormal and disabling steady state persists also.

The newborn animal resembles its parents in that it has the same temperature at birth, the same

* The Leonard Parsons Lectures delivered in Birmingham on May 12 and 13, 1959.

general make-up and the same osmolar concentrations of electrolytes in its plasma, but in other respects its composition is not altogether the same. There is relatively more fluid outside its cells, for example (Flexner, Wilde, Proctor, Cowie, Vosburgh and Hellman, 1947; Friis-Hansen, 1954), and correspondingly more sodium and chloride in its body (Stapleton, 1958), for these are the main ions in extracellular fluid, and there are many less striking differences in chemical composition. There is, for example, a higher concentration of inorganic phosphate in the plasma (Murtagh, Videla, Marenzi and Braegger, 1957) and there may be a higher concentration of potassium (Widdowson and McCance, 1956). Some of the 'steady states', in other words, so highly characteristic of the adult, may not necessarily be the same in the newborn animal.

Birth is generally regarded as a physiological upheaval, and so it is, but mainly for what may be described as the supply services and sewage departments, and a successful entry into the new world should involve no major loss of internal stability. The great reorganizations in the vascular, pulmonary and digestive systems are all directed towards maintaining the services and steady states which had been in existence before.

It is not generally realized to what extent the foetus, with its 'adnexa', maintains its own steady states and internal stability. The foetus creates and maintains its own large volumes of extracellular fluids and then gradually reduces them in that part of itself destined to become the newborn animal. Work of our own has shown that birth makes no break in this process. The creation and functional efficiency of other foetal fluids are also the work of the foetus. The maintenance and composition of the allantoic and amniotic fluids, for instance, are the work of its kidney (Ahlfeld, 1906; Makepeace, Fremont-Smith, Dailey and Carroll, 1931; Bates, 1933; Potter, 1952; Baird, 1957; Davies and Routh, 1957; Alexander, Nixon, Widdas and Wohlzogen, 1958a, b) and of the membranes themselves (Dickerson and McCance, 1957; McCance and Dickerson, 1957; Jeffcoate and Scott, 1959), but unfortunately we know very little about all this at present. The high concentration of amino acids in foetal plasma, and of certain vitamins (Baker, Ziffer, Pasher and Sobotka, 1958), the accumulation of immune bodies (Brambell, 1954), and variations in placental blood flow (Nyberg and Westin, 1957; Westin, 1957) must be regarded as regulations of the foetus for its own welfare, and many of these foetal steady states are carried forward for weeks or months by the newborn animal. Some, the high concentrations of fructose, for example (Goodwin, 1957), and of creatinine (Zweymüller, Widdowson and McCance, 1959) in the plasma of some ungulate foetuses are not, and some of the changes which do take place in the infantile steady states are part, specifically, of the physiology of the newly born (Bangham, Ingram, Roy, Shillam and Terry, 1958; McCance and Widdowson, 1959a).

The chemical stability of the body in the newly born depends mainly upon the same organs as in later life. As in adults, moreover, cells all over the body may participate in maintaining the stability of the internal environment by sacrificing some of their own (Schwartz, Jenson and Relman, 1954; Leaf and Newburgh, 1955; Elkinton and Danowski, 1955), and the stability of the internal environment can be destroyed with fatal results if the cells are not able to maintain themselves in a state of functional efficiency. Nevertheless the newborn animal is not just a little adult. Its stability may be threatened or upheld in ways without counterpart in adults. Some of these are important practically, all theoretically.

The object of these lectures is to examine a few of these stabilizing mechanisms and steady states; why some of them are particularly vulnerable in the first few days of life and what happens if they fail. Comparison with adults will be necessary and also a study of several species, for only thus is it possible to grasp the complexities of the subject and arrive at any useful generalizations. Our knowledge is not great enough to solve any of these problems satisfactorily, even those on which most work has been done. Nevertheless, enough is known to demonstrate its importance and the desirability of extending this knowledge.

The Arterial Tension of Oxygen

Acute deprivation of oxygen constitutes an immediate hazard to every steady state within the body, and indeed to life itself, but adults and newborns react to it rather differently. Elderly people may never recover their mental poise after what may seem to the onlooker to have been a trifling incident, such as a minor anaesthetic (Bedford, 1957; Bourne, 1957). If the lack of oxygen has encouraged overbreathing in an atmosphere containing little or no carbon dioxide the respiratory alkalosis thus created may have contributed to the results, for this has been shown to reduce cerebral blood flow (Kety, 1950).

When adult dogs are placed in nitrogen, or the air surrounding them is suddenly decompressed, their blood pressure, their respiration rate and consequently the *p*H of their blood all rise within the first minute, but by about the second or third minute their blood pressure has begun to fall rapidly, and respiration may cease. The *p*H of the blood falls as death approaches, but remains within normal limits, and is usually not far from its initial level at the end. When puppies are suddenly deprived of oxygen, their blood pressure, respiration rate and blood *p*H do not rise, but all fall progressively. Respiratory efforts may be made for 16-20 minutes and the heart may go on beating feebly for twice this time. Anoxia raises the cardiac output to about four times its previous level in adult sheep, whereas it leaves it unchanged in the newborn lamb (Cross, Dawes and Mott, 1958a, 1959). Puppies have recovered after 26 minutes without oxygen when their blood pressure had fallen to 5·2/3·7 mm. Hg and the *p*H of their blood to 6·5 (Swann and Brucer, 1949; Swann, 1953; Swann, Brucer and King, 1953; Swann, Christian and Hamilton, 1954); puppies' brains are also very tolerant of anoxaemia (Kabat, 1940), and some primitive respiratory centre can continue to initiate gasps for many minutes even when the heads of many newborn animals are removed from their bodies and placed in nitrogen, but this ability fades away as the animals grow (Selle, 1941; Thoms and Hiestand, 1947).

Prolonged survival of this kind, relative to that of an adult, and a useful life thereafter, seem to depend on the ability of the newborn animal to make extensive use of anaerobic glycolysis to provide the energy required to maintain its life processes and in particular to synthesize the high energy phosphate bonds which maintain the proper structure and function of its brain (Stone, Marshall and Nims, 1941; Fazekas and Himwich, 1941; Fazekas, Alexander and Himwich, 1941; Čapek, Hahn, Křecek and Martínek, 1956). If glycolysis is prevented by iodoacetate or fluoride, newborn rats die in a few minutes in nitrogen, although they can still live on for 50 minutes in oxygen, presumably by utilizing their available carbohydrate in other ways, as will later be discussed (Fazekas and Himwich, 1941; Conference, 1958). The effects of anoxia on the brain can be mitigated by an adequate supply of circulating glucose or made worse by hypoglycaemia and insulin (Himwich, Fazekas and Alexander, 1941; Himwich, Bernstein, Herrlich, Chesler and Fazekas, 1942; Gellhorn and Kessler, 1942). It is possible, however, that the quantity of glycogen available to the heart muscle may sometimes set the seal on the survival time (Dawes, Mott and Shelley, 1959). As might have been anticipated, this resistance to oxygen deprivation has been shown to vary with the species and the maturity of the animal at birth, but particularly with the state of development of the brain at this time. Guinea-pigs, for example, which are highly developed at birth, succumb much more quickly than rats in a reduced supply of oxygen (Fazekas *et al.*, 1941), and the brain seems to be the most vulnerable organ, even in the undeveloped rat (Adolph, 1948; Čapek *et al.*, 1956; Conference, 1958).

The transition from uterine to atmospheric respiration does not always go as smoothly as one could wish (Editorial, 1957a, b; Turnbull and Baird, 1957), and some investigators have taken a very serious view of respiratory failure and oxygen deficiencies in the newborn baby (Darke, 1944; Preston, 1945; Evans, 1948; Bernstein, 1958). Others admittedly have not (Campbell, Cheeseman and Kilpatrick, 1950; Usdin and Weil, 1952; Apgar, Girdany, McIntosh and Taylor, 1955) and the resistance of newborn animals to a shortage of oxygen is undeniably great (Adolph, 1948; Smith, 1959; Swann *et al.*, 1954), partly perhaps because they do not as a rule over-ventilate (Cross, Tizard and Trythall, 1955), and also because they can make such good use of anaerobic glycolysis to supply all their physiological needs (Dawes, Mott and Shelley, 1958). Signs of anaerobic metabolism may be found after normal birth, even in man (Gonzales and Gardner, 1957). Kittens and rats have been delivered in good shape after their mother had died of anoxaemia (Fazekas *et al.*, 1941), and it is common knowledge how difficult it is to drown these animals. The whole matter has been the subject of experiment since the time of Boyle (1672), and there are many records of healthy infants being born alive up to 20 minutes after the death of their mothers (Harvey, 1651; Hellman, 1953). The case recorded by Bullough (1958) shows what a newborn infant can withstand in the way of asphyxia and still survive to win a baby competition nine months later.

In spite of this tolerance, if an infant is born in an advanced stage of asphyxia and if respiration does not begin when the cord is cut (perhaps because of the asphyxia), an acute emergency may develop in a few moments. The crisis may appear later in a more chronic form, particularly in premature infants, as part of the so-called 'respiratory distress syndrome'. Whatever the cause, the primary and secondary changes in the chemistry of the internal environment are now becoming clear, and are common to all species (Dawes and Mott, 1959). The failure of the supply of oxygen may not be so immediately fatal to the newborn baby as it would be to an adult because of the ability of the newly born to make good for a time with anaerobic glycolysis, but this results in the accumulation of lactic and to some extent other non-volatile acids in the body. The stabilizing systems in the plasma and cells respond to this, and mitigate the effects, but the *p*H falls and the available 'buffer base' is reduced. If CO_2 can be eliminated there is a fall in the plasma bicarbonate. In human infants the plasma bicarbonate is normally lower than the values accepted as normal for adults (Reardon, Baumann and Haddad, 1954), but in line with those found in late pregnancy (Goodland, Reynolds and Pommerenke, 1954), with which the foetal bicarbonate has been in equilibrium *in utero* (Weisbrot, James, Prince, Holaday and Apgar, 1958). In respiratory failure, however, the elimination of CO_2 is interfered with to the same extent as the delivery of oxygen. Consequently the pressure of CO_2 rises, and this intensifies the acidosis, but as the compensation for it is a rise in the plasma bicarbonate it is impossible to interpret single determinations of plasma bicarbonate, and a figure quite normal for a pregnant or non-pregnant adult might be found in the presence of a serious fall of plasma *p*H, much too high a pressure of CO_2 and a much reduced buffer base (Singer and Hastings, 1948).

The incidence of asphyxia in full term infants has been investigated by Miller, Behrle, Smull and Blim (1957), and more recently by James, Weisbrot, Prince, Holaday and Apgar (1958) and James (1958). These investigators have employed very beautiful and delicate techniques to follow the chemical changes in the serum for the first hours or days of life. An abstract of their findings has been given in Table 1 and their results are very well worth thoughtful consideration. Firstly, these workers have found that, although there are great individual variations, which make it difficult to generalize, few infants are delivered without some signs of asphyxia. This may be partly the natural course of events, but there are strong reasons for believing that much of it is man-made and preventable. Few babies are born today as nature intended them to be. Anaesthetics are given to the mother which are known to reduce the blood pressure and to prolong the dangerous second stage of labour. If they are volatile anaesthetics the methods of administration may interfere with maternal gas exchange in the lungs and give rise to some deficiency of maternal oxygenation. Women are frequently delivered lying on their backs which must interfere with the venous return from the uterus and lower limbs, and drugs are used which depress the respiratory centres in the infant and make resuscitation more difficult (James *et al.*, 1958; Shields and Taylor, 1957; Henderson, Mosher and Bittrich, 1957). Secondly, changes in the tensions of oxygen and CO_2 and signs of an acidosis are not the only, or perhaps the most serious, results of asphyxia. The serum potassium may rise; this may be due to hydrogen-potassium exchange across the cell boundary, more commonly seen in reverse during potassium deficiencies, or it may be due to the acidosis preventing the cells in some part of the body maintaining the normal gradient between themselves and their surroundings (Schwarz, Cohen, Lubash and Rubin, 1959). Thirdly, in spite of all these handicaps, once respiration is established the full term infant shows great powers of recuperation, restores the chemical abnormalities in its serum to normal and establishes its own internal stability on a physiological basis.

TABLE 1

RECOVERY FROM NEONATAL ASPHYXIA IN 'NORMAL' BABIES

	*p*H	P CO_2 mm. Hg	Plasma Bicarbonate mEq./l.	Buffer Base mEq./l
Birth ..	7·23	58	25	41
1 hr. ..	7·30	39	21	42
3 hr. ..	7·34	38	22	44
24 hr. ..	7·41	34	21	45

The premature infant can do the same. Usher (1958) has followed some of these infants carefully and watched the clinical and chemical signs of asphyxia develop with the onset and progress of respiratory distress. He has emphasized the rise in the serum potassium and attributed to it the gross abnormalities he has found in the electrocardiogram, and to it also possibly the immediate cause of death. He has also succeeded in reversing some of these signs of chronic asphyxia by glucose and alkaline infusions. Similar beneficial effects on the serum potassium and the cardiogram have been obtained by the administration of bicarbonate to adults suffering from the severe acidosis of uraemia (Schwarz *et al.*, 1959).

Asphyxia therefore constitutes the first great threat to somatic stability in the newly born. Infants are very tolerant of anoxaemia and asphyxia, but both of these affect their chemical stability and, as will later be shown, their thermal balance, and everything should be done to prevent them or minimize their effects. Once respiration is established or re-established, however, the infant can safely be left to recover and maintain all the steady states which depend upon an adequate supply of oxygen (Kaiser and Goodlin, 1958).

The Level of Circulating Bilirubin

Some yellowness of the skin is so common in the days following birth and usually so transient and apparently harmless that it came to be termed physiological jaundice of the newborn. In premature babies, however, it may be much more severe (Crosse, Meyer and Gerrard, 1955) and indeed pathological. The dangerous limits for circulating bilirubin are of the order of 20 mg./100 ml. of serum (Lucey and Dolan, 1959). This concentration is a direct threat to the stability of the internal environment, and the whys and wherefores for this are among the most interesting developments of modern paediatrics (Editorial, 1958). The pigment is always of the 'indirect' type according to the van den Bergh nomenclature. This pigment is relatively non-toxic, but it was found by Day (1954) and by Walters and Bowen (1955) that as its concentration rose the pigment interfered with the uptake of oxygen by rat brain tissue *in vitro*. Chopped tissues and homogenates were used and the inhibition was much greater in newborn than in adult preparations. The inhibition was removed by adding cytochrome or methylene blue. Zetterström and Ernster (1956) then showed on mitochondria isolated from the liver that the pigment 'uncoupled' the processes of oxidation from those of the phosphorylation of adenosine diphosphate. The evidence is, therefore, that if bilirubin accumulates to any extent the proper uptake of oxygen will cease and with it the normal production of heat so necessary to maintain the body temperature at this age. Furthermore, the metabolism which does go on will be functionally less valuable.

The pigment produced by the degradation of haemoglobin is normally prepared for excretion by the liver. The process is rather a complicated one and is illustrated diagrammatically in Fig. 1. The final step is the conjugation of the pigment with glucuronic acid and its transportation from the serum to the bile, but the evidence at present is that this can only be brought about in a certain way. Uridine triphosphate is a pyrimidine nucleotide used in many reactions in the body. These uridine compounds are involved for instance in the metabolism of galactose in the mammary gland (Malpress, 1958), and galactosaemia, the hereditary disorder of metabolism (Holzel and Komrower, 1955), is caused by a failure in the development of the enzyme in the liver which catalyses the conversion of uridine diphosphate glucose (Anderson, Kalckar and Isselbacher, 1957; Collip and Donnell, 1959) to uridine diphosphate galactose. The compound may also be involved in the transport of amino acids across the renal tubules since this is one of the mechanisms disorganized in galactosaemia (Cusworth, Dent and Flynn, 1955). In the preparation for bilirubin conjugation the uridine triphosphate combines with glucose 1 phosphate to give uridine diphosphate glucose and pyrophosphate which need not be further considered. The uridine diphosphate glucose is then oxidized by a dehydrogenase enzyme to uridine diphosphate glucuronic acid. These are the compounds from which two glucuronic acid mole-

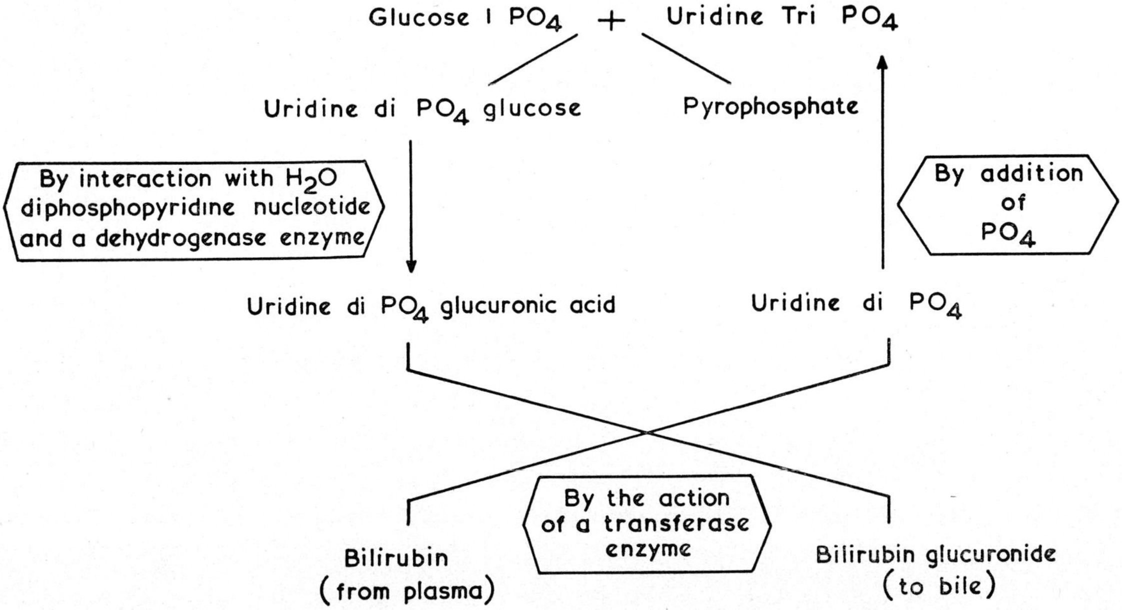

FIG. 1.—The conjugation of bilirubin with glucuronic acid in the liver cell.

cules are transferred to one bilirubin molecule and the reaction is catalysed by an enzyme which is called a transferase. The uridine diphosphate is then reconverted to uridine triphosphate by a process involving adenosine triphosphate and subsequent oxidation, and the cycle starts again. The reaction, however, goes much more slowly in the newborn animal or human infant than in adults of the same species because of the immaturity of the enzyme systems in the liver at birth (Brown and Zuelzer, 1958; Lathe, Claireaux and Norman, 1958). The activities of the dehydrogenase and of the transferase are both very small by adult standards, but they increase very rapidly (Lathe and Walker, 1957; Dutton, 1959). Bilirubin is not the only compound conjugated with glucuronic acid, and other compounds can be used to test the activity of the enzymes. Para-aminophenol has been used, and Vest (1958) used acetanilide in his work on human infants. According to him the activity increased rapidly after birth, but did not reach the adult level until the babies were about 3 months old. Evidence is strong that the enzyme systems are less developed in infants born before than at full term, which is in keeping with clinical observations all over the world on the effect of prematurity on jaundice (Shnier and Levin, 1959). Holman (1958) examined a group of white and negro premature infants in Baltimore, for instance, and found that both the incidence and the severity of the jaundice were increased by prematurity, and that it tended to be worse in the white infants than in the negro ones, probably because of the recognized racial differences between the degree of maturity of white and black infants at birth. Here then is an example of chemical stability which is threatened mainly by virtue of immaturity, and a most interesting discovery about it has recently been made by Cremer, Perryman and Richards (1958). These authors have found that the bilirubin in serum is highly photosensitive, and the levels in the body can be greatly reduced by exposing infants to sunlight or artificial light. This would appear to be the first time that light has been shown to have a stabilizing effect on the internal environment. It may have been much more important to primitive man living in equatorial Africa than to infants nowadays, but the authors suggest that treatment with light may remove the necessity for a certain number of the exchange transfusions now being carried out, admittedly with some risk (Walker and Mollison, 1957; Farquhar and Smith, 1958), as a method of treating hyperbilirubinaemia in premature infants (Editorial, 1958).

Danoff, Boyer and Holt (1958, 1959) have tried treating hyperbilirubinaemia by the administration of glucuronic acid, and have found the concentration of bilirubin in the serum to fall. Although such treatment might seem an obvious one, it does not appear to be fundamentally sound if the chain of reactions illustrated in Fig. 1 is correct, and it has been heavily criticized (Jeliu, Schmid and Gellis, 1959). Treatment of hereditary jaundice with glucuronic acid in the Gunn strain of rats also reduces the serum bilirubin, but the bilirubin is not excreted and appears to accumulate in the cells. The conclusions of Danoff *et al.* (1958, 1959) were cautious and restrained, and further experimental work on the subject will no doubt decide the issue one way or the other.

It has been recognized for some years (Allison, 1955; Bound and Telfer, 1956; Meyer and Angus, 1956; Willi, 1956) that there was some reason to suppose that the vitamin K analogues, particularly Synkavit, tended to cause a haemolytic anaemia and to increase the incidence of hyperbilirubinaemia in premature infants. This is a matter of importance because premature infants or their mothers are often given vitamin K as a protection against haemorrhagic diseases of the newly born. Synkavit is a sodium diphosphate compound of menadione, and another analogue called Hykinone, which is menadione sodium bisulphite, has now been found to be rather more dangerous than Synkavit (Lucey and Dolan, 1959). It is uncertain at present how and why exhibition of these vitamin K analogues constitutes such a risk to chemical stability. It is possible that it is due to an effect on the red blood cells and enhanced by a vitamin E deficiency (Allison, 1955). It may also be due to some unknown toxic action on the liver. Another explanation is based upon the fact that these analogues are to some extent excreted as glucuronides. This means that they must be conjugated like bilirubin. They may therefore compete with bilirubin for the transferase enzyme. If they are preferentially absorbed on to the enzyme molecule and not so easily removed, a little menadione may prevent the conjugation of a great deal of bilirubin, for this is how the sulphonamides and other compounds act upon bacteria.

Renal Function, Food and Growth

Fig. 2 shows the course of the blood urea in three species of animals during the first days of life. All were fed on mother's milk. In each of them the concentration of urea in the serum rose for a short time and then fell again to a lower level (McCance and Otley, 1951; Joppich and Wolf, 1958). It was at first supposed that the rise was an indication of functional immaturity of the kidney, and the fall due to its rapid development at this age, for the general

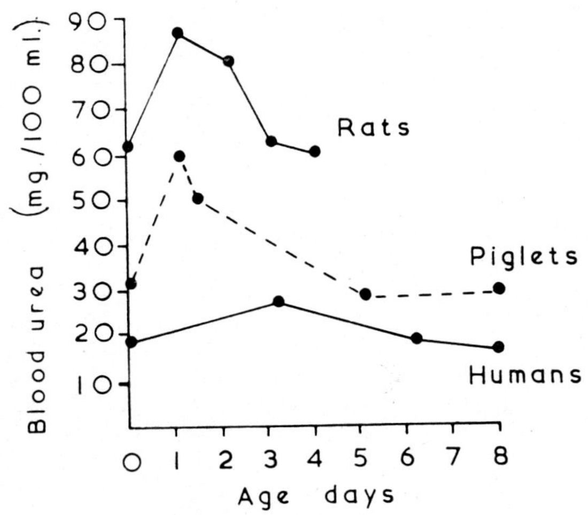

FIG. 2.—Changes in the concentration of urea in the blood during the early days of life.

work on renal function in early life seemed to suggest this. Aspects of this development have been reviewed in some detail by McCance (1950), Barnett and Vesterdal (1953), McIntosh (1957), Adolph (1957) and Vesterdal (1959), and only the general principles of infantile renal function need be considered here.

Before doing so, however, it is necessary to point out that there are certain difficulties in interpreting the results of work on the function of the kidney just after birth. These have arisen because of a natural desire to compare the findings with those in adults which were much better known. The comparison of some functions presents no difficulty. The ability to concentrate the urine for example, is among these, and some results, which were obtained by McCance and Widdowson (1954a), indicate that the kidney of the newborn does not raise the osmolar concentration of the urine to the same extent as it does in adults. When studies of glomerular filtration rates and urea clearances began to be made, however, some method of eliminating the effects of size had to be devised, for the results of these tests are given as the number of ml. of extracellular fluid passing through the glomeruli or cleared of urea per minute, and it is evident that a field mouse could never hope to compete with an elephant in this regard, although it might have a much more effective kidney. Difficulties due to size were therefore eliminated by adopting the practice used in metabolic work and expressing the results per unit of surface area. At first this seemed satisfactory to most people interested in babies, but those who worked on animals mostly expressed their results on the basis of body weight. By both methods (McCance and Young, 1940) the human newborn infant appears to have sub-normal renal function by adult standards but, whereas on the basis of surface area functions such as glomerular filtration rate rise progressively after birth and reach the adult level at about 2 years of age, on the basis of body weight they pass through a phase well above the adult level at this time of life (McCance and Widdowson, 1952). These bases of comparison cannot both be 'right' and others have been suggested from time to time. The matter has been further confused by those who have administered their test doses on one basis and compared the results on another, and the only correct and proper thing to do now is to study the renal function of the newborn and immature animal in its own right and to establish the proper normal for every age. This is gradually becoming recognized, and the paper of Edelmann, Troupkou and Barnett (1959) shows how the study of the concentrating power of the kidney in infancy is now being approached. There is, nevertheless, plenty of evidence on all bases of comparison that the kidney of the newborn animal is functionally immature. The glomerular filtration rates and urea clearance show this, and so do some of the tubular functions such as the excretion of diodone and para-amino hippuric acid, and the reabsorption of glucose. Interesting confirmation of this which does not depend upon any arbitrary basis of comparison came from the work of Rennick and Hamilton (1958) on the ability of isolated kidney slices to pick up para-amino hippurate and tetra-ethyl ammonium from the surrounding medium and concentrate them in tubule cells. The rat provides particularly good examples of renal immaturity, for just after birth its kidney varies its rates of excretion little in response to substances administered as tests. The kidneys of other species, however, have been shown to be little better. The excretion of water (McCance and Wilkinson, 1947; Heller, 1947; Ames, 1953; McCance and Widdowson, 1955; Falk, 1955; Hoy and Adolph, 1956; Adolph, 1957; Ziskind and Gellis, 1958), sodium chloride (Dean and McCance, 1949; McCance and Widdowson, 1957), and ammonium ions (Cort and McCance, 1954; Widdowson and McCance, 1958; Hatemi, 1959) have all been shown to be less efficient than the corresponding functions in adults.

Other signs of immaturity are provided by a certain lack of balance between glomerular and tubular function. Some of the excretory functions of the tubules appear to be more undeveloped than the glomerular filtration rates whereas others, such as the reabsorption of sodium and chloride, are more highly developed. Responses, moreover, which rely upon the integration of a detector as well as the effector organ, such as the regulation of the volume and osmolar concentration of the extracellular fluids, will later be shown also to be defective, and although all newborn animals will suck milk, many will not take water by mouth till they are a certain age in response to somatic dehydration, and only 'learn' to do so as they develop (Adolph, 1957). An example of still more remote control of ren al function in the newborn period is provided by those animals like the puppy, kitten and rat which can only empty their bladders during early suckling if the mother animal licks the perineum at appropriate intervals (McCance and Wilkinson, 1947; Cort and McCance, 1954). Yet the volume and composition of the body fluids remain within normal limits from birth onwards and the steady states proper to the infant are adequately maintained. The rise in the blood urea shown in Fig. 2 is trifling and its fall is not, as was originally thought, due to the rapid maturation of the urea clearance, for this takes place much too slowly. No basis of comparison can explain this discrepancy between experience and experiment, and we worried about it for years. We began to search for stabilizing mechanisms other than the kidney, and for a more constructive approach to the study of the internal stability and steady states of the developing organism.

Much of the protein nitrogen in the food of a freely growing animal is incorporated directly or indirectly into tissue protein and never appears in the form in which it is excreted by the kidney. This relieves the kidney of any such animal of much of the work which it is called upon to do in adult life. Minerals in the food are absorbed also and retained in a growing organism in the tissues and bones. Edwards (1824) fully recognized the overwhelming importance of growth in relationship to every function of the body: 'Dans la jeunesse tout paraît tendre au développement et à l'accroissement du corps.' It was emphasized by Stransky and Bálint (1920) as an aspect of renal function, but the possible implications of these wise remarks were not appreciated at the time and have only recently been demonstrated experimentally (McCance and Widdowson, 1956). Table 2 gives results which were obtained in a study of the newborn pig. Half the animals were given no food and the others were fed by hand on the kind of diet provided by the sow at this age. The intake and excretion of nitrogen was followed. Comparison of the two groups shows that nine-tenths of the protein nitrogen in the food was incorporated into the tissues and never presented

TABLE 2

NITROGEN BALANCES OF NEWBORN PIGLETS WHICH WERE 'FED' OR 'NOT FED'

	Animals Given: Milk	Animals Given: Water
N intake (mg./kg./24 hr.) ..	3,500	0
N output (mg./kg./24 hr.) ..	350	250
N 'balance' (mg./kg./24 hr.)..	+3,150	−250

itself to the kidney for excretion as urea. The same is true to a lesser, but still to a surprising, extent of the more slowly growing human baby aged 7 days. Immature, therefore, as the kidney of the newborn may appear to be when some such test as the urea clearance or the excretion of para-amino hippuric acid is applied to it, it is quite capable of maintaining the blood urea and creatinine within normal limits, provided growth is taking place as it should, and there is no forced degradation of tissue protein. The effect of this on the blood urea has been demonstrated by the heights to which it may rise in human infants which have survived a protracted and difficult labour (McCance and Widdowson, 1954b) or in animals kept without food in a cold environment (McCance and Widdowson, 1959b), and it could certainly be demonstrated again by giving the newborn animal some food which could not for some reason promote growth. Correspondingly, anything which can delay the breakdown of tissue protein can actually reverse the usual rise in the serum urea after birth demonstrated in Fig. 2. Glucose has been shown to do this experimentally in the starving newborn pig (McCance and Widdowson, 1956).

The stabilizing effects of growth have also been demonstrated in another way (McCance and Widdowson, 1958a). Newborn piglets were given 26 mEq./kg. body weight of potassium per 24 hours over the first 40 hours of their lives (Table 3). Some

TABLE 3

EFFECT OF GIVING KCl AND WATER OR KCl AND MILK TO NEWBORN PIGLETS

	KCl+Water	KCl+Milk
K intake (mEq./kg./24 hr. ..	26	27
K retained (mEq./kg./24 hr.)	+2·9	+10·5
Serum K (mEq./l.)	9·3	5·9
Signs of toxicity	Paralysed	None
Change in body weight (g./kg. birth weight)	−104	+103

of the piglets were given this potassium dissolved in water, others in a volume of sow's milk so adjusted that all the animals received the same amount of water as well as potassium. The animals getting the potassium in water lost weight and did not excrete the potassium fast enough to prevent a major rise in its concentration in their sera and they became paralysed. The blood sugars also rose, which surprised us very much at the time, although the result might have been expected from the work of Silvette, Britton and Kline (1938). The other piglets gained weight, for they grew rapidly and incorporated much of the potassium into their cells. The concentrations in the sera rose relatively little, although the urine volumes were comparatively small, and the piglets appeared perfectly normal at the end.

Table 4 shows the effect of giving large but quite reasonable amounts of water unbalanced by food to newborn puppies (McCance and Widdowson, 1958b). These animals differ from piglets in that they tend to excrete water much less freely and sodium chloride more freely at this time of life. The puppies which received milk grew satisfactorily and maintained a perfectly normal internal concentration of sodium and chloride, whereas those given water only excreted a relatively small fraction of the quantity which had been administered. They gained considerable weight although they were getting no food, and their body fluids became diluted to an extent which was clearly pathological. It is probably true to say that many, if not most, of these effects were appreciated and demonstrated in rather different settings nearly 30 years ago by Kerpel-Fronius and his associates in Hungary (Kramár, 1927; Kerpel-Fronius and Leövey, 1931; Csapó and Kerpel-Fronius, 1933; Kerpel-Fronius, 1933), but the implications were missed by everyone who read the papers at the time, and by most people since.

Yet one more example of the stabilizing effects of growth is provided by a study of the metabolism of phosphate in newborn infants. Table 5 illustrates this (Widdowson and McCance, 1959). During the first 48 hours of their lives these babies were given no food, and the serum phosphorus rose somewhat and phosphorus began to be excreted. This rise appears to be due to starvation and the liberation of phosphorus from organic combination, and it is shown in a more exaggerated form in the newborn pig. By the seventh day, however, when the intake of phosphorus had been raised by mother's milk from nothing to 25 mg./kg./day and the infants were growing, so much phosphorus was being incorporated into the tissues that the serum phosphorus had fallen and virtually none was being excreted.

The capacity for growth can be saturated only by an optimum diet, and the percentage of protein, fat and carbohydrate in the mother's milk has long been known to be correlated with the growth requirements of the newborn animal (Bunge, 1898). The inorganic constituents of the diet must also be correlated with the function of the kidney and growth. The amount of calcium and phosphorus in human milk, for example, would never support the bone growth of a healthy piglet. The whole principle of feeding in the newborn period, and indeed later, must be to saturate the growth requirements of the animal in question if rapid growth is desired, but at the same time to provide the stabilizing organs with the minimum amount of work. This principle has many implications. A suitable environmental temperature, for example, may considerably reduce the requirements for food.

TABLE 4

EFFECT OF FOOD AND GROWTH ON OSMOLAR HOMOEOSTASIS IN THE NEWBORN PUPPY

	Water Alone	Water and Milk Solids
Fluid given (ml./kg. birth weight /24 hr.)	256	256
Urine volume (ml./kg. birth weight/24 hr.)	135	37
Visible water balance (ml./kg. birth weight/24 hr.) ..	+121	+219
Serum Na (mEq./l.)	120	141
Serum osmolar conc. (mEq./l.)	243	310
Gain of body weight (g./kg. birth weight/24 hr.)	69	178

TABLE 5

EFFECT OF FOOD AND GROWTH ON PHOSPHORUS HOMOEOSTASIS IN NEWBORN INFANTS

	1st Day	2nd Day	7th Day
P intake (mg./kg./24 hr.) ..	0	Traces	25
P output in urine (mg./kg./24 hr.)	0·05	3·24	0·02
	At birth	At 48 hr.	7th day
Serum P (mg./100 ml.)	6·03	7·28	6·04

A good example of the necessity for integrating food and renal function is the effect of raising the intake of sodium chloride in the newborn infant or piglet by adding salt to the milk. Owing to the very large intake of fluid by the newborn animal quite a small percentage of salt in the milk can lead to the ingestion of more salt than an adult would normally take. Given the corresponding amount of water, however, an adult would excrete both without a breakdown in the stability of the body fluids. Not so the human infant. Fig. 3 shows the effect of making up the milk for three premature babies so that it contained 0·7% of sodium chloride. In each one the normal gain in weight from day to day

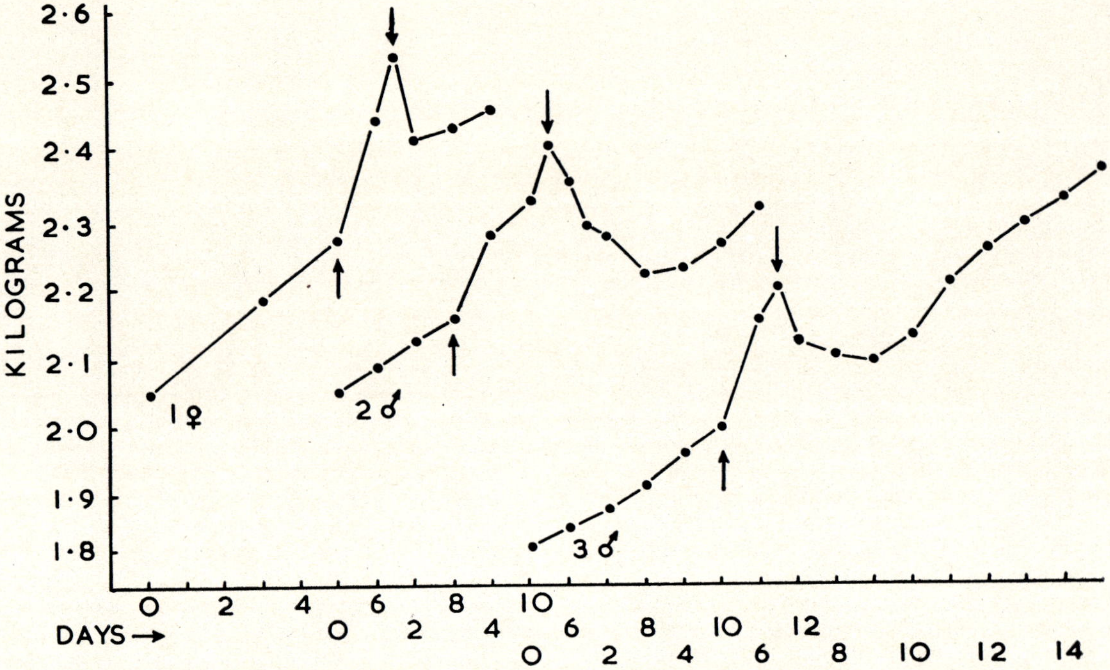

FIG. 3.—The weight charts of three infants before, during and after the period of salt administration.

altered to a more rapid one, which was in fact pathological. In a short time the babies became oedematous and sick, but on putting them back on to their proper intake of water and salt their weights fell and they began to gain weight again at their previous and more satisfactory rate (McCance and Widdowson, 1957).

Table 6 shows exactly the same effect in piglets to which no food was given but only water or salted water. The gain of weight on the solution of salt without food was quite clearly pathological. Table 6, however, shows other features. Firstly, although the amount of water retained in the body was large, it was not large enough to prevent a rise in the concentration of sodium in the serum. This also happened in the babies, and in both species the administration of the salt led to hypertonic expansion of the extracellular fluids. Secondly, the administration of the salt solution led to a fall in the serum urea and this in turn was the result of a smaller breakdown of tissue protein in the starving newborn animal. This result has always been obtained in these experiments. It is difficult at present to say why. It is tempting to suppose that a large volume of extracellular fluid in some way inhibits the breakdown of tissue protein, which can be regarded as one way of promoting growth, and that therefore the rapid growth of the foetus and newborn animal is associated in some way with the large volume of extracellular fluids in its body, but it is perhaps more probable that the effect is due to an alteration in the rate of secretion of one of the suprarenal hormones brought about in response to the pathological increase of these fluids, and part of a stabilizing mechanism. There for the moment the matter must rest.

TABLE 6

EFFECTS OF GIVING NEWBORN PIGLETS WATER OR AN EQUAL VOLUME OF 0·9% SODIUM CHLORIDE SOLUTION

	Water Alone	Water+Salt
Change of weight in 40 hr. (g./kg. birth weight)	−53	+96
Percentage of water in bodies ..	82·7	87·4
Na balance (mEq./kg./24 hr.) ..	−0·3	+35·5
Serum Na (mEq./l.)	138	147
Serum urea (mg./100 ml.) ..	42·2	23·6

(To be continued)

The references for Parts 1 and 2 will be printed together at the end of Part 2 which will appear in the December issue of *Archives*.

THE RELATIONSHIP BETWEEN CALCIUM-PHOSPHORUS METABOLISM, THE 'KREBS CYCLE' AND STEROID METABOLISM

BY

ETTORE DE TONI, Jr. and SERGIO NORDIO

From the Department of Paediatrics, Gaslini Children's Hospital, Genoa University School of Medicine, Italy

(RECEIVED FOR PUBLICATION MARCH 6, 1959)

It has been shown in the course of the last few years that the number of factors playing a part in calcium-phosphorus (Ca-P) metabolism is far greater than had been known. It was found that the calcification of bones depends in the first place on the 'citric acid cycle' and on adenosine triphosphate (ATP) (oxidative phosphorylation) (Dickens, 1941; Albaum, Hirshfeld and Sobel, 1952; Dixon and Perkins, 1952; Marks, Hiatt and Shorr, 1953). Alkaline phosphatase intervenes chiefly in the processes concerned with the formation of the organic substance of the skeleton.

Some factors as yet unknown (citrates ?) similarly regulate the action of the parathyroid hormone, an action which has not yet been accurately defined (Zweymüller, 1958). The role played by the parathyroid in classical and in vitamin D resistant rickets is still uncertain (Lamy, Royer, Frézal and Lestradet, 1958). Similarly, the action of vitamin D seems to be dependent on factors which regulate the sensitivity of the organism to its effect (Fanconi and Spahr, 1956). The suprarenals have acquired some degree of importance, as was shown in studies on idiopathic hypercalcaemia, on tetany occurring in newborn infants of diabetic mothers and on hypercalcaemia with osteosclerosis found in a number of cases of myxoedema (Gittleman, Pincus, Schmerzler and Saito, 1956; Winberg and Zetterström, 1956; Anderson, Brewis and Taylor, 1957; Royer, Lestradet and Habib, 1958; Zetterström and Arnhold, 1958). Cortisone acts as an antagonist of vitamin D by impairing the absorption of calcium from the intestines; another action of cortisone is to reduce the rate of tubular reabsorption of phosphorus (Roberts and Pitts, 1953). It is possible that there is a relationship between the suprarenals and the parathyroid glands, as suggested by cases of hypoparathyroidism associated with Addison's disease (Leonard, 1946; Papadatos and Klein, 1954; Whitaker, Landing, Esselborn and Williams, 1956).

We have become conversant in recent years with the importance of the relationship between ossification, parathyroid hormone, vitamin D and the 'Krebs cycle' (Glanzmann, Meier and Walthard, 1946; Heinz, Müller and Rominger, 1947; Harrison and Harrison, 1952a; Nordio, Semach and Grego, 1956; de Toni, 1957). In rickets the citric acid level in the blood and urine is diminished (Harrison, 1954; Nordio *et al.*, 1956). The same phenomenon is observed in idiopathic hypercalcaemia (Forfar, Balf, Maxwell and Tompsett, 1956; Nordio *et al.*, 1956). Administration of vitamin D and, although less regularly, of parathormone leads to a rise in the citric acid level in blood and urine (Harrison and Harrison, 1952a; Steenbock and Bellin, 1953; Nordio *et al.*, 1956). Considerable importance is attributed to the 'citric acid cycle' in the renal tubules in connexion with the regulation of the acid-base balance and the reabsorption of phosphorus, amino acids and glucose (Harrison and Harrison, 1941; Durand, Manzini, Bruni and Semach, 1956; Nordio *et al.*, 1956). As is known, the synthesis of steroids has the 'Krebs cycle' as its starting point, and it may be possible to interpret the various disturbances of calcium-phosphorus metabolism also in terms of the Krebs cycle.

Classical Rickets Treated with ATP

We have studied the following four cases of classical rickets in the florid stage, no treatment with vitamin D ever having been given.

Case 1 was a boy aged 2 years 4 months; **Case 2** was a girl aged 4 years 1 month (sister of Case 1); **Case 3** was a boy aged 19 months, and **Case 4** was a girl aged 13 months.

Treatment. All four cases received ATP intramuscularly, the dosage being, in Cases 1 and 2, 5 mg. daily for a period of 50 days and 10 mg. daily for a further period of 25 days; in Case 3, 5 mg. daily for a period of 20 days and 10 mg. daily for a further period of 10 days; and in Case 4, 5 mg. daily for a period of 40 days.

These were cases of classical rickets with hyperamino-aciduria and slight changes in the acidification of the urine. Results of treatment are shown in Table 1. The citrate content of the blood was markedly lowered in two cases only, in contrast to the other cases studied by Harrison (1954) and Nordio, Segni and Massaccesi, 1957. The citric acid content of the urine was not markedly lowered and in Case 2 it was even raised, whilst the figures for blood citric acid were low. Administration of ATP led to a definite improvement in the radiological picture of the bones (Figs. 1-4), to a rise in blood phosphorus, and in three instances to a lowering of the phosphatase figures. The changes in phosphaturia and in the citric acid levels in the urine and blood did not conform to any regular pattern, and the changes in urinary amino acids were only slight.

Rickets and Sensitivity to Vitamin D

Case 5. This boy, aged 18 months, had radiological and clinical signs of severe rickets. The main biochemical features were as follows: the blood citric acid level was markedly lowered with a comparative increase of urinary output of citric acid; there was a moderate lowering of the blood phosphorus level with normal urinary output of phosphorus, and a moderate rise in phosphatase (Table 2).

TREATMENT. After daily administration of 10,000 i.u. of vitamin D_2 over a period of 40 days the following findings were noted. There was an increase in calcification of the bones but severe deformities of the metaphyses were still present. There was a return to normal of the blood phosphorus but no change in phosphatase or citrate. After two months' treatment with ATP (10 mg. daily) the radiological picture became normal and there was some improvement in the phosphatase level. This case shows partial resistance to vitamin D but complete clinical and radiological cure with ATP.

Cases 6 and 7. These twins, aged 17 months, had severe clinical and radiological signs of rickets. One sister had suffered from rickets and still showed signs of the disease. The radiological and biochemical findings in both twins were more or less identical.

The biochemical findings showed: a moderately low blood phosphorus level with slightly increased phosphaturia; a marked increase in phosphatase, increased amino-aciduria, considerable lowering of the blood citric acid level and marked hypercitruria (Table 2). Table 3 gives the blood and urine citric acid levels compared with normals.

In contrast to findings in normal subjects, intravenous loading with citric acid did not lead to any marked rise in the citric acid content of the blood (Fig. 5). The citric acid content of the urine before citric acid administration was 6·75 mg. per hour; after loading it was 32·4 mg. per hour.

By simultaneous determination of the endogenous creatinine clearance, we were able to show that the glomerular filtration rate of citrate was less than the final urinary excretion rate (Table 4). In a number of normal subjects of different ages and in other cases of rickets of the classical type we have always found the urinary excretion per minute of citric acid to be smaller than the glomerular filtration per minute. Our findings suggest a lowering of the renal threshold for citric acid in the twins. It appears that in these cases the renal tubules excrete rather than reabsorb citric acid. These studies show the existence in certain forms of rickets of a 'citric renal diabetes'.

The mother of the twins showed a very low blood citric acid level and a very high urinary citric acid output. Similarly, the sister of the twins, who was affected by rickets, showed a very low blood citric acid level (Table 5). The father and brothers, who were free from rickets, had normal blood citric acid levels. It seems that the marked familial predisposition to rickets was associated with a change in citrate metabolism.

TREATMENT. Case 6, following a single injection of 15 mg. (600,000 i.u.) of vitamin D_2, was given 5,000 i.u. daily by mouth over a period of two months. We noted only a slight improvement in the radiological picture but the phosphorus content of the blood became normal

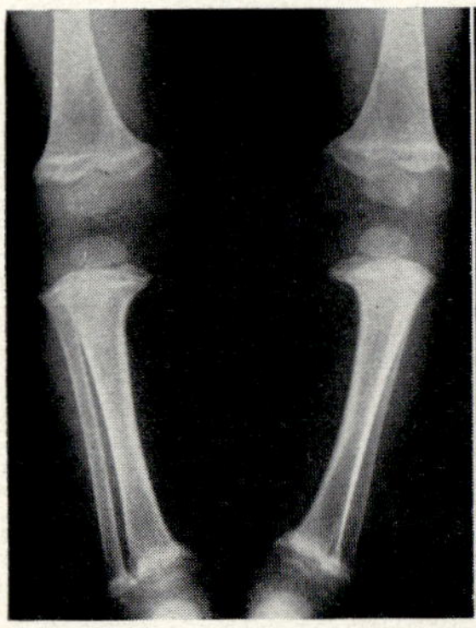

FIG. 1

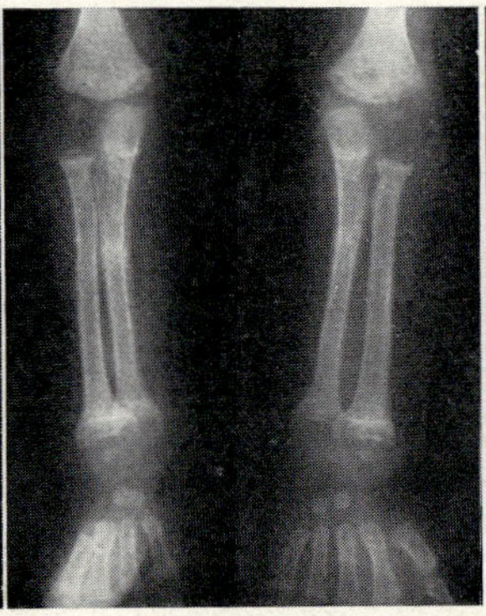

FIG. 2

FIGS. 1 and 2.—Case 3. Before ATP treatment.

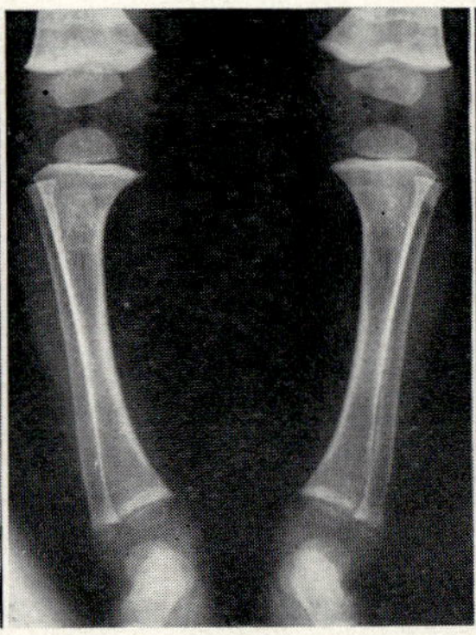

FIG. 3

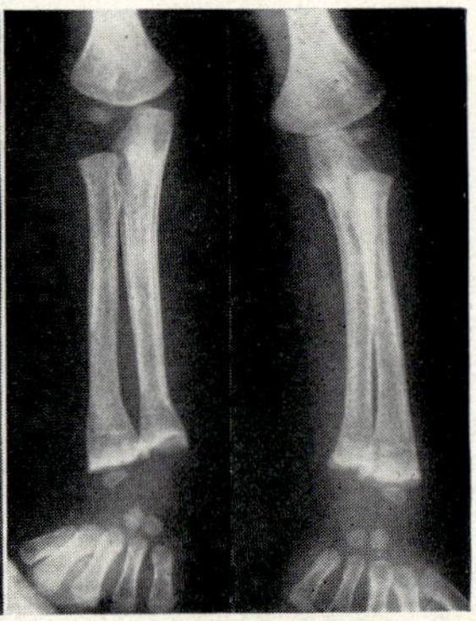

FIG. 4

FIGS. 3 and 4.—Case 3. After ATP treatment.

TABLE 1

CLASSICAL RICKETS TREATED WITH ATP

	Case 1			Case 2			Case 3			Case 4		
	A	B	C	A	B	C	A	B	C	A	B	C
		(50 days)	(75 days)		(50 days)	(75 days)		(20 days)	(30 days)		(25 days)	(40 days)
Blood												
Ca (mg. %)	9·3	9·6	10·6	9	11·4	11·4	11·8	12·4	11·8	11·6	10·8	12·2
P (mg. %)	2·5	1·8	4·2	2·9	4·6	6·1	3·8	3·4	4·2	3·6	3·6	4·1
Citric acid (mg. %)	1	0·5	0·3	0·5	0·6	0·3	2·5	2	2·5	3	2	3
Phosphatase (K.A. units)	58	52·8	31·2	56·2	32	23·2	40·4	50·4	44·8	38	27·6	20·2
Cl (mEq./l.)	109·4			106			106·2			104·2		
Na (mEq./l.)	132·6			137			145·6			139·1		
K (mEq./l.)	4·8			4·6			5·1			6·1		
CO_2 (vol. %)	41·4			42·7			49·2			48·2		
Urine												
P (mg./kg./24 hr.)	50	63	22	14	38	37	54	16	60	15	22	18
Citric acid (mg./kg./24 hr.)	7·5		10	12·5	27	14	7	5	6·7	17	5·6	2·2
Sulkowitch reaction	+	+	+	+	+	+	+−	+	++	+	++	+++
*p*H	6·5–8			7–8			6–8			6·5–7·5		
Amino acids												
Glycine	++++++		++++++	++++		++++	++++++		+++++	++++++		++++
Taurine	++++++		++++	++++		++++	++		++			+
Glutamic acid	++++		++++	+		+	++			+		
α-alanine	+++++		++++	++++		+++			++++	++++		+++
Serine	+++		++	+++		++	++++++		+++	+++		++
Leucine	++		+++				+			+		
Proline	+		+				+					
Proline derivatives	+		+									
Tyrosine	+		+	+		+	+		+	++		+
Threonine				+		++	+++			++		+
Glutamine				+++		+++	+++		++++	++++		++
Aspartic acid				+		+			+			
Glucosamine				++++								

A = before treatment; B = after treatment with ATP; C = end of treatment with ATP.

TABLE 2

BIOCHEMICAL FINDINGS

	Case 5			Case 6	Case 7
	A	B	C	A	A
Blood					
Ca (mg. %)	9·2	10·4	10·2	9·6–11·5	9·2–9·5
P (mg. %)	3·3	7	6·6	3–3·5	3–3·6
Citric acid (mg. %)	0·2	0·35	0·25	0·15–0·2	0·15–0·25
Phosphatase (K.A. units)	27·4	26·8	20·2	53·2	84
Cl (mEq./l.)	101·4			105	101·4
Na (mEq./l.)	145			141·3	139·4
K (mEq./l.)	5			6·4	5
CO_2 (ml. %)	45			53·2	47
Urine					
P (mg./kg./24 hr.)	23	37	30	44–56	38–55
Citric acid (mg./kg./24 hr.)	11	5·5	9	58–94	64–75
Sulkowitch reaction	+	+	+	++	+
Cl (mg./kg./24 hr.)				4,170	3,300
Na (mg./kg./24 hr.)				2,200	2,750
K (mg./kg./24 hr.)				85	150
*p*H	6–7·5			5–8	5–8
Aminoacids					
Glutamine				++++++	++++++
α-Alanine				++++++	++++++
Glycine				++++++	++++++
Istidine				++++++	++++++
Serine				++++++	++++++
Tyrosine				+++	++++
Threonine	Normal	Normal	Normal	++	++++
Valine				++	++
β-Aminoisobutyric acid				++	+++
Leucine				++	++
Asparagine				++	
Phenylalanine				+	++
Proline					++
Glutamic acid					++

A=before treatment; B=after treatment with Vitamin D_2; C=after treatment with ATP

TABLE 3

BLOOD AND URINE CITRIC ACID LEVELS COMPARED WITH THOSE IN NORMAL CONTROLS

	Normal Controls	Case 6	Case 7
Citric acid (mg. %) in blood	1·5–5·5	0·15–0·20	0·15–0·25
Citric acid (mg./24 hr.) in urine	100–600	760–800	550–645
Citric acid (mg./kg./24 hr.) in urine	4–16	89–94	64–75
Rate citric acid (mg. %) in urine / citric acid (mg. %) in blood	3–15	660–800	516–733

TABLE 4

	Case 6	Case 7
Glomerular filtrate (creatinine)	86/1·72 sq. m./min.	85/1·72 sq.m./min.
Glomerular filtrate for citric acid	0·070/min.	0·11/min.
Urinary output citric acid	0·84/min	0·85/min.

TABLE 5

BIOCHEMICAL FINDINGS IN MOTHER AND SISTER OF CASES 6 AND 7

	Blood Citric Acid (mg. %)	Urine Citric Acid
Mother	0·20	1900 mg./24 hr. (31·6 mg./kg./24 hr.)
Sister	0·30	

(4·5 mg. per 100 ml.); the blood citric acid level remained very low (0·20 mg. per 100 ml.).

Case 7 received orally over a period of two months 5,000 i.u. of vitamin D_2 daily. There was a slight deterioration in the radiological picture, but again the blood phosphorus level became normal (4·5 mg. per 100 ml.), and the citric acid level in the blood remained very low (0·30 mg. per 100 ml.).

Thereafter we started ATP treatment (5 mg. intramuscularly daily over a period of 4 months) in both children. The radiological findings were checked three times during those four months, and a progressive improvement was noted, which culminated in complete

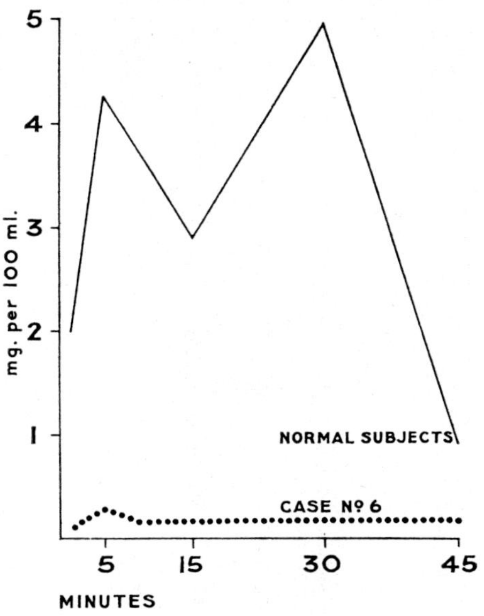

FIG. 5.—Case 6. Blood citric acid levels after intravenous loading with citric acid.

cure at the end of the period of ATP treatment. It was, however, not possible to undertake biochemical follow-up studies.

These cases show (1) a much greater involvement of the citric acid and amino acid levels with lowering of the renal threshold in comparison with the changes in the calcium and phosphorus levels, and (2) a relative resistance to vitamin D_2 therapy contrasted with good therapeutic results obtained with ATP.

Review of the Seven Cases

There is a similarity between Cases 5, 6 and 7 in their poor sensitivity to vitamin D_2. These are intermediate forms between normal sensitivity and severe resistance to the antirachitic vitamin of Fanconi and Spahr (1956). This resistance shows itself in the first place in the poorness or absence of radiological improvement and in the citric acid levels. On the other hand, the blood phosphorus levels became normal under treatment with vitamin D_2. This is a different phenomenon from that observed in classical rickets, in which high doses of vitamin D_2 frequently lead to an improvement in the radiological findings without improvement in the blood phosphorus level. It may well be that in such cases the correction of the blood phosphorus level proves insufficient, in the presence of changes in citric acid and amino acid metabolism, to ensure normal bone development.

A study of the therapeutic action of ATP in all seven cases confirms the importance of the part played by 'oxidative phosphorylation' (synthesis of ATP in the Krebs cycle) in the pathogenesis of rickets. The lowered renal threshold for citrates and amino acids provides evidence that the changes in 'oxidative phosphorylation' take place predominantly in the renal tubules. The therapeutic action of ATP represents a substitutive effect at the level of the bones, given the fact that the biochemical changes are not uniform in nature. The reduction in phosphatase is a more or less regular feature of an improved skeletal condition. In vitamin D resistant rickets Hoffmann-Credner, Rupp and Swoboda (1955) have demonstrated a deficiency in the synthesis of ATP.

Rickets and Steroid Metabolism

In Cases 1, 2, 3 and 4 we studied the urinary output of 17-ketosteroids, the Thorn test (with adrenaline) and the blood sugar levels after insulin administration. In three cases the 17-ketosteroid output in the urine showed a rise before onset of treatment (average for that age not higher than 1 mg. per day). The drop in eosinophils following administration of adrenaline showed an insufficient reduction in two cases only (Cases 5 and 6). The lowering of blood sugar levels following injection of insulin was not very marked (maximum reduction 25%). ATP led to a change in the excretion of 17-ketosteroids and in the results of the Thorn test (Fig. 6).

These findings show that rickets is also associated with disturbances of steroid metabolism. It appears that in the pathogenesis of rickets hyperadrenocorticism plays an important part, representing a contrast to the condition prevailing in idiopathic hypercalcaemia. Future investigations directed towards the total range of suprarenal hormones, especially the 11-oxycorticoids, will lead to further clarification of these problems. It is likely that a disturbance in steroid metabolism may have some bearing on the action of vitamin D and that there exists some relationship between such metabolic disturbance and the sensitivity or resistance of organisms to antirachitic vitamins.

In Case 5 administration of vitamin D_2 led to a rise in output of 17-ketosteroids without significant radiological improvement; this may represent an example of the above-mentioned relationship. ATP, apart from effecting a cure of the rachitic condition, has also exerted an influence on that metabolic-hormonal sphere, probably an action directed towards synthesis of the steroids (ATP-acetylCoA-steroids).

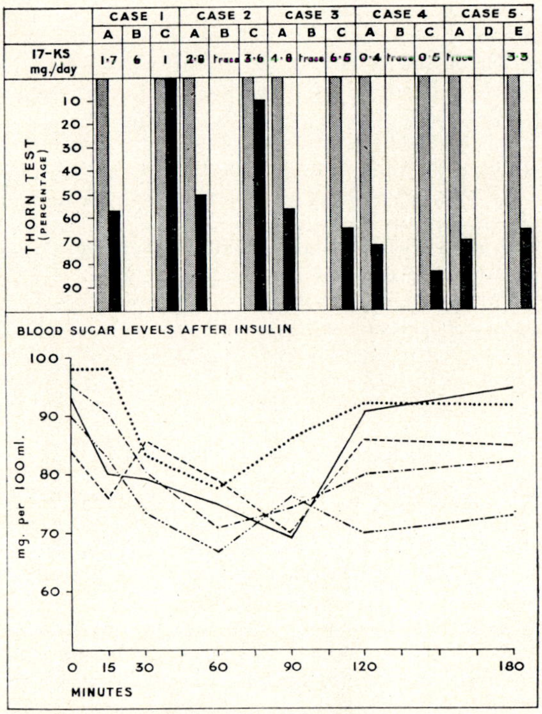

FIG. 6.—Cases 1—5.

A = before therapy		Case 1	————————
B = during ATP therapy		,, 2	— — — — — —
C = after ATP therapy		,, 3	. . . .
D = during vitamin D therapy		,, 4	— . — . —
E = after vitamin D therapy		,, 5	. . . — . . . —

Renal Rickets with Renal Gluco-phospho-amino Acid Diabetes (de Toni-Debré-Fanconi Syndrome)

Case 8. This was a girl aged 6 years 2 months. At the age of 4 months enlargement of the liver was found, a finding which was confirmed frequently at subsequent examinations. At the age of 8 months a diagnosis of rickets was made and treatment with vitamin D_2 in massive doses was started (Ostelin-800). At the age of 2 years glycosuria was detected for the first time. From the age of 4 years the patient complained of pains in the bones and joints and of difficulty in walking. From that time on she was subjected, without any satisfactory results, to various therapeutic procedures, the details of which were not given. The statural development was normal for her age ("pachysomia" according to de Toni's classification). There were severe clinical and radiological signs of rickets with a tendency to recurrences, especially in the long bones, and enlargement of the liver and spleen. Plain radiological examination as well as radiographs taken after insufflation of air into the retroperitoneal space showed enlargement of both kidney shadows. Results of blood and urine examinations are given in Table 6.

After treatment with ATP (10 mg. per day over a period of two months) we found that the glycosuria, phosphaturia and aminoaciduria were practically unchanged (Table 7), and there was no change on radiological examination of the skeleton.

In the course of a determination of the endogenous creatinine glomerular filtrate before therapy we were able to establish the clearance values for citric acid and phosphorus shown in Table 8.

Such results demonstrate that the tubular reabsorption of phosphorus corresponds to 92·7% of the glomerular filtrate. The glomerular filtrate per minute of citric acid was smaller than the urinary flow per minute. It is possible that the renal tubule secretes 0·29 mg. citric acid per minute.

Case 8 is a case of 'renal rickets with renal gluco-phospho-amino acid diabetes' without dwarfism and with enlargement of the kidneys. There are no reports in the literature of cases of de Toni-Debré-Fanconi syndrome without dwarfism and with nephromegaly. The case is difficult to interpret with regard to the enlarged kidneys. The blood sugar curve following injection of adrenaline and loading with glucose does not suggest any hepatorenal glycogen storage disease. The spleen contracted following adrenaline injection. Apart from glucose, the urine contained pentose, as in the case of Aballí, Montero, Escobar Acés and Jimenez (1944); it also contained in larger or smaller quantities all the amino acids which are commonly found in the de Toni-Debré-Fanconi syndrome. The output of urinary phosphatase was increased. The Ellsworth-Howard test was negative (Fig. 7), showing that the tubular reabsorption of phosphorus was impaired to such a degree that no subsequent modification could take place. There was only a slight change in the acidification of the urine without true acidosis and with a slight increase in the blood chlorides. The polyuria, which was not marked, responded to pitressin administration (Fig. 8). We were unable to do a liver biopsy, but the liver function tests failed to reveal the presence of a cirrhotic condition such as that found by Dent (1947) in other cases of the syndrome.

The citric acid levels were very low in the blood and high in the urine. The glomerular filtrate of citric acid was lower than the urinary flow. In this particular case the 'gluco-phospho-amino acid renal diabetes' proved to be associated with 'citric acid renal diabetes'. An increase in organic acids (keto-bodies, pyruvic acid, uric acid) was found in cases of 'de Toni-Debré-Fanconi syndrome' by Aballí *et al.* (1944), van Creveld and Arons (1949) and Sirota and Hamerman (1954).

Our findings show that a disturbance of the 'Krebs cycle' occurs in the renal tubules in some cases of 'de Toni-Debré-Fanconi syndrome'. Nordio

TABLE 6

BLOOD AND URINE ANALYSIS IN CASE 8

	Blood		
	1	2	3
Ca (mg. %)	10·8	10·2	10·4
P (mg. %)	1·7	1·8	2·2
Citric acid (mg. %)	0·05		
Phosphatase (K.A. units)	52·8	49·4	49
Cl (mEq./l.)	106		
Na (mEq./l.)	147·8		145·6
K (mEq./l.)	4·8		4·2
CO_2 (ml. %)	40·8	42·6	
Amino acids (mg. %)	7		
Glucose (mg. %)	90	91	
Nitrogen (mg. %)	47		
Cholinesterase	2·1		
Transaminase SGO/SGP	18/40		
Bilirubin (mg. %)	0·7		
Cholesterol (mg. %)	Est. 75/Free 44		
Maclagan	Negative		
Hanger	Negative		
Takata-Ara	Negative		
Blood sugar curve (glucose)	high and prolonged		
Blood sugar curve (adrenaline)	normal		
Blood pressure	Between 115/60 and 130/65		
Metabolic rate	Between +12% and +25%		
E.C.G.	Normal		
Thorn test (adrenaline)	143/59 (−58%)		
Cystine	Absent in eyes and bone marrow		
	Urine		
	1	2	3
Sulkowitch reaction	+++	+++	+++
P (mg./kg./24 hr.)	20·4		
Citric acid (mg./kg./24 hr.)	19·4		
Cl (mg./kg./24 hr.)			
Na (mg./kg./24 hr.)	3,900	4,300	4,800
K (mg./kg./24 hr.)	2,500	1,400	1,800
*p*H	7–7–6–6–5–6–7–6–7–6–6–6–7–6–7		
Amino acids			
Glycine	++++++	++++++	
Tyrosine	++++++	++++++	
α-alanine	++++	++++	
Glutamine	+++	++++	
Taurine	+++		
Threonine	+++	+++	
Lysine		+++	
Hydroxyproline		+++	
Valine		++	
Leucine	++	++	
Aspartic acid		++	
Phenyl-alanine	++		
Glutamic acid	++	+	
Histidine		+	
17-Ketosteroids (mg./24 hr.)	3·6		8·9
11-Oxysteroids γ/sq.m./body surf.	2,790		
Glucose (g./l.)	Between 0 and 6·25		
Other sugars (aldopentose)	Frequently present (+)		
Urine examination	Always negative		
Specific gravity	Max. 1027		
Dilution test	Max. 1000		
P.S.P. test	Total urinary output: 41%		
Glomerular filtrate (endog. creatinine)	83/min./1·72 sq.m. body surface		
Intravenous pyelography	Normal		

TABLE 7

BLOOD ANALYSIS IN CASE 8 AFTER TWO MONTHS' TREATMENT WITH ATP

Citric acid (mg. %)	0·5
Calcium (mg. %)	11·8
Phosphorus (mg. %)	2
Phosphatase (K.A. units)	34·8

TABLE 8

CASE 8

	Glomerular Filtrate/min.	Urinary Output/min.
Citric acid	0·16	0·31
Phosphorus	2·2	0·23

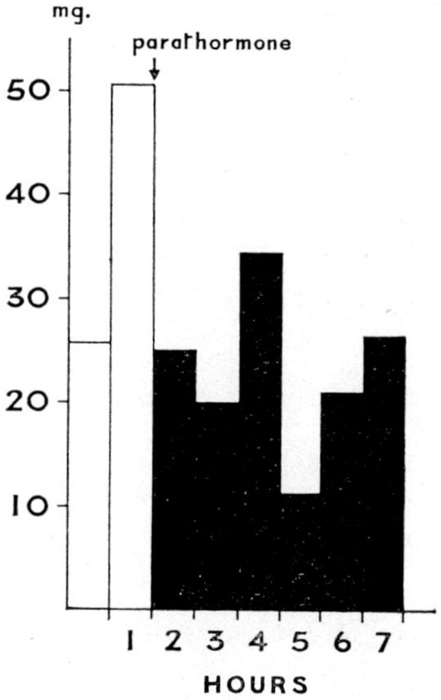

FIG. 7.—Case 8. Ellsworth-Howard test showing tubular parathormone resistance.

et al. (1956) have produced experimentally in rabbits a 'de Toni-Debré-Fanconi syndrome' by means of the administration of succinates (metabolites originating in the 'Krebs cycle'). In animals subjected to this treatment they found swelling of the mitochondria in the cells of the renal tubules, indicating a probable uncoupling of the oxidative phosphorylation process. The hypothesis was suggested, and supported also by Freudenberg (1954), that the synthesis of ATP had undergone some disturbance. Schwarz-Tiene, Careddu and Cabassa (1957) showed the existence of an analogous condition in cases of 'de Toni-Debré-Fanconi syndrome' produced experimentally by means of the administration of cystine. Harrison (1954) and subsequently Durand *et al.* (1956) produced an experimental 'de Toni-Debré-Fanconi syndrome' by administration of maleic acid (an antimetabolite of malic acid, the tricarboxylic acid of the 'Krebs cycle'). Durand *et al.* (1956) also noted, in animals treated in this way, a disappearance of the glycosuria following administration of ATP.

For these reasons we treated a rabbit with alpha-

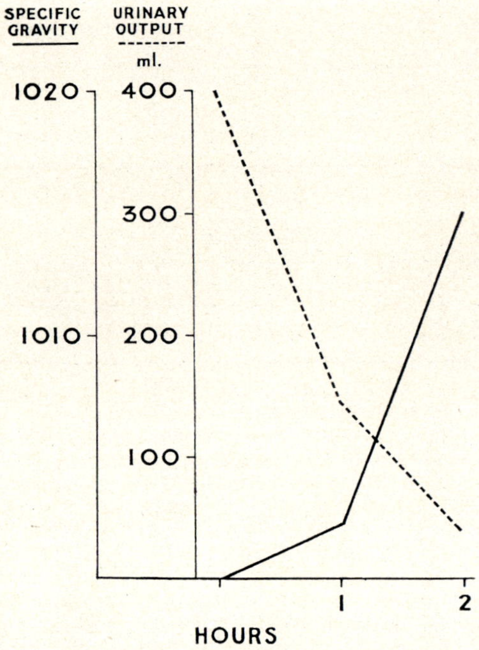

FIG. 8.—Case 8. Pitressin test showing a tubular pitressin sensitivity.

dinitrophenol (DNP), which leads to an uncoupling of oxidative phosphorylation; however, we did not succeed in producing a 'de Toni-Debré-Fanconi syndrome' (Table 9). After treatment there was some osteofibrosis in the juxtametaphyseal region similar to that observed by Nordio *et al.* (1956) after treatment of the rabbit with succinates.

As regards the relationship between the 'de Toni-Debré-Fanconi syndrome' and the 'uncoupling of oxidative phosphorylation', we must draw attention to the fact that, in contrast with the other cases of rickets which we have investigated, ATP had no therapeutic effect in our case, apart from a moderate increase in the citric acid and phosphorus levels of the blood and a drop in the phosphatase levels. The patient was subjected to combined treatment with ATP and vitamin D_2.

The increased urinary output of 17-ketosteroids and of 11-oxysteroids, which we observed in our case, shows that there exists in the 'de Toni-Debré-Fanconi syndrome' an additional disturbance in steroid metabolism. The latter may be associated with the metabolic disturbance of the 'Krebs cycle'.

Tetany with Hyperadrenocorticism and (?) Hypoparathyroidism

Case 9. This girl was 13 months old. From the age of 6 months she had been subjected to continuous treatment with vitamin D_2. She was admitted to our clinic with signs of tetany and radiological examination failed to show any evidence of rickets or of osteosclerosis (Figs. 9 and 10).

Treatment consisted of 20 i.u. of parathormone daily for five days, 20,000 i.u. of vitamin D_2 daily for five days and AT_{10} (Calcamina Wander 0·5% oily solution) 10 to 60 drops daily over a period of 50 days (combined with 20 mg. of prednisolone daily over a period of eight days). After an interruption of one month, during which calcium was administered, treatment with AT_{10}, 15 drops daily, was resumed and continued without interruption during the whole course.

This was a case of tetany with hypocalcaemia, hyperphosphataemia and lowered blood phosphatase (Table 10). Renal function was normal, there was no intestinal stasis and no radiological evidence of rickets. The low blood citric acid and urinary citric acid levels correspond to the findings in other forms of tetany with hypocalcaemia. These findings are characteristic of a certain form of 'hypoparathyroidism'. The results of the Howard test showed a drop in urinary phosphate excretion, which was already low before the test, indicating that the parathyroid function, which was depressed before the test, was susceptible to further depression as a result of the intravenous infusion of calcium (Fig. 11). In view of the difficulty in taking blood samples every hour, determinations were made only in the urine.

The patient's response to the various forms of treatment was abnormal, a relative resistance to AT_{10} developing during a certain period.

Of special importance are the results of the studies of suprarenal function which showed an all-round increase. Radiological examination after insufflation of air into the retroperitoneal space revealed no enlargement of the suprarenals (Fig. 12). The presence of hyperaldosteronism was confirmed by the rather high urinary output of potassium (Fig. 13) and by the occurrence of hypopotassaemic crises

TABLE 9

BLOOD AND URINE ANALYSIS IN A RABBIT FOLLOWING TREATMENT WITH DNP

	Before Treatment	After 4 Days	After 10 Days
Blood			
CO_2 (ml. %) ..	55·2	58·7	47·6
P (mg. %) ..	2·6	1·6	2·9
K (mg. %) ..	16	17	24
Glucose (mg. %)	111	130	148
Urine			
CO_2 (ml. %) ..	149	800	31·4
P (mg. %) ..	6·2	7·5	10
Fehling test ..	Negative	Negative	Negative
Aminoaciduria ..	Normal	Normal	Normal

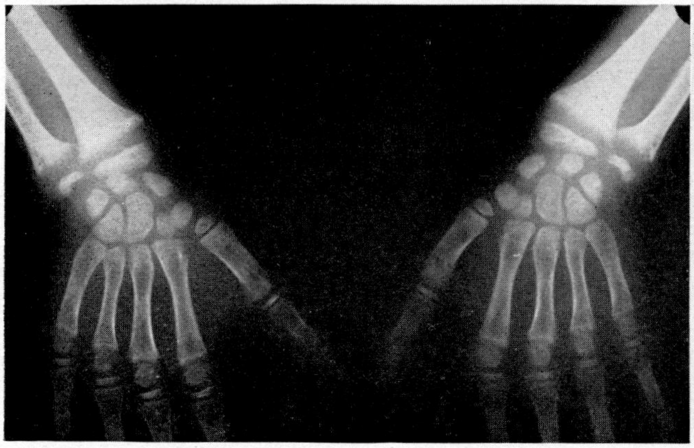
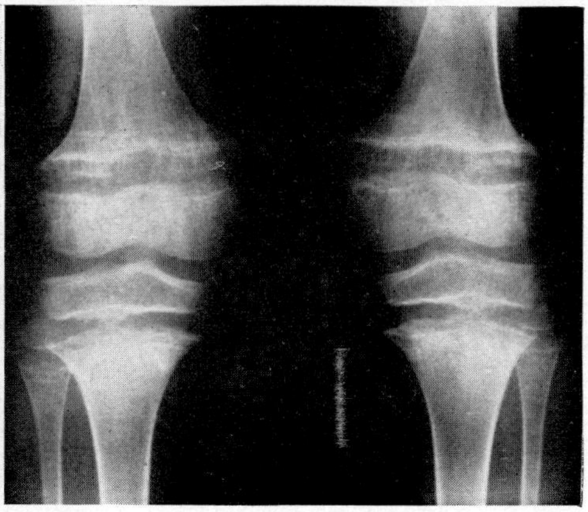

FIGS. 9 and 10.—Case 9.

TABLE 10

BIOCHEMICAL FINDINGS IN CASE 9

Blood	
Ca (mg. %)	7·2– 8
P (mg. %)	8–11
Citric acid (mg. %)	0·5
Phosphatase (K.A. units)	2·2
Na (mEq./l.)	145·6
Cl (mEq./l.)	102·8
K (mEq./l.)	4·7
CO_2 (ml. %)	59·3
Urine	
P (mg./kg./24 hr.)	3·1–1·7
Citric acid (mg./kg./24 hr.)	4·9
Sulkowitch reaction	Between + and ++
Na (mg./kg./24 hr.)	125
Cl (mg./kg./24 hr.)	225
K (mg./kg./24 hr.)	124
*p*H	Between 5 and 7
Amino acids	Normal

Renal functions (blood nitrogen, urine examination, concentration test, P.S.P. test)	Normal
Neuromuscular hyperexcitability	+++
E.C.G. Phonocardiogram: Typical for hypocalcaemia with increased mechanical systole	
Galvanic stimulation (Erb's sign): Typical of hypocalcaemia	
Thorn test (adrenaline)	50–0·3 (−150%)
17-Ketosteroids in the urine (mg./24 hr.)	2·5–6·2
11-Oxysteroids (γ/24 hr.)	346
Aldosterone (γ/24 hr.)	10
Blood cholesterol (mg. %)	Est. 93/Free 40
Cultures for *Candidae* (stools, urine, pharynx)	Negative
Bones and urinary tract x-ray examination	Negative
Ophthalmological examination (lens and fundus)	Negative
E.E.G. examination	Negative

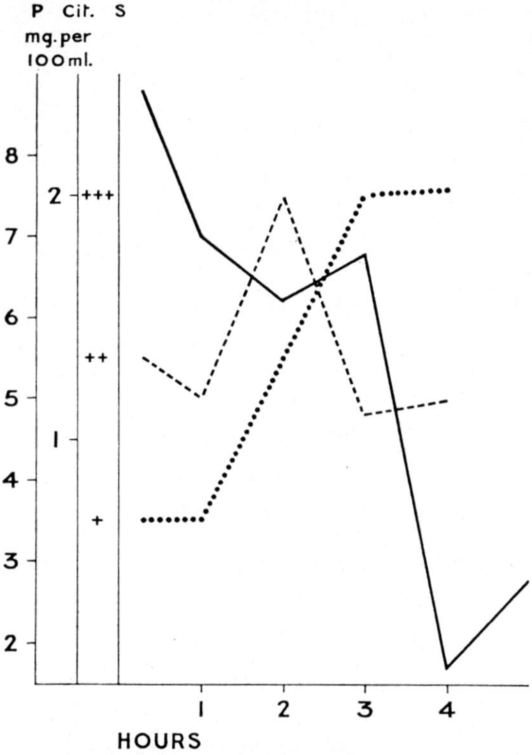

FIG 11.—Case 9. Intravenous calcium-gluconate infusion (Howard test).
—— Phosphates; — — — citrates; · · · · Sulkowitch reaction

during treatment with AT_{10}. It seems likely that the hypopotassaemia was associated with a state of alkalosis (for technical reasons it was impossible to determine the CO_2 levels in the blood plasma), for in a subsequent case the levels of CO_2 in the blood plasma proved to be rather high following a return to normal of the blood potassium levels.

Interpretation of this case is difficult. The hyperadrenocorticism might account for the hypocalcaemia but not for the hyperphosphataemia. In the absence of renal disturbances one suspects 'hypoparathyroidism associated with hyperadrenocorticism'. It may therefore be a case of two different endocrine disturbances both exerting a negative influence on the calcium balance of the organism.

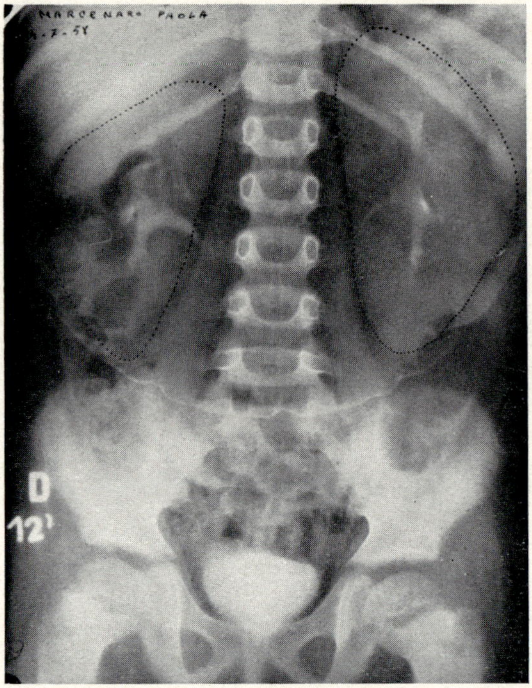

FIG. 12.—Case 9.

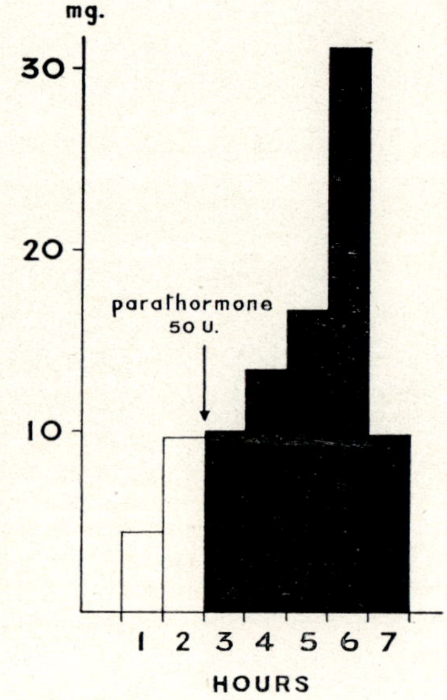

FIG. 13.—Case 9. Ellsworth-Howard test showing increased P output in urine.

A functional relationship between the parathyroid and suprarenal glands is demonstrated in these cases by a return to normal of the 17-ketosteroids output during treatment with parathormone (Fig. 14). The changes in 17-ketosteroid excretion after treatment with vitamin D_2 and AT_{10} provide further evidence of a complete change in the steroid balance.

Rachitogenous Tetany

Case 10. A girl, aged 10 months, was admitted to our clinic following an attack of tonic and clonic convulsions. All clinical signs of tetany were positive. Erb's test as well as an electrocardiogram were characteristic of hypocalcaemia. Radiological examination showed evidence of fresh rickets. There was evidence of a disturbance in citric acid metabolism in tetany caused by rickets.

In view of the fact that there was no decrease in citric acid excretion in the urine, and especially in view of the low citric acid levels in the blood (Table 11), it is possible that in this case also there was a lowering of the renal threshold. In contrast to the other case of tetany (Case 9) and to some cases of classical rickets, the urinary output of 17-ketosteroids proved to be normal. On the other hand, the Thorn test suggested an impaired function of the pituitary and suprarenals.

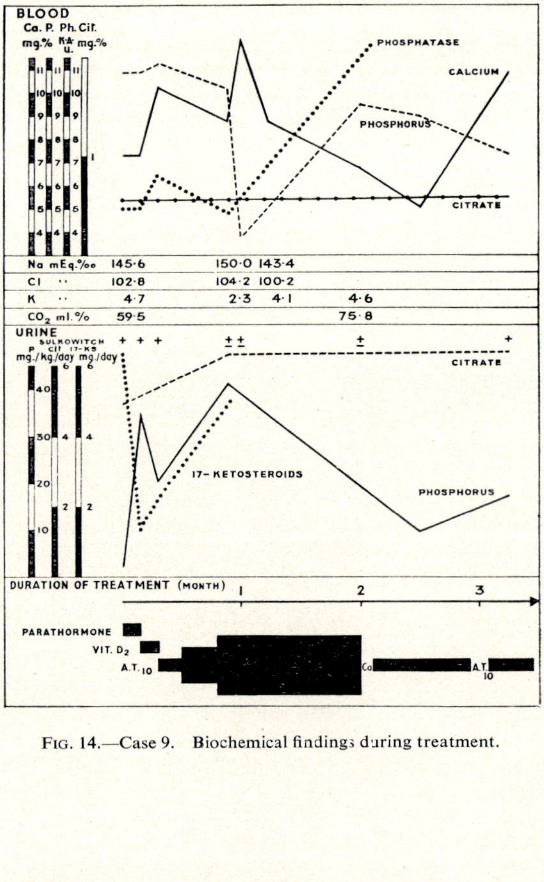

FIG. 14.—Case 9. Biochemical findings during treatment.

TABLE 11

BIOCHEMICAL FINDINGS IN CASE 10

Blood	
Ca (mg. %)	5·2
P (mg. %)	3·2
Citric acid (mg. %)	0·3
Phosphatase (K.A. units)	30
Na (mEq./l.)	136·4
Cl (mEq./l.)	103·4
K (mEq./l.)	5·3
Urine	
P (mg./kg./24 hr.)	50
Citric acid (mg./kg./24 hr.)	12
Na (mg./kg./24 hr.)	75
K (mg./kg./24 hr.)	17
Cl (mg./kg./24 hr.)	125
Sulkowitch reaction	+
*p*H	Between 5 and 6
Thorn test	46–13 (−25%)
17-Ketosteroids	Trace

Discussion

The cases reported show clearly that isolated investigation of data relating to calcium, phosphorus and phosphatase do not provide a comprehensive picture of the pathogenesis of disturbances of calcium-phosphorus metabolism and ossification. Cases 5, 6 and 7 also provide evidence that the radiological picture of the skeleton does not necessarily run parallel to the blood calcium and phosphorus levels.

We have confirmed the importance in pathogenesis of the metabolism of citrates as well as of their renal threshold not only in classical rickets but also in cases of tetany associated with rickets, in cases of vitamin D resistant rickets, in the 'de Toni-Debré-Fanconi syndrome' and in a special form of 'hyperadrenocorticism-hypoparathyroidism'. The changes in citric acid metabolism and the therapeutic action of ATP indicate that disturbances affecting the process of 'oxidative phosphorylation' can play an important part in the pathogenesis of rickets. Such a concept finds confirmation in the therapeutic action exerted by Pantetine in classical rickets (Coenzyme A) (Nordio *et al.*, 1957). Some disturbance of 'oxidative phosphorylation' occurs also in the 'de Toni-Debré-Fanconi syndrome'. The absence or weakness of any therapeutic action of ATP in a case of that disease and the fact that it has not been possible to produce the condition experimentally by administration of DNP show clearly that certain differences, not yet accurately defined, exist between the biochemical disturbance underlying classical rickets and that leading to vitamin D resistant rickets or the de Toni-Debré-Fanconi syndrome. The increased urinary output of steroids in some cases of rickets and in the 'de Toni-Debré-Fanconi syndrome' may be due to a disturbance of the whole steroid metabolism, as in idiopathic hypercalcaemia. There is probably a very close relationship between the disturbances of citric acid metabolism on the one hand and steroids on the other.

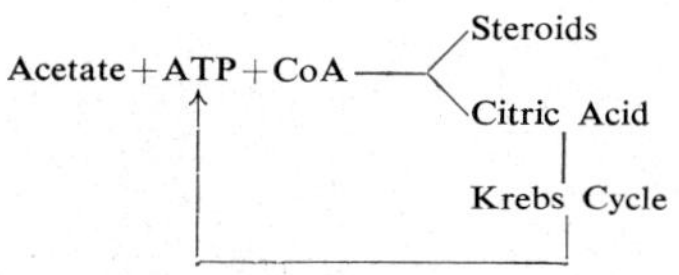

Evidence of such connexions can be found in a case in which an endocrine disturbance, probably caused by a suprarenal tumour, was associated with changes in the blood and urine levels of citric acid. This was in a boy, aged 3, who showed clear evidence of precocious puberty of adrenal type (enlarged penis, pubic and axillary hair, and testicles of normal size). Radiological examination following insufflation of air into the retroperitoneal space showed an enlargement of the right suprarenal gland with some calcification. Before we were able to complete all necessary investigations and to submit the boy to laparotomy the parents decided to take him home (Table 12). In Case 9 we believe that a more detailed study of the relationship between the parathyroid and suprarenal glands would be of considerable interest.

TABLE 12

BIOCHEMICAL FINDINGS IN A CASE OF PRECOCIOUS PUBERTY OF ADRENAL TYPE

17-Ketosteroids (mg./24 hr.)	7·86–11·3
Chromatography of the steroids	γ
Fraction I	1124
Fraction II-III	1800
Fraction IV-V	1200
Fraction VI-VII	1800
Fraction VIII	1500
Citric acid in blood (mg. per 100 ml.)	0·5
Citric acid in urine (mg./kg./24 hr.)	3

Conclusions

We consider that, for an elucidation of the disturbances of calcium and phosphorus metabolism and of ossification, the function of the 'citric acid cycle', which is closely correlated with the action of the parathyroid hormone, and that of vitamin D and AT_{10}, is of considerable importance (Harrison and Harrison, 1952a; Nordio *et al.*, 1956). It is likely that the sensitivity and resistance of the organism to vitamin D and AT_{10} are closely related to steroid metabolism and the 'Krebs cycle' in the renal tubules. Special importance is attached to the function of the 'Krebs cycle' in the renal tubules. It controls the reabsorption of amino acids, glucose and phosphorus and regulates the acid-base equilibrium, as shown in the studies of Cooke, Segar, Darrow, Reed, Etzwiler, Brusilow and Vita (1953), Harrison (1954), Durand *et al.* (1956) and Nordio *et al.* (1956) and in the investigations carried out in our case of 'de Toni-Debré-Fanconi syndrome'. In view of certain biochemical disturbances common to these pathological conditions, some relationship may also exist between the 'de Toni-Debré-Fanconi syndrome', classical rickets and vitamin D resistant rickets. In some cases of rickets it was also possible to demonstrate the presence of hyperphosphaturia, hyperaminoaciduria, renal acidosis and eventually glycosuria (Jonxis, 1955; Jeune, Charrat, Cotte and Freycon, 1958; Bickel, 1958), and a fall in blood citric acid levels with hypo- or hypercitruria.

The changes affecting the 'Krebs cycle' may be related to similar disturbances of steroid metabolism found in some types of rickets, in our case of 'de Toni-Debré-Fanconi syndrome' and in that of hypoparathyroidism. These observations suggest the possibility of a unified pathogenesis for this varied group of pathological conditions.

Methods Used

Citric acid: Pucher-Sherman-Vickery modified by Bonsignore and Ricci
Sodium and potassium: flame photometry
Calcium: precipitation according to Powell and estimation by flame photometry
Phosphorus: Gomory
Alkali reserve: van Slyke
Alkaline phosphatase: King-Armstrong
Creatinine: Folin-Wu
Blood sugar: Hagedorn-Jensen
Blood amino acids: Böhm-Grüner
Bilirubin: Jendrassik-Grof
17-Ketosteroids in urine: acid hydrolysis and extraction according to Pincus and Balter; colorimetric estimation according to Zimmerman modified by Callow
11-Oxysteroids: Gornall and McDonald
Aldosterones: Neher-Wettstein
Transaminase: Thonhazy-White-Umbreit
Cholinesterase: Hall-Lucas

Summary

A new approach to the mechanism regulating calcium/phosphorus metabolism and the process of ossification has been suggested. In classical and vitamin D resistant rickets as well as in the 'de Toni-Debré-Fanconi syndrome' evidence has been found of a disturbance of citric acid metabolism and of the suprarenal steroids; the same disturbances have been shown in a case of tetany with hyperadrenocorticism: such biochemical disturbances are probably related to one another. It seems possible that an alteration in the 'Krebs cycle' operating in the renal tubules plays an important part. In one case of 'de Toni-Debré-Fanconi syndrome' and in two cases of rickets, which did not respond to the usual treatment with vitamin D_2, the renal threshold for citric acid was lowered ('renal citrate diabetes'). These findings suggest the possibility of a unified pathogenesis for the various disturbances of calcium/phosphorus metabolism.

We are indebted to the Zilliken Co. of Genoa for putting at our disposal the ATP used in our therapeutic studies.

References

Aballí, A. J., Montero, R., Escobar Acés, A. and Jimenez, J. (1944). *Bol. Soc. cubana Pediat.* 16, 3.
Albaum, H. G., Hirshfeld, A. and Sobel, A. E. (1952). *Proc. Soc exp. Biol. (N.Y.)*, 79, 238.
Anderson, J., Brewis, E. G. and Taylor, W. (1957). *Archives of Disease in Childhood*, 32, 114
Bickel, H. (1958). International Symposium on Carbohydrates. Berne.
Cooke, R. E., Segar, W. E., Darrow, D. C., Reed, C., Etzwiler, D., Brusilow, S. and Vita, M. (1953). *A.M.A. Amer. J. Dis. Child.*, **86**, 611.
Dent, C. E. (1947). *Biochem. J.*, **41**, 240.
de Toni, G. (1957). *Int. Z. Vitaminforsch.*, **28**, 57.
de Toni, E. jr. and Giordano, S. (1957). *Minerva pediat. (Torino)*, **9**, 903.
Dickens, F. (1941). *Biochem. J.*, 35, 1011.
Dixon, T. F. and Perkins, H. R. (1952). *Ibid.*, **52**, 260.
Durand, P., Manzini, W., Bruni, R. and Semach, F. (1956). *Minerva pediat. (Torino)*, **8**, 1073.
Fanconi, G. and Spahr, A. (1956). *Helv. paediat. Acta.* **10**, 156.
Forfar, J. O., Balf, C. L., Maxwell, G. M. and Tompsett, S. L. (1956). *Lancet*, **1**, 981.
Freudenberg, E. (1954). *Ann. Pediat.*, **182**, 85.
Gittleman, I. F., Pincus, J. B., Schmerzler, E. and Saito, M. (1956). *Pediatrics*, **18**, 721.
Glanzmann, E., Meier, K. and Walthard, B. (1946). *Z. Vitaminforsch.*, 17, 159.
Harrison, H. E. (1954). *Pediatrics*, **14**, 285.
—— and Harrison, H. C. (1941). *J. clin. Invest.*, **20**, 47.
——, —— (1952a). *Yale J. Biol. Chem.*, **24**, 273.
——, —— (1952b). *J. Pediat.*, **41**, 756.
Heinz, E., Müller, E. and Rominger, E. (1947). *Z. Kinderheilk.*, **65**, 101.
Hofmann-Credner, D., Rupp, W. and Swoboda, W. (1955). *Arch. Kinderheilk.*, **150**, 221.
Jeune, H., Charrat, A., Cotte, Y. and Freycon, M. (1958). Personal communication.
Jonxis, J. H P. (1955). *Helv. paediat. Acta*, **10**, 245.
Lamy, M., Royer, P., Frézal, Y. and Lestradet, H. (1958). *Arch. franç. Pédiat.*, **15**, 1.
Leonard, M. F. (1946). *J. clin. Endocr.* **6**, 493.
Marks, P. A., Hiatt, H. H. and Shorr, E. (1953). *J. biol. Chem.*, **204**, 175.
Nordio, S., Semach, F. and Grego, M. (1956). *Minerva pediat. (Torino)*, **8**, 868.
——, Segni, G. and Massaccesi, R. (1957). *Ibid.*, **9**, 1569.
Papadatos, C. and Klein, R. (1954). *J. Clin. Endocr.*, **14**, 653.
Roberts, K. E. and Pitts, R. F. (1953). *Endocrinology*, **52**, 324.
Royer, P., Lestradet, H. and Habib, R. (1958). *Arch. franç. Pédiat.*, **15**, 896.
Schwarz-Tiene, E., Careddu, P. and Cabassa. N. (1957). *Minerva pediat. (Torino)*, **9**, 231.
Sirota, J. H. and Hamerman, D. (1954). *Amer. J. Med.*, **16**, 138.
Steenbock, H. and Bellin, S. A. (1953). *J. biol. Chem.*, **205**, 985.
van Creveld, S. and Arons, P. (1949). *Ann. paediat. (Basel)*, 173, 299.
Whitaker, J., Landing, B. H., Esselborn, M. and Williams, R. R. (1956). *J. clin. Endocr.*, **16**, 1374.
Winberg, J. and Zetterström, R. (1956). *Acta paediat. (Uppsala)*, **45**, 96.
Zetterström, R. and Arnhold, R. G. (1958). *Ibid.*, **47**, 107.
Zweymüller, E. (1958). *Mod. Probl. Pädiat.*, 3, 433.

For further details on these studies and further literature the authors wish to refer to their paper (*Minerva pediat. (Torino)*, **11**, 129 (1959)).

FAMILIAL VITAMIN D-RESISTANT RICKETS

METABOLIC STUDIES IN ONE FAMILY CONCERNING AETIOLOGY AND TREATMENT, AND INDICATING THE SEPARATE ACTIONS OF VITAMIN D

BY

C. P. DANCASTER* and W. P. U. JACKSON

From the Endocrine Group, Department of Medicine, Groote Schuur Hospital and University of Cape Town, South Africa

(RECEIVED FOR PUBLICATION FEBRUARY 2, 1959)

Rickets which is refractory to ordinary doses of vitamin D was first recognized when vitamin preparations of high potency became available (Albright, Butler and Bloomberg, 1937). As an isolated metabolic disorder it is commonly known as 'vitamin D-resistant rickets', also as 'phosphate diabetes' (Fanconi, 1936a, b) and phosphate losing (or renal tubular) rickets, type 1 (Dent, 1952). Whereas it was originally regarded as a rare condition—Freeman and Dunsky (1950) found only some 30 cases in the literature up to 1950—Dent and Harris (1956) consider it the most common form of rickets in England at present. Possible explanations of its apparent increase are the diminished incidence of ordinary rickets in England following fortification of various foodstuffs with vitamin D, and an awareness of the family trait and the possible association of renal dysfunction with the resistant type.

Vitamin D-resistant rickets in many ways resembles true rickets (e.g. the changes in blood chemistry and histological appearance). However, there are differences between these conditions. The resistant type is familial (in the large family described by Winters, Graham, Williams, McFalls and Burnett (1958), it appeared as a sex-linked dominant characteristic), the serum calcium is never low enough to cause tetany, the level of urine calcium in some is normal and the muscular weakness and hypotonia, so typical in classical rickets, is not very conspicuous. In addition, the patients usually appear well nourished and generally healthy. Very large doses of vitamin D or dihydrotachysterol (AT 10) are necessary to initiate mineralization. Furthermore, radiographs may show very little rachitic change at the bone ends, despite pronounced dwarfing and typical biochemistry. There is no excess amino-aciduria.

* Senior Bursar, Council for Scientific and Industrial Research.

The aetiology of the condition is not fully understood. It is not a dietary deficiency of any known factor, nor is it due to lack of intestinal absorption of vitamin D, since intravenous vitamin D fails to evoke a response, and blood levels of vitamin D have been normal (Freeman and Dunsky, 1950). A defect in renal function with resultant hyperphosphaturia has been suggested by Fanconi (1936a, b), Robertson, Harris and McCune (1942), Dent (1952) and Jackson and Linder (1953). This hypothesis has much to commend it. Familial defects in renal tubular function associated with bony abnormalities of rachitic and osteomalacic type are recognized syndromes. Diminished tubular reabsorption can affect numerous substances and produce various clinical pictures. It is postulated that phosphorus reabsorption alone may be affected, resulting in a clinical condition resembling rickets but resistant to ordinary doses of vitamin D. It has been shown that in cases of Fanconi's syndrome (in which there is deficient tubular reabsorption of phosphorus, glucose, amino-acids, water and potassium) large doses of vitamin D, in addition to correcting skeletal deformities and phosphorus excretion, can improve tubular reabsorption of other substances, so that diminished glycosuria and amino-aciduria result. In vitamin D-resistant rickets, renal tubular reabsorption of phosphorus has also improved after very large doses of vitamin D. Dent (1952) has reported two brothers with the disease, one of whom had renal glycosuria while the other did not.

However, Albright *et al.* (1937) believed that there was an intrinsic resistance to the primary effect of vitamin D. According to their view, deficient absorption of calcium from the gastro-intestinal canal resulted in a low serum calcium and this caused parathyroid hyperplasia. Increased parathyroid secretion led to hyperphosphaturia and a lowering of the serum phosphorus. Any effects from vitamin D therapy were interpreted as being due to reduction of the parathyroid hypersecretion as the absorption of calcium became normal.

Case Histories

A family of bow-legged children (Fig. 1) presented at the out-patient department. There were four children, three males aged 7, 9 and 11 years and one female aged 3 years. All were dwarfed but well nourished. As can be seen (Table 1) the dwarfing is mainly accounted for by the lack of growth of the lower segment. They had all been exposed to a great deal of sunlight and two of them (James and Elizabeth) had had 1 drachm of Vidaylin (=800 units vitamin D) daily for two months before being seen by us. Skeletal changes, which were strikingly similar in each, had first been noticed when they started to walk. There was anterior and lateral bowing of the tibiae and femora. The skull was normal and no protuberance could be felt in the ribs and wrists. There were no other abnormal findings clinically. The mother of these children had had an osteotomy at the age of 13, because of bowed legs, and the residual deformity was still apparent. We were unable to establish any other family history.

TABLE 1
MEASUREMENTS AND WEIGHTS OF FAMILY

	Height (in.)	Weight (lb.)	Span (in.)	Lower Segment	Upper Segment	Age (years)
James ..	46 (54)*	62 (67)	49 (53·4)	21½ (27)	25½ (27)	10
Henry ..	45¾ (51)	55 (58)	48½ (51)	21½ (25)	24¼ (26)	9
Peter ..	44 (47·2)	44 (48)	46 (46)	20 (22·5)	24 (24¾)	7
Elizabeth ..	33½ (37)	30 (32)	33½ (36)	15½ (16)	18 (21)	3
Mother ..	62	136¾	65¼	31½	30½	38

* Normal figures in brackets. (Adapted from Engelbach, Endocrine Medicine, Springfield, Illinois. Charles C. Thomas, 1932.)

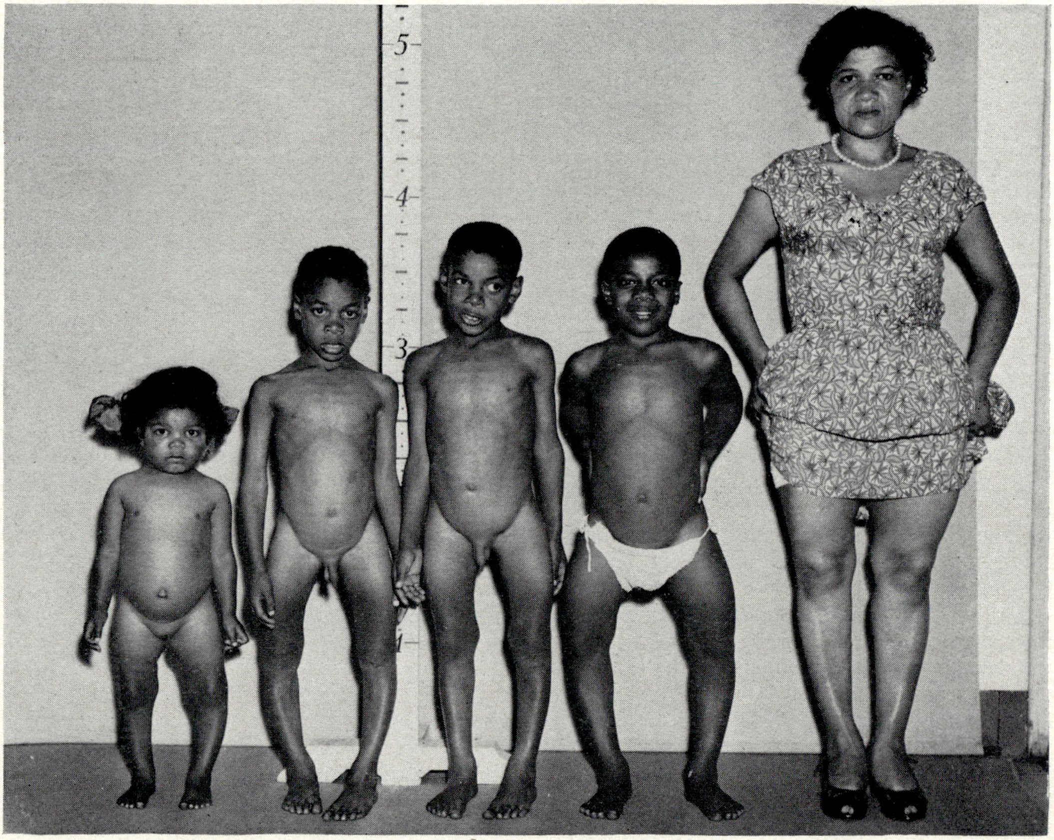

FIG. 1.—Family showing vitamin D-resistant rickets.

Radiography. The bowing of the tibiae and femora is common to all four children. Only Elizabeth, the youngest, had typically rachitic epiphyseal changes present at the wrist. In the others the most marked changes occurred in the tibial epiphyses (Fig. 2). A lack of calcification particularly affecting the medial half of the epiphyses is characteristic of vitamin D-resistant rickets (Dent, 1958). This is well seen in Elizabeth with subsequent calcification after therapy (Fig. 2c, d). There was no radiological evidence of secondary hyperparathyroidism.

Initial Laboratory Investigations. Biochemical examination revealed low serum inorganic phosphorus, raised alkaline phosphatase and normal (or slightly reduced) serum calcium figures (Table 2). Other electrolytes were normal. James' serum phosphorus readings ranged from 2·0 to 4·5 mg. per 100 ml. (11 estimations). Potassium was 3·6 mEq./l., sodium 150 mEq./l., chloride 106 mEq./l. and blood urea 26 mg. per 100 ml. His blood count was normal except that there was an unexplained eosinophilia of 20%.

TABLE 2
BIOCHEMICAL INVESTIGATIONS

	Calcium (mg./100 ml.)	Inorganic Phosphorus (mg./100 ml.)	Alkaline Phosphatase*
Henry . .	9·1	2·6	22·5
Elizabeth	9·6	1·8	34·6
Peter . .	9·4	2·2	22·5
James . .	9·4	2·1	41·6
Mother . .		2·7	6·5

* Shinowara-Bodansky

The findings thus far indicated that we were dealing with a type of familial rickets. There was no glycosuria, polyuria or amino-aciduria, but the amount of phosphorus excreted in the 24 hours was high in relation to the serum level, and there was a diminished tubular reabsorption of phosphorus (Table 3).

It was decided to employ large doses of vitamin D after control studies and metabolic balances had been performed on two of the children, Elizabeth and James. In addition, the effect of parathormone was observed (Ellsworth-Howard test) and renal function was investigated (creatinine clearance studies).

Methods

Response to Vitamin D using Metabolic Balance Studies. Eight consecutive five-day metabolic balance studies were performed on James while he was receiving a normal diet. The dose of vitamin D was gradually increased during this time up to a maximum of 1 million units daily (supplied as Ostelin Forte, 50,000 units per tablet by Glaxo.)

Three consecutive five-day metabolic balance studies were performed on Elizabeth, one a control and the others during the administration of large doses of vitamin D (400,000 and 1 million units daily).

Food and stools were homogenized and these and the urine were analysed for calcium, phosphorus, nitrogen and potassium content. Faecal collections ran from mid-day to mid-day and stool markers were not used. Food and urine collections went from 7 a.m. to 7 a.m. Bowels were kept regular by bland non-metabolic laxatives when necessary. Results are shown in Figs. 3 and 5, charted after the manner of Reifenstein, Albright and Wells (1945). Serum levels of calcium, phosphorus and alkaline phosphatase were taken at frequent intervals in order to detect any effect of vitamin D, either therapeutic or toxic, and to correlate any variation in the blood with other metabolic changes.

Ellsworth-Howard Test. Parathyroid hormone in the dosage of 200 U.S.P. was injected intravenously after three control periods of one hour each. The urine was collected by catheter and the phosphorus content estimated in three periods before and for three similar periods after injection.

Creatinine Clearance Studies. The 24-hour urinary excretion of creatinine and phosphorus were calculated and the serum level of these substances was estimated during this collection. From these figures the percentage of phosphorus reabsorbed by the tubules was calculated.

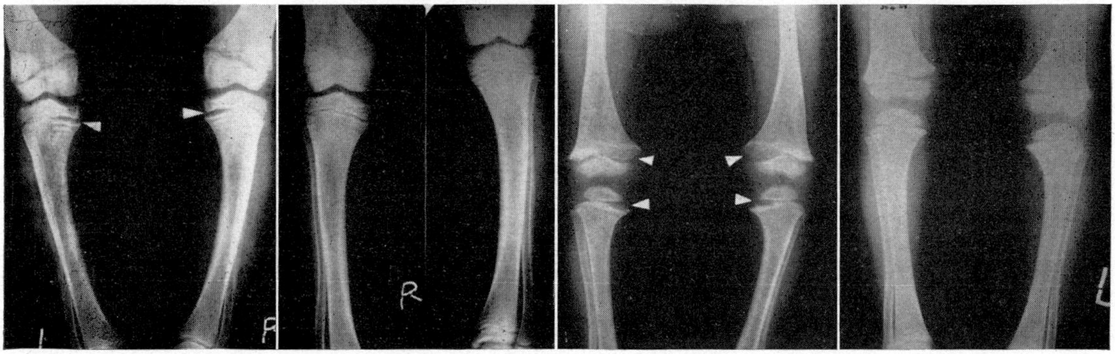

(a) (b) (c) (d)

FIG. 2.—(*a*) James' radiograph showing (1) lack of calcification particularly of medial aspect of growing bone at upper end of tibiae (arrows); (2) obliquity of epiphyses; (3) Harris' lines at upper and lower tibia. (*b*) James: healing four months later. (*c*) Elizabeth: radiograph showing lack of calcification particularly of medial aspect of growing bone at upper tibial and lower femoral epiphyses (arrows). *d*) Elizabeth: healing four months later.

TABLE 3

RENAL FUNCTION STUDIES

Date (1958)	Vit. D (units)	GFR* (uncorrected)	Fp	UVp (mg./min.)	TRP	Reabsorbed (%)
			James			
January						
23	Control	27	·71	·38	·33	46
25	,,	22	·63	·27	·36	57
27	,,	22	·59	·33	·26	44
March						
13	1 million	35	1·37	·4	·97	70
14	,,	26	·92	·4	·52	57·6
17	,,	31·2	1·17	·4	·77	66
18	400,000	24·5	1·07	·31	·76	71
21	,,	26·8	1·74	·31	1·43	82
25	200,000	28	1·64	·24	1·4	85
			Elizabeth			
March						
10	Control	13	·448	·434	·014	3·1†
14	400,000	13	·35	·25	·10	29
15	,,	8·7	·29	·24	·05	17
17	,,	13·3	·40	·25	·15	37
19	1 million	14	·78	·48	·3	38·5
20	,,	16·6	·78	·48	·3	38·5

* GFR = Glomerular filtration rate (ml./min.). Fp = Filtered phosphorus (mg./min.).
UVp = Urinary phosphorus (mg./min.). TRP = Tubular reabsorption of phosphorus (mg./min.).
† This low figure is accounted for by the high daily urinary phosphorus excretion, 624 mg., when the total filtered phosphorus was 645 mg.

Results

Renal Function Studies. The 24-hour creatinine clearance was estimated in two patients (Elizabeth and James) before and during therapy with vitamin D, to observe whether there was a diminished tubular reabsorption of phosphorus and whether this would be corrected by treatment. In both cases there was an improvement in tubular reabsorption of phosphorus after therapy. Results are shown in Table 3. There was possibly a slight increase in glomerular filtration rate.

Response to Parathyroid Extract (Parathormone, Lilly). In view of the alleged tubular defect in this condition and the possible secondary hyperparathyroidism, the response to parathyroid extract was investigated (Table 4). There was a poor phosphorus diuresis after the intravenous administration of 200 I.U. parathormone. However, the interpretation of this finding is obscure since we have found that not all normal subjects respond to intravenous parathormone (Dancaster, Schendel and Jackson 1959).

Metabolic Balance Studies

James (Figs. 3 and 4). CALCIUM METABOLISM. The difference between the faecal excretion of calcium in period 1 and periods 2 and 3 is probably due to incomplete collection in period 1. For this reason an average of the faecal excretions over the first three periods is considered more accurate. The gastro-intestinal absorption was poor during this time, resulting in a negative balance. The dose of calciferol was increased to 100,000 units but this had no effect on faecal excretion of calcium. However, an increase to 400,000 units daily in period 5, and to 1 million units daily in period 6 improved gastro-intestinal absorption. Again, an

TABLE 4

ELLSWORTH-HOWARD TEST: MARCH 30, 1958

	Urinary Phosphorus (mg./hr.)	Serum Phosphorus (mg. %)
Specimen 1	9·43	Period 2:2·63
2	29·39—Av. 16·5	
3	10·63	
Parathormone 200 units intravenous		
Specimen 4	34·90	
5	13·11—Av. 24·3	Period 5: 2·50
6	24·98	

average of faecal excretions in periods 5 and 6 is probably more accurate than their separate representations. In spite of improved absorption the patient remained in negative balance during this time, and it was only after a month that the gastro-intestinal absorption improved sufficiently to produce a positive balance (periods 7 and 8).

In agreement with earlier workers we found the urinary excretion of calcium to be low (10-25 mg./day), in spite of normal and even high serum figures. Calciferol administered in doses of 100,000 and 400,000 units daily had no effect on the urinary excretion and it was not until calciferol administration was increased to 1 million units daily that urinary calcium rose to abnormal figures (800 mg. daily in period 6). This extraordinary rise in urinary calcium preceded any marked improvement in gastro-intestinal absorption. The serum level exceeded 11 mg. per 100 ml. in period 5 and remained elevated till the end of the balance study. On account of this, calciferol administration was temporarily discontinued after period 8. The rise in serum calcium preceded any marked improvement in gastro-intestinal absorption and did not alter the very low urinary excretion of calcium in period 5.

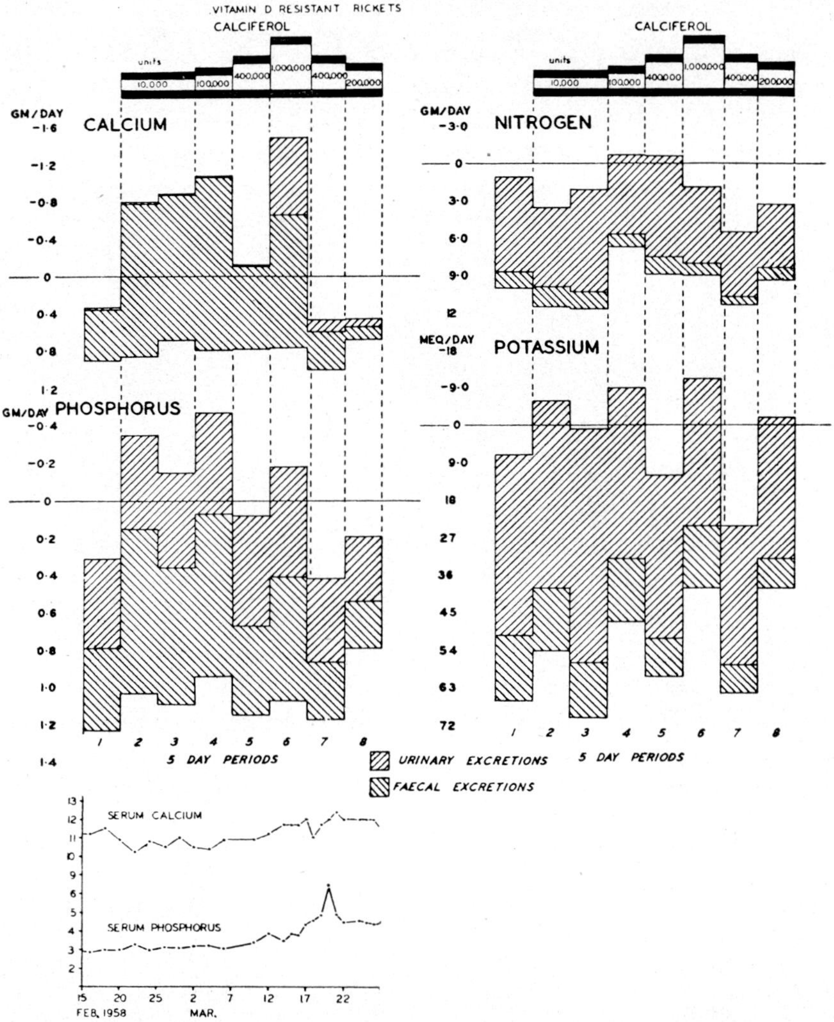

FIG. 3.—James: metabolic balance.

PHOSPHORUS METABOLISM. An average of the faecal phosphorus over the first three periods indicated a very slight negative phosphorus balance at this time.

An increased dose of calciferol resulted in improvement in gastro-intestinal absorption comparable to that achieved with calcium. A definite positive balance was observed only in the final two periods but improvement in absorption was first evident in period 5, while the patient was taking 400,000 units of calciferol. The urinary excretion of phosphorus remained constant during the first six periods in spite of increasing serum figures. There was a small decrease in urinary phosphorus in periods 7 and 8.

Before therapy was commenced, serum phosphorus was estimated on 11 occasions and was usually between 2-3 mg. per 100 ml. However, it was twice above 3 mg. per 100 ml. (3·9 and 4·5 mg. per 100 ml.). The daily variations in serum phosphorus level are noteworthy and are not unusual in this condition.

During therapy the serum phosphorus remained at about 3 mg. till period 6, when, on 1 million units of calciferol, it started to rise.

Elizabeth (Figs. 5 and 6). The discrepancy in the faecal excretion of calcium and phosphorus between the first two balance periods may have been due to incomplete faecal collections in period 1. After calciferol administration had been increased to 1 million units daily (period 3) the gastro-intestinal absorption of calcium improved. Increased urinary excretion occurred during the same period.

A marked improvement in gastro-intestinal absorption

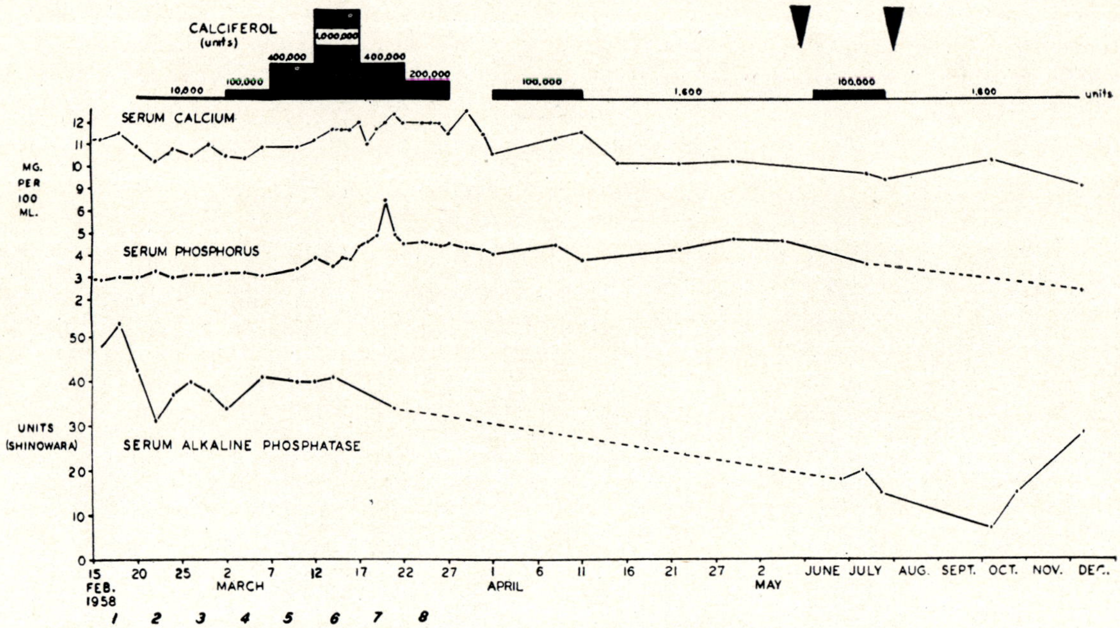

FIG. 4.—James: blood chemistry. (Arrows indicate osteotomies.)

of phosphorus occurred in period 3. Both the serum calcium and phosphorus were elevated at this time.

Nitrogen balances did not vary much, being mostly positive in both children. The faecal potassium seemed to fall in the latter periods of both children on vitamin D therapy (as was noticed by Henneman, Dempsey, Carroll and Albright, 1956, in sarcoidosis).

Discussion

Actions of Vitamin D. We believe that vitamin D has three main actions on calcium metabolism (discussed in greater detail elsewhere) (Jackson and Dancaster, 1959): (1) increasing absorption of calcium from the intestinal tract (Albright and Reifenstein, 1948); (2) increasing the serum calcium, presumably by drawing calcium from the bone and so tending to lead to decalcification (Dent, 1954); (3) increasing the urinary calcium by diminution in renal tubular reabsorption or possibly change in the form of the serum calcium. This is often the earliest action of all (Dent, 1954; Howard and Connor, 1954 ; Jackson, Hoffenberg, Linder and Irwin, 1956; Litvak, Moldawer, Forbes and Henneman, 1958).

These actions may appear separately or in different order in different patients. Thus we have seen the serum calcium rise without change in urinary calcium or intestinal absorption in patients with sarcoidosis given vitamin D. Dent has actually found a large fall in urine calcium in one case of osteomalacia under treatment while the serum calcium rose. We have seen the urine calcium rise without or before change in faecal or serum calcium in normal and in hypoparathyroid subjects.

The separate effects of vitamin D stand out clearly from the balance studies of James. The serum, and particularly the urinary calcium, rose markedly in period 6 without any change in intestinal absorption: the serum calcium then rose further while the urinary calcium fell vastly (periods 7 and 8). In the case of Elizabeth, the serum calcium appeared to rise before there was any fall in faecal calcium or a rise in urinary calcium, but this is less clear-cut.

In both children the initial urinary calcium was exceedingly low (7 and 25 mg./day) despite a normal or even high-normal serum calcium. This presumably indicates a specific depression of renal excretory mechanism for calcium (? increased tubular reabsorption), possibly a part of the 'resistance' to the action of normal amounts of circulating vitamin D. In ordinary D-lack rickets, one frequently finds the same thing; i.e. an almost absent urinary calcium, with normal serum levels, further supporting the view that vitamin D has a specific action in maintaining the urinary excretion of calcium.

Mechanisms in Resistant Rickets and Its Treatment with Vitamin D. Pre-treatment balance studies, especially in James, indicate defective absorption of both calcium and phosphorus from the gut. In both children large doses of vitamin D (period 7 in James and period 3 in Elizabeth) plainly increased the intestinal absorption of both elements. In James we also have evidence of a distinct increase in phosphorus reabsorption by the renal tubules under the same treatment.

The mechanism of improved tubular reabsorption of phosphorus by vitamin D is not certain. Albright has shown that patients with idiopathic hypoparathyroidism have an increased renal excretion of phosphorus after vitamin D, but if the parathyroids are intact the tubular reabsorption may be improved and the urine phosphorus may fall (Albright and Reifenstein, 1948). He interprets this as being due to secondary hypoparathyroidism following increase in serum calcium. In James the increase in serum calcium occurred on the same day as the improved tubular reabsorption, but in Elizabeth serum calcium elevation preceded any change in phosphorus reabsorption by four days. However, as the serum calcium did not remain consistently elevated during this time we do not consider this is evidence in favour of Albright's hypothesis. It may be that vitamin D really increases tubular reabsorption of phosphorus by direct action on the kidneys in the resistant rickets syndrome.

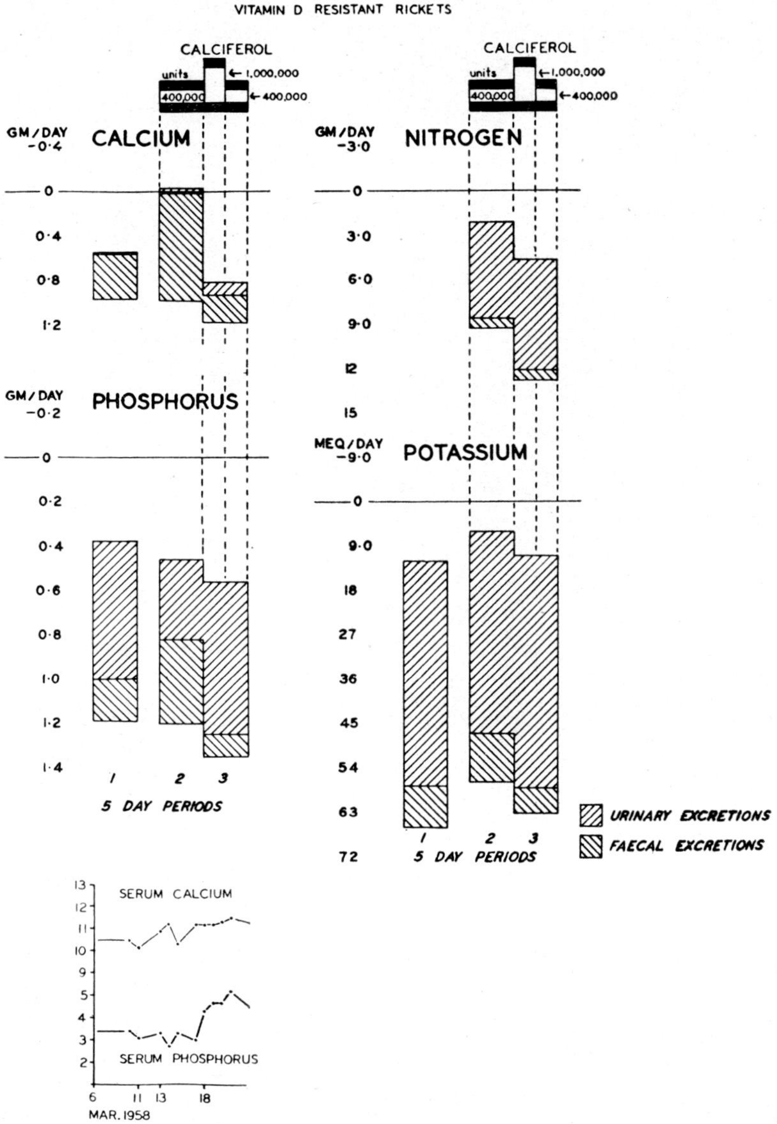

FIG. 5.—Elizabeth: metabolic balance.

As we found in a patient with adolescent osteomalacia with raised resistance to vitamin D, there appears to be evidence, at least in some cases, that both defective absorption of calcium from the gut and a 'phosphate leak' into the urine may be implicated in the aetiology of 'resistant rickets' (Jackson, Dowdle and Linder, 1958).

Subsequent Treatment and Control

As the aetiology of this condition is not completely understood, treatment must aim at correcting abnormal findings. With large doses of vitamin D the serum phosphorus and alkaline phosphatase may return to normal, as may the radiological appearances of the epiphyses. It is important to know to what extent treatment can prevent progression and aggravation of existing deformities and how best to assess cessation of activity of the rachitic process. While gross deformities of the shafts of long bones will have to be corrected surgically, the normal calcification of epiphyseal osteoid after

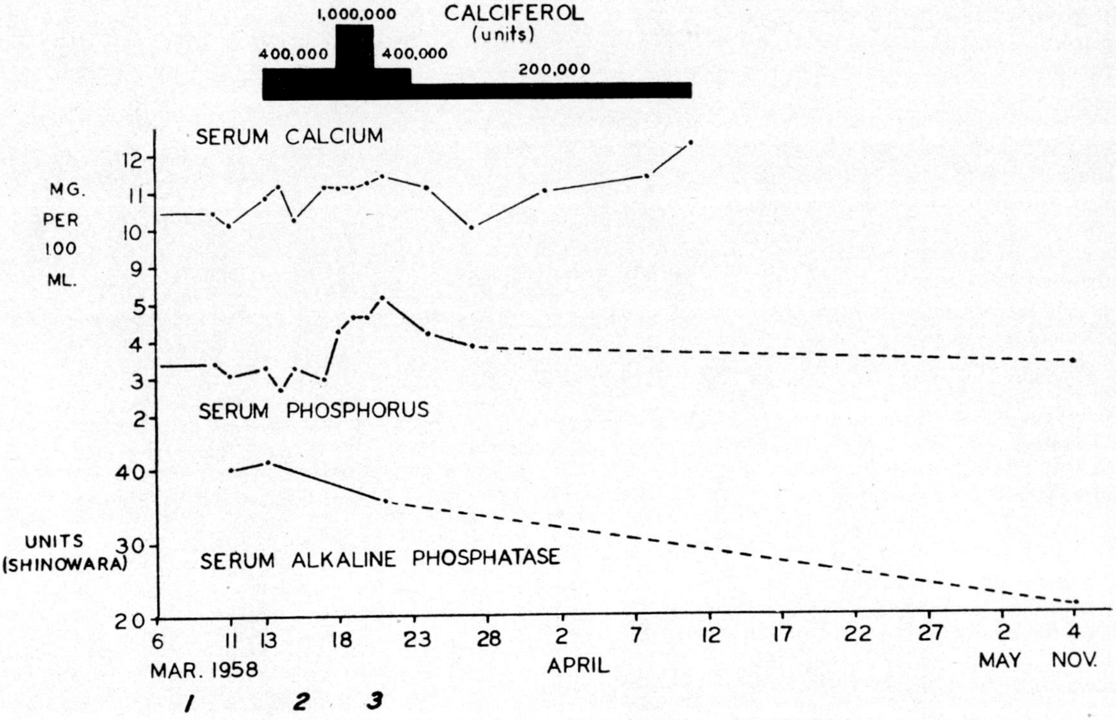

FIG. 6.—Elizabeth: blood chemistry. (No vitamin D after April 12, 1958.)

vitamin D prevents progression of the deformity and enables growth to occur (a patient has been reported as growing 12 inches in six years (Albright, Burnett, Parson, Reifenstein and Roos, 1946). Radiological control is probably the most satisfactory way of assessing progress because in some cases the abnormal changes in serum alkaline phosphatase and phosphorus may persist in spite of healing. In both our patients, the serum phosphorus returned to normal before there was any change in alkaline phosphatase, and there was radiological evidence of healing while the alkaline phosphatase was still elevated.

The length of time during which therapy has to be continued is often difficult to assess. Most cases heal spontaneously at puberty. However, even after radiological evidence of healing, relapses have occurred after puberty (Christiansson, 1958). The biochemical abnormalities may persist many years after epiphyseal closure. James has shown both radiological and biochemical healing after nine months therapy with large doses of vitamin D (200,000 units daily). However, after therapy had been discontinued for two months the alkaline phosphatase became elevated again (Fig. 4).

Although mineralization of the skeleton can be effected with vitamin D, there is still a lack of normal compact bone histologically (Engfeldt, Zetterström and Winberg, 1956). It would seem that vitamin D is not curative and that it is therefore extremely important to have regular radiological and biochemical assessment of progress. Any radiological evidence of regression would be an indication for further treatment, but whether complete biochemical cure (i.e. normal serum alkaline phosphatase and phosphorus) is essential, is debatable.

Although the therapeutic dose of vitamin D is increased in this condition, the toxic threshold is apparently unaltered and the margin of safety therefore small. In fact some cases may be impossible to treat, since the curative dose from the point of view of the rickets may be toxic with regard to the serum calcium level.

If osteotomy is to be performed, it is usually done at puberty once the condition has been controlled with vitamin D. Discontinuance of therapy for a period of two weeks before surgery and during the period of bed rest has been advised in view of the possible complication of renal calculi. In James the serum calcium went up to 12·4 mg. per 100 ml.

during treatment. By reducing the dose of vitamin D from 400,000 to 250,000 units daily the serum calcium level was reduced to 11·5 mg. per 100 ml., but reduction of the dose of vitamin D to 100,000 units daily had little effect in reducing the calcium further. However, four days after discontinuance of all vitamin D therapy the serum calcium returned to normal at 10·0 mg. At one stage the blood urea rose from 31 mg. to 51 mg. while on vitamin D. There was hypercalcaemia (11·6 mg./100 ml.) and a hypercalcuria of 840 mg./day at this time. When the dose was reduced from 1 million to 400,000 units the blood urea fell to 26 mg. and the hypercalcuria diminished although the hypercalcaemia persisted.

In Elizabeth, although the serum calcium went above 12 mg. on one occasion and was frequently between 11-12 mg., the urinary calcium did not exceed 110 mg. per day. A reduction in dose of vitamin D had little effect on hypercalcaemia, but after its discontinuance the serum calcium returned to normal within four days.

From these findings it appears that routine testing of the urine with Sulkowitch's reagent is not sufficiently accurate in this condition. There were no clinical findings to suggest hypercalcaemia in our children despite serum levels above 12 mg. per 100 ml., so that periodic estimations of serum calcium are essential.

Note on Genetics. The appearance of 'resistant rickets' in a mother, three sons and one daughter is compatible with a dominant sex-linked inheritance, the responsible gene being situated on the non-homologous portion of the X chromosome. An affected father cannot pass on the condition to his sons, but the mother can pass it to both sons and daughters.

In the present family, of course, simple autosomal dominance would equally well fit, but sex-linked dominance seems more likely in this condition, judging from the work of Winters *et al.* (1958) and the data of Dent (1958).

Summary

A family of bow-legged children are described whose clinical features fitted the syndrome known as 'vitamin D-resistant rickets'. Metabolic balances and renal clearance studies were performed on two of them. An elevation of serum calcium and phosphorus followed the use of vitamin D in high dosage. This occurred in spite of continued poor gastro-intestinal absorption, which in one case persisted for 25 days after therapy was commenced and then improved.

It was considered that the source of the calcium which accounted for the hypercalcaemia and hypercalcuria on vitamin D was bone, but that the increase in serum phosphorus was accompanied by an improved renal tubular reabsorption. The three actions of vitamin D on calcium metabolism appeared nicely separated in these patients. Their disorder seemed to be caused by a mixture of poor intestinal absorption of calcium and increased renal loss of phosphorus.

Our thanks are due to Professor F. Ford for enabling us to investigate Elizabeth, to Professor G. Linder and staff for alkaline phosphatase determinations, and to Professor F. Forman for constant interest and advice; also to Staff Nurse Schoonraad for his help in the metabolic ward. The work here reported is part of the programme of the Endocrine Research Group supported in the Department of Medicine, University of Cape Town, by the Council for Scientific and Industrial Research.

References

Albright, F. and Reifenstein, E. C. (1948). *The Parathyroid Glands and Metabolic Bone Diseases.* Williams and Wilkins, Baltimore.
——, Burnett, C. H., Parson, W., Reifenstein, E. C. and Roos, A. (1946). *Medicine (Baltimore)*, **25**, 399.
——, Butler, A. M. and Bloomberg, E. (1937). *Amer. J. Dis. Child.*, **54**, 529.
Christiansson, G. (1958). *Acta paediat. (Uppsala)*, **47**, 288.
Dancaster, C. P., Schendel, H. and Jackson, W. P. U. (1959). In the press. *Clin. Sci.*
Dent, C. E. (1952). *J. Bone Jt Surg.*, **34B**, 266.
—— (1954). In *Ciba Foundation Symposium on the Kidney*, p. 242 Churchill, London.
—— (1958). Personal communication.
—— and Harris, H. (1956). *J. Bone Jt Surg.*, **38B**, 204.
Engelbach, W. (1932). *Endocrine Medicine.* Thomas, Springfield, Ill.
Engfeldt, B., Zetterström, R. and Winberg, J. (1956). *Ibid.*, **38A**, 1323.
Fanconi, G. (1936). Quoted by McCune, D. J., Mason, H. H. and Clarke, H. T. (1943). *Amer. J. Dis. Child.*, **65**, 81.
—— (1936a). *Dtsch. med. Wschr.*, **62**, 1169.
—— (1936b). *Jb. Kinderheilk.*, **147**, 299.
Freeman, S. and Dunsky, I. (1950). *Ibid.*, **79**, 409.
Henneman, P. H., Dempsey, E. F., Carroll, E. L. and Albright, F. (1956). *J. clin. Invest.*, **35**, 1229.
Howard, J. E. and Connor, T. B. (1954). *Trans. Ass. Amer. Phycns*, **67**, 199.
Jackson, W. P. U. and Dancaster, C. P. (1959). *J. Clin. Endocr.* **19**, 658.
——, Dowdle, E. and Linder, G. C. (1958). *Brit. med. J.*, **1**, 1269.
——, Hoffenberg, R., Linder, G. C. and Irwin, L. (1956). *J. Clin. Endocr.*, **16**, 1043.
—— and Linder, G. C. (1953). *Quart. J. Med.*, **22**, 133.
Litvak, J., Moldawer, M. P., Forbes, A. P. and Henneman, P. H. (1958). *Ibid.*, **18**, 246.
Reifenstein, E. C., Albright, F. and Wells, S. L. (1945). *Ibid.*, **5**, 367.
Robertson, B. R., Harris, R. C. and McCune, D. J. (1942). *Amer. J. Dis. Child.*, **64**, 958.
Winters, R. W., Graham, J. B., Williams, T. F., McFalls, V. W. and Burnett, C. H. (1958). *Medicine (Baltimore)*, **37**, 97.

ELECTROPHORETIC STUDIES OF SERUM PROTEIN PATTERNS IN NEWBORN INDIAN INFANTS

BY

B. S. KULKARNI, R. S. SATOSKAR, M. N. PARIKH and R. G. CHITRE

From the Department of Pharmacology, Seth G.S. Medical College and Nowrosjee Wadia Maternity Hospital, Bombay 12, *India*

(RECEIVED FOR PUBLICATION MARCH 17, 1959)

The concentration of gamma globulin in the serum of apparently healthy adults from tropical areas is considerably higher than that of residents in temperate zones (Holmes, Stanier, Semambo and Jones, 1951; Satoskar and Lewis, 1954; Deegan, Gilles and McGregor, 1956; Kulkarni, 1957b; Edozien, 1957). In studies of plasma protein patterns in 100 Indian medical students (Satoskar and Lewis, 1954) gamma globulin and albumin levels were found to be twice as high as those among non-tropical residents. Furthermore there was no obvious correlation between past illness and the plasma proteins. Although some correlation was noticed between the dietary protein source and the level of gamma globulin, a definite cause for this rise could not be found. It would therefore be interesting to study the serum protein patterns of umbilical cord blood to see whether the newborn Indian infant also has a high level of globulin, particularly the gamma fraction, as compared with infants born in temperate zones.

Studies in the U.S.A. have shown the serum gamma globulin of cord blood to be as high as, or even higher than, that of maternal blood (Longsworth, Curtis and Pembroke, 1945; Orlandini, Sass-Kortsak and Ebbs, 1955; Saito, Gittleman, Pincus and Sobel, 1956; Jencks, Smith and Durrum, 1956). But similar studies on African infants showed the serum gamma globulin of cord blood to be lower than that of the maternal blood at delivery (Stanier and Thompson, 1954). Our previous studies on plasma proteins in normal pregnant women at term showed a lower serum albumin level than that reported by foreign workers; however the serum gamma globulin in these women was much higher (Coryell, Beach, Robinson, Macy and Mack, 1950; Mack, Robinson, Wiseman, Schoeb and Macy, 1951; Brown, 1954; Purandare, Satoskar and Lewis, 1954). The average birthweight of Indian newborn infants is considered to be lower than the Western birthweight standard. Since the diet of the average Indian is qualitatively and quantitatively low in protein content, it would be of interest to find out if this is in any way related to birthweight and levels of the different protein fractions of the newborn.

In the present study serum protein fractions of the newborn infants and their correlations with birthweights and with the protein pattern of maternal blood at delivery have been investigated. The effect of pre-eclampsia in the mother on the protein pattern of infants has also been studied.

Materials and Method

The subjects of this study were divided into two main groups according to their economic status. Group A consisted of mothers admitted to Nowrosjee Wadia Maternity Hospital and belonged to a class with a low income, representing a sample from the majority of the population of Bombay. More than 80% were Hindus, who ate meat or meat products only occasionally. Group B included mothers from a private maternity hospital and belonged to a class with a much higher economic status. Moreover, these women were Indian Christians who had had meat and fish in their daily diet. They, however, represented a sample from the minority of the population.

Blood from the umbilical cord was collected in clean dry test tubes at the time of delivery from infants born normally. Clear, non-haemolysed serum was separated by centrifugation. The weight of the infant was recorded immediately after birth. Blood samples from the mothers were collected at the time of delivery and treated in the same way. The total protein content was determined by the copper sulphate specific gravity method (Phillips, Van Slyke, Dole, Emerson, Hamilton and Archibald, 1943). Paper electrophoretic separation, staining of electrophoretograms and the quantitative estima-

TABLE 1

ANALYSIS OF BIRTH WEIGHTS OF INDIAN NEWBORN INFANTS

Weight Group (lb.)	Low Income Group A			High Income Group B		
	Males (No.)	Females (No.)	Total (No.)	Males (No.)	Females (No.)	Total (No.)
3·00–3·99	61	44	105	1	1	2
4·00–4·99	162	163	325	2	3	5
5·00–5·99	445	461	906	13	18	31
6·00–6·99	489	474	963	45	57	102
7·00–7·99	171	117	288	47	35	82
8·00–8·99	36	22	58	19	10	29
9·00–9·99	4	4	8	3	1	4
10·00–10·99	0	0	0	1	0	1
Total	1,368	1,285	2,653	131	125	256
Mean weight for all groups (lb.)	5·90	5·83	5·87	6·98	6·63	6·81
S.D.	1·05	1·00	1·03	1·05	0·95	1·01
S.E.	0·030	0·028	0·020	0·092	0·085	0·063
No. of babies weighing below 4·84 lb.	205 (15%)	192 (15%)	397 (15%)	3 (2·3%)	4 (3·2%)	7 (2·7%)
No. of premature babies according to W.H.O. Standard	410 (30·0%)	422 (32·8%)	832 (31·3%)	10 (7·6%)	13 (10·4%)	23 (9·1%)

tion of proteins were carried out as described previously (Kulkarni, 1957a).

Results

Infant's Birth Weight and Mother's Socio-economic Status. In order to establish an average normal Indian birth weight standard the weights of 2,653 infants (51·6% males and 48·4% females) born of mothers belonging to group A were analysed. The results are presented in Table 1. The average birth weight of males was 5·90+1·06 (S.D.) lb. and that of females 5·83±1·00 (S.D.) lb., the average for the whole group being 5·87±1·03 (S.D.) lb. Though the average weight of males was slightly more than that of females, this difference was not statistically significant ($p>0·05$). A histogram shows the frequency distribution of the infants in various weight groups (Fig. 1). The birth weights of the majority of normal Indian infants from the general population varied between 4·84 and 6·90 lb. and this range is taken as normal. According to this standard, 15% of the infants studied were below normal average weight. However, according to World Health Organization Standards, 31·3% of the infants were premature (below 5·5 lb.).

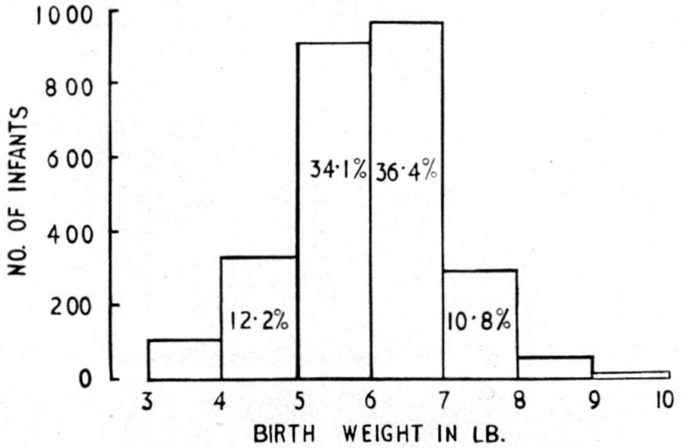

FIG. 1.—Frequency distribution of Indian infants, born of mothers with low economic status, according to their birth weights.

Table 1 includes an analysis of the birth weights of infants from the private maternity hospital (group B). Of the 256 infants studied, 51·1% were males and 48·9% were females. The average birth weight of males (6·98±1·05 lb.) in this group was higher than that of females (6·63±0·95 lb.), the difference being statistically significant ($p<0·01$). The mean birth weight for the whole group was 6·81±1·01 (S.D.) lb. The difference between the average birth weights of infants in this group and those in group A is highly significant ($p<0·001$). Furthermore only 2·7% of the infants in group B were below the normal Indian birth weight standard mentioned above and only 9·1% of them were below the standard laid down by W.H.O., as compared to the high percentage of prematurity observed in group A.

Serum Protein Pattern and Infant's Birth Weight. Table 2 shows the mean figures of different protein fractions of (1) group A infants with higher weights and their mothers, (2) group A infants with lower weights and their mothers, and (3) group B infants and their mothers.

The total protein content of infants with higher weights from group A was more than that of infants with lower weights ($p<0·01$), and this difference was mainly at the expense of a significant rise in

TABLE 2

MEAN SERUM PROTEIN FRACTIONS (G./100 ML.) OF CORD AND MATERNAL BLOOD WITH STANDARD DEVIATION AND STANDARD ERROR

Group	No.	Birthweight (lb.)	Total Proteins	Albumin	Globulin			
					Alpha 1	Alpha 2	Beta	Gamma
Infants group A, weights above 4·84 lb...	20	6·13 0·61 0·14	5·64 0·58 0·13	3·67 0·38 0·09	0·14 0·03 0·01	0·30 0·06 0·01	0·39 0·09 0·02	1·14 0·23 0·05
Mothers of above	20	— — —	5·94 0·56 0·13	2·69 0·42 0·09	0·27 0·06 0·01	0·66 0·11 0·02	0·92 0·16 0·04	1·40 0·29 0·06
Infants group A, weights below 4·84 lb...	21	3·87 0·86 0·19	5·09 0·67 0·15	3·15 0·44 0·10	0·18 0·04 0·01	0·33 0·06 0·01	0·44 0·10 0·02	0·99 0·31 0·07
Mothers of above	21	— — —	5·76 0·45 0·10	2·50 0·28 0·06	0·28 0·05 0·01	0·65 0·13 0·03	0·92 0·11 0·03	1·41 0·32 0·07
Infants group B	10	7·09 0·82 0·26	6·21 0·78 0·25	3·93 0·47 0·15	0·17 0·06 0·02	0·35 0·14 0·04	0·50 0·17 0·06	1·26 0·26 0·08
Mothers of above	10	— — —	6·77 0·45 0·14	3·46 0·43 0·14	0·29 0·07 0·02	0·68 0·20 0·06	0·93 0·17 0·05	1·41 0·32 0·10
Infants of pre-eclamptic mothers group A	11	4·69 1·74 0·53	5·13 0·44 0·13	3·09 0·45 0·14	0·16 0·06 0·02	0·32 0·06 0·02	0·47 0·24 0·07	1·09 0·15 0·05
Mothers of above	11	— — —	5·09 0·64 0·19	1·92 0·46 0·14	0·30 0·08 0·03	0·67 0·16 0·05	0·84 0·22 0·07	1·36 0·37 0·11

serum albumin ($p<0·01$). However, on comparing the serum protein patterns of mothers from both the higher and lower weight groups, no significant difference was noticed.

The infants born of mothers with higher economic status had higher serum total protein content than those of the low income group ($p<0·05$). This was due to a small rise in all the serum protein fractions. The mothers with high economic status had 0·8 g. of total proteins more than that observed in mothers with low economic status. It should be emphasized that this rise was due solely to a 30% increase in the albumin fraction. As there was no significant change in the globulin fraction in either group, the A:G ratios were $0·82\pm0·06$ (S.E.) and $1·04\pm0·12$ (S.E.) in groups A and B respectively, the difference being highly significant ($p<0·001$).

The correlation of the birth weight with the total proteins, albumin, total globulins and gamma globulin values is shown in Fig. 2. The serum total proteins and albumin showed a considerable rise with the increase in birthweight. The regression analysis confirmed that this rise in total proteins and albumin with increasing birthweight is highly significant ($p<0·001$). Gamma globulin also revealed a similar rise but to a lesser extent ($p<0·005$). However, the total globulins did not show any significant change.

Correlation of Mother's Serum Protein Pattern with that of the Infant. Fig. 3 shows the correlation of the total proteins, albumin and total globulins of cord blood with those of maternal blood. Serum total proteins of cord blood showed a progressive rise with the increase in the total protein content of maternal blood ($p<0·01$). A similar trend was also observed in total globulin values ($p<0·002$), but the albumin fraction did not show a significant change ($p>0·1$).

Pre-eclampsia in Mother and Infant's Serum Protein Fractions. The average values of different protein fractions of pre-eclamptic mothers at delivery and their newborn infants are shown in Table 2. The pre-eclamptic mothers had notably low serum total proteins. This drop was mainly due to 30% reduction in serum albumin; the respective globulin fractions were not significantly different. The protein pattern of infants in this group was very similar to that of infants in the low weight group.

Serum Protein Fractions in Twins. Table 3 shows the values of different protein fractions of the cord blood obtained from twin infants born of mothers from group A. The average birth weight and the mean serum protein pattern of twins were very

TABLE 3

SERUM PROTEIN FRACTIONS (G./100 ML.) OF CORD BLOOD FROM TWINS

	First Baby							Second Baby						
				Globulins							Globulins			
Pair No.	Birth weight (lb.)	Total Proteins	Albumin	Alpha 1	Alpha 2	Beta	Gamma	Birth weight (lb.)	Total Proteins	Albumin	Alpha 1	Alpha 2	Beta	Gamma
1	3·13	4·7	2·82	0·15	0·32	0·42	0·99	2·12	4·6	2·82	0·15	0·29	0·37	0·97
2	4·31	3·6	2·20	0·12	0·24	0·36	0·68	3·75	4·7	3·01	0·16	0·34	0·42	0·77
3	2·25	4·3	2·51	0·17	0·43	0·53	0·66	2·50	4·0	2·60	0·17	0·26	0·33	0·64
4	4·00	5·0	2·66	0·13	0·34	0·53	1·34	2·00	4·7	2·40	0·24	0·49	0·60	0·97
5	3·00	4·0	2·64	0·17	0·27	0·25	0·67	2·87	3·5	2·06	0·17	0·25	0·40	0·62
6	3·19	5·1	3·19	0·18	0·27	0·30	1·16	3·94	5·3	3·15	0·22	0·36	0·38	1·19
7	4·25	5·0	3·03	0·14	0·29	0·47	1·07	3·87	4·7	3·16	0·13	0·30	0·33	0·78
8	3·19	4·9	2·47	0·25	0·52	0·76	0·90	2·75	5·3	2·84	0·30	0·44	0·61	1·11
9	6·00	4·9	2·81	0·23	0·37	0·42	1·07	5·12	5·3	2·89	0·23	0·38	0·59	1·21
10	4·50	5·5	3·29	0·25	0·31	0·43	1·22	3·62	5·3	2·85	0·23	0·35	0·53	1·34
Mean	3·78	4·70	2·76	0·18	0·34	0·45	0·97	3·25	4·74	2·78	0·20	0·35	0·45	0·96
S.D.	1·07	0·54	0·32	0·05	0·09	0·14	0·24	0·97	0·61	0·34	0·05	0·08	0·11	0·25
S.E.	0·34	0·17	0·10	0·01	0·03	0·05	0·08	0·31	0·19	0·11	0·02	0·02	0·04	0·08

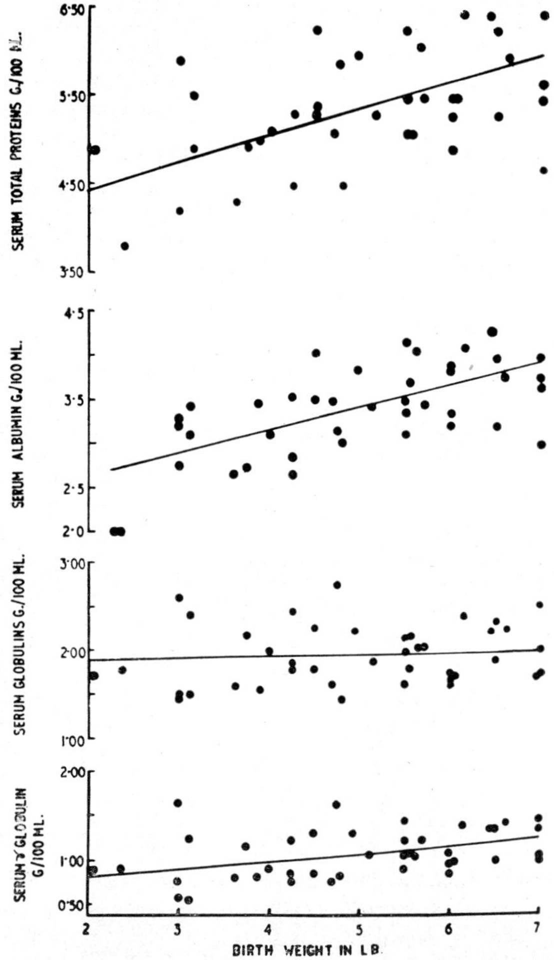

FIG. 2.—Relationships of serum total proteins, albumin, total globulins and gamma globulin with the birth weights of Indian infants.

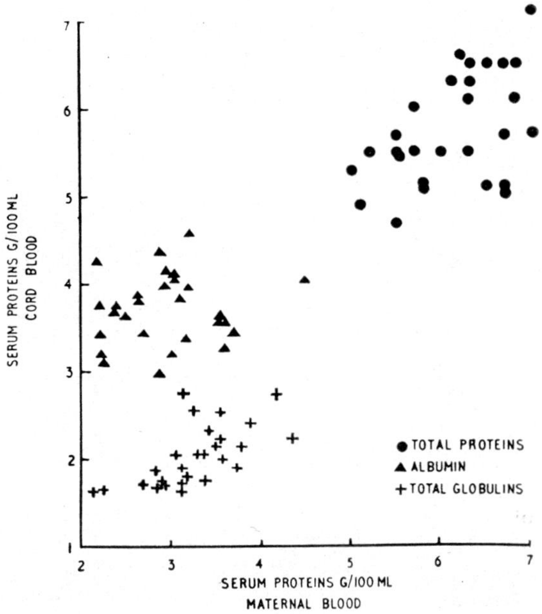

FIG. 3.—Relationship of serum total proteins, albumin and total globulin content of maternal blood with those of cord blood.

similar to those of infants with low birthweights. Statistical analysis showed that the differences in the protein fractions between each pair were not significant.

Discussion

That the definition of prematurity based on weight alone is unsatisfactory is demonstrated in the National Survey on 'Maternity in Great Britain' where 29% of infants weighing 5·5 lb. or less at birth were not considered premature by length of gestation (Douglas, 1950). Our results show that the average birth weight of the newborn Indian infant is much lower than the reported Western standard of 7·3 lb. (Bowes, 1950; Humphreys, 1954). Furthermore about 32% of Indian infants will have to be considered premature according to the W.H.O. standard.

The effect of the mother's socio-economic and nutritional status on the infant's birth weight has been noted previously (Drillien, 1957). The nutritional and socio-economic status of the average Indian is lower than that in Western countries, and this is reflected in lower levels of serum total protein and albumin observed during pregnancy in Indian women (Purandare *et al.*, 1954; Kulkarni, 1957b). Judged by the Registrar General's 'Classification of Occupations', 1950 (quoted by Drillien, 1957), our group consisting of mothers with low incomes corresponds to classes IV and V, whereas mothers in group B belonged to classes I and II. The average birth weight of an Indian infant born of a mother belonging to a low income group was about 5·9 lb., and this figure is in good agreement with that reported from other parts of India (Tampan, 1955; Sen, 1955; Bhonsale, 1955). The low levels of serum protein and albumin in the cord blood from infants born of mothers in the low income group are probably explained by the low level of the dietary protein which is prevalent in India. This is supported by the fact that the mothers with high economic status as well as their infants had serum protein and albumin values very similar to those reported by Western workers (Table 4). Also the average birth weight of these infants was similar to the reported Western standard; while the prematurity rate in this group was only 9·1%. As the serum total protein and albumin were correlated with the birth weights, the low weights observed in infants born of mothers with low economic status indicate the low nutritional status of their mothers.

The average concentrations of different protein fractions in infants with weights below 4·84 lb. were lower than those in infants weighing above 4·84 lb. from the same group. This finding is in general agreement with the observations of Saito *et al.* (1956).

The increase in gamma globulin level of the apparently normal Indian adult (Satoskar and Lewis, 1954; Kulkarni, 1957b) suggested the possibility that this represented a continuation into adult life of an infantile trait. This study indicates that Indian infants are born with higher gamma globulin levels than those reported in temperate zones (Table 4). Furthermore, this gamma globulin level shows very little further rise up to adult age, so that no significant difference has been observed between the gamma globulin level of an infant and an adult of 30 years of age (Kulkarni, unpublished). Another difference is that the Indian infant is born with a lower gamma globulin level than its mother, whereas the Western infant is born with a gamma globulin level higher than its mother. Similar findings in African infants have been reported by Stanier and Thompson (1954).

In contrast to the differences in serum total protein and albumin values, the gamma globulin levels observed in infants of groups A and B were very similar, irrespective of their mothers' nutritional and socio-economic status. The gamma globulin levels of mothers in these two groups were also very similar and definitely higher than that reported by foreign workers. It is concluded therefore that the increased gamma globulin level observed in Indian infants is due to a high gamma globulin level in the maternal blood. The direct transmission of homo-

TABLE 4

SERUM PROTEIN FRACTIONS (G./100 ML.) OF CORD AND MATERNAL BLOOD, REPORTED FROM VARIOUS COUNTRIES

Subjects	No.	Country	Method	Total Proteins	Albumin	Globulins: Alpha 1	Alpha 2	Beta	Gamma	Author
Newborn infants	11	U.S.A.	E	6·18	3·82	0·29	0·49	0·60	0·97	Longsworth *et al.* (1945)
Mothers at delivery	11			7·17	3·56	0·47	0·79	1·62	0·72	
Newborn infants	14	Africa	E	5·31	3·26	0·73		0·26	1·03	Stanier *et al.* (1954)
Mothers at delivery	9			5·61	2·45	0·98		0·75	1·42	
Newborn infants	28	Canada	C	6·24	3·63				0·90	Orlandini *et al.* (1955)
Mothers at delivery	28			6·68	3·50				0·82	
Newborn infants	14	U.S.A.	PE	5·44	3·31	0·28	0·50	0·51	0·84	Saito *et al.* (1956)
Newborn infants	41	U.S.A.	PE	5·70	3·94	0·14	0·41	0·44	0·77	Jencks *et al.* (1956)
Mothers at delivery	325			6·60	3·80	0·33	0·73	0·90	0·84	
Newborn infants	20	India	PE	5·64	3·67	0·14	0·30	0·39	1·14	
Mothers at delivery	20			5·94	2·69	0·27	0·66	0·92	1·40	This paper

E=Electrophoresis. PE=Paper electrophoresis. C=Chemical.

logous maternal albumin and gamma globulin to the foetal circulation has recently been demonstrated in rhesus monkeys; furthermore, it was found that the gamma globulin was transmitted some 15 to 20 times more easily than albumin, whereas the alpha and beta globulins did not reach the foetal circulation (Bangham, Hobbs and Terry, 1958).

The serum proteins of infants born of pre-eclamptic mothers showed a pattern similar to that seen in infants with weights below 4·84 lb. However, the serum total proteins and albumin in these mothers were considerably lower than those in normal mothers from the same group. Similar protein patterns have been reported previously in pre-eclamptic women at term (Purandare *et al.*, 1954). These changes in the protein pattern of mothers are attributed to probable liver damage. It seems however that this liver damage, if any, in the mother, does not considerably affect the serum protein pattern of her infant. Slight lowering of the total proteins and albumin observed in infants of pre-eclamptic mothers, as compared with those of infants with higher weights, might be due to their premature births.

Summary

The birth weights and serum protein patterns of Indian newborn infants and their mothers have been studied. Infants of mothers of low income group had lower birth weights and serum total protein and albumin than those born of mothers with high economic status. The serum total globulins of these infants showed a definite relation to that of their mothers. The gamma globulin levels in these infants were higher than the corresponding figures reported from temperate zones. This rise could not be correlated with the nutritional status of the mothers.

The serum protein patterns revealed no significant difference in each pair studied.

The serum protein pattern of infants born of pre-eclamptic mothers resembled that of infants in the low weight group, although the pre-eclamptic mothers had considerably lower serum total protein and albumin content.

The implications of these findings are discussed.

We sincerely thank Professor U. K. Sheth, professor of pharmacology, Seth G.S. Medical College, for his encouragement and valuable criticism, and Dr. K. M. Masani, honorary principal medical officer, Nowrosjee Wadia Maternity Hospital, for his co-operation in this study. Our thanks are also due to Dr. E. J. Sequeira for supplying us with the blood samples from his private maternity hospital.

References

Bangham, D. R., Hobbs, K. R. and Terry, R. J. (1958). *Lancet*, **2**, 351.

Bhonsale, I. (1955). VIII All India Obstetric and Gynaecological Congress. Summary of papers, p. 44. Bombay, March, 1955.

Bowes, K. (1950). *Modern Trends in Obstetrics and Gynaecology*, p. 59. Butterworth, London.

Brown, T. (1954). *J. Obstet. Gynaec. Brit. Emp.*, **61**, 781.

Coryell, M. N., Beach, E. F., Robinson, A. R., Macy, I. G. and Mack, H. C. (1950). *J. clin. Invest.*, **29**, 1559.

Deegan, T., Gilles, H. M. and McGregor, I. A. (1956). *Ann. trop. Med. Parasit.*, **50**, 451.

Douglas, J. W. B. (1950). *J. Obstet. Gynaec. Brit. Emp.*, **57**, 143.

Drillien, C. M. (1957). *Ibid.*, **64**, 161.

Edozien, J. C. (1957). *J. clin. Path.*, **10**, 276.

Holmes, E. G., Stanier, M. W., Semambo, Y. B. and Jones, E. R. (1951). *Trans. roy. Soc. trop. Med. Hyg.*, **45**, 371.

Humphreys, R. C. (1954). *J. Obstet. Gynaec. Brit. Emp.*, **61**, 764.

Jencks, W. P., Smith, E. R. B. and Durrum, E. L. (1956). *Amer. J. Med.*, **21**, 387.

Kulkarni, B. S. (1957a). *Indian J. med. Sci.*, **11**, 320.

—— (1957b). Thesis. Bombay University.

Longsworth, L. G., Curtis, R. M. and Pembroke, R. H. (1945). *J. clin. Invest.*, **24**, 46.

Mack, H. C., Robinson, A. R., Wiseman, M. E., Schoeb, E. J. and Macy, I. G. (1951). *Ibid.*, **30**, 609.

Orlandini, T. O., Sass-Kortsak, A. and Ebbs, J. H. (1955). *Pediatrics*, **16**, 575.

Phillips, R. A., Van Slyke, D. D., Dole, V. P., Emerson, K. Jr., Hamilton, P. B. and Archibald, R. M. (1943). *Bull. U.S. Army med. Dept.*, No. 71, p. 66.

Purandare, B. N., Satoskar, R. S. and Lewis, R. A (1954). Tirage à part du volume "La prophylaxie en gynécologie et obstétrique" tome I, Conférences et Rapports du Congrès international de gynécologie et d'obstétrique, Genève.

Saito, M., Gittleman, I. F., Pincus, J. B. and Sobel, A. E. (1956). *Pediatrics*, **17**, 657.

Satoskar, R. S. and Lewis, R. A. (1954). *Indian J. med. Sci.*, **8**, 663.

Sen, S. C. (1955). VIII All India Obstetric and Gynaecological Congress. Summary of papers, p. 39. Bombay, March, 1955.

Stanier, M. W. and Thompson, M. D. (1954). *Archives of Disease in Childhood*, **29**, 110.

Tampan, R. K. K. (1955). VIII All India Obstetric and Gynaecological Congress. Summary of papers, p. 38. Bombay, March, 1955.

TETANUS IN AFRICAN CHILDREN

BY

A. B. TOMPKINS

From the Children's Department, University College Hospital, Ibadan, Nigeria

(RECEIVED FOR PUBLICATION APRIL 20, 1959)

This paper is based upon part of a thesis accepted by the University of London for the M.D. degree in 1957, but it now includes the experience of the Children's Department of University College Hospital, Ibadan, Nigeria, in treating 79 children with tetanus between April, 1953, and August, 1958. Patients with neonatal tetanus are not included as they were the subject of a previous paper (Tompkins, 1958).

Publication is thought to be justified for three reasons: (1) The methods of treatment employed were simple, such as can be carried out with limited staff and equipment, so the results may be useful for comparison with those obtained by more elaborate means, such as muscle relaxants. (2) A wide range of doses of tetanus antitoxin was employed in the hope of obtaining definite information about its value in treatment. (3) The importance of the middle ear as a source of infection is stressed and the characteristic type of tetanus arising from this source is described.

Site of Infection

It was seldom possible to be certain of the site of infection owing to the high incidence of tropical ulcer, guinea-worm and infected abrasions of the legs from which few of the poorer Nigerian children are ever completely free. One patient developed post-operative tetanus after a laparotomy and in 21 patients the source of infection was thought to be the middle ear.

Seasonal Incidence

Seasonal incidence is shown in Fig. 1, prepared from the records of 77 patients admitted between August, 1953, and August, 1958. It shows the incidence to be rather lower during the wet season (June to October) than during the dry. The peak in March and the low incidence recorded for November are probably sampling errors.

Mortality

Of the 79 patients 25 died, a mortality of 31·6%. The mortality reported by other writers is set out in Table 1.

Dietrich (1940) and Silverthorne (1947) both attributed the lower mortality among the later patients in their series to abandoning the intrathecal route of antitoxin administration, and Silverthorne also thought that the replacement of the intravenous by the intramuscular route of administration may have been a further contributory factor.

Forbes and Auld (1955) considered that the lower mortality among their patients, when compared with those previously treated in the same hospital, was due to the greater attention they paid to the maintenance of a good airway.

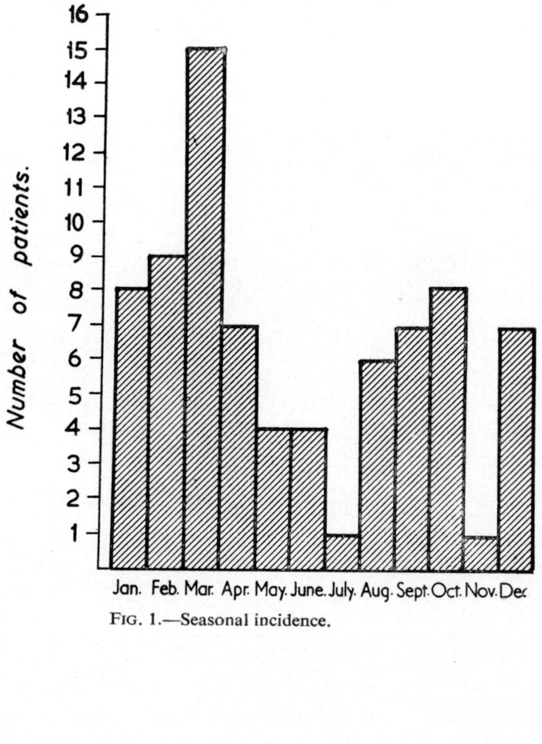

FIG. 1.—Seasonal incidence.

TABLE 1
MORTALITY REPORTED BY OTHER WRITERS

Author	Year	Place	Age Group (yr.)	Number	Mortality (%)
Calvin and Goldberg (1930)	1917–30	Chicago	1–5	12	83
			6–10		34
			11–15	171	65
			Adults	—	65
Paterson (1930)	—	Australia	—	26	26·9
Yodh (1937)	1931–35	Bombay	1–10	78	44·8
			11–20	89	50
Cole (1940)	—	Cambridge	0–5	5	60
			6–10	8	35
Dietrich (1940)	1921–32	California	—	15	80
	1933–38		—	13	8
Spaeth (1940)	—	U.S.A.	0–5		12·5
			6–10	30	40
			11–15		30
			Over 15		20
Vener and Bower (1941)	—	California	1–4	14	50
			5–9	29	14
			10–14	16	7
Silverthorne (1947)	1921–46	Toronto	3–13		47
	1921–28			70	66
	1936–46				28·5
Noel and McSwain (1950)	—	Tenessee	0–9	50	48
Segar, Littlefield and Walcher (1952)	—	Indiana	3½–14	10	0
Forbes and Auld (1955)	1945–49	Texas	—	19	47
	1950–53		0–11	15	0

Age Incidence, and Mortality in Relation to Age. The age distribution of the patients ranged between 4 months and 13 years and is shown in Fig. 2 which

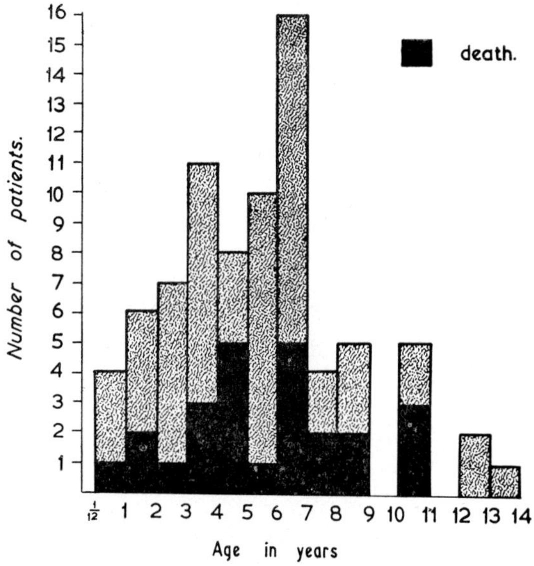

FIG. 2.—Age distribution and mortality.

also shows the percentage mortality for each age group. It shows that the incidence is highest during the middle years of childhood with a sudden decrease after the age of 7 years, though this might be due to a higher proportion of the older children being admitted to the adult wards.

Most writers consider the mortality of tetanus to be lowest during the middle years of childhood but the figures quoted in Table 1 do not give definite confirmation of this view. The present series shows a fairly uniform mortality for all ages and if a comparison is made between the mortality during the first four years of life (28 patients with seven deaths) and that during the second four years (38 patients with 13 deaths) χ^2 (with Yate's correction)$=0\cdot28$, $P=0\cdot6$, which is not significant.

Sex Incidence. The sex incidence and the mortality in relation to it are shown in Table 2.

TABLE 2
MORTALITY IN RELATION TO SEX INCIDENCE

	Male (No.)	Female (No.)
Patients	50	29
Deaths	13	12
Mortality	26%	41·4%

Comparing the mortality of the two sexes, χ^2 (corrected)$=1\cdot36$, $P=0\cdot25$, i.e. no significant difference. Cole (1940) considered the prognosis to be better in female patients. Vener and Bower (1941) reported a mortality of 14% among boys and 37·5% among girls, but Pratt (1945), on the other hand, found the mortality among boys and girls to be 46% and 35% respectively.

Incubation Period. This could only be estimated in 22 cases. Of these the 13 patients who survived had an average incubation period of 7·3 days with a range of two to 15 days, while the nine who died had an average of 8·2 days and a range of five to 12 days.

It is generally agreed that the length of the incubation period is one of the most important factors determining the prognosis in tetanus and that the longer the incubation period the greater the chance of survival. The fact that the above figures do not conform to this principle may be due either to a sampling error or to the general inaccuracy of the uneducated African's idea of time.

In Calvin and Goldberg's (1930) series the mortality when related to incubation period was as follows: one to five days, 84%; five to 10 days, 83%; 10 to 14 days, 37%; two to three weeks, 25%; three to four weeks, 33%; more than four weeks, 10%.

Cole (1940) described 38 patients in whom the incubation period was known. The average incubation period of those who died was 6·5 days, and of those who recovered, 11·0 days. Only two of his patients who recovered had incubation periods of less than seven days. He stresses that the incubation period is measured from the time of infection, which is not necessarily the time of injury.

Spaeth (1940), among the patients he had treated personally, found an average incubation period of 12 days among the patients who recovered and six days for those who died.

Forbes and Auld's (1955) series of patients had an average incubation period of 9·6 days. All of them recovered, but of the eight patients having incubation periods of 10 days or less six were graded as severe, but the four whose incubation period exceeded 10 days included only one severe case with an incubation period of 30 days.

In the present series nine of the patients, whose incubation periods were known, were graded as severe and these had an average incubation period of 6·7 days while 11 who were graded as mild had an average of 8·6 days (two patients had to be excluded from this calculation because of insufficient information about the severity of the illness).

Onset Interval. This is the period which elapses between the appearance of the first symptoms, usually muscle stiffness, and the onset of tetanic spasms. It is of considerable prognostic importance because the mortality of tetanus has been found to vary inversely with the length of the onset interval.

Cole (1938, 1940) drew attention to this relationship. Among 13 patients who died he found the onset interval to be 48 hours or less in 12 and 72 hours in one, while among 16 patients who recovered the period of onset was more than 72 hours in 12, 48 hours in three and 18 hours in one. He also mentioned that in the patients who died the time of survival increased with the length of the onset interval but was never more than four times its duration.

Díaz-Rivera, Deliz and Berio-Suárez (1948) estimated the onset interval in 35 of their 59 patients. Ten patients developed convulsions on the first day of the illness with six deaths (60%); six developed them on the second day with three deaths (50%); three on the third day with one death (33·3%) and 16 on the fourth day or later with no deaths.

Johnstone (1958), working with adult patients in Ibadan, found a mortality of 69% among his patients having an onset interval of 48 hours or less, and only 30% among those with an onset interval of more than 48 hours, the difference being statistically significant.

In the present series an estimate of the onset interval could be made in 18 cases. Of those patients with an onset interval of 24 hours or less, four survived and three died, while of those whose onset interval exceeded 24 hours, nine survived and two died (χ^2 (corrected)$=0\cdot36$, $P=0\cdot6$, i.e. no significant difference).

Clinical Features

As a rule the patients were not brought to hospital until the onset of spasms but they generally gave a history in which the earliest symptom was either trismus or stiffness of the neck and back. Trismus and abdominal rigidity were the most constant physical signs. The spasms did not appear to be painful.

Most of the patients were pyrexial at some stage of their illness and the relation between fever and mortality is shown in Table 3. Spaeth (1940, 1941a, b) considered pyrexia to be a bad prognostic sign. In his series of patients between 1 and 15 years of age,

TABLE 3

MAXIMUM AND MINIMUM RECORDED TEMPERATURES AND MORTALITY BASED ON THE RECORDS OF 42 PATIENTS

Temperature (°F.)	Patients (No.)	Deaths (No.)
Maximum:		
98–100	15	1
100–102	9	1
102–104	8	5
Over 104	10	6
Minimum:		
Less than 95	1	0
95–96	20	0
96–98	14	6
98–100	6	6
Over 100	1	1

no deaths occurred among the 21 patients who were consistently apyrexial. The present series does not reveal such a constant relationship but suggests, as did the temperature records of the neonatal patients, that a high minimum temperature is of more serious significance than a high maximum one.

The following case history is typical of severe tetanus with recovery.

Case 1. O.D., a male, aged 2 years, was admitted on December 15, 1953, with a history and physical signs suggesting an intussusception. A laparotomy was carried out soon after admission when the terminal ileum was found to be packed with roundworms. The bowel was opened and the worms removed.

He did not receive any prophylactic antitoxin but was given procaine penicillin 300,000 units daily. His progress was uneventful until December 26 when a nurse noticed that he was unable to open his mouth. He was immediately given 100,000 units of antitoxin intramuscularly, but next day he showed fully developed tetanus with opisthotonus and frequent severe spasms.

Fairly good control of the spasms was obtained with sodium amytal, 2 gr. intramuscularly as required, but his condition gave rise to anxiety for about a week. The last recorded spasm took place on January 7 when he received a further 20,000 units of antitoxin without ill effect.

By January 15 he was able to stand and he was discharged on January 28 with no residual signs except for some rigidity of the abdominal wall. He has been seen repeatedly since discharge and is perfectly normal.

Complications

The most important complications were respiratory obstruction and bronchopneumonia which might have been avoided in many cases had tracheotomy been carried out as recommended by recent authors (Turner and Galloway, 1949; Godman and Adriani, 1949; Creech, Woodhall and Ochsner, 1950; Biehl and Helm, 1951; Herzon, Killian and Pearlman, 1951; Segar *et al.*, 1952; Díaz-Rivera, Trilla and Pons, 1954; Forbes and Auld, 1955).

Compression fracture of the vertebrae is a well known complication of tetanus. Dietrich (1940) encountered this in nine out of 13 patients and stressed the importance of a radiological examination of the spines of all tetanus patients before discharge. Routine radiography of the spine was not part of our practice and compression fractures were only diagnosed in two patients.

One of these patients appeared quite well on discharge from the hospital but returned to the out-patient clinic a few days later complaining of pain in the back. Radiographs then showed compression fractures of the bodies of four of the dorsal vertebrae. A radiograph of the other patient, in the absence of any symptoms, showed a series of compression fractures. He received no treatment and now appears to be perfectly normal.

Otogenous Tetanus. It is well known that the middle ear may be the site of infection in tetanus, but references to it are scattered and few writers describe more than one patient.

In 21 patients of the present series tetanus of a distinctive clinical type was associated with otitis media. In no case was full bacteriological confirmation obtained, but in 13 patients in whom bacteriological examinations were carried out the following organisms were isolated:

Escherichia coli (4); *Staphylococcus saprophyticus* (1); *Pseudomonas* (1); *Proteus* (1); *Bacillus subtilis* (3); *Pleurococcus pyocyanea* (4); diphtheroids (2); terminal spore-bearing *Clostridia* (2); other *Clostridia* (1). In many cases a mixed growth of organisms was obtained.

These patients presented a distinctive clinical picture in which trismus and risus sardonicus were severe in proportion to spasms and generalized rigidity which were usually mild, but two of them died. One of these had mild tetanus of the type described and died of bronchopneumonia. The other started with a mild cephalic type of tetanus but two days after admission she developed generalized severe spasms. A swab from her ear showed the presence of terminal spore-bearing *Clostridia* so it is likely that the ear was the true source of infection.

Case 2. S.A., a male, aged 2½ years, was admitted on January 4, 1954, with a five-day history of pain in the left ear and occasional muscular spasms. The day before admission the ear had begun to discharge.

On admission the child had a temperature of 99° F. There was well marked trismus and risus sardonicus, with generalized muscular rigidity but no spasms. The tongue had been bitten slightly. There was a copious purulent discharge from the left ear. Other systems were normal. A direct smear of pus from an aural swab showed the presence of 'drumstick' bacilli morphologically resembling *Cl. tetani*, but culture and virulence tests were not carried out.

He was given tetanus antitoxin 200,000 units intramuscularly on admission and procaine penicillin 600,000 units daily. After admission he began to have mild spasms for which sedation with sodium amytal, gr. 2 intramuscularly, was given as required.

The spasms ceased after two days although the trismus, risus sardonicus and muscular rigidity persisted and he used to stand all day leaning stiffly against the side of his cot. He was able to take food by mouth throughout the illness.

He was quite well on discharge although the left otorrhoea persisted and the pus still contained tetanus-like organisms.

Corcoran (1938) described the case of an Irish adult who showed trismus and minimum muscular rigidity associated with chronic suppurative otitis media. *Cl. tetani* was not isolated from the ear. The patient died of bronchopneumonia.

Stonham (1938) described a more severe case in an Indian adult who recovered, but again *Cl. tetani* was not isolated from the ear.

Magarey (1947) described tetanus developing in a boy aged 9 with chronic otitis media and in this case *Cl. tetani* was successfully isolated from the aural discharge. The disease was mild although general spasms occurred and the boy recovered. This case closely resembles that described above.

Rosa Febles, Ramirez, Armaiz and Torregrosa (1950) described a girl of 19 who developed mild tetanus with trismus but no spasms 16 days after an injury to her ear which caused it to discharge. *Cl. tetani* was present in the aural pus.

Ghosh (1950) mentioned that the ear was the source of infection in 70% of the children he treated, but did not give any details, and Khosla and Bhatt (1952), in a series of 88 Indian patients of all ages, found that in children under 4, excluding the newly born, smallpox vaccination and the middle ear were the commonest sites of infection.

Jelnes (1955) gives the case of a 45-year-old Norwegian man who developed trismus and spasm of the left facial muscles. He had undergone a left radical mastoidectomy 20 years before with satisfactory results except for occasional slight discharge. The cavity was re-opened and necrotic material removed from which *Cl. tetani* was grown. The patient never had any generalized spasms and made a good recovery.

Treatment

General. All writers recommend that tetanus patients should be nursed in a quiet, darkened room, but no such accommodation is available at the Adeoyo Hospital and the patients had to be nursed in the general children's ward. Even now, in University College Hospital, where cubicle accommodation is available, the writer prefers to keep these patients in the open ward where they can be supervised by the nurses more closely than is possible in the cubicles.

Treatment of the Wound. As the site of infection was usually unknown, no local treatment was carried out except for simple dressings to any lesion requiring them.

Authorities are divided on the question of the local treatment of the wound in cases of tetanus, some recommending wound excision, others only such treatment as appears to be necessary according to ordinary surgical standards. Creech *et al.* (1950) carried out excision of the wound in all cases, even when it was healed, packing it after excision with peroxide gauze. Segar *et al.* (1952) carried out wound debridement only when it was necessary for surgical reasons, when the area around the wound was first infiltrated with antitoxin; most other writers make similar recommendations. Forbes and Auld (1955) considered that the mortality was lower in patients whose wounds were not given any specific treatment, but this may reflect the tendency for severe wounds to be associated with a severe type of tetanus.

All these workers obtained good results, but one of Creech's six patients died, while Segar's 10 and Forbes' and Auld's 15 patients all recovered so the balance of evidence favours the view that wound excision in tetanus is unnecessary and is possibly even harmful.

Feeding. Most of the patients were able to take a liquid diet by mouth from the time of admission but some required intravenous fluids for the correction of dehydration and electrolyte imbalance.

Tube feeding after an initial trial was largely discarded as it was found to provoke spasms. Forbes and Auld (1955) abandoned it for the same reason, but during the past year, thanks to the more efficient sedation afforded by chlorpromazine and phenobarbitone, it has been used again more successfully to give a high-protein mixture composed of milk, Casilan and egg which has proved very valuable in protracted cases with inability to swallow.

Penicillin. All the patients received an aqueous suspension of procaine penicillin in doses of 300,000 to 600,000 units daily. Penicillin is now an accepted part of the treatment of tetanus but no critical assessment of its value has yet been made. Altemeier (1946), from a study of 16 patients, concluded that it was only of value in the prevention and treatment of complications, but had no effect on the course of tetanus itself. Díaz-Rivera, Ramirez, Pons and Torregrosa (1951) took swabs from the suspected sites of infection in 17 patients with tetanus. Cultures were positive for *Cl. tetani* in eight of these. After the swabs had been taken penicillin treatment was started and serial cultures taken from the wounds. *Cl. tetani* disappeared from five of the wounds within 24 hours, from six within 48 hours and from seven within 72 hours. In only one wound did it persist for longer than 72 hours and from this it was eventually cleared by the use of local penicillin.

Cortisone. This was not used in the treatment of any patient in this series and has not been used at all extensively in the treatment of tetanus though Lewis, Satoskar, Joag, Dave and Patel (1954) carried out a controlled trial on two groups of 20 patients and found that the mortality was significantly lower in the cortisone-treated group. Intramuscular cortisone was thought to be harmful, but oral cortisone and hydrocortisone had beneficial effects in reducing fever and spasms.

Antitoxin. Eight of the patients received no antitoxin, the others received it in doses of 10,000 to 500,000 units. In three cases there is no record of the amount given so these have been excluded from the subsequent calculations.

The whole amount was given as a single intramuscular injection at the time of admission and only two children received extra doses later in the illness. No patient was given antitoxin intravenously or intrathecally and the intramuscular injections were given without hyalase.

Table 4 shows the results obtained with the different doses, the extra doses mentioned above being excluded.

Comparing the results obtained by giving doses of 0-20,000 units with those obtained from doses of more than 20,000 units, $\chi^2=2\cdot6$, $P=1\cdot0$, i.e. no significant difference. If those receiving more or less than 70,000 units are similarly compared, $\chi^2=1\cdot1$, $P=0\cdot3$, again without significance.

TABLE 4

MORTALITY IN RELATION TO ANTITOXIN ADMINISTERED

	Units of Antitoxin		
	0–20,000	20–70,000	Over 70,000
No. of patients ..	16	25	35
No. of deaths ..	7	8	8
Mortality ..	43·7%	32%	20·3%

The value of antitoxin in the treatment of tetanus is still undetermined and, though many series of patients have been treated without antitoxin, the writer can find no reference to the crucial experiment now being carried out here in which a large number of patients are allocated at random into two groups, one receiving adequate doses of antitoxin and the other none, all other treatment being standardized for both groups. Such a trial is now in progress here but it will take time for a large enough series of patients to be collected to give a conclusive result. So far 44 patients have been included in the trial, 29 with neonatal tetanus and 15 older children. The results and their significance are set out in Table 5 which shows no significant difference in mortality between the group which received antitoxin and that which did not.

TABLE 5

MORTALITY FIGURES FOR 44 PATIENTS TREATED WITH AND WITHOUT ANTITOXIN

	Antitoxin	No Antitoxin
Neonates:		
Recovered	4	1
Died	11	13
χ^2 (corrected)$=0\cdot8$, $P=0\cdot4$		
Older children:		
Recovered	2	5
Died	4	4
χ^2 (corrected)$=0\cdot1$, $P=0\cdot7$		
Total:		
Recovered	6	6
Died	15	17
χ^2 (corrected)$=0\cdot2$, $P=0\cdot8$		

Calvin and Goldberg (1930) analysed the results obtained in treating 136 patients. Of these, 26 received doses of antitoxin of 25,000 units or less with 23 deaths, and 110 patients doses of more than 25,000 units with 63 deaths ($\chi^2=8\cdot8$, $P=$less than $0\cdot01$ (present writer's calculation)). This means that there is a significant difference in favour of the group of patients who received the larger dose, but the patients received daily doses of antitoxin and, as the authors point out, those who survived would necessarily have received larger amounts of antitoxin than those who died early in the illness.

Huntington, Thompson and Gordon (1937) collected the records of 642 patients from a group of hospitals in the United States. The control group consisted of 72 patients who were treated before antitoxin was available and of these 47 died. Of the 570 patients who received antitoxin all but 228 received intrathecal antitoxin and are excluded from the present analysis. Of this antitoxin-treated group of 228 patients 142 died. Comparing the mortality in these two groups, $\chi^2=0\cdot21$, $P=0\cdot6$ (present writer's calculation), i.e. no significant difference.

Bryant and Fairman (1940), working in the Sudan, treated 22 patients with sulphapyridine and sodium evipan and did not use antitoxin. Their mortality rate of 27% achieved under very primitive conditions compares favourably with most series treated with antitoxin.

Spaeth (1940) treated his series of patients with doses of antitoxin ranging from 11,000 to 82,000 units, the whole amount being given as a single intravenous injection soon after admission and after preliminary skin testing. Seven patients received doses of 20,000 units or less with one death, and 25 received more than 20,000 units with seven deaths ($\chi^2=0\cdot06$, $P=0\cdot80$ (present writer's calculation), i.e. no significant difference).

Spaeth also collected the records of 570 patients who had received no antitoxin and of whom 462 (81%) died, and compared them with 1,917 patients who had been treated with antitoxin and of whom 1,088 (56·7%) died ($\chi^2=110$, P=less than 0·01, i.e. significantly in favour of the antitoxin-treated group).

Spaeth does not say whether the patients in his group who did not receive antitoxin were treated before antitoxin was available. Cole (1940) points out a fallacy in comparing series treated before and after the advent of antitoxin. In general, severe wounds lead to a severe form of tetanus with a high mortality. Patients with severe wounds now usually receive prophylactic antitoxin and most cases of tetanus which occur nowadays are associated with minor wounds and tend to be mild in consequence. Besides this, patients treated since the introduction of antitoxin have the advantage of many other improved methods of treatment which create a bias against the earlier group. These considerations add weight to the findings of Huntington *et al.* (1937), who found no significant difference in mortality in spite of these sources of bias acting against their pre-antitoxin group.

In another paper Spaeth (1941) reported the results of titrations of the antitoxin levels in the blood of 14 patients with tetanus at periods of six to 42 days after the administration of 20,000 to 100,000 units of antitoxin intravenously or intramuscularly. He concluded from his findings that from 30,000 to 50,000 units should be sufficient for routine use, but recommended 60,000 units for patients during the first five days of the illness and 40,000 units for patients with mild tetanus admitted more than five days after onset.

The best results in the treatment of tetanus in children have been those of Segar *et al.* (1952) and Forbes and Auld (1955) who treated 10 and 15 patients respectively without a death. Segar gave a single dose of 40,000 to 80,000 units intramuscularly after preliminary skin testing while Forbes and Auld gave from 40,000 to 340,000 units as a single dose on admission. Sensitivity tests were first carried out and the dose was given half intravenously and half intramuscularly. The total dose given was not related to the child's weight.

Sedation. The object of drug treatment in tetanus is to diminish the frequency and severity of the spasms, lessen the muscular rigidity and so prevent exhaustion. This can be done either by the use of sedatives to depress sensory excitability or by the use of muscular relaxants to prevent the excessive muscular response.

The sedatives most commonly used in the treatment of tetanus have been magnesium sulphate, now largely abandoned, chloral hydrate, the barbiturates, bromethol and paraldehyde. Recently the use of chlorpromazine has been investigated extensively (Cole and Robertson, 1955; Kelly and Laurence, 1956).

The earlier patients in the series were given sodium amylobarbitone gr. 1-3 intramuscularly as required. This was replaced later by paraldehyde given in doses of 2-6 ml. intramuscularly as often as necessary, which was thought to cause less respiratory depression then amylobarbitone. It then became the practice to give sodium phenobarbitone gr. 1-2 on admission as a basal sedative which was not repeated until two or three days later and supplemented by 2-3 ml. of paraldehyde given intramuscularly as required.

The method of sedation now employed was suggested by Dr. J. P. Puthumana (personal communication). Phenobarbitone gr. ½-1 and chlorpromazine 12·5-25 mg. are given every six to eight hours, by mouth if the patient can swallow or is being tube-fed, otherwise intramuscularly, with supplementary intramuscular injections of paraldehyde if required. This has been found to give better control of the spasms and less respiratory depression than any other combination of drugs.

Segar *et al.* (1952) treated their 10 patients with metubine iodide 1-2 mg. intramuscularly every two to three hours, giving just enough to prevent convulsions and severe spasms without abolishing rigidity, and giving supplementary sedation with barbiturates when necessary.

Forbes and Auld (1955) used thiopentone given by continuous intravenous infusion to abolish convulsions and opisthotonus but not to produce rigidity. They considered relaxation of the abdominal muscles in the presence of a cough response to tracheal suction to be the desirable level of sedation.

Tracheotomy. According to Herzon *et al.* (1951) this operation was first advocated for the treatment of tetanus by Thomas Curling in 1837 and first performed by G. M. Humphry in 1856, but it did not take its place in routine treatment until recently. Most authors who have written about tetanus during the past few years stress the importance of tracheotomy as a means of maintaining a good airway in patients with respiratory difficulty (Harris, McDermott and Montreuil, 1948; Turner and Galloway, 1949; Creech *et al.*, 1950; Herzon *et al.*, 1951; Segar *et al.*, 1952; Díaz Rivera *et al.*, 1954; Forbes and Auld, 1955).

Tracheotomy was not employed in any of the patients in the present series, but considering them in retrospect the writer considers that life might have been saved in several cases had the operation been carried out.

Summary

The experience gained in treating tetanus in 79 children whose ages ranged from 4 months to 13 years is described. The total mortality was 31·6% and this was fairly uniformly distributed throughout the age groups. No significant difference in the mortality rates for the two sexes could be demonstrated.

In the sample available the average incubation period for the patients who died was found to be slightly longer than that for those who recovered, in contradiction to the generally accepted rule that the longer the incubation period the better the prognosis, but this finding is thought to be accidental. The incubation period in the mild cases was found to be slightly longer than in the severe cases, being 8·6 and 6·7 days respectively. No significant association between the onset interval and the mortality could be demonstrated.

The clinical features are described and show no unusual features, but in 21 of the patients the site of infection was thought to be the middle ear and these showed a typical mild form of the disease in which trismus and risus sardonicus were prominent but spasms and generalized rigidity slight.

No special local treatment was employed. It was usually possible to give the patients an adequate fluid diet by mouth, but tube-feeding had to be employed in some cases and parenteral fluids in others. All patients received penicillin.

Most of the patients received tetanus antitoxin in varied doses up to 500,000 units, but eight patients received none. Analysis of the results obtained does not suggest that antitoxin is of any value in treatment, but no conclusion has yet been reached.

A combination of phenobarbitone and chlorpromazine was found to be greatly superior to any other sedative.

Tracheotomy was not employed but its value in treatment is acknowledged.

My thanks are due to Professor A. W. Woodruff, for his advice on the preparation of this paper, to Mr. D. L. N. Sly, for help with the statistics, and to Dr. R. W. F. Collis and Dr. R. G. Hendrickse, for permission to include their patients.

References

Altemeier, W. A. (1946). *J. Amer. med. Ass.*, **130**, 67.
Biehl, J. P. and Helm, R. A. (1951). *J. Lab. clin. Med.*, **38**, 791.
Bryant, J. and Fairman, H. D. (1940). *Lancet*, **2**, 263.
Calvin, J. K. and Goldberg, A. H. (1930). *J. Amer. med. Ass.*, **94**, 1977.
Cole, A. C. E. and Robertson, D. H. H. (1955). *Lancet*, **2**, 1063.
Cole, L. (1938). *Proc. roy. Soc. Med.*, **31**, 1205.
—— (1940). *Lancet*, **1**, 164.
Corcoran, J. (1938). *Brit. med. J.*, **1**, 1004.
Creech, O., Woodhall, J. P. and Ochsner, A. (1950). *Surgery*, **27**. 62.
Díaz-Rivera, R. S., Deliz, L. R. and Berio-Suárez, J. (1948). *J. Amer, med. Ass.*, **138**, 191.
——, Ramirez, E., Pons, E. R. and Torregrosa, M. V. (1951). *Ibid.*, **147**, 1635.
——, Trilla, F. and Pons, E. R. (1954). *Ann. intern. Med.*, **40**, 563.
Dietrich, H. F. (1940). *Amer. J. Dis. Child.*, **59**, 693.
Forbes, G. B. and Auld, M. (1955). *Amer. J. Med.*, **18**, 947.
Ghosh, S. M. (1950). *J. Indian med. Ass.*, **19**, 328.
Godman, H. E. and Adriani, J. (1949). *J. Amer. med. Ass.*, **141**, 754.
Harris, R. C., McDermott, T. F. and Montreuil, F. L. (1948). *Pediatrics*, **2**, 175.
Herzon, E., Killian, E. and Pearlman, S. J. (1951). *A.M.A. Arch. Otolaryng.*, **54**, 143.
Huntington, R. W., Thompson, W. R. and Gordon, H. H. (1937). *Ann. Surg.*, **105**, 93.
Jelnes, K. (1955). *Acta oto-laryng. (Stockh.)*, **45**, 398.
Johnstone, D. D. (1958). *Brit. med. J.*, **1**, 12.
Kelly, R. E. and Laurence, D. R. (1956). *Lancet*, **1**, 118.
Khosla, H. L. and Bhatt, A. N. (1952). *J. Indian med. Ass.*, **22**, 52.
Lewis, R. A., Satoskar, R. S., Joag, G. G., Dave, B. T. and Patel, J. C. (1954). *J. Amer. med. Ass.*, **156**, 479.
Magarey, I. (1947). *Clin. Rep. Adelaide Child.Hosp.*, **1**, 39.
Noel, O. F. and McSwain, B. (1950). *Sth. Med. Surg.*, **33**, 67.
Paterson, A. E. (1930). *Med. J. Aust.*, **1**, 832.
Pratt, E. L. (1945). *J. Amer. med. Ass.*, **129**, 1243.
Puthumana, J. P. (1958). Personal communication.
Rosa Febles, C., Ramirez, E., Armaiz, G. and Torregrosa, M. V. (1950). *Bol. Asoc. méd. P. Rico*, **42**, 243.
Segar, W. E., Littlefield, P. A. and Walcher, D. N. (1952). *J. Pediat.*, **40**, 772.
Silverthorne, N. (1947). *Ibid.*, **30**, 195.
Spaeth, R. (1940). *Amer. J. Dis. Child.*, **60**, 130.
—— (1941a). *Ibid.*, **61**, 1146.
—— (1941b). *Arch. intern. Med.*, **68**, 1133.
Stonham, F. V. (1938). *Brit. med. J.*, **1**, 386.
Tompkins, A. B. (1958). *Ibid.*, **1**, 1382.
Turner, V. C. and Galloway, T. C. (1949). *Arch. Surg. (Chicago)*, **58**, 478.
Vener, H. I. and Bower, A. G. (1941). *J. Amer. med. Ass.*, **116**, 1627.
Yodh, B. B. (1937). *Brit. Med. J.*, **1**, 855.

THREE CASES OF NIEMANN PICK'S DISEASE IN CHILDREN

BY

W. I. FORSYTHE, E. F. McKEOWN and D. W. NEILL

From the Departments of Pathology and Child Health, The Queen's University, Belfast

(RECEIVED FOR PUBLICATION MARCH 23, 1959)

The classical description of Niemann Pick's disease is a disorder of lipoid metabolism, which is believed to occur almost invariably in infancy and to prove fatal within the first two years of life. The following three cases are recorded as unusual examples of the disease in patients, still alive, aged 19, 9 and 10 years respectively.

Clinical Summaries

Case 1. A girl, aged 19 years, was seen at the age of 3, when her spleen was found to be enormously enlarged and her liver palpable four fingerbreadths below the costal margin. The heart and lungs were normal, and the superficial lymph nodes were not enlarged. There was no abnormal skin pigmentation. A moderate anaemia and leucopenia were present. The platelet count was normal and a bone marrow biopsy did not reveal any abnormal cells. At the age of 7 years a radiograph of the chest showed miliary mottling throughout the lung fields. Repeated tuberculin skin tests were negative. During the next 11 years this miliary appearance was replaced by a coarser mottling and reticulation of most of the lung fields (Fig. 1). At the age of 10 the patient was only 4 ft. 2 in. in height. The spleen was larger and extended to the brim of the pelvis. The blood picture was normal. No abnormal cells were found in bone marrow biopsy, but splenic puncture performed by Dr. M. G. Nelson revealed many large cells 20-30μ in diameter, with a small eccentric nucleus and abundant foamy cytoplasm. These had all the characteristics of Niemann Pick cells.

The patient was examined at intervals and by the age of 14 bone marrow biopsy showed many Niemann Pick cells. Liver function tests were repeatedly within normal limits, there was no radiological evidence of bone involvement and an electrocardiogram was normal. Apart from these findings the patient remained very well and had no respiratory or other complaints. At the age of 17, however, she noticed a greatly increased sense of weight in her abdomen and was now conscious of her abdominal swelling which was causing her a certain amount of social embarrassment. Clinical examination showed a marked splenomegaly. She had an epistaxis, and blood examination showed W.B.C. count of 4,900/c.mm. and platelets 72,000/c.mm. These findings suggested a hypersplenic effect on the blood with thrombocytopenia and a tendency to bleeding. Splenectomy was advised and carried out on May 3, 1957. Following operation the W.B.C. count rose to 13,500/c.mm. and platelets to 258,000/c.mm. At the last follow-up examination on December 8, 1958, the patient was in good health with Hb 94%, W.B.C. 17,700/c.mm. and platelets 264,000/c.mm.

FAMILY HISTORY. Her father, mother and two sisters are alive and well, and have no splenic enlargement. There is no history of Jewish ancestry.

Case 2. This patient, now aged 9 years 2 months, was first seen at the age of 4, when she had a sudden attack of abdominal pain, which persisted for 24 hours. Her mother felt her abdomen and found a lump 'as big as a grapefruit on the left side of her tummy'.

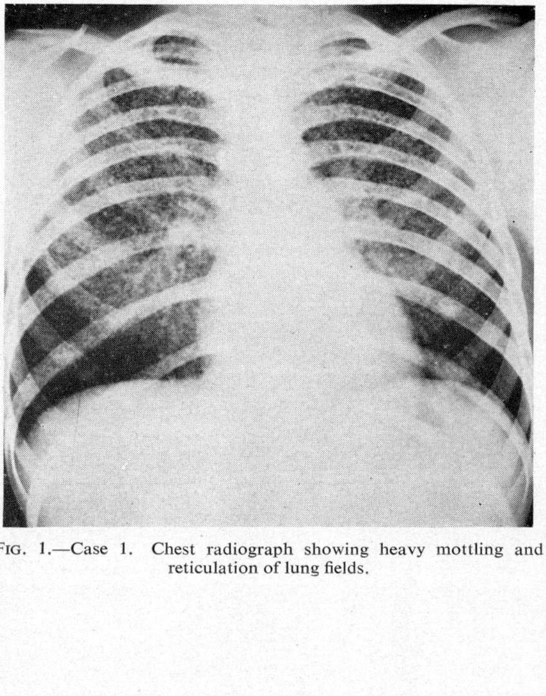

FIG. 1.—Case 1. Chest radiograph showing heavy mottling and reticulation of lung fields.

Physical examination revealed an enlarged spleen, with the lower pole extending to the umbilicus, and the liver edge was palpable two fingerbreadths below the costal margin. Skin pigmentation was absent, and radiographs of the long bones were normal. A radiograph of the chest showed a soft mottling symmetrically distributed in both lung fields (Fig. 2). A bone marrow biopsy revealed large cells up to 40μ in size, with finely vacuolated cytoplasm and small nuclei, suggesting a diagnosis of Niemann Pick's disease (Fig. 3).

By the age of 7 a peripheral pancytopenia was noted, bone marrow biopsy showed a hyperplastic picture, and the spleen had increased considerably in size. Splenectomy was therefore advised and carried out on July 11, 1956. At the last follow-up examination on December 2, 1958, the patient, then aged 9 years, had a Hb of 95%, W.B.C. 10,700/c.mm. and platelets 438,000/c.mm., and felt perfectly well, although a radiograph of the chest at this time showed considerably increased mottling.

FAMILY HISTORY. The mother and father and their five other children were examined and subjected to bone marrow biopsy. No sign of Niemann Pick's disease was found except in an older sister (Case 3). There is no history of Jewish ancestry.

Case 3. This patient, a girl now aged 10 years 3 months, is a sister of Case 2. She was admitted to hospital at the same time, at the age of 5, and was found to have an enlarged spleen palpable three fingerbreadths below the left costal margin, and the liver edge palpable two fingerbreadths below the right costal margin. The peripheral blood picture was normal and remained so during the next three years. Bone marrow biopsy showed numerous Niemann Pick cells. A radiograph of the chest revealed a fine diffuse mottling in both lung fields. Frequent examinations showed no other abnormal physical signs and at the last follow-up on December 2, 1958, the child was in good health with Hb 80%, W.B.C. 4,800/c.mm. and platelets 106,000/c.mm. There are as yet no definite indications for splenectomy although the platelet count has fallen.

Pathology of Splenectomy Specimens. The spleen in Case 1 weighed 1,080 g. and in Case 2, 875 g. The pathological findings in both were identical and need not be described separately. Macroscopically the capsule was tense, and on section the pulp was firm and salmon pink in colour (Fig. 4). The Malpighian bodies and other structural markings were indistinct. Histologically the pulp was packed with large cells 20-40μ in diameter (Fig. 5). A few appeared to lie within the sinusoids, and not infrequently some occupied the centre of the Malpighian bodies. The cells had abundant foamy cytoplasm and rather small eccentric nuclei. A few were binucleated. They stained a delicate pink with H. and E., bright red with Scharlach R, pale blue with Mallory's aniline blue and blue-black with Smith Dietrich (Fig. 6).

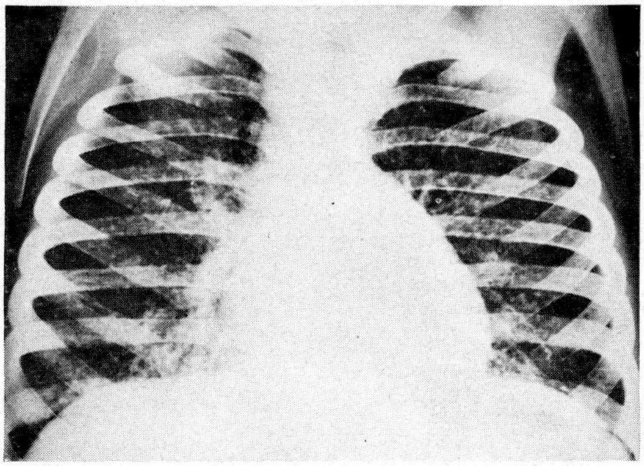

FIG. 2.—Case 2. Chest radiograph with coarse mottling of both lungs.

Phospholipid estimations were carried out on formalin-fixed material.

METHOD. Fixed spleen in 10 g. portions was homogenized for 10 minutes in 50 ml. 0·9% sodium chloride, using a domestic type of homogenizer, and 5 ml. portions of the homogenate were added drop by drop to 50 ml. alcohol-ether mixture (5:1), which was then brought to the boil in a water bottle, made to 100 ml. and filtered. The filtrate (representing 0·05 g. spleen) was carefully evaporated to dryness in 5 ml. aliquots in tubes marked at 6 ml., 0·5 ml. 60% perchloric acid was added, and digestion allowed to proceed until colourless. After cooling, the contents of the tubes were diluted with 5 ml. water, when 0·4 ml. 5% ammonium molybdate and 0·2 ml. 1% ascorbic acid were added and mixed. The colours of the contents of the tubes were measured absorptiometrically at 700 m.μ against that produced in a standard 0·02 mg. phosphorus solution similarly treated. The results are shown in Table 1.

TABLE 1
PHOSPHOLIPID ESTIMATION

Spleen	Thannhauser (mg./100 g.)	Present Series (mg.)
Normal	5·5–11	19·5
Gaucher	9·4	13·8
Niemann Pick	42·5	Case 1: 88
		Case 2: 54

From these findings it is evident that there is a greatly elevated phospholipid concentration in both spleens.

Comment

The occurrence of Niemann Pick's disease outside the period of infancy is exceptional, and for that reason the present cases are of some interest. According to Thannhauser (1950), only four verified cases in adults had been reported. Two of these were described by Dusendschon (1872) who confirmed the diagnosis by chemical analysis of the

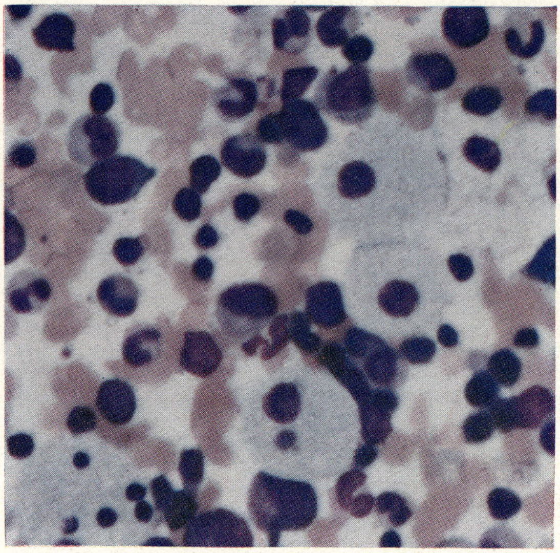

FIG. 3.—Case 2. Bone marrow smear showing several Niemann Pick cells with abundant foamy cytoplasm. (Leishman × 650.)

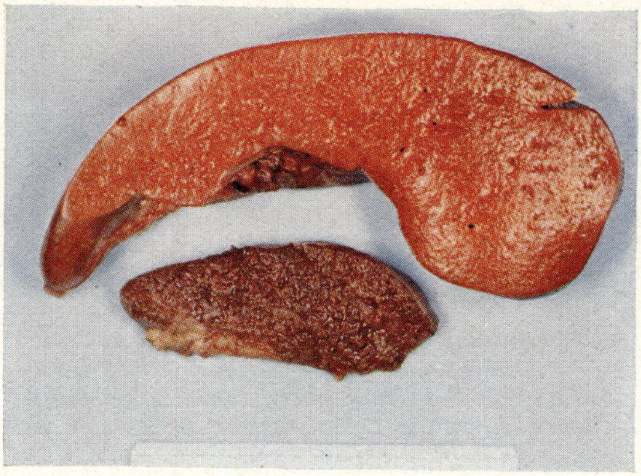

FIG. 4.—Splenectomy specimen with normal control showing great enlargement, and salmon pink coloration of cut surface.

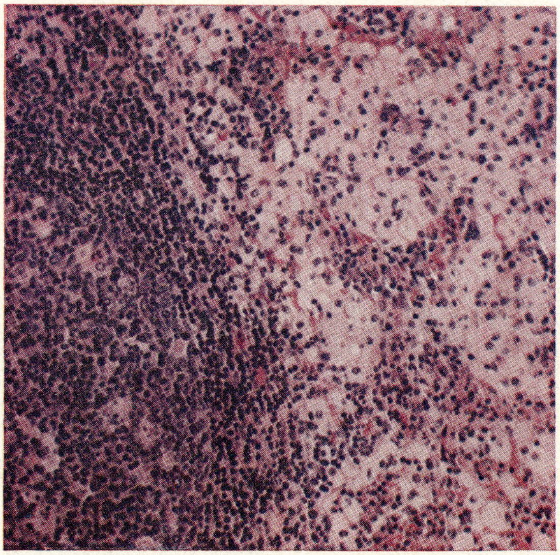

FIG. 5.—Spleen, with accumulation of Niemann Pick cells in the pulp. (H. and E. × 250.)

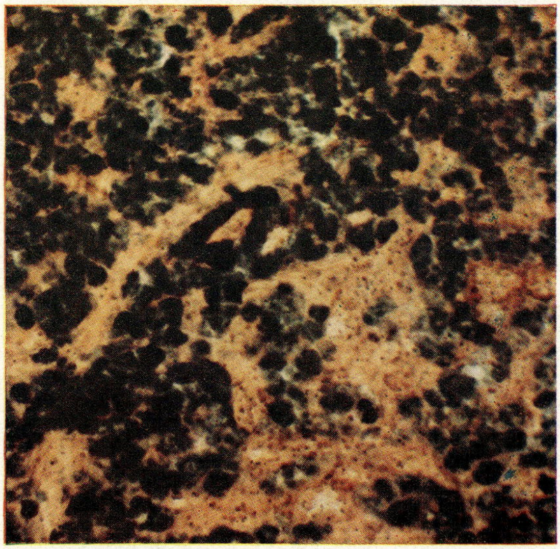

FIG. 6.—Spleen, showing Niemann Pick cells staining blue-black due to presence of phospholipids. (Smith Dietrich × 350.)

organs in two brothers aged 29 and 33. Glanzmann (1943) reported the third case in an 8-year-old girl, and Farber and Thannhauser (1950) the fourth in an 8-year-old boy. In 1954, Terry, Sperry and Brodoff published a possible further case of adult lipoidosis of Niemann Pick type developing in a man of 52. Histologically the infiltrations in lungs, liver and spleen showed cells which resembled Niemann Pick cells in structure and staining characters, but chemical analysis of the affected tissues, though revealing increased amounts of phosphosphingosides, showed levels which did not come within the range generally found in infantile cases.

However, a recent review by Crocker and Farber (1958) presents data from 18 cases, five of whom died between the age of 3-6 years, three between 12-20 years and one patient was still alive at 18 years, with the diagnosis made at 4 months of age. These writers emphasize the importance of recognizing that Niemann Pick's disease has a broader range of biological behaviour than is usually stated, and that it may not have an invariably rapid and fatal course with death in early infancy. They suggest that if the early critical phase of the disease can be survived a non-progressive state may be entered with long survival.

The occurrence of these adolescent and adult types of the disease tends to allow of a correlation with the other diseases of lipoid metabolism. Thus Gaucher's disease may present as an infantile, adolescent or adult type. Letterer-Siwe's disease is also recognized in infancy and adult life, whilst the cerebral lipoidosis described by Tay Sachs may also present in infancy or adolescence.

The clinical diagnosis in the present three cases rested on the finding of the characteristic large foam cells in the bone marrow and in the spleen. These cells, varying in size from 20-40μ, stained lightly acidophilic with H. and E., pale blue with Mallory's aniline blue, to some extent bright red with Scharlach R and heavily blue-black with Smith Dietrich. The latter stain is specific for phospholipids. Since the disease is a disturbance of lipid metabolism in which large quantities of phospholipids, and in particular the diaminophosphatide, sphingomyelin, accumulate within the affected organs, the final diagnosis depends on demonstrating by chemical analysis a significant increase in the amount of sphingomyelin present. In both splenectomy specimens a very high content of phospholipid was found, far above normal, and even above the range generally recorded in most cases of Niemann Pick's disease. It is worth noting that the weights of the spleen in these two cases greatly exceed that of any recorded case, the heaviest being 480 g.

The value of splenectomy in this condition is doubtful. In some patients it has been carried out merely for relief of pressure symptoms. In others, as in two of the present cases, there may be a 'hypersplenic' blood picture, and splenectomy has led to improvement. According to Crocker and Farber (1958) at least there is no evidence that the procedure hastens the progression of the disease or subsequently lowers resistance to infection.

The prognosis in these non-infantile cases is uncertain. As a metabolic disorder the disease is likely to be chronically progressive. Nevertheless in spite of evidence of involvement of lungs, liver, spleen and bone marrow over a period of years in the three cases here recorded, each patient is in excellent health. Since a radiograph of the lungs shows a heavy miliary mottling and obviously denotes extensive infiltration with Niemann Pick cells, it is possible that increasing pulmonary fibrosis, which is usually associated with these infiltrations, may lead to right ventricular failure. This occurred in one of Dusendschon's cases (1872). The pulmonary lesions may also render the patients more liable to intercurrent infection. On the other hand, the hepatic infiltrations may later be associated with cirrhosis. This was described in both of Dusendschon's cases. However, his patients were alcoholics and it is doubtful which was the decisive factor, as cirrhosis has not been reported in the adult form of Gaucher's disease. With pulmonary, hepatic, splenic and bone marrow involvement in the three present cases it is difficult to envisage the disease being other than progressive.

Summary

Niemann Pick's disease is generally confined to early infancy, but its occurrence in three patients, still alive, aged 19, 9 and 10 years respectively, is described. In spite of evidence of pulmonary, hepatic, splenic and bone marrow involvement, the general health of the patients is good. It is possible that the form of Niemann Pick's disease in older subjects may run a chronic and relatively benign course.

We are indebted to Dr. R. Marshall and Dr. W. A. B. Campbell for permission to study Case 1 and Cases 2 and 3 respectively, to Mr. D. Mehaffey for the illustrations and to the Northern Ireland Hospitals Authority for a grant towards research work.

References

Crocker, A. C. and Farber, S. (1958). *Medicine (Baltimore)*, 37, 1.
Dusendschon, A. (1872). Thèse, Faculté de Médecine, Genève.
Farber, S. and Thannhauser, S. J. (1950). Unpublished. Cited by Thannhauser, S. J. (1950). *Lipidoses*, 2nd ed. p. 564.
Glanzmann, E. (1943). *Schweiz. med. Wschr.*, 73, 1414.
Terry, R. D., Sperry, W. M. and Brodoff, B. (1954). *Amer. J. Path.*, 30, 263.
Thannhauser, S. J. (1950). *Lipidoses*, 2nd ed. Oxford University Press, New York.

A STUDY OF CONGENITAL HEART DEFECTS IN MONGOLISM

BY

M. C. LIU and K. CORLETT

From the Fountain Hospital, London, S.W.17

(RECEIVED FOR PUBLICATION MARCH 11, 1959)

Mongolism has aroused widespread interest since the days of Langdon Down's pioneer work in 1866. Numerous hypotheses relating to its aetiology and mechanism have appeared, but none can be regarded as conclusive or final, further observations and research being necessary before a full understanding is possible.

Of the many anomalies found in mongolism, affecting nearly every system, that of congenital heart disease is the most remarkable and least understood, certainly, as Abbott (1936) stated, 'calling for an explanation'.

The life span of mongol children has already been extended by chemotherapy and antibiotics, and a further prolongation will follow the recent advances in cardiac surgery. For this reason congenital heart disease in mongols has ceased to be of mere post-mortem interest and has become a stimulus to further understanding. The cause of the cardiac abnormality, the stage of foetal life at which it occurs and the pathological processes involved are problems of considerable interest which are difficult to solve.

Among the early observations were those of Abbott, who has stressed the frequent combination of mongolism and persistent ostium primum. Taussig (1947) emphasized the high correlation between mongolism and persistent atrioventricularis communis. Esen (1957) found a similar high correlation, but Evans (1950), in his study of cardiac anomalies in mongolism, showed a preponderance of ventricular and atrial septal defects. Benda (1946) stated that about 75% of mongoloid infants who die in the first two years of life have congenital heart disease, and 35% of the survivors thereafter. In Evans' series 50% died before 5 years of age. Keith, Rowe and Vlad (1958), in their study of 18 mongoloid infants who died at the Hospital for Sick Children, Toronto, mentioned that few die in the first month of life, and two-thirds die between 4 weeks and 1 year. On clinical evidence, those with the most severe cardiac anomalies die young, and so, as the age group progresses, the incidence of severe cardiac anomaly becomes less. This largely accounts for the comparatively low incidence found by other observers. This point is well illustrated in the two different age groups studied at the Fountain Hospital, the percentage of cardiac anomalies in the 3-year age group being much higher than that in the 10-year group.

Southwick (1939) and Ingalls (1947) were interested in the causation and time of origin of the cardiac anomalies. Ingalls postulated that the latter was between the sixth and ninth week of foetal life. This hypothesis has been well supported by many pathologists from necropsy material as well as from embryological evidence. The higher incidence, about to be discussed, of maternal illness in the early part of pregnancy in the congenital heart defect group than in the control group, suggests that the time of development of the anomalies must be early. The frequent combination of congenital heart defect and mongolism suggests that the cause and time of development of congenital heart defect are similar to, if not identical with, that of mongolism as a whole.

Among the many factors involved in the aetiology of mongolism, advanced maternal age (Davenport and Allen, 1925; Penrose, 1934; Bleyer, 1938), and maternal illness (Ingalls, Babbott and Philbrook, 1957) are considered here. Engler (1949) stressed the influence of an unfavourable intrauterine environment. Maternal rubella as a cause of congenital heart defect was mentioned by Gregg (1941) and Swan, Tostevin, Moore, Mayo and Black (1943). So far rubella has not been recorded in the literature as a cause of congenital heart defect in mongolism.

Present Study

The present work is an attempt to assess the incidence, aetiology and type of congenital heart defect in 216 mongoloid imbeciles admitted to the Fountain Hospital in the 14 years between September, 1944, and July, 1958. It is based on social and clinical assessments and, in some cases, on autopsy findings. Forty-three cases have been discharged and excluded from this survey and 51 died, leaving a total of 122 children, whose mean age was 10 years, still in the hospital. Eleven of the 122 cases had a congenital heart defect, the diagnosis being made on the clinical history, physical findings and radiological and cardiological investigations. In another 17 cases, a variable soft precordial systolic murmur had been reported during earlier life, but in only seven of these was it present at the time of investigation; radiology then revealed a heart of normal size and shape and the electrocardiogram was normal. An analysis of the findings in the 111 children with normal hearts is given in Table 1.

In nine of the 11 cases with congenital heart defect cardiac catheterization, cine angiography and other necessary investigations were carried out in the cardiac department of St. George's Hospital. The following case reports illustrate the two more frequent types of cardiac anomaly.

Case 2 (Table 2). B.J., a mongol girl, was born on August 20, 1945, of normal intelligent parents, the father aged 40 and the mother 39 years at the birth. This was the mother's fourth pregnancy, the second resulting in a stillbirth due to malpresentation, the first and third producing children of normal health and intelligence. The mother's health was good during this pregnancy and the birth was rapid. The birthweight was 8·5 lb. There was no unusual neonatal history and mongolism was diagnosed at birth.

The child was admitted to the Fountain Hospital aged 6½ years. She had all the usual mongoloid characteristics with a shy, docile and co-operative temperament. Her speech was poor and her I.Q. was 30 on the Stanford-Binet (T.M. Rev.) Form L. She had repeated attacks of respiratory illness each year; during these her peripheral circulation, never very good, was poor and her extremities became cold and cyanotic. She was breathless on exertion but there was no evidence of heart failure. The femoral pulses were present and her B.P. was 115/70. An ejection systolic murmur and a fixed splitting of the second sound were heard over the pulmonary area. Radiography suggested a right heart enlargement. The electrocardiogram showed an rsR pattern in V_1 and an atrial septal defect was diagnosed and confirmed by cardiac catheterization.

Case 5. L.P., a boy 9 years old, was born on August 26, 1948, the mother's age being 43, the father's 42 years at the birth. He was the second child, the first being a girl of average intelligence. The pregnancy and birth were said to have been normal. The birthweight was 8·5 lb. There was no unusual neonatal history except

TABLE 1

AN ANALYSIS OF 111 MONGOLS WITH NORMAL HEARTS

Age range (yr.)	1–5	6–10	11–15	16–20	21–25	Mean 10
Patients (No.)	14	46	34	15	2	Total 111

Birthweights (lb.)	2·8–4	4·1–5	5·1–6	6·1–7	7·1–8	8·1–9	9·6	Mean 6·57
Patients (No.)	2	8	22	21	16	6	1	Total 76

Prenatal history	Maternal illness before four months gestation	Maternal illness throughout period of gestation	Total
Cases (No.)	26	4	30

I.Q.	5–10	11–15	16–20	21–25	26–30	31–35	36–40	41–45	46–50	51–55	Mean 30
Patients (No.)	5	7	12	12	17	21	17	7	7	3	Total 108

Parents' age ranges at patient's birth (yr.)	20–25	26–30	31–35	36–40	41–45	46–50	51–55	56–60	Mean	Total No. of cases
Father	14	20	12	25	15	9	1	1	35	97
Mother	(16–25) 20	17	11	32	17	3			33·6*	100

* Ages are calculated in decimals in all Tables to facilitate statistical analysis.

CLINICAL DETAILS OF 11 M

Case No.	Age (yr.)	Sex	History		Birth-weight (lb.)	Cyanosis	Clubbing	Polycythaemia	Cardiac Murmurs		Radiolog
			Prenatal	Neonatal					Types	First detected (yr.)	
1	10·2	F	Haemorrhage	Cyanosed	9·0	–	–	–	S.M.	At birth	Heart enlarg globular sha
2	12·9	F	N	N	8·5	–	–	–	S.M.	6·5	Rt. heart sl.
3	16·9	F	N	Cyanosed	7·25	–	–	–	S.M.	At birth	Heart enlarg
4	18·3	F	Hyperemesis gravidarum	Jaundiced	5·5	+	+	+	S.M.	2	R.V.++; b ectasis
5	9·9	M	N	N	8·5	–	–	–	S.M.	At birth	Globular he pulm. pletho
6	13·3	F	N	Jaundiced	7·0	–	–	–	S.M.	At birth	Heart promi border
7	17·3	F	N	Difficult sucking	7·0	–	–	–	S.M.	11	Enlarged hea R.A.++; plethora
8	5·9	M	N	Jaundiced; difficult sucking	8·0	+	+	–	S.M.	4	Enlarged hea plethora
9	4·5	M	N	Cyanosed; difficult sucking	6·0	–	–	–	S.M.	At birth	Rt. heart
10	2·0	M	N	Cyanosed; difficult sucking	6·8	+	–	–	S.M.	At birth	Heart round
11	11·8	F	Show 4 mth.	N	8·1	+	+	+	S.M.	3·7	Heart enlarg bronchiectasi
Mean	11·2				7·4						

N=normal S.M.=systolic murmur R.V.=right ventricle L.V.=left ventricle P.A.=pulmonary artery R.B.A.=right brachi
I.V.C.=inferior vena cava R.A.=right auricle P.V.=pulmonary vein A.S.D.=atrial septal defect V.S.D.=ventricular sep
P.S.=pulmonar

that a cardiac murmur was heard when he was 1 week old. He suffered from bronchitis, pneumonia and meningococcal meningitis in infancy. However, his general health has gradually improved since admission to this hospital aged 2 years 10 months, and at present he enjoys better health than most of his fellow patients. He is a pleasant, co-operative boy. His I.Q. was 31 on the Stanford-Binet Scale (T.M. Rev.) Form L. On examination he appeared to be in good general health with a good peripheral circulation and no signs of heart strain. The radial pulses were strong and full, with a rate of 82 per minute, and the B.P. was 120/80. A loud systolic murmur was heard at the apex. Radiography revealed a slightly globular-shaped heart, and the electrocardiogram was within normal limits. Both cardiac catheterization and selective cine angiography demonstrated a left to right shunt at ventricular level, and a ventricular septal defect was diagnosed.

Autopsy Cases. Among the 51 patients who died, autopsies were performed on 44, of whom 16 had congenital heart defects (Table 3). Six patients had patent foramen ovale and were not included in the number of those with congenital anomalies, leaving a total of 22 in whom autopsy showed a normal heart. Table 4 illustrates the causes of death of the latter.

The tentative diagnosis of congenital heart defect was initially based on clinical examination (e.g. cardiac murmurs, cyanosis, etc.). There were six patients with cardiac anomalies which had not been detected during life. Possible reasons for this include the observers' inexperience, difficulty in examination owing to an unco-operative patient, lack of full examination, murmurs not being present

:ARDIAC DEFECTS

C.G.	Catheterization and Other Cardiac Investigations			Diagnosis
	Pressure (mm. Hg)	Blood O_2 Saturation	Others	
V.+	R.V.=47/4 P.A.=50/30	R.V.=57% R.P.A.=62% Main P.A.=63% L.P.A.=60%	Pulm. resistance 6 units	I.P.H.*; persistent L. S.V.C.
V.+	P.A.=37/17		Pulm. systemic flow=2·2:1	A.S.D.
V.+	R.V.=105/5	Aorta=80%	Cine-angio. showed simultaneous flow to aorta and pulmonary artery; A.S.D. ; ? V.S.D.	Eisenmenger's syndrome ; A.S.D. ; ? V.S.D.
V.+	P.A.=118/80	R.B.A.=94% Thoracic A.=83%	Pulmonary flow 2 l./min.; pulm. resistance 28 units	P.D.A.; pulm. hypertension
mal	R.V.=25/5 P.A.=25/8	R.V.=153 ml./l. S.V.C.=141 ml./l. I.V.C.=R.A.	P=5·7 l./min.; S=4·5 l./min.; P:S=1·3:1; cine-angio. showed lt. to rt. ventricular shunt; pulm. resistance 2 units	V.S.D.
V.+	R.V.=62/2		Cine-angio. showed valvular type pulm. stenosis and A.S.D. shunt at 2·4 l./min.	P.S.; A.S.D.
V.+	R.V.=110/0 P.A.=37/12	S.V.C.=I.V.C.=63% R.A.=74%; R.V.=89%; B.A.=86% P.V.=94%	P:S=2·4:1 Pulm. resistance 5 units	V.S.D.+; P.S.+; A.S.D. ?
V.+ V.+	R.V.=130/0 L.B.A.=100/60	L.B.A.=74%	Evans blue showed rt. to lt. shunt; cine-angio. showed V.S.D.	Eisenmenger's syndrome ; V.S.D.
mal				V.S.D.
V.+ V.+				V.S.D.; P.S.; over-riding great vessels
V.+	R.V.=80/0 Aorta=80/40		Bi-directional shunts at atrioventricular levels	Atrioventricular canal ; pulm. hypertension

L.B.A.=left brachial artery R.P.A.=right pulmonary artery L.P.A.=left pulmonary artery S.V.C.=superior vena cava
pulmonary flow S=systemic flow I.P.H.=idiopathic pulmonary hypertension P.D.A.=patent ductus arteriosus

at the time, excessive noise in the thoracic cavity, pulmonary infection and pericardial effusion. (There were two cases of pericardial effusion containing more than 100 ml. of straw-coloured fluid.) A comparison was made of the types of cardiac anomalies diagnosed on clinical grounds and at autopsy and is summarized in Tables 2, 3 and 6.

An analysis of the various types of lesions showed that ventricular septal defect was the most common and occurred in 10 cases, of which six were in the clinical group. Atrial septal defect was the next most frequent, a total of eight cases, four of which were in the clinical group. Patent ductus arteriosus was the third most frequent, occurring in seven cases, of which six were in the autopsy group. Vessel anomalies occurred in four cases and were equally distributed in both groups. Pulmonary stenosis occurred in three cases of the clinical group and none in the autopsy group. Atrioventricularis communis occurred in three instances, Fallot's tetralogy, Eisenmenger's syndrome and valvular anomalies each occurred in two instances. Other rare defects had the same frequency; idiopathic pulmonary hypertension occurred in one case only in the clinical group.

Associated anomalies of the general systemic organs may be as numerous and variable as the outward manifestations of mongolism, and a comparative study of their relative development in time would lead towards an understanding of both the stage of foetal life at which cardiac anomalies occur and their aetiology. Unfortunately, such a study

TABLE 3

CLINICAL DETAILS AND AUTOPSY FINDINGS IN 16 MONGOLS WITH CONGENITAL CARDIAC DEFECTS

Case No.	Age at death (yr.)	Sex	History: Prenatal	History: Neonatal	Birth Wt. (lb.)	Birth Rank	I.Q.	Age at Patient's Birth (yr.): Mother	Age at Patient's Birth (yr.): Father	Cyanosis	Clubbing	Cardiac murmurs	At Death: Wt. (lb.)	At Death: Ht. (in.)	Cause of Death	Type of Cardiac Anomalies
a. 1	3·8	M	Dysentery	N*	6·6	5	48	40	37	–	–	S.M.	36		Laryngitis	P.D.A.
a. 2	7·2	F	Fall at 3 mth.	Morbis cordis	7·5	1	46	37	56			S.M.	36		Subacute infective endocarditis; thrombosis of superior sagittal sinus	V.S.D. P.D.A.
a. 3	1·0	F	Hydramnios (?)	Vomiting; 'Bad breather'	6·5	2	50	25	26	+	+	S.M.	15	25	Bronchopneumonia; heart failure	Atrioventricularis communis P.D.A.
a. 4	3·5	M	N	N	5·6	2	9	29	32				16	34	Bronchopneumonia	A.S.D. of ostium secundum type; persistence of left superior vena cava
a. 5	1·7	F	N	Jaundiced	7·0	2	36	30	30	+		S.M.	18	30	Bronchopneumonia; enteritis	Atrioventricularis communis
a. 6	2·3	F	Sick	N	8·0	2	–	32	32			S.M.	24·5		Fibrillation; heart failure	A.S.D. of ostium secundum type
a. 7	27·0	F	Bad health	Morbis cordis	7·5	3	32	32	35	+	+	S.M.	118·5		Bronchopneumonia; heart failure	P.D.A.; V.S.D.; right heart hypertrophy
a. 8	1·9	F	Pleurisy	N	6·8	1	32	23	23	–	–	M	16	32	Bronchopneumonia	V.S.D.; right heart hypertrophy; coronary sinus opens into rt atrium
a. 9	1·5	F	Threatened abortion 3 mth.	Morbis cordis	7·2	1	–	24	27	+		S.M.	20	31	Bronchopneumonia; cerebral embolism	Fallot's tetralogy
a.10	3·0	M	N	?	5·5	2	27	26	26	+	+	S.M.	19	33	Acute bronchitis; pulmonary collapse	Fallot's tetralogy
a.11	1·3	F	N	N	6·8	3	33	34	33				16	28	Bronchopneumonia; meningitis	V.S.D.; P.D.A.; rt. heart hypertrophy
a.12	2·9	M	Oedema of legs	N	8·0	9	5	50	50				34	37·5	Bronchopneumonia	A.S.D. of ostium secundum type; rt. heart enlarged
a.13	7·8	F			6·3	2	30	31	36				44		Acute laryngotracheobronchitis	P.D.A.; heart enlarged
a.14	2·7	M	Hypertension		4·5	3	27	25	22				10·5	28·7	Bronchopneumonia	Bicuspid aortic valve and fenestration
a.15	2·6	M	V.D.		9·4	4	65	39	38				20	32	Bronchopneumonia R.V.H. (pericardial effusion)	A.S.D. of ostium secundum type
a.16	4·3	F	Haemorrhage			2	13	38	46				20	32	Acute bronchitis R.V.H. (pericardial effusion)	Tricuspid valve malformation
Mn.	3·2				6·9	2·8	32	33	36				23	31		
Mean of Tables 2 and 3					7·11											

* See abbreviations used in Table 2.

has not been possible with the records available for discussion in this paper.

CAUSE OF DEATH. The high mortality rate in children with congenital heart defect has been reduced recently by the introduction of chemotherapeutic and antibiotic drugs. More recently still, advances in cardio-surgical techniques have led to the promise of a completely new outlook.

The major cause of death in this series was chest infection, chiefly bronchopneumonia. The high incidence of cardiac complications in the congenital heart defect group is worth mentioning. Two cases had pericardial effusion, one had infective endocarditis and another cerebral embolism. From the study of these cases it seems obvious that if the condition were recognized early enough, precautions against current infections could be taken or special surgical measures could be provided, enabling most of these complications to be prevented or treated.

MEAN AGE OF DEATH. The mean age at death of the congenital heart defect group is 3·2 years, and that of the mongols without congenital heart defect is 3·3 years (Tables 3 and 4). These figures are almost identical, and the difference is probably too small to be of any statistical significance (not including

TABLE 4

CLINICAL DETAILS AND AUTOPSY FINDINGS IN 22 MONGOLS WITH NORMAL HEARTS

Case No.	Age (Yr.)	Sex	History		B.W. (lb.)	B.R.	I.Q.	Age at Patient's Birth (yr.)		At Death		Cause of Death
			Prenatal	Neonatal				M.	F.	Wt. (lb.)	Ht. (in.)	
a.17	3·0	F				1	56	20		22·5	33	Bronchopneumonia
a.18	4·3	M	Familial poor health			3		41	41	29·8		Acute bronchitis
a.19	2·7	F	N	N	8·5	2	21	28	30	21		Bronchopneumonia; gastro-enteritis
a.20	2·5	M	N	N	7·1	3	23	25	22	25		Otitis media; cerebral oedema; congestion of lungs; pyonephrosis (one kidney only)
a.21	4·3	M	N	N*	5·0	1	10	25	26	28	42	Inhalation pneumonia; renal haemorrhage
a.22	1·3	F				2				24	29	Bronchopneumonia
a.23	0·9	M	N	N		3	33	37	38	14		Bronchopneumonia
a.24	2·4	M	N	N	6·8			36	41	30	35	Peritonitis; perforation of Meckel's diverticulum
a.25	3·8	M	N	N	6·0	9	31	46	50	31·5		Acute laryngotracheo-bronchitis
a.26	2·9	M			4·8	1	50	25	40	17	30	Bronchopneumonia; thrombocytopenic purpura
a.27	9·0	M			7·0	2	24	39	38	51		Purulent bronchitis; measles
a.28	3·8	M	N	N	5·2	1	27	39	41	20	30	Bronchopneumonia
a.29	5·3	F	N	N		3	20	35	34	26·5	36·5	Acute bronchitis
a.30	4·3	F	N	N	7·0	7	19	48	30	18	34	Bronchopneumonia
a.31	3·2	F					26			24	34	Bronchopneumonia
a.32	3·5	M	Swollen ankles		7·0	3	9	38	39	11·5	30	Bronchopneumonia; hydronephrosis
a.33	2·0	M	Poor health Fainting	*		3	42	26	34	28	29·5	Bronchopneumonia
a.34	1·6	F	N	N		3	55	32	42	2·1	34	Otitis media; pulmonary collapse
a.35	2·5	F					36	37		26·5		Bronchopneumonia
a.36	5·6		N	N	7·6	4	44	41	41	35	39	Bronchopneumonia
a.37	3·2	M			6·0	3	26	23	25	22	34	Lobar pneumonia
a.38	1·3	M				2		25		18	29	Acute tracheobronchitis
Mean	3·3				6·5	2·9	31	34·4	37·2	24·7	33·3	

* Premature.

Case a.7). Experience suggests that after the first year of life, mongols with congenital heart defect have an equal chance of survival with those having a normal cardiovascular system.

Ingalls, as already mentioned, was of the opinion that the cause of mongolism operates before the end of the third month of foetal life and it is generally believed that the processes leading to the associated cardiac defects originate during the same period. This being accepted, a knowledge of early foetal environment might throw considerable light on the aetiology of these defects, but unfortunately little objective information of importance is available in most cases. However, since mongolism is of overriding importance to the mother compared with her reaction to the presence of congenital heart defect in her mongol child, it is felt that information obtained from her concerning her health during pregnancy might lead to the recognition of significant differences between the foetal environment in cases with and without congenital heart defect. The following information includes, therefore, a social history as well as points from hospital reports where these are available.

For the purpose of analysis, special emphasis is placed on the following aspects of prenatal history.

Parental Age (Tables 1 and 3-5). The mean age of the fathers at the birth of the 111 patients without congenital heart defect was 35 years, and that of the mothers 33·6 years. The mean age of the fathers for the 11 clinically diagnosed congenital heart defect cases was 36·7 years and that of the mothers was 34·5 years, the controls being 34·9 and 34 for the fathers and mothers respectively. Those for the autopsied congenital heart defect group were 36 years and 33 years, and for the group with normal hearts, 37·2 years and 34·4 years for fathers and mothers respectively. All these results showed no appreciable difference between the various groups.

Maternal Illness. This was recorded in three instances in the 11 clinical cases of congenital heart defect: for instance, in Case 1 (Table 2) there was a history of haemorrhage at two months of gestation which lasted four weeks. In Case 4, maternal 'ill-health' and sickness and excessive worry persisted throughout the pregnancy, and in Case 11 there was a history of vaginal bleeding before the fourth month of gestation.

Among the 16 autopsy cases with congenital heart defect (Table 3) there were 11 with a history of maternal illness, and where possible a definite date has been shown. One had amoebic dysentery and developed a liver abscess at the third month of pregnancy. She also suffered from severe anaemia. In the second case, the mother had a bad fall at the third month of gestation. Three cases suffered from 'ill-health' and one of these had hydramnios. In Case a.8 the mother had pleurisy during the first three months of pregnancy; in Case a.9 she had a threatened miscarriage at the third month; in Case a.12 she suffered from 'ill-health' and swelling of the legs; in Case a.14 she had high blood pressure, in Case a.15 venereal disease and in Case a.16 the mother was very ill with tertian malaria. She had a 'stroke' (details unknown) with vomiting and haemorrhage.

Maternal illness affected only 30 of the 111 mothers (Table 1) whose infants had no congenital heart defect. Twenty-six of these occurred before the fourth month of pregnancy. A few were unwell throughout. The nature of the illnesses more or less followed the same pattern as those mentioned above. These were haemorrhage in eight, symptoms of 'toxaemia' in eight, feverish illnesses in five, trauma in five, attempted abortion in four, and a history of shock and previous miscarriages in three. These give a total incidence of 51·5% (14/27) of maternal illness in early pregnancy in the congenital heart defect group, and 27% (30/111) in the group with normal hearts. These differences are statistically significant ($\chi^2=6\cdot16$, P0·02<>0·01 dfi.).

Prematurity. This was present in 13 cases (11·7%) in the group with normal hearts. Among the 22 autopsied patients with normal hearts (Table 4) two had a history of prematurity. Case a.21 was six to seven weeks premature and the birthweight was 5 lb. Case a.33 resulted from an eight months' gestation, the birthweight not being recorded. There was no instance of prematurity among the 11 clinically diagnosed cases of congenital heart defect (Table 2). Of the 16 autopsied cases with congenital heart defect, prematurity was mentioned in Case a.6, but the birthweight was 8 lb. (Table 3) and prematurity was therefore excluded.

Birth Rank. This was compared in the two groups. Table 5 shows 3·4 for the congenital heart defect group and 2·9 for the control group, while Tables 3 and 4 show 2·8 for the congenital heart defect group and 2·9 for the group with normal hearts.

Neonatal History. In Table 5 the neonatal history of the 11 clinical cases of congenital heart defect is compared with 11 controls consisting of mongoloid patients with normal hearts, their ages and sexes being matched as closely as possible. Four of the congenital heart defect group were cyanosed

TABLE 5

A COMPARISON OF 22 MONGOLS, 11 WITH AND 11 WITHOUT CONGENITAL CARDIAC DEFECTS

Case No	Age (Yr.)	Sex	Birth Rank	Birth Wt. (lb.)	History		I.Q.	Wt. (lb.)	Ht. (in.)	Parents' Age	
					Prenatal	Neonatal				Mother	Father
Mongolism with C.H.D.											
1	10·2	F	3	9·0	Haemorrhage 2 mth.	Cyanosed	32	42·7	46·5	35	35
2	12·9	F	4	8·5	N	N	30	56·8	49·0	39	40
3	16·9	F	1	7·25	N	Cyanosed	28	126·1	55·8	34	41
4	18·3	F	1	5·5	Familial	Jaundiced	42	98·6	57·5	20	19
5	9·9	M	2	8·5	N	N	31	70·3	52·0	43	42
6	13·3	F	5	7·0	N	Jaundiced	32	64·3	49·5	34	39
7	17·3	F	6	7·0	N	Sucking difficulty	22	84·8	55·5	44	43
8	5·9	M	4	8·0	N	Sucking difficulty. Jaundiced	40	42·1	36·5	32	36
9	4·5	M	4	6·0	N	Sucking difficulty. Cyanosed	25	28·4	32·5	30	27
10	2·0	M	4	6·8	N	Sucking difficulty. Cyanosed	21	14·3	24·4	28	29
11	11·8	F	3	8·1	Show 4 mth.	N	36	56·1	49·3	41	53
Mean	11·2		3·4	7·4			30·8	67·6	47·5	34·5	36·7
Mongolism without C.H.D.											
1	9·8	F	3	7·2	N	N	18	56·6	48·5	37	38
2	13·6	F	4	8·0	N	N	26	58·5	52·5	43	49
3	16·5	F	3	6·5	Familial	Poor feeder	30	98·8	58·3	35	34
4	20·0	F	2	6·0	Familial	N	40	98·5	56·7	32	31
5	9·1	M	2	5·4	? Toxaemia	Jaundiced	16	42·5	48·3	36	36
6	14·1	F	4	7·0	N	N	22	84·7	52·3	41	39
7	16·0	F	6	7·6	N	Sucking difficulty	26	70·6	54·5	38	42
8	5·6	M	1	7·4	N	'Blue' asphyxia	50	42·0	36·5	27	25
9	4·9	M	1	9·0	N	N	32	28·1	31·0	23	24
10	2·9	M	3	6·6	Threatened abortion 3 mth.	N	34	14·8	28·0	26	29
11	11·8	F	3	6·2	N	N	45	70·4	54·5	36	37
Mean	11·3		2·9	7·0			30·8	69·2	48·4	34	34·9

at birth, and another three were 'jaundiced'. Of another four cases (Table 2) with a history of difficulty in sucking, one has been diagnosed as having a ventricular septal defect, pulmonary stenosis and a possible atrial septal defect, one as a ventricular septal defect, pulmonary stenosis and overriding great vessels, the third as a ventricular septal defect and Eisenmenger's syndrome and the fourth as a ventricular septal defect alone. Only three of the 11 cases with congenital heart defect had a normal neonatal history. In six of the 11 cases congenital heart defect was diagnosed at birth.

In the control group one case was cyanosed, one was jaundiced, one was a poor feeder and another had sucking difficulty, while seven had a normal neonatal history.

Birthweight. The mean birthweight of 76 of the 111 cases without cardiac anomalies was 6·57 lb. (Table 1). The mean weight of the 26 cases with cardiac anomalies was 7·11 lb. (11 clinical cases, with mean birthweight of 7·4 lb., and 15 autopsied cases, 6·9 lb.). These mean differences are statistically significant at the ·05 level (t=2·260).

Growth and Development. In Table 5 growth and development are compared in the clinical congenital heart defect group and in the controls. The mean age of the congenital heart defect group was 11·2 years, while that of the control group was 11·3 years. The mean weights, 67·6 and 69·2 lb., and mean heights, 47·5 and 48·4 in., respectively, show that there were no significant differences in these respects between the two groups.

In Tables 3 and 4 similar comparisons are made for the autopsied groups. In Table 4 only 15 of the patients without congenital heart defect had their heights measured at the time of death, the mean being 33·3 in. The age range was from 11 months (0·9 year) to 9 years (mean 3·3 years), and the mean weight was 24·7 lb. The mean height and weight for the 16 autopsied cases with congenital heart defect was 31 in. and 23 lb., the mean age being 3·2 years and age range from 1 year to 7 years and 10 months (7·8 year). Case a.7 was not included because of age (27 years).

Intelligence Quotient. In Table 5 the I.Q. is compared in the clinical congenital heart defect and control groups, both averaging 30·8. In the autopsied groups the I.Q. averages 32 for the congenital heart defect group (Table 3) and 31 for the group with normal hearts (Table 4). This finding is consistent with the general opinion that a congenital heart defect has no effect on the intellectual capacity, hence mongolism associated with congenital heart defect still falls within the imbecile range common to the general mongoloid population. However, Mossberger (1949) has shown that heart malformation causing insufficient blood supply to the brain can cause mental retardation.

Discussion

Among all the possible factors so far postulated relating to the causation of mongolism, advanced maternal age has been most frequently incriminated. Jenkins (1933), Penrose (1934) and Bleyer (1938) all arrived at a critical maternal age of 32 years for the production of mongolism. They attached no importance to the father's age. Lahdensuu (1937) did not agree that maternal age plays a very important part in causing mongolism.

Parents' age in relation to congenital cardiac anomalies in mongolism has not previously been mentioned. In the present series there was no marked difference between parents' ages in the congenital heart defect group and in the group with normal hearts.

Birthweight needs further investigation and more consideration.

Southwick (1939), after comparing the birthweight of mongols and normal infants, concluded that there was no significant difference. On the other hand, Smith and McKeown (1955) found that prematurity was more frequent among mongol infants. A mean birthweight of 6·38 lb. for 103 mongols was lower than that of 7·10 lb. for the 4,931 controls. The former figure is similar to that arrived at in our present analysis of the group with normal hearts, but a mean birthweight of 7·11 lb. is found in our congenital heart defect group, which is higher than that of their controls.

Taussig (1947), in her chapter on transposition of the great vessels, mentioned that non-mongol infants so affected may have a normal weight curve at birth. In our series this anomaly was not seen. In the present series vessel anomalies were suggested in four cases, for instance, Case 1 in Table 2 had a persistent left superior vena cava, the birthweight being 9 lb. Case 10 had an over-riding of the great vessels combined with other anomalies, the birthweight being 6·8 lb. In Table 3 Case a.4 had a persistent left superior vena cava combined with ostium secundum, the birthweight being 5·6 lb., and in Case a.8 there was a persistence of the sinus venosus combined with a ventricular septal defect, the birthweight being 6·8 lb. These give a mean birthweight of 7·05 lb.

The large percentage of higher birthweights in the congenital heart defect group needs further explanation. Birthweight in general offers significant and valuable information regarding viability and subsequent growth and development. Obviously there are many factors operating in prenatal growth : heredity, maternal health, unusual intrauterine environment, order of birth, etc., may all play some part.

In the present series, a higher birthweight is noted in the mongols with congenital heart defect than in those without. Although the number of cases is small, the high birthweight in both clinical and autopsy groups is significant. As Taussig has said, certain types of congenital heart defect may not affect the intrauterine circulation and consequently play no part in foetal growth. The high birthweight in the congenital heart defect group raises the possibility that the cardiac anomaly may be favourable to foetal growth, but, on the other hand, the increased birthweight may be related to some degree of tissue oedema due to circulatory disturbance. Unfortunately, no studies of subsequent development and rate of growth of the neonatal period have yet been made in this group of patients, so the usual causes of high birthweight cannot be excluded and this highly interesting and controversial finding cannot adequately or satisfactorily be explained.

Davenport and Allen (1925) found a tendency for mongolism to occur in later pregnancies, and in Lahdensuu's (1937) series 28·3% were first-born. Our series shows that there is a slight suggestion of later birth rank in the clinical congenital heart defect group, but among the autopsied cases the birth rank is slightly higher in the group without congenital heart defects. On the other hand, of the 27 cases in the congenital heart defect group, five or 18·5% were first-born, and in the control groups (11 clinical controls and 22 autopsy cases with normal hearts) six or 18·2% were first-born. The difference between these two groups is too small for statistical assessment, but it seems reasonable to conclude that there is no evidence of a higher birth rank for mongols with congenital heart disease than for those without.

Table 6 summarizes the different cardiac abnormalities occurring in 27 mongols, but owing to the incidence of multiple lesions in some cases there were 42 defects.

TABLE 6

TYPES OF CONGENITAL CARDIAC DEFECTS FOUND IN 27 MONGOLS

Types of Congenital Cardiac Anomalies	Clinical Group	Autopsy Group	Total No. of Lesions (No.)	(%)
Ventricular septal defect	6	4	10	24
Atrial septal defect	4	4	8	19
Patent ductus arteriosus	1	6	7	17
Vessel anomalies	2	2	4	9
Pulmonary stenosis	3		3	7
Atrioventricularis communis	1	2	3	7
Fallot's tetralogy		2	2	5
Valvular anomalies		2	2	5
Eisenmenger's syndrome	2		2	5
Idiopathic pulmonary hypertension	1		1	2
Total			42	100

The result of the present survey agrees with Leech's (1935) observation that persistent atrioventricularis communis is not the most common cardiac anomaly in mongolism in the age ranges studied, and supports Evans' finding that ventricular septal defect is the most common, atrial septal defect the second, and patent ductus arteriosus the third in frequency. Others, such as vessel anomalies, pulmonary stenosis, atrioventricularis communis, Eisenmenger's syndrome and Fallot's tetralogy, etc. are less common.

Summary

Congenital heart disease has been studied in a group of 173 mongoloid imbeciles admitted to the Fountain Hospital during a period of 14 years. Fifty-one died and autopsies were performed on 44 of them (mean age 3·3 years), 36·4% (16/44) showing congenital heart defects. Of the 122 patients still in hospital (mean age 10 years), 9% (11/122) have proved to have congenital heart defects.

The high proportion of maternal illness in the congenital heart defect group suggests that maternal health during pregnancy may have a direct bearing on the heart malformation.

No difference was found in parental age and birth rank between the groups with and without congenital heart defect.

Higher birthweights and no prematurity were found in the mongols with congenital heart disease.

Congenital heart defect has no influence on the I.Q.

Ventricular and atrial septal defects are the commonest congenital heart anomalies in mongolism.

We wish to express our thanks to the Physician Superintendent and the Director of the Research Committee of the Fountain Hospital for their permission to undertake this study, and to Dr. A. Leatham and his colleagues in the Cardiac Department of St. George's Hospital for all their help. Our thanks are due also to our Pathology Department for allowing us free use of their autopsy material and notes, to all our colleagues for their constant encouragement and helpful criticism, and to the Medical Records Department for their cordial co-operation.

REFERENCES

Abbott, M. E. (1936). *Atlas of Congenital Cardiac Disease.* American Heart Association, New York.
Benda, C. E. (1946). *Mongolism and Cretinism.* Grune and Stratton, New York.
Bleyer, A. (1938). *Amer. J. Dis. Child.*, **55**, 79.
Davenport, C. B. and Allen, G. (1925). *J. Psycho-Asthenics.*, **29**, 266.
Engler, M. (1949). *Mongolism*, p. 48. Wright, Bristol.
Esen, F. M. (1957). *Arch. Pediat.*, **74**, 243.
Evans, P. R. (1950). *Brit. Heart J.*, **12**, 258.
Gregg, N. M. (1941). *Trans. ophthal. Soc. Aust.*, **3**, 35.
Ingalls, T. H. (1947). *Amer. J. Dis. Child.*, **73**, 279.
——, Babbott, J. and Philbrook, R. (1957). *Amer. J. Obstet. Gynec.*, **74**, 572.
Jenkins, R. L. (1933). *Amer. J. Dis. Child.*, **45**, 506.
Keith, J. D., Rowe, R. D. and Vlad, P. (1958). *Heart Disease in Infancy and Childhood.* The MacMillan Co., London.
Lahdensuu, S. (1937). *Acta paediat. (Stockh.)*, **21**, 256.
Leech, C. B. (1935). *J. Pediat.*, **7**, 802.
Mossberger, J. I. (1949). *Amer. J. Dis. Child.*, **78**, 28.
Penrose, L. S. (1934). *Proc. roy. Soc. B.*, **115**, 431.
Smith, A. and McKeown, T. (1955). *Archives of Disease in Childhood*, **30**, 257.
Southwick, W. E. (1939). *Amer. J. Dis. Child.*, **57**, 68.
Swan, C., Tostevin, A. L., Moore, B., Mayo, H., and Black, G. H. B. (1943). *Med. J. Aust.*, **2**, 201.
Taussig, H. B. (1947). *Congenital Malformation of the Heart.* Oxford University Press.

THE ELECTRICAL CONDUCTIVITY OF ELECTROLYTES FOUND IN THE SWEAT OF PATIENTS WITH FIBROCYSTIC DISEASE OF THE PANCREAS

BY

ALLAN BLOXSOM

From the University of Texas Postgraduate School of Medicine, Houston, Texas

(RECEIVED FOR PUBLICATION MARCH 31, 1959)

A search of the available medical literature reveals no study of the electrical conductivity relative to NaCl of the electrolytes found in the sweat of patients with fibrocystic disease of the pancreas.

Methods of Study

Simultaneous chemical and electrical conductivity studies have been done on the blood serum and sweat of five children with proven fibrocystic disease of the pancreas. The electrical conductivity tests were made by means of a modified Wheatstone bridge previously described (Bloxsom, 1959). These electrical conductivities in equivalent mEq./l. of sodium chloride, together with the chemical analyses of the serum and sweat, are compared with the normal (Table 1).

Comment

The electrolytes in sweat are sodium, chloride, potassium and lactic acid, with sodium chloride being the major constituent (Best and Taylor, 1950). The electrical conductivities of the electrolytes present in sweat vary considerably, and in this study ranged from 15 to 60 mEq./l. solutions of sodium chloride in the normal children. In the patients with fibrocystic disease of the pancreas the electrical conductivities ranged from 80 to 150 mEq./l. solutions of sodium chloride. The electrical conductivities of normal and abnormal sweat parallel closely the electrolyte content.

Lundgren, Ramanathan, Sen Gupta and Chakravarti (1955) report that, in 25 samples of sweat obtained from 12 normal subjects, the chloride con-

TABLE 1

ELECTROLYTE CONDUCTIVITIES OF NORMAL SWEAT AND ABNORMAL SWEAT (FIBROCYSTIC DISEASE OF THE PANCREAS)

Patient	Chemical Values in mEq./l.				Electrical Conductivity in Equivalent mEq./l. NaCl Sweat
	Blood Serum		Sweat		
	Na	Cl	Na	Cl	
Normal:					
Hill	169		48	45	60
Hill	165	109	13	31	45
Shepherd	144	101	28	14	20
Shepherd	146	102	28	15	20
Radcliffe	144	121	31	24	38
Poinflick	154	112	15	7	15
Loekin			17	15	20
Gibson	144	110	10	10	16
Herde	146	110	26	19	25
Lee	148	107	37	32	35
Wagner	146	103	75	56	55
Mattfield	141	112	40	37	37
		Mean	31	25	32
Fibrocystic Disease of the Pancreas:					
Marsh	144	112	91	105	80
Hill	144	110	110	100	100
Williams	144	105	100	142	120
Lundgren	144		144	137	150
Emde	139	112	108	117	120
		Mean	130	120	114

centration varied from 8 to 80 mEq./l., with the majority of readings between 25 and 40 mEq./l. and an average of 35·9 mEq./l., these readings being made on a modified Philips conductivity bridge, model GM 4249. These investigators state that the procedure for determination of the specific conductivity of small amounts of sweat was found to give results which correlated with the chloride concentration ($r = 0{\cdot}90$) and the sodium concentration ($r = 0{\cdot}78$). They conclude that the electrical conductivity method can therefore be used for estimation of the concentration of sodium chloride which is the major electrolyte in sweat. The main requirements in determining electrical conductivity are that such a procedure is simple and rapid, can be applied to minute volumes of sweat (less than $\frac{1}{6}$ ml. (Lundgren *et al.*, 1955)) and is relatively free of error.

In this study there was no overlapping of the electrical conductivities of normal and abnormal sweat. The determination of the electrical conductivity of sweat is a simple, rapid laboratory procedure, relatively free of error.

Summary

Electrical conductivities of normal and abnormal sweat, expressed relative to standard solutions of NaCl, parallel the concentrations of the electrolytes present and their determination constitutes a quick, simple and inexpensive, error-free laboratory procedure that can be used in the study of fibrocystic disease of the pancreas.

References

Best, C. H. and Taylor, N. B. (1950). *The Physiological Basis of Medical Practice*, 5th ed., pp. 494-495. Williams and Wilkins Co , Baltimore.

Bloxsom, A. P. (1959). *J. Lab. clin. Med.*, **54**, 136.

Lundgren, Nils P. V., Ramanathan, N. L., Sen Gupta, A. and Chakravarti, H. S. (1955) *Indian J. med. Res.*, **43**, 157.

THE RELATIONSHIP BETWEEN DECREASED 5-HYDROXYINDOLE METABOLISM AND MENTAL DEFECT IN PHENYLKETONURIA

BY

C. M. B. PARE, M. SANDLER* and R. S. STACEY

From the Bethlem Royal and Maudsley Hospitals, the Royal Free Hospital and St. Thomas's Hospital, London

(RECEIVED FOR PUBLICATION APRIL 15, 1959)

In 1957 we demonstrated a defect of 5-hydroxyindole metabolism in 10 patients with phenylketonuria and suggested that, in view of the probable importance of 5-hydroxytryptamine (5HT) in normal brain function, this deficiency might be a factor in the mental defect (Pare, Sandler and Stacey, 1957). In the work described below, the previous findings are extended and the relationship of the 5-hydroxyindole deficiency to the mental defect is examined further.

Methods

In all, 49 patients with phenylketonuria and 32 mental defective controls were seen. All the controls and 26 of the phenylketonurics came from one hospital and these groups were comparable for weight, age and intelligence. The remaining phenylketonurics were drawn from four different hospitals. Tests of intelligence used included the Stanford-Binet (Terman-Merrill revision), the Merrill-Palmer and the Vineland Social Maturity scale. Serum 5HT was estimated on all children with the exception of one control, and urinary 5-hydroxyindoleacetic acid (5HIAA) and creatinine were estimated on early morning specimens of urine from all. Methods used have been described previously (Pare *et al.*, 1957).

Results

5-Hydroxyindole Estimations. The 5-hydroxyindole deficiency in phenylketonuria was confirmed (Fig. 1). The mean value for urinary 5HIAA in 49 phenylketonurics was 2·2 mg./g. creatinine compared with 7·2 mg./g. for 32 mental defective controls. The difference between the two groups is shown by there being only one phenylketonuric with 5HIAA values greater than 4·2 mg./g. creatinine and only two controls with values below this. Similar results were found for serum 5HT, where the mean level in 49 phenylketonurics was 71·2 ng./ml. compared with 283 ng./ml. in 31 controls. Six phenylketonurics had values greater than, and five controls less than, 120 ng./ml.

Relationship between 5-Hydroxyindole Values and Intelligence in Phenylketonurics. This assessment was made on patients in one hospital to exclude inter-hospital variability in estimation of intelligence and possible dietary or other effects acting on 5-hydroxyindole metabolism. As the estimation of intelligence in low-grade defectives can only be approximate, a straightforward product-moment correlation could not reasonably be applied. Instead, patients were grouped into three categories with respect to intelligence, and the mean values for age, 5HT and 5HIAA estimated for each group (Table 1). This showed there was no significant association between intelligence and either 5HT or 5HIAA.

TABLE 1

MEAN VALUES FOR AGE (YEARS), 5-HYDROXYTRYPTAMINE (5HT) (NG./ML.) AND 5-HYDROXYINDOLEACETIC ACID (5HIAA) (MG./G. CREATININE) IN 26 PHENYLKETONURICS GROUPED ACCORDING TO INTELLIGENCE (I.Q.)

I.Q.	Patients (No.)	Age	Serum 5HT	Urinary 5HIAA
<20	16	13·5±1·7	79·5±12·9	2·48±0·24
20–34	7	4·3±0·9	76·0±20·3	2·79±0·50
>34	3	3·9±1·6	83·0±34·4	2·53±0·66
>20	10	4·2±0·8	78·1±16·5	2·71±0·39
Total	26	9·9±1·4	79·0±9·9	2·57±0·23

Relationship between Age, 5HT and 5HIAA in Phenylketonurics and Other Mental Defectives. The product-moment correlation coefficient was computed for the following in both phenylketonurics and

* Present address: Queen Charlotte's Maternity Hospital, London, W.6.

mental defective controls: age with 5HIAA, age with 5HT and 5HT with 5HIAA (Table 2). In both groups of patients there was a small negative correlation between age and 5HIAA. There was no correlation between age and 5HT but a small positive correlation between 5HT and 5HIAA.

TABLE 2

CORRELATION BETWEEN AGE–5HIAA, AGE–5HT, AND 5HT–5HIAA IN 26 PHENYLKETONURICS AND 32 MENTAL DEFECTIVE CONTROLS

Diagnosis	Variables	Cases (No.)	'r'
Phenylketonuria ..	Age–5HIAA	26	−0·18
Controls	Age–5HIAA	32	−0·33
Phenylketonuria ..	Age–5HT	26	+0·01
Controls	Age–5HT	31	−0·10
Phenylketonuria ..	5HT–5HIAA	26	+0·14
Controls	5HT–5HIAA	31	+0·40

Abnormality of 5-Hydroxyindole Metabolism in Non-phenylketonuric Mental Defectives. The variability of 5HIAA and 5HT values in normal children is not completely known. It will be seen from Fig. 1 that some of the patients had values for serum 5HT which were as high as those found in patients with the carcinoid syndrome. Many have been repeatedly examined over a period of two to three years and remain consistently high. These children, who present certain interesting features, have been further investigated and form the subject of a separate communication (Pare, Sandler and Stacey, 1959).

Discussion

The small negative correlation between age and 5HIAA excretion was to be expected, for 5HIAA was estimated as mg./g. creatinine and the excretion of creatinine/kg. body weight increases with age (Harding and Gaebler, 1922).

The small correlation only between 5HT and 5HIAA should not occasion surprise; for although 5HIAA is the major metabolite of 5HT, 5HT follows other metabolic pathways (Chadwick and Wilkinson, 1958; McIsaac and Page, 1958; Weissbach, Redfield and Udenfriend, 1958). Likewise, some 5HIAA may be derived from other sources. The concentration of 5HT in serum is almost wholly a measure of platelet-bound 5HT (Hardisty and

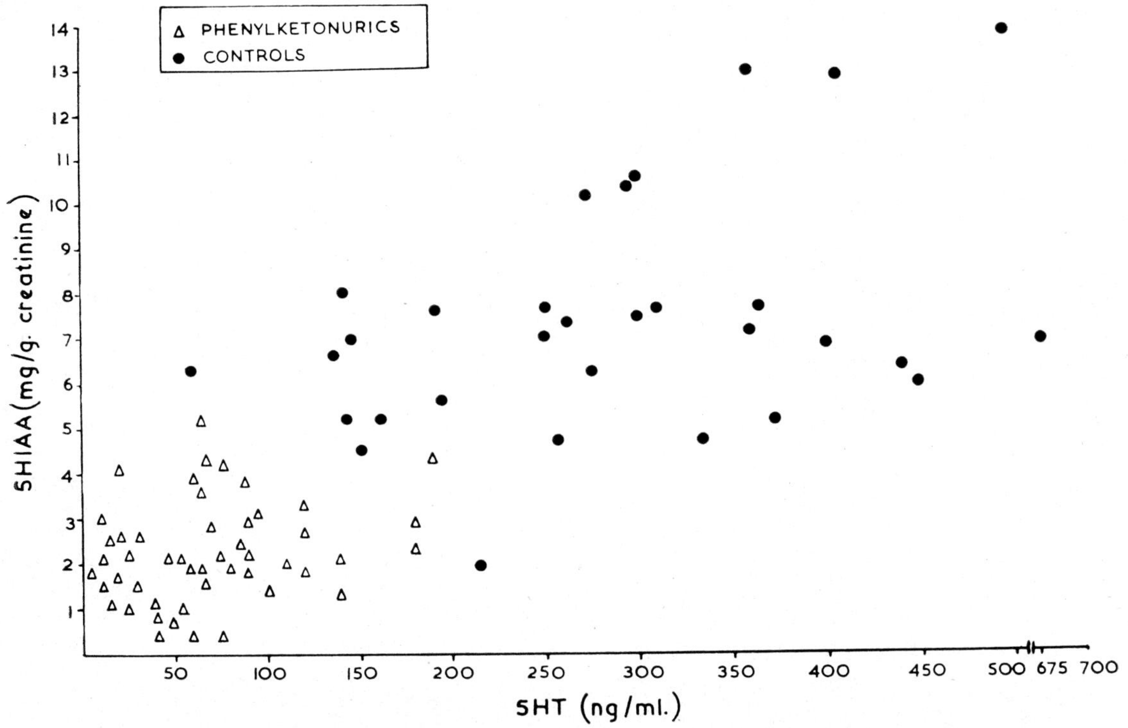

FIG. 1.—Serum 5-hydroxytryptamine (5HT) (ng./ml.) and urinary 5-hydroxyindoleacetic acid (5HIAA) (mg./g. creatinine) values in 49 phenylketonurics and 31 non-phenylketonuric mentally defective controls.

Stacey, 1955). Levels will depend on the number of circulating platelets and their ability to take up 5HT which in turn varies with platelet adenosine triphosphate concentration (Born, Ingram and Stacey, 1958).

Relationship between 5-Hydroxyindole Deficiency and the Mental Defect. We have been able to confirm our previous finding (Pare *et al.*, 1957) of decreased 5-hydroxyindole production in a considerably augmented series. One of the reasons for starting this investigation was the possibility that the defect in hydroxylation of phenylalanine to tyrosine, which is known to be the primary fault in phenylketonuria, might be associated with a similarly abnormal hydroxylation of tryptophan. Little is known of the latter reaction and its further investigation is hampered, as the site in mammals of an enzyme able to carry it out has not yet been demonstrated. Recent work has indicated, however, that some aromatic acid metabolites of phenylalanine, produced in large quantities in phenylketonuria, are able to depress the synthesis of 5HT. Davison and Sandler (1958) have shown, by *in vitro* studies, that phenylpyruvic acid, phenylacetic acid and phenyllactic acid inhibit 5-hydroxytryptophan (5HTP) decarboxylase, the enzyme responsible for the production of 5HT from its precursor 5HTP, and evidence has also accrued to indicate that at least phenylacetic acid has a similar action *in vivo* (Davison, Ruthven and Sandler, 1959; Sandler and Close, 1959; Sandler, Davies and Rimington, 1959). The finding of a decreased 5HTP decarboxylase activity in phenylketonuria by Pare, Sandler and Stacey (1958) must probably be interpreted then as a result of inhibition of this enzyme by aromatic acid metabolites of phenylalanine, and decarboxylase inhibition now seems a likely cause of the abnormal 5-hydroxyindole metabolism reported above. The situation, however, is still by no means clear.

5HTP decarboxylase is not the only enzyme system so affected by these phenylalanine metabolites. Fellman (1956) has shown that DOPA decarboxylase, which may be identical with 5HTP decarboxylase (Westermann, Balzer and Knell, 1958) and is essential in the synthesis of catechol amines, is similarly inhibited, and data suggesting that this might happen *in vivo* are also to be found. Thus, Weil-Malherbe (1955) has demonstrated a deficiency of a substance with the biochemical characteristics of adrenaline in platelets from phenylketonurics; Cawte (1954, 1957) has described an abnormal sensitivity to adrenaline in these patients, and Armstrong (1958) has found a decreased output of 3-methoxy-4-hydroxymandelic acid, the major metabolite of adrenaline and noradrenaline (Armstrong, McMillan and Shaw, 1957), in a small number of affected children he investigated. It is likely that catechol amines play as important a part in the normal functions of the central nervous system as 5HT.

Another biologically active amine which is likely to prove of great importance in brain physiology is γ-aminobutyric acid (Elliott, 1958). It is of interest that the enzyme responsible for its formation, glutamic acid decarboxylase, may also be inhibited *in vitro* by this group of aromatic acid metabolites of phenylalanine (Hanson, 1958).

Viewed in this light, it is possible that there is a multiple deficiency in phenylketonuria. If so, it is hardly surprising that we failed to demonstrate any correlation between the degree of 5-hydroxyindole deficiency and I.Q. Nor is it to be wondered at that Kirman, Pare, Sandler and Stacey (1958) were unable to show any improvement in I.Q. during a controlled trial of 5HTP in affected children. If a decreased brain concentration of biologically active amines, singly or in combination, is responsible in some degree for the mental defect in phenylketonuria, then any method of increasing their total concentration in the brain might provide a rational therapy. This can probably be achieved by treating affected children with iproniazid, which inhibits monoamine oxidase, the enzyme responsible for much of the further metabolism of biologically active monoamines (Blaschko, 1952; Davison, 1958). We are carrying out such a trial at present (Kirman, Pare, Sandler and Stacey, 1959).

Summary

The low serum 5-hydroxytryptamine and urinary 5-hydroxyindoleacetic acid previously reported in phenylketonuria has been confirmed in a larger series. There was no relationship between 5-hydroxyindole levels and intelligence.

We are grateful to Dr. F. H. Corbitt of Stallington Hall Hospital, Dr. B. H. Kirman of the Fountain Hospital, Dr. A. Shapiro of Harperbury Hospital and Dr. D. H. H. Thomas of Cell Barnes Hospital for their kind co-operation and for allowing us access to their patients; to Miss Lilith Emslie and Miss Doreen Crabtree of the Royal Free Hospital for skilled technical assistance, and to the Royal Free Hospital Endowment Fund and Roche Products Limited for defraying their respective salaries.

References

Armstrong, M. D. (1958). Personal communication.
——, McMillan, A. and Shaw, K. N. F. (1957). *Biochim. biophys. Acta*, **25**, 422.
Blaschko, H. (1952). *Pharmacol. Rev.*, **4**, 415.
Born, G. V. R., Ingram, G. I. C. and Stacey, R. S. (1958). *Brit. J. Pharmacol.*, **13**, 62.
Cawte, J. E. (1954). *Med. J. Aust.*, **2**, 15.
—— (1957). *J. ment. Defic. Res.*, **1**, 111.

Chadwick, B. T. and Wilkinson, J. H. (1958). *Biochem. J.*, **68**, 1P.
Davison, A. N. (1958). *Physiol. Rev.*, **38**, 729.
——, Ruthven, C. R. J. and Sandler, M. (1959). In preparation.
—— and Sandler, M. (1958). *Nature* (*Lond.*), **181**, 186.
Elliott, K. A. C. (1958). *Rev. canad. Biol.*, **17**, 367.
Fellman, J. H. (1956). *Proc. Soc. exp. Biol.* (*N.Y.*), **93**, 413.
Hanson, A. (1958). *Naturwissenschaften*, **45**, 423.
Harding, V. J. and Gaebler, O. H. (1922). *J. biol. Chem.*, **54**, 579.
Hardisty, R. M. and Stacey, R. S. (1955). *J. Physiol.* (*Lond.*), **130**, 711.
Kirman, B. H., Pare, C. M. B., Sandler, M. and Stacey, R. S. (1958). Proceedings of the First International Meeting of Neuropsychopharmacology, Rome. In the press.
——, ——, ——, —— (1959). To be published.
McIsaac, W. M. and Page, I. H. (1958). *Science*, **128**, 537.
Pare, C. M. B., Sandler, M. and Stacey, R. S. (1957). *Lancet*, **1**, 551.
——, ——, —— (1958). *Ibid.*, **2**, 1099.
——, ——, —— (1959). In preparation.
Sandler, M. and Close, H. G. (1959). *Lancet*, **2**, 316.
——, Davies, A. and Rimington, C. (1959). *Lancet*, **2**, 318.
Weil-Malherbe, H. (1955). *J. ment. Sci.*, **101**, 733.
Weissbach, H., Redfield, B. G. and Udenfriend, S. (1958). *Fed. Proc.*, **17**, 418.
Westermann, E., Balzer, H. and Knell, J. (1958). *Arch. exp. Path. Pharmakol.*, **234**, 194.

HONEYCOMB LUNGS WITH PERICHOLANGITIS

BY

S. SIVANESAN

From the Department of Pathology, University of Malaya, Singapore

(RECEIVED FOR PUBLICATION APRIL 3, 1959)

Cystic lungs are diverse both morphologically and aetiologically. One form of cystic lungs characterized by multiple air-containing thin-walled cysts, having a maximum diameter of 1 cm., scattered more or less uniformly throughout both lungs, was described by Fowler and Godlee (1898) as 'honeycomb' or 'worm-eaten' in appearance.

Honeycomb lungs have been found only in association with other disorders (Heppleston, 1956). These may take the form of granulomata such as eosinophilic granuloma, tuberose sclerosis (Oswald and Parkinson, 1949), tuberculosis, sarcoidosis (Heppleston, 1956) and pericholangitis or allied hepatic disorders.

This disease occurred especially in children (Sharkey, 1894; Tooth, 1897; Fletcher, 1901; Bernstein, 1905). Were it not for the confusing terminology in the literature, such as foetal bronchiectasis (Sandoz, 1907), congenital bronchiectasis, congenital cyst formation of lung (Koontz, 1925), alveolar cystic disease and cystic emphysema (Willis and Almeyda, 1943; Paliard, Plauchu, Galy and Papillon, 1946), this condition might well have been reported more often under the name of honeycomb lungs.

A case of honeycomb lungs with pericholangitis is presented here.

Case History

A 2-year-old Chinese boy was admitted to the paediatric unit of the General Hospital, Singapore, with dyspnoea, cough, sweating and fits. He was apparently well till the evening before the day of admission, when the parents noticed difficulty in breathing, a slight cough and sweating. At noon on the day of admission the child began to have fits.

He was the seventh child of normal parents, the siblings being normal and well. Birth was normal, the patient then weighing 7½ lb. Mental and physical growth were normal.

On examination the patient was having fits. The eyes were rolling upwards and there was frothing at the mouth. He had a temperature of 103° F. and had generally been very toxic with dyspnoea and cyanosis. The throat was injected, and the tongue dry and coated. The trachea was central, respiratory rhythm was normal and on auscultation harsh breath sounds were heard. The pulse rate was 130 per minute, and no abnormality was detected in the cardiovascular system. The liver was three fingerbreadths palpable below the right costal margin. The spleen and lymph nodes were not palpable. There were no abnormalities detectable in the central nervous system or skeletal system. The child died within one hour of admission.

Autopsy. The body was that of a cyanosed, undernourished Chinese boy. There were no external deformities.

The trachea and bronchi contained a fair amount of frothy fluid. Both lungs were fully expanded. There were no pleural adhesions nor exudate. The surface of both lungs was studded with numerous cysts varying from 0·1 cm. or less to 1·0 cm. (Fig. 1). The larger cysts had thin transparent walls and were raised above the general surface of the lungs while others were within the substance of the lungs. A group of confluent cysts was conspicuous at the apical segment of the right lower lobe. Cysts were also seen in both lungs on all aspects of the visceral pleura. The right interlobular fissure dividing the apex and mid-lobe was deficient and represented by a fibrous septum.

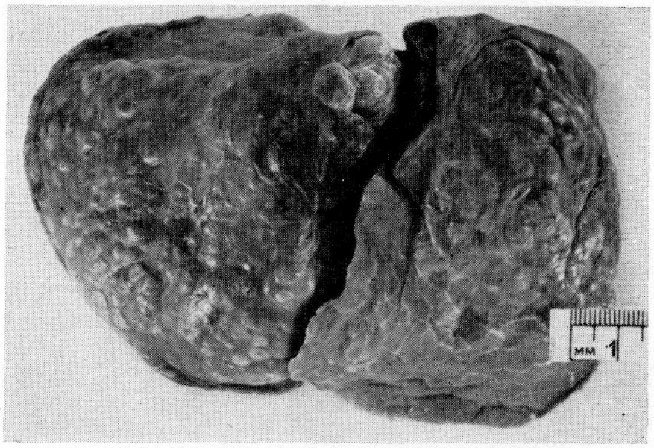

FIG. 1.—P.M. 2034/58. Shows the surface of the right lung studded with numerous cysts.

The cut surface showed the lungs to be studded with cysts scattered diffusely throughout and extending from

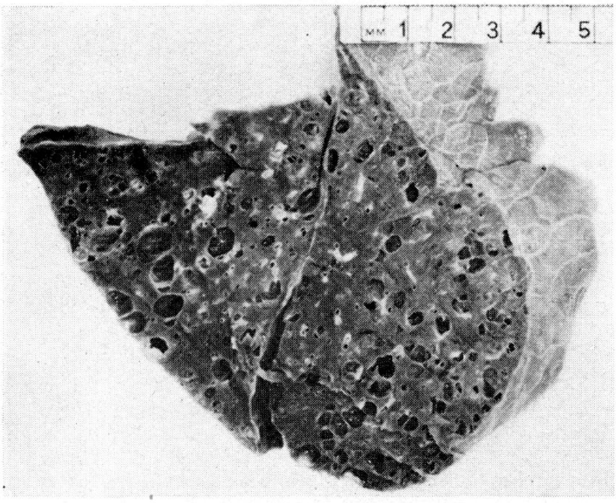

FIG. 2.—P.M. 2034/58. Cut surface of the left lung studded with diffusely scattered cysts.

the hilum to the periphery (Fig. 2), giving them a honeycomb appearance. The cysts varied in size and shape. Most of the cysts had a rounded outline whereas others were polygonal and irregular. They contained air and had a smooth lining. Numerous thin-walled septa protruded into most of the cysts. Some of these septa had pores in them. Some of the cysts were also seen to communicate with other large or smaller ones. The intervening lung tissue was relatively airless and had a fleshy homogeneous appearance.

The liver was enlarged, weighing 570 g. It was firm, had a smooth surface and sharp borders. It was cut with difficulty. The cut surface showed that there were islands of inspissated bile in dilated bile ducts surrounded by a thick dense rim of fibrous tissue (Fig. 3). The intervening parenchyma was apparently normal.

The gall bladder and biliary passages were normal. The pancreas appeared normal. No cysts were seen.

The Peyer's patches were conspicuous, but mesenteric nodes were not enlarged. There was one ascaris worm in the small intestine. The brain was congested. The heart appeared normal in size. There was an oval (5 × 3 mm.) auricular septal defect. The valves were

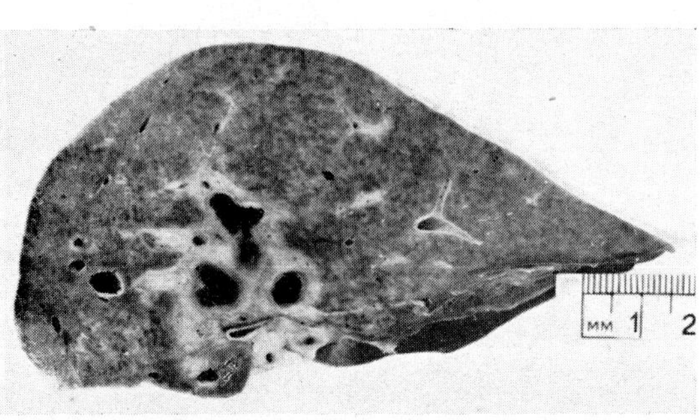

FIG. 3.—P.M. 2034/58. Cut surface of the liver showing islands of inspissated bile surrounded by a thick dense rim of fibrous and granulomatous tissue.

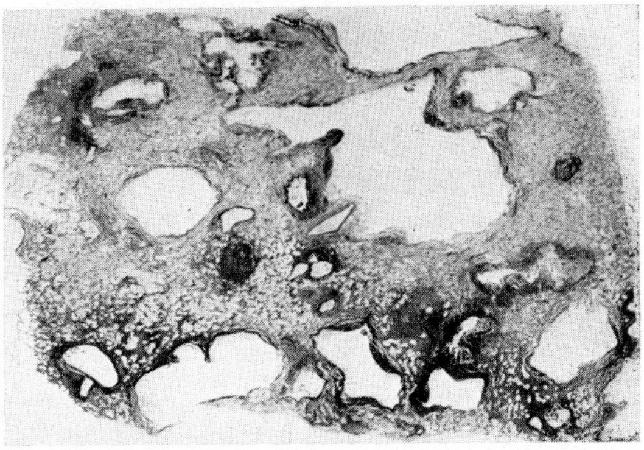

FIG. 4.—P.M. 2034/58. Photomicrograph of cysts and granulomatous tissue. H. and E. × 8.

normal. The spleen, stomach and kidneys appeared normal.

Microscopic Appearances. The only organs to show variations from normal were the lung and liver.

In the lung the most striking features were cysts and granulomatous tissue (Fig. 4). The cysts were of varying size and shape. Larger cysts had a fairly rounded outline and did not communicate freely with other cysts. Smaller cysts had irregular outlines and communicated freely with one another. Thick septal projections were found in some of the cysts. The cysts had no constant lining. Some cysts were partly or wholly lined with granulomatous tissue, others by compressed alveoli and, rarely, flattened epithelium (Fig. 5). No cyst was found to have a complete lining of epithelium.

The distribution of cysts was in close relation to bronchioles and blood vessels (Fig. 6). These included all orders of bronchioles. The larger bronchioles remained discrete, surrounded by several larger and smaller cysts, whilst smaller bronchioles were compressed by the

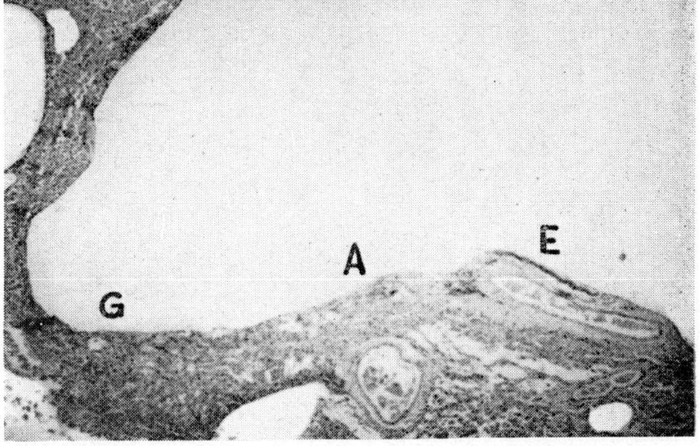

FIG. 5.—P.M. 2034/58. Part of a cyst lined by compressed alveoli (A), granulomatous tissue (G) and epithelium (E). H. and E. × 26.

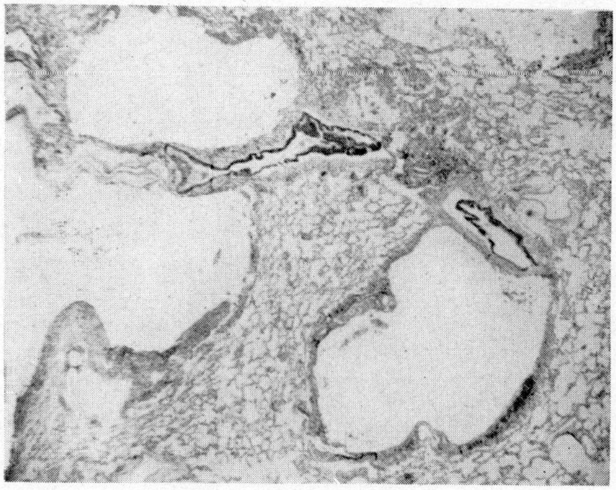

FIG. 6.—P.M. 2034/58. Shows the distribution of cysts to be in close relation to bronchioles and blood vessels H. and E. × 25.

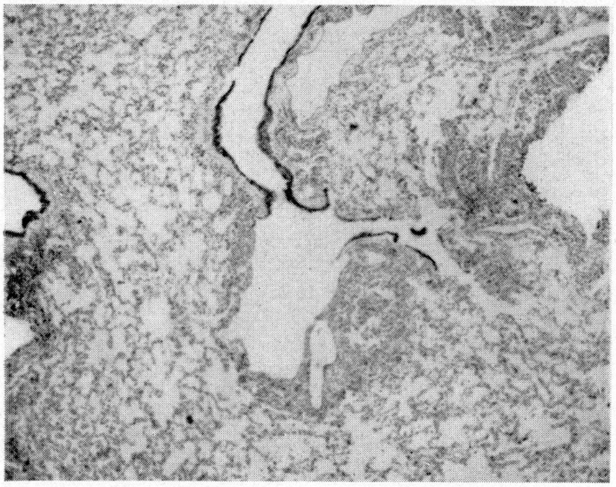

FIG. 7.—P.M. 2034/58. Bronchiole communicating with cyst with bronchiolar epithelium continuing to line part of it. H. and E. × 35.

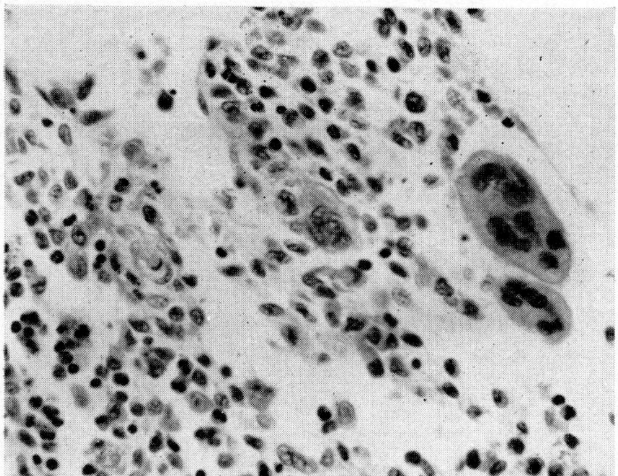

FIG. 8.—P.M. 2034/58. Granulomatous tissue consisting mainly of histiocytes, occasional eosinophils and giant cells. H. and E. × 400.

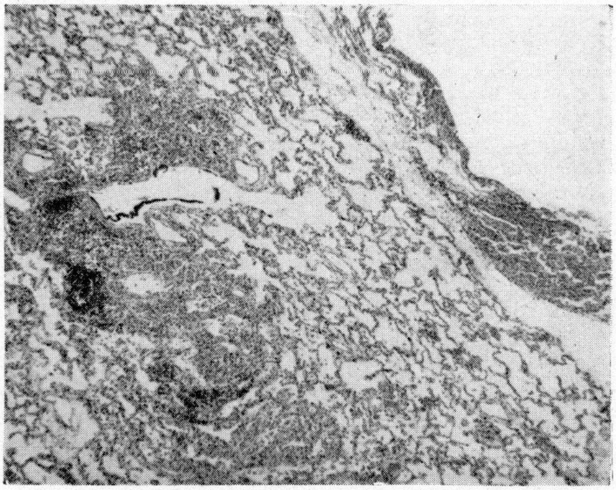

FIG. 9.—P.M. 2034/58. Granulomatous foci in relation to cyst and bronchiole. H. and E. × 35.

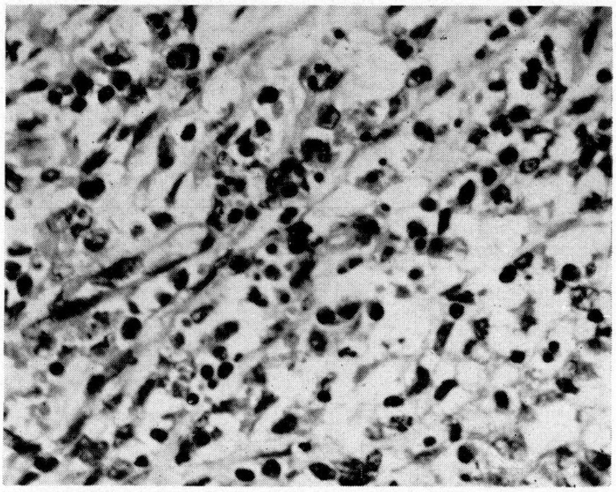

FIG. 10.—P.M. 2034/58. Granulomatous tissue consisting of histiocytes and eosinophils found in relation to bile ducts. H. and E. × 400.

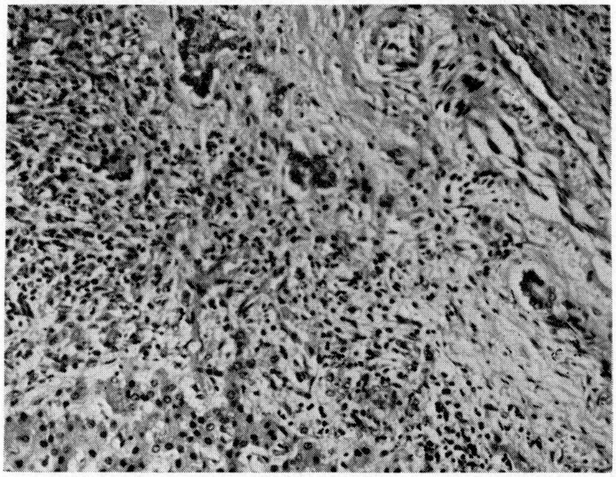

FIG. 11.—P.M. 2034/58. Shows reduplicated bile ducts surrounded by fibrous and granulomatous tissue at the margins of liver lobules. H. and E. × 118.

cysts. Serial sections showed communication between cysts and respiratory bronchioles. Where such communication existed the bronchiolar epithelium continued to line part of the cyst (Fig. 7).

The interstitial tissue in cystic areas showed accumulations of granulomatous tissue. Granulomata, consisting mainly of histiocytes, occasional eosinophils and giant cells (Fig. 8), were found to exist as discrete rounded foci in close relation to cysts and bronchioles sometimes abutting on them (Fig. 9). Granulomatous tissue also formed part or whole of the lining of the cysts.

Non-cystic areas of lung showed normal alveolar tissue. A few patches of early bronchopneumonia were seen. There was no abnormal fibrosis or increase in smooth muscle as shown by Van Gieson and picro-Mallory stains.

The bile ducts contained inspissated bile and were found to be dilated. They were surrounded by a thick rim of granulomatous and fibrous tissue. In some parts these were replaced by scar tissue. There was proliferation of bile ducts in the portal tracts. Granulomatous tissue, consisting mainly of histiocytes and a few eosinophils (Fig. 10), was either found as scattered islands in the fibrous tissue or surrounding some of the bile ducts. The liver parenchyma was unaffected except at the margins of the portal tracts where fibrous tissue and reduplicated bile ducts were found infiltrating margins of the lobules (Fig. 11).

Discussion

The association of honeycomb lungs with pericholangitis is rare. The only other cases in the literature were reported by Fletcher (1901), Bernstein (1905) and Oswald and Parkinson (1949).

The first case reported was a boy, aged 3½ years. Two weeks before admission there was abdominal pain which was followed by breathlessness and cough. On examination the respiratory rate was increased; there were râles and rhonchi over both lungs. The liver was enlarged. He died with extreme dyspnoea five days after admission. At post-mortem examination the lungs had a honeycomb appearance, and the liver was enlarged (weight 600 g.) with cystic dilatation of the bile ducts.

The second case was a girl, aged 3 years, admitted to Westminster Hospital with a history of pain in the back and cough for one month. She was cyanosed, febrile and severely breathless, and she died very soon after admission. Necropsy revealed a right-sided pneumothorax and both lungs had a honeycomb system of cavities throughout. The liver was enlarged (500 g.) and on section yellow nodules the size of a pin's head were seen. Microscopy of the liver showed small round and oval cells surrounding the bile ducts.

The third case in the series was a boy, aged 2 years, admitted with severe dyspnoea, cough and cyanosis. He had clubbing of the fingers, and the percussion note over the chest was hyper-resonant. Rhonchi were present throughout the lungs. During the next two weeks his condition deteriorated and he died from progressive heart failure. At post-mortem examination diffuse cystic changes were found throughout the lungs. The liver was studded with pale nodules. On microscopic examination the cysts were irregular in size and contained varying degrees of epithelial lining, and the liver showed widespread, subacute and chronic inflammation of the mucosa of the large bile ducts with concentric fibrosis. The inflammatory cells were mostly mononuclear.

Earlier discussions on the nature of honeycomb lungs stressed a congenital cause for this condition. This explains terminology such as foetal bronchiectasis, congenital cyst formation of lung, congenital cyst malformation of lung, congenital bronchiectasis and honeycomb lungs, which were all used synonymously (Koontz, 1925). Some of the views put forward to support a congenital basis were faulty development of alveoli from the small end bulbs of the bronchial tree in the embryo (Sandoz, 1907), aplasia of the alveoli (Hueter, 1914) and foetal atelectasis (Adami and Nicholls, 1911).

These explanations suggest that the negative intrapleural pressure, which at birth would cause normal alveoli to expand, exerts its pull on the bronchioles in these cases, leading to the so-called foetal bronchiectasis. It is interesting to note that a congenital heart defect, such as was found in the case described above, is a factor contributing to foetal atelectasis (Sutherland, 1913). To meet the criteria for a congenital origin the cysts should be more than mere distensions of alveoli, such as those found in emphysema. In the case presented, cysts with a partial epithelial lining continuous with that of respiratory bronchioles were seen. This and the fact that cysts were found close to and surrounding the bronchioles suggest a congenital defect of respiratory bronchioles and proximal portions of alveolar ducts which predispose them to cyst formation.

It is becoming increasingly evident that honeycomb lung is a manifestation of many disorders. Heppleston (1956) regards pulmonary fibrosis or granulomata as the usual antecedents of honeycomb lungs. Cunningham and Parkinson (1950) studied in detail nine cases of honeycomb lungs and came to the conclusion that six of these showed varying degrees of a granulomatous process resulting in fibrosis.

In the case described here there was granulomatous tissue consisting predominantly of histiocytes and a few eosinophils in the lungs and the liver. Fibrosis was seen only in the liver. This granulomatous tissue is the result of an inflammatory reaction which may be due to allergy, a chronic infection or even ascariasis.

Cyst formation in the lungs probably resulted from stenosis caused by granulomatous foci abutting on bronchioles and thereby preventing egress of air. Destruction of areas of normal lung by the granulomatous process may lead to distension of the adjacent unaffected alveoli.

Marked periportal fibrosis has been seen in schistosomiasis and to a lesser degree in cases of chronic biliary obstruction. Liver involvement with honeycomb lungs has been reported in eosinophilic granuloma (Rowland, 1928; Farber, 1942; Oswald and Parkinson, 1949). In the present case there were no foam cells and staining of frozen section with Sudan black did not reveal abnormal lipoid content. The histological evidence here suggests that either cholangiectasis with stagnation of bile caused reactionary changes in the portal tracts or that the bile ducts were affected by an inflammatory process with consequent weakening of their walls.

Summary

A case of honeycomb lungs associated with liver lesions is presented.

In this case and in the three cases previously reported the disease occurred in children between 2 and $3\frac{1}{2}$ years of age, with an onset of dyspnoea, cough, bizarre findings in the lungs on auscultation and enlarged liver. At autopsy both lungs showed honeycombing and there was an enlarged liver with pericholangitis.

The nature of the lesion is discussed. It is concluded that in the pathogenesis both congenital and acquired factors are involved.

I wish to thank Professor R. Kirk for his kind encouragement, Dr. K. Shanmugaratnam and Dr. C. S. Muir for their valuable criticisms and Mr. V. Nalpon for the photomicrographs.

References

Adami, J. G. and Nicholls, A. G. (1911). In *The Principles of Pathology*, 2nd ed., Vol. 2. H. Frowde, London.
Bernstein, J. M. (1905). *Trans. path. Soc. Lond.*, **56**, 330.
Cunningham, G. J. and Parkinson, T. (1950). *Thorax*, **5**, 43.
Farber, S. (1942). *New Engl. J. Med.*, **226**, 394.
Fletcher, H. M. (1901). *Trans. path. Soc. Lond.*, **52**, 193.
Fowler, J. K. and Godlee, R. J. (1898). *The Diseases of the Lung*, p. 143. Longmans, Green, London.
Heppleston, A. G. (1956). *Thorax*, **11**, 77.
Hueter, C. (1914). *Beitr. path. Anat.*, **59**, 520.
Koontz, A. R. (1925). *Bull. Johns Hopk. Hosp.*, **37**, 340.
Oswald, N. and Parkinson, T. (1949). *Quart. J. Med.*, **18**, 1.
Paliard, Plauchu, Galy and Papillon, (1946). *Poumon*, **2**, 205.
Rowland, R. S. (1928). *Arch. intern. Med.*, **42**, 611.
Sandoz, E. (1907). *Beitr. path. Anat.*, **41**, 495.
Sharkey, S. J. (1894). *St. Thom. Hosp. Rep.*, **22**, 33.
Sutherland, G. A. (1913). In *Diseases of Children*, ed. by A. E. Garrod, F. E. Batten and H. Thursfield, p. 340. Arnold, London.
Tooth, H. H. (1897). *Trans. path. Soc. Lond.*, **48**, 30.
Willis, F. E. S. and Almeyda, J. (1943). *Tubercle (Lond.)*, **24**, 27.

SPLENIC AGENESIS AND MULTILOBULATE SPLEEN

BY

C. S. MUIR

From the Department of Pathology, University of Malaya, Singapore

(RECEIVED FOR PUBLICATION MARCH 20, 1959)

Agenesis of the spleen has for many years been held to be extremely rare, and of interest only to the morbid anatomist. Since it was shown (Gasser and Willi, 1952; Willi and Gasser, 1955) that diagnosis *in vivo* is possible, interest in the lesion, and in the cardiac anomalies usually found with it, has increased.

This paper records the incidence of splenic agenesis, and of the closely allied condition of multilobulate spleen, in the past 22,500 autopsies performed at the General Hospital, Singapore.

Of these, 520 died with some form of congenital heart disease. In this latter group seven cases of splenic agenesis and one of multilobulate spleen were found. Splenic agenesis without cardiac malformation occurred in one instance: a case of multilobulate spleen associated with hydranencephaly and a normal heart has been reported elsewhere (Muir, 1959) and is not included in this series.

Splenic Agenesis

Case 1. Chinese male, aged 6 weeks. Complaint: cyanosis and diarrhoea. P.M. 731/51. There was dextrocardia, the aortic arch being right-sided. From a biloculate heart a large common trunk arose, the lungs being supplied by a patent ductus arteriosus. There was a congenitally short oesophagus, most of the stomach being intrathoracic. The duodenum and pancreas were situated normally; the liver was central, the gall bladder being found on the right lobe. There was a central mesentery.

Case 2. Chinese male, aged 1 year. Complaint: cyanosis and gangrene of left leg. P.M. 769/52. There was dextrocardia. Both interventricular and interauricular septa were rudimentary. A four-cusped atrioventricular valve was inserted into the apex of the common ventricle. The aortic arch and aorta were left-sided. There was adherent greyish thrombus at the bifurcation of the left common iliac vessel and in the right-sided superior vena cava. Both lungs showed three lobes. The liver was symmetrical. The stomach was left-sided, the mesentery central, the caecum in the left flank, and the descending colon in the right.

Case 3. Chinese female, aged 1 month. Complaint: dyspnoea, cyanosis and refusal of feeds. P.M. 2135/53. The venae cavae opened into the left atrium, the pulmonary veins draining into the superior vena cava as it entered the atrium. There was a large atrio-septal defect, allowing blood to enter the right atrium. The pulmonary artery arose normally from a thick-walled dilated right ventricle. Each lung showed three lobes. A small diaphragmatic hernia contained the fundus of the stomach. Stomach, pancreas and duodenum were transposed.

Case 4. Chinese male, aged 1 month. Complaint: dyspnoea and cyanosis. P.M. 1578/54. There was a single hypertrophied dilated ventricle from which a right-sided aorta arose. The pulmonary artery arose from the same chamber. The ductus arteriosus was widely patent; there was a large atrio-septal defect. The tricuspid valve was larger than normal, the mitral valve showing complete atresia. The right lung showed three lobes, the left six. The liver was transposed as were stomach, pancreas and duodenum.

Case 5. Chinese male, aged 2 months. Complaint: fever. The child was dead on arrival at hospital. P.M. 439/55. There was a biloculate heart, exhibiting a corrected transposition of the great vessels. The liver was symmetrical, the gall bladder being in the left lobe. Stomach, pancreas and duodenum were transposed. There was an abnormally long central mesentery.

Case 6. Chinese female, aged 4 months. Complaint: cough, dyspnoea and cyanosis. P.M. 1332/56. There was a very large ventricular and several small atrio-septal defects. A common truncus arose, over-riding the septal defect and giving off a common pulmonary artery which later divided to supply each lung. Both lungs showed four imperfectly formed lobes and were the seat of a lobar type of pneumonia. There was complete transposition of all the abdominal viscera.

Case 7. Chinese male, aged 18 months. Complaint: cyanosis and fever. P.M. 1877/58. There was a cor triloculare biventriculare. The lungs showed a purulent bronchitis. Apart from absence of the spleen no other intra-abdominal abnormalities were detected.

The first case of splenic agenesis in a child with concomitant cardiac anomalies was recorded by Martin in 1826. At autopsy he found the stomach to be right-sided, the liver to be central, the aorta and pulmonary artery transposed, the left superior vena cava present, and a cor triloculare biatriatum, or, as he remarked, 'the heart of a fish'. By 1952 Polhemus and Schafer were able to collect from the literature 26 cases in infants and 10 in adults, including four infants of their own. They tabulated the defects most commonly found, and noted atrioventricularis communis in 11 of the infants. The adults showed no heart lesions and seemed quite unaffected by the absence of the spleen, one indeed living to her seventy-third year (Sternberg, 1903). Gilbert, Nishimura and Wedum (1958) feel that the spleen has probably been destroyed in those who show no cardiac defects and who die from prolonged chronic infection or neoplasia.

Ivemark (1955) collected 65 cases in children from the world literature and noted that splenic agenesis is usually associated with incomplete fusion of the A-V cushions. Of his cases 61 had some form of cono-truncus lesion, the most common being persistent truncus arteriosus, transposition of the great vessels, pulmonary atresia, cor biloculare and cor triloculare biatriatum. In 33 there was transposition of the stomach, and many showed anomalous lobulation of the lungs.

The most recent review is that of Gilbert *et al.* (1958), who tabulate the morbid findings in 104 adults and children.

The majority of the reported cases with concomitant heart disease have been in persons of white race, although the lesion has been observed in a Chinese (Hu, 1929), a Japanese (Kimura, 1930) and in five Negroes (Shapiro, 1930; Leikin, 1951; Gilbert *et al.*, 1958).

Bush and Ainger (1955) describe with clarity the blood findings in their case. The peripheral blood showed anisocytosis and hypochromia of the red cells. Numerous target cells were present. At the age of 1 year there were 5,000 normoblasts per c.mm. They noted numerous Howell-Jolly bodies. There was a marked increase of resistance to haemolysis by hypotonic saline solutions. The plasma iron was low, the plasma copper high, features characteristic of iron deficiency in infancy (Lahey, Gubler, Cartwright and Wintrobe, 1953). Siderocytes were not present, although the administration of iron resulted in a brisk siderocyte and reticulocyte response; the Howell-Jolly bodies, normoblasts and target cells persisted. They were unable to demonstrate the Heinz bodies that Gasser and Willi (1952, 1955) felt were pathognomonic for the condition. Nihoyannopoulos, Zannos, Oeconomou-Mavrou and Statherou (1956) found normoblasts, target cells and Heinz bodies in the peripheral blood of a 2-month-old Greek girl, but no siderocytes or Howell-Jolly bodies were seen. Gilbert *et al.* (1958) found normoblasts in the peripheral blood of their five cases, but make no mention of Howell-Jolly or Heinz bodies. It appears that the blood picture is not as characteristic as Gasser and Willi (1952) have claimed; rather, it is very like that found after splenectomy. The haemoglobinopathies and haemolytic anaemias must be excluded before the diagnosis is made.

Instances of asplenia with a normal heart are relatively few, Gilbert *et al.* (1958) collecting 28 from the literature. A further case is recorded below.

Case 8. Chinese female, aged 4 years. Complaint: convulsions and fever. On lumbar puncture gram positive diplococci were demonstrated. P.M. 268/59. The heart was normal; the ductus arteriosus was closed. The lungs were congested. The peritoneal cavity contained about 200 ml. of faintly turbid fluid. The mesenteric glands were enlarged and congested. Apart from absence of the spleen there was no other intra-abdominal abnormality. The splenic vessels were present although slightly smaller than normal. The brain was thinly covered, particularly over the vertex, by a greenish-yellow pus from which pneumococci were grown. The middle ears were normal.

King and Shumacker (1952) have drawn attention to the relative frequency of infections generally, and of meningitis in particular, in those who have undergone splenectomy in infancy. Ivemark (1955) found five cases of meningitis in 66 cases of asplenia, including a 9-month-old female child without cardiovascular anomaly.

Multilobulate Spleen

Although agenesis is relatively rare, the association of mutilobulation of the spleen with congenital heart disease is even rarer. The writer has been able to trace only 17 such cases in the literature (Lochte, 1898; Geipel, 1903; Royer and Wilson, 1908; Miller, 1925; Putschar, 1934; Ivemark, 1955; Greenberg, 1957).

In the majority the cardiac abnormalities found were of a much more sophisticated nature than those seen in simple agenesis. Lochte (1898) describes transposition of the great vessels, pulmonary stenosis and transposed A-V valves in a left-sided heart. The tricuspid valve was irregular and malformed, and there were anomalous systemic and venous connections.

In the case of Royer and Wilson (1908) there were five transposed spleens, levocardia, transposition of the great vessels and malformed A-V valves.

Miller (1925) found that in addition to the presence of six small dextroposed spleens, the common iliac and hemiazygos veins passed posteriorly behind the aorta to empty into a very large normally placed azygos vein. The inferior vena cava was represented by a small trunk running from the liver to the right auricle. The left innominate vein did not join the right but passed down to join a much enlarged coronary sinus. The aorta and pulmonary artery were transposed. There was persistence of the common A-V canal. The lungs were atypically lobed and fissured.

Greenberg (1957) found that the four pulmonary veins, the venae cavae and the coronary sinus emptied into a large common atrium, which possessed two distinct auricular appendages. There was a single four-leaflet A-V valve attached to the apex of a common ventricle. The liver was normal. The stomach, pancreas and spleen were transposed. The splenic tissue weighed 6 g. and consisted of 16 lobules held together by delicate bands of connective tissue. In view of the rarity of the lesion the following case is recorded in some detail.

Case 9. C.K.J., an 8-month-old Hokkien Chinese boy was admitted to the General Hospital, Singapore, on September 3, 1958, with five days' history of cough and fever. The tonsils were enlarged and inflamed. There was a diffuse systolic murmur over most of the praecordium. The liver was palpable two and a half fingerbreadths below the right costal margin. Numerous crepitations were heard over both lung bases. A radiograph showed the apex of the heart to be tilted, and the cardiac outline to be enlarged to both left and right of the sternum. The pulmonary vascular markings were prominent.

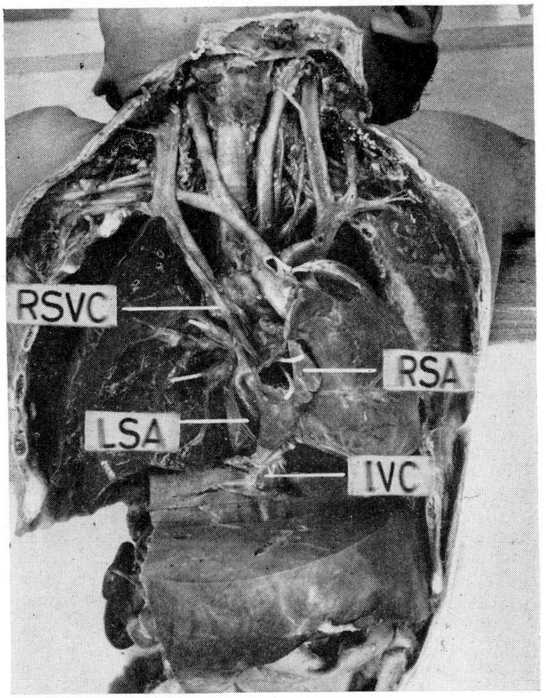

FIG. 2.—The heart has been displaced to the left. The plastic rods are in the two anomalous pulmonary veins which drain into the right-sided atrium. The junction of the right superior vena cava and the left-sided atrium is seen.

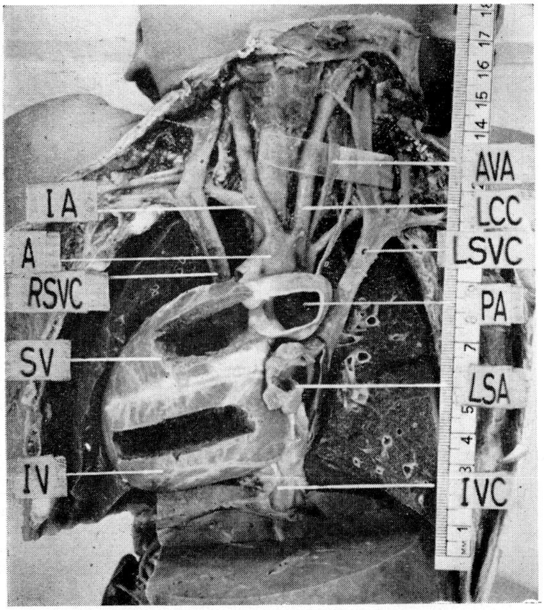

FIG. 1.—Shows the dissected thoracic organs. The symbols used are explained in the text.

The child died three days after admission and an autopsy was performed (P.M. 1767/58). The right testicle was noted to be lower than the left. The heart was enlarged, lay transversely and was, for the most part, in the right side of the chest (Fig. 1).

There were twin superior venae cavae (RSVC and LSVC). That on the left drained into the apex of a left-sided atrium (LSA), receiving, just before doing so, a left-sided vena azygos. Both the myocardium and endocardium of this chamber were thickened. It was larger than usual, measuring 4·0 cm. in the saggital plane and 2·0 cm. in the coronal. At its mid-point posteriorly it received two pulmonary veins from the right lung, and at a comparable point nearer the left lateral border two left pulmonary veins. Lying more medially and above the pulmonary veins was a patent foramen ovale 0·8 cm. in diameter, which was covered in part by a valvular septum. Passing behind the ventricles the RSVC entered the LSA posteriorly at a point midway between the entrance of the pulmonary veins and the junction of the inferior vena cava (IVC) with the LSA (Fig. 2). Anteriorly, between the point of junction of the RSVC and IVC, the coronary sinus drained into the LSA.

Blood flowed from the LSA through a normal tricuspid

valve into a large inferiorly lying ventricle (IV). This chamber was dilated; the wall was 0·9 cm. thick. Blood then passed almost vertically through a large ventricular septal defect 1·7 cm. in diameter to gain a much smaller superiorly placed ventricle (SV) whose wall was 0·8 cm. thick. At the apex of this chamber a muscular septum divided the pulmonary artery (PA) from the posteriorly placed aorta (A).

The right-sided atrium (RSA) was small, lay posteriorly and received two pulmonary veins from the right lung (Fig. 2). Blood left the RSA, which lay anterior to the RSVC, through a normal three-cusped valve to gain the SV.

The PA was dilated, being 2·2 cm. in diameter. The pulmonary valves were normal. There was a small patent ductus arteriosus. The aorta was of normal calibre and was left-sided. A large coronary artery arose behind the posteromedial aortic cusp to pass between the ventricles. A very small coronary artery arose behind the most anterior aortic cusp to pass between the RSA and SV. The aorta gave off four vessels from its arch. From right to left they were: (1) the innominate artery (IA) which divided normally; (2) the left common carotid artery (LCC); (3) an accessory vertebral artery (AVA), which passed posteriorly to lie behind the left internal carotid artery and which disappeared into a foramen of a transverse process at the level of the thyroid cartilage (C4); and, (4) the left subclavian artery which gave off a very small vertebral vessel which entered its vertebral foramen normally at the level of C6. The vertebral artery on the right side was normal.

The lungs were irregularly fissured and both showed two major lobes. The right lung, as noted previously, showed an anomalous distribution of the pulmonary veins and had a well marked cardiac impression.

The stomach, duodenum and pancreas were transposed. The splenic vessels ran normally beyond the tail of the pancreas, breaking up to supply an aggregation of nine splenunculi. These masses of splenic tissue were enveloped in a loose connective tissue network and taken together made up a normal sized spleen (Fig. 3). The individual splenunculi varied in diameter from 2·5 to 0·5 cm. The caecum and appendix were central, being attached by a long central mesentery. The descending colon was on the right side.

It will be apparent from the case recorded above, and the brief descriptions of a few of the other specimens, that the cardiac lesions associated with multilobulate spleen may be very complex. It is worth remembering that portions of tissue which grossly resemble splenunculi may on histological examination prove to be accessory livers (Ivemark, 1955; Cases 9 and 11).

The association of cardiac malformation with splenic anomaly may be explained by the assumption that the teratogenic agent, which affects the developing heart, damages the developing spleen at one and the same time. The splenic primordium has been shown by Ivemark (1955) to appear when the embryo is in Horizons XV-XVII. At this time contact between the dorsal and ventral endocardial cushions has just been established, and separation of the truncus arteriosus into its aortic and pulmonary components is under way, hence the predominance of cono-truncus lesions.

Broman (1921) has shown that late in the third embryonal month a series of notches ('Inscisuren') appear in the splenic primordium. Should the noxious agent strike at this time, an arrest of fusion may occur, the partitioned spleen continuing to grow, making up on aggregate the normal bulk of splenic tissue. Damage to the heart at this time would result in the more complex type of lesion seen with multilobulate spleen. It is probable that multilobulation may occur at an earlier date as Ivemark (1955) found notches in the splenic primordium of an embryo in Horizon XVI, which would correspond to an ovulation age of 32-34 days (Streeter, 1948).

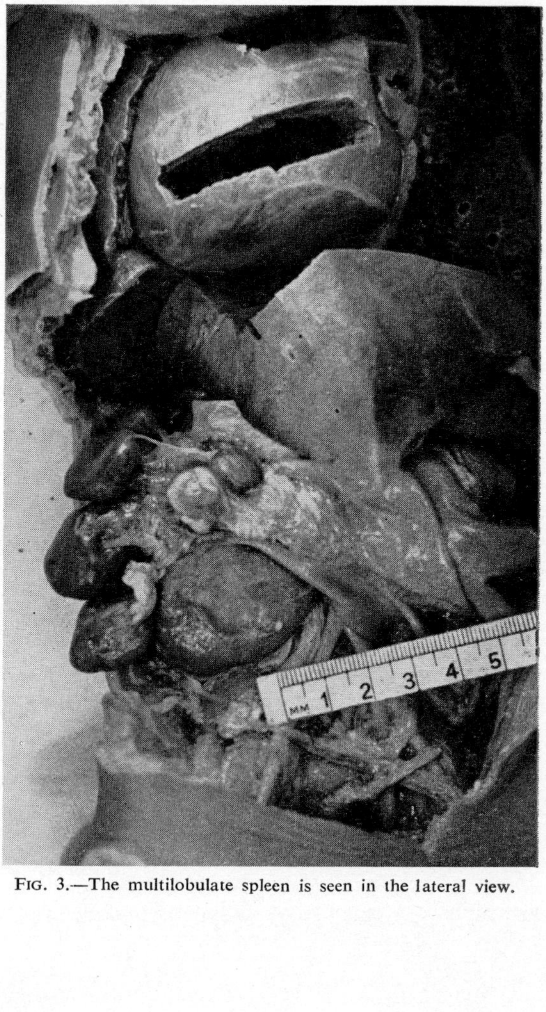

FIG. 3.—The multilobulate spleen is seen in the lateral view.

It may be asked why splenic agenesis should be so rare when congenital heart disease is so common. Gasser and Willi (1952) consider it quite certain that the causative factor is endogenous, a lethal factor with pleiotropic effects. This hypothesis, although difficult to prove, would explain the discrepancy. It may be that the noxious agent which damages the heart destroys a large part of the splenic tissue present. Should none survive, then 'agenesis' would be the end result. However, should a small amount of splenic material survive the initial assault, a rapid increase in the remainder would make good the damage done, as the spleen is known to have excellent regenerative powers.

Summary

Seven cases of splenic agenesis associated with cono-truncus heart lesions, occurring in Chinese children in Singapore, are briefly described.

A single case of asplenia, without cardiac malformation, dying from pneumococcal meningitis, and a case of multilobulate spleen with gross cardiac anomalies are reported.

The embryological significance of the association of congenital heart disease with asplenia. and with multilobulate spleen, is discussed.

I wish to thank Professor R. Kirk for many useful suggestions, Dr. T. Balasingham and Dr. E. B. La'Brooy for access to their autopsy notes and material, Dr. C. Elaine Field of the Paediatric Unit, General Hospital, Singapore, for permission to quote briefly from case records, Mr. V. Nalpon for the photographs, and Mr. P. A. Samuel who typed the script.

References

Broman, I. (1921). Quoted by Ivemark (1955) *loc. cit.*
Bush, J. A. and Ainger, L. E. (1955). *Pediatrics*, **15**, 93.
Gasser, C. and Willi, H. (1952). *Helv. paediat. Acta*, **7**, 369.
Geipel, P. (1903). *Arch. Kinderheilk.*, **35**, 112.
Gilbert, E. F., Nishimura, K. and Wedum, B. G. (1958). *Circulation*, **17**, 72.
Greenberg, S. D. (1957). *A.M.A. Arch. Path.*, **63**, 333.
Hu, C. H. (1929). *Amer. J. Path.*, **5**, 389.
Ivemark, B. I. (1955). *Acta paediat.* (*Uppsala*), **44**, suppl. 104.
Kimura, H. (1930). *Jap. med. World*, **10**, 63.
King, H. and Shumacker, H. B. (1952). *Ann. Surg.*, **136**, 239.
Lahey, M. E., Gubler, C. J., Cartwright, G. E. and Wintrobe, M. M. (1953). *J. clin. Invest.*, **32**, 329.
Leikin, S. L. (1951). *Clin. Proc. Child. Hosp. Wash.*, **7**, 236. Quoted by Bush and Ainger (1955).
Lochte (1898). *Beitr. path. Anat.*, **24**, 187.
Martin, G. (1826). *Bull. Soc. anat. Paris*, **1**, 39.
Miller, A. J. (1925). *Amer. J. Path.*, **1**, 467.
Muir, C. S. (1959). *Archives of Disease in Childhood*, **34**, 231.
Nihoyannopoulos, J., Zannos, L., Oeconomou-Mavrou, C. and Statherou, E. (1956). *J. clin. Path.*, **9**, 323.
Polhemus, D. W. and Schafer, W. B. (1952). *Pediatrics*, **9**, 696.
Putschar, W. (1934). Quoted by Ivemark (1955).
Royer, B. F. and Wilson, J. D. (1908). *Arch. Pediat.*, **25**, 881.
Shapiro, P. F. (1930). *Arch. Path.* (*Chicago*), **9**, 54.
Sternberg, C. (1903). *Virchows Arch. path. Anat.*, **173**, 571.
Streeter, G. L. (1948). *Carnegie Contrib. to Embryol.*, **32**, 133.
Willi, H. and Gasser, C. (1955). *Ét. néonatal.*, **4**, 25.

BIRTH TRAUMA TO THE VERTEBRAL ARTERIES

BY

P. O. YATES

From the Department of Pathology, University of Manchester

(RECEIVED FOR PUBLICATION APRIL 11, 1959)

Birth is a very traumatic event. This is particularly emphasized by the frequency of intracranial haemorrhage and cerebral damage in the newborn infant. However, the greatest manipulative strain in all methods of delivery is imposed on the infant's neck and it is therefore surprising that there have been very few investigations of this region except following breech delivery. Moreover none of the reports records the effects of trauma on the cervical portions of the vertebral arteries, two of the principal vessels supplying the brain. It is the purpose of this paper to draw attention to traumatic lesions in the necks of infants delivered by a variety of methods who died round about the time of birth, and to indicate their possible significance in the production of damage to the brain.

Material and Methods

The infants examined were selected during one year from 213 stillborn and neonatal deaths occurring in 2,800 births. The only cases excluded were malformed foetuses, such as hydrocephalics or anencephalics, and those who, judging by the degree of maceration, had been dead *in utero* before labour started. With these exceptions the necks were removed from 60 foetuses chosen at random and were examined without any knowledge of the findings in the rest of the autopsy or of the method of delivery.

The 60 cases included eight breech deliveries and three by caesarean section. Twenty were more than two weeks premature and eight had Rhesus antibody disease; 16 were stillborn.

The cervical vertebrae were removed intact, usually from C7 to the foramen magnum. Occasionally lower vertebrae were included and the foramen magnum itself. The specimen was fixed in 10% formol saline after which it was placed in 6% nitric acid for 24-48 hours to allow decalcification. It was divided in horizontal planes into five to seven blocks, which were then embedded in paraffin wax. Histological sections stained by a variety of methods were examined from different levels. Occasionally serial sections were examined.

Since it was not possible to examine every joint, ligament or nerve root histologically, the lesions described below must be considered the minimum number present.

Results

Evidence of distortional trauma to the cervical spine was found in 27 cases. The lesions were of three main types: extradural and subdural haemorrhages which lay commonly beneath the ligaments of the arch and were often very extensive (Fig. 1); haemorrhages into joint capsules and synovial villi (Fig. 2); torn ligaments and dura (Fig. 3). These changes were present following all methods of delivery including caesarean section. They were in general most severe after breech delivery.

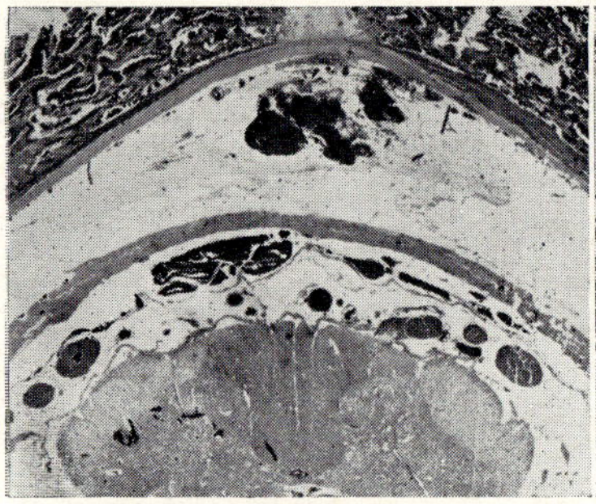

FIG. 1.

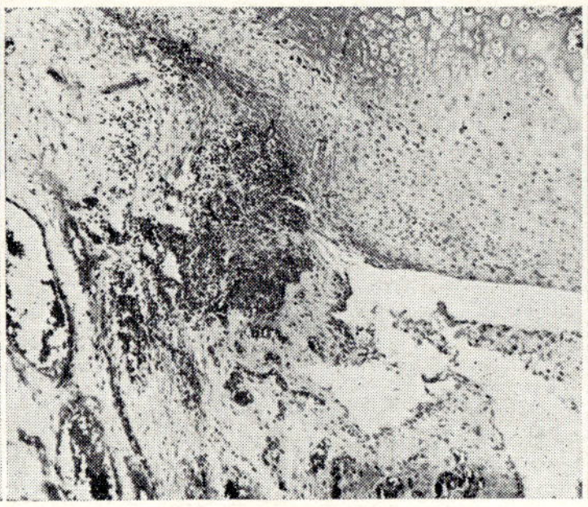

FIG. 2.

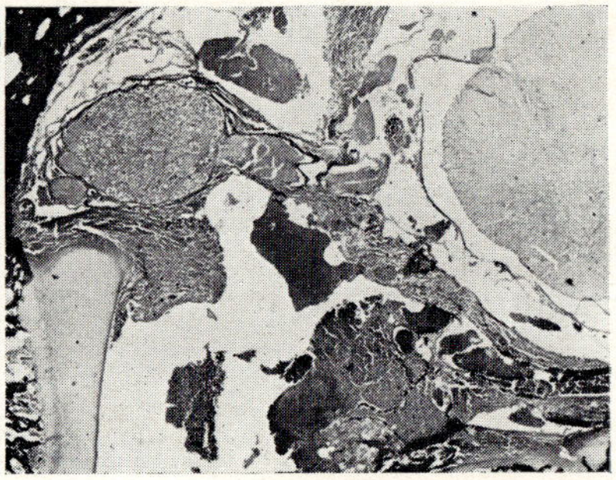

FIG. 3.

FIG. 1.—Transverse section of cervical spine showing subdural haemorrhage and haemorrhage into the tissues beneath the vertebral arch.
FIG. 2.—Joint capsule showing haemorrhage and some tearing. × 20.
FIG. 3.—A disrupted ligament lies beneath the posterior nerve root.

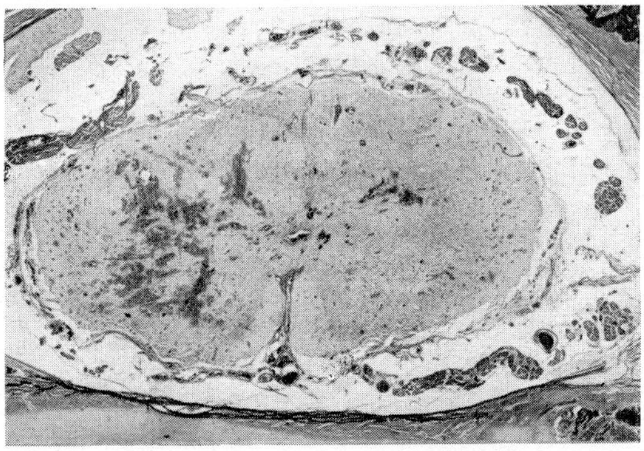

FIG. 4.—Spinal cord showing contusion.

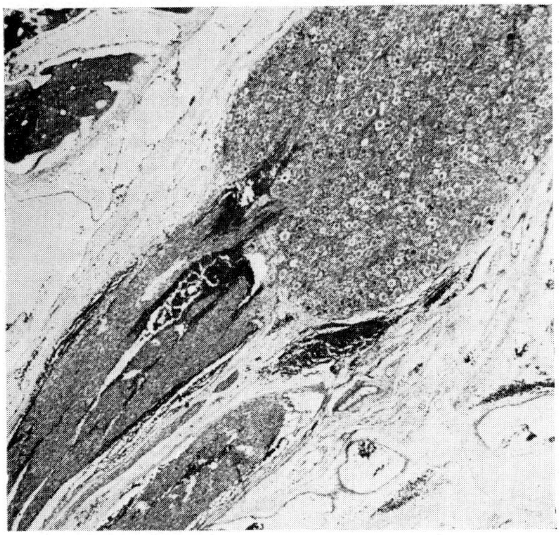

FIG. 5.—The dorsal nerve root has been partially torn as it leaves the posterior root ganglion. × 30.

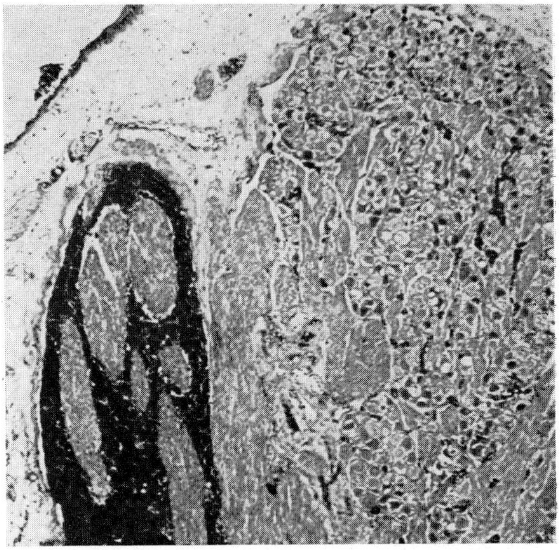

FIG. 6.—Extensive haemorrhage into torn anterior nerve root. × 50.

Direct damage to the spinal cord was not common. In only two cases, both breech deliveries, was there extensive bruising and destruction of the cord (Fig. 4). Occasional haemorrhages of no obvious significance *per se* were found in other cases. On the other hand, bruising and tearing of spinal nerve roots was found in nine cases, the anterior root being slightly more frequently affected than the posterior. In general the nerve roots of one side only were affected (Figs. 5 and 6).

Since the vertebral arteries are of vital importance to the brain, evidence was sought of damage or obstruction to these vessels in their course through the transverse processes of the cervical vertebrae. In 24 cases there were haemorrhages in the adventitial coat of one or both arteries. These varied in size, some small and crescentic, others large and either surrounding the vessel or reducing its lumen by compression from one side (Figs. 7, 8 and 9). They extended for up to 1 cm. along the wall of the vessel. The vertebral artery in its canal is accom-

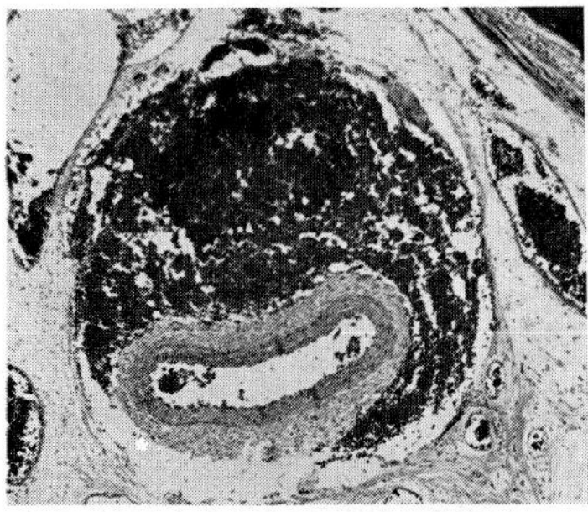

FIG. 7.

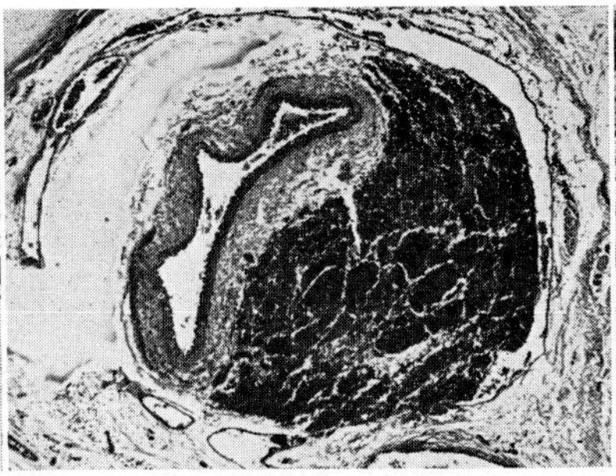

FIG. 8.

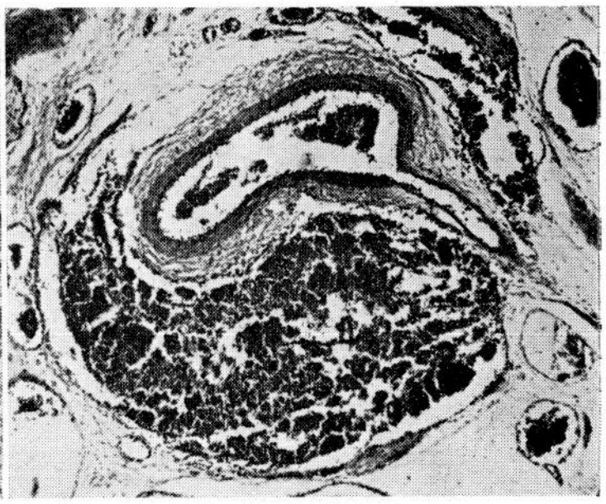

FIG. 9.

FIG. 7.—Haematoma almost surrounding a vertebral artery. × 20.
FIG. 8.—Compression of a vertebral artery by a large crescentic haematoma. × 20.
FIG. 9.—Haematoma extending from the neighbourhood of the origin of a branch from a vertebral artery. × 20.

panied by many large thin-walled venous sinuses. These also were ruptured in some cases with haemorrhage into loose connective tissue of the transverse foramen. However, the haematomas in the wall of the artery were usually enclosed within a collagenous outer adventitial layer. This outer adventitia is important in preventing over-distension of the vessel and it may therefore be expected to resist any outward expansion required to accommodate a haematoma. Serial sections of some of these mural haematomas indicated that they arose from tearing of the branches of the vertebral artery at their junction with the major trunk (Figs. 9 and 10). Nowhere in the sections examined was the main vessel itself torn.

In one baby, who died 12 days after birth, the left vertebral artery was found to be completely occluded by thrombus as it passed around the first cervical vertebra (Fig. 11). This thrombus showed evidence of early organization and appeared to be about three to four days old. It is not possible therefore to attribute the thrombosis to birth injury with any certainty, though other evidence of trauma was present in the neck.

Discussion

It is not the intention in this paper to correlate the findings closely with a detailed analysis of the techniques of delivery or with the pathological changes in the rest of the autopsy, but to emphasize the frequency of the lesions described in a random group of perinatal deaths.

Direct Trauma to Spinal Cord. The occurrence of birth injury to the brain and its clinical effects

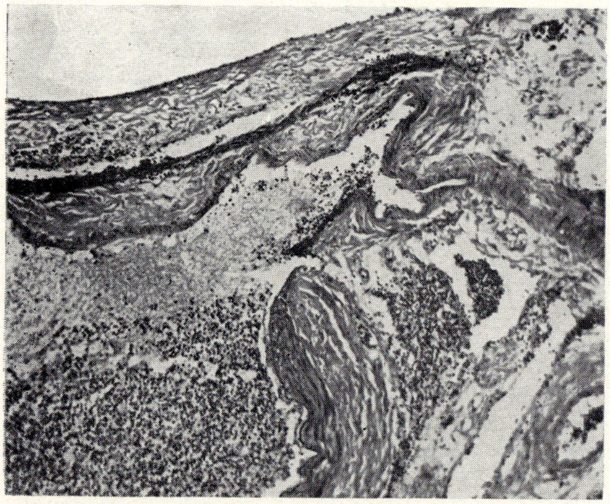

FIG. 10.—A tear in the wall of a branch of a vertebral artery at its origin from the parent vessel. Blood has escaped into the angle between the vessels and is continuous with a much larger haematoma in this section. × 70.

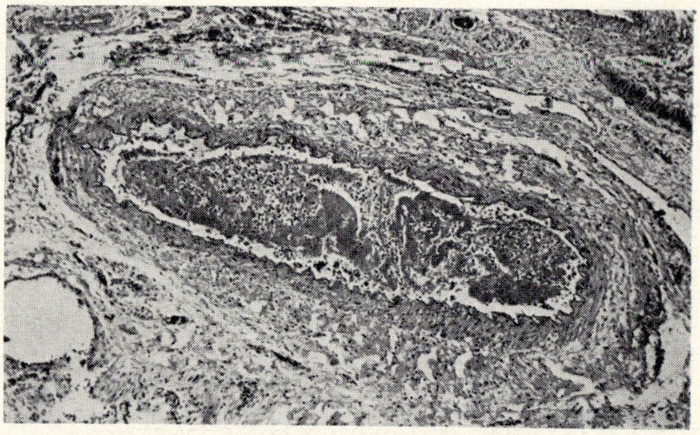

FIG. 11.—Vertebral artery occluded by thrombus. × 30.

were well appreciated a century ago by Radford (1834) and Little (1843). Little (1862) was aware also of damage more particularly to the brain stem and spinal cord and stated that difficulty in deglutition and respiration resulted from damage to the medulla. Injury to the neck is especially liable to occur during breech delivery, and Pierson (1923) recorded 17 cases of fracture or dislocation of vertebrae in 36 deaths. Disruption of the spinal cord itself was reported by Ford (1925) in six cases of breech delivery. In contrast Crothers and Putnam (1927), reviewing birth injuries to the spinal cord, concluded that serious cord damage was rare after vertex presentation. However, minor haemorrhages into the substance of the cord have been found after all methods of delivery. Hausbrandt and Meier (1935) examined the spinal cord in 103 premature and full-time foetuses for whom there was either no obvious cause of death or a clinical diagnosis of intra-uterine asphyxia or inhalation of liquor had been made. They found petechial haemorrhages in 30% of the spinal cords, especially in the upper cervical region. Hirvensalo (1949) found that small haemorrhages were present in medulla and pons in 37% of all premature and 50% of full-term foetuses.

In the present series a significant degree of traumatic bruising of the cervical cord was found in only two cases, both breech deliveries (Fig. 4). The mode of origin of smaller petechial haemorrhages is not clear. Whilst they may be a manifestation of general anoxic damage to capillaries, Baar (1946) has pointed out that such 'asphyxial' haemorrhages are often indistinguishable from those produced by the great intra- and extra-vascular pressure differences in the presenting parts during labour, a factor which would account for their frequent occurrence after vertex presentation.

Damage to Spinal Nerve Roots. In nine cases tearing and bruising of spinal nerve roots was found and occasional arterial twigs from the vertebral arteries supplying the nerve roots were found to be torn. Such lesions may of course result in a fully developed Erb or Klumpke type of paralysis. Where the third and fourth cervical roots are disrupted then a complete phrenic palsy may be obvious; simple bruising or ischaemic damage would result in temporary respiratory difficulty through dysfunction of the diaphragm.

It is widely held that congenital torticollis is the result of tearing of the muscle belly of the sternomastoid during delivery. This was evidently not the opinion of Little (1862) whose Cases 48 and 49 had wrynecks. He thought the condition was due to spasm of the muscle following injury to the neck. Chandler (1948) treated 225 cases surgically, 26 of whom were under 4 months of age. In the excised specimen he found degenerating muscle and fibrosis but no evidence of an old haematoma. Roemer (1954) followed up 44 cases and found four with persistent associated palsies. One had an Erb's palsy, one a facial paralysis and two had scoliosis. It is possible in many cases that the underlying lesion in congenital torticollis is partial denervation of the sternomastoid muscle with spasm and subsequent muscular atrophy and contracture.

Damage to the Vertebral Arteries. The intramural haematomas found in the vertebral arteries of 24 foetuses may be a very important cause of perinatal morbidity and mortality. Where the arterial obstruction is of moderate degree the infant may survive to show later evidence of ischaemic cerebral damage.

It is clear that in normal circumstances intramural haemorrhages, since they cannot be formed at more than systolic blood pressure, only compress the lumen significantly if a valve pocket is produced by dissection of the wall from the lumen. However, the situation during delivery of the head and neck of an infant is quite different. The presenting parts may be at or near atmospheric pressure whilst the rest of the body is subject to the additional pressure of the contracting uterus, perhaps 200 mm. Hg. The blood pressure is therefore raised from the normal 90/50 to 290/250 mm. Hg, the pulse pressure remaining the same. With the tissues of the neck and head at normal atmospheric pressure and the intravascular pressures very considerably raised any slight tear of vein or artery will produce a haematoma. If the haemorrhage has occurred within the tough adventitia of the vertebral artery the haematoma will be unable to disperse rapidly. On completion of delivery the intravascular arterial pressure returns to normal levels, which may be inadequate to maintain the lumen of the artery past a tense intramural haematoma formed at a pressure of 290 mm. Hg. By such a mechanism vertebral bloodflow may be seriously embarrassed for a period of minutes or hours, which is sufficient for permanent cerebral ischaemic damage to be caused. Furthermore, disruption of the adventitial coat may affect the autonomic innervation of the vertebral artery producing for a time spasmodic and irregular contractions.

The vertebral arteries are unique in that they unite to form a common basilar arterial trunk which then gives off bilaterally symmetrical branches. Because of this arrangement obstruction of one vertebral artery may be sufficient to produce bilateral lesions of the brain stem, cerebellum and occipito-temporal regions (Hutchinson and Yates, 1957).

Obstruction to the vertebral arterial flow is particularly significant at the time of birth since it is at this period that the vegetative functions of the brain stem are established. This is emphasized by the observation of Himwich and Fazekas (1941) that in neonatal dogs the metabolic activity, as measured by oxygen demand *in vitro*, was much lower in the cerebral hemisphere than in the cerebellum or medulla. In later life the reverse was true. Similar observations were made on tissue from human infants by Racker (1942).

The effects of ischaemia of the brain stem may be evident as cardio-respiratory failure; in the words of Radford (1834) 'the difficulty of commencing respiration does not depend upon a mechanical obstruction, from mucus in the trachea; but on the injury which the brain has suffered'. This may be associated with difficulty in deglutition (Little, 1862).

It is likely that some cases of facial palsy are not due to pressure of the forceps blade on the nerve but rather to ischaemic damage within the facial nucleus; Gaisford (1953) has pointed out that this palsy may occur after normal delivery. Central ischaemic damage may also be the cause of congenital facial diplegia for which no adequate explanation has ever been offered other than agenesis of the brain stem, presumably genetic in origin (Murphy and German, 1947). It is pertinent that Hellström (1949) found other cranial nerves to be involved frequently in this condition. In 64% the abducent and in 23% the hypoglossal were affected. In 10% there was some mental defect.

At the upper end of the brain stem the nuclei of the third, fourth and sixth nerves will be damaged by vertebral arterial ischaemia, providing an explanation for the observation of Guibor (1950) that over half the patients with cerebral palsy have imbalance of extra-ocular muscles. This might be a fully developed squint or a latent lesion, as in the cases reported by Breakey (1955) who found esotropia in 25% and exotropia in 7% of 100 spastics. Guibor (1953) reported a case of fixed bilateral nasal squint associated with hypotonicity of the limbs suggesting a concomitant cerebellar lesion. A clear history of trauma resulting from rotation of the neck during forceps delivery was found by Lebensohn (1955) in an infant with Perinaud's syndrome. The fixed pupils and loss of upward gaze probably resulted from ischaemia of the quadrigeminal plate region.

The vertebral arteries supply not only the auditory and vestibular nuclei of the brain stem but via the internal auditory arteries they supply the inner ear; some degree of deafness may be expected in those who survive birth injury to the cervical portion of these vessels. Auditory function is certainly disturbed in many spastics.

There is considerable evidence to suggest that stenosis or occlusion of the vertebral arteries at birth is an important factor in the production of cerebral palsy. Analogy with the lesions found in vertebral arterial occlusion in adults (Hutchinson and Yates, 1956, 1957) indicates that bilateral symmetrical lesions of calcarine occipital cortex might be expected. Indeed Norman (1953) found that five out of 45 cases of cerebral palsy had been characterized clinically by cortical blindness and showed bilateral calcarine occipital gyral damage. Jéquier, Dufour and Rabinowicz (1957) reported the findings in a 10-year-old blind spastic idiot. In this case also, bilateral calcarine cortical ulegyria and sclerosis of the pulvinar were observed but were attributed to a lesion of the vein of Galen. The symmetry of some of the lesions in cerebral palsy has been interpreted in a variety of ways. Penrose (1949) felt that it must indicate a genetically determined hereditary cause. Benda (1952) stated that 'the symmetry of lesions depended on the one common structure which is equally shared by both hemispheres—the venous drainage into the great vein of Galen'. Many of the findings would be better explained by a consideration of the unique arterial union of the vertebral arteries which, as mentioned earlier, results in symmetrical blood supply of the brain stem, cerebellum and via the posterior cerebral arteries, the occipito-temporal cerebral cortex.

There is a sub-group of cerebral palsy, known as the atactic-cerebellar type, who commonly show normal mental function and in whom the pathological changes are confined to cerebellum and brain stem. It is difficult to find any alternative explanation for such a condition other than vertebral arterial occlusion produced by birth trauma.

Epilepsy is common in cerebral palsy. Faber (1947) reported its occurrence in 48% of 99 cases. In general a large proportion of epilepsy has been attributed to lesions in the temporal lobe (Bailey and Gibbs, 1951). Falconer (1958) reported scarring of the ammon's horn, uncus and amygdala in 21 of 50 cases operated on for temporal lobe epilepsy. The age of onset of attacks in this group was 4½ years and it has been suggested that natal injury is responsible for the damage in epilepsy of this type (Earle, Baldwin and Penfield, 1953). These authors demonstrated that compression of the brain at birth produced herniation of parts of the temporal lobe through the tentorial opening with damage and scarring of the hippocampal region. Lindenberg (1955) emphasized that arterial ischaemia resulting from compression of branches of the posterior cerebral artery might be important. Much of the pathological change found in these cases of epilepsy lies within territory ultimately dependent on the vertebral arteries. It is possible therefore that bruising of these vessels in their cervical course may be an additional factor in producing such scars.

Summary

The necks of 60 infants dying in the perinatal period were examined histologically for evidence of birth trauma. The cases were selected at random from 213 stillborn and neonatal deaths occurring in 2,800 births. They included eight breech deliveries and three by caesarean section; 16 were stillborn.

In 27 cases evidence was found of distortional trauma to the cervical spine in the form of extra- and sub-dural haemorrhage, haemorrhage into joint capsules and torn ligaments and dura.

A significant degree of traumatic damage to the spinal cord was found in only two cases, both breech deliveries.

In nine cases there was bruising and tearing of spinal nerve roots.

In 24 cases, following all methods of delivery, there were haemorrhages into the adventitial coat of one or both vertebral arteries. These haematomas were often of considerable size, narrowing the lumen of the vessel. They were thought to arise from tearing of the arterial twigs, supplying nerve roots and spinal cord, at their origins from the vertebral arteries.

In one infant, who died 12 days after birth, the left vertebral artery was occluded by thrombus.

The significance of stenosis of the cervical part of the vertebral arteries is discussed in relation to ischaemic damage to the brain stem and as a probable cause of cerebral lesions in many cases of cerebral palsy.

I would like to thank Dr. F. A. Langley and Dr. T. Wade-Evans for allowing me to carry out this special examination of cases on which they were performing a general autopsy.

REFERENCES

Baar, H. S. (1946). *Brit. med. Bull.*, **4**, 178.
Bailey, P. and Gibbs, F. A. (1951). *J. Amer. med. Ass.*, **145**, 365.
Benda, C. E. (1952). *Developmental Disorders of Mentation and Cerebral Palsies.* Grune and Stratton, New York.
Breakey, A. S. (1955). *A.M.A. Arch. Ophthal.*, **53**, 852.
Chandler, F. A. (1948). *J. Bone Jt Surg.*, **30A**, 566.
Crothers, B. and Putnam, Marian, C. (1927). In *Birth Injuries of the Central Nervous System*, by Ford, F. R., Crothers, B. and Putnam, M. C. Medicine Monographs XI. Baillière, Tindall and Cox, London.
Earle, K. M., Baldwin, M. and Penfield, W. (1953). *A.M.A. Arch. Neurol. Psychiat.*, **69**, 27.
Faber, H. K. (1947). *Amer. J. Dis. Child.*, **74**, 1.
Falconer, M. A. (1958). *Proc. roy. Soc. Med.*, **51**, 613.
Ford, F. R. (1925). *Arch. Neurol. Psychiat. (Chicago)*, **14**, 742.
Gaisford, W. (1953). In *Paediatrics for the Practitioner*, Vol. 1, p. 80. Ed. by W. Gaisford and R. Lightwood. Butterworth, London.
Guibor, G. (1950). *Med. Clin. N. Amer.*, **34**, 283.
—— (1953). *Amer. J. Ophthal.*, **36**, 1719
Hausbrandt, F. and Meier, A. (1935). *Frankfurt. Z. Path.*, **49**, 21.
Hellström, B. (1949). *Acta paediat. (Stockh.)*, **37**, 464.
Himwich, H. E. and Fazekas, J. F. (1941). *Amer. J. Physiol.*, **132**, 454.
Hirvensalo, M. (1949). *Acta paediat. (Stockh.)*, **37**, Suppl. 1.
Hutchinson, E. C. and Yates, P. O. (1956). *Brain*, **79**, 319.
——, —— (1957). *Lancet*, **1**, 2.
Jéquier, M., Dufour, R. and Rabinowicz, T. (1957). *Schweiz. Arch. Neurol. Psychiat.*, **79**, 170.
Lebensohn, J. E. (1955). *Amer. J. Ophthal.*, **40**, 738.
Lindenberg, R. (1955). *J. Neuropath. exp. Neurol.*, **14**, 223.
Little, W. J. (1843). *Lancet*, 1843-44, **1**, 318.
—— (1862). *Trans. obstet. Soc. Lond.*, 1861, **3**, 293.
Murphy, J. P. and German, W. J. (1947). *Arch. Neurol. Psychiat (Chicago)*, **57**, 358.
Norman, R. M. (1953). *Proc. roy. Soc. Med.*, **46**, 627.
Penrose, L. S. (1949). *J. ment. Sci.*, **95**, 373.
Pierson, R. N. (1923). *Surg. Gynec. Obstet.*, **37**, 802.
Racker, E. (1942). *Fed. Proc.*, **1**, 69.
Radford, T. (1834). *Lond. Med. Surg. J.*, **5**, 144.
Roemer, F. J. (1954). *Amer. J. Obstet. Gynec.*, **68**, 1146.

ACUTE INTESTINAL OBSTRUCTION DUE TO MESENTERIC LYMPHANGIOMA

BY

B. M. L. UNDERHILL

From the Government Hospital, Bahrain

(RECEIVED FOR PUBLICATION MARCH 18, 1959)

The rarity of abdominal lymphangiomata is emphasized by Raiford (1932) who found only one example in 11,500 necropsies.

Willis (1953) quotes one case in a 4-year-old girl who had a history of recurrent abdominal pain for eight months. MacNab and Menzies (1950) found an example in an 18-year-old recruit and Wood (1955) reports two cases from Leicester, both in males, one 29 and one 8 years old. Standeven (1953) and Callaghan and Farley (1958) each describe one case of multiple mesenteric lymphatic cysts.

A comprehensive review of the condition was given by Levene, Walker and White (1956) when they published an account of two male children, one 12 and one 4 in whom a mesenteric lymphangioma gave rise to acute abdominal symptoms. These children presented with abdominal colic of one or two days' duration but in only one of the cases mentioned above was there complete intestinal obstruction.

This unusual mode of presentation makes the following case worthy of record.

Case Report

A 7-year-old Arab boy was admitted to the Bahrain Government Hospital on March 23, 1958. His father said that he had been thin for some time but had been ill only for three days during which there had been vomiting and constipation and the child's abdomen had increased to an enormous size. The father was adamant in his statement that the boy's abdomen had been of normal size until three days previously.

The patient presented a bizarre appearance. He was a thin, desperately ill little boy adherent to the back of a vast distended abdomen over which the skin was tightly stretched. Veins of the abdominal wall were grossly distended. There appeared to be two very large coils of intestine crossing the abdomen from left to right but no peristalsis could be seen in them though bowel sounds were loud and tinkling. In fact, these 'coils' proved to be the cyst bisected across its middle by a band of ileum.

Transfusion with dextrose-saline solution was begun and gastric suction instituted through a Ryle's tube. After a few hours of this treatment, the child's condition had improved and laparotomy was undertaken.

The abdomen was opened through a long right paraumbilical incision and the swelling was found to consist of an enormous purple mesenteric cyst approximately 10 by 8 in. (25 by 20 cm.). Over the cyst a tape-like loop of ileum was tightly stretched. Obstruction was complete and proximal coils of intestine were distended. The loop of stretched gut and the cyst were excised as a V wedge and end-to-end anastomosis was performed. No other abnormalities were found.

Apart from a mild and transient wound infection, convalescence was uncomplicated. The child began to put on weight and became a gay and happy little boy. He was discharged on the sixteenth post-operative day. Unfortunately, as he was taken straight back to his home in Saudi Arabia, follow-up has been impossible.

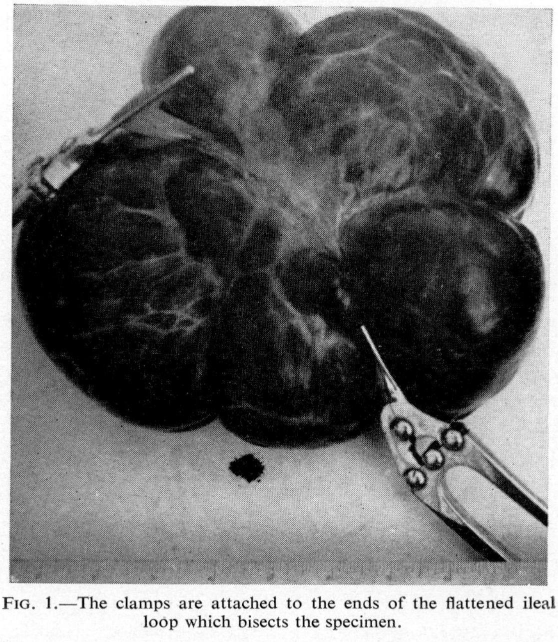

FIG. 1.—The clamps are attached to the ends of the flattened ileal loop which bisects the specimen.

Histological Report (Dr. Stallybrass). 'The specimen consists of a multilocular thin-walled cyst containing brown fluid and many cholesterol crystals. The intestinal wall is normal except for numerous lymph spaces in the sub-serosa. The sub-serosa is continuous with the cyst lining. There are many lipoid crystals in the wall and the appearance is characteristic of mesenteric lymphangioma.'

The gross appearance of the specimen is shown in Fig. 1.

Discussion

Willis (1953) regards these tumours as being congenital rather than neoplastic in nature and considers that fluid accumulation and progressive formation of collateral channels with supervening thrombosis and organization are enough to account for their increase in size. Very rapid increase in volume is not unusual due to dilatation of the abdominal spaces following torsion, inflammation or pressure changes. Such dilatation must have taken place in this case bringing about complete obliteration of the ileal lumen as it passed over the cyst.

Fortunately these lesions are completely benign so that excision is curative. A length of intestine has usually to be excised with the cyst which cannot be shelled out without vascular destruction.

REFERENCES

Callaghan, R. P. and Farley, D. L. B. (1958). *Brit. J. Surg.*, **45**, 655.
Levene, M., Walker, P. A. and White, T. A. (1956). *Arch. Dis. Childh.*, **31**, 502.
MacNab, T. and Menzies, T. (1950). *Brit. J. Surg.*, **37**, 294.
Raiford, T. S. (1932). *Arch. Surg. (Chicago)*, **25**, 122.
Standeven, A. (1953). *Brit. J. Surg.*, **41**, 102.
Willis, R. A. (1953). *Pathology of Tumours*, 2nd ed. Butterworth, London.
Wood, K. (1955). *Brit. J. Surg.*, **43**, 304.

A DESCRIPTION AND CLASSIFICATION OF THE COMMON DISORDERS OF SPEECH IN CHILDREN

BY

T. T. S. INGRAM

From the Department of Child Life and Health, University of Edinburgh and the Royal Hospital for Sick Children, Edinburgh

(RECEIVED FOR PUBLICATION MARCH 9, 1959)

The full assessment of children suffering from speech defects requires a team consisting of speech therapist, paediatrician, psychologist and otologist. The additional services of a phonetician, neurologist, orthodontist, plastic surgeon, radiologist, social worker or psychiatric social worker and child psychiatrist are often helpful.

Unfortunately the majority of descriptions and classifications of speech disorders in childhood are by speech therapists working without much medical co-operation and advice. With honourable exceptions, they tend to regard speech disorders as rather isolated phenomena, dissociated from the other behavioural and psychological characteristics of the child. In the present paper an attempt is made to describe and classify the disorders of speech most frequently encountered in a hospital speech clinic from the point of view of the paediatrician of a diagnostic team.

Case Material and Methods of Examination

The descriptions of speech disorders are based largely on experience in the Speech Clinic of the Royal Hospital for Sick Children, Edinburgh, in the last three years. During this time a total of 348 patients were referred, though for various reasons it was possible to investigate only 189 of them fully. The patients are not representative of an unselected sample of children in the community as judged by the figures for all live births given by the Registrar General for Scotland (1951). There is an excess of patients in Social Classes I and II, possibly because of the greater attention paid to speech defects in these classes (Table 1). The greater excess of patients in Social Classes I and II over the age of 5 than under the age of 5 is probably the result of the fact that children in the lower social classes attend corporation schools where there is a very comprehensive speech therapy service. In private fee-paying schools, where more attention is usually paid to speech defects, speech therapy is rarely provided. Children with speech defects attending these schools were frequently referred to the Speech Clinic in the Hospital.

Detailed family, birth and developmental histories were taken, with particular emphasis on the rate, and any abnormalities, of speech development. The children were subjected to a detailed paediatric and neurological examination, and behaviour in play was observed for as long as possible in each case. The child's speech was studied jointly by the paediatrician and the speech therapist, and detailed notes were made of its intelligibility and of the particular defects which were observed. In many cases tape recordings were made, though it is always easier, in fact, to examine speech for defects of articulation in the presence of the patient. Speech was studied from the points of view of level of language ability and defects of articulation.

Attempts were made to assess the child's ability to understand what was said to him by his parents

TABLE 1

DISTRIBUTION OF 189 PATIENTS WITH SPEECH DISORDERS BY AGE AND SOCIAL CLASS

Age	Social Class I	II	III	IV	V	Total
Under 3	1	1	10	2	1	15
3–5	25	16	48	13	9	111
5–10	12	11	20	5	2	50
10+	3	3	3	2	2	13
All ages	41	31	81	22	14	189
Under 5	43		58	25		126
Over 5	29		23	11		63
All ages	72		81	36		189
Approx. %	39		42	19		100
Registrar General Scotland 1951 %	12·5		58·3	29·2		100

and by other people. Any apparent tendency for the child to rely unduly on gesture, or on watching people talking to him, was noted. Rough tests of hearing were used during the general examination of the patient, his responses to whistles of various pitches, bells, the rustling of paper, vibration forks, whispering, talking and shouting being observed. Full audiometry was performed on all children as soon as they were co-operative enough for this examination to be performed. Handedness was tested rather unscientifically by noting the hand which the child used in each of four performance tests carried out three times. Each patient was asked to turn a door handle, break a stick, throw and catch a ball. Patients not using a single hand for nine or more of the total of 12 tests were classified as being ambidextrous. Eyedness and footedness were also tested (Ingram and Reid, 1956).

A psychiatric social worker, seconded to the Clinic, was asked to investigate the home situation of 41 patients in whom psychological stress appeared to be important. Thirty-one patients were further assessed in the Department of Psychological Medicine. The opinion of an otolaryngologist was asked in 34 cases, of a plastic surgeon in five, and of an orthodontist in eight. Eleven patients were admitted to hospital on account of physical conditions noted at the time of assessment. These included patients suffering from cretinism, epilepsy, enuresis, phenylketonuria, fibrocystic disease of the pancreas and Sjøgren's syndrome.

Classification

The classification is by clinical findings. Categories are defined in the first place by the form of the major speech defect. Thus distinctions are made between disorders affecting the voice predominantly (dysphonia), those whose main effect is to alter the rhythm of speech (dysrhythmia) and those in which abnormalities of articulation are the presenting feature.

It must be admitted that classification on the basis of the major defect of speech is somewhat arbitrary and crude (as are most classifications), and it is necessary to ignore a number of significant clinical findings in many cases for the purpose of giving the speech condition a name. For example, many patients suffering from a stammer will have minor abnormalities of articulation; some patients with 'specific developmental speech disorders' will have minor stammer (speech dysrhythmia). It is impossible to take account of these subsidiary defects in the major categories.

Further classification is by associated clinical findings. When direct interference with the function of the articulatory organs can be demonstrated the disorder is considered to be 'dysarthric'. When the abnormalities of articulation are part of a more general disorder and no direct interference with the function of the articulatory organs can be demonstrated they are considered to be 'secondary'. When disorders apparently confined only to the functions of speech are present, unassociated with direct interference with the articulatory organs, they are classified as 'specific developmental' or 'functional speech disorders' (Table 2).

TABLE 2

CLASSIFICATION OF SPEECH DISORDERS FOUND IN 189 CHILDREN

(1) Disorders of Voicing (Dysphonia) (4)	
a. With demonstrable disease of the larynx	1
b. Without demonstrable disease of the larynx . .	3
(2) Disorders of Rhythm (Dysrhythmia) (29)	
a. Clutter	3
b. Stammer	26
(3) Disorders of Articulation with Demonstrable Dysfunction of Articulatory Apparatus (Dysarthria) (30)	
a. Due to neurological abnormalities	7
b. Due to local abnormalities	23
(4) Disorders of Articulation without Demonstrable Dysfunction of Articulatory Apparatus (Secondary Speech Disorders) (41)	
a. Secondary to hearing defect	8
b. Secondary to mental retardation	29
c. Secondary to psychogenic disorders	3
d. Secondary to aphasia due to brain damage . .	1
(5) Specific Developmental Speech Disorders (Functional Speech Disorders) (80)	
a. Involving language development and articulation	40
b. Involving articulation only	40
(6) Mixed Cases (4)	4
(7) Unclassified and Other (1)	1
Total	189

In some cases there are contributory causal factors in the speech disorder. For example, a child with brain damage secondary to encephalitis or trauma may have a disorder of articulation which is partly secondary to aphasia and partly the result of inco-ordination of the organs of articulation. Such patients may conveniently be placed in the category of 'mixed cases'. They are relatively few.

Categories

Disorders of Voicing. Disorders of voicing are relatively uncommon in childhood, amounting to no more than 4% in most large series of patients with speech defects. In the present series there were four patients with disorders of the voice (approximately 2% of the series).

The only disorder of voicing considered in the present classification is chronic lack of voice, which makes the child sound as if he is hoarse. This is similar in quality to the 'loss of voice'' suffered by adults with laryngitis. It must be distinguished from the effects of excessive nasal escape (hyperrhinophonia) or nasal obstruction (hyporhinophonia). In these conditions difficulty of articulation is the striking abnormality. They have therefore been included under the heading of 'dysarthria'.

Dysphonia affects girls rather more frequently than boys, or at any rate is complained of more frequently by the parents of girls. It may occur at any age and has been observed in a child of 6 months, but more commonly it begins between the ages of 2 and 8 years. Its onset is commonly gradual. Often there is a period of weeks or months during which the condition is intermittent, being present for a day or two at a time and then recovering. Even when finally established, the severity of dysphonia varies from week to week, from day to day and even from hour to hour. Frequently the child is able to shout, and sometimes to sing, but not to speak with normal voice.

A number of inflammatory, traumatic and neoplastic laryngeal conditions interfering with the function of the vocal cords may cause dysphonia in childhood. I have seen it personally following traumatic laryngoscopy and inhalation of caustic, complicating chronic bronchitis and laryngitis, associated with nodules of the vocal cords and papillomata of the larynx, and occurring in the course of Sjøgren's syndrome (Birrell, 1954).

In many cases, however, no abnormalities of the larynx can be found. The immediate assumption is commonly made that the dysphonia is therefore of 'psychological origin'. It seems to be equally likely that there are abnormalities of the vocal cords in these patients, which cannot be recognized by our present crude methods of investigation.

There are no well recognized methods of treating dysphonia in childhood by 'speech therapy'. Rest of the voice for a period of four to six weeks will often result in a marked improvement in voicing. Unfortunately this is often transient, and relapse occurs as soon as the child begins to shout again. A proportion of children with dysphonia, more boys than girls, show improvement at the time of adolescence, whether the larynx is obviously abnormal or not. Such improvement is impossible to predict, however, and many patients continue to have abnormalities of voicing into adult life.

Speech Dysrhythmias. Involuntary interference with the normal rhythm of speech is one of the commonest disorders of speech in childhood. Two main types may be recognized.

Clutter consists of a more or less sudden irregular acceleration of speech which results in a shift of stress and syllable division in speech. The words sound 'run into one another' and sometimes speech may be so disturbed as to be incomprehensible. Many children aged between 2 and 4 years may show clutter transiently for a period of weeks or months without any associated or subsequent abnormality of speech. When clutter occurs after the age of 5 it is more often associated with stammer or hesitation (Van Riper, 1947).

Involuntary temporary arrest of the flow of speech may be manifest as hesitation, a transient inability to produce the next expected syllable resulting in a period of no speech. Stammer consists of the involuntary repetition of a sound as well as an inability to move beyond it. It is unrewarding to distinguish too cleverly between hesitation and stammer. They are often associated. Many patients' dysrhythmia first takes the form of hesitation, and months or years later they begin to stammer. Others stammer first and then show hesitation.

Hesitation or stammer is found more often in children whose fathers are in Social Classes I and II (Registrar General) than in the lower social classes. There appears to be no difference in the observed and expected birth order of patients. Males are more frequently affected than females, the ratio being as high as four to one in some series (Wilson, 1954). In the family history a high proportion of relatives stammer, 44% according to Johnson, Brown, Curtis, Edney and Keaster (1948). There is a higher proportion of ambidexterity and left-handedness amongst relatives than expected (Travis, 1931). Of the present small series of 29 patients, 38% had parents or siblings with speech defects. These were dysrhythmic in type except in one instance. The parents and/or siblings of 27% were left-handed or ambidextrous.

The birth history and motor milestones of patients tend to be within normal limits. Speech development is not significantly retarded. The majority of children are of average intelligence or better, and show no neurological defects.

A relatively high proportion of patients will be found to be left-handed or ambidextrous, the proportion depending largely on the methods of testing used (Orton, 1937; Morley, 1957). In the present series, 12 of the 29 patients were found to show little laterality of handedness, and one was sinistral.

A high proportion of patients show abnormalities of behaviour. These were present in 21 of the 29 patients studied in this series. They included temper tantrums in four, excessive dependence in five, excessive excitability or tearfulness in five, night terrors in four, enuresis in three and habit spasms in three. Nine of the patients were disturbed enough to merit psychiatric treatment. The extent to which the speech dysrhythmia is an aetiological factor in causing anxiety symptoms is probably overestimated. In many cases symptoms of abnormal behaviour preceded the appearance of the speech defect, and both could be related to the same emotional stresses. Parents related the onset of symptoms to maternal separation before the age of 4 years in five instances (the child being hospitalized in three), to physical accidents in two, to severe whooping cough in two and to crippling accidents to the father in two.

The modes of onset and course of dysrhythmia in childhood are relatively consistent. The majority of cases of uncomplicated clutter recover normal speech before they are 5 years of age. Hesitation or stammering appears in most persistent stammerers for the first time between the ages of 2 and 4 years. In only five of 25 patients with stammer or hesitation in this series did symptoms appear after 5 years of age. It is difficult to know how many children showing definite persistent stammering at this period recover completely and how many later have dysrhythmic speech symptoms. Of children who present with persistent stammer, two-thirds (17 of 25 in this series) have never been really free of the symptoms for more than four weeks at most from the time of its onset.

True remissions of stammer lasting for more than six months are more frequent in those where first symptoms occur under the age of 5 years, but the statement made in text-books that a stammer occurring in a pre-school child is likely to be of little significance requires qualification. Of the eight remissions of stammer which occurred in this series, all but one of them occurred before the age of 5 years. Only three of the remissions lasted longer than three years. The remaining five patients began to stammer again shortly after going to school. It is too early to know if the other three remissions are permanent or not.

The subsequent course of stammer varied greatly according to the reaction of the patient to his symptom. Some children adjusted to quite a severe dysrhythmia and were surprisingly undisturbed by its presence. Others began to avoid speaking and making social contact whenever possible. They attempted to avoid words on which they believed they would stammer, and restricted their activities in an attempt to hide their speech defect. In time the fear of stammering may become the most potent cause of stammer.

It is extremely doubtful if speech therapy *per se* is helpful in speech dysrhythmia. A mother confessor or a child psychiatrist (either of which roles speech therapists may be found adopting) occasionally seems to benefit the patient's attitude to his speech defect. There appear to be no reliable comparative figures on which to base conclusions about the proportion of patients with stammer who spontaneously improve at adolescence or in early adult life with the help of, in spite of, or without speech therapy.

My clinical impression is that patients in whom it has taken very severe emotional stresses to precipitate stammering tend to have a better prognosis than those who stammered without much evident emotional stress being necessary. This impression, like so many concerning speech disorders, requires confirmation.

Dysarthric Speech Disorders. In this category are included those disorders of articulation which are the result of organic disease causing interference with or failure of the normal mechanical functions of part or parts of the articulatory apparatus. Thirty-one of the 189 patients were in this category.

The category is divided into two sub-categories. Patients whose articulatory difficulties are due to neurological abnormalities are included in the first. In these there is rarely much deformity of the articulatory organs themselves. In the second are those disorders of articulation which are the result of local abnormalities affecting the articulatory apparatus. Deformity of the articulatory organs may often be observed.

In general, speech defects in this category are characterized by their consistency. They vary relatively little from day to day or from hour to hour, and the same sounds as are abnormal during spontaneous speech are found on testing to be defective. For example, the sounds requiring nasopharyngeal closure will be consistently defective in patients with cleft palate.

Apart from the six patients with cerebral palsy, motor milestones were within normal limits, and only one of the other 24 patients had retarded language development, though in many cases it was a long time before people outside their immediate families could understand what the children said. Three of the six patients with cerebral palsy failed to walk without support before 18 months, and all of them failed to say recognizable first words by 18 months and phrases by 30 months (Table 3). Again with the exception of those patients with cerebral palsy, the children in this category appeared to be of average intelligence. A relatively high proportion, 14 of the 30 patients, suffered from abnormalities of behaviour, however. In five cases there was immaturity of behaviour, manifest as excessive attachment to the mother, inability to play with other children of similar age, inability to accept a school situation at the normal age or play

TABLE 3

WALKING AND SPEECH DEVELOPMENT OF 30 CHILDREN WITH DEMONSTRABLE DYSFUNCTION OF ARTICULATORY APPARATUS (DYSARTHRIA)

Walking and Speech Development	Cerebral Palsy	Hypomandibulosis and Malocclusion	Other	Total
Walking before 18 months ..	3	7	15	25
Walking after 18 months ..	3	1	1	5
Total	6	8	16	30
Words before 18 months and phrases before 30 months	0	6	8	14
Words before 18 months and phrases after 30 months; Words after 18 months and phrases before 30 months	0	2	3	5
Words after 18 months and phrases after 30 months ..	6	0	1	7
Unknown	0	0	4	4
Total	6	8	16	30

characteristic of a younger age level. Enuresis was present in six patients, thumb or hand sucking in three. Three patients were excessively tearful, fearful, or unusually withdrawn. Three patients showed a characteristic form of overactive behaviour often found in children with cerebral damage, especially when it affects the temporal lobe (Ingram, 1956). The extent to which these abnormalities of behaviour could be regarded as other symptoms of the underlying disturbance which was responsible for the speech defect, and how much they were the result directly and indirectly of the speech defect, is extremely difficult to assess.

The neurological lesions in this category are conveniently divided into those affecting the brain, those affecting the brain stem and those affecting the lower motor neurone (Table 4). Cerebral palsy is by far the commonest cause of neurological lesions, but it is worth emphasizing that dysarthria is not the commonest form of speech defect in cerebral palsy. Though dysarthria is relatively frequently found in severe diplegia, severe ataxia, dyskinesia and bilateral hemiplegia, it is uncommon in mild diplegia (especially paraplegia) and hemiplegia. In the latter disorders defective speech is more frequently part of a general retardation of development, or is secondary to aphasia. In patients with dyskinesia following kernikterus, abnormalities of articulation are commonly the result of a combination of articulatory inco-ordination and hearing defect.

TABLE 4

CLASSIFICATION INTO SUB-CATEGORIES OF 30 PATIENTS SUFFERING FROM DISORDERS OF ARTICULATION WITH DEMONSTRABLE DYSFUNCTION OF ARTICULATORY APPARATUS (DYSARTHRIA)

a. Due to Neurological Abnormalities (7)		
Cerebral palsy	.. ..	6
Suprabulbar palsy	.. ..	1
Lower motor neurone lesions	.. ..	0
b. Due to Local Abnormalities (23)		
Jaws and Teeth	Hypomandibulosis	6
	Other malocclusion	2
Tongue	Tie	1
	Tongue thrust	4
Lips	Cleft lip (only)	0
	Other	1
Palate	Cleft (with or without cleft lip) ..	5
	Other	0
Pharynx	Large pharynx (palatal disproportion)	3
	Acquired disease	1
Total	.. ..	30

Suprabulbar paresis (facial diplegia, Moebius' syndrome) is easily recognized when it is severe and especially when it affects eye movements (Henderson, 1939; Evans, 1955). Minor manifestations of the condition may be more difficult to recognize, however, and a number of patients have been observed in whom poor voluntary movements of the lips, tongue and soft palate were present without obvious voluntary paralysis of these organs. The trained phonetician can be of great help in the accurate diagnosis of these disorders by his interpretations of the child's speech in terms of tongue, lip and palatal movements.

Though no cases occurred in the present series, lower motor neurone lesions affecting articulation have been seen occasionally following poliomyelitis and diphtheria, but they are more commonly the result of peripheral nerve damage during tonsillectomy. The history in patients who have suffered damage to a palatal nerve is typical. Following discharge from hospital the speech is noted to be abnormal and fluids may come down the nose when the child tries to drink. Though the ability to drink is recovered after a few weeks the child continues to speak 'down the nose', and defects of the plosives, vowels and 's' 'Θ' and 'ʃ' sounds are noted.

Since a single local abnormality of the mouth or pharynx may affect a number of the organs of articulation it is more convenient to classify dysarthric speech disorders by the nature of the abnormality rather than by the type of speech defect which they cause. Thus whilst hypomandibulosis prevents correct dental occlusion and sometimes apposition of the lips, involuntary protrusion of the tongue during speech, 'tongue thrust', is often a more important cause of disordered articulation.

Other forms of malocclusion and dental abnormalities cause abnormalities of articulation less frequently than hypomandibulosis. The commonest of them are the result of an undue prominence of the lower jaw, associated with open bite, wide separation of the incisors, or missing teeth. These conditions are most frequently associated with 'lisping' due to the lateral or central protrusion of the tongue between the teeth when sibilants are produced.

In a few children the wide separation or anterior protrusion of the upper incisors appears to be attributable to excessive finger or thumb sucking. In others there is associated 'tongue thrust', though the extent to which this can be regarded by itself as the cause of dental abnormalities must remain in doubt.

Tongue tie is an uncommon cause of articulatory difficulties, though it is often blamed for them. A commoner abnormality of the function of the tongue which does cause articulatory difficulties is 'tongue thrust'. This condition may be associated with cerebral palsy or congenital abnormalities of the mouth, as have been described. It is often found in association with chronic tonsillitis and adenoiditis. But it may be present as the only obvious abnormality in many cases. In children showing it the pattern of swallowing is often observed to be immature in type and on stroking the lips gently a mild sucking reflex associated with opening of the mouth and some tongue protrusion is not infrequently observed (Francis, 1958). Abnormalities of the lips alone are not a common cause of articulatory difficulty, though one case occurred in the present series in which the upper lip was abnormally high and fixed.

Malformations of the palate are relatively frequent causes of severe articulatory difficulties. The commonest malformation is an actual cleft in the soft palate. Less commonly a midline defect in the muscular elements without a defect in the mucous membrane (submucous cleft palate) may be diagnosed if the cleft palate is gently palpated. The articulatory defect is similar in type, though less severe than that found in a true cleft palate.

The excessive nasal escape which results when the palate is cleft impairs all vowel and consonant sounds, with the exception of 'm', 'n' and 'ŋ' in which considerable nasal outflow of air is usually required. Substitutions for particularly defective sounds are frequent. For example glottal stops may replace plosives. Associated abnormalities also contribute to the speech defect. Especially in children with bilateral clefts of the palate there is frequently marked deformity of the alveolar bony structure, especially after operation, and dental malocclusion results. The upper lip is all too often rather functionless (Morley, 1954).

A relatively small number of patients present with 'cleft palate speech' with nasal escape, in whom no abnormalities of palatal movement can be found. In the majority speech has been 'through the nose' from the earliest years, and in a few there is a history of escape of fluids through the nose when drinking in infancy. In others a change from normal speech has been noted following adenoidectomy. On examination many of these patients show marked anterior prominence of the maxillary bones and the pharynx appears to be unusually deep, so that the length of the palate is inadequate for its posterior margin to reach the posterior nasopharyngeal wall. Radiological investigation will often confirm that the pharynx is, in fact, abnormally deep and the palate inadequate in size, in spite of full movement, to close the nasopharynx. Many of these patients can be helped by operations designed to reduce the size of the pharyngeal aperture (Calnan, 1957; Gibb, 1958). In a few patients nasal escape appears to be due to impaired palatal movement, the result of inflammatory peri-tonsillar induration, or scarring following tonsillectomy.

Tonsillitis and enlargement of the adenoids are much less common single causes of significant persistent dysarthria in childhood than is often stated. In the present series only one patient was included in the sub-category of dysarthria due to 'acquired disease of the pharynx'.

Secondary Speech Disorders. These are disorders of articulation which are not due to direct interference with the mechanics of the articulatory organs, but are secondary to other physical, mental or psychiatric conditions. Often it may be demonstrated that these organs can be moved normally, and frequently that sounds not used in spontaneous speech can in fact be produced by the child. The most important causes of articulatory disorders of this type are hearing defects and mental retardation.

Children with hearing defects have never heard or have ceased to hear speech sounds correctly, and therefore cannot be expected to reproduce them in speech. A study of the behaviour and articulatory abnormalities shown by the child will often give a clue to the type of hearing defect. Children with some loss of hearing for high tones only will commonly show failure in articulating 'f' 'Θ', 'p', 't', 'ʃ' and 's'. Children with more severe hearing loss for all frequencies will often only produce sounds requiring much lip movement, which they can see when they watch people talking to them. This is not always the case, however, and a number of patients have been seen with retarded speech development and poor performance on intelligence tests whose hearing was found to be significantly defective on audiometry, to the surprise of the examiner. Once they have learnt how to use a suitable hearing aid the children have often improved markedly in their performance on intelligence tests. This emphasizes the need for routine audiometry in all children with speech defects.

Children with mental retardation present more complex disturbances of articulation. Often there appears to be a failure to perceive and discriminate speech sounds accurately, possibly because of a reduced span of attention. Even when 'parrotting' what has just been said to them, their articulation will often be quite inaccurate. Speech development is usually considerably retarded, and the patients show errors of articulation commonly found in much younger normal children. In these patients the later acquired sounds are usually abnormal, especially 'r', 'Θ', 'ʃ', 'tʃ' and 'dʒ'.

Defects of articulation are often inconsistent and vary from sentence to sentence of spontaneous speech. There may also be language disorder with the omission of small words, especially prepositions, auxiliary verbs and conjunctions. There may be a general innaccuracy in the articulation of practically all speech sounds, which almost justifies the loose description of 'clumsy speech' which is often given by the parents of these patients. There is often a failure to develop normal patterns of intonation and stress, so that speech is curiously monotonous.

Whilst in aphasia the defect of language is (by definition) the most important cause of interference with speech, the importance of articulatory abnormalities has been rather under-estimated (Critchley, 1952). Especially in children whose cerebral damage has been sustained before speech development has been completed, there is often gross disturbance of the ability to articulate words and their component individual syllables correctly. In many cases it is difficult to draw a line between the language difficulties and difficulties in articulation; omission of small words, conjunctions, prepositions, auxiliary verbs and pronouns may be associated with the omission of syllables, especially the terminal parts of words; reversals and confusion of word order may be associated with reversals and the confusion of the order of syllables in individual words and in the distortion and mispronunciation of syllables which are spoken. There may also be quite bizarre alterations of rhythm and stress, making the patient sound as if he were speaking a foreign language rather well, as in a case of Monrad-Krohn (1947).

As might be expected, the milestones of motor and speech development were very retarded amongst patients in the category of 'secondary speech disorders', largely due to the high proportion of mentally retarded patients. Major and minor physical abnormalities were relatively common. Epilepsy was present in six cases. Hyperteleorism, syndactyly, hypospadias, congenital heart disease and hemiplegia were each observed in two patients. There was one untreated cretin amongst the mentally retarded patients.

Behaviour abnormalities were also common, occurring in 31 of the 41 patients. Twenty-two children were described as being excessively dependent or immature by their parents. Three were over-active and showed the typical behaviour shown by some brain-damaged children described by Ounsted (1955) and Ingram (1956). In two cases behaviour was classified as autistic by child psychiatrists.

Specific Developmental Speech Disorders ('Functional Speech Disorders'). In this category are placed those patients who show disorders of articulation from the time they first attempt formed speech, and in which the speech disorder is neither associated with obvious abnormalities of articulatory function, nor secondary to demonstrable disease. Eighty of the 189 patients who were fully examined were placed in this category.

Patients in this category are characterized by the unexpectedly slow development of intelligible speech, though their milestones of motor development are usually within normal limits and their intelligence is within average limits, or not sufficiently impaired to account for the degree of retardation of speech development. This is shown in Table 5 in which it will be observed that 49, or 61·25%, of the 80 patients said their first recognizable words (excepting Mum, Mam, Mama, Da, Dad, Dada) after the age of 18 months and first joined words together after the age of 30 months. Fifteen, or almost 19%, did not say their first words until after 30 months and phrases until 42 months or later. Yet, in spite of its slow development, speech is almost invariably perfectly intelligible by the age of 7 or 8 years in these patients.

Of the 80 patients in this category 58 were boys and 22 were girls, giving a male to female sex ratio which is comparable to other hospital series of children with specific developmental speech and related disorders (Hallgren, 1950). The high proportion of patients (46·25%) with fathers in Social Classes I and II is striking, and probably reflects the greater attention paid by parents in these classes to retarded speech development rather than any greater prevalence of the disorders in the higher social classes. The prospects of their undergoing competitive entrance interviews in order to obtain a place in private schools often exacerbated parents' anxieties about their children's speech.

The majority of the children referred were under the age of 5, as might be expected in view of the tendency for specific developmental disorders of speech to remit as the patient grows older. Only

15 of the 80 patients were over the age of 5, and in the majority of these the speech disorder, though a nuisance in school, had ceased to be a major cause of anxiety to the parents. The fact that only three of the patients were over the age of 7 illustrates that in the majority of patients speech is perfectly comprehensible by this age.

The distribution of children by their birth order was not significantly different from the expected random distribution. The fact that 43 of the 73 patients were last-born is unremarkable in view of their youth. Their parents had not had time to produce subsequent children, especially those staid middle-class Scots with planned families. Seven of the patients were illegitimate.

A family history of retarded speech development is often found in cases of specific developmental speech disorders. Thirty-seven of the 73 legitimate patients (about half) had parents or siblings whose speech development was known to have been slow. Since it was common on examination to find siblings with speech disorders who had been stated by the parents to be 'rare talkers' or 'lovely speakers', this is probably an under-estimate. Parents were known to have retarded speech development in 19 cases, and one or more siblings in 21.

Fifteen patients were born after pregnancies, labours or deliveries which were in some way abnormal, 11 of them being born prematurely by weight. No convincing evidence of birth injury was found in any of them, however, and neurological examination failed to reveal any clinical signs of cerebral injury.

Ambidexterity, as assessed by the tests which have been described, was noted in half of the 80 patients. Only one patient was strongly left-handed. Parents reported left-handedness or ambidexterity in themselves in 22 cases, and in the patients' siblings in 16 cases. Thus 38, or approximately 52%, of 73 legitimate patients had an immediate family history of sinistrality or ambidexterity.

Seven children had intelligence quotients of more than 120 on the Terman Merrill scale, and only two were considered to be dull and backward. It was interesting to observe, however, that specific educational difficulties (dysgraphia or dyslexia) were present in seven of the 15 patients over the age of 5. In these cases it seemed legitimate to conclude that the children were having specific difficulties with the written word which might be related to the troubles they had previously had with the spoken word (Ingram and Reid, 1956; Drew, 1956).

Two forms of retarded development may be recognized in patients coming into this category. About half of the children are described by their parents as having 'names' for objects within their environment which are not intelligible to observing strangers at quite an early age, though they may be comprehensible to the patient's siblings and parents. Their vocabulary is often considerable, but their articulation of the words they know is so defective that they cannot be understood. Frequently the ends of words are much less well articulated than their beginnings. When the children begin to join words together the defects of articulation tend to become more prominent, and a frequent complaint from baffled mothers is that 'he says plenty and he's anything but stupid, but I can understand only a few words of what he says'. In these patients the major disability is imperfect articulation. The development of language may not be much retarded, but what the child says is so imperfectly spoken that much of it cannot be understood.

The articulatory difficulties of children with specific developmental speech disorders are complex, and at first hearing quite baffling when one tries to analyse them. The sounds most often poorly articulated are shown in Table 6. (It should be pointed out that this was the result of study by the author and by speech therapists, not that of properly trained phoneticians.) In general the sounds which are the last to be correctly articulated by normal children are the ones which cause most difficulty. They may be omitted, faultily pronounced, or substituted by other sounds. The substitutions employed vary with the context of the sound which is defective. Sounds are more often omitted or faultily articulated at the ends than at the beginnings or middle portions of words, and more frequently at the beginnings than the middles. It is characteristic that words which the child has had in his vocabulary for a long time are articulated with more faults than words more recently acquired. Thus a child may say 'goggie' for 'doggie', 'wa-wa' for 'water' and 'ba' for 'bath', but be able to say 'Dalgleish', 'wetter' and 'with' quite well. That the articulatory difficulties appear to be so inconsistent often leads parents to accuse their children of laziness. Their observation that many patients can produce sounds correctly on request, which are abnormal in spontaneous speech, further infuriates them.

About half of the patients in the category have language difficulties. They are slow in acquiring new words and often the rate of vocabulary gain is so poor that they have to use gestures to indicate their simplest needs until the age of 3 years or older. When sentences are eventually formed, inversion of word order, omission of consonants, prepositions, auxiliary verbs and some personal pronouns are commonly noted. Many of these children will use, quite unwittingly, a completely inappropriate word in a sentence in place of a similarly sounding one which would have been appropriate. They suffer from classical 'developmental aphasia' (Orton, 1937).

Of the 80 patients suffering from developmental speech disorders in the present series, 40 had obvious language (aphasic) difficulties of the type which has been described, and in the other 40 the speech defect appeared to be predominantly of articulation and did not affect the development of language so severely.

Difficulty in comprehending what was said to them was frequently observed in children suffering from specific developmental speech disorders. In severe cases the child's inability to understand what is said is severe enough to make the parents suspect deafness, though they will often give circumstantial accounts of why they think this unlikely; for example, 'he hears the whistle of the television set when it goes off, and looks up at aeroplanes'. In less severe cases parents were often irritated by the child's tendency to demand repetition of everything which was said to him by saying 'Eh', 'Beg pardon', 'What', or the child would look blank. Mothers and fathers would often complain of their partner's tendency to gesture to the child, though they are unaware of their own tendency to do so. On examination a distinct lapse of time may be observed before the child comprehends what is said to him, though his reactions when he has understood are often intelligent. The tendency of some patients to look at faces and rely on gesture rather than on speech is frequently evident.

In the present series 30 patients appeared to have comprehension difficulties of this type. In 23 they were associated with marked retardation of language development, and language difficulties characteristic of developmental aphasia were observed on examination. In seven language difficulties were not apparent at the time of examination. In general, children with obvious difficulties in comprehension had the most retarded development of speech and the most severe defects of articulation and language, as is seen in Table 5.

TABLE 5

SPEECH DEVELOPMENT OF 80 CHILDREN SUFFERING FROM SPECIFIC DEVELOPMENTAL SPEECH DISORDERS†

Speech Development	Total	Receptive Difficulty		Language Difficulty	
		With	Without	With	Without
Words before 18 mth. and phrases before 30 mth.	21	5	16	4	17
Words before 18 mth. and phrases after 30 mth. .. .. Words after 18 mth. and phrases before 30 mth.	10	4	6	7	3
Words after 18 mth. and phrases after 30 mth.	49*	21	28	29	20
Total ..	80	30	50	40	40

* Of these 49 children: words came after 24 mth. and phrases after 36 mth. in 22 cases; words came after 30 mth. and phrases after 42 mth. in 15 cases.

† All but nine children walked before 18 months.

TABLE 6

MOST FREQUENTLY MISPRONOUNCED, SUBSTITUTED OR OMITTED SOUNDS IN 80 CHILDREN WITH SPECIFIC DEVELOPMENTAL SPEECH DISORDERS

Sounds	Group 1* % with defective sounds	Group 2† % with defective sounds
r	78	37
ʃ (sh)	74	15
θ (*th*ing)	66	31
s	63	5
l	62	1
k	36	12
ʃ (*ch*ur*ch*)	34	13
dʒ (he*dg*e)	34	13
g	26	9
f	20	6
v	17	–
p	17	1
b	17	–

* 80 children with specific developmental speech disorders.

† Sample group of 112 unselected children aged 3½ years (Morley, 1957).

TABLE 7

LOCAL ABNORMALITIES OF THE ARTICULATORY APPARATUS IN 80 PATIENTS WITH SPECIFIC DEVELOPMENTAL SPEECH DISORDERS

Abnormalities	Associated with Abnormal Palatal Movements	Associated with Abnormal Tongue Movements	Associated with Abnormal Palatal and Tongue Movements	Not Associated with any Local Interference	Total
Enlarged tonsils only	1	0	1	5	7
Enlarged adenoids only	1	1	1	0	3
Enlarged tonsils and adenoids	1	2	1	7	11
Hypomandibulosis	0	2	0	0	2
Other malocclusion and dental abnormalities, e.g., open bite, diastasis of incisors	0	2	0	2	4
Tongue thrust only	0	1	0	0	1
Total	3	8	3	14	28

Frequently minor abnormalities of the articulatory apparatus are observed in patients with specific developmental speech disorders. Those found in the present series are shown in Table 7. In many patients (14 of the 28 with local abnormalities) no interference with the function of the articulatory organs could be demonstrated. In the remainder it required only a rudimentary knowledge of phonetics to realize that the local abnormalities could not be held responsible for the complex speech disturbance, often affecting language as well as articulation of a wide variety of sounds.

Abnormalities of behaviour are frequent in patients with specific developmental speech disorders. In the majority of cases they appear to be secondary to the speech defect. Obviously the situation in which an intelligent child with a speech defect often finds himself is stressful. He is deprived of the means to communicate his ideas, frequently in social circumstances where much attention is paid to language and articulation. Later on specific educational difficulties may also be present.

His reactions to this situation may be by withdrawal. Solitariness, inability to play with other children, day-dreaming, excessive dependence on the mother, and fearfulness were complained of in 18 of the patients. Four others seemed unusually tense, excitable and tearful. Four reacted to frustration by severe temper tantrums. Three (over the age of 4 years) were enuretic.

Mixed Cases and Unclassified Cases. In a classification whose categories are defined in terms of the single major speech disability it is inevitable that a small number of patients with multiple defects could fall into more than one of the major categories. Provision is made for them by having a category for 'mixed cases'. There were only four such patients in the present series. They included one child with severe hypomandibulosis, cerebral diplegia causing impaired voluntary movement of the articulatory organs and mental defect. Another had a cleft palate and suffered from nerve deafness following tuberculous meningitis.

A few patients resist classification even after full investigation and they are provided for in the category of 'other and unclassified cases'. This category may be compared to a basket of correspondence marked 'pending', from which cases will be taken and placed in other categories when more accurately diagnosed.

Discussion

That there is a need for an adequate description of speech disorders in childhood cannot be doubted by anyone who has to deal with children suffering from speech defects, or by anyone acquainted with the currently accepted literature on the subject (Seth and Guthrie, 1935; Van Riper, 1947). Unfortunately the amount of clinical investigation devoted to disorders of children's speech has been relatively small. Much of it has been the result of speech therapists, phoneticians, linguists, otologists, neurologists or psychologists working in isolation. Yet the problems of accurate diagnosis cannot be solved by a lone worker from one of these disciplines, however expert he may be. Classification based on the clinical findings which seem to be important to a worker in any one of these sciences is bound to be inadequate for other workers with differing points of view.

The benefits of a team approach to speech problems in childhood have not been sufficiently realized, though the work of Miss Muriel Morley and her colleagues shows that it may be rewarding (Morley, Court and Miller, 1950; Morley, Court and Miller, 1954; Morley, Court, Miller and Garside, 1955; Morley, 1957). Their pioneer descriptions and classification of speech defects in childhood mark a significant advance on previous work and deserve close study and criticism (Table 8).

TABLE 8

CLASSIFICATION OF SPEECH DEFECTS IN CHILDHOOD BY MORLEY (1957)

Delayed Development of Speech:
Due to psychogenic retardation
Due to mental retardation
Due to hearing defects
Due to developmental aphasia
Defective Articulation:
Developmental dysarthria
Developmental articulatory apraxia
Dyslalia
Due to partial hearing loss
Due to structural (local) abnormalities
Stammering

It will be seen that an attempt is made to distinguish between 'delayed development of speech' and 'defective articulation' as major categories. Unfortunately this ignores the fact that a high proportion of patients with 'delayed development of speech' have defective articulation, and a significant number with 'defective articulation' have retarded speech development.

The definition of a number of the sub-categories is unsatisfactory, and sometimes misleading. Thus 72 of her 74 patients considered to suffer from 'developmental aphasia' are regarded as suffering from 'executive aphasia' because they showed no difficulty in comprehending speech at the time of examination, though their speech development was retarded. The term 'executive aphasia' has a very specific meaning in adult neurology. It is misused when it is applied to children with retardation of language development merely because they have no obvious difficulties of comprehension. If speech were merely the issuing through the mouth of sequences of sounds which had been poured into the child's ear, as if through a pipeline, there might be some justification for using the term in this way. But the processes involved in the perception, comprehension and utterance of speech are incredibly complicated and still poorly understood. To assume that a child suffers from 'executive' or even 'expressive aphasia' because the end result of this process is defective, though the child appears to comprehend speech, is an unjustified simplification of an extremely complicated problem.

The term 'developmental articulatory apraxia' is open to severe criticism. It implies that appreciation of the movements made by the articulatory organs during speech is so defective that accurate articulation is impossible. Yet it is usually impossible to demonstrate any abnormality of movement on examination, as the author admits. The assumption she makes that apraxia is troublesome only with fine movements required by speech is more ingenious than convincing. The use of the term 'apraxia', a descriptive neurological term, is probably best avoided until means of testing for apraxia of tongue, lips and palate during speech are available.

The fact that five of 12 children with 'developmental articulatory apraxia' who were closely studied by Morley and her colleagues had 'some delay in the first use of words; and phrases were not attempted before 4 years', suggested similarities to histories of patients she classifies as suffering from 'developmental aphasia'. Nine of the 15 children with 'developmental aphasia' had 'defective articulation'. There seems to be a good case for grouping together patients with these two conditions into a single major category of 'specific developmental speech disorders', in which retardation of the development of language and articulation are the major characteristics. This suggestion is followed in the present classification.

It will be noted that the classification dispenses with the category of 'dyslalia' which occurs in Miss Morley's classification. The term dyslalia is used very indiscriminately by clinicians to refer to a wide variety of speech disorders in childhood. Even Morley (1957) does not provide a satisfactory definition though most of the patients she includes in the category appear to suffer from transient, usually mild, disorders of articulation not associated with obvious abnormalities of the movements of the articulatory organs or with retardation of speech development. She suggests that 'dyslalia' may be associated with mental defect, 'environmental and psychogenic factors', and imitation or persistence of faulty patterns of articulation. Many of the cases in this category could obviously be placed in other of her categories. In view of this and the wide misuse of the term dyslalia, it has been thought best to discard it.

The term 'developmental dysarthria' is misleading. The adjective 'developmental' implies that the disorder will disappear or be very much ameliorated with maturation. Yet many of the patients in the category of 'developmental dysarthria' suffer from cerebral palsy and other neurological abnormalities. In them the improvement in speech tends to be extremely disappointing, especially after the age of 5 or 6 years. In this sense their speech disorders cannot be regarded as being 'developmental'.

The aim in the present classification has been to define the categories of children's speech disorders in terms of the major abnormality of speech which is present, and by the child's associated clinical and psychological abnormalities. Clearly such a classification requires that patients shall be fully studied from a number of different points of view. This requires a team approach in modern conditions, similar to that used in cerebral palsy and child guidance clinics. If such a team approach cannot be adopted, accuracy of diagnosis of speech defects suffers, and the classification accordingly becomes less useful.

Summary

Descriptions of the commoner defects of speech encountered in a hospital speech clinic largely devoted to the treatment of pre-school children have been presented.

A new classification of speech disorders in childhood based on the major defect of speech and on associated clinical and psychological findings is given. It is emphasized that accurate diagnosis and classification of speech defects requires a team consisting of speech therapist, psychologist, paediatrician and otologist. The help of a social worker, neurologist, phonetician, child psychiatrist and other hospital staff may be required in both diagnosis and treatment.

Criticisms are made of the classification of speech defects proposed by Morley (1957) on the grounds of the imprecise use of a few neurological terms and the lack of clear definition of some of the categories proposed, in terms of clinical findings.

I have to thank Miss Morrison, Speech Therapist to the Royal Hospital for Sick Children, Edinburgh, and her assistants for their co-operation and interest during the investigation. I am indebted to Miss Mason, lately of the Psychology Department, University of Edinburgh, and Miss Mary Waller for the psychological examinations, Miss Sylvia Massey of the Department of Psychological Medicine for her psychiatric social reports, and Dr. Margaret Methven of the same Department for her consistent co-operation and help. Dr. Werner Schutt examined many of the patients from the paediatric point of view. I must thank Professor R. W. B. Ellis for his stimulus and encouragement of this work, and the physicians and surgeons of the Royal Hospital for Sick Children for their interest and co-operation during it. I am grateful to Mr. Ian Catford, Director of the School of Applied Linguistics, University of Edinburgh, who was good enough to criticize this paper.

References

Birrell, J. F. (1954). *Speech*, **18**, 40.
Calnan, J. (1957). *Ibid.*, **21**, 59.
Critchley, M. (1952). *J. Laryng.*, **66**, 1.
Drew, A. L. (1956). *Brain*, **79**, 440.
Evans, P. R. (1955). *Archives of Disease in Childhood*, **30**, 237.
Francis, T. R. (1958). *Speech Path. and Therapy*, **1**, 70.
Gibb, A. G. (1958). *J. Laryng.*, **72**, 433.
Hallgren, B. (1950). *Acta psychiat. scand.*, Suppl. 65.
Henderson, J. L. (1939). *Brain*, **62**, 381.
Ingram, T. T. S. (1956). *J. ment. Sci.*, **102**, 550.
—— and Reid, J. F. (1956). *Archives of Disease in Childhood*, **31**, 161.
Johnson, W., Brown, S. F., Curtis, J. F. Edney, C. W. and Keaster, J. (1948). *Speech Handicapped School Children.* Harper, New York.
Monrad-Krohn, G. H. (1947). *Acta psychiat. scand.*, Suppl. **46**, 204.
Morley, M. E. (1954). *Cleft Palate and Speech*, 3rd ed. Livingstone, Edinburgh.
—— (1957). *The Development and Disorders of Speech in Childhood.* Livingstone, Edinburgh.
——, Court, D. and Miller, H. (1950). *Brit. med. J.*, **1**, 574.
——, ——, —— (1954). *Ibid.*, **1**, 8.
——, ——, —— and Garside, R. F. (1955). *Ibid.*, **2**, 463.
Orton, S. T. (1937). *Reading, Writing and Speech Problems in Children* Chapman and Hall, London.
Ounsted, C. (1955). *Lancet*, **2**, 303.
Registrar General for Scotland (1951). Ninety-seventh Annual Report. H.M.S.O.
Seth, G. and Guthrie, D. (1935). *Speech in Childhood: Its Development and Disorders.* Oxford University Press, London.
Travis, L. E. (1931). *Speech Pathology*. Appleton, New York.
Van Riper, C. (1947) *Speech Correction—Principles and Methods*, 2nd ed. Prentice-Hall, New York.
Wilson, S. A. Kinnier (1954). *Neurology*, 2nd ed. Edited by A. N Bruce. Butterworth, London.

BOOK REVIEWS

Dégénérescence Hépato-Lenticulaire. By G. BOUDIN and B. PÉPIN. (Pp. vii+250. 46 figures; Fr. fr. 3,500). Paris: Masson. 1959.

Metabolic disorders are at present very popular subjects for articles and neurological metabolic abnormalities occupy a very special place in present day literature. One such disease, which is particularly suitable for a monograph, is hepato-lenticular degeneration in which an abnormality of copper metabolism is a feature. Recently, numerous articles have been published on this disorder and it has occupied a well merited prominent place in international neurological meetings. It is therefore a pleasure to be able to review a monograph by two well-known French writers, that will rank in the French language with that written by Hall on the same subject in 1921.

The two authors have seen and recorded their findings in nine cases and have reviewed much of the literature of the subject. After a short historical survey and discussion on general aetiological factors a full and wide discussion of the clinical features is given. A rather undue stress is perhaps laid on the results of the liver disorder in comparison with the neurological features. The anatomical aspects are well recorded, and this is followed by some account of the biochemical disorders. The various modes of therapy available are mentioned with the results obtained in the patients seen. Finally there is a section concerning some personal observations on nine cases of which four had not previously been recorded.

More than 700 references are mentioned, a full bibliography even though not all are references to hepato-lenticular degeneration.

Few mistakes are present, apart from the unfortunate spelling of two names in the preface. An index would have been an advantage together with a slightly more critical approach to the reports of other writers whose clinical acumen is always taken for granted, but these, however, are minor faults.

This volume should be read by all neurologists and those interested in copper metabolism.

La Psychoanalyse des Enfants. By MELANIE KLEIN. (Pp. 320; Fr. fr. 1,600.) Paris: Presse Universitaire de France. 1959.

In this translation into French of Melanie Klein's classic book *The Psycho-analysis of Children*, the text, as in the fourth English edition, is unchanged from the original published in 1932. Dr. Boulanger makes it clear that great trouble has been taken to give an accurate presentation, and Mrs. Klein has herself checked the entire translation.

Although Mrs. Klein has added to and extended her observations and theories in a number of later papers and books, the fact that no revision has been necessary in this basic work is a testimony to the accuracy, penetration and fundamental nature of Mrs. Klein's observations and theoretical arguments. This, in turn, is in a large measure due to the fact that everything she says in her books is founded on extensive clinical analytic work with children whose ages ranged from 2¾ years to 14 years.

Mrs. Klein describes how she evolved her play technique on the basis of her conviction that play is the child's natural means of expression, just as speech is that of the adult. She provided a play room with table, chairs, couch or sofa, and a basin with running water, plus small toys of varied and primitive kind.

Mrs. Klein points out that 'even a child that is usually inhibited in its play will at least glance at the toys, or touch them, and will so give me a glimpse into its complexive life by the way it begins to play with them or lays them aside, or by its general attitude towards them'.

She makes it clear that her method of analysis of children differs from the psycho-analytic treatment of adults in technique but not in principle. As opposed to certain other analysts, and to most child guidance therapists, Mrs. Klein has studiously avoided all educational measures and relies entirely on interpretation of the material the child presents in his play, his drawings, and his general attitude and behaviour towards the analyst. She thus gained access to the child's unconscious mind, and she has always made his anxieties the centre of her attention.

The first part of the book deals with the varied technique of child analysis at different ages, and contains also chapters on 'Neuroses in children' and 'The sexual activities of children' which paediatricians should find particularly useful. She shows, for example, how neurosis in childhood is not always recognized as such, and may be regarded as excessive naughtiness, or be passed over completely in an unusually 'good' child, and she shows how these characteristics are related to adult difficulties which are more generally recognized as symptoms. She gives criteria for the recognition of severe difficulties, and shows how the common factor of anxiety underlies all the varying manifestations of disorder.

In the second part of her book Mrs. Klein deals in great detail with the effects of early anxiety situations on all aspects of the development of the child, and illustrates her material with extensive clinical examples.

Le Sommeil de l'Enfant. By ROBERT DEBRÉ and ALICE DOUMIC. (Pp. xii+195; 24 figures. Fr. fr. 800.) Paris: Presse Universitaire de France. 1959.

In this book the authors discuss sleep disorders in children under 3 years of age. The subject matter is divided into five sections. The first two sections are devoted to a review of the physiology and normal pattern of sleep (including E.E.G. findings). Physical, intellectual and emotional development are summarized in the third section.

In the fourth section, the authors consider the reasons for sleep disturbances at this age based on a clinical study of 72 patients. Illustrative case reports are quoted in support of their findings. They conclude that during the first three months sleep disorders are common and almost always due to one of three causes, hunger, discomfort or maternal over-anxiety. By contrast, sleep disturbances are rarely encountered between 3 and 9 months. After 9 months wakefulness at night is again a matter of frequent concern. At this age the cause is often complex and obscure; teething is rarely an important aetiological factor.

Diagnosis and treatment are considered in the final section. The importance of considering the day-time management when evaluating the cause and treatment is emphasized.

Although sleep disturbances in the very young are a common cause of parental concern, it is a subject which has received little attention. The recorded experience of these authors is a welcome contribution towards a better understanding of this important aspect of child care.

Nursing of Children, 5th ed. By R. A. LYON and E. M. WALLINGER. (Pp. xv.+554; 156 figures. 35s.) Philadelphia and London: W. B. Saunders. 1959.

It should be noted that the title of this book from the U.S.A. is *Nursing of Children*, which implies a more comprehensive approach than the more usual title of 'Sick Children' or 'Children's Diseases'; it is a better title and carries with it expanded thought in line with the progressive outlook in the care, guidance and management of children in sickness and in health. The care of the child in its broadest interpretation calls for an increasing knowledge of the physiology of growth and development and of the mind and its relationships to health and disorder. This book wisely interprets these needs for the nurse and places before her a sensible sequence of ideas, facts and opinions.

The first 200 pages are used for applied physiology and practical care of infants and children. It is notable that there is a good detailed description of breast feeding, a distinct encouragement for those nurses who might, in some places, think that lactation and its maintenance is of relative unimportance. Good descriptions are to be found in the book: 'the care of the well child', 'training and education' and 'prevention of disease' are well thought out chapters. Poisonings and accidents receive very proper emphasis. A section on 'Children in the Home' is followed immediately by 'Children in the Hospital' and there are many sensible remarks on the social aspects, ward arrangements, toys and books and other diversional amenities: strangely enough, there is hardly a line on parents' visiting and the part they might play in the care and treatment of their own child in hospital. Some mention could usefully have been made about liaison with almoners or the domiciliary team.

The nurse as a health educator is given due prominence. Some nursing procedures are well illustrated by clear line drawings, but it is doubtful if tight strapping is really necessary for umbilical hernia. There is good systematic writing on diseases as seen in infancy and childhood and most of the statements are succinct and to the point. Coeliac disease, however, is a notable exception: it is poorly related and indicates nothing of the remarkable story of gluten and the essentials of dietetic treatment. But a few pages further on there is a much more sensible commentary on 'Tonsils and Adenoids'.

The nurse who reads this book will gather a harvest of general and allied information on 'The Convalescent Child', 'Mental Health and Child Guidance', and the values of infant welfare. Physical handicaps are discussed and ways and means of dealing with special groups are included with some special remarks on cerebral palsy. Finally, the tables at the end are very useful and surprisingly contain lists of 'Best Books for Children'. The index is good and the book is well and topically illustrated. A nurse who has really absorbed the sense and science and the spirit and humanity in this volume will not fail to create a favourable impression on the child who is placed under her care.

Survey of Clinical Pediatrics, 3rd ed. By LAWRENCE B. SLOBODY. (Pp. viii+554. 156 figures. 85s. 6d.) London: McGraw-Hill. 1959.

It has been suggested that a textbook ought properly to be reviewed by one who is intended to learn from it, and this is hardly ever done. Dr. Slobody has written and revised a book which is intended to 'help the student and practitioner focus on the highlights of pediatrics'. In reading it I have tried to put myself in the place of a student approaching paediatrics for the first time, which is not easy.

The book is not a complete work of reference but, on the other hand, it is not a synopsis; it is a fairly concise account of the whole subject including some surgical aspects, and fitting this into 550 moderately small pages has meant oversimplifying and even skimping some parts at the expense of others.

There are no pictures, which saves a great deal of space, but may make the book rather forbidding to the average student at first sight; nor are there references or bibliography, but at the end of each chapter there is a page or two of questions by which the reader may test his newly gained knowledge.

The chapter on growth and development of the normal child is particularly good and this is something one does not find well written in most paediatric textbooks of the size. Breast feeding, though encouraged, is dealt with in a mere two pages. In the short chapter on psychological problems I would have liked more emphasis on the sort of things which lead to these problems (e.g. long separation of mother and child) rather than the usual division into sections on tics, masturbation, enuresis and the like. Incidentally enuresis, which takes up so much of the paediatrician's time, is granted only half a page. Fluid and electrolyte balance is dealt with at length

(15 pages) and great detail is included in the section on treatment of its disorders.

Throughout the book, where medical treatment is described, the exact dosage or concentration of therapeutic agents is given, which is admirable. The passing reference to avoidance of wheat gluten in coeliac disease (almost, it seems, put in as an afterthought) is in line with most other American textbooks.

On the whole the book shows evidence of having been carefully written and, if one is prepared to pass quickly over such verbs as 'suctioning', it makes pleasant reading. I do not think many undergraduate medical students in this country will find the time to read it, but for the postgraduate student seeking, perhaps, the Diploma of Child Health, it may be confidently recommended.

Röntgendiagnostik beim Neugeborenen und Säugling. By HERMANN G. WOLF. (Pp. 317; 370 figures. £8 7s. 5d.) Wien-Bonn-Bern: Wilhelm Maudrich Verlag. 1959.

A textbook on diagnostic radiology confined to the first year of life is justified by the very particular aspect that congenital abnormalities, and the rapid growth and development of infants, imposes on abdominal, heart, lung and bone radiology. Dr. Wolf draws his material from the Vienna University Children's Clinic, and has as his predecessors such men as Escherich, Wimberger, Chiari and Swoboda, which ensures its high quality. The book is divided into three sections dealing with the skeletal system, chest and the abdomen respectively. Within each section various conditions are briefly discussed in the text, followed by radiographs and, at times, by diagrams, each with its own explanatory note. The book claims to be comprehensive, and on the whole the range is very wide indeed, though there are some rather obvious omissions. Thoracic tuberculosis is deliberately left out. Fractures are also not dealt with at all, presumably because of their rarity in the first year of life, and there is no mention of thoracic tumours or cysts, nor of abdominal neoplasms. It is obvious that Dr. Wolf confines his attention almost entirely to the newborn baby, and it would have been better if this had been made clear by omitting the word 'infant' (Säugling) from the title. There is at times also a lack of balance in the space devoted to different conditions: pyloric stenosis, for instance, gets 10 pages and no less than 27 very beautiful radiographs; diaphragmatic hernia gets eight pages and 22 illustrations, whereas congenital heart disease is encompassed in four pages and 13 illustrations, and rickets in just three illustrations. Other less important criticisms might be that there is no systematic use of erect and prone, or even AP and PA views of the chest; that a chronological series of ossification centres might have been included; that a clearer exposition of the interpretation encephalo- and ventriculograms would have been appreciated. However, perhaps almost all these failures are redeemed by the standard of radiology and the quality of reproductions which are uniformly high throughout, and at times almost unbelievably good. In the abdomen some of the radiographs have an almost three-dimensional appearance. This is to some extent due to the practice of reproducing positives rather than negatives, and is one which might well be copied in monthly periodicals. This pictorial excellence and the quality of the paper and the binding make it a pleasurable as well as a useful book to possess, and is the only textbook on radiology devoted to the newborn infant known to the reviewer.

THE MAINTENANCE OF STABILITY IN THE NEWLY BORN*

2. THERMAL BALANCE

BY

R. A. McCANCE

From the Medical Research Council Department of Experimental Medicine, Cambridge

Thermal stability, which is one of the hall marks of mammalian efficiency, must always be associated with metabolism and chemical stability, for the production of heat depends largely on biological oxidations and these in turn depend upon the supply of oxygen. Anything which interferes with this constitutes an immediate threat both to chemical stability and thermal stability, but the temperature of the body also plays a vital part in regulating the metabolic rate and hence the demand for oxygen, so that each reacts upon the other.

The Basis of Thermal Control

The maintenance of thermal balance rather than a constant internal temperature may be the real basis of temperature control (Glaser and Newling, 1957), for both the central and superficial temperatures do vary as part of their participation in the overall stability of the adult body, but these are among the finer points at present. Thermal stability is brought about by the production of heat and the loss of heat being kept about the same. Heat production is the result of the metabolic activity of all the cells of the body when it is at rest, together with the additional production due to muscular exertion. The basal production is extensively modified by thyroid activity and affected by the environmental temperature (Osiba, 1957). Heat is lost mainly from the body surface, and if a person were completely insulated against heat loss his temperature would go up at a rate which would bring it to boiling point in about two days if the mechanisms for heat production were not, as of course they would be, inactivated long before this temperature had been reached. The amount of heat lost from the surface of the body would tend to vary only in accordance with air movement and the surrounding temperature, were it not that the rate of loss can be greatly reduced at low temperatures by constricting the blood supply to the periphery and extremities and allowing them to take up temperatures far below the central parts and not much above those of the surroundings. Animals with fur and birds with feathers can modify their heat losses to some extent by erecting their hair or fluffing out their feathers, and some large animals which live in a cold environment are very well protected against heat loss by long hair and a thick layer of subcutaneous fat. Heat is also lost from the lungs by the evaporation of water and by warming the inspired air, but in man these losses are linked to the metabolic needs and are not varied apart from them. At high environmental temperatures the rate of heat loss in man is adjusted to the requirements of the body by sweating, which deposits a film of water on the skin. The evaporation which follows keeps down the body temperature even when the environmental temperature is higher. In animals without sweat glands this way of losing heat may be replaced by passing air very rapidly in and out over the large wet surfaces provided by their tongues.

Animals vary greatly in their response to a change in their environmental temperature, but there are features common to all. There is a fast response followed by a much slower one if the change persists, and the whole constitutes the process of acclimatization which enables the animal to become master of its new surroundings. A rapid increase in metabolic rate is the immediate response in all warm blooded animals to a fall in environmental temperature, and this is indeed the chief response of mice and other small rodents, for they do little to reduce their loss of heat by varying their insulation or vasomotor control. It is a biological impossibility that they should do so to any extent, for the weight of the insulating material required for such small animals

* The Leonard Parsons Lectures delivered in Birmingham on May 12 and 13, 1959.

at low temperatures would immobilize them. Some strains of mice increase their oxygen consumption by as much as four times when they are transferred from a temperature of 21°C. to −3°C. By doing so and making for themselves good nests (Barnett and Manly, 1958) they are able to maintain a normal body temperature, but they require just that much more food, which in nature they have to find (Barnett, 1956, 1959; Barnett and Manly, 1956; Barnett, Coleman and Manly, 1959). Increased tone and shivering constitute the first line of defence against a sudden fall in the environmental temperature, and this is the role of the skeletal muscles. It is initiated by reflexes from the skin, and if the shivering thus initiated is not enough to maintain the 'core' temperature, the fall in the latter greatly intensifies the muscular response (Giaja and Gelineo, 1931; Pickering, 1958). After the process of acclimatization is complete the metabolic rate remains high, although the animals are no longer shivering. This is usually attributed to increased 'tone' in the skeletal muscles, but what this means in terms of mechanical work and tissue metabolism nobody knows (Baker and Sellers, 1953; Burton and Edholm, 1955; Scholander, 1958). The basal metabolic rate also rises after a time, and this rise persists and can be demonstrated after the animal has been restored to a higher environmental temperature once more (Engelmann, 1930; Sellers and You, 1950). The liver participates in this (Burton and Edholm, 1955) as well as the muscles and heart, but not, it seems, the thymus, testis or brain (Hart, 1958).

A fundamental point in thermal control at all ages, but particularly in the newly born, is the environmental temperature at which the metabolic rate of the animal is at its lowest. This is variously termed the critical temperature or the point of thermal neutrality. It is really a band or range of temperature within which variations in heat loss enable the animal to maintain a normal body temperature with the least possible expenditure of energy. Departure from it in either direction raises the metabolic rate. If the environmental temperature has fallen the rise in metabolic rate will serve a useful purpose in maintaining the temperature in the body desirable for that species, but if the reverse has taken place the body temperature will rise and it is this which produces the rise in metabolic rate (see later). The critical temperature varies with the age of the animal (Cairnie and Pullar, 1957) and the plane of nutrition (Graham, Wainman, Blaxter and Armstrong, 1959), and is considerably higher soon after birth than it is in later life. It also varies from one species to another.

The laws of physics and chemistry provide that the rates at which chemical reactions proceed vary directly with the temperature of the system in which they are taking place. The metabolic rate of an animal without temperature control, therefore, varies closely and directly with the environmental temperature. If the temperature of an animal with any semblance of temperature control is lowered sufficiently there comes a time when its metabolic rate and oxygen consumption fall in spite of the increase in metabolism which was tending to prevent it, and this can be enormously facilitated by abolishing the normal adaptive response. This is the way in which the body temperature is lowered (Hellings, 1958; Pickering, 1958) in order to reduce the metabolism for therapeutic or experimental purposes, but a subnormal temperature in a newborn baby or any other young animal is no proof that it has a lower metabolic rate than it would have at its critical temperature. In fact, the reverse is much more probable if it is making any adaptive response (Giaja and Gelineo, 1931; Krog, Monson and Irving, 1955; Hart, 1958).

The response of an adult to a change in the environmental temperature is a very complicated one (Scholander, 1958), integrated at various levels and depending upon the central nervous system (Pickering, 1958), and a co-ordinating 'centre' in the hypothalamus (Ranson, 1940; Kennedy, 1953). Successful adaptation depends upon the hypophysis (Thibault, 1949), and the suprarenal glands participate at two stages. Part of the immediate increase in metabolic rate is almost certainly due to the release of adrenalin and nor-adrenalin, although precisely how these operate is obscure (Griffith, 1951). Their effects are not abolished by curare (Hsieh and Carlson, 1957), and they are intensified in an animal which has become fully acclimatized to cold. Thyroidectomy reduces them (Swanson, 1956). The cortex of the suprarenal is also essential for successful acclimatization to a lowered environmental temperature (Ingle, 1958), and is thought to be one of the organs responsible for the higher metabolic rate which develops slowly and persists for some time. The thyroid is also involved in this (You, You and Sellers, 1950).

The energy derived from the oxidation of protein, fat and carbohydrate is used for the synthesis of compounds such as adenosine triphosphate and creatine phosphate, which contain high energy phosphate bonds and with which the cell is able to carry out the work required of it. Some of the energy is 'wasted' and dissipated as heat which the homoeotherm also requires *per se*, but it is generally thought that in the healthy and intact cell most of the oxidation is coupled with the synthesis of these high energy phosphate bonds and limited by the amount of work required for functional efficiency. Bilirubin and a number of other poisons, such as cyanide, interfere with many of the oxidation processes in a less specific way and reduce the coupling as well. Others, such as dinitrophenol and possibly thyroxin, also interfere with the coupling, but in a different way, for they allow the oxygen consumption and heat production to rise to high levels without the performance of any visible or invisible work. Some such uncoupling, if physiological, or some purposeful deviation of the metabolic pathways to bypass the coupling mechanisms, would produce the heat required by the body for acclimatization more economically than any other way, and the possibilities of this happening in the processes of acclimatization are being actively explored (Depocas, MacLeod and Hart, 1957; Hart, 1958; Potter, 1958; Smith, 1958). Adaptive changes in the enzyme systems are well recognized to take place in the kidney, at any rate in some animals (Rector, Seldin, Roberts and Copenhaver, 1954; Rector and Orloff, 1959), and some such deviation from the more usual metabolic pathways is now accepted as a cause of hereditary obesity in mice (Tepperman, 1958; Zomzely and Mayer, 1958) and possibly in human obesity (Pawan, 1959).

Whatever its size, the body temperature of an adult is largely a matter of its own genetics and biophysical efficiency. The white rhinoceros or the hippopotamus, which both live in equatorial Africa where the temperature may be 32°C. in the shade, and which both weigh upwards of 3,000,000 g., have body temperatures of the order of 35°C. (Allbrook, Harthoorn, Luck and Wright, 1958; Luck and Wright, 1959), whereas a mouse living at −3°C. and weighing about 30 g. has a body temperature around 37·5°C. (Barnett, 1956).

The matter of size, however, is an important one in temperature regulation because small bodies have relatively greater surface areas than large ones and therefore cool more quickly in surroundings below the temperature of their bodies. This has been compensated for, however, in nature by the arrangement that birds and animals, large and small, have metabolic rates in proportion to their surface areas rather than to their weights. This is one of the great biological generalizations, but how it is brought about is quite unknown. Why each cell in a mouse has so much higher a metabolic rate than each one in an elephant is unknown, but the solution of this problem should help us to understand the processes of acclimatization.

The Newborn Animal

Whatever it may do towards maintaining its own chemical stability *in utero*, the unborn animal has no responsibilities for its body temperature, and most animals are born before they have acquired all the integrated mechanisms they will later require for the control of their body temperatures. The newborn rat is almost poikilothermic at birth and takes up the temperature of its surroundings. Puppies and kittens have little more thermal stability, but less is known about them. The lamb and the pig are both examples of animals with a good measure of temperature control at birth, and so within limits is the human infant. Edwards (1824, 1832), the great pioneer in this subject, showed that this was not just a matter of size, but also one of immaturity. By choosing adults and newborn animals from different species he found out that tiny adult birds like wrens had far greater thermal stability than newly hatched birds such as hawks which were much larger, when both were exposed to an external temperature of 17°C. Edwards also realized that many newborn animals would never survive unless a special environment had been created for them by nature. He pointed out that the proximity of the rest of the litter huddled together in a nest protected each member of the litter from the cold they would have to face in isolation. With this shelter of the nest and the warmth of the mother's body, to which the newborn animal always tends to move, even the newborn rat can achieve a body temperature high enough to enable it to feed and grow, and mice can be reared by their mothers in a good nest at −3°C. (Barnett, 1956) and breed in cold meat stores at much lower temperatures, even down to −21°C. (Laurie, 1946). If the mother of an animal without temperature control leaves the nest and fails to return for some time the temperature of the newborn animals must fall and with it their demands for oxygen. This is probably no disadvantage for a time, for it reduces the consumption of energy material within the body without doing the newborn any harm (Fairfield, 1948). The survival time of eviscerated, and therefore poikilothermic, adult rats is reduced if the temperature is raised from 26° to 38°C., but this effect can be countered to a large extent by the administration of glucose (Ingle and Nezamis, 1950).

The metabolic rate of a poikilothermic animal like the newborn rat varies with its environmental and consequently its body temperature. The oxygen consumption of the newborn lamb, however, rises three to four times between the last days *in utero*, when it has an oxygen consumption in keeping with its mother's surface area, and the second day of life when it has one more in line with its own (Dawes and Mott, 1958, 1959). Pigs have not been investigated *in utero* but their oxygen consumption also rises rapidly in the first days after birth (Mount, 1958a). With the knowledge available to us at the moment we must regard this rise in oxygen consumption as the response of struggling but still imperfect homoeotherms to a fall in their environmental and also, probably, in their somatic temperature, for after birth pigs have been shown to raise their oxygen consumption steadily as the ambient temperature falls below that of their own point of thermal neutrality (Holub, Forman and Ježková, 1957; Mount, 1958b). Giaja (1925a, b), another pioneer, put forward a way of expressing all this quantitatively and of comparing the response of one young animal with that of another.

Man certainly, and most large animals also, regulate their thermal balance to a large extent by 'physical' methods, i.e. by varying the dissipation and conservation of the heat produced within them by their natural activities, but there is evidence that this is not so to any great extent in the newborn human infant or animal (Hahn, 1956c; McIntyre and Ederstrom, 1958). Piglets (Mount, 1959) and many other newborn animals with similar possibilities open to them (Baccino, 1935) increase their effective size by huddling together and so reducing their cooling surface, but speaking generally the newborn animal achieves what measure of thermal control it may possess (if in isolation) by 'chemical' methods, i.e. by varying its heat production, and this is not possible before the neurones in the hypothalamus are myelinated (Reynolds, 1953). Adult rodents and particularly mice (Barnett, 1959; Barnett *et al.*, 1959) certainly employ chemical rather than physical methods, particularly in isolation, and this is what makes them a valuable study for those interested in the newborn of larger species. Barnett and Manly (1958) have given an account of the ability of young mice of various ages and strains to survive transference from 21°C. to −3°C., and in this work investigations were made of the role of the thyroid and adrenal glands in various ways.

On the analogy of what happens in adults, it may be presumed that the greater part of any increase in the oxygen consumption registered during the hours following birth or subsequently in response to a fall in the ambient temperature takes place in the skeletal muscles. The lamb and pig may shiver violently soon after birth, but a great increase in the metabolic rate can take place without it (Dawes and Mott, 1958, 1959). It is not known why the oxygen consumption does not reach the level at which it stabilizes for some days, but if the skeletal muscles are as poorly equipped with respiratory enzyme systems as the liver of the rat would appear to be (Dawkins, 1959) it is fully understandable. The liver of all animals develops many of its functions with great rapidity after birth (Driscoll and Hsia, 1958), and this may contribute something to the increased heat production, but it can have little to do with the thermal regulation of the body, for the respiratory enzymes in the liver of the newborn rat mature in a matter of days, whereas thermal stability is not attained for several weeks and the liver is not the centre of it.

Wherever it takes place, the increased metabolic rate which follows birth in animals with some measure of thermal control at that time can only be brought about by the combustion of protein, fat and carbohydrate. These may have been in the body at birth or be supplied as food. In either case they are the price which the newborn animal has to pay for thermal stability outside the uterus. The newborn poikilothermic rat pays no such price; the mother provides the whole service, and nearly all the food can be used for somatic development. It is worth a thought, therefore, that every degree below their critical temperature at which the pig, lamb or human baby may be held, reduces the amount of material available for survival or growth. This is no doubt why the young rat 10 days old lives no longer without food at an environmental temperature of 20°C. than at 30°C. although it has had a lower body temperature all the time it has been exposed to the lower environmental one (Braun and Mosinger, 1958). We have been able to put a quantitative figure on this by keeping newborn pigs in metabolism cages without food or water for the first 24 hours of their lives. At an ambient temperature of 31°C. these animals lived quite comfortably for at least 48 hours and had blood sugars and body temperatures within normal limits at the end. At an ambient temperature of 12°C., however, the animals could only maintain reasonably normal body temperatures for 8-12 hours. Their temperatures fell more and more rapidly after this and by about 24 hours were usually 20-22°C., their blood sugars were very low and the animals were *in extremis* (Fig. 1). Hypoglycaemia has been observed before in newborn piglets who were at the point of death (Morrill, 1952; Goodwin, 1957) and the administration of glucose is said to have been beneficial (Morrill and Sampson, 1952). Table 1 shows the way in which the ambient temperature affected the breakdown of protein, fat and carbohydrate within the body. In these animals glycogen was the main source of energy, for newborn pigs contain practically no fat, and the Table shows to what extent lowering the environmental temperature increased their rate of utilization. This is not the whole story, however. Once the body temperature falls, deviations from the normal metabolic

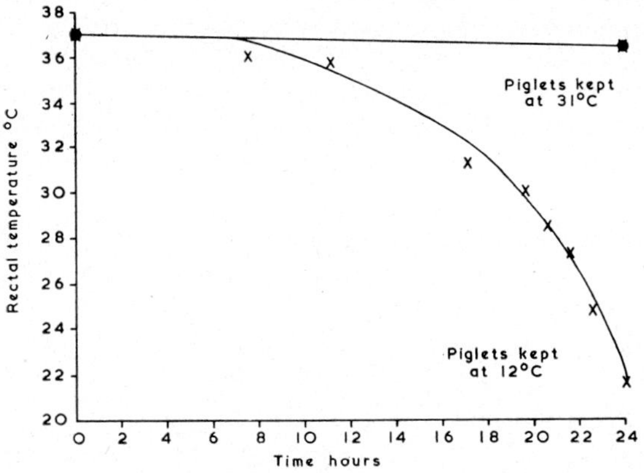

FIG. 1.—Rectal temperatures of piglets kept at 12°C. and 31°C. for 24 hours.

TABLE 1

EFFECT OF AMBIENT TEMPERATURE ON BREAKDOWN OF TISSUE SOLIDS IN STARVING NEWBORN PIGLET

	Solids Catabolized			
	(g./kg./24 hr.)		Percent of Total	
	Hot	Cold	Hot	Cold
Total solids	13·4	28·6	—	—
Protein	0·6	1·7	4·9	6·7
Fat	2·9	3·9	21·5	13·6
Carbohydrate 'by difference'	9·9	23·0	74	80
Glycogen directly determined	9·0	19·8	67	69

pattern may follow (Wynn, 1954, 1956), and we have ourselves encountered some of them (McCance and Widdowson, 1959b). A suggestive side issue has opened up in the course of this work. The amount of weight lost and volume of urine formed were similar at 31° and 12°C., but the animals kept at 12°C. metabolized so much more of their body solids that they became more watery than the others and actually developed oedema. Premature babies may do the same even when they are given nothing by mouth. This oedema may have a similar origin.

The development of temperature control after birth can be studied most completely and easily in animals which have very little control when they are born. The puppy has recently been investigated (McIntyre and Ederstrom, 1958) and the mouse (Barnett and Manly, 1958), but the rat has had most attention. Adolph (1948, 1957), Fairfield (1948) and others in America have worked at it extensively and so have a group of active investigators in Czechoslovakia (Hahn, 1956a, b, c, d; Hahn, Křeček and Křečková, 1956; Křeček, Křečková and Martínek, 1957; Hahn and Koldovský, 1958a, b, 1959). Many of the conclusions so far are based upon results obtained after removing the thyroid or adrenal glands which may be a rather crude technique (Astwood, 1957), and some of them may have been confused by the effects of restraint (Bartlett, Bohr and Inman, 1955; Hahn and Koldovský, 1958b). Full temperature control is not acquired till the animals are about 26 days old. Only at 14 days does the thyroid begin to play any part, and although the newborn animals soon begin to grow hair, this does not improve their thermal control till they are 18 days old. The adrenal glands may also be involved (Tyslowitz and Astwood, 1942; Hubble, 1957). Jailer (1953) thought that they only began to respond to the stimulus of cold about the sixteenth day of life although they were capable of reacting to ACTH and adrenalin before this time. More recent work (Hahn and Koldovský, 1958a) suggests that a response can be detected by the fifth day if the stimulus is not too severe. To what extent these glands function in the newborn pig or man is still unsolved, in spite of all the work which has been put into their investigation by paediatricians (Gardner, 1956; Harlem and Myhre, 1957).

With such poor control of their own body temperatures few animals would live through their first days in the world were it not for the fact that they can tolerate and survive a much greater fall in body temperature than adults of the same species (Adolph, 1951). In that investigation Adolph showed that some adult guinea-pigs, rabbits and cats survived body temperatures of 18°C., and rats 14°C., whereas golden hamsters could be cooled with impunity to much lower body temperatures. Newborn guinea-pigs were cooled successfully only to 15°C., but these animals are very mature at birth. Newborn kittens and rabbits were cooled to 6°C. and rats and hamsters survived after their temperatures had been as low as 0°C. Work on hypothermia in adults has gone forward very rapidly since Adolph's publication (Andjus and Smith, 1954; Goldzveig and Smith, 1956; Colloquium, 1957), and it is now known that by taking the right precautions remarkably low body temperatures can be achieved even in man (Drew and Anderson, 1959; Drew, Keen and Benazon, 1959). Rats and monkeys have been cooled to 5°C. with recovery (Niazi and Lewis, 1954, 1957). The concentration of carbon dioxide in the tissues may be important for survival (Miller and Miller, 1958), as it is in oxygen deficiency. A young woman, who was found in the snow with a body temperature of about 16°C., has recovered although extensively injured by frostbite (Laufman, 1951). Other examples of accidental hypothermia in man, not quite so severe, and not complicated by frostbite have been recorded by Rees (1958).

The Human Infant

Physiologically the human infant born at term seems to fall into the natural scheme of things so far as its thermal stability is concerned. In cold surroundings it can maintain a normal body temperature better than the puppy, kitten, rabbit or rat but probably not as well as the guinea-pig, and certainly not as well as the lamb. The full term infant is so much larger than the newborn pig that the control of its body temperature must always be easier, but it seems to have about the same measure of thermal control. It has been known for many years (Preyer, 1885; Raudnitz, 1888; Burnard and Cross, 1958; Smith, 1959) that the body temperature tends to fall soon after birth and then to rise again within the next 12 hours to a more normal adult level. This is exactly what one would expect from work on the rise in oxygen consumption which follows birth in the pig or lamb, and the way in which newborn infants respond to a change in their environmental temperature (Mordhorst, 1932). In all respects the premature infant has much less stability (Blackfan and Yaglou, 1933). In all infants much depends on the ambient temperature, but the chances of hypothermia must always be high so long as the basal metabolic rates remain below those of adults per unit of surface area. This has always been found to be the case (Marsh and Murlin, 1925; Du Bois, 1936; Day, Curtis and Kelly, 1943; Boekelman, 1957), and these rates would certainly have been lower had they been measured in the zone of thermal neutrality.

Like all other newborn animals the human infant is very tolerant of low body temperatures, and moderate hypothermia has been advocated for premature infants with the idea that it would reduce their metabolic rate and oxygen requirements. This must remain *sub judice* at present and each case will always require separate assessment, but the work of Silverman, Fertig and Berger (1958) indicates that hypothermia is not good paediatrics. Uncontrolled exposure to cold is certainly an insidious and dangerous enemy (Mann and Elliott, 1957). Babies born in very cold weather in homes that are inadequately heated are sometimes admitted to hospital suffering from the effects of this. By the time these babies reach the eye and the touch of an expert they may have passed from a physiological to a pathological state, and present with some superadded infection. They always feel cold, but in spite of this they may appear surprisingly well, with red face and hands. Sometimes the external cold has made the extremities oedematous and the skin hard and white. The protracted exposure lowers their body temperature internally and makes them apathetic and unwilling to take food, and perhaps because of this they sometimes have blood sugars low enough to cause convulsions. They may die before or during treatment from what appears to be respiratory failure, and pulmonary haemorrhage has often been found after death.

From what is known about animals one must suppose that the thyroid and suprarenal glands are integral parts of the stabilizing mechanisms, but our knowledge of their role in thermal regulation or anything else at birth is woefully small (Gardner, 1956; Harlem and Myhre, 1957; Khalil, 1958), and there is scope for some imaginative work on this subject in animals and then in mankind.

Once a baby has become pathologically chilled, glucose should probably be given cautiously before the temperature is raised, for hypoglycaemia may be expected, and warming without giving glucose may precipitate convulsions in piglets.

Up to this point one may say that newborn animals have very variable but always poor temperature control, and in their usual surroundings tend to get cold. Life in nature must always be a compromise, in this instance between the well-being of the mother and the newborn. Young animals tolerate a subnormal body temperature extremely well, but there is no evidence that it is ever in itself beneficial or should be allowed, and there is good evidence that newborn animals might benefit if they could spend the first critical days of their lives within their range of thermal neutrality. Such ambient temperatures, however, would sometimes be harmful to the maternal organism.

The Lesser of Two Evils

The lethal effects of a complete or partial failure of the respiratory exchanges have already been described. The tolerance of the newborn for a lack of oxygen has also been discussed, the reasons for it and its results in terms of chemical stability. A change-over from aerobic to anaerobic metabolism has, however, got other important consequences, for anaerobic metabolism produces much less heat. The complete oxidation of a molecule of glucose to CO_2 and water, for example, provides at least 10 times more heat than its conversion to lactic acid, which is as far as the process can go in nitrogen (Hendricks, 1957). This fall in heat production makes no difference to the body temperature of a poikilotherm such as the newborn mouse, but it tends to lower the body temperature of others (unless they are in very warm surroundings), particularly of those with imperfect control of their body temperature. As already described, if adaptation is not taking place, any fall in body temperature slows down all the chemical processes of the body, including the utilization of the glycogen stores and the accumulation of acid metabolites, either of which may be fatal. Notwithstanding any bad effects which hypothermia itself may have, many experiments have demonstrated the survival value of a fall of body temperature when the animal is facing immediate extinction from anoxaemia. Thus Fazekas, Alexander and Himwich (1941) and Himwich (1953) found that the survival time of day-old and therefore still poikilothermic rats in nitrogen was raised from 20 minutes to 50 minutes by lowering their body temperature from 34°C. to 24°C. (see also Adolph, 1948, 1957). Selle and Witten (1941) made some experiments with a bearing upon this. They showed that the isolated heads of newborn rats gave more gasps per minute when the temperature was raised, but not more gasps *in toto*. Consequently, raising the temperature reduced the time for which the heads went on gasping. Cooling the heads had the opposite effect. More recent and more extensive experiments on newborn guinea-pigs have shown that cooling the animals in ice water up to the neck prolongs their life when they are made to breathe a mixture of 95% nitrogen and 5% carbon dioxide (Miller and Miller, 1953, 1954; Miller, 1954).

A reduction in the partial pressure of oxygen in respired air has been a common enough human experience since men began to mountaineer, and the effects have been well investigated; respiratory failure and distress are dangers at all times of life. Cardiac failure and abnormalities may produce very similar end results. It is generally recognized in adults that there is rarely, if ever, any reduction in oxygen consumption when the pressure of oxygen in the ambient air falls, even to the low levels met with at very high altitudes (Barcroft, Elliott, Fraser, Herkel, Matthews and Talaat, 1934; Houston and Riley, 1947; Rothschuh, 1947; Frank and Wezler, 1948; Pugh, 1957). The oxygen tension falls in the arterial blood, but a sustained increase in respiration and alveolar ventilation helps to maintain the supply of oxygen to the tissues. This is true also of the adult dog (Cordier and Mayer, 1935; Gorlin and Lewis, 1954) and to a somewhat lesser extent of the rabbit (Hamon, Kolodny and Mayer, 1935), and no doubt of most other adult mammals over a certain size (Cross, Dawes and Mott, 1959). A reduction in the percentage saturation of the arterial blood, therefore, does not materially affect the heat production of adult men, sheep or dogs. The smaller mammals, however, do not react in this way (Béhague, Garsaux and Richet, 1927; Gellhorn and Janus, 1936), except when they are held within their range of thermal neutrality (Lintzel, 1931), and at usual environmental temperatures the oxygen consumption and with it the body temperature of mice begin to fall when the percentage of oxygen in the surrounding air is reduced to about 16% (Chevillard and Mayer, 1935), with a corresponding fall in the percentage saturation of the arterial blood. The fall in body temperature so diminishes the demands of the tissues for metabolic exchange that it prolongs the survival time of these animals (Strughold, 1954), and this has repeatedly been demonstrated experimentally in a number of ways (Campbell, 1936, 1938). It is possible that the thyroid is involved in this fall of temperature (Smith, Emmens and Parkes, 1946-1948).

Newborn animals, including the human infant, behave like the small adult rodents. This was first observed by Cross, Tizard and Trythall (1955, 1958), who showed that when the oxygen in the ambient air of a newborn baby was reduced from the normal 21% to 15% there was only a trifling increase in ventilation rate, and the consumption of oxygen fell by some 17%. The respiratory effects in infants have also been observed by Behrle and Smull (1957), and it has been claimed that reducing the oxygen in the ambient air has a place in the management of infants (Sjöstedt and Rooth, 1957). The fall in oxygen consumption was confirmed by Moore (1956a, b), who used puppies and kittens as his experimental animals. Similar effects have been noted in the lamb (Acheson, Dawes and Mott, 1957; Cross, Dawes and Mott, 1958b). Hill (1958) has reconfirmed all these results in kittens, and added the important point that the oxygen consumption only falls to any extent if the animals are being held below their critical temperature. This suggests that the decrease in oxygen consumption takes place mainly in those organs in which it is thought to increase when the environmental temperature falls below the critical one. The organs mainly involved are probably the skeletal muscles, and work on the lamb supports this suggestion (Cross *et al.*, 1958b, 1959). It is known that animals do not shiver when they are anoxic. If the reflex circuit required for shivering and tone in the skeletal muscles at this age could operate only when the tension of oxygen in the tissues was sufficiently high, a great deal of these facts could be very simply explained, for then the thermoregulatory metabolism of the skeletal muscles would virtually cease when the tension of oxygen fell. Alternatively, one of the oxidizing enzymes in the muscles may become inoperative when the tension of oxygen in the tissues falls. It is impossible to decide between these suggestions at present, even if either is right, for it has not yet been shown, and this is a vital theoretical point, whether the reduction in aerobic metabolism is replaced by an equivalent amount of anaerobic metabolism. The second theory suggests that it would be. At all events, as might have been predicted on either theory, all the investigators are agreed that a fall in body temperature follows the reduction in oxygen consumption (Moore, 1956b; Brodie, Cross and Lomer, 1957). Burnard and Cross (1958) showed this in experiments which had been arranged for them by nature in a group of full-term infants who had suffered from some degree of asphyxia at birth. Other things being equal, one must suppose that a fall in oxygen consumption *per se* will mitigate the effects of partial asphyxia or hypoxaemia if they are prolonged, and at most environmental temperatures any reduction in oxygen consumption, whatever its cause, must be followed by a fall in the production of heat, particularly in those organs which are responsible for maintaining the temperature of the body above that of its surroundings. Everything which is known suggests that the fall in body temperature, which will invariably follow, will further mitigate the effects of the deficiency of oxygen and prolong the period of survival. Within the zone of thermal neutrality hypoxaemia did not lead to the same reduction of oxygen consumption (Hill, 1958) and consequently there should have been less fall in body temperature. One would expect both these statements to be true of the foetus *in utero* yet, strangely enough, progressive hypoxaemia in the foetus does lead to a progressive reduction in its consumption of oxygen and the same seems to be true of the newborn animal immediately after birth (Dawes, 1959; Cross *et al.*, 1959; Dawes and Mott, 1959). In these experiments on the foetus the lamb was being maintained at a constant temperature in a saline bath, but its body temperature must be equally well maintained *in utero*, so there can be no fall in it there.

The pathological sequence is now clear enough to indicate that if anoxaemia has been a cause of a fall in the body temperature of the human infant, treatment should begin with the administration of glucose. This will enable the anaerobic metabolism to go on as long as possible, and the acidosis which will inevitably be created by it should be countered by simultaneous administration of bicarbonate. There is no concrete evidence at present whether the hypothermia should be put right before, during or after the relief of the anoxaemia, but there are many indications that one should begin by correcting the hypoxaemia.

When I was privileged to give the Goulstonian lectures at the College of Physicians in 1936 I waxed very enthusiastic about the future of biochemistry. I recalled Prout's discoveries in it over 100 years before and I suggested that its influence on medicine was still only beginning to be felt and that there was no reason why neurology might not become just as chemical a subject as nutrition, or that certain problems of psychology and even of human behaviour might not be solved in the future by the biochemists (McCance, 1936). As I sat down the President rose to his feet and castigated me properly for my presumption, and in particular for supposing that anything which came out of a test tube could ever influence the psyche of man. I felt utterly crushed and went home that night feeling that I had been a very silly young man. Times have changed very rapidly, and biochemistry has been acclaimed by all to be one of the great conquering forces in the world of medicine of today. More and more biochemists are trying to isolate functions, cells, even parts of cells and enzyme systems, and to study them apart from their natural surroundings. This is most valuable work and no one could admire it more than I do, although I am not able to keep up with the pace, but many of the adaptations to extra-uterine life will not be solved by organic chemistry. Most of them involve the integration of several functions, and sometimes the co-ordinated responses of mother and young. I do not wish to go back now on one word which I said in 1936 and I am not yet as old as the President was at that time, nor will I ever have his wisdom, but I can see the dangers now and I am inclined to think that no army of biochemists, equipped with all the photometers and chromatography in the world, will ever solve these problems by themselves. The study of isolated systems can be very misleading and it tends to breed isolated minds. There will always be a place in physiology and in medicine for men like Sir Leonard Parsons who are interested in the study of the whole animal and have the breadth of vision necessary for it. The study is a specialization in itself, and perhaps the most difficult one of all. Those who attempt it will never any more be able to understand all the biochemistry behind the isolated functions they are trying to co-ordinate. They must always be prepared to talk humbly to the experts (other experts!) for the best information available about it, and use the knowledge to further the welfare of the animal to which they are devoting their lives.

I have received help over these lectures from people who work all over the world and I have visited some of them in places as far apart as Prague and Vancouver. It would be difficult to acknowledge them all. I must, however, single out our secretaries, the nurses, the hospital staff, the animal attendants, and all those past and present members of the department who have made the lectures possible at all. They are my joint authors, in fact, if not in name.

REFERENCES (Parts 1 and 2)

Acheson, G. H., Dawes, G. S. and Mott, J. C. (1957). Oxygen consumption and the arterial oxygen saturation in foetal and newborn lambs. *J. Physiol* (*Lond.*), **135**, 623.
Adolph, E. F. (1948). Tolerance to cold and anoxia in infant rats. *Amer. J. Physiol.*, **155**, 366.
—— (1951). Responses to hypothermia in several species of infant mammals. *Ibid.*, **166**, 75.
—— (1957). Ontogeny of physiological regulations in the rat. *Quart. Rev. Biol.*, **32**, 89.
Ahlfeld, F. (1906). Fruchtwasserschwund in der zweiten Schwangerschaftshälfte, eine typische Form der Oligohydramnie. *Z. Geburtsh. Gynäk.*, **57**, 67.
Alexander, D. P., Nixon, D. A., Widdas, W. F. and Wohlzogen, F. X. (1958a). Gestational variations in the composition of the foetal fluids and foetal urine in the sheep. *J. Physiol.* (*Lond.*), **140**, 1.
——, ——, ——, —— (1958b). Renal function in the sheep foetus. *Ibid.*, **140**, 14.
Allbrook, D. B., Harthoorn, A. M., Luck, C. P. and Wright, P. G. (1958). Temperature regulation in the white rhinoceros. *Ibid.*, **143**, 51P.
Allison, A. C. (1955). Danger of vitamin K to newborn. *Lancet*, **1**, 669.
Ames, R. G. (1953). Urinary water excretion and neurohypophysial function in full-term and premature infants shortly after birth. *Pediatrics*, **12**, 272.
Anderson, E. P., Kalckar, H. M. and Isselbacher, K. J. (1957). Defect in uptake of galactose-1-phosphate into liver nucleotides in congenital galactosemia. *Science*, **125**, 113.
Andjus, R. K. and Smith, A. U. (1954). Revival of hypothermic rats after arrest of circulation and respiration. *J. Physiol.* (*Lond.*), **123** 66P.
Apgar, V., Girdany, B. R., McIntosh, R. and Taylor, H. C. (1955). Neonatal anoxia. 1. A study of the relation of oxygenation at birth to intellectual development. *Pediatrics*, **15**, 653.
Astwood, E. B. (1957). The adrenal cortex and energy metabolism. In *Hormonal Regulation of Energy Metabolism.* Ed. L. W. Kinsell, p. 223. Thomas, Springfield, Illinois.
Baccino, M. (1935). La température optimum de croissance des jeunes homéothermes. Diverses méthodes de determination. *C.R. Soc. Biol.* (*Paris*), **119**, 1246.
Baird, D. (1957). *Combined Textbook of Obstetrics and Gynaecology*, 6th ed. Livingstone, Edinburgh.
Baker, D. G. and Sellers, E. A. (1953). Carbohydrate metabolism in the rat exposed to a low environmental temperature. *Amer. J. Physiol.*, **174**, 459.
Baker, H., Ziffer, H., Pasher, I. and Sobotka, H. (1958). A comparison of maternal and foetal folic acid and vitamin B_{12} at parturition. *Brit. med. J.*, **1**, 978.
Bangham, D. R., Ingram, P. L., Roy, J. H. B., Shillam, K. W. G. and Terry, R. J. (1958). The absorption of ^{131}I-labelled serum and colostral proteins from the gut of the young calf. *Proc. roy. Soc. B*, **149**, 184.
Barcroft, J., Elliott, R. H. E., Fraser, F. R., Herkel, W., Matthews, B. H. C. and Talaat, M. (1934). A case of deficient acclimatization to low oxygen pressure. *J. Physiol.* (*Lond.*), **82**, 369.
Barnett, H. L. and Vesterdal, J. (1953). The physiologic and clinical significance of immaturity of kidney function in young infants. *J. Pediat.*, **42**, 99.
Barnett, S. A. (1956). Endothermy and ectothermy in mice at −3°C. *J. exp. Biol.*, **33**, 124.
—— (1959). The skin and hair of mice living at a low environmental temperature. *Quart. J. exp. Physiol.*, **44**, 35.
——, Coleman, E. M. and Manly, B. M. (1959). Oxygen consumption and body fat of mice living at −3°C. *Ibid.*, **44**, 43.
—— and Manly, B. M. (1956). Reproduction and growth of mice of three strains, after transfer to −3°C. *J. exp. Biol.*, **33**, 325.
——, —— (1958). Adaptation to cold in young mice. *Physiol. bohemoslov.*, **7**, 19.
Bartlett, R. G., Bohr, V. C. and Inman, W. I. (1955). Relationship of oxygen consumption to body temperature in the restrained rat. *Canad. J. Biochem.*, **33**, 654.
Bates, G. S. (1933). Bilateral renal agenesis in the fetus, associated with oligohydramnios. *Amer. J. Obstet. Gynec.*, **25**, 41.
Bedford, P. D. (1957). Cerebral damage from shock due to disease in aged people with special reference to cardiac infarction, pneumonia and severe diarrhoea. *Lancet*, **2**, 505.
Béhague, P., Garsaux and Richet, C. (1927). Modifications thermiques observées sur le lapin, soumis à la dépression atmosphérique. *C.R. Soc. Biol.* (*Paris*), **96**, 766.
Behrle, F. C. and Smull, N. W. (1957). Differences of somatic and respiratory response to hypoxia in newly born and older infants. *Pediatrics*, **20**, 601.
Bernard, Claude (1865). *Introduction à l'Etude de la Médecine Expérimentale.* Baillière, Paris.
Bernstein, J. (1958). Renal tubular and pancreatic islet necrosis in newly born infants. *A.M.A. J. Dis. Child.*, **96**, 705.
Blackfan, K. D. and Yaglou, C. P. (1933). The premature infant. A study of the effects of atmospheric conditions on growth and on development. *Amer. J. Dis. Child.*, **46**, 1175.
Boekelman, T. (1957). Diaferometrische gasstogwisselingsbepalingen bij verschillende proepen Zuigelingen. Thesis. Groningen University.
Bound, J. P. and Telfer, T. P. (1956). Effect of vitamin-K dosage on plasma-bilirubin levels in premature infants. *Lancet*, **1**, 720.
Bourne, J. G. (1957). Fainting and cerebral damage: a danger in patients kept upright during dental gas anaesthesia and after surgical operations. *Ibid.*, **2**, 499.
Boyle, R. (1672). *The works of Robert Boyle*, **3**, 355. London.
Brambell, F. W. R. (1954). Transport of proteins across the fetal membranes. *Cold Spr. Harb. Symp. quant. Biol.*, **19**, 71.
Braun, T. and Mosinger, B. (1958). Effect of hypothermia on death by starvation. *Nature* (*Lond.*), **181**, 968.
Brodie, H. R., Cross, K. W., and Lomer, T. R. (1957). Heat production in new-born infants under normal and hypoxic conditions. *J. Physiol.* (*Lond.*), **138**, 156.
Brown, A. K. and Zuelzer, W. W. (1958). Studies on the neonatal development of the glucuronide conjugating system. *J. clin. Invest.*, **37**, 332.
Bullough, J. (1958). Protracted foetal and neonatal asphyxia. *Lancet*, **1**, 999.
Bunge, G. (1898). *Lehrbuch der physiologischen und pathologischen Chemie*, 4th ed., p. 118. Leipzig. Quoted by Lusk, G. (1928). *The Elements of the Science of Nutrition*, 4th ed. Saunders, Philadelphia.
Burnard, E. D. and Cross, K. W. (1958). Rectal temperature in the newborn after birth asphyxia. *Brit. med. J.*, **2**, 1197.
Burton, A. C. and Edholm, O. G. (1955). *Man in a Cold Environment.* Edward Arnold, London.
Cairnie, A. B. and Pullar, J. D. (1957). The metabolism of the young pig. *J. Physiol.* (*Lond.*), **139**, 15P.
Campbell, J. A. (1936). Body temperature and oxygen poisoning. *Ibid.*, **89**, 17P.
—— (1938). Oxygen-want and its alleviation. *Lancet*, **1**, 914.
Campbell, W. A. B., Cheeseman, E. A. and Kilpatrick, A. W. (1950). The effects of neonatal asphyxia on physical and mental development. *Arch. Dis. Childh.*, **25**, 351.
Čapek, K., Hahn, P., Křeček, J. and Martínek, J. (1956). Studie o fysiologii novorozenych mlád 'at. *Rozpr. české Akad.*, **66**, 1.
Chevillard, L. and Mayer, A. (1935). Recherches sur l'influence de la tension d'oxygène sur les échanges. 3. Influence de la tension de l'oxygène contenu dans l'air inspiré sur les échanges gazeux de la souris. *Ann. Physiol. Physicochim. biol.*, **11**, 225.
Collipp, P. J. and Donnell, G. N. (1959). Galactosemia presenting with gangrene. *J. Pediat.*, **54**, 363.
Colloquium (1957). A discussion on viability of mammalian cells and tissues after freezing. *Proc. roy. Soc. B.*, **147**, 424.
Conference (1958). Aerobic and anaerobic metabolism in the fetus and newborn. *Trans. Josiah Macy Foundation Conferences on Physiology of prematurity*, **2**, 9.
Cordier, D. and Mayer, A. (1935). Recherches sur l'influence de la tension d'oxygène sur les échanges. 1. Influence de la tension de l'oxygène contenu dans l'air inspiré sur la consommation d'oxygène des mammifères . . . Étude sur le chien. *Ann. Physiol. Physicochim. biol.*, **11**, 199.
Cort, J. H. and McCance, R. A. (1954). The renal response of puppies to an acidosis. *J. Physiol.* (*Lond.*), **124**, 358.
Cremer, R. J., Perryman, P. W., and Richards, D. H. (1958). Influence of light on the hyperbilirubinaemia of infants. *Lancet*, **1**, 1094.
Cross, K. W., Dawes, G. S. and Mott, J. C. (1958a). Changes in the cardiac output of the lamb after birth and during anoxia. *J. Physiol.* (*Lond.*), **144**, 16P.
——, ——, —— (1958b). A change in regional oxygen consumption during anoxia in the new-born lamb. *Ibid.*, **143**, 71P.
——, ——, —— (1959). Anoxia, oxygen consumption and cardiac output in new-born lambs and adult sheep. *Ibid.*, **146**, 316.
——, Tizard, J. P. M. and Trythall, D. A. H. (1955). The metabolism of newborn infants breathing 15% oxygen. *Ibid.*, **129**, 69P.
——, ——, —— (1958). The gaseous metabolism of the new-born infant breathing 15% oxygen. *Acta paediat.* (*Uppsala*), **47**, 217.
Crosse, V. M., Meyer, T. C. and Gerrard, J. W. (1955). Kernicterus and prematurity. *Arch. Dis. Childh.*, **30**, 501.
Csapó, J. and Kerpel-Fronius, E. (1933). Zur Pathologie der Säuglingstoxikose. 1. Über das Säure-Basen-Gleichgewicht bei der experimentellen Exsikkose. *Mschr. Kinderheilk.*, **58**, 1.
Cusworth, D. C., Dent, C. E. and Flynn, F. V. (1955). The aminoaciduria in galactosaemia. *Arch. Dis. Childh.*, **30**, 150.
Danoff, S., Boyer, A. and Holt, L. E. (1958). The treatment of bilirubinemia with glycuronic acid. *Trans. Ass. Amer. Phycns.* **71**, 120.
——, ——, —— (1959). The treatment of hyperbilirubinemia of the newborn with sodium glucuronate. *Pediatrics*, **23**, 570.
Darke, R. A. (1944). Late effects of severe asphyxia neonatorum. *J. Pediat.*, **24**, 148.
Davies, J. and Routh, J. I. (1957). Composition of the foetal fluids of the rabbit. *J. Embryol. exp. Morph.*, **5**, 32.
Dawes, G. S. (1959). *Arch. Dis. Childh.*, **34**, 281.
—— and Mott, J. C. (1958). A threefold increase in O_2 consumption at birth. *J. Physiol.*(*Lond.*), **143**, 7P.

Dawes, G. S. and Mott, J. C., (1959). The increase in oxygen consumption in the lamb after birth. *Ibid.*, **146**, 295.
——, ——, and Shelley, H. (1958). The ability of the foetal and new-born animal to withstand total anoxia. *Ibid.*, **144**, 18P.
——, ——, —— (1959). The importance of cardiac glycogen for the maintenance of life in foetal lambs and new-born animals during anoxia. *Ibid.*, **146**, 516. See also Dawes, G. S. (1959). Frederick Still Lecture to British Paediatric Association.
Dawkins, M. J. R. (1959). Respiratory enzymes in the liver of the newborn rat. *Proc. roy. Soc. B*, **150**, 284.
Day, R., Curtis, J. and Kelly, M. (1943). Respiratory metabolism in infancy and childhood. 27. Regulation of body temperature of premature infants. *Amer. J. Dis. Child.*, **65**, 376.
Day, R. L. (1954). Inhibition of brain respiration *in vitro* by bilirubin; reversal of inhibition by various means. *A.M.A. Amer. J. Dis. Child.*, **88**, 504.
Dean, R. F. A. and McCance, R. A. (1949). The renal response of infants and adults to the administration of hypertonic solutions of sodium chloride and urea. *J. Physiol.* (*Lond.*), **109**, 81.
Depocas, F., MacLeod, G. K. and Hart, J. S. (1957). Studies on glucose metabolism of warm and cold acclimatized rats at −5°C. *Rev. canad. Biol.*, **16**, 83.
Dickerson, J. W. T. and McCance, R. A. (1957). The composition and origin of the allantoic fluid in the rabbit. *J. Embryol. exp. Morph.*, **5**, 40.
Drew, C. E. and Anderson, I. M. (1959). Profound hypothermia in cardiac surgery. *Lancet*, **1**, 748.
——, Keen, G. and Benazon, D. B. (1959). Profound hypothermia. *Ibid.*, **1**, 745.
Driscoll, S. G. and Hsia, D. Y-Y. (1958). The development of enzyme systems during early infancy. *Pediatrics*, 22, 785.
Du Bois, E. F. (1936). *Basal Metabolism in Health and Disease*, 3rd ed. Baillière, Tindall and Cox, London.
Dutton, G. J. (1959). Glucuronide synthesis in foetal liver and other tissues. *Biochem. J.*, **71**, 141.
Edelmann, C. M., Troupkou, V. and Barnett, H. L. (1959). Renal concentrating ability in newborn infants. *Fed. Proc.*, **18**, 40.
Editorial (1957a). Effects of foetal anoxia. *Lancet*, **1**, 572.
—— (1957b). The newborn infant's oxygen-supply. *Ibid.*, **1**, 1338.
—— (1958). Neonatal hyperbilirubinaemia. *Ibid.*, **2**, 1162.
Edwards, W. F. (1824). *De l'Influence des Agents Physiques sur la Vie.* Crochard, Paris.
—— (1832). *On the Influence of Physical Agents on Life.* (Translated from the French by Dr. Hodgkin and Dr. Fisher). Highley, London.
Elkinton, J. R. and Danowski, T. S. (1955). *The Body Fluids.* Williams and Wilkins, Baltimore.
Engelmann, B. (1930). Anhaltende Grundumsatzverminderung durch Wärmeeinwirkung. *Arbeitsphysiologie*, 2, 387.
Evans, P. R. (1948). Antecedents of infantile cerebral palsy. *Arch. Dis. Childh.*, **23**, 213.
Fairfield, J. (1948). Effects of cold on infant rats: body temperatures, oxygen consumption, electrocardiograms. *Amer. J. Physiol.*, **155**, 355.
Falk, G. (1955). Maturation of renal function in infant rats. *Ibid.*, **181**, 157.
Farquhar, J. W. and Smith, H. (1958). Clinical and biochemical changes during exchange transfusion. *Arch. Dis. Childh.*, **33**, 142.
Fazekas, J. F., Alexander, F. A. D. and Himwich, H. E. (1941). Tolerance of the newborn to anoxia. *Amer. J. Physiol.*, **134**, 281.
—— and Himwich, H. E. (1941). The significance of a pathway of carbohydrate breakdown not involving glycolysis. *J. biol. Chem.*, **139**, 971.
Flexner, L. B., Wilde, W. S., Proctor, N. K., Cowie, D. B., Vosburgh, G. J. and Hellman, L. M. (1947). The estimation of extracellular and total body water in the newborn human infant with radioactive sodium and deuterium oxide. *J. Pediat.*, **30**, 413.
Frank, E. and Wezler, K. (1948). Der Gaswechsel in O_2-Mangel bei Behaglichkeitstemperatur. *Pflüg. Arch. ges. Physiol.*, **250**, 320.
Friis-Hansen, B. (1954). The extracellular fluid volume in infants and children. *Acta paediat.* (*Uppsala*), **43**, 444.
Gardner, L. I. (1956). Adrenocortical metabolism of the fetus, infant and child. *Pediatrics*, **17**, 897.
Gellhorn, E. and Janus, A. (1936). The influence of partial pressure of O_2 on body temperature. *Amer. J. Physiol.*, **116**, 327.
—— and Kessler, M. (1942). The effect of hypoglycemia on the electroencephalogram at varying degrees of oxygenation of the blood. *Ibid.*, **136**, 1.
Giaja, J. (1925a). Le métabolisme de sommet et le quotient métabolique. *Ann. Physiol. Physicochim. biol.*, **1**, 596.
—— (1925b). La marge de la thermogénèse et le quotient métabolique au cours du développement embryonnaire et de la croissance. *Ibid.*, **1**, 628.
—— and Gelineo, S. (1931). La thermogénèse aux températures inférieures à celle de la résistance homéotherme. *Ibid.*, **7**, 152.
Glaser, E. M., and Newling, P. S. B. (1957). The control of body temperature in thermal balance. *J. Physiol.* (*Lond.*), **137**, 1.
Goldzveig, S. A. and Smith, A. U. (1956). A simple method for reanimating ice-cold rats and mice. *Ibid.*, **132**, 406.
Gonzales, R. F. and Gardner, L. I. (1957). Concentration of pyruvic acid in the blood of the newborn infant: demonstration of differences in concentration between maternal and cord circulation. *Pediatrics*, **19**, 844.
Goodland, R. L., Reynolds, J. G. and Pommerenke, W. T. (1954). Alveolar carbon dioxide tension levels during pregnancy and early puerperium. *J. clin. Endocr.*, **14**, 522.
Goodwin, R. F. W. (1957). The relationship between the concentration of blood sugar and some vital body functions in the newborn pig. *J. Physiol.* (*Lond.*), **136**, 208.
Gorlin, R. and Lewis, B. M. (1954). Circulatory adjustments to hypoxia in dogs. *J. appl. Physiol.*, **7**, 180.
Graham, N. McC., Wainman, F. W., Blaxter, K. L. and Armstrong, D. G. (1959). Environmental temperature, energy metabolism and heat regulation in sheep. 1. Energy metabolism in closely clipped sheep. *J. agric. Sci.*, **52**, 13.
Griffith, F. R. (1951). Fact and theory regarding the calorigenic action of adrenalin. *Physiol. Rev.*, **31**, 151.
Hahn, P. (1956a). The development of thermoregulation. 2. The participation of the thyroid gland in the development of thermoregulation in rats. *Physiol. bohemoslov.*, **5**, 291.
—— (1956b). The development of thermoregulation. 4. Carbohydrate metabolism and thermoregulation in infant rats. *Ibid.*, **5**, 432.
—— (1956c). The development of thermoregulation. 3. The significance of fur in the development of thermoregulation in rats. *Ibid.*, **5**, 428.
—— (1956d). Effect of environmental temperatures on the development of thermoregulatory mechanisms in infant rats. *Nature* (*Lond.*), **178**, 96.
—— and Koldovský, O. (1958a). Significance of the adrenal glands during the post-natal development of thermoregulation in the rat. *Ibid.*, **181**, 847.
——, —— (1958b). The effect of restraint on rats with special reference to their post-natal development. *Physiol. bohemoslov.*, **7**, 515.
——, —— (1959). Some factors affecting the level of glycogen in the heart during fasting in rats at various ages. *Ibid.*, **8**, 180.
——, Křeček, J. and Křečková, J. (1956). The development of thermoregulation. 1. The development of thermoregulatory mechanisms in young rats. *Ibid.*, **5**, 283.
Hamon, F., Kolodny, S. and Mayer, A. (1935). Recherches sur l'influence de la tension d'oxygène sur les échanges. 2. Influence de la vie à basse tension d'oxygène sur les échanges du lapin. *Ann. Physiol. Physicochim. biol.*, **11**, 211.
Harlem, O. K. and Myhre, E. (1957). Congenital adrenal hypoplasia. *A.M.A. J. Dis. Childh.*, **94**, 696.
Hart, J. S. (1958). Metabolic alterations during chronic exposure to cold. *Fed. Proc.*, **17**, 1045.
Harvey, W. (1651). *De generatione animalium.* Translated by Willis, R. (1847). The works of William Harvey. Sydenham Society, London.
Hatemi, N. (1959). Personal communication.
Heller, H. (1947). The response of newborn rats to administration of water by the stomach. *J. Physiol.* (*Lond.*), **106**, 245.
Hellings, P. M. (1958). Controlled hypothermia. *Brit. med. J.*, **2**, 346.
Hellman, L. M. (1953). Fetal tolerance of anoxia. In Proceedings of a Conference sponsored by the Association for the Aid of Crippled Children: 'Prematurity, congenital malformation and birth injury', p. 240.
Henderson, H., Mosher, R. and Bittrich, N. M. (1957). Oxygen studies of the cord blood of cesarean-born infants. *Amer. J. Obstet. Gynec.*, **73**, 664.
Hendricks, C. H. (1957). Studies on lactic acid metabolism in pregnancy and labor. *Ibid.*, **73**, 492.
Hill, J. R. (1958). The relation between oxygen consumption, hypoxia and environmental temperature. *J. Physiol.* (*Lond.*), **143**, 64P.
Himwich, H. E. (1953). The maturation of the respiratory enzymes in the central nervous system of experimental animals. In Proceedings of a Conference sponsored by the Association for the Aid of Crippled Children: 'Prematurity, congenital malformation and birth injury', p. 59.
——, Bernstein, A. O., Herrlich, H., Chesler, A. and Fazekas, J. F. (1942). Mechanisms for the maintenance of life in the newborn during anoxia. *Amer. J. Physiol.*, **135**, 387.
——, Fazekas, J. F. and Alexander, F. A. D. (1941). Hypoglycemia in the infant rat. *Ibid.*, **133**, 328.
Holman, G. H. (1958). Studies on physiologic hyperbilirubinemia of negro and white premature infants. *Pediatrics*, **22**, 1115.
Holub, A., Forman, Z. and Ježková, D. (1957). Development of chemical thermoregulation in piglets. *Nature* (*Lond.*), **180**, 858.
Holzel, A. and Komrower, G. M. (1955). A study of the genetics of galactosaemia. *Arch. Dis. Childh.*, **30**, 155.
Houston, C. S. and Riley, R. L. (1947). Respiratory and circulatory changes during acclimatization to high altitude. *Amer. J. Physiol.*, **149**, 565.
Hoy, P. A. and Adolph, E. F. (1956). Diuresis in response to hypoxia and epinephrine in infant rats. *Ibid.*, **187**, 32.
Hsieh, A. C. L. and Carlson, L. D. (1957). Role of adrenaline and noradrenaline in chemical regulation of heat production. *Ibid.*, **190**, 243.

Hubble, D. (1957). Some principles of homoeostasis. *Lancet*, **2**, 301.

Ingle, D. J. (1958). Endocrine mechanisms in adaptation to cold. *Fed. Proc.*, **17**, 1064.

—— and Nezamis, J. E. (1950). Effect of temperature upon survival of the eviscerate rat. *Amer. J. Physiol.*, **160**, 122.

Jailer, J. W. (1953). Pituitary and adrenal responsiveness in the newborn. In Proceedings of a Conference sponsored by the Association for the Aid of Crippled Children: 'Prematurity, congenital malformation and birth injury', p. 84.

James, L. S. (1958). Personal communication.

——, Weisbrot, I. M., Prince, C. E., Holaday, D. A. and Apgar, V. (1958). The acid-base status of human infants in relation to birth asphyxia and the onset of respiration. *J. Pediat.*, **52**, 379.

Jeffcoate, T. N. A. and Scott, J. S. (1959). Polyhydramnios and oligohydramnios. *Canad. med. Ass. J.*, **80**, 77.

Jeliu, G., Schmid, R. and Gellis, S. (1959). Administration of glucuronic acid to icteric newborn infants. *Pediatrics*, **23**, 92.

Joppich, G. and Wolf, H. (1958). Reststickstofferhöhungen im Blut von Frügeboronen in den ersten Lebenstagen. *Klin. Wschr.*, **36**, 616.

Kabat, H. (1940). The greater resistance of very young animals to arrest of the brain circulation. *Amer. J. Physiol.*, **130**, 588.

Kaiser, I. H. and Goodlin, R. C. (1958). Alterations of pH, gases and hemoglobin in blood and electrolytes in plasma of fetuses of diabetic mothers. *Pediatrics*, **22**, 1097.

Kennedy, G. C. (1953). The role of depot fat in the hypothalamic control of food intake in the rat. *Proc. roy. Soc. B*, **140**, 578.

Kerpel-Fronius, E. (1933). Chloropenie und Osmoregulation. *Z. ges. exp. Med.*, **90**, 676.

—— and Leövey, F. (1931). Über die Störung der Osmoregulation bei der experimentellen Exsikkose. *Arch. Kinderheilk.*, **94**, 9.

Kety, S. S. (1950). Circulation and metabolism of the human brain in health and disease. *Amer. J. Med.*, **8**, 205.

Khalil, M. (1958). The circulating eosinophil level in the newborn infant following normal and difficult labor. *J. Pediat.*, **53**, 662.

Kramár, E. (1927). Untersuchungen über die Pathologie der Säuglingsintoxikation. 2. Die Rolle des Eiweisses. *Jb. Kinderheilk.*, **115**, 289.

Křeček, J., Křečková, J. and Martínek, J. (1957). The development of thermoregulation. 5. Effect of rearing under cold and warm conditions on the development of thermoregulation in young rats. *Physiol. bohemoslov.*, **6**, 329.

Krog, H., Monson, M. and Irving, L. (1955). Influence of cold upon the metabolism and body temperature of wild rats, albino rats and albino rats conditioned to cold. *J. appl. Physiol.*, **7**, 349.

Lathe, G. H., Claireaux, A. E. and Norman, A. P. (1958). In *Recent Advances in Paediatrics*, 2nd ed. Ed. D. Gairdner. p. 87. Churchill, London.

—— and Walker, M. (1957). An enzyme defect in human neonatal jaundice and in Gunn's strain of jaundiced rats. *Biochem. J.*, **67**, 9P.

Laufman, H. (1951). Profound accidental hypothermia. *J. Amer. med. Ass.*, **147**, 1201.

Laurie, E. M. O. (1946). The reproduction of the house-mouse (*Mus musculus*) living in different environments. *Proc. roy. Soc. B*, **133**, 248.

Leaf, A. and Newburgh, L. H. (1955). *Significance of the Body Fluids in Clinical Medicine*, 2nd ed. Thomas, Springfield, Illinois.

Lintzel, W. (1931). Über die Wirkung der Luftverdünnung auf Tiere. 5. Gaswechsel weisser Ratten. *Pflüg. Arch. ges. Physiol.*, **227**, 693.

Lucey, J. F. and Dolan, R. G. (1959). Hyperbilirubinemia of newborn infants associated with the parenteral administration of a vitamin K analogue to the mothers. *Pediatrics*, **23**, 553.

Luck, C. P. and Wright, P. G. (1959). The body temperature of the hippopotamus. *J. Physiol. (Lond.)*, **147**, 53P.

McCance, R. A. (1936). Medical problems in mineral metabolism. *Lancet*, **1**, 643, 704, 765, 823.

—— (1950). Renal physiology in infancy. *Amer. J. Med.*, **9**, 229.

—— and Dickerson, J. W. T. (1957). The composition and origin of the foetal fluids of the pig. *J. Embryol. exp. Morph.*, **5**, 43.

—— and Otley, M. (1951). Course of the blood urea in newborn rats, pigs and kittens. *J. Physiol. (Lond.)*, **113**, 18.

—— and Widdowson, E. M. (1952). The correct physiological basis on which to compare infant and adult renal function. *Lancet*, **2**, 860.

——, —— (1954a). Normal renal function in the first two days of life. *Arch. Dis. Childh.*, **29**, 488.

——, —— (1954b). The influence of events during the last few days *in utero* on tissue destruction and renal function in the first two days of independent life. *Ibid.*, **29**, 495.

——, —— (1955). The response of puppies to a large dose of water. *J. Physiol. (Lond.)*, **129**, 628.

——, —— (1956). Metabolism, growth and renal function of piglets in the first days of life. *Ibid.*, **133**, 373.

——, —— (1957). Hypertonic expansion of the extracellular fluids. *Acta paediat. (Uppsala)*, **46**, 337.

——, —— (1958a). The response of the newborn piglet to an excess of potassium. *J. Physiol. (Lond.)*, **141**, 88.

McCance, R. A. and Widdowson, E. M. (1958b). The response of the newborn puppy to water, salt and food. *Ibid.*, **141**, 81.

——, —— (1959a). The effect of colostrum on the composition and volume of the plasma of new-born piglets. *Ibid.*, **145**, 547.

——, —— (1959b). The effect of lowering the ambient temperature on the metabolism of the new-born pig. *Ibid.*, **147**, 124.

—— and Wilkinson, E. (1947). The response of adult and suckling rats to the administration of water and hypertonic solution or urea and salt. *J. Physiol. (Lond.)*, **106**, 256.

—— and Young, W. F. (1940). The secretion of urine by newborn infants. *Ibid.*, **99**, 265.

McIntosh, R. (1957). On growth and development. *Arch. Dis. Childh.*, **32**, 261.

McIntyre, D. G. and Ederstrom, H. E. (1958). Metabolic factors in the development of homeothermy in dogs. *Amer. J. Physiol.*, **194**, 293.

Makepeace, A. W., Fremont-Smith, F., Dailey, M. E. and Carroll, M. P. (1931). The nature of the amniotic fluid. A comparative study of human amniotic fluid and maternal serum. *Surg. Gynec. Obstet.*, **53**, 635.

Malpress, F. H. (1958). The biosynthesis of lactose. *Proc. roy. Soc. B*, **149**, 362.

Mann, T. P. and Elliott, R. I. K. (1957). Neonatal cold injury due to accidental exposure to cold. *Lancet*, **1**, 229.

Marsh, M. E. and Murlin, J. R. (1925). Energy metabolism of premature and undersized infants. *Amer. J. Dis. Child.*, **30**, 310.

Meyer, T. C. and Angus, J. (1956). The effect of large doses of 'Synkavit' in the newborn. *Arch. Dis. Childh.*, **31**, 212.

Miller, F. S. and Miller, J. A. (1953). Effects of hypothermia on neonatal asphyxia and its sequelae. *Bull. Ga Acad. Sci.*, **11**, 54.

Miller, H. C., Behrle, F. C., Smull, N. W. and Blim, R. D. (1957). Studies of respiratory insufficiency in newborn infants. 2. Correlation of hydrogen-ion concentration, carbon dioxide tension, carbon dioxide content and oxygen saturation of blood with trend of respiratory rates. *Pediatrics*, **19**, 387.

Miller, J. A. (1954). Effects of variations in body temperature upon resistance to asphyxia in the neonatal guinea pig. *Cold Spr. Harb. Symp. quant. Biol.*, **19**, 152.

—— and Miller, F. S. (1954). Factors in neonatal resistance to anoxia. 2. Effects of elevated and reduced temperature upon survival and recovery by neonatal guinea pigs. *Surgery*, **36**, 916.

——, —— (1958). Effects of drugs and anaesthetics on reanimation of ice-cold mice. *J. Physiol. (Lond.)*, **140**, 23P.

Moore, R. E. (1956a). The effects of hypoxia on the oxygen consumption of newborn dogs. *Ibid.*, **131**, 27P.

—— (1956b). Hypoxia, oxygen consumption and body temperature in newborn kittens. *Ibid.*, **133**, 69P.

Mordhorst, H. (1932). Über die chemische Wärmregulation frühgeborener Säuglinge. *Mschr. Kinderheilk.*, **55**, 174.

Morrill, C. C. (1952). Studies on baby pig mortality. 10. Influence of environmental temperature on fasting newborn pigs. *Amer. J. vet. Res.*, **13**, 322.

—— and Sampson, J. (1952). Studies on baby pig mortality. 12. A note on the influence of ingestion of distilled water, physiological saline, and glucose solutions on fasting newborn pigs. *Ibid.*, **13**, 327.

Mount, L. E. (1958a). Changes in oxygen consumption with age in piglets during the first week of life. J. *Physiol. (Lond.)*, **142**, 57P.

—— (1958b). Change in oxygen consumption of the new-born pig with a fall in environmental temperature. *Nature (Lond.)*, **182**, 536.

—— (1959). The effect on rate of heat production of grouping newborn pigs together. *J. Physiol. (Lond.)* (Not yet published.)

Murtagh, J. J., Martinez Castro Videla, C. E., Marenzi, A. D. and Braegger, E. (1957). Plasma electrolytes during the neonatal period. *Ét. néo-natal*, **6**, 150.

Niazi, S. A. and Lewis, F. J. (1954). Tolerance of adult rats to profound hypothermia and simultaneous cardiac standstill. *Surgery*, **36**, 25.

——, —— (1957). Profound hypothermia in the monkey with recovery after long periods of cardiac standstill. *J. appl. Physiol.*, **10**, 137.

Nyberg, R. and Westin, B. (1957). The influence of oxygen tension and some drugs on human placental vessels. *Acta physiol. scand.*, **39**, 216.

Osiba, S. (1957). The seasonal variation of basal metabolism and activity of thyroid gland in man. *Jap. J. Physiol.*, **7**, 355.

Pawan, G. L. S. (1959). The possible conversion of fat into carbohydrate in the obese human. *Biochem. J.*, **72**, 20P.

Pickering, G. (1958). Regulation of body temperature in health and disease. *Lancet*, **1**, 1, 59.

Potter, E. L. (1952). *Pathology of the Fetus and the Newborn*. Year Book Publishers, Chicago.

Potter, V. R. (1958). Possible biochemical mechanisms underlying adaptation to cold. *Fed. Proc.*, **17**, 1060.

Preston, M. I. (1945). Late behavioral aspects found in cases of prenatal, natal and postnatal anoxia. *J. Pediat.*, **26**, 353.

Preyer, W. (1885). *Specielle Physiologie des Embryo*. Grieben, Leipzig.

Pugh, L. G. C. E. (1957). Resting ventilation and alveolar air on Mount Everest: with remarks on the relation of barometric pressure to altitude in mountains. *J. Physiol.* (*Lond.*), **135**, 590.

Ranson, S. W. (1940). Regulation of body temperature. In *The Hypothalamus and Central Levels of Autonomic Function. Res. Publ. Ass. nerv. ment. Dis.*, **20**, 342.

Raudnitz, R. W. (1888). Die Wärmeregelung beim Neugeborenen. *Z. Biol.*, N.S. **24**, 423.

Reardon, H. S., Baumann, M. L. and Haddad, E. J. (1954). Respiratory alkalosis—a frequent phenomenon observed in newborn infants. *A.M.A. Amer. J. Dis. Child.*, **88**, 371.

Rector, F. C., Jr. and Orloff, J. (1959). The effect of the administration of sodium bicarbonate and ammonium chloride on the excretion and production of ammonia. The absence of alterations in the activity of renal ammonia-producing enzymes in the dog. *J. clin. Invest.*, **38**, 366.

——, Seldin, D. W., Roberts, A. D. and Copenhaver, J. H. (1954). Relation of ammonia excretion to urine pH. *Amer. J. Physiol.*, **179**, 353.

Rees, J. R. (1958). Accidental hypothermia. *Lancet*, **1**, 556.

Rennick, B. R. and Hamilton, B. (1958). Accumulation of para-amino-hippurate and tetraethylammonium by renal slices of the newborn puppy and piglet. *Fed. Proc.*, **17**, 131.

Reynolds, S. R. M. (1953). Maturation of respiratory enzymes. In Proceedings of a Conference sponsored by the Association for the Aid of Crippled Children : 'Prematurity, congenital malformation and birth injury', p. 75.

Rothschuh, K. E. (1947). Zur Frage eines 'Sparstoffweshsels' bei kurzdauerndem Sauerstoffmangel. *Pflüg. Arch. ges. Physiol.*, **249**, 175.

Scholander, P. F. (1958). Studies on man exposed to cold. *Fed. Proc.*, **17**, 1054.

Schwartz, W. B., Jenson, R. L. and Relman, A. S. (1954). The disposition of acid administered to sodium depleted subjects: the renal response and the role of the whole body buffers. *J. clin. Invest.*, **33**, 587.

Schwarz, K. C., Cohen, B. D., Lubash, G. D. and Rubin, A. L. (1959). Severe acidosis and hyperpotassemia treated with sodium bicarbonate infusion. *Circulation*, **19**, 215.

Selle, W. A. (1941). Influence of age on survival of respiration, spinal reflexes, pupillary responses and heart action. *Proc. Soc. exp. Biol.* (*N.Y.*), **48**, 417.

—— and Witten, T. A. (1941). Survival of the respiratory (gasping) mechanism in young rats subjected to anoxia. *Ibid.*, **47**, 495.

Sellers, E. A. and You, S. S. (1950). Role of the thyroid in metabolic responses to a cold environment. *Amer. J. Physiol.*, **163**, 81.

Shields, L. V. and Taylor, E. S. (1957). Serial oxygen saturation studies of newborn infants following obstetrical complications, difficult deliveries, and cesarian section. *Amer. J. Obstet. Gynec.*, **73**, 1011.

Shnier, M. H. and Levin, S. E. (1959). Hyperbilirubinaemia and kernicterus in premature and full-term Bantu newborn infants. *Brit. med. J.*, **1**, 1004.

Silverman, W. A., Fertig, J. W. and Berger, A. P. (1958). The influence of the thermal environment upon the survival of newly born premature infants. *Pediatrics*, **22**, 876.

Silvette, H., Britton, S. W. and Kline, R. (1938). Carbohydrate changes in various animals following potassium administration. *Amer. J. Physiol.*, **122**, 524.

Singer, R. B. and Hastings, A. B. (1948). An improved clinical method for the estimation of disturbances of the acid-base balance of human blood. *Medicine* (*Baltimore*), **27**, 223.

Sjöstedt, S. and Rooth, G. (1957). Low oxygen tension in the management of newborn infants. *Arch. Dis. Childh.*, **32**, 397.

Smith, A. U., Emmens, C. W. and Parkes, A. S. (1946-48). A simple mammalian test for thyroidal activity. *J. Endocr.*, **5**, xxxii.

Smith, C. (1959). *The Physiology of the Newborn Infant*, 3rd ed. Thomas, Springfield.

Smith, R. E. (1958). In discussion. *Fed. Proc.*, **17**, 1069.

Stapleton, T. (1958). Mineral metabolism. In *Modern Trends in Paediatrics*. Butterworth, London.

Stone, W. E., Marshall, C. and Nims, L. F. (1941). Chemical changes in the brain produced by injury and by anoxia. *Amer. J. Physiol.*, **132**, 770.

Stransky, E. and Bálint, A. (1920). Die Nierenfunktion im Säuglingsalter. Die Stickstoffverteilung im Blute und Harne im Säuglingsalter. *Jb. Kinderheilk.*, **93** [3 ser., 43], 350.

Strughold, H. (1954). Hypoxia, hypoxidosis, hypoxidation, hibernation, apparent death and suspended animation. *J. Aviat. Med.*, **25**, 113.

Swann, H. G. (1953). The principles of resuscitation. *Anesthesiology*, **14**, 126.

—— and Brucer, M. (1949). The cardiorespiratory and biochemical events during rapid anoxic death. *Tex. Rep. Biol. Med.*, **7**, 511.

——, —— and King, B. R. (1953). Assay of resuscitation procedures. *J. appl. Physiol.*, **5**, 421.

——, Christian, J. J. and Hamilton, C. (1954). The process of anoxic death in newborn pups. *Surg. Gynec. Obstet.*, **99**, 5.

Swanson, H. E. (1956). Interrelations between thyroxin and adrenalin in the regulation of oxygen consumption in the albino rat. *Endocrinology*, **59**, 217.

Tepperman, J. (1958). Etiologic factors in obesity and leanness. *Perspectives in Biol. Med.*, **1**, 293.

Thibault, O. (1949). Les facteurs hormonaux de la régulation chimique de la température des homéothermes. *Rev. canad. Biol.*, **8**, 3.

Thoms, R. K. and Hiestand, W. A. (1947). Relation of survival time of respiratory gasping mechanism of the isolated mouse head to age. *Proc. Soc. exp. Biol.* (*N.Y.*), **64**, 1.

Turnbull, E. P. N. and Baird, D. (1957). Maternal age and foetal oxygenation. *Brit. med. J.*, **2**, 1021.

Tyslowitz, R. and Astwood, E. B. (1942). The influence of the pituitary and adrenal cortex on resistance to low environmental temperatures. *Amer. J. Physiol.*, **136**, 22.

Usdin, G. L. and Weil, M. (1952). Effect of apnea neonatorum on intellectual development. *Pediatrics*, **9**, 387.

Usher, R. (1959). The respiratory distress syndrome of prematurity. 1. Changes in potassium in the serum and the electrocardiogram and effects of therapy. *Pediatrics*, **24**, 562.

Vest, M. (1958). Insufficient glucuronide formation in the newborn and its relationship to the pathogenesis of icterus neonatorum. *Arch. Dis. Childh.*, **33**, 473.

Vesterdal, J. (1959). Glomerular filtration and renal water excretion. In *Die physiologische Entwicklung des Kindes*. Springer-Verlag, Berlin-Göttingen-Heidelberg p. 204.

Walker, W. and Mollison, P. L. (1957). Haemolytic disease of the newborn. *Lancet*, **1**, 1309.

Walters, W. J. and Bowen, W. R. (1955). Bilirubin encephalopathy; studies related to cellular respiration. *A.M.A. J. Dis. Child.*, **90**, 603.

Weisbrot, J. M., James, L. S., Prince, C. E., Holaday, D. A. and Apgar, V. (1958). Acid-base homeostasis of the newborn infant during the first 24 hours of life. *J. Pediat.*, **52**, 395.

Westin, B. (1957). Technique and estimation of oxygenation of the human fetus in utero by means of hystero-photography. *Acta paediat.* (*Uppsala*), **46**, 117.

Widdowson, E. M. and McCance, R. A. (1956). The effect of development on the composition of the serum and extracellular fluids. *Clin. Sci.*, **15**, 361.

——, —— (1958). The development of acid-base control. *Ciba Foundation Colloquia on Ageing*, **4**, 209.

——, —— (1959). The effect of food and growth on the metabolism of phosphorus in the newly born. *Acta paediat.* (*Uppsala*), **48**, 383.

Willi, H. (1956). Synkavit-Schädidung bei Frühgeborenen. *Helv. paediat. Acta*, **11**, 325.

Wynn, V. (1954). Electrolyte disturbances associated with failure to metabolise glucose during hypothermia. *Lancet*, **2**, 575.

Wynn, V. (1956). The metabolism of fructose during hypothermia in man. *Clin. Sci.*, **15**, 297.

You, S. S., You, R. W. and Sellers, E. A. (1950). Effect of thyroidectomy, adrenalectomy and burning on the urinary nitrogen excretion of the rat maintained in a cold environment. *Endocrinology*, **47**, 156.

Zetterström, R. and Ernster, L. (1956). Bilirubin, an uncoupler of oxidative phosphorylation in isolated mitochondria. *Nature* (*Lond.*), **178**, 1335.

Ziskind, A. and Gellis, S. S. (1958). Water intoxication following tap-water enemas. *A.M.A. J. Dis. Child.*, **96**, 699.

Zomzely, C. and Mayer, J. (1958). Levels of serum cholesterol in obese mice. *Nature* (*Lond.*), **182**, 1738.

Zweymüller, E., Widdowson, E. M. and McCance, R. A. (1959). The passage of urea and creatinine across the placenta of the pig. *J. Embryol. exp. Morph.*, **7**, 203.

FOETOMATERNAL TRANSFUSION AS A CAUSE OF NEONATAL ANAEMIA*

BY

WILLIAM KRIVIT,† ROBERT GOODLIN,‡ NEWELL ZIEGLER§ and ROGER LIENKE†
From the Departments of Pediatrics,† Obstetrics‡ and Bacteriology and Immunology,§ University of Minnesota Medical School, Minneapolis

(RECEIVED FOR PUBLICATION MAY 1, 1959)

After Levine, Burnham, Katzin and Vogel (1941) had described iso-immunization to the Rh factor, they postulated that sensitization might occur by passage of foetal red cells into the maternal circulation. Wiener (1948) first reported such a clinical example. Later Chown (1954) presented convincing evidence that foetomaternal transfusion was a definite entity.

Chown (1955) utilized three methods in his case for demonstrating passage of foetal cells into the maternal circulation. First he observed an elevated level of foetal type haemoglobin in the mother's blood. Second, by differential serum agglutination, he showed that red cells with foetal type antigen were present in the maternal circulation. Third, he observed a progressive rise in anti-D indirect Coombs titre in the mother.

Since Chown's proof of foetomaternal transfer, Colebatch, Pitt and Maddison (1956), Borum, Loyd and Talbot (1957), Gunson (1957), Shiller (1957), Goodall, Graham, Miller and Cameron (1958), McGovern, Driscoll, DuToit, Grove-Rasmussen and Bedell (1958), and Pearson and Diamond (1959) have reported further examples. Chown's case report is the only one thus far in which all three methods enumerated above were used to prove that foetomaternal transmission had taken place.

The case reported here includes proof of such foetomaternal red cell transfer by determination of elevated levels of foetal haemoglobin, by a rising anti-D titre and by detection of infant's cells in the mother's circulation using differential agglutination. The observations are submitted to confirm those of Chown.

Case History

Infant Q. was born on November 28, 1958. No signs of foetal or maternal distress had been noted. At delivery, however, the infant was pale and listless.

On examination, except for the marked pallor and listlessness, the infant was normal (length 18 in., head circumference 12½ in., weight 6 lb. 8 oz.). The liver was palpable 2 cm. below the costal margin. The spleen was not palpable. No petechiae were noted. There were no signs of foetal distress at this time.

Haemoglobin by skin prick shortly after birth was 6·7 g.%. The direct Coombs test was negative. There were 108 normoblasts per 100 white cells. Total bilirubin was 0·4 mg. %. The infant's blood cells were O (Rh+).

Because of the pallor and anaemia, the infant received 54 ml. of group O (Rh−) blood which was well tolerated. The haemoglobin on the second day of life was 11·8 g.%. Subsequent growth and development of the infant have been normal.

Maternal History. The pregnancy had been normal. One previous pregnancy had resulted in a normal infant who was Coombs negative and had a haemoglobin of 18·5 g.% at birth. The mother was group A Rh negative and no anti-D (Rh_o) had been found during either pregnancy. She had no postpartum complications and specifically did not have any fever or chills or other signs of blood incompatibility. Blood samples from the mother were available on days 1, 10, 17, 22, 40, 60 and 88 postpartum.

Evidence of Transfer of Foetal Cells into Maternal Circulation

Foetal Haemoglobin. The amount of foetal haemoglobin noted in the maternal circulation is shown in Fig. 1. The specimen obtained on the first postpartum day contained 6·6% of foetal haemoglobin. Thereafter there was a gradual decline to the normal range of 0·5% at 60 days postpartum. The infant's foetal haemoglobin at birth was 61%.

The methods used in this laboratory were those of Singer, Chernoff and Singer (1951). The range in the normal postpartum period for foetal haemoglobin was 0·5-1·0%.

Indirect Coombs Titre. The mother was group A Rh negative. Serum from day 1 revealed no antibodies to D antigen or to any other of a group of 22 antigens with which this serum was tested. However, subse-

* Supported in part by grants from the Graduate School of the University of Minnesota and U.S.P.H.S. Grant H-3107.

quently, as shown in Fig. 1, there was a definite rise in anti-D titre by the indirect microscopic Coombs test. This rise from zero on day 1 to 1:8 on day 8 and to 1:128 in 60 days is characteristic of events following the introduction of a large amount of antigen. No other antibodies were found in any of the later specimens.

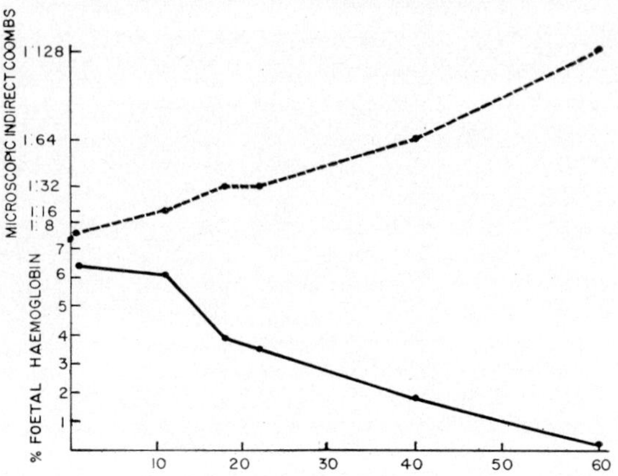

FIG. 1.—Indirect Coombs titre and foetal haemoglobin from mother.

Differential Agglutination Studies. The infant's blood group was O DCe/dce; $Fy^{a}+$; M+ N+; K−. The mother was group A dce/dce; $Fy^{a}+$; M+ N+; K−.

Therefore, direct differential agglutination was done by addition of anti-D serum to an aliquot of the mother's cells. By this method the infant's cells were agglutinated. The difference between the number of cells originally present and those cells remaining after addition of anti-D was considered to represent the cells of the infant.

The direct agglutination method, when first done, revealed that approximately 11% of the cells were of the Rh positive type. The percentage of the cells that were of the infant's type decreased gradually during the next 60 days to 3% at 30 days and 0 at 88 days.

Later, the indirect agglutination method was used. In this method the mother's cells, group A, were agglutinated by addition of anti-A serum and this left only the infant's cells, group O. By this method, cells that were antigenically like the infant's were identified in the maternal circulation. The percentage of surviving infant's cells, as determined by differential agglutination, parallels the foetal haemoglobin but at a slightly higher level.

Discussion

This article supports the thesis that foetal red cells can pass the placental barrier and enter the maternal circulation. The finding of infant's red cells, foetal type haemoglobin and a significant rise in anti-D titre in the blood of the mother indicates that a foetomaternal transfusion had occurred. These findings confirm those of Chown (1954) and others.

Recognition of the entity of foetomaternal transfusion provides a basis for the abnormal clinical condition existing in the infant. Furthermore, knowledge that foetomaternal transfusion can occur provides an understanding of a mechanism for iso-immunization.

Levine *et al.* (1941) and Wiener (1948) had postulated that infant's red cells escaped into the maternal circulation. Until the entity of foetomaternal transfusion had been established the placental passage of foetal red cells had been considered impossible.

Physiological data now indicate that the foetal venous pressure is higher than that in the intervillous space. This pressure differential provides an explanation for the expulsion of infant's cells into the maternal system after a breech in the placental barrier has occurred.

The problem remains to determine how often and to what extent foetomaternal transfusion occurs. In answer to the problem, several methods have been devised.

Foetal type haemoglobin has been measured by O'Connor, Shields, Kohl and Sussman (1957) in mothers whose infants had cord blood haemoglobin levels below normal. Foetal haemoglobin was above average in these women. It was concluded that the anaemia of their babies was due to transfusion of foetal cells into the mother.

Another study by Creger and Steele (1957) has indicated that foetal red cells of group O infants are significantly increased in the circulation of group A women. For controls the unagglutinable cell counts in women of group A who had infants of group A were used.

A fuller understanding of the placental dysfunction that allows these transfusions to occur may evolve a means of preventing the clinical disease of erythroblastosis foetalis.

Summary

A case report of foetomaternal transfusion is presented.

Positive identification of the infant's cells in the mother's circulation was made by direct agglutination technique.

An increased level of foetal haemoglobin was noted in the maternal circulation.

A rising titre of anti-D was observed in the maternal circulation.

References

Borum, A., Loyd, H. O. and Talbot, T. R. (1957). Possible fetal hemorrhage into maternal circulation. *J. Amer. med. Ass.*, **164**, 1087.

Chown, B. (1954). Anaemia from bleeding of the foetus into the mother's circulation. *Lancet*, **1**, 1213.

—— (1955). The fetus can bleed. Three clinico-pathological pictures. *Amer. J. Obstet. Gynec.*, **70**, 1298.

Colebatch, J. H., Pitt, D. and Maddison, T. G. (1956). Foeto-maternal transfusion: another cause of post haemorrhagic anaemia in the newborn. *Med. J. Aust.*, **2**, 209.

Creger, W. P. and Steele, M. R. (1957). Human feto-maternal passage of erythrocytes. *New Engl. J. Med.*, **256**, 158.

Goodall, H. B., Graham, F. S., Miller, M. C. and Cameron, C. (1958). Transplacental bleeding from the fetus. *J. clin. Path.*, **11**, 251.

Gunson, H. H. (1957). Neonatal anemia due to fetal hemorrhage into maternal circulation. *Pediatrics*, **20**, 3.

Levine, P., Burnham, L., Katzin, E. M. and Vogel, P. (1941). The role of iso-immunization in the pathogenesis of erythroblastosis fetalis. *Amer. J. Obstet. Gynec.*, **42**, 925.

McGovern, J. J., Driscoll, R., DuToit, C. H., Grove-Rasmussen, M. and Bedell, R. F. (1958). Iron-deficiency anemia resulting from fetomaternal transfusion. *New Engl. J. Med.*, **258**, 1149.

O'Connor, W. J., Shields, G., Kohl, S. and Sussman, M. (1957). The occurrence of anemia of the newborn in association with the appearance of fetal hemoglobin in the maternal circulation. *Amer. J. Obstet. Gynec.*, **73**, 768.

Pearson, H. A. and Diamond, L. K. (1959). Fetomaternal transfusion. *A.M.A. J. Dis. Child.*, **97**, 267.

Shiller, J. G. (1957). Shock in the newborn caused by transplacental hemorrhage from fetus to mother. *Pediatrics*, **20**, 7.

Singer, K., Chernoff, A. I. and Singer, L. (1951). Studies on abnormal hemoglobins. II. Their identification by means of the method of fractional denaturation. *Blood*, **6**, 429.

Wiener, A. S. (1948). Diagnosis and treatment of anemia of the newborn caused by occult placental hemorrhage. *Amer. J. Obstet. Gynec.*, **56**, 717.

MEDIASTINAL DUPLICATION OF THE GUT

BY

J. STANLEY ELWOOD

From the Department of Pathology, The Royal Liverpool Children's Hospital

(RECEIVED FOR PUBLICATION APRIL 24, 1959)

Duplication cysts of the mediastinum are not common. Morrison (1958) includes six in a series of 332 mediastinal cysts and tumours; in his Table 1 (which includes his own series) 15 gastric and enterogenous cysts were found in a total of 1,055 published cases of mediastinal cysts and tumours, an incidence of 1·5%.

Although cases have been described (Mixter and Clifford, 1929; Gross, Neuhauser and Longino, 1950; Gross, Holcomb and Farber, 1952; Dickson, Clagett and McDonald, 1946; McLetchie, Purves and Saunders, 1954), it is unusual for duplications of the gut to extend from the abdomen through the diaphragm into the mediastinum.

Details of two cases of mediastinal duplication of the gut occurring in childhood are presented in this communication to illustrate a possible aetiological mechanism.

Case Reports

Case 1 (R.L.C.H. 14002). This boy attended at the age of 18 months because of pallor and anorexia of recent onset. His left shoulder had drooped since he had started to walk. On physical examination some fullness of the left side of the chest was observed, and dullness and diminished air entry were found posteriorly to the left of the vertebrae. Severe anaemia (9·6 g. %) was present.

A radiograph of the chest (Fig. 1) revealed (1) a developmental abnormality with hemivertebrae in the mid-dorsal region; scoliosis with concavity to the right, and a slight developmental abnormality of the upper and middle ribs; (2) a rounded opaque shadow situated posteriorly and medially in the upper half of the left side of the chest; and (3) shadowing in the anterior portion of the superior mediastinum (? thymus).

Further radiological examination showed that the oesophagus and whole length of the gut was normal. A small left cervical rib was present and spina bifida of the fifth lumbar and first and second sacral vertebrae was detected. The skull and cervical vertebrae were normal.

A diagnosis of duplication cyst of the gut was made and thoracotomy advised.

At operation a large cystic tumour was found behind the pleura lying on, and closely applied to, the necks of the left ribs, vertebral bodies and the aorta; no localized attachment to the vertebrae was noted. The cyst was removed without difficulty. Convalescence was uneventful and subsequent progress has been satisfactory.

PATHOLOGY. The cyst was received fixed in formalin; it measured 3 × 2 × 2 cm.; its outer surface was shaggy in places but smooth elsewhere. The interior was pale,

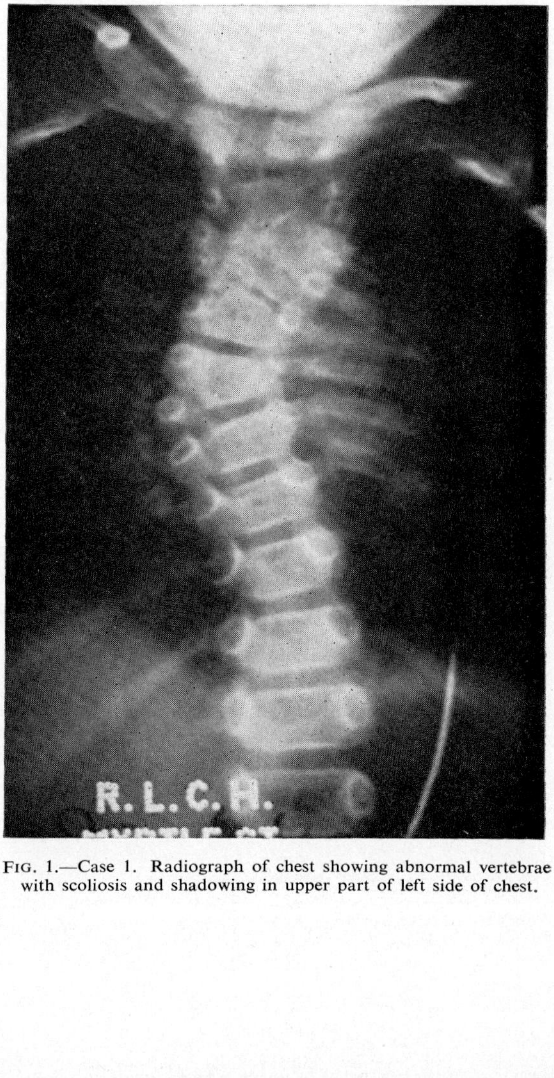

FIG. 1.—Case 1. Radiograph of chest showing abnormal vertebrae with scoliosis and shadowing in upper part of left side of chest.

smooth and velvet-like over the greater part; in places it was covered by a slough. Microscopic examination of the contents, a reddish-yellow viscous fluid, showed many red cells and some leucocytes but no organisms. The *p*H was 7·6.

Histological examination (Fig. 2a) showed the wall to be composed of two layers of muscle arranged at right-angles to each other, Auerbach's and Meissner's plexuses being identified. The appearance of the mucosa was variable: over the greater part it was thick, lined by columnar epithelium thrown into short thick villous processes, with racemose glands in its deeper part, sometimes containing oxyntic cells. There was a well developed muscularis mucosae separated from the muscular layers by the submucosa in which were many lymphocytes, sometimes focally aggregated. In one small area the mucosa was reduced to a single layer of columnar cells lying on a thin submucosa and was here devoid of a muscularis mucosae. A single area of ulceration was found in which there was fibrosis of the muscle underlying a slough and fusion of it with the muscularis mucosae as seen in typical peptic ulcers (Fig. 2b).

External to the muscle layers was a thick fibrous layer which showed evidence of haemorrhage and chronic inflammation.

Case 2 (R.L.C.H. 33286). This female infant, weighing 9 lb. 6 oz., was born by normal delivery at home. She was the seventh child of healthy parents, the siblings being well. Shortly after birth she was transferred to hospital because of dyspnoea and cyanosis.

A radiograph of the chest (Fig. 3) showed translucency of the right side of the chest with displacement of the heart to the left. Spina bifida of the seventh cervical and upper four dorsal vertebrae was present.

A tentative diagnosis of congenital cystic lung was made and a right thoracotomy was performed 16 hours after birth.

At operation a large mass was discovered deep to the pleura, occupying the postero-inferior portion of the right chest and compressing the right lung, which itself appeared normal. On opening the pleura the mass was seen to be a segment of gut which disappeared from view as it passed through the diaphragm in the right paravertebral fossa. Its upper end thinned out into an elongated process which passed upwards close to and behind the oesophagus to its attachment on the anterior surface of the second dorsal vertebral body, slightly to the left of the midline.

Aspiration of the lesion showed it to contain air and bile. It was freed from its attachments, its upper end being divided between ligatures, but in view of the poor condition of the patient, it was divided and sutured at the diaphragm without exploring its abdominal extension.

Shortly afterwards the child died. Complete radiological examination of the vertebrae after death did not show additional abnormalities.

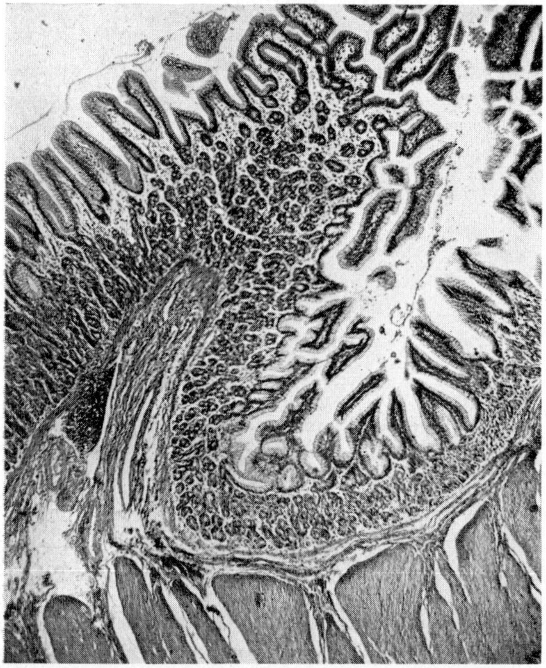

FIG. 2a.—Case 1. Photomicrograph of wall of duplication cyst showing thick mucous membrane containing many oxyntic cells. Note well-developed muscularis mucosae. (× 70)

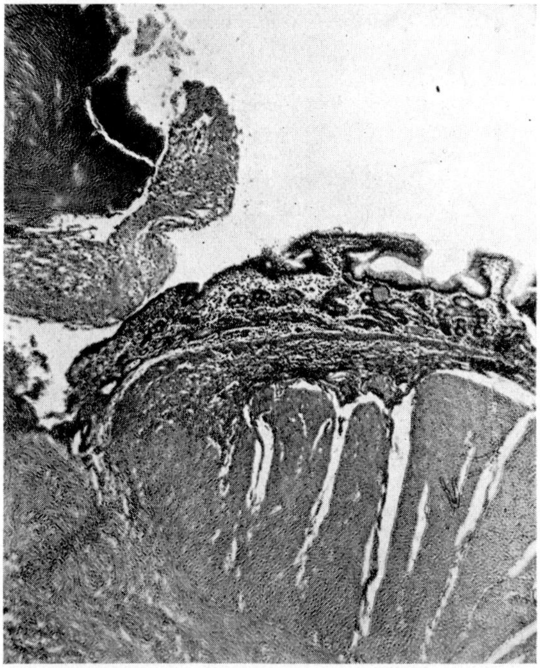

FIG. 2b.—Another area from the same cyst as in Fig. 2a showing ulceration of mucosa which here is devoid of oxyntic cells. (× 75)

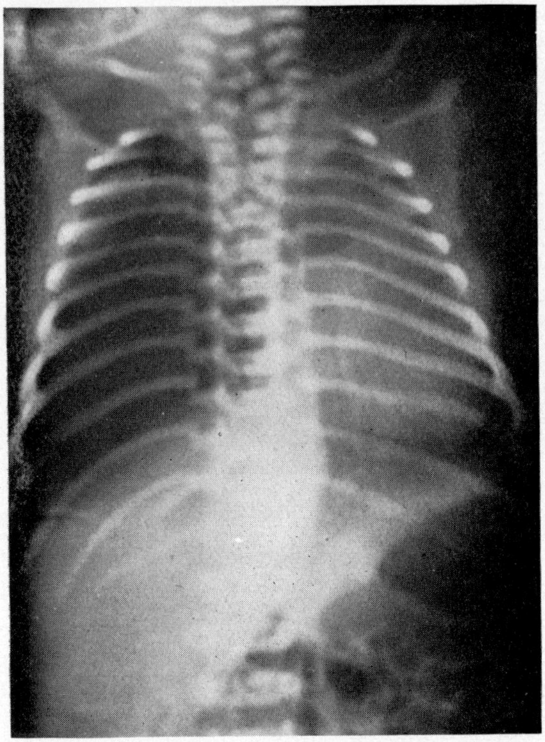

FIG. 3.—Case 2. Radiograph of chest showing translucence on right side and deformity of vertebrae.

AUTOPSY FINDINGS. The immediate cause of death was haemorrhage into the right thorax, about 50 ml. of blood being present.

The oesophagus and stomach were normal in shape and position, the duodenum was normal in its first part but the second part was unduly short and the duodeno-jejunal flexure was at the ampulla of Vater just to the right of the midline. The ascending colon had a short mesentery which allowed the colon and appendix to lie in the right hypochondrium. The descending and transverse colon were normal.

Thirty-three centimeters from the pylorus a duplication of the gut arose from its mesenteric border and passed upwards in front of the duodenum and colon to end as a sutured stump under the right cupola of the diaphragm. This duplication was identical in size and appearance to the adjacent jejunum and its stoma admitted a half-centimeter probe.

The upper ligated stump of the duplication was seen on the anterior aspect of the second thoracic vertebra and, when freed by blunt dissection, passed through this to its attachment on the anterior surface of the spinal cord between the roots of the second thoracic spinal nerves (Fig. 4).

The part of the duplication excised at operation was roughly spherical, 4 cm. in diameter. Externally it was rough, its lower end showing the impress of forceps and its upper end being constricted by a ligature. Its wall was 2 mm. thick and was composed of a thick mucosa lying on muscle.

The hole in the second thoracic vertebra was lined by dura. A coronal section through this part of the vertebral column (Fig. 5) showed the body of T4 to be complete but narrow at its lateral edges; T3 had two wedges of cartilage indenting the sides of its body and T2 was formed by four fragments of bone isolated by cartilage, the hole through which the stump of the diverticulum passed being an elongated vertical median cleft. T1 was likewise formed by four bony fragments incompletely separated by cartilage. C7 was divided horizontally by a plate of cartilage.

The brain and its membranes were normal; the spinal cord showed a slight localized expansion in the region of the stump of the duplication. The remaining organs were normal.

Histological examination of the duplication (Fig. 6) showed it to be formed of two layers of muscle arranged as in normal gut, Auerbach's and Meissner's plexuses being present. The submucosa was simple connective tissue without cellular infiltration. The mucosa, limited externally by a muscularis mucosae, was thrown into villous folds with occasional simple gland acini at their bases. The epithelium was a single layer of tall columnar cells with occasional goblet cells. Its appearance was

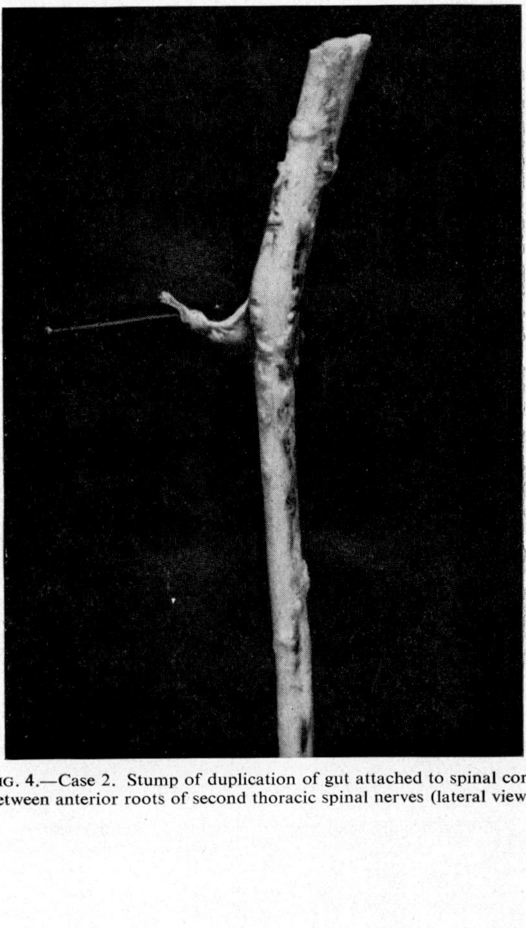

FIG. 4.—Case 2. Stump of duplication of gut attached to spinal cord between anterior roots of second thoracic spinal nerves (lateral view).

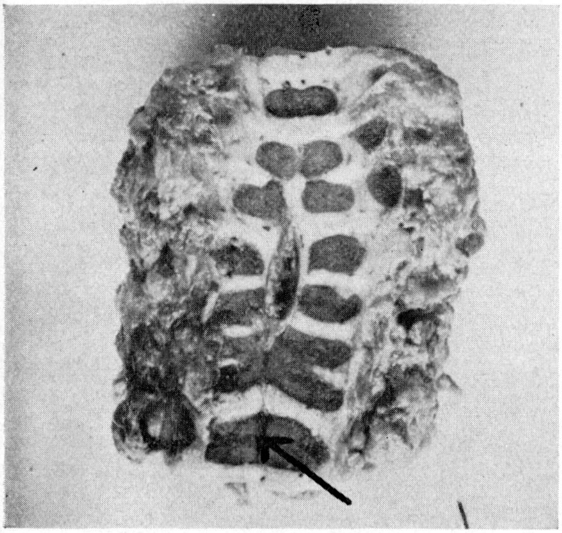

FIG. 5.—Case 2. Coronal section of vertebrae showing cartilage plates dividing the bodies; and median vertical fissure through which the stump of duplication of gut passed to its attachment on spinal cord. Arrow indicates fourth thoracic vertebra.

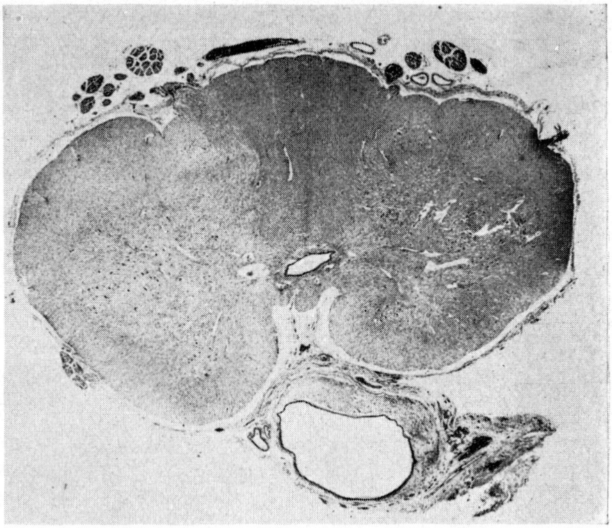

FIG. 7a.—Case 2. Photomicrograph of attachment of duplication of gut to anterior surface of spinal cord. Note mantle of nervous tissue surrounding dorsal aspect of lumen and scattered bundles of smooth muscle in ventral part. (× 10.)

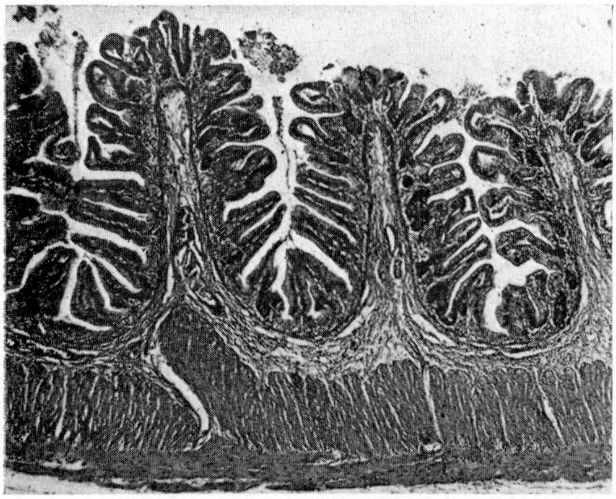

FIG. 6.—Case 2. Section of wall of duplication of gut showing typical appearances of normal jejunum. (× 70)

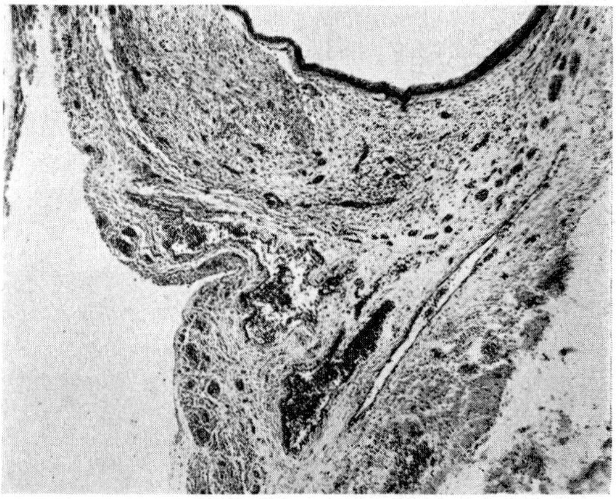

FIG. 7b.—Case 2. Higher power photomicrograph of lumen of diverticulum with mantle of nervous tissue and muscle bundles adjacent to its lumen. (× 40.)

typical of jejunum, and its structure was constant throughout its length.

The stump, attaching the duplication to the spinal cord, contained a small lumen, lined by squamous epithelium up to four cells thick, which lay ventrally on connective tissue rich in capillaries and sparsely infiltrated with lymphocytes, and containing scattered bundles of smooth muscle (Figs. 7a and b). Dorsally this epithelial-lined lumen was covered with a mantle of nervous tissue in which nerve cells, nerve fibres and neuroglia were identified, and was continuous with the white matter of the spinal cord. The pia mater of the spinal cord was continuous with a similar covering of the stump.

Serial section of the spinal cord over the extent of the attachment of the duplication failed to show communication between the central canal of the spinal cord and the lumen of the duplication. At the lower end of this attachment the ependyma of the central canal had disappeared and nervous tissue of the duplication projected into its lumen.

The jejunum adjacent to the diverticulum showed a normal microscopic structure.

Discussion

The clinical and surgical features of mediastinal duplications of the gut have been discussed by several writers recently and little is to be gained by repetition. Interest centres in the mode of development rather than in the intricacies of diagnosis and treatment of the condition. Five theories which have been advanced to explain its development will be briefly outlined, full accounts being given in the references cited.

I. Incomplete Separation of the Notochord. During the third week of embryonic development the notochord separates from the roof of the entodermal vesicle (yolk sac) and later becomes enveloped by paraxial mesoderm which segments and forms the vertebrae. It has been postulated (Fallon, Gordon and Lendrum, 1954) that in some cases separation of the notochord from the entoderm is incomplete and adhesions between it and the parent entoderm prevent mesodermal envelopment around the notochord, so giving rise to vertebral abnormalities. Medial migration of the mesoderm causes the notochord and entoderm to separate and any adhesion between them would give rise to a traction diverticulum of the entoderm.

II. Ectoderm-entoderm Adhesion. McLetchie *et al.* (1954) suggest that in the presomite stage a cleft occurs in the notochord, thus permitting the entoderm to become attached to the ectoderm, and in this way a 'neurenteric band' develops which prevents proper medial migration of paraxial mesoderm and so leads to vertebral abnormalities. A traction diverticulum of the entoderm occurs as the entodermal vesicle and ectoderm are separated by medial migration of the paraxial mesoderm. Bremer (1952) postulates that an adhesion between the entoderm and the neural ectoderm gives rise to an 'accessory neurenteric canal' around which the midline structures (notochord, spinal cord and vertebrae) must develop. Vertebral abnormalities of necessity occur and a traction diverticulum of the entoderm develops as the entoderm and ectoderm are separated by medial migration of the paraxial mesoderm.

III. Vacuolation Theory. During development of the gut its epithelium proliferates rapidly and the lumen becomes obliterated, never from end to end but only focally (solid stage). Vacuoles filled with secretion from the cells form and later coalesce to reform the lumen, or sometimes, several lumina. With lengthening of the gut its epithelium thins out to cover the increasing surface and vacuoles formed earlier disappear.

Persistence of a vacuole results in a mucosal cyst, and if the epithelium between it and the true lumen breaks down at one point only a mucosal diverticulum results. Development of muscle in its wall is assumed to follow migration of mesoderm into a fissure of the epithelium forming in the neighbourhood of the vacuole; now the wall can become intestinal in structure, not simply mucosal (Evans, 1929; Bremer, 1944; Ladd and Scott, 1944; Gross *et al*, 1952).

IV. Sequestration of Cells from a Lung Bud. The respiratory tract develops as an out-pouching from the primitive digestive tube, and the lungs form as separate buds on this larger out-pouching. This theory postulates that during the development of the lung bud (or by formation of a similar but separate bud) some cells become sequestrated in the mesoderm and there develop into cystic structures with either enteric, gastric, intestinal or bronchial epithelium (Mixter and Clifford, 1929; Olenik and Tandatnick, 1946; Bickford, 1949; Wooler, 1950).

V. Mucosal Diverticula. Lewis and Thyng (1908) observed diverticula of the mucosa of the intestine, especially in its distal parts, in embryos of pigs, rabbits and in some human embryos. They suggest that these diverticula, although normally disappearing, may occasionally give rise to pathological diverticula.

The majority of authors consider either the vacuolation theory or the theory of sequestration of cells from a lung bud to be the most probable explanation for duplications of the gut occurring in the mediastinum. Only a few favour the mucosal diverticulum theory.

These theories would explain the formation of a duplication closely related to and sharing the muscle coats of the parent gut as has been described in the oesophagus (Ladd and Scott, 1944; Williams and Johnson, 1952). It is unlikely, however, that the muscular wall of a duplication so formed would consist of two layers over the whole of its circumference. But these theories do not offer any explanation for the frequent association of vertebral abnormalities with mediastinal duplications of the gut; this frequent co-existence has been stressed by Veeneklaas (1950) who, visualizing by tomography abnormalities not seen on straight films of the vertebrae, suggests that the association of the two abnormalities is even more frequent than the study of the literature indicates.

Both the theory of incomplete separation of the notochord and the ectoderm-entoderm adhesion theory give a satisfactory explanation of the association of vertebral abnormalities with mediastinal duplications of the gut. If the former theory is correct, one would not expect to find any connexion between the duplication and the central nervous system but when such connexion is found the latter theory provides a more satisfactory explanation for the simultaneous development of both abnormalities.

On the basis of the ectoderm-entoderm adhesion theory one would expect to find, in extreme cases, a fistula between the gut and the skin in the midline of the back passing through the vertebrae and spinal cord; such cases have, in fact, been described by Saunders (1943) and Bremer (1952). In less complete examples a tubular extension or solid cord passes from the apex of the duplication to the skin, spinal cord, meninges or vertebrae, traversing midline structures between its attachment and the duplication. Neuhauser, Harris and Berrett (1958) have described three cases of duplication of the gut with vertebral abnormalities and with a solid cord connecting it with the spinal cord; and also one case with a solid process of the duplication attached to the meninges. Budde (1911) recorded a case where a long solid cord, composed of nervous and muscular tissue, traversed abnormal vertebrae to connect the apex of a gastric duplication with the medulla. Case 2 of this communication is a further example of a partly solid cord passing through abnormal vertebrae to connect the spinal cord with the apex of an intestinal duplication.

Although, in some cases, the abdominal connexion of the duplication is retained, all trace of its connexion with midline structures may be lost, as in the cases of Gross *et al.* (1952); here the vertebral abnormalities are strong presumptive evidence of previous connexion with midline structures.

Finally the abdominal connexion of the duplication may disappear and a single cyst or several cysts may be found at the site of the original duplication. In these cases the dense adhesion of the duplication cyst to the bodies of the vertebrae, themselves frequently abnormal, is a significant fact and is frequently mentioned in case reports.

It must be admitted that no case report of purely abdominal duplication of the gut associated with abnormal vertebrae has been found. If such duplications arise from ectoderm-entoderm adhesions, one must assume that the adhesion has not persisted long enough to prevent envelopment of the notochord by paraxial mesoderm. This is most improbable and such duplications are more reasonably explained by the vacuolation theory or the mucosal diverticulum theory.

In the opinion of the writer, duplications of the gut associated with vertebral abnormalities are most satisfactorily explained by assuming that, early in embryonic development, an adhesion occurring between ectoderm and entoderm produces a traction diverticulum of the entoderm and also prevents proper covering of the notochord by paraxial mesoderm. The final anatomical form of the duplication will be influenced by whether or not its original connexions with the alimentary tract and midline structures are retained and to what extent its lumen remains patent. Its length will be determined to some extent by the site of origin; when arising from entoderm destined to become upper alimentary tract it will lengthen as this descends from the cervical region to its final subdiaphragmatic site. Various epithelial linings are to be expected in the duplication as the primitive fore-gut entoderm can differentiate into squamous, columnar, ciliated or acid-secreting epithelium.

Summary

Two cases of mediastinal duplications of the gut are described, one an isolated mediastinal cyst, and the other a jejunal duplication which, passing through the diaphragm into the mediastinum, terminated in a neuromuscular strand attached to the spinal cord. In both cases gross vertebral abnormalities were present.

Several theories explaining the development of this abnormality are briefly reviewed and it is concluded that the most probable assumes that, early in embryonic life, an adhesion, occurring between the ectoderm and entoderm, prevents proper covering of the notochord with paraxial mesoderm and also results in a traction diverticulum of the entoderm.

Due acknowledgment is made to my clinical colleagues, Professor J. D. Hay, Dr. H. G. Farquhar and Dr. Olive Scott, for clinical details of the cases; to Mr. B. J. Bickford, for details of the operative findings; and to Dr. Norah Walker, for reproductions of the radiographs.

The photographs were taken by Miss M. A. Fisher and the photomicrographs by Mr. W. Lee; Mr. Arthur Knowlson prepared many histological sections. To all I record my thanks.

References

Bickford, B. J. (1949). *Brit. J. Surg.*, **36**, 410.
Bremer, J. L. (1944). *Arch. Path. (Chicago)*, **38**, 132.
—— (1952). *A.M.A. Arch. Path.*, **54**, 132.
Budde, M. (1911). *Beitr. path. Anat.*, **52**, 91.
Dickson, J. A., Clagett, O. T and McDonald, J. R. (1946). *J. thorac. Surg.*, **15**, 318.
Evans, A. (1929). *Brit. J. Surg.*, **17**, 34.
Fallon, M., Gordon, A. R. G. and Lendrum, A. C. (1954). *Ibid.*, **41**, 520.
Gross, R. E., Neuhauser, E. B. D. and Longino, L. A. (1950). *Ann. Surg.*, **131**, 363.
——, Holcomb, G. W. and Farber, S. (1952). *Pediatrics*, **9**, 449.
Ladd, W. E. and Scott, H. W. (1944). *Surgery*, **16**, 815.
Lewis, F. T. and Thyng, F. W. (1908). *Amer. J. Anat.*, **7**, 505.
McLetchie, N. G. B., Purves, J. K. and Saunders, R. L. de C. H. (1954). *Surg. Gynec. Obstet.*, **99**, 135.
Mixter, C. G. and Clifford, S. H. (1929). *Ann. Surg.* **90**, 714.
Morrison, I. M. (1958). *Thorax*, **13**, 294.
Neuhauser, E. B. D., Harris, G. B. C. and Berrett, A. (1958). *Amer. J. Roentgenol.*, **79**, 235.
Olenik, J. L. and Tandatnick, J. W. (1946). *Amer. J. Dis. Child.*, **71**, 466.
Saunders, R. L. deC. H. (1943). *Anat. Rec.*, **87**, 255.
Veeneklaas G. M. H. (1950). *Amer. J. Dis. Child.*, **83**, 500.
Williams, M. H. and Johnson, J. F. (1952). *A.M.A. Arch. Surg.*, **64**, 138.
Wooler, G. H. (1950). *Brit. J. Surg.*, **37**, 356.

INTESTINAL OBSTRUCTION IN A CASE OF DUPLICATION OF THE TERMINAL ILEUM

BY

J. A. WILLIAMS
From the Children's Hospital, Birmingham

(RECEIVED FOR PUBLICATION MAY 22, 1959)

Duplication of the alimentary tract is a rare but well-known condition, the aetiology of which is imperfectly understood. The present knowledge and theories are discussed by Willis (1958). Duplications occur on the dorsal or mesenteric aspect of the normal alimentary tract and may or may not communicate with it. Often they do not communicate and the secretions of the epithelial lining lead to cyst formation, giving rise to a variety of symptoms. Such cysts are found throughout the alimentary tract but are most common in the terminal ileum. They are lined by epithelium, which resembles the adjacent bowel but which may contain any type of intestinal epithelial cell. The muscular coat is intermingled with that of the adjacent bowel and their blood supply is common, making operative dissection of the cyst impossible (Gross, 1953).

Intestinal obstruction may result from pressure on the adjacent bowel when it and the cyst lie where movement is restricted. Duodenal duplications are particularly prone to give rise to obstruction in infancy, showing a picture akin to that seen in pyloric stenosis. Duplications in the rest of the bowel are not likely to give rise to early obstruction as the bowel can be displaced by the growing cyst.

A case is described in which an anatomical structure was seen to be the cause of the neonatal intestinal obstruction.

Case Report

N.S., a male child, was admitted aged 15 days. Delivery had been normal at full term and his birth weight was 9 lb. He had been fed with National Dried Milk. Meconium was passed and a normal stool was seen on the fourth day. The bowels continued to be open until the fourteenth day, when vomiting, which had been occasional and mild, became marked and changed from milk curds to brown fluid.

On examination the child was slightly dehydrated but in good general condition. Peristalsis was visible and bowel sounds were excessive.

In the right iliac fossa there was a smooth well defined cystic swelling, which was mobile in both directions. On rectal examination the lump could be felt bimanually and its smooth surface and cystic nature were confirmed. It was also noted to be grooved rather like a plum.

A plain radiograph of the abdomen showed distended loops of small intestine. The appearance of the chest and spine were normal on the antero-posterior radiograph (see Fallon, Gordon and Lendrum, 1954).

A diagnosis of low small bowel obstruction was made and was thought to be due to the palpable cystic mass. It was felt that this must therefore be a duplication of the ileum. The significance of the groove was not appreciated.

Rehydration was begun and the child was submitted to laparotomy. Through a right lower rectus-splitting incision the abdomen was entered and the ileo-caecal region was exposed. The terminal ileum was obstructed by a cystic swelling on the mesenteric border, the normal bowel being compressed against a firm vascular band running to the caecum. The diagnosis of duplication was therefore confirmed and a resection of the ileum adjacent to the cyst and the caecum was performed. A two-layer end-to-end anastomosis was made between the ileum and ascending colon, and the mesentery was repaired.

The bowel sounds returned on the second post-operative day and normal feeding was resumed on the fourth day. He was discharged on the twentieth post-operative day having been delayed by a persistent oral thrush.

Ths specimen removed at operation consisted of a cystic mass 5 cm. in diameter on the mesenteric border of the ileum at the ileo-caecal angle (Fig. 1). The normal ileum was shown to be patent by passing a probe into the caecum but the lumen was compressed by a cyst. Acute obstruction occurred where the vascular fold of the caecum formed an unyielding structure on the anti-mesenteric border of the bowel (Fig. 2). This fold is a normal anatomical structure and contains the anterior caecal branch of the ileo-colic artery. This formed the

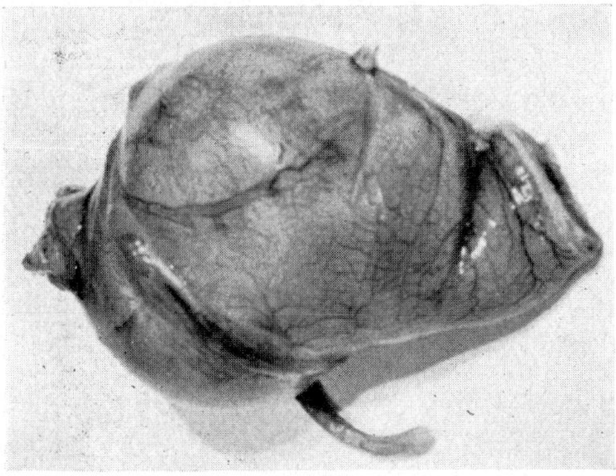

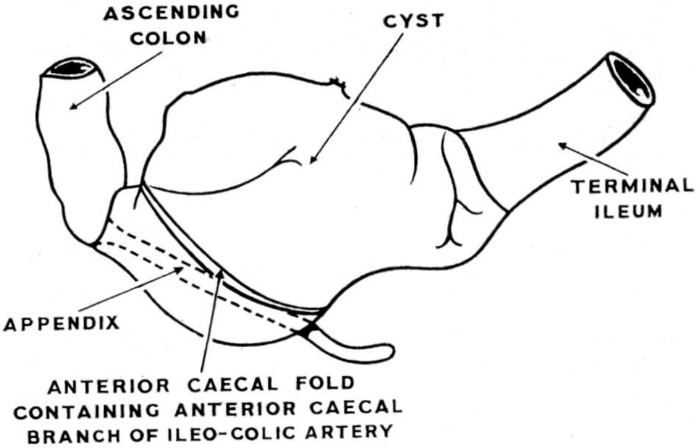

FIG. 1.

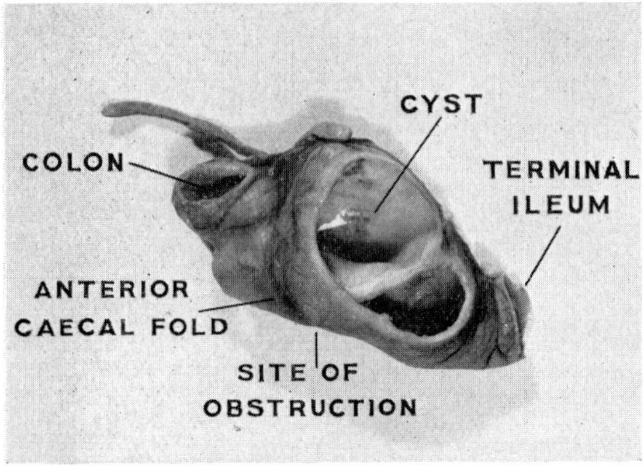

FIG. 2.

groove which was palpable per rectum. Microscopically the cyst was lined by flattened epithelium of the small bowel type. In some areas groups of cells were seen similar to Brunner's glands of the duodenum.

Discussion

A reduplication cyst of the terminal ileum is a rare cause of intestinal obstruction. These cysts may cause obstruction due to intussusception and a number of such cases have been described. It is less common for obstruction to be caused by obstruction of the ileo-caecal valve, although Gross (1953) mentions six cases. In the case here recorded I suggest that intestinal obstruction occurred early in life because the ileum was compressed against the vascular fold of the caecum. Pachman (1939) and Hardaway, Wedgwood, Swartley and Rudman (1952) record similar cases at the ages of 2 and 5 days respectively. They do not mention the presence of the caecal fold though in both cases the description and photographs lead one to suspect that this may have been the cause of the obstruction.

I wish to thank Dr. W. H. P. Cant for permission to publish this case and Dr. A. H. Cameron for the pathological examination and his advice. I also wish to thank Mr. J. W. Williamson for the photographs and Miss V. D. Whissell for her assistance.

REFERENCES

Fallon, M., Gordon, A. R. G. and Lendrum, A. C. (1954). *Brit. J. Surg.*, **41**, 520.
Gross, R. E. (1953). *The Surgery of Infancy and Childhood*, p. 232. W. B. Saunders, Philadelphia and London.
Hardaway, R. M., Wedgwood, R. J., Swartley, R. N. and Rudman, T. (1952). *Ann. Surg.*, **136**, 296.
Pachman, D. J. (1939). *Amer. J. Dis. Child.*, **58**, 485.
Willis, R. A. (1958). *The Borderland of Embryology and Pathology*, p. 188. Butterworth, London.

THE INCIDENCE OF INGUINAL HERNIA IN NEWCASTLE CHILDREN

BY

GEORGE KNOX

From the Department of Child Health, University of Durham, King's College, Newcastle upon Tyne

(RECEIVED FOR PUBLICATION APRIL 27, 1959)

The intensive investigations of recent years into the incidence of congenital malformations have largely ignored inguinal hernia. This is surprising in view of its common occurrence and the generally accepted belief that it is congenital in origin even when not apparent at birth.

This paper gives an estimate of the present incidence of inguinal hernia in children in Newcastle upon Tyne and considers certain factors which may influence the risk of its occurrence.

Material

Almost all children in Newcastle who require hospital care, together with many from surrounding districts, receive it in one of the units associated with the University Department of Child Health. The main material for the present analysis consists of all Newcastle children who had not reached their twelfth birthday and who were admitted to one of these units between 1953 and 1957 for surgical repair of an inguinal hernia. Secondary repair following recurrence and operations in the same child upon a second hernia were excluded, together with femoral, incisional, hiatal and other types of hernia. Surgical repair is therefore part of the definition used for the present purpose. This main group supplied a measure of incidence and of the variation of the risk with age.

One unit recorded with sufficient consistency for analysis the birth rank and birth weight of the affected child and the age of the mother. A consecutive series of 200 children treated for inguinal hernia at this unit was used in assessing the relevance of these factors; 40 of these were also included in the main group and the remaining 160 were from outside the city or, if from Newcastle, were admitted before 1953.

Finally, since there was uncertainty about the existence of a seasonal variation in the birth dates of affected children, the date of birth was reviewed in a much larger number of children treated for hernia and falling outside the two groups described above.

Results

Incidence. There were 229 Newcastle children treated for inguinal hernia before their twelfth birthday in the five years 1953 to 1957. They are presented according to the year of operation and year of birth in Table 1.

TABLE 1

YEAR OF OPERATION AND YEAR OF BIRTH IN 229 NEWCASTLE CHILDREN WITH SURGICALLY TREATED INGUINAL HERNIA

Year of Birth	Year of Operation 1953	1954	1955	1956	1957	Oblique Totals
1957	—	—	—	—	2	13
1956	—	—	—	2	7	56
1955	—	—	0	11	10	44
1954	—	3	11	14	3	17
1953	6	12	8	5	5	33
1952	15	9	5	7	4	18
1951	3	3	6	2	3	13
1950	1	7	4	2	0	5
1949	8	2	6	2	1	7
1948	6	0	2	0	0	6
1947	2	0	1	1	2	9
1946	1	3	1	3	0	4
1945	2	2	1	2	1	4
1944	2	1	0	1	—	
1943	2	1	1	—	—	
1942	1	1	—	—	—	
1941	0	—	—	—	—	
Totals	49	44	46	52	38	229

The last column of this table, giving the oblique totals, shows the time relationships between the calendar year of birth and the calendar year of operation. The highest rates of operation were in the first and second calendar years after the year of birth.

This presentation is used because it is the basis on which the incidence of the disease has been calculated. A complementary table (not given) can be constructed from the Registrar-General's reports in which the cells contain the number of children at risk. These figures can be taken as the number of live births in the appropriate year, minus the infant deaths in that year. Thus it follows, for example, that the oblique total 44 in Table 1 represents a number of child years at risk equivalent to the live births of the years 1951 to 1955 less the infant deaths in those years. For the first and last totals (see Table 2) these denominators are halved.

TABLE 2

HERNIA OPERATIONS AND CHILDREN AT RISK BY CALENDAR YEAR OF OPERATION RELATIVE TO THE CALENDAR YEAR OF BIRTH

Year of Birth plus :	Hernia Operations	Children at Risk	Rate/1,000
0	13	23,793/2	1·093
1	56	23,558	2·377
2	44	23,353	1·884
3	17	23,722	0·716
4	33	24,110	1·368
5	18	24,816	0·724
6	13	26,290	0·494
7	5	27,533	0·181
8	7	27,171	0·258
9	6	27,188	0·221
10	9	25,991	0·346
11	4	23,880	0·168
12	4	21,840/2	0·366
Totals	229	—	10·198

When this has been carried out for each of the oblique totals, the results may be added to give an overall estimate of incidence which is unaffected to any serious extent by interaction between the age incidence of operation and the waxing and waning of the birth rate over the period concerned. The details are given in Table 2 where it is shown that the incidence of repaired inguinal hernia in Newcastle children surviving to the age of 12 is 10·2/1,000. The 95% confidence limits of this estimate are 9·0/1,000 and 11·4/1,000. Since the disease occurs much more frequently in boys than in girls (M/F approx. 12/1) an alternative expression of incidence would be 19 per 1,000 boys. Clearly, these estimates refer to the number of children who survive for 12 years and get a hernia, and the proportion of children under 12 affected at any one time will be less.

Age Incidence. The dates of operation, birth and reputed onset of the hernia were recorded with sufficient accuracy to state the exact age at operation in 226 of the 229 children, and the exact age at onset in 191. The distributions are given in Table 3

TABLE 3

AGE DISTRIBUTION OF ONSET AND OF OPERATION IN INGUINAL HERNIA

Age		Onset (No.)	Operation (No.)	Cumulative Incidences of: Onset	Operation
Months	— 1	31	2	1·66	0·09
	— 3	23	5	2·89	0·31
	— 6	12	7	3·52	0·64
	—12	12	17	4·17	1·40
Years	— 2	24	60	5·45	4·10
	— 3	18	29	6·41	5·42
	— 4	23	20	7·64	6·32
	— 5	14	31	8·38	7·72
	— 6	7	16	8·76	8·44
	— 7	5	6	9·03	8·71
	— 8	7	8	9·40	9·07
	— 9	5	5	9·66	9·29
	—10	4	10	9·88	9·75
	—11	5	4	10·15	9·93
	—12	1	6	10·20	10·20
		191	226	—	—

together with the calculated cumulative incidences by age both for onset and for operation. These figures are derived by equating the number recorded with the overall incidence.

Fig. 1 demonstrates the relationship between the

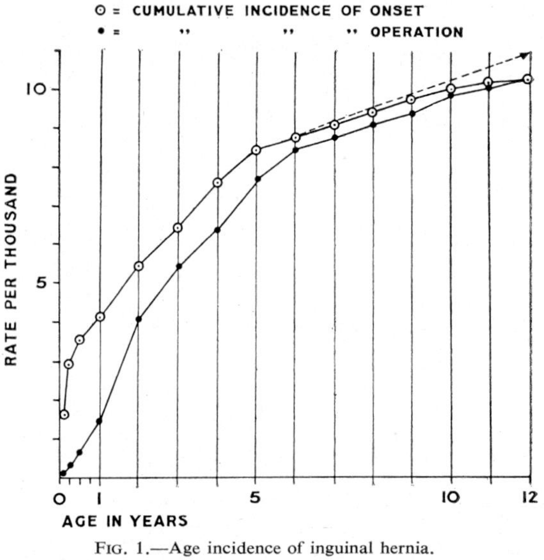

FIG. 1.—Age incidence of inguinal hernia.

cumulative incidence of onset and the cumulative incidence of operation and shows that the waiting time between onset and operation was about one year. The convergence of the lines towards the twelfth year is of course a consequence of the definition used but the picture is such as to give

TABLE 4

PROPORTIONAL (%) DISTRIBUTION OF LIVE BIRTHS AND OF CHILDREN WITH INGUINAL HERNIA BY MATERNAL AGE

	Maternal Age at Delivery in Years							
	–19	–24	–29	–34	–39	–44	45+	Total
Tyneside (1952) %	3·5	28·4	32·0	22·1	10·7	3·1	0·3	100·1
Northern Region (1952) %	3·9	29·3	31·5	21·5	10·4	3·1	0·2	99·9
200 Children with Hernia (No.)	9	46	51	30	19	9	0	164 (plus 36 NR)
(%)	5·5	28·0	31·1	18·3	11·6	5·5	0	100·0

some confidence that at ages under 10 years the estimate of incidence is not greatly short of the true figure. The interrupted line in the figure indicates how the line might proceed if the mean waiting time to operation were consistent by age after starting school and suggests that the true incidence at 12 years might be about a tenth greater than the estimate derived.

Influence of Sex. Among 200 consecutive cases seen at one unit 15 were female. The male/female ratio was 12·3:1.

The Side Affected. Among the same 200, 58 were on the left side, 127 on the right and 15 were bilateral when seen. The ratio right/left among the 215 individual hernias was 142/73 = 1·95:1. This pattern was similar in both sexes, the figures for girls being 10 on the right and six on the left.

Maternal Age. The maternal age at the time of admission was recorded in 164 of the 200 cases and the age at delivery was calculable. The distribution is given in Table 4 and compared with proportional distributions for the area in 1952 (Registrar-General, 1952); there are no obvious discrepancies.

Birth Rank. The number of previous live births was recorded for 192 of the 200 consecutive cases at one unit. This distribution is given in Table 5 and compared with figures for England and Wales in 1952 (Registrar-General, 1952). Here there is some suggestion of an increased proportion of first babies among those with inguinal hernia although it does not reach formal significance.

Birthweight. Birthweights as recalled by the mother were recorded in 184 of the 200 cases. The data are presented in Table 6 grouped according to

TABLE 5

PROPORTIONAL (%) DISTRIBUTION OF LIVE BIRTHS AND CHILDREN WITH INGUINAL HERNIA BY NUMBER OF PREVIOUS LIVE BIRTHS

	Previous Live Births						
	0	1	2	3	4 or more	Total	Mean
England and Wales: %	39·5	30·1	15·6	7·2	7·6	100·0	1·24
200 Children (No.)	84	61	24	10	13	192 (plus 8 NR)	1·07
(%)	43·7	31·8	12·5	5·2	6·8	100·0	

TABLE 6

BIRTHWEIGHT DISTRIBUTIONS OF CHILDREN WITH INFANTILE HERNIA AND LATER HERNIA

	Birthweight (last complete recorded pound)										
	2	3	4	5	6	7	8	9	10	11	Total (No.)
Infantile hernias	1	2	4	5	22	11	12	4	0	1	62
Later hernias	0	1	3	6	27	40	32	7	4	2	122
All hernias	1	3	7	11	49	51	44	11	4	3	184 (plus 16 NR)

Mean Birthweights		
Infantile hernia	6·97	
Later hernia	7·62	
	7·40	F = 8·6; P < 0·005

the last complete recorded pound, and the mean weight for each group is taken as half a pound more than this value. The mean weight for the 184 children at birth was 7·40 lb. Table 6 also compares in terms of birthweight children whose hernias were first noted before the first birthday with those noticed afterwards. The mean birthweight of the first group was 6·97 lb. and of the second group 7·62 lb. The difference of 0·65 lb. is statistically significant ($P<0·005$).

We can compare this group with 429 normal boys born in Newcastle who were the subject of another investigation (Miller, Court, Walton and Knox, 1959), and whose mean birthweight was 7·43 lb. Considering differences in the method of recording, this is reasonably close to the higher of the previous two figures, but well above the lower one. We can therefore fairly conclude that a high risk of infantile hernia is associated with a low average birthweight.

Birthweight is known to rise with birth rank and this recalls the apparent (although not significant) increased risk of hernia in early birth ranks (see Table 5). It is natural to ask if either the birth weight or birth rank association could be secondary to the other. There is evidence on this point from two sources.

First we have the data of the 429 normal boys analysed by birth rank; in this sample the mean weight of first children was 7·23 lb. and of later children 7·58 lb. The difference between mean birthweights detected by analysis in terms of the timing of a hernia (0·65 lb.) was therefore greater than that detected in a normal sample by means of birth rank (0·35 lb.). This suggests that birthweight rather than birth rank was the factor more directly associated with altered risk of infantile hernia.

Secondly, and more directly, the children with hernias did not demonstrate a correlation between birth rank and the timing of the hernia. The distribution by birth rank and time of onset in the children in whom both were recorded is given in Table 7. There are therefore double grounds for regarding the association between low birthweight and increased risk of infantile hernia as primary.

TABLE 7

BIRTH RANK AND AGE AT ONSET OF INGUINAL HERNIA

	Age at Onset		
	First Year	Later	Total
Birth rank:			
First or second	47	98	145
Third or greater	19	32	51
Total	66	130	196
% First or second	71·2	75·4	

Season. The possibility of a seasonal variation in dates of birth was examined. Figures are given in Table 8 for children in the samples already described together with a supplement of extra children whose notes were scanned in the course of extracting data but who were rejected because they fell outside the time and geographical limits set. There was no evidence of a seasonal variation.

Discussion

There are two aspects of the technique of measurement used in this assessment which might have affected the result. The first is a presumed existence at the age of 12 years of hernias which have not yet come to operation, but reasons for regarding the number as small have been given. The second is that hernia defined in terms of repair precludes those which might have disappeared spontaneously. Most paediatricians and surgeons in Newcastle believe that inguinal hernias do not often resolve spontaneously and so most children reaching hospital come to operation. But general practitioners and parents may not all share this belief and in some children reaching an out-patient department with a symptomless hernia treatment may well be postponed until they have reached a more suitable age for hospital admission. We cannot therefore ignore the possibility that the natural history of the disease may be such that as an estimate of total incidence the present figure is too low. Paterson and Gray (1927), for example, stated that as many as 24% of hernias in children resolved spontaneously.

This possibility must also be taken into account in our interpretation of the inverse correlation between birthweight and the risk of hernia in infancy. It may be as valid to interpret the effect of birthweight

TABLE 8

MONTH OF BIRTH OF 655 CHILDREN WITH INGUINAL HERNIA

	Month of Birth												
	Jan.	Feb.	Mar.	Apl.	May	June	July	Aug.	Sept.	Oct.	Nov.	Dec.	Total
Children ..	65	41	67	62	51	64	49	59	48	54	43	52	655

as expressing a reduced rate of remission as a high rate of occurrence.

There do not seem to be any recent estimates of incidence in known populations of children with which the present estimate can be compared. Keith (1923) estimated that the prevalence of hernia among males of all ages was 20 per 1,000 living, a figure which is reached in Newcastle at the present time among boys surviving to early adult life. Keith's statement of age incidence is difficult to follow but suggests that his estimate of incidence in children is very much less than the current one. Edwards' more recent (1943) estimate of the incidence in adult males (143 of 1,300 service recruits aged 35 to 36) strongly suggests that Keith's estimates were based on a low degree of ascertainment.

Collins (1938) supplies some relevant information and from his data may be calculated cumulative incidences of 2·7, 6·2 and 7·1 per thousand children at ages 5, 10 and 12 respectively. These rates, however, were based on only 43 hernia operations at all ages, and the number occurring in childhood, although not given, is obviously small.

Landers (1938), estimating the incidence of hernia in adults, found an incidence of 16 per 1,000 males aged 16 to 20 years, but once more this was based on small numbers, five cases among 320 examined.

The present estimates of age incidence therefore show no serious discrepancies from the few valid estimates which have already been made, and are presented with some confidence in their relative precision. The only serious objections are the methodological ones which have already been presented; but the figures given stand firmly as minimum incidences and for most purposes, certainly at the earlier ages, can be regarded as absolute measures.

I have not been able to find any previous examination of possible relationships between hernia and the factors tested here except the sex ratio of the disease, which is of course well known, and the preponderance of right over left sided hernias. Paterson and Gray (1927) in their series found 696 males and 77 females and quote another earlier survey with 906 males and 94 females. The M/F ratio in these two series combined is 9·4:1. The same two series included 1,344 right and 647 left hernias, a ratio of 2·1:1 compared with the present estimate of 1·95:1.

Summary

The incidence of inguinal hernia coming to operation was measured in Newcastle children between 1953 and 1957 and found to be 10·2 per 1,000 children of both sexes surviving to their twelfth birthday. The highest rate of onset was in infancy and it fell steadily in succeeding years.

Among possible aetiological factors tested, maternal age and season of birth had no detectable effect and birth rank a doubtful one. The latter may have been secondary to an effect of birthweight: low birthweight was associated with a high incidence of onset in infants but not in older children.

References

Edwards, H. (1943). *Proc. roy. Soc. Med.*, **36**, 186.
Collins, S. D. (1938). *Publ. Hlth Rep. (Wash.)*, **53**, 587.
Keith, Sir A. (1923). *Brit. J. Surg.*, **11**, 455.
Landers, M. B. (1938). *Indust. Med.*, **7**, 671.
Miller, F. J. W., Court, S. D. M., Walton, W. S. and Knox, E. G. (1959). *Growing Up*. Oxford University Press, London (in press).
Paterson, D. and Gray, G. M. (1927). *Archives of Disease in Childhood*, **2**, 328.
Registrar-General (1952). The Registrar General's Review of England and Wales, 1952, Part II. H.M.S.O., London.

A LONGITUDINAL STUDY OF THE GROWTH AND DEVELOPMENT OF PREMATURELY AND MATURELY BORN CHILDREN

PART V. PATTERNS OF MATERNAL CARE (A STUDY OF CHILD REARING IN SCOTLAND)

BY

CECIL MARY DRILLIEN

From the Department of Child Life and Health, University of Edinburgh

(RECEIVED FOR PUBLICATION MAY 1, 1959)

In previous papers in this series (Drillien, 1958, 1959a, b) reference has been made to maternal efficiency and maternal grading in relation to physical and mental development and morbidity. In this final paper, dealing with the progress of prematurely and maturely born children in the first two years of life, patterns of maternal care in different types of home are described for 368 singleton children. Working class mothers, who form 90% of the total, are divided into superior working class, with husbands mainly in the Registrar General's Social Class III, where standards of child care and household management approximate closely to those found in homes with fathers in Social Classes I and II, average and poor working class. In the last group there is a predominance of mothers of low intelligence and fathers who are sporadically employed on labouring work. In the subsequent discussion, mothers with husbands included in the Registrar General's Social Classes I and II are described as maternal grade 1. Superior working class are described as grade 2, average and poor working class, 3 and 4. The numbers included in these four groups are shown in Table 1. The social class distribution of the sample does not differ significantly from that of all singleton children born in Edinburgh during the same period. The patterns of care described in this paper probably give a reasonably accurate picture of child care in the general population of this city.

TABLE 1

COMPOSITION OF SAMPLE BY MATERNAL GRADE

Maternal Grade	Birthweight (lb. oz.)				Total	
	5·8 and under		5·9 and over			
	No.	%	No.	%	No.	%
1	16	6·4	22	18·5	38	10·3
2	70	28·1	47	39·5	117	31·8
3	107	43·0	40	33·6	147	39·9
4	56	22·5	10	8·4	66	18·0
Total	249	100·0	119	100·0	368	100·0

Table 2 gives the maternal grading for working class mothers in the survey by the Registrar General's social classification, for different birthweight groups. In the mature control group there are more better type mothers of like social class than in the premature groups. Assuming that children included in the survey are a fair sample of all children born during the same period of like birthweight and social class, it is possible to estimate the incidence of maternal grade for all children born in Edinburgh during the same period, using basic data previously published (Drillien, 1956). The figures are set out in Table 3. The birthweight distribution of legitimate singletons in the general population was

TABLE 2

MATERNAL GRADING BY REGISTRAR GENERAL'S SOCIAL CLASSIFICATION

Maternal Grade	Registrar General's Social Classification					
	3			4 and 5		
	Birthweight (lb. oz.)			Birthweight (lb. oz.)		
	<4·1	4·1–5·8	>5·8	<4·1	4·1–5·8	>5·8
	(%)	(%)	(%)	(%)	(%)	(%)
2	36·4	37·9	62·1	7·2	12·0	14·8
3	50·0	47·4	31·8	35·7	39·7	63·0
4	13·6	14·7	6·1	57·1	48·3	22·2
Total	100·0	100·0	100·0	100·0	100·0	100·0

TABLE 3

ESTIMATED MATERNAL GRADING FOR ALL SINGLETON LEGITIMATE BIRTHS IN EDINBURGH (1953-55)

Maternal Grade	Birthweight (lb. oz.)			All Births
	<4·1	4·1–5·8	>5·8	
	(%)	(%)	(%)	(%)
1	20·5	11·6	22·4	21·8
2	20·5	26·0	37·5	36·7
3	37·2	39·6	31·7	32·2
4	21·8	22·8	8·4	9·3
Total	100·0	100·0	100·0	100·0

4 lb. or less at birth, 1·2%; 4 to 5½ lb., 5·2%; and over 5½ lb., 93·6%. There is probably an under-estimate of the poorer types of mothers, as the survey contains an excess of first births in the mature control group, and it has been shown in the discussion on morbidity that standard of maternal care is highly correlated with parity (Drillien, 1959a, b).

Reference will be made to over-anxious and over-protective mothers. A mother was not classified as over-anxious when her fears arose as a result of failure to thrive or other difficulties in the child's progress, but only when anxiety was present from the earliest months in the absence of any obvious reason.

Feeding and Diet

Breast Feeding. As would be expected, the incidence of breast feeding varies with birthweight. Of the mature controls, 70% were discharged from hospital partially or fully breast fed. Only 53% continued with breast feeding for longer than two weeks after discharge. By 3 months of age, 30% of the total were still on the breast and 24% were fully breast fed for six months or longer. Of those who were 4 lb. or less at birth, only one was breast fed on discharge from hospital. Of those between 4 and 5 lb., 40% were discharged on breast feeding, 25% continued to breast feed for longer than two weeks, 17% continued for three months and 13% for six months or longer. The reasons given by the mothers for changing to bottle feeding are set out in Table 4.

TABLE 4

REASONS GIVEN FOR DISCONTINUING BREAST FEEDING

Reason for Stopping	Duration of Breast Feeding (mth.)		
	<1	1–3	3–6
	(%)	(%)	(%)
Insufficient lactation	70·3	80·5	62·4
Mastitis or breast abscess	18·5	11·1	—
Illness of mother	5·6	5·6	18·8
Other causes	5·6	2·8	18·8
Total	100·0	100·0	100·0

The commonest reason given was that the baby was not satisfied on the breast, but it was apparent that in many cases the mother had no real desire to breast feed, and gave this as a suitable excuse. The incidence of breast feeding varied with maternal grade, as is shown in Fig. 1. Of those who were

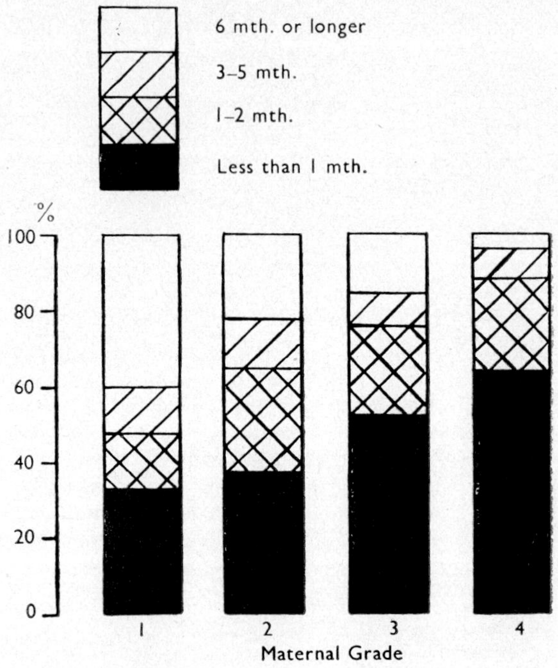

FIG. 1.—Duration of breast feeding, by maternal grade.

discharged from hospital as full breast feeding, more than one-half of mothers in maternal grade 1 continued for three months or longer, whereas two-thirds of poor working class mothers had changed to the bottle within two weeks.

In general, it was observed that breast fed babies suffered from less illness and were easier to manage than bottle fed babies, but this would be expected, owing to the predominance of better type mothers in the breast fed group. Table 5 gives mean weight

TABLE 5

AVERAGE WEIGHT INCREMENT (OZ.) AT 1 YEAR FOR BREAST AND BOTTLE FED BABIES, BY MATERNAL GRADE

Breast Feeding	Maternal Grade		
	1 and 2	3	4
	(oz.)	(oz.)	(oz.)
Six months or longer	239	230	176
Less than one month	258	245	236

increments at 1 year for those babies who were breast fed for six months or longer, compared with those who were breast fed for less than one month, by grade of mother. In each maternal grade group weight increment at 1 year is greater for bottle fed babies.

Table 6 gives the incidence of infective illness

TABLE 6

INFECTIVE ILLNESS IN FIRST YEAR FOR BREAST AND BOTTLE FED BABIES, BY MATERNAL GRADE AND FAMILY PLACING

	Infective Illness in First Year					
	Little or None		Some		Frequent	
Breast Feeding	6 months	<1 month	6 months	<1 month	6 months	<1 month
Maternal Grade	First born children:					
	(%)	(%)	(%)	(%)	(%)	(%)
1 and 2	78·3	74·2	21·7	22·6	0·0	3·2
3	61·5	57·6	23·1	27·3	15·4	15·2
4	—	42·9	—	28·6	—	28·6
	Later born children:					
1 and 2	72·8	50·0	27·3	43·8	0·0	6·2
3	—	37·8	—	41·4	—	20·9
4	—	20·0	—	20·0	—	60·0

(classified as little or none, some, frequent) in the first year, by grade of mother, for those breast fed for six months or longer, and less than one month. Here the cases have been divided into first and later born. There is little evidence that first born breast fed babies are any less susceptible to infection than bottle fed babies from a similar environment. Where there are other children in the family the proportion of breast fed babies in maternal grades 1 and 2 having little or no infective illness in the first 12 months (72·7%) is significantly higher than the 50·0% for those on the bottle. However, it should not be assumed that this significant relationship is necessarily a causal one, although it is suggestive. So few poor working class mothers or average working class mothers with other children breast feed for as long as six months that comparisons cannot be made between the incidence of infection in bottle and breast fed babies in these groups.

The incidence of behaviour problems in the first two years was found to be significantly higher amongst breast fed babies but, as will be shown in a later section, these problems are related to anxiety in the mother. Over-anxious mothers were found more frequently in maternal grades 1 and 2. After the exclusion of these mothers, the percentages reporting no marked problem of behaviour in the first two years were 82% for breast fed and 88% for bottle fed babies in middle and superior working class homes, 63% for breast and 68% for bottle fed babies in average working class homes. These small differences are not statistically significant.

In all there is not much concrete evidence from the experience of this sample that breast feeding carries any special advantages over bottle feeding when the type of home is taken into account.

Age of Weaning to Mixed Feeding. As would be expected, the age at which babies are first introduced to solid food and finally weaned from breast and bottle differs considerably in different types of home. Prematurely born children were usually later both in starting solids and in changing completely to spoon and cup feeding. There is an excess of prematurely born children in the poorest homes; therefore in Tables 7 and 8, which give the ages at which spoon

TABLE 7

AGE OF WEANING TO MIXED FEEDING, BY MATERNAL GRADE

Maternal Grade	Age of Weaning (mth.)				No. of Cases
	<7	7–9	10–12	13–15	
	(%)	(%)		(%)	
1 and 2	89·6	10·4	—	—	153
3	76·2	21·0	—	2·8	143
4	60·1	35·4	—	4·5	67

TABLE 8

AGE BY WHICH WEANING WAS COMPLETED, BY MATERNAL GRADE

Maternal Grade	Age Weaning Completed (mth.)			1–2 Bottles at 2 yr.	All Fluid by Bottle at 2 yr.	No. of Cases
	<13	13–18	19–24			
	(%)	(%)	(%)	(%)	(%)	
1 and 2	52·7	37·4	8·6	1·2	—	152
3	29·9	43·3	19·4	6·0	1·5	134
4	23·1	23·9	16·6	10·2	25·5	62

feeding commenced and bottle feeding ceased, the figures have been standardized to give the expected figures if birthweight composition was similar for all maternal grade groups. In maternal grades 1 and 2 there was little difference in the average age of weaning for babies of different birthweights. In the poorest homes the average age of weaning for maturely born babies did not differ significantly from that for the higher maternal grades, but in two-thirds of the cases of those prematurely born, no solids were given until the eighth month or later. When solids were introduced, cereal and pudding predominated often well into the second year.

In maternal grades 1 and 2, 90% of children were completely weaned by 18 months, whereas in maternal grade 4 one-quarter of the children were still taking all fluids by the bottle at the age of 2 years.

Diet at 1 Year. Table 9 shows the proportion of children considered to be receiving a restricted diet

TABLE 9
RESTRICTED DIET AT 1 YEAR, BY MATERNAL GRADE AND BIRTHWEIGHT

Maternal Grade	Percentage Receiving Restricted Diet		
	Birthweight (lb. oz.)		
	<4·9	4·9–5·8	>5·8
1 and 2	11·1	13·7	10·1
3	62·5	36·2	26·3
4	63·2	47·1	40·0

at 1 year, by maternal grade and birthweight. Apart from bottle feeds, these children were receiving mainly starchy foods, such as baby cereal and puddings, with some soup or strained vegetables and sometimes a taste of egg. Tinned baby foods were given frequently in maternal grades 1 and 2. In the best maternal grade the incidence of restricted diet is very low and is much the same for all birthweight groups. In average and poor working class homes the proportion of children receiving an inadequate diet is much higher for prematurely born children, especially those who were 4½ lb. or less at birth. This may be part of the explanation of a previous finding (Drillien, 1958) that a low standard of maternal efficiency had a more marked effect on the growth of premature than of maturely born children.

Diet at 18 Months. When the children reached the age of 18 months a number of mothers were asked to keep a detailed diary for seven days of everything which the child was given to eat or drink, including main meals and all in-between meal snacks. Mothers were selected whose husbands were in employment, who had not more than one other child, who were in good health and not pregnant, and who occupied their own house. Mothers who had asked for advice on diet at 1 year were excluded. Of the 110 mothers who satisfied these requirements, 99 completed and returned the diaries. All were kept in considerable detail. Table 10 gives the average weekly score, by maternal

TABLE 10
DIET SCORES AT 18 MONTHS, BY MATERNAL GRADE

	Average Weekly Score		
Maternal Grade	Variety	Protein	Fruit and Vegetables
1	31	16	19
2	31	15	18
3	25	14	14
4	17	11	5

grade, for variety of diet (each different item of food being scored once) and for each occasion on which the child was given a first-class protein food (excluding milk) and fruit and vegetables (excluding potatoes). This Table does not include a number of children who had feeding problems at the time at which the diary was completed. In these cases diet was often quite severely restricted, more often as a result of refusal to eat what was proffered, than an inadequate diet being presented. It was found that in homes with mothers graded as 1 and 2, diets were very similar, the children being offered most of the normal adult diet with cereal for breakfast, a two- or three-course dinner and a cooked tea. Meat, eggs, fish and cheese were given twice daily as well as fresh and cooked fruit and vegetables. In homes where the mother was considered a poor working class type there was a noticeable lack of variety and lower intake of protein, fruit and vegetables apart from potatoes. In these homes the level of protein intake often seemed to depend on whether the child would take boiled eggs. If these are taken readily, the child may get one daily, thus compensating for the negligible quantities of other first-class protein offered. In these homes the typical diet consisted of cereal and a roll for breakfast, soup (often tinned or made with a meat cube) and custard pudding for dinner, and chips, beans or perhaps an egg for tea, with frequent sweets, ice-cream, biscuits and buns between meals.

Feeding Problems. Feeding problems are here defined as refusal to eat or excessive faddiness, usually accompanied by regular meal-time battles, lasting for three to six months or longer. Temporary difficulties in getting the child on to solids at the beginning of weaning or after some illness have not been included. Feeding difficulties were not associated with maternal grade or birthweight once allowance had been made for the excess of over-anxious mothers of prematurely born children and in maternal grades 1 and 2.

Of 59 mothers who were considered over-anxious, 30 children showed marked feeding problems (50·8%), mainly in the second year of life, compared with an incidence of 7·9% for children whose mothers were not over-anxious. No difference could be demonstrated in weight or height increments at 2 years between those who had and those who had not exhibited feeding problems, even when the refusal to eat had been prolonged for more than six months. Most of these children drank one and a half to two pints of milk daily and took fruit readily which seemed to compensate for the otherwise inadequate diet.

Vitamin Supplements. Table 11 gives the proportion of infants, by maternal grade, who were given vitamin supplements regularly during the first year.

TABLE 11

ADMINISTRATION OF VITAMIN SUPPLEMENTS IN FIRST YEAR, BY MATERNAL GRADE

Maternal Grade	Vitamin Supplements			
	Nil	A & D, C	A & D only	C only
	(%)	(%)	(%)	(%)
1	6·7	93·3	—	—
2	11·7	79·3	4·5	4·5
3	30·4	59·4	7·2	2·9
4	68·8	25·0	6·2	—

The mothers' reports may not have been accurate, especially as regards regularity of administration, but care was taken in posing the question to avoid any implied criticism if the answer should be in the negative. As would be expected, those whose diet was most inadequate in other respects were least likely to be given vitamin supplements. In maternal grade 4, vitamin supplements were given only to prematurely born infants. In the other maternal grades there was no difference between premature and maturely born babies. No cases showing evidence of vitamin deficiency were found in this group. The majority of babies, especially in the poorer homes, were fed on National Dried Milk, which at that time contained a minimum of 280 i.u. per ounce of powder. The vitamin D level has now been dropped to an average of 100 i.u. per ounce.

Clinic Attendance

Table 12 gives the proportion of children, by maternal grade, reported as attending infant welfare clinics during the first year of life, divided into first and later born. There was little difference in the incidence of clinic attendance for premature and maturely born children. Again it appears that those who are most in need of advice in bringing up their children are least likely to avail themselves of the facilities offered.

TABLE 12

CLINIC ATTENDANCE, BY MATERNAL GRADE AND FAMILY PLACING

Maternal Grade	Family Placing	Clinic Attendance			
		Never	Regularly to 6 mth.	Regularly to 12 mth.	Occasionally
		(%)	(%)	(%)	(%)
1	First born	20·0	10·0	50·0	20·0
	Later born	30·8	7·7	46·2	15·4
2	First born	16·4	8·2	69·9	5·5
	Later born	36·6	7·3	46·3	9·8
3	First born	30·9	12·3	53·1	3·7
	Later born	45·5	10·9	38·2	5·5
4	First born	45·5	18·2	15·1	21·2
	Later born	75·8	3·0	6·1	15·2

Protective Immunization

Table 13 gives the proportion of children, by maternal grade, who were protected against smallpox, diphtheria and whooping cough before the second birthday, and shows the expected differences for maternal grade.

TABLE 13

PROTECTIVE IMMUNIZATION BEFORE SECOND BIRTHDAY, BY MATERNAL GRADE

Maternal Grade	Protective Immunization against			No. of Cases
	Smallpox	Diphtheria	Whooping Cough	
	(%)	(%)	(%)	
1	86·8	97·4	97·4	38
2	90·5	90·5	87·9	116
3	77·4	76·7	73·7	133
4	52·2	59·7	50·7	67

Toilet Training

As would be expected, habits of toilet training varied considerably according to the type of home. Table 14 gives the age of starting toilet training, by maternal grade. Nearly 90% of mothers graded as middle or superior working class had instituted regular toilet training before the first birthday, whereas in the poorest homes no attempt at toilet training had been made by 2 years in over one-quarter of the total. The incidence of marked resistance to toilet training, lasting for six months or more, was the same for maternal grades 1, 2 and 3 (28%). A lower incidence of 20% in the poorest homes is accounted for by the fact that attempts at training were usually discontinued at once if the child resisted. A highly significant difference was found between the sexes, 33% of boys showing marked resistance compared with 20% of girls. Little difference was found in incidence of resistance by age at which training was first started, being 22% when training was instituted in the first six months

TABLE 14

AGE OF STARTING REGULAR TOILET TRAINING, BY MATERNAL GRADE

Maternal Grade	Age at Start of Training (mth.)				No Training	No. of Cases
	1–6	7–12	13–18	19–24		
	(%)	(%)	(%)	(%)	(%)	
1 and 2	54·8	34·2	8·4	2·6	—	155
3	25·7	40·7	21·4	7·9	4·3	140
4	1·6	25·0	29·6	17·2	26·6	64

and 28% when delayed until after the first birthday. Regular potting from the early months does not appear to influence the incidence of toilet training problems later on. There was no appreciable difference in the incidence of toilet problems between the premature and maturely born children.

Excluding those cases where no toilet training had been attempted, 67% of girls and 49% of boys were reliable by day before the second birthday. At night 36% of girls were dry, compared with 23% of boys. These differences between the sexes are highly significant. There was no difference in the incidence of later feeding troubles or of other behaviour problems between those who were potted from an early age and those who did not begin regular training until after the first birthday, once the excess of over-anxious mothers, who begin training early, had been accounted for. The smaller premature infants of $4\frac{1}{2}$ lb. or under were much later in acquiring bladder control, 36% being reliable by day at the age of 2 years and 16% at night, compared with 67% by day and 34% by night for those over $4\frac{1}{2}$ lb. at birth When these smaller premature infants had been excluded, little difference was found between the ages at which children became reliable in different types of home, where regular training had been started during the same period.

The age at which bladder control was acquired was compared for children over $4\frac{1}{2}$ lb. at birth whose training had started at different ages, and the results are set out in Table 15. Regular potting from early infancy does not appear to have any marked effect on the age at which the child becomes reliable by day, though more of these children are dry at night by 2 years. Very few children in the sample were dry at night at this age without being lifted, and mothers who had carried out energetic toilet training from an early age were the most likely to lift their children at night.

TABLE 15

ACQUISITION OF BLADDER CONTROL, BY AGE AT WHICH TRAINING STARTED

Age at Start of Training	Dry at 2 Years	
	By Day	By Night
	(%)	(%)
Birth– 6	71	55
7–12	69	34
13–18	60	21
19–24	42	8

Sleeping Problems

It was not possible to estimate the sleep requirements of these children with any accuracy owing to the absence of regular routine in many cases, especially in maternal grades 3 and 4 where the child's bed-time was often regulated by the social commitments of the family, and day-time sleep depended largely on the time at which the child had gone to bed the previous night.

Sleeping problems were relatively common in the second year of life, and took the form of refusal to settle when put to bed, often until 10 or 11 p.m. or later, or frequent waking and demanding attention throughout the night. Temporary disturbances of sleep, due to teething or illness, have not been included. Of a total of 344 children about whom a reliable history could be obtained, 91 exhibited sleeping problems lasting for six months or longer during the second year of life. In no case did there appear to be any deleterious effect on the child due to lack of sleep, although the effect on the mother was often marked. Sleeping problems were found to be associated with maternal grade and the presence of over-anxiety previously noted in the mother. It was surprising to find that the type of housing appeared to have little effect. Only in maternal grades 3 and 4 were there sufficient numbers living in poor accommodation to make comparisons. In maternal grade 3 the incidence of sleeping problems in good housing, where the child had a separate bedroom, was 25% compared with 31% for one-room houses. For maternal grade 4 the comparable figures were 33% and 36%. These small differences are not significant. After the exclusion of over-anxious mothers, the incidence of sleeping problems, by maternal grade, was: (1) 7·7%; (2) 7·7%; (3) 25·9% and (4) 35·3%. It seems likely that the much lower incidence of problems in the better homes is due to the regular routine practised at bed-time.

Where the mother had previously been noted as over-anxious, the incidence of sleeping problems was very much higher and similar for all maternal grades, being 46·2% for grade 1, 54·5% for grade 2 and 53·3% for grade 3.

The commonest solution of sleeping problems in the 1- to 2-year-old was to take the child into the parents' bed and, having once started, there was often considerable difficulty in stopping the habit. In maternal grades 1 and 2 no children other than those with sleeping problems slept with their parents, though in maternal grade 4 30% of those without problems and 45% of the total regularly slept with their parents, this being the case even when accommodation was adequate for separate beds. Of those with sleeping problems 48% in maternal grades 1 and 2 and 70% in maternal grades 3 and 4 either slept with their parents or were taken in regularly during the night.

Other Behaviour Problems

In the first two years of life a behaviour problem from the mother's point of view means a type of behaviour which she considers abnormal or which causes her anxiety and embarrassment. Many mothers, especially those with a first child, are worried about forms of behaviour which could be considered a phase of normal development, and these cases are not included in the subsequent discussion.

Apart from problems of feeding, sleeping and toilet training, two forms of behaviour were commonly encountered in the second year of life, which might be considered as problems, being temper tantrums and excessive timidity.

Temper Tantrums. Temper has been classified as excessive only in those cases where tantrums occurred several times a day and whenever the child did not immediately get his own way. The mother would state that when thwarted the child would throw himself on the floor, kicking and screaming, or hurl the nearest object that came to hand. Head banging and breath holding were common manifestations of temper, the latter causing great anxiety to the mother especially in the few cases in which it was carried to the extent of unconsciousness. Several children would induce vomiting when in a temper. Such manifestations were most common after the age of 15 months.

Excessive Timidity. In these cases the mother stated that she could never leave the child: he always cried and clung to her if strangers were present or if spoken to in a shop. He could not be left, even with grandparents, and if she wished to go out at night she must wait until the child was sleeping.

Temper and timidity were often co-existent. The incidence of these problems was again related to the maternal grade and over-anxiety. Little difference was found in incidence in first or later born children or between those who were premature or mature at birth when over-anxious mothers, who predominated amongst those with a first or prematurely born child, had been excluded. There was a higher incidence, but not significantly so, in the smallest prematures (those of $3\frac{1}{2}$ lb. or less at birth). Numbers in this group are small.

Fig. 2 shows the relative incidence of those who had no serious behaviour problems in the second year of life, by grade of mother and presence or absence of maternal anxiety, also of those who exhibited excessive temper or timidity for six months or longer during this period. In maternal grade 4 only three mothers were considered over-anxious and these have not been included. It will be seen that the incidence of excessive temper and timidity is much commoner in the poorer homes and also where the mother was considered over-anxious. The mother's anxiety, though aggravated by the child's behaviour, was not caused by it, as all these mothers had been noted as over-anxious from the first visit at 6 months, before any problems had arisen.

The decrease in proportion of children free from any marked behaviour problem with decreasing maternal standards is statistically highly significant, as is the increase in excessive temper and timidity in

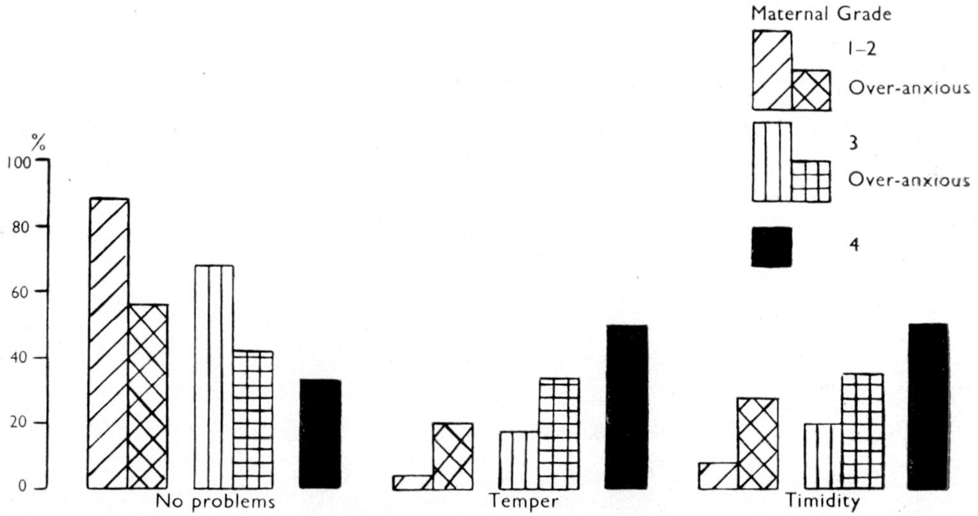

FIG. 2.—Incidence of behaviour problems, by maternal grade and maternal over-anxiety.

the children of over-anxious mothers from the same type of home. It will be interesting to see whether these children, who have exhibited behaviour problems in early childhood, show other problems when they reach school age.

Summary and Discussion

This paper describes different patterns of child rearing in the first two years of life in an unselected group of premature and maturely born infants born in Edinburgh hospitals. Comparison with all births in Edinburgh during the same period suggests that of working class mothers nearly one-half observed standards of household management and child care which approximate closely to those found in middle class homes, and that in approximately one working class home in 10 standards appear to be definitely below the level required for good health and normal development of the young child. The incidence of prematurely born infants is highest in these poor homes and, as previous papers have shown (Drillien, 1958, 1959a, b), the proportion of undersized, retarded children, who suffer from frequent ill health, is also highest in this group.

Contrary to the findings of other investigators, which are summarized by Illingworth (1953), no striking advantage could be demonstrated for breast feeding, as opposed to bottle feeding, in similar types of home. The reported lower incidence of infection in breast fed babies (e.g. Robinson, 1951) is almost certainly due largely to the predominance of better type mothers in the breast fed group. Underfeeding appeared to be commoner in breast fed babies, especially in the poorer working class homes. National Dried Milk was the food of choice for the majority of bottle fed babies, and even in the poorest homes most mothers sterilized bottles and teats regularly, no doubt as a result of supervision and instruction from health visitors. The incidence of gastro-intestinal infection was low in all types of home in the first six months and reached a peak in the second half of the first year when the child was being introduced to solids.

There was no evidence that behaviour problems in the first two years were any less common in babies who had been breast fed. There was, however, a marked association between behaviour problems and over-anxiety in the mother. It seems likely that the contented baby is the satisfied baby, whether breast or bottle fed, and that the contented baby is more likely to produce a contented, confident mother, who is calm in her handling. Hytten, Yorston and Thomson (1958) studied a group of 106 primiparae and found that mothers who continued to lactate for three months were more often unwell and worried than those who abandoned breast feeding soon after leaving hospital, and conclude that there is little justification for pressing the mother to continue when she is either unwilling or apparently unable to breast feed efficiently.

Apart from the incidence of breast feeding, the most marked differences in feeding habits in the best and worst homes were the later age of weaning to mixed feeding and finally stopping bottle feeds in the latter; a predominance of starchy foods at 1 year; lack of variety and lower intake of protein, fruit and vegetables in the second year of life.

No evidence could be obtained from the sample that early toilet training has an adverse effect on the child at a later date, once it is recognized that the rigid, over-conscientious and over-anxious mother is more likely to practise rigorous toilet training. Behaviour problems of all types were much commoner in the children of these mothers, whether or not there had been early toilet training. A significantly higher incidence of resistance to potting was found in boys, who also were significantly later in acquiring sphincter control.

The incidence of prolonged feeding battles and sleeping problems was five times as high in the children of mothers previously noted as being over-anxious. Sleeping problems were also much more common in poorer homes and seemed to be associated with the lack of regular routine at bed-time, rather than with inadequate accommodation.

Other behaviour problems, notably excessive temper and timidity, were also found most frequently in the poorest homes, and in good homes where the mother was over-anxious.

It is a pleasure to thank Professor R. W. B. Ellis for his help and encouragement throughout.

This investigation is being supported by a grant from the Scottish Hospitals Endowments Research Trust.

REFERENCES

Drillien, C. M. (1956). *Arch. Dis. Childh.*, **31**, 390.
—— (1958). *Ibid.*, **33**, 423.
—— (1959a). *Ibid.*, **34**, 37.
—— (1959b). *Ibid.*, **34**, 210.
Hytten, F. E., Yorston, J. C. and Thomson, A. M. (1958). *Brit. med. J.*, **1**, 310.
Illingworth, R. S. (1953). *The Normal Child.* Churchill, London.
Robinson, M. (1951). *Lancet*, **1**, 788.

MASCULINIZATION OF A FEMALE FOETUS WITH OESTROGENIC EFFECT

BY

G. H. VALENTINE

From the St. Thomas Elgin General Hospital, St. Thomas, and the Department of Paediatrics, University of Western Ontario, Canada

(RECEIVED FOR PUBLICATION MAY 20, 1959)

Masculinization of a female foetus by androgenic hormones produced by an arrhenoblastoma in the mother during pregnancy was described by Brentnall (1945). Masculinization and pseudohermaphroditism caused by the administration of 17-methyltestosterone to the mother during pregnancy was reported by Hayles and Nolan (1957), Grunwaldt and Bates (1957) and others.

Since Wilkins, Jones, Holman and Stempfel (1958) described masculinization of the female foetus attributed to the administration of progestins with androgenic activity, an increasing number of cases of non-adrenal pseudohermaphroditism are being recognized. Their paper reports 21 cases of non-adrenal masculinization of the external genitalia. In 15 cases the oral progestin 17-ethinyl-testosterone (ethisterone or anhydrohydroxyprogesterone) had been given, in two cases the mother had received intramuscular injections of progesterone, in one case the progesterone had been given together with oral methyltestosterone and in three cases no steroid had been administered.

Since the publication of their paper the number of cases observed by them or collected from colleagues' reports has risen to 60. The mothers of 25 had received 17-ethinyltestosterone; the mothers of 28 had been given 17-ethinyl-19-nortestosterone (norethindrone, norlutin) (Wilkins, 1959).

The clinical picture resembles the more familiar pseudohermaphroditism of the adrenogenital syndrome. Phallic enlargement varies according to the degree of labio-scrotal fusion. Complete fusion and a penile urethra may occur, though the formation of a urogenital sinus or phallic enlargement alone is more usual. The baby is chromatin positive. The mother has been given a progestin early in the pregnancy, usually with the intention of preventing a miscarriage. There is no increase in the urinary 17-ketosteroids and no abnormality of the internal genitalia. The condition is not progressive once the baby has been removed from the influence of the administered progestin and, apart from surgical correction of the external abnormality, if necessary, for psychological, cosmetic or reproductive purposes, no treatment is required. The outlook for child-bearing is good.

Our case is believed to be unique in that, although there was masculinization, there is also strong evidence of a potent oestrogenic effect.

Case History

After two miscarriages the mother was given by mouth the synthetic progestin steroid 17-ethinyl-19-nortestosterone (norlutin) from the time when she missed her first period. She received 5 mg. twice daily throughout the pregnancy except at the times when the first three periods were due when she was given 5 mg. four times daily. About the third month she noticed that her voice was becoming deep and she was seen by an otolaryngologist who found only some oedema of the vocal cords. The significance of the deepening of the voice was not appreciated at that time. She noticed also that the hair on her head appeared to grow more rapidly than formerly, but she noted no other abnormality. The delivery was normal at term.

The baby appeared superficially to be a normal female. She developed quite deep jaundice eight hours after birth, but no blood group incompatibility haemolytic disease could be demonstrated. The jaundice soon faded. At 5 days the baby had slight vaginal bleeding, but this was not considered very unusual. She made excellent progress. During the next few weeks the mother noticed a good deal of mucous vulval discharge which did not cause her any concern.

When 10 weeks old the child had vaginal bleeding lasting six days, and this prompted further investigation. The nipples were abnormally prominent and slightly pigmented and there was a small button of breast tissue beneath. The labia majora were large, slightly wrinkled and very slightly pigmented. The clitoris was very definitely enlarged with a small palpable corpus cavernosum and a small visible glans. The appearance was similar to that in the case illustrated by Hillman (1959).

There was no posterior fusion at the fourchette and a vaginal orifice at the usual site was visible. The hymen was fleshy and redundant, overlying and partly obscuring the urethral opening. The appearance of the vulval lining was quite unusual for a baby of this age. There was a copious mucoid colourless discharge and the mucosa was obviously thickened and pale. These changes themselves suggested the possibility of an oestrogenic effect. The depth of the vagina was 1¾ in. and a normal uterus could be felt per rectum. No ovarian tumour was palpated.

A buccal mucosal smear showed that the chromosomal pattern was that of a genetic female. Radiography showed that the bone age was normal for the chronological age. Two 24-hr. specimens of urine showed 17-ketosteroid levels of 0·19 and 0·14 mg. A 48-hr. specimen was examined for gonadotrophic follicle-stimulating hormone and, although conducted at the most sensitive level, no such hormone was detected. A vaginal smear was made by aspirating a small amount of the initially copious discharge from high in the vagina. This showed that 28% of the cells were cornified. This is a high index of cornification and is comparable to that found in a woman in the reproductive age. Although Wilkins *et al.* (1958) recommend that investigation should include radiography and endoscopic examination of the urogenital sinus or vagina and also laparotomy and gonadal biopsy, it was felt that the baby should simply be watched in spite of the unusually high cornification index.

The baby thrived normally. Examinations and vaginal smears were made at frequent intervals. The vulval mucosa became more obviously delicate over the next three months and the mucoid secretion more scanty so that the preparation of satisfactory smears became increasingly difficult. The cornification index is shown in Fig. 1.

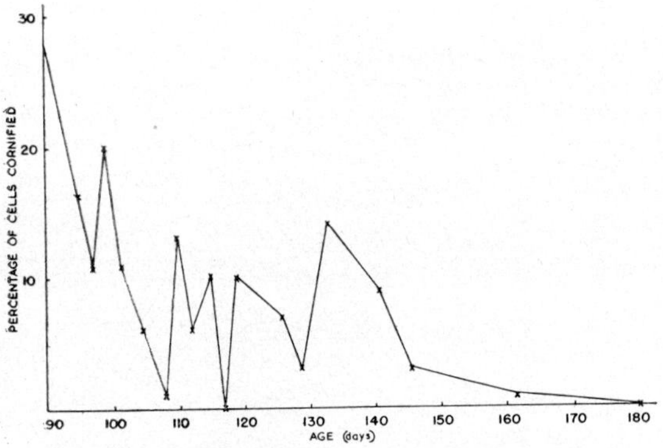

FIG. 1.—Vaginal smear cornification index.

Finally, the appearance of the vulva became normal, apart from the enlarged clitoris which did not change. There was no further bleeding. Along with the return toward normal of the vulval mucosa the nipple prominence and pigmentation and the slight breast enlargement disappeared, and by the age of 6 months the breasts appeared normal.

The mother's voice, though less deep than at the end of the pregnancy, is still rather husky.

Discussion

It now seems well established that certain of the synthetic progestins, and even progesterone itself, may have androgenic activity. In 15 of the cases described by Wilkins *et al.* (1958) the oral progestin 17-ethinyl-testosterone was incriminated. This steroid is said to have 7% of the androgenic activity of testosterone, as judged by its effect on the prostate and seminal vesicles of the castrated rat (Vollmer, 1958). The steroid in question in this case, 17-ethinyl-19-nortestosterone, is stated by the same authority to possess 20% of the activity of testosterone, when judged by its effect on the prostate, and 113% of the activity of testosterone, when judged by its effect on the seminal vesicles of castrated rats. The androgenic activity of the steroid used in this case is thus considerable. Moreover it was administered from the time when the first menstrual period was missed and was continued throughout the pregnancy. It seems reasonably certain that the masculinization of this baby was due to the effect of the progestin used.

The oestrogenic effect as shown by the vaginal smears is not easy to explain. Its association with the masculinization can scarcely be coincidence. There was no reason to suspect that the baby had received oestrogens from vitamin drops, cosmetic preparations or the like. There was the possibility that a pituitary-activated temporary precocious puberty had occurred as a form of rebound overactivity of a gland depressed for a time by the steroid administered to the mother. That no follicle-stimulating hormone was detected in the urine does not vitiate this possibility. By the time that the estimation was made at 12 weeks of age the gonadotrophin level might have dropped a great deal. Even if present, the estimation might not have been of sufficient sensitivity to detect it. This possibility of pituitary over-activity certainly remains.

The possibility of an ovarian or even an adrenal oestrogen-producing tumour was considered but was rejected when the cornification index was seen to be falling and when no ovarian tumour could be palpated.

Most plausible of all is the hypothesis that part of the androgenic progestin administered to the mother became converted to an oestrogen. Oestrogens do not protect the foetus from the masculinization effect (Wilkins *et al.*, 1958) whereas there is good evidence that androgens can be converted to oestrogens which result in cornification of the vagina (Steinach and Kun, 1937; Nathanson and Towne, 1939; Heard, Jellinck and O'Donnell, 1955).

If, as seems probable, such a conversion was responsible for the oestrogenic effect shown in this case, the question then arises: Did the conversion occur in the mother with transfer of both androgen and oestrogen to the baby, or was the conversion from androgen to oestrogen entirely in the baby? I do not think one can answer this. In any case it certainly seems that the source of oestrogen persisted in the baby for some months, but the storage of androgen or oestrogen (or both) seems unlikely.

Nevertheless it might have been quite possible for the developing foetal tissues, exposed as they were for nearly nine months to the administered progestin, to store sufficient for a diminishing effect to be shown for many weeks. Oestrogens, like bilirubin and a number of other substances, require conjugation before they can be removed as active agents (Kretchmer, 1959). Conjugation of this kind is known to be extremely ineffective in newborn infants. Failure of this conjugation mechanism might well have perpetuated the activity of the oestrogen. It is also possible that the early onset of jaundice, which raised the possibility of haemolytic disease, might have resulted from competition by the oestrogen with bilirubin for the conjugation pathway. Perhaps such competition for the glucuronide-conjugating mechanism explains why sulfisoxazole (Gantrisin), which also requires conjugation for its excretion, may cause hyperbilirubinaemia in the newborn premature baby.

Summary

A case of non-adrenal pseudohermaphroditism in a female newborn baby is described. In addition to the masculinization, an oestrogenic activity was demonstrated. The masculinization is attributed to the administration to the pregnant mother of an androgenic progestin. There is speculation as to the cause of the oestrogenic effect.

My thanks are due to Dr. J. Walters and Dr. Earl Plunkett, both of the University of Western Ontario and the Ontario Cancer Foundation. The former generously examined the many vaginal smears and the latter kindly arranged for the hormonal estimations in the Collip Laboratory. The help of both is gratefully acknowledged. Dr. Murray Barr kindly determined the chromosomal pattern. Dr. J. F. Curtis, of St. Thomas, referred the case to me.

References

Brentnall, C. P. (1945). *J. Obstet. Gynaec. Brit. Emp.*, **52**, 235.
Grunwaldt, E. and Bates, T. (1957). *Pediatrics*, **20**, 503.
Hayles, A. B. and Nolan, R. B. (1957). *Proc. Mayo Clin.*, **32**, 41.
Heard, R. D. H., Jellinck, P. H. and O'Donnell, V. J. (1955). *Endocrinology*, **57**, 200.
Hillman, D. A. (1959). *Canad. med. Ass. J.*, **80**, 200.
Kretchmer, N. (1959). *Pediatrics*, **23**, 638.
Nathanson, I. T. and Towne, L. E. (1939). *Endocrinology*, **25**, 754.
Steinach, E. and Kun, H. (1937). *Lancet*, **2**, 845.
Wilkins, L. (1959). Personal communication.
Wilkins, L., Jones, H. W., Holman, G. H. and Stempfel, R. S. (1958). *J. clin. Endocr.*, **18**, 559.
Vollmer, E. P. Personal communication cited by Wilkins *et al.* (1958).

ADDISON'S DISEASE WITH HYPOFUNCTION OF THE PARATHYROID GLANDS

BY

H. SZCZEPAŃSKA and J. SAPIECHA
From the Clinic for Infectious Diseases of Childhood, Warsaw, Poland

(RECEIVED FOR PUBLICATION APRIL 2, 1959)

Addison's disease is an extremely rare disease in childhood, especially in girls. Since 1855, 92 cases have been reported in children under 15; 26 were 10-15 years old, so that under 10 years of age there are only 66 cases (the figures for 1855-1946 are from Jaudon (1946a, b, c), quoted by White and Sutton (1950); those for 1946-1957 are from Welch (1957)).

Case Record

Z.B., No. 6661/118, a girl born in 1952, was the second child of elderly healthy parents; siblings aged 6, 3, 2 and 1 year were healthy, and no contact with tuberculosis or other infectious diseases was known. She was normally developed, and had never been ill before. She had not been vaccinated nor had B.C.G.; the tuberculin reaction was not known. She was a very active child, good-tempered and liked to take care of the younger children.

She became ill about two months before admission. The disease developed gradually without fever. She became weak, inactive, and tired quickly. Brown stains appeared on the skin, first on the face, and then on the body and extremities. She lost her appetite and vomited after meals, and a general decline set in. Her temper changed visibly: she became hypersensitive, cried often and never smiled. As these symptoms got worse, the child was admitted to a hospital where she was in contact with pertussis and was therefore brought to Warsaw and admitted to our clinic on December 12, 1957 with suspected Addison's disease.

On admission she appeared acutely ill. She lay motionless on one side with her knees pulled up to her chin, and moaned from time to time. She took no interest in her surroundings and, though conscious, would only answer in monosyllables. She greedily accepted liquids and frequent small feeds but vomited them immediately.

There were no constitutional anomalies except for clubbing of the fingers (Fig. 1). Her height was 3 ft. 5 in. (104 cm.) and weight 2 st. 8 lb. (16·5 kg.).

She had marked inanition, atrophy of the subcutaneous tissues, oedema of the lumbar region and ankles and marked dehydration. The skin was dry, rough and cold with patches of brown-grey pigmentation (Fig. 2). The face, neck, elbows, knees, dorsal surface of the fingers and toes and inguinal areas were dark brown, and in some places nearly black. The soles and palms of the hands were of a lighter colour. The mucous membrane of the mouth was pink and unpigmented. The tongue was smooth. Though there was no evidence of muscular atrophy the muscles were flaccid and weak.

Heart sounds were dull and the rate was regular at 120 per minute. The pulse was weak and soft. The internal organs and nervous system were normal.

The following investigations were performed:

B.P. 90/60; blood sedimentation rate 25/50; Hb 81%; R.B.C. 4,130,000; colour index 1·0; W.B.C. 6,600 (polymorphs 51%, eosinophils 9%, lymphocytes 40%); blood group O Rh+; serum albumin 7·1 g.%; sodium 310 mg.%; potassium 16·5 mg. %; chlorine (as NaCl) 546 mg.%; calcium 5·5 mg.%; phosphorus 7·5 mg.%; sugar 54·7 mg.%; blood Wassermann negative.

Examination of the capillaries showed the flow to be slow and intermittent; there was dilatation of the loops at the apex and pallor; the number of loops was lessened and they were uneven; the efferent vessels were dilated. Professor J. Bogdanowicz confirmed that there was capillary stasis and lessened tension of the vessel walls.

The Thorn test was negative. Electrocardiography showed dysfunction of the blood flow of the heart muscle and a heart muscle lesion.

Urine: chemical and microscopical examination of the sediment showed no abnormality; Cl 220 mg.%; sodium 266 mg.%; potassium 117 mg.%; daily (24 hr.) 17-ketosteroids 2·8 mg.%.

A radiograph of the thorax was normal, but the ossification centres of the hands were similar to those found in a 3-year-old child.

The tuberculin reaction (Moro, Mantoux 1:1,000) was negative. The basal metabolic rate was slightly increased. There was nothing frankly abnormal in the electroencephalogram (Koślacz). Cerebrospinal fluid was normal and the culture sterile. The gastric contents showed free hydrochloric acid, 35·6; total acidity 57·2. Examination of the larynx revealed a marked ozaena (Borkowska). Ophthalmological and neurological examination disclosed no abnormality (Naróg and Kirkow).

From the history and the clinical manifestations we diagnosed Addison's disease.

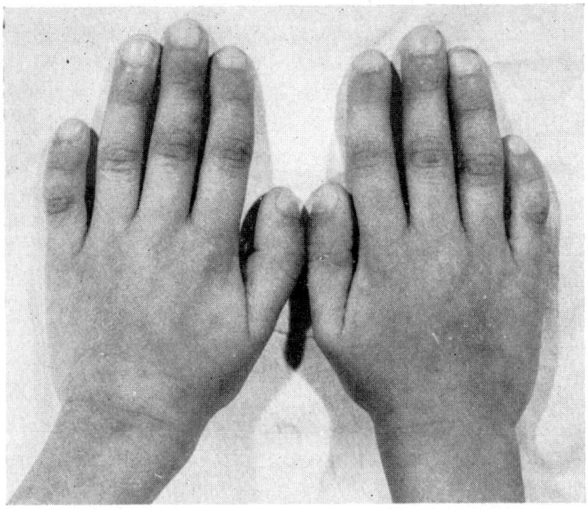

FIG 1.

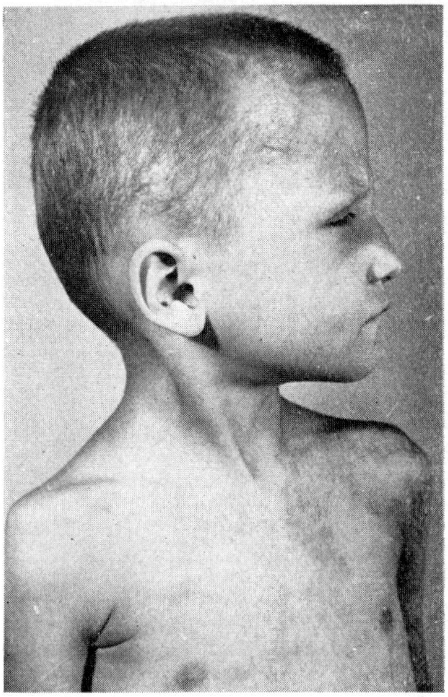

FIG 2.

Though we had no doubt of the diagnosis, there were some perplexing points; for example, the dysfunction of the other endocrine glands: hypofunction of the parathyroid (Leonard, 1946; Fargašová, 1958) was indicated by the lowered blood serum calcium and the increased phosphorus levels, by the normal renal function, the lack of change in the osseous system, and by the clinical picture of a dry, rough skin, onychorrhexis, poor dentition, numbness of the extremities, sensation of cold and a positive Chvostek test. The delay in ossification of the long bones suggested a concomitant thyroid dysfunction.

The diagnosis of acute Addison's disease called for energetic treatment. The patient was given desoxycorticosterone in oily solution intramuscularly in a dose of 10 mg.; then 5 mg. every day, every second day, and finally every third day. Simultaneously we added 4-5 g. salt daily to the child's food to increase the effect of the desoxycorticosterone. In addition she received 100 mg. of cortisone daily, with the dose reduced successively to 50 and 25 mg. We tried three times to give her prednisone instead of cortisone, but each time the child's condition deteriorated with vomiting and general weakness. The deterioration was probably due to the effect of the prednisone on the electrolyte balance.

We have not found any report in the literature in which cortisone was ineffective in Addison's disease. Because of the persistent vomiting in this case, sometimes 30 times during 24 hours, the marked dehydration, vascular collapse and grave heart condition, we administered from the outset a continuous intravenous drip of 5% glucose in physiological salt solution, a blood and plasma drip, oxygen and a vitamin complex in addition to the desoxycorticosterone and cortisone. Later on the child received thyroid orally in a dose of 0·06 g. daily. After eight to 10 days' treatment the child gradually began to recover. She took an interest in her surroundings, she smiled and was glad to have her toys. The discoloration of her skin gradually became less marked, she vomited less and began to gain weight.

Three months after the child's admission a marked improvement was noted: she was good-tempered, smiling and active. However, in the fourth month her condition visibly worsened and, although a blood examination showed normal sugar, albumin and electrolyte values, she passed into a convulsed and insensible state which persisted for 35 hours. This was followed by an increasing dementia.

Our attempts to control her condition by transfusions and by hormone treatment were ineffective. Finally, in spite of prophylactic antibiotics, the child developed pneumonia and died on September 8, 1958, after eight months' treatment in the clinic. The clinical diagnosis was Addison's disease, hypoparathyroidism, bilateral lobar pneumonia, ozaena, dementia, cachexia and myocarditis.

At autopsy we found a confluent lobar pneumonia, mucopurulent tracheobronchitis, hypertrophy of the left heart, cortical atrophy of the suprarenal gland, hypertrophy of the clitoris, leptomeningeal oedema, inflammatory enlargement of the spleen and cachexia.

Microscopical examination revealed that in the suprarenals the medulla was unaffected, but the cortex showed extreme atrophy. The hypophysis was normal. The ovaries were normal, as were the thyroid and the pancreas. The thymus was atrophic with few Hassall's corpuscles. The brain was normal (Rosnowski).

We might have treated this case with greater success if the newest drugs, such as aldosterone and α-fluorohydrocortisone had been available.

It is worth pointing out that, although the albumin-carbohydrate balance and the electrolyte balance were restored to normal, it proved impossible, finally, to control the mental deterioration, to restore the child's weight or to master the increasing prostration.

The autopsy confirmed the clinical diagnosis of Addison's disease, but there is no doubt that there was also some disturbance of the parathyroid glands, though, as they were not found at autopsy (? atrophy), it was impossible to examine them histopathologically.

The autopsy did not throw any light on the mental deterioration and psychical disorders which persisted for a few months; they should probably be related to persistent and increasing anoxia of the cerebral cortex and to its abnormal carbohydrate metabolism.

Ozaena and clubbed fingers are extremely rare signs in Addison's disease.

References

Fargašová, Irena (1958). Primary idiopathic hypoparathyroidism and Addison's disease in a 12-year-old girl. *Čsl. Pediat.*, **13**, 539.
Jaudon, J. C. (1946a). Addison's disease in children. *J. Pediat.*, **28**, 737.
—— (1946b). Hypofunction of the adrenals in early life. *Ibid.*, **29**, 696.
—— (1946c). Addison's disease in an infant. *J. clin. Endocrin.*, **6**, 558.
Leonard, Martha F. (1946). Chronic idiopathic hypoparathyroidism with superimposed Addison's disease in a child. *Ibid.*, **6**, 493.
Welch, R. G. (1957). Addison's disease in a nine-year-old girl. *Brit. med. J.*, **1**, 980.
White, F. P. and Sutton, L. E. (1950). Addison's disease in a negro child. *J. Pediat.*, **37**, 778.

THE EFFECT OF CALOMEL ON PLASMA EPINEPHRINE IN THE RAT AND THE RELATIONSHIP TO MECHANISMS IN PINK DISEASE*

BY

DONALD B. CHEEK† and FANNIE WU

From the University of Texas Southwestern Medical School, Dallas, Texas

(RECEIVED FOR PUBLICATION MAY 4, 1959)

Zahorsky (1922) stated that he was inclined to the view that calomel was the causative agent in pink disease. However, some patients were encountered having no history of calomel ingestion, so the idea was dismissed. Lesesne Smith of South Carolina considered that mercury was involved. His belief led Davison (1938) to include mercury as the aetiological agent in the 1938 edition of his current text. Ten years later scientific evidence for the involvement of mercury was furnished by the work of Warkany and Hubbard (1948, 1953) and by Fanconi and Botsztejn (1948).

The mode of action of mercury has not been understood, especially by workers investigating the autonomic dysfunction. They have tried to determine the nature of the dysfunction either by indirect physiological studies (Day, Smith and Klingman, 1939; Vulliamy, 1952; Bower, 1954; Farquhar, Crawford and Law, 1956) or by observation of the therapeutic effect of antisympathetic drugs (Gillespie, 1952; Bower, 1954; Peterson and Laughmiller, 1954). Their work supports the contention that excessive action of the sympathetic division exists. This contention is also supported by the findings that basal metabolic rate and venous pressure are increased in pink disease (Cheek, 1957). The methods involved in earlier attempts to measure blood epinephrine in this disease (Cheek, Hetzel and Hine, 1951) are now known to be inadequate.

Other work (Cheek and Hicks, 1950; Cheek, 1953) drew attention to the role of 'stress' in pink disease, to the failure of patients to withstand intercurrent infections, atmospheric heat, and intravenous hypotonic solutions, and of further electrolyte loss. Preliminary work (Cheek and Hicks, 1950) indicated a state of salt loss. A significant reduction of the total body chloride and extracellular volume was demonstrated subsequently (Cheek, 1957). Since extracellular volume is intimately related to the production of aldosterone (Bartter, Liddle, Duncan, Barber and Delea, 1956), a state of functional adrenal insufficiency is thought to be present (Cheek, 1953). Urine 17-ketosteroid excretion is high and sweat sodium concentration is low, so that the production of steroids is adequate if not high. Since sweat water loss contains steroids and approximates or exceeds urine water loss, it seems impossible to measure accurately 11-oxysteroid excretion. A resistance to sodium-retaining steroids also has been demonstrated (Cheek, 1954) while the increase in red cell water (Cheek, 1957) may reflect a similar state of affairs in other tissue cells.

For the most part, all these electrolyte findings can be related to the actions of mercury. Calomel, the major offender, is a mercurial diuretic of bygone days. Mercurial diuretics produce an increase in cell hydration in rats, while calomel causes loss of body Cl and Na and retention of body K without change in renal structure (Cheek, Bondy and Johnson, 1959). Resistance to sodium-retaining steroids is compatible with the action of mercurial diuretics (Weston, Escher, Grossman and Leiter, 1952).

By contrast, the clinical features of hypertension, tachycardia, sweating and hypotonia do not appear, on the surface, to be related to the role of mercury. A study of the problem was undertaken by observing the effects of calomel and epinephrine on the young rat. It was found (Cheek *et al.*, 1959) that the ordinary effects of epinephrine (haemoconcentration, increased insensible water loss, hypertension, tachycardia) were perpetuated and intensified if the rat had received 10 mg. of calomel. Whether these

* Paper read in part at the International Pediatric Congress, Montreal, July, 1959. The expenses for this work were defrayed by a grant from Mead Johnson & Company, Illinois.

† Present address: Royal Children's Hospital, Melbourne, Australia.

results were due to an increased tissue response to epinephrine or to the maintenance of a high level of epinephrine in the rat is the subject of the present study.

Experimental Procedures and Methods

Male albino rats weighing 80 g. were divided into two equal groups, experimental and control. The experimental group received 10 mg. of calomel suspended in water by tragacanth, which was introduced into the stomach by a rubber catheter. Food and water were available, and the rats were placed in individual cages. After 22 hours the animals were lightly anaesthetized with ether and bled from the aorta, using a syringe containing 0·5 ml. of sodium thiosulphate-fluoride mixture to preserve the catecholamines, according to the technique of Weil-Malherbe and Bone (1952). In the second experiment the 'calomel' and control rats were placed in a refrigerated room (4°C.) with water but without food and left for 21 hours. Then they were anaesthetized and bled as before. In subsequent experiments 0·5 mg. of epinephrine in oil was injected intramuscularly into control and calomel rats. The calomel rats received their injection four hours after the administration of the mercurous chloride. Food and water was available. Twenty to 21 hours from the beginning of the experiment the animals were sacrificed as described. Before the injection of epinephrine in oil, the solution was taken from several ampoules and mixed thoroughly so as to ensure uniformity of dosage. The potency of epinephrine in oil varies slightly from ampoule to ampoule. The determination of epinephrine was carried out using the method described by Weil-Malherbe and Bone (1952) with the aid of a Coleman photofluorometer.

Results

In Table 1 the data for the plasma levels of epinephrine in the calomel and control rats are listed. Twenty-one hours after mercurous chloride administration there was a slight increase in plasma epinephrine as compared with the control group. When the two groups of rats were subjected to stress from cold (4°C.), a fourfold increase in epinephrine level was seen in the calomel rats. In the subsequent experiments epinephrine in oil was injected 16 to 18 hours before sacrifice. Since epinephrine in oil was slowly liberated into the circulation, the results reflected the rate of destruction of the epinephrine concentration. Clearly, rats exposed to calomel had a concentration two or three times as high as control animals. These data from all experiments are statistically highly significant ($P<0·01$).

TABLE 1
PLASMA EPINEPHRINE LEVELS (μg./l.)

Experiment	No. of Rats per Group	Remarks	Control Rats ±S.D.	Calomel Rats ±S.D.
1	7	22 hr. after 10 mg. calomel	2·15±0·33	4·01±0·54
2	5	20-21 hr. after calomel; stress of 4°C.	2·34±0·21	9·18±0·72
3	5	20-21 hr. after calomel; 16 hr. after 0·5 mg. epinephrine	14·89±1·55	31·72±5·10
4	8	20-21 hr. after calomel; 16 hr. after 0·5 mg. epinephrine	8·37±1·60	23·20±3·60
5	6	20-21 hr. after calomel; 18 hr. after 0·5 mg. epinephrine	2·60±0·20	7·04±1·47

S.D.=standard deviation.

Discussion

The present findings and those of the previous study (Cheek *et al.*, 1959) demonstrate the ability of calomel to augment the activity of the sympathetic branch of the autonomic nervous system. Stimulation of the sympathetic division by cold stress or by the direct injection of epinephrine gave rise to a higher level of plasma epinephrine if calomel was also present in the body. During the course of the present study a possible explanation for this phenomenon came to hand.

Axelrod and Tomchick (1958) found that epinephrine is destroyed in body tissues mainly by methyl transferase and not by mono-oxidase, as was believed previously. For this enzyme, methyl transferase, to work, a substrate adenosyl methionine is necessary. The latter substrate contains sulphhydryl groups and is inhibited by inorganic mercury.

Calomel is the source of mercury in pink disease in most instances (calomel disease), and it seems reasonable to believe that the same potentiation of sympathetic activity can occur in the clinical situation.

Evidence has accumulated that the formation of haem from iron and protoporphyrin is enzyme-dependent (Schwartz, Cartwright, Smith and Wintrobe, 1959). The enzyme requires sulphhydryl groups for its action, and it is possible that the high reticulocyte count noted in some patients with pink disease, and the slightly increased porphyrin excretion in the urine (Cheek *et al.*, 1951) are due to the fact that mercury inhibits sulphhydryl groups.

From the present data and from previous work it is possible to suggest the mechanisms which are active in pink disease, and to explain the role of mercury (Fig. 1).

If activity of the sympathetic branch of the autonomic nervous system is enhanced in the infant by previous illness or by environmental or other factors, the response of the sympathetic division will tend to

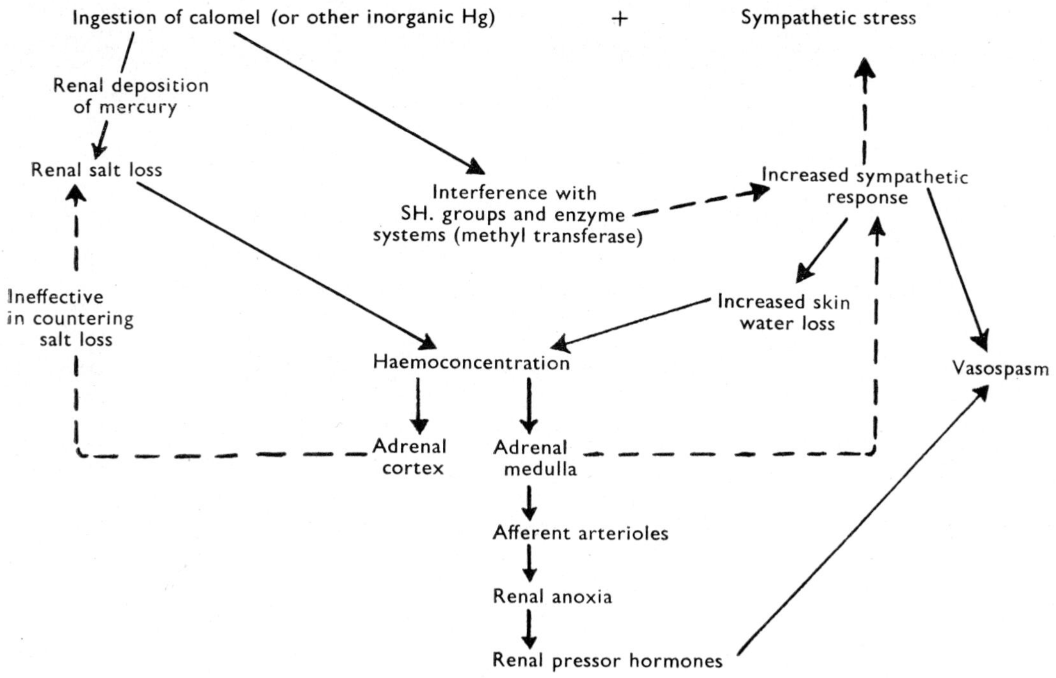

FIG. 1.—Suggested mechanisms in pink disease.

be perpetuated if calomel or another inorganic mercurial is present. Calomel can also act as a mercurial diuretic and can reduce body NaCl and extracellular volume, which in turn would produce endogenous sympathetic activity.

In earlier years, when a high salt intake and desoxycorticosterone was used experimentally, a dramatic improvement was observed in some patients but not in others (Cheek and Hicks, 1950; Murray, 1950; Cheek *et al.*, 1951; Forman, 1951; Williams, MacDonald and Callow, 1951). It is possible that some patients do respond to steroid with expansion of extracellular volume, a result which could break a vicious cycle (Fig. 1).

Stimulation of the sympathetic branch of the autonomic nervous system by the injection of epinephrine produced damage to the cortico-medullary junction of the rat kidney if calomel was also present (Cheek *et al.*, 1959). Renal pressor factors may also be important in pink disease in the maintenance of vasospasm.

The sympathetic division of the autonomic nervous system seems to be more active in infants than in adults. Perhaps this accounts for the clearly defined age incidence of the disease. In earlier years it was suggested that functional adrenal cortical insufficiency was present in pink disease, and to this we can now add maximal activity of the adrenal medulla. It is agreed generally by adrenal physiologists that if sympathetic activity overrides adrenal cortical activity there is a failure of adaptation or failure to meet added stresses (Ramey and Goldstein, 1957). It seems that the nature of pink disease includes a predominating adrenal medullary action together with a functional cortical insufficiency, all of which is related to the presence of inorganic mercury in the body. This disease should find a place adjacent to pheochromocytoma in the current texts.

Removal of as much mercury as possible from the body seems important, together with the administration of anti-sympathetic drugs and efforts to restore extracellular electrolyte. It may also be important to supply additional sulphhydryl groups in the form of methionine.

Summary

Previous experiments on young rats, by indirect methods, demonstrated that calomel potentiates the effect of epinephrine on the body. The present study presents direct data on the plasma epinephrine concentration. Rats subjected previously to a small dose of calomel had higher plasma epinephrine concentrations than control animals. The difference in plasma epinephrine concentrations would be magnified by subjecting the animals to cold stress, or by the injection of 0·5 mg. of epinephrine in oil.

It is suggested that in the clinical counterpart, pink disease or calomel disease, there is the same potentiation of sympathetic activity. In the light of the present and previous work, the mechanisms operating in pink disease are suggested.

Attention is drawn to the possibility that stress or a previously activated sympathetic system may be aetiologically important in pink disease.

We are grateful to Dr. Marvin Siperstein and Dr. T. Shires for their help with the method of epinephrine determination.

REFERENCES

Axelrod, J. and Tomchick, R. (1958). *J. biol. Chem.*, **233**, 702.
Bartter, F. C., Liddle, G. W., Duncan, L. E., Barber, J. K. and Delea, C. (1956). *J. clin. Invest.*, **35**, 1306.
Bower, B. D. (1954). *Quart. J. Med.*, **23**, 215.
Cheek, D. B. (1953). *J. Pediat.*, **42**, 239.
—— (1954). *Med. J. Aust.*, **1**, 822.
—— (1957). *Pediatrics*, **19**, 68.
——, Bondy, R. K. and Johnson, L. R. (1959). *Ibid.*, **23**, 302.
——, Hetzel, B. S. and Hine, D. C. (1951). *Med. J. Aust.*, **2**, 6.
—— and Hicks, C. S. (1950). *Ibid.*, **1**, 107
Davison, W. C. (1938). *The Compleat Pediatrician.* 2nd ed. Durham, N. C., Duke University Press.
Day, R., Smith, J. R. and Klingman, W. O. (1939). *Amer. J. Dis. Child.*, **57**, 269.
Fanconi, G. and Botsztejn, A. (1948). *Helv. paediat. Acta.* **3**, 264.
Farquhar, J. W., Crawford, T. B. B. and Law, W. (1956). *Brit. med. J.*, **2**, 276.
Forman, H. (1951). *Ibid.*, **1**, 1144.
Gillespie, A. E. (1952). *Canad. med. Ass. J.*, **67**, 418.
Murray, F. (1950). *Brit. med. J.*, **2**, 1116.
Peterson, J. C. and Laughmiller, R. (1954). *Acta. paediat.*, **43**, Suppl. 100, p. 517.
Ramey, E. R. and Goldstein, M. S. (1957). *Physiol. Rev.*, **37**, 155.
Schwartz, H. C., Cartwright, G. E., Smith, E. L. and Wintrobe, M. M. (1959). *Blood*, **14**, 486.
Vulliamy, G. D. (1952). *Lancet*, **2**, 1248.
Warkany, J. and Hubbard, D. M. (1948). *Ibid.*, **1**, 829.
——, —— (1953). *J. Pediat.*, **42**, 365.
Weil-Malherbe, H. and Bone, A. D. (1952). *Biochem. J.*, **51**, 311.
Weston, R. E., Escher, D. J. W., Grossman, J. and Leiter, L. (1952). *J. clin. Invest.*, **31**, 901.
Williams, H., MacDonald, W. B and Callow, V. (1951). *Med. J. Aust.*, **1**, 363.
Zahorsky, J. (1922). *Med. Clin N. Amer.*, **6**, 97.

A CASE OF ARTHROGRYPOSIS MULTIPLEX CONGENITA WITH LESIONS IN THE NERVOUS SYSTEM

BY

MALCOLM FOWLER

From the Adelaide Children's Hospital, Adelaide, South Australia

(RECEIVED FOR PUBLICATION MAY 19, 1959)

Although clinical descriptions of arthrogryposis multiplex congenita are not uncommon, very few reports of the pathological findings are available. In 1932 Sheldon reviewed the literature and stated that there had been no autopsies on these cases up to that time. Since then descriptions of autopsy material have been published, including those by Price (1933), Gilmour (1946), Brandt (1947) and Adams, Denny-Brown and Pearson (1953), but the part played by abnormalities of the nervous system is not fully established by these reports. Recently, Ek (1958) has emphasized on clinical grounds the possible importance of brain damage in this disease. The present report concerns a case showing gross abnormalities in the brain and spinal cord.

Clinical Findings

The patient, a first-born female, was admitted to the Adelaide Children's Hospital at the age of 1 week. The pregnancy had been normal until the last week when, because of breech presentation, the baby had been turned. She was born as a face presentation.

On examination she was very small, weighing 4 lb. 10 oz., but in no respiratory distress. The head circumference was 12½ in. and the anterior fontanelle was small. The lower jaw was asymmetrical and small. The limbs showed little spontaneous movement and all joints had a limited range of passive movement. The head was retracted and a torticollis was present, the face being turned to the left. The wrists were flexed with ulnar deviation of the hands. The fingers were extended but the metacarpo-phalangeal joints were flexed, the thumbs being adducted across the palm. The elbows were flexed. A moderate range of shoulder movements was possible, largely because of the mobility of the scapulae. The left humerus was fractured and slightly angulated near the mid-shaft; this had apparently occurred during extraction at birth. The legs showed no spontaneous movements. Although both hips and knees were kept flexed they had a moderate range of passive movement. Bilateral talipes equino-varus was present. Muscle development was very poor. A diagnosis of arthrogryposis multiplex congenita was made and because of the obscurity surrounding this clinical condition a muscle biopsy was undertaken. At operation for removal of a piece of gastrocnemius muscle great difficulty was experienced in finding anything resembling muscle tissue, and microscopical examination revealed that the material removed consisted mainly of fat and fibrous tissue with a few small bundles of tiny muscle fibres.

Under treatment in the physiotherapy department both range of movements and muscle power in the arms slowly improved but no response was obtained in the legs. After a few months she showed some ability to flex her neck when attracted by a rattle. The consultant ophthalmologist reported that there was some optic atrophy and that there was little co-ordination of eye movements. She developed little awareness of the people around her and it was concluded that she was mentally defective. Because there was no sucking ability she was fed by gavage throughout her life. During her course in hospital she had several periods of fever, accompanied by dyspnoea and signs of consolidation in the lungs, and suffered from recurrent otitis media requiring myringotomies. She died during an attack of pneumonia at the age of 11 months.

Pathological Examination

Autopsy (A.C.H. No. 120/58) was performed 36 hours after death. The body was plump and showed the deformities previously described. The anterior fontanelle was closed, the head circumference being 16½ in.

Muscles. The left leg was opened from the inferior iliac spine to the heel, revealing complete absence of normal muscles, which were replaced by fat. On closer inspection a few pale pinkish-yellow gelatinous strands of tissue resembling muscle bundles were found in the mid-thigh posteriorly and in the calf. The posterior upper part of the left arm was incised where the triceps could be easily identified, but it was very small, flabby, pale and gelatinous. The erector spini group was slightly smaller than normal. The iliacus muscles were replaced by fat. Other muscles, such as the latissimus dorsi, the psoas, neck and abdominal muscles, were all hypoplastic, pale and soft. The diaphragm was firm but slightly pale. Microscopically, changes varied from a minimal accumulation of sudanophilic lipoid droplets in the striations to complete absence of muscles and replacement by adipose tissue. In one of the two sections from the buttock and thigh one small group of muscle fibres was found, most of these being very small with a few hypertrophied fibres (Fig. 1).

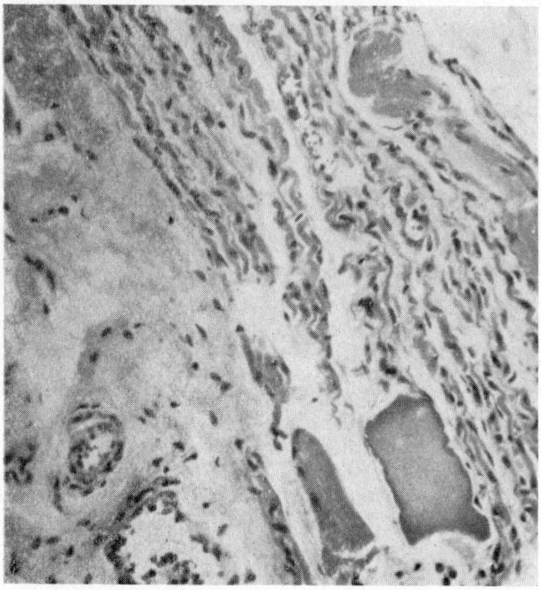

FIG. 1.—Tissue from thigh showing a group of small muscle fibres and a few hypertrophied fibres. H and E. × 160.

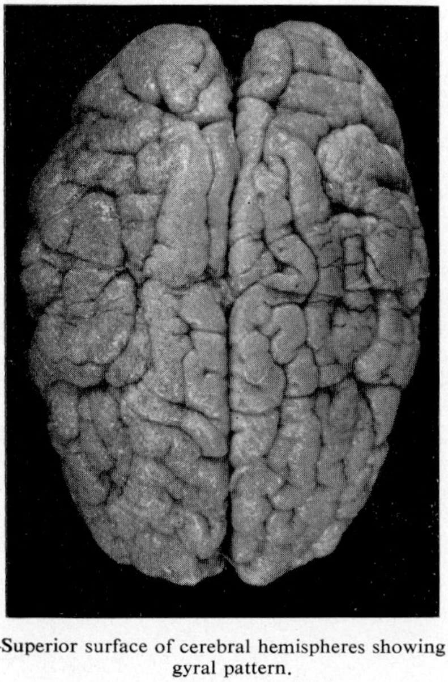

FIG. 2.—Superior surface of cerebral hemispheres showing abnormal gyral pattern.

In the less affected muscles, bundles of small fibres were very scanty but there was patchy endomysial and perimysial replacement by adipose tissue. The number of muscle spindles appeared to be increased in all muscles except in the leg specimens where none was seen, either in the small island of muscle fibres or in the surrounding adipose tissue. The diaphragm showed no abnormality apart from fatty droplets in the striations. Increase in nuclei was found only where there were groups of small fibres. There was no evidence of phagocytic activity.

The sciatic nerve appeared normal macroscopically, but microscopically there was an increase in perineural collagen and large fibres were very scanty. The only joint examined was the left knee, where the femoral articular surface was seen to be very small and flat without any curve onto the anterior and posterior surfaces of the bone. The joint capsule was normal and there were no intra-articular adhesions.

Nervous System. The brain was small, weighing 585 g. The cerebral hemispheres were narrow and had a grossly abnormal convolutional pattern. The Sylvian fissures were short and the central sulci were not identifiable. A sulcus roughly in the region of the inferior two-thirds of the central sulcus could be seen, but it did not continue to the medial edge of the hemisphere. Running along the edge of the sagittal sulcus and parallel to it were two gyri extending from the occipito-parietal region towards the frontal pole. The lateral convolution of the pair curved down and became continuous with the inferior temporal gyrus. The superior and middle temporal gyri, the parietal gyri and the posterior frontal gyri were firm, and irregular in shape, some parts being very large with smooth or finely granular surfaces, other parts being minutely convoluted or bossed. The occipital gyri, the anterior and inferior parts of the frontal lobes and the inferior temporal gyrus were relatively normal. All these cortical changes were bilateral and roughly symmetrical (Figs. 2 and 3). When the arachnoid was being stripped, it was noted that the blood vessels entered the crowns of the gyri more frequently than is normal and

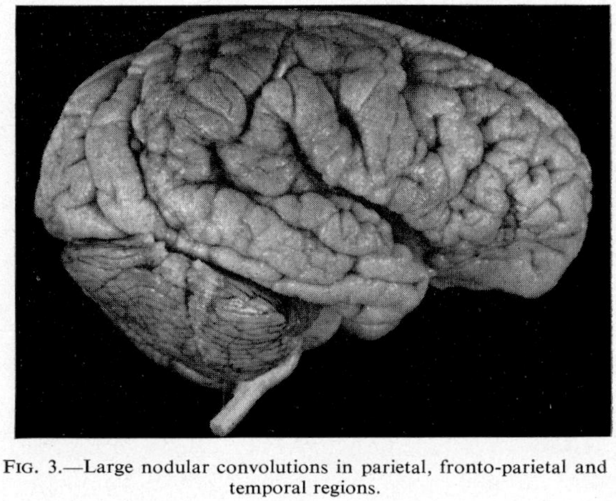

FIG. 3.—Large nodular convolutions in parietal, fronto-parietal and temporal regions.

then ran obliquely into the cortex, particularly in the malformed gyri. The uncus was large, the optic tracts, pons and pyramidal tracts small. On incision the lateral ventricles were seen to be large and the central white matter of the hemispheres was reduced. The cortical grey matter, particularly in the areas of convolutional irregularity, was thick. Nodular masses of heterotopic grey matter projected from the lateral walls of the lateral ventricles. The thalamus was small; the hippocampus appeared normal. The spinal cord was slender and the lumbo-sacral enlargement inconspicuous.

Macroscopic examination of large coronal sections stained for myelin (Fig. 4) showed in addition a very small internal capsule containing, despite its small size, a conspicuous thalamo-cortical bundle. The internal capsule at most levels ran more horizontally than normally and the putamen was of normal size and was depressed. A few irregularly disposed islands of grey matter in the white matter of the insula apparently represented the claustrum. The temporal horn of one lateral ventricle was greatly narrowed by the protrusion of an elongated amygdaloid nucleus into it. A few small nodules of heterotopic grey matter were present under the ependyma of both temporal horns.

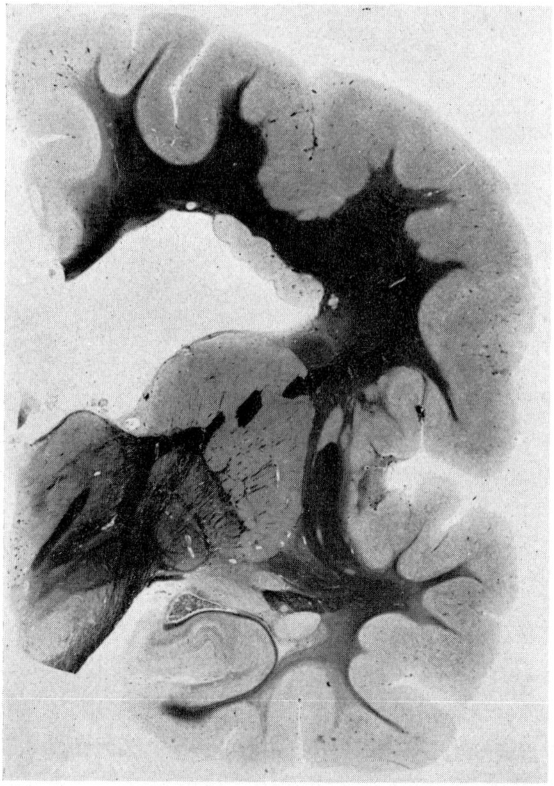

FIG. 4.—Coronal section of a hemisphere, stained by Weil's method for myelin, showing thickened areas of cortex, reduction in amount of central white matter, malformed insula and claustrum and heterotopic grey matter in wall of lateral ventricle.

Microscopically the abnormally thick cortical grey matter in the bossed areas showed no lamination although occasionally the neurones were arranged for short distances in irregular festoons. Small bundles of myelinated fibres penetrated amongst them here and there but cores of white matter did not regularly appear so that a miniature gyral pattern was not obvious. The small depressions on the pial surface were found to correspond with the site of fusion of molecular layers of adjacent abortive gyri. Sometimes the molecular layer was very thick and formed rounded masses encroaching on the underlying nerve cell layer. No giant neurones of the Betz type were found, nor were large pyramidal neurones present, the cells being small or moderate in size with relatively large nuclei. Even in areas where normal lamination of the cortical grey matter had occurred the range of variation in size of the neurones was reduced. Apart from its location, the amygdaloid nucleus was normal, as was the hippocampus.

The vessels in the abnormal cortex were numerous and often ran as quite large channels parallel to the surface. The pia contained areas of glial and fibrous thickening which often fused with the molecular layer.

There was no evidence of calcification, microglial activity or infiltration by other inflammatory cells.

Apart from the very small size of the pyramidal tracts (Fig. 5) the medulla oblongata and cerebellum were normal.

Macroscopic examination of myelin-stained sections of the spinal cord showed a reduction in size of the lateral columns, due presumably to absence of the cortico-spinal tracts. The anterior and posterior horns were therefore closer together. Lateral expansion of the anterior horns in the lumbar region was absent, the horns having an elliptical shape in cross section. The anterior columns were reduced in size but the posterior columns were normal. The substantia gelatinosa appeared to be situated just lateral to the central canal but on microscopic

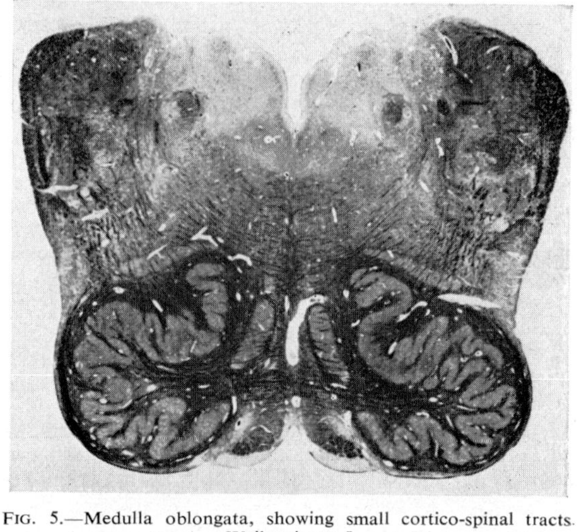

FIG. 5.—Medulla oblongata, showing small cortico-spinal tracts. Weil stain × 5.

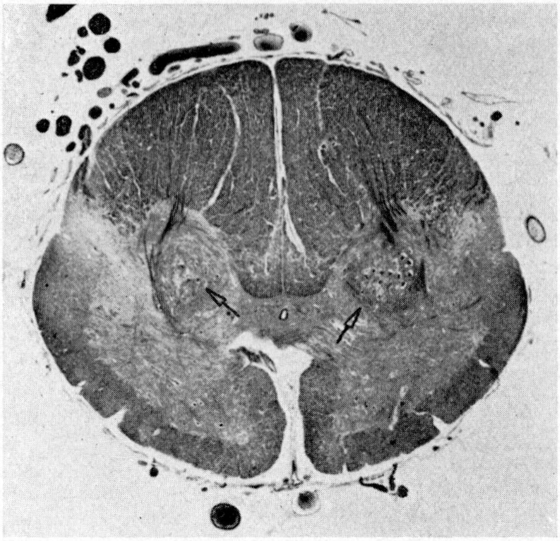

FIG. 6.—Lumbar spinal cord showing reduction in size of lateral columns, abnormal disposition of anterior and posterior horns, rounded nucleus of motor cells, indicated by arrows, and minute size of anterior nerve roots. Weil stain × 9.

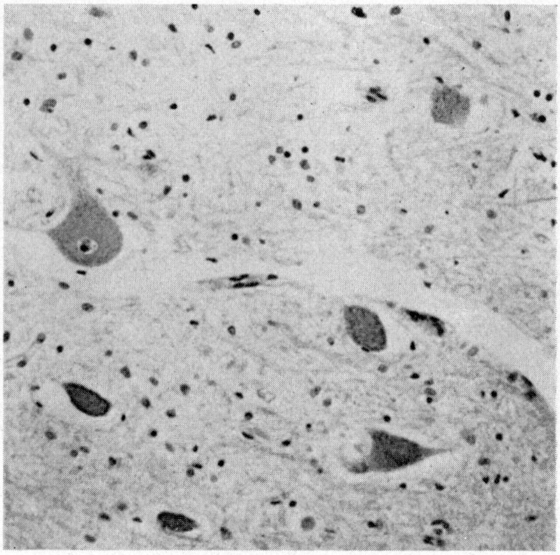

FIG. 7.—Lumbar cord showing neurones from dorsally situated nucleus. H. and E. × 190.

examination this structure was found to have been replaced by a rounded group of large motor cells (Figs. 6 and 7), the real substantia gelatinosa being compressed inconspicuously lateral to these motor neurones. In the sacral cord this group of large cells was absent, suggesting the possibility that they represented Clarke's column of the higher lumbar region, but, apart from other morphological differences, their large size seemed to exclude this. The cells of Clarke's column in the thoracic cord were normal. In the cervical region the shape of the horns was less abnormal and here a dislocated group of large motor cells was not found.

Throughout the cord the number of neurones in the anterior horns was reduced, approximating 25% of the normal population in the cervical region and showing an even greater reduction in the lumbo-sacral cord. Most of those remaining were small and angular, sometimes elongated, but with well-marked Nissl substance (Fig. 8); a few large neurones of normal size were present. There were many vacuoles in the myelin sheaths of decussating fibres in the region of the anterior horns, but apart from some central chromatolysis in the dislocated motor cells, which was consistent with post-mortem change, the bodies of the neurones showed no evidence of degeneration.

In the anterior horns there was an excess of glial tissue, mainly astrocytic, in proportion to the number of neurones present. In the position of the lateral corticospinal tracts, particularly in the thoracic and cervical regions, a few myelinated fibres were found widely separated by 'ground substance' containing scattered glial cells. No empty cell beds were found in the anterior horns and there was no abnormal sudanophilia or hyperplasia of microglia nor were perivascular cellular infiltration or capillary proliferation present.

The anterior nerve roots were very small but showed no evidence of recent demyelination.

There was a widespread bronchopneumonia, *H. influenzae* being cultured from lung swabs. Centrilobular necrosis of the liver was accompanied by an infiltration with neutrophil polymorphonuclear leucocytes and there were focal necroses in the suprarenal cortex. A blood culture was not made, but it was thought that the changes

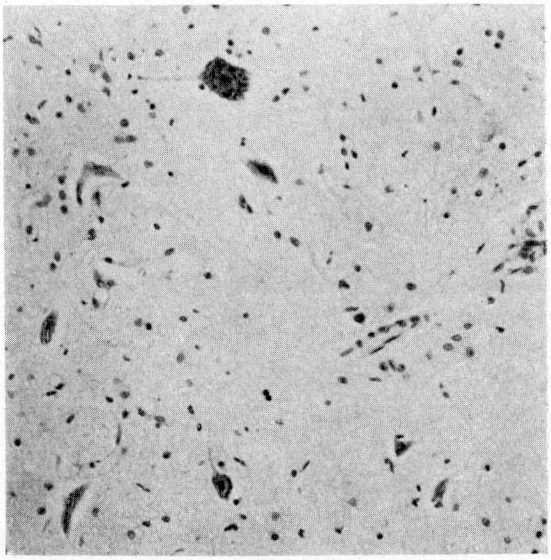

FIG. 8.—Lumbar cord showing small neurones from the most anterior part of an anterior horn. H. and E. × 148

in the liver were most likely due to septicaemic spread of the organisms.

Discussion

Since the earlier descriptions of arthrogryposis multiplex congenita (Stern, 1923), accounts of the condition have been uniform as far as the main clinical aspects are concerned. The affected child is born with a restricted range of movement in multiple joints, usually bilateral. The degree and distribution of the deformities are variable, but a common pattern is seen in extension of the elbows, ulnar deviation of the hands and flexion of the fingers, flexion of the hips and talipes equino-varus. Dislocation of the hips is common and fractures of the limbs, mostly resulting from difficult extractions at birth, have frequently been reported. Muscular development, particularly in relation to the most severely affected joints, is poor, and muscle biopsy has shown small muscle fibres and occasionally some adipose tissue replacement. Often the mother has noticed that foetal movements were slight or absent. When information is sought on the occurrence of neurological changes and mental deficiency, on the other hand, it is only in the last two decades that clinical observations implicating the nervous system have begun to accumulate (Ek, 1958).

The interpretation of the muscular changes and of the lesions in the central nervous system has been delayed to a large extent by the lack of a complete autopsy. Price (1933) found the brain normal whereas sections of the spinal cord showed degeneration of the neurones in both anterior and posterior horns and also degenerative changes in the white columns, but her photographs do not illustrate these points with any certainty. The arm muscles were reduced in size and intermingled with fatty tissue; some were absent. Dissection of the elbow joint revealed circumscribed articular surfaces on the lower end of the humerus. Gilmour's case (1946), a foetus, stillborn at 30 weeks' gestation, was studied in more detail. He found 'slight hydrocephalus of unexplained cause', a reduction in the number of anterior horn cells in the thoracic cord and a reduction in size of those in the seventh cervical segment. Most muscles were greatly reduced in size; some were absent. The articular surfaces of the knee joint were smaller than normal.

Brandt (1947) found no gross structural alterations in the central nervous system, but there were 'profound' changes in the motor neurones of the anterior horns of the spinal cord. As pointed out by Adams *et al.* (1953), the changes shown in the illustrations could be due to post-mortem artefacts. Biopsy of a quadriceps muscle in Brandt's case showed extreme atrophy. The muscles were not apparently examined microscopically post mortem, and no joints were mentioned.

Adams *et al.* (1953) reported two cases, one being incompletely examined. In one case they found a disappearance of anterior horn cells in the lumbo-sacral region and a reduction in their number and size at higher levels. The brain was small and had an abnormal convolutional pattern and large lateral ventricles, but further details of the brain are not given. In their other case they found a reduction in the number and size of anterior horn cells in the lumbo-sacral segments of the spinal cord.

Kanof, Aronson and Volk (1956) described three patients, one of whom came to autopsy. The muscles were in various degrees reduced in size; one knee joint was examined and found to be normal. A normal number of anterior horn cells was seen in the lumbar cord, but a decrease in number had occurred in the lower cervical region. Their photograph of the lumbar cord, illustrating what they have interpreted as demyelination of the lateral cortico-spinal tracts, could represent absence or reduction of the tracts with disturbed relations of the anterior and posterior horns.

One of the cerebral abnormalities found in the present case has been called 'micropolygyria' (Norman, 1958), the abnormal cortex consisting of large gyri often with a granular surface resembling cobblestoning. In some cases the internal arrangement suggests incompletely separated small gyri, but in this case, although there was fusion of the molecular layers, the thick zone of neurones was rarely penetrated by miniature cores of white matter. In addition, as is sometimes found with micropolygyria, nodules of grey matter were present in the walls of the lateral ventricles. The large fissures of the brain were abnormal, the central sulcus, if present at all, being incomplete. No Betz cells were identifiable and the pyramidal tracts were minute. Apart from deducing that these findings are due to an arrest of neuronal migration with subsequent abnormal development, there is nothing to indicate whether the aetiology is genetic or acquired. Except for occasional foci of pial thickening by glial and, to a lesser extent, fibrous tissue there was nothing which could reasonably be construed as evidence of an inflammatory reaction, nor were there any remains of past softening or haemorrhage. Bertrand and Gruner (1955), in a detailed description of micropolygyria, which they call 'status verrucosus', emphasize the abnormality in the course of the small cortical blood vessels such as that observed in the present case, and Norman (1958) mentions that this finding is compatible with

Bielschowsky's view (1917) that micropolygyria is a consequence of abnormal vascularization of the cortex.

The findings in the anterior horns indicated a loss of neurones, with hypoplasia of a large proportion of the remainder. Since the posterior horns merged with the anterior horns it was not certain how many of these small neurones were rightful members of the anterior horns, but their angular shape and well-developed Nissl substance indicated that most of them were of motor type. Although the abnormal disposition of the horns of the spinal cord may be attributed to the virtual absence of the lateral cortico-spinal tracts, the abnormality of the anterior horn cells is unlikely to be an example of trans-synaptic atrophy, but rather a defect in development contemporaneous with that in the brain. That the absence of the cortico-spinal tracts does not necessarily lead to congenital muscular hypoplasia is evident from the well-developed musculature in anencephalic monsters.

Adams *et al.* (1953) have pointed out that arthrogryposis multiplex congenita might well have a multiple aetiology. Recently Banker, Victor and Adams (1957) reported two cases which were due to muscular dystrophy and they refer to several others reported in the literature. In spite of the small number of cases submitted to autopsy it is evident that lesions in the nervous system may also produce this clinical syndrome, that under such conditions the muscle changes are secondary to neural abnormalities, and that the changes in the joints can be attributed, as Gilmour suggested (1946), to lack of movement during the early stages of their development *in utero*.

Summary

A female baby was born with arthrogryposis multiplex congenita; she never sucked and there were no spontaneous movements of the legs. Mental development was thought to be impaired and there was some optic atrophy. Autopsy at the age of 11 months revealed micropolygyria, hypoplasia of the cortico-spinal tracts and a great reduction in the number of anterior horn cells. Voluntary muscles were virtually absent in the legs and small elsewhere, the microscopic appearances being consistent with neurogenic atrophy.

The pathological findings in some previously reported cases are briefly reviewed. Although the aetiology of arthrogryposis multiplex congenita is multiple, it is concluded that lesions in the nervous system account for a significant proportion of cases.

Thanks are due to the Board of the Adelaide Children's Hospital and to Dr. Eric Sims for permission to publish details of this case. I am grateful to Mrs. Helga Thiede for technical assistance and to Mr. R. Boyd for the preparation of the illustrations.

References

Adams, R. D., Denny-Brown, D. and Pearson, C. M. (1953). *Diseases of Muscle.* Hoeber, New York.
Banker, B. Q., Victor, M. and Adams, R. D. (1957). *Brain*, **80**, 319.
Bertrand, I. and Gruner, J. (1955). *J. Neuropath. exp. Neurol.*, **14**, 331.
Bielschowsky, M. (1917). *J. Psychol. Neurol (Lpz.)*, **22**, 1. Quoted by Norman, R. M. (1958).
Brandt, S. (1947). *Acta paediat. (Stockh.)*, **34**, 365.
Ek, J. I. (1958). *Ibid.*, **47**, 302.
Gilmour, J. R. (1946). *J. Path. Bact.*, **58**, 675.
Kanof, A., Aronson, S. M and Volk, B. W. (1956). *Pediatrics*, **17**, 532.
Norman, R. M. (1958). In *Neuropathology*, by Greenfield, J. G. *et al.* Chapter 5. Arnold, London.
Price, D. S. (1933). *Arch. Dis. Childh.*, **8**, 343.
Sheldon, W. (1932). *Ibid.*, **7**, 117.
Stern W. G. (1923). *J. Amer. med. Ass.*, **81**, 1507.

THE EFFECT OF A BRONCHODILATOR AEROSOL ON VENTILATORY CAPACITY IN FIBROCYSTIC DISEASE OF THE PANCREAS

BY

BRYAN GANDEVIA and CHARLOTTE ANDERSON

From the Clinical Research Unit, Royal Children's Hospital, Melbourne

(RECEIVED FOR PUBLICATION APRIL 27, 1959)

Wheezing is a relatively common symptom or sign in patients with fibrocystic disease of the pancreas and the obstructive nature of their breathing is frequently obvious. Nevertheless, bronchodilator therapy is often not dramatic in its effect and its role has not been clearly defined despite the increasing use of aerosol therapy for the pulmonary aspects of this disease. The aerosol usually contains several constituents, including a bronchodilator drug. As yet no objective evidence has been provided as to the efficacy of the combined therapy or of any individual component.

Modern single-breath tests of ventilatory capacity, which are readily applicable to children, afford accurate and sensitive indices of response to bronchodilator drugs. We have therefore studied the ventilatory capacity of 16 patients immediately before and after a potent bronchodilator aerosol, our aim being to assess the proportion of potentially reversible bronchoconstriction.

Methods

A spirometer of the pattern described by Bernstein, D'Silva and Mendel (1952) and a kymograph with a paper speed of 1·5 cm. per second were used. With the subject seated, the vital capacity (VC) was estimated in the conventional manner and a tracing then made of maximum forced expiration after a full inspiration. The volume of gas expired in the first second of the forced expiration (forced expiratory volume at one second* or $FEV_{1\cdot0}$) was measured, the mean of three observations being recorded. The percentage of the vital capacity expired in the first second ($FEV_{1\cdot0}$ %) was then calculated. Predicted values for VC and $FEV_{1\cdot0}$ were derived from normal standards for children prepared by one of us (Gandevia, 1960). Predictions were based on height; values calculated for age take no account of the small stature of children suffering from fibrocystic disease of the pancreas. In one instance (Case 1), a boy of 17 years, an adult prediction formula based on surface area was used; the study of normal children mentioned above showed this to be appropriate for boys of this age.

An aerosol of 1:1,000 isoprenaline (isopropyl-noradrenaline) was administered for one and a half to two minutes, using an effective nebulizer producing a fine mist with an oxygen flow of about 8 l./minute. Approximately two minutes later the tests of ventilatory capacity were repeated. Previous observations in adults have indicated that isoprenaline is a powerful and quick-acting bronchodilator agent and that this duration of administration is adequate to produce a maximum effect* (Hume and Gandevia, 1957a, b; Hume, 1957). Subsequent experience with children has not altered these conclusions. In normal children and in children with funnel chest but no pulmonary symptoms, a bronchodilator aerosol has not produced an increase of more than 5% in VC of $FEV_{1\cdot0}$.

Clinical Material

The 16 children studied had been for the most part under observation by one of us (C.A.) for a number of years, their ages ranging from 6 to 17 years. They represented at the time of examination the majority of surviving patients over 5 years of age with fibrocystic disease of the pancreas known to the hospital and may be considered a representative series in this age group. At the time of testing no patient was suffering an exacerbation of pulmonary disease; several were having long-term antibiotic therapy. Individual case histories are summarized in the appendix with particular reference to the severity of pulmonary symptoms. In all cases the diagnosis was considered proven from clinical and investigational data. All but one patient (Case 1) had pancreatic achylia as determined by duodenal intubation; all but this patient also had impaired fat absorption as shown by fat balance studies, and

* The terminology used in this paper is that adopted by the Thoracic Society of Great Britain (Gandevia and Hugh-Jones, 1957).

* We do not wish to imply that isoprenaline is the best preparation for clinical use. Its potency and rapidity of action are responsible for its selection for the present investigation. Therapeutically, its disadvantages when used alone are the frequency of annoying side-effects and the relatively short duration of its action.

all but one (Case 2) had raised levels of sodium and chloride in the sweat as determined by the method of Anderson and Freeman (1958). Case 1 showed impaired pancreatic secretion by duodenal intubation but he had a 'positive' sweat test and three siblings with the disease.

On clinical grounds, the patients were divided into groups according to their pulmonary symptoms by one of us (C.A.) without reference to the results of ventilatory capacity studies.

Group 1 (five patients). No persistent cough or sputum was present but there were occasional mild bouts of bronchitis of no greater severity or frequency than might be expected in normal children; there was normal exercise tolerance, and no wheezing was recorded during the years of observation.

Group 2 (six patients). There was clinical evidence of mild persistent or recurrent pulmonary infection with purulent sputum, but little impairment of exercise tolerance or general health. Intermittent wheezing was recorded during the period of observation.

Group 3 (five patients). Severe persistent pulmonary infection was present with purulent sputum, moderately or severely restricted exercise tolerance and intermittent or persistent wheezing.

The children in each group are listed in Table 1 in order of increasing severity of chest symptoms as judged clinically.

Results

The results of the initial ventilatory capacity studies, together with the change produced by the isoprenaline aerosol, are set out in Table 1, which also shows the age, sex and height for each subject in the three groups. The pre-aerosol values are also shown as a percentage of predicted values; the following summary of the results is most conveniently based chiefly on these figures.

As anticipated on clinical grounds, the overall pattern of abnormality is that of an obstructive ventilatory defect with a normal or low VC, a reduced $FEV_{1\cdot 0}$ and a lowered $FEV_{1\cdot 0}$ %. In Group 1 three patients (Cases 3, 4 and 5) have normal values for all three indices, but in two of these, as with the group as a whole, there is significant increase in $FEV_{1\cdot 0}$ after the aerosol. Case 1 is an exception to the comparative normality of this group in that an $FEV_{1\cdot 0}$ % of 59·3% is unequivocally below the normal range, although the $FEV_{1\cdot 0}$

TABLE 1

EFFECT OF BRONCHODILATOR AEROSOL ON VENTILATORY CAPACITY OF 16 SUBJECTS WITH FIBROCYSTIC DISEASE OF THE PANCREAS

					Before Aerosol		Initial Values as % of Predicted Values†		After Aerosol: % increase on pre-aerosol values		
Group	No.*	Sex	Age (yr.)	Height (in.)	FEV 1·0 (l.)	FEV 1·0%	FEV 1·0	VC	FEV 1·0	VC	FEV 1·0%
1	1	M	17	66·0	2·35	59·3	75·8	98·8	4·7	4·3	0·2
	2	F	10¼	51·5	1·30	84·4	80·7	80·8	8·4	11·0	−2·0
	3	F	11½	52·5	1·67	84·3	99·3	99·0	5·4	1·0	5·7
	4	F	8	46·0	1·36	83·4	113·3	123·3	8·1	8·0	1·1
	5	M	8½	46·5	1·25	75·8	105·0	113·8	16·0	1·2	10·9
	Means‡ for Group 1					77·4§	94·§	103·1	8·5	5·1	3·2
2	6	M	9¼	52·0	1·32	73·3	83·3	91·3	15·2	12·2	1·9
	7	M	12	60·5	1·58	57·5	67·2	93·7	17·1	8·0	4·8
	8	F	10¼	53·0	0·97	72·4	55·6	65·3	22·9	21·7	0·6
	9	M	7¾	47·5	1·12	71·8	87·3	102·6	8·6	2·1	3·5
	10	M	11¼	56·5	1·32	55·5	65·3	94·8	18·2	−1·3	10·8
	11	M	15	55·0	1·21	54·0	63·9	95·2	9·8	7·1	0·9
	Means‡ for Group 2					64·1§	70·4	90·5	15·3	8·3	3·8
3	12	M	10	47·5	0·52	54·2	40·7	63·2	21·2	22·8	−0·8
	13	M	13½	52·0	1·03	57·1	62·3	89·0	4·9	6·1	−0·6
	14	M	6	41·0	0·81	68·7	83·5	98·3	9·9	4·2	3·7
	15	M	9½	50·5	0·75	59·1	49·4	67·8	9·3	11·2	−1·7
	16	F	14¼	52·0	0·42	65·6	25·5	32·7	9·4	3·8	3·6
	Means‡ for Group 3					60·9§	52·3	70·2	10·9	9·6	0·8
					Gas volumes at BTPS						

* The children are listed in approximate order of increasing severity of pulmonary symptoms as judged clinically.

† The adult prediction formula for vital capacity was used in this instance (2·5 l./sq. m. of body surface).

‡ The means are quoted to help rapid assessment; no purpose is served by attempting to show statistically significant differences between these groups.

§ Strictly speaking, it is invalid to calculate the mean $FEV_{1\cdot 0}$% directly because the predicted values vary slightly with age (Gandevia, in preparation). However, as this variation is small (78% to 84% for the age range of this series), its effect is insignificant for present purposes.

(2·35 litres) indicates a maximum breathing capacity of over 80 litres per minute. This patient has no clinical evidence of 'bronchitis' or asthma and no restriction of exercise tolerance.

The ventilatory defect is more apparent in Group 2, and is best exemplified by Cases 7, 10 and 11. The group shows little or no reduction in VC, but a considerable fall in $FEV_{1\cdot0}$ and hence $FEV_{1\cdot0}$ %. The ventilatory capacity of all members of the group is improved after the bronchodilator aerosol; this is best seen in the striking increase in $FEV_{1\cdot0}$ in Cases 6, 7, 8 and 10. Case 8 indicates one of the fallacies of considering any of the three indices of ventilatory capacity in isolation; $FEV_{1\cdot0}$% is only slightly lowered but there is considerable reduction in both VC and $FEV_{1\cdot0}$.

In Group 3 ventilatory capacity is further reduced. The impairment is manifest not only in a further fall in the mean $FEV_{1\cdot0}$ to about half the normal value but also in a marked lowering of the VC. $FEV_{1\cdot0}$ % thus shows a less striking decrease. With the exception of the least severe case in this group (Case 12) the response to the isoprenaline aerosol was disappointing although significant in three instances. The almost normal results for all indices in Case 14 may be related to inaccurate prediction of the normal values for so short a child.

Comparison of the clinical ranking in the whole series with ranking according to $FEV_{1\cdot0}$, $FEV_{1\cdot0}$ % and VC yields correlation coefficients of 0·586, 0·516 and 0·414; the first two are significant at the 5% level and approach significance at 1%. The correlation between the increase in $FEV_{1\cdot0}$ after the aerosol and clinical assessment is negative and of the same order of significance.

Discussion

In summary, the results show a reasonably good correlation of clinical assessment with ventilatory capacity, although there are individual discrepancies. $FEV_{1\cdot0}$ and $FEV_{1\cdot0}$ %, and to a much lesser extent VC, tend to diminish progressively according to the clinical evaluation of severity of pulmonary symptoms and disability. The response to a bronchodilator aerosol is consistently in the direction of improvement; it is most impressive in several children in the intermediate, moderately affected group and least apparent in the most disabled children.

There is little or no improvement in $FEV_{1\cdot0}$ % after a bronchodilator aerosol, even in the presence of moderate increases in $FEV_{1\cdot0}$. This finding, which appears anomalous at first sight, is in accord with experience in adults with emphysema or asthma. Thompson and Hugh-Jones (1958) found a sharp increase in $FEV_{1\cdot0}$ % after a bronchodilator aerosol only in asthmatic subjects who were already nearly normal at the time of testing; in emphysematous patients or patients severely asthmatic at the time of testing little or no change in $FEV_{1\cdot0}$ % was found, irrespective of the degree of improvement in $FEV_{1\cdot0}$ and VC. It is of interest in this connexion that in the present series there is no correlation between change in $FEV_{1\cdot0}$ and the initial findings of $FEV_{1\cdot0}$ or VC (expressed as percentages of predicted values). In patients with uncomplicated asthma and comparable ventilatory capacity findings a greater response in $FEV_{1\cdot0}$ and VC to isoprenaline might be anticipated. The comparative lack of such response and the failure of $FEV_{1\cdot0}$ % to improve to a normal level (in all but one patient) suggest that the decreased ventilatory capacity in the present series, at least in Groups 2 and 3, is due partly to changes other than reversible bronchoconstriction. Probable factors are bronchial or bronchiolar occlusion by tenacious mucus, organic bronchiolar narrowing or obliteration and structural emphysema.

In addition to the development of structural changes in the more severely affected patients, two other factors may play a part in determining the relative responsiveness of patients in Group 2. The first is that the series as a whole may reflect the same pattern of response to a bronchodilator aerosol as Hume and Gandevia (1957a, b) found in individual patients with asthma, namely a small response (expressed in absolute units) in periods of exacerbation and of remission but a large (absolute) response in the intermediate stages. The second possibility is that the three groups reflect successive phases in the natural history of the pulmonary lesion in fibrocystic disease, Group 2 representing an intermediate phase characterized by a comparatively large component of reversible bronchoconstriction. We can offer no evidence as to the relative importance of these factors in the present series, and it must be noted that clinical wheeze was one of the criteria used to differentiate our Groups 1 and 2.

West, Levin and Di Sant' Agnese (1954) found no improvement in ventilatory capacity after Vaponefrin in the six patients whom they describe in detail. Only one other reference to the objective assessment of bronchodilator therapy is known to us: Royce (1956) referring to a 'representative' series of pulmonary function studies on one child, observed that a bronchodilator agent increased ventilatory capacity 'to a significant degree'.

In the absence of objective measurement the varying opinions to be found in the literature as to the value of bronchodilator drugs are attributable to several factors, the chief of which is perhaps the inadequacy of clinical methods of assessment. Audible wheezing, often taken as clinical evidence of bronchospasm, may also be due to mechanical factors such as mucous plugging, expiratory invagination of the posterior tracheal wall and bronchial collapse. This wheezing may remain after 'bronchospasm' has been reduced by a bronchodilator drug and its persistence does not necessarily mean that no alteration in the degree of bronchial constriction has taken place. Conversely, in some patients with no audible wheeze at the time of testing, considerable subjective and objective improvement may follow bronchodilator therapy, as in fact occurred in some patients in the present series.

The absence of a striking response in over half the present series should not be interpreted as indicating that bronchodilator therapy is neither indicated nor useful; even 10% improvement is worth while to a patient whose initial ventilatory capacity is a half or a third of normal. Furthermore the tests may not fully reflect an improved ability to cough up phlegm, a point which may be particularly relevant to the therapeutic use of complex aerosols. Our results in an 'acute experiment' indicate a significant though in some instances small response to isoprenaline, and a more comprehensive long-term trial of aerosol therapy is currently being undertaken.

Summary

The ventilatory capacity of 16 patients with fibrocystic disease of the pancreas was assessed immediately before and after a bronchodilator aerosol. A uniform trend towards improvement was found, more particularly in the intermediate group of children with moderate pulmonary disability as judged clinically. Improvement was less marked in children with mild or severe pulmonary symptoms. In perhaps a third of the children studied the improvement might be considered striking. The significance of these findings is briefly reviewed, and the difficulties of clinical assessment in the evaluation of bronchodilator therapy and its role are outlined.

References

Anderson, C. M. and Freeman, M. (1958). A Simple Method of Sweat Collection with Analysis of Electrolytes in Patients with Fibrocystic Disease of the Pancreas, and their Families. *Med. J. Aust.*, 1, 419.

Bernstein, L., D'Silva, J. L. and Mendel, D. (1952). The Effect of the Rate of Breathing on the Maximum Breathing Capacity Determined with a New Spirometer, *Thorax*, 7, 255.

Gandevia, B. (1960). *Arch. Dis. Childh.* In the press.

—— and Hugh-Jones, P. (1957). Terminology for Measurements of Ventilatory Capacity. *Thorax*, 12, 290.

Hume, K. M. (1957). Personal communication.

—— and Gandevia, B. (1957a). Ventilatory Capacity in Chronic Bronchitis after Oral Ephedrine. *Tubercle (Lond.)*, 38, 199.

——, —— (1957b). Forced Expiratory Volume Before and After Isoprenaline. *Thorax*, 12, 276.

Royce, S. W. (1956). Cardiac and Pulmonary Complications in Fibrocystic Disease of the Pancreas. In *Report of the Eighteenth Ross Pediatric Research Conference*, Ross Laboratories, Ohio, p. 79.

Thompson, W. B. and Hugh-Jones, P. (1958). Forced Expiratory Volume as a Test for Successful Treatment of Asthma. *Brit. med. J.*, 1, 1093.

West, J. R., Levin, S. M. and Di Sant' Agnese, P. A. (1954). Pulmonary Function in Fibrocystic Disease of the Pancreas. *Pediatrics*, 13, 155.

APPENDIX

A brief summary of the clinical history of each patient is given with particular reference to the severity of pulmonary symptoms.

Group 1

Case 1. K.R., a male of 17 years, weighing 110½ lb., was diagnosed at 9 years of age following an attack of pneumonia slow to resolve. There has been no persistent chest infection since then and he is now well grown, at work, has normal exercise tolerance, a clinically normal chest and no clubbing of the fingers. He has a palpable and firm liver.

Case 2. K.M., a female of 10 years 3 months, weight 58 lb., was diagnosed at 6 years of age. She had had abnormal stools since birth, recurrent bronchitis in winter and occasional pneumonia but no permanent cough. During the years of observation there has been no attack of pneumonia. At present she is well, has no cough, no abnormal clinical signs in the chest and no finger clubbing. She attends school regularly and has normal exercise tolerance.

Case 3. L.W., a female, sister of Case 4, 11 years 6 months, weighing 71 lb., had had abnormal stools since birth with prolapse of the rectum at times. Intermittent colds with slight cough were easily cleared by an occasional short course of an antibiotic. There has been no episode of pneumonia, her chest has been clinically clear; slight clubbing of the fingers is present. School attendance has been regular, and exercise tolerance normal.

Case 4. D.W., a female, sister of Case 3, aged 8 years, weighing 49 lb., had shown abnormal stools since early life, prolapse of the rectum and a large appetite. She has been subject to mild bronchitis in winter but has not had pneumonia nor any persistent cough. The chest has been clinically normal but slight clubbing of the fingers is present. School attendance is regular and exercise tolerance normal.

Case 5. A.P., a male aged 8 years 6 months, weighing 42 lb., was diagnosed at 6 years, having had abnormal motions and a distended abdomen since birth. There were intermittent bouts of wheezing with an attack of pneumonia at 5 years, and he had another attack of pneumonia which cleared readily at 7 years. There was no cough or wheezing at recent examinations and he had had no antibiotic therapy for one year. The chest was clinically normal. School attendance and exercise tolerance have been good.

Group 2

Case 6. J.A., a male, aged 9 years 3 months, weighing 66½ lb., was diagnosed at 6 years 11 months following abnormal motions for 15 months with cough and sputum for two months. The chest symptoms cleared with antibiotics and since then there has been only intermittent mild chest infection. Some cough and sputum were present at the time of examination but school attendance has been regular and exercise tolerance is normal.

Case 7. D.W., a male of 12 years, weighing 87½ lb., was diagnosed at 7 years following abnormal stools since birth, recurrent bronchitis and attacks of bronchopneumonia. His chest symptoms improved with antibiotics and he is now free of cough and sputum for months at a time. When tested, some cough and sputum were present with rhonchi and rales scattered over his chest. He is a well grown boy but has finger clubbing. School attendance is fair and exercise tolerance normal.

Case 8. M.B., a female, aged 10 years 3 months, weighing 52 lb., had had offensive stools since birth and recurrent attacks of pneumonia with severe cough until the age of 2½ years when the diagnosis was made. She has improved gradually since then but still has some persistent cough and sputum despite continuous antibiotic therapy. Occasional rhonchi and rales are heard in the chest but were absent at the time of testing. School attendance is regular and exercise tolerance normal.

Case 9. G.P., a male, aged 7 years 9 months, weighing 43 lb., had had abnormal stools since birth with intermittent attacks of bronchitis. The diagnosis was made at the age of 4 years when he had some cough and sputum, slight clubbing of the fingers and some signs of emphysema. He improved and was relatively free of cough and sputum with continuous antibiotic therapy. At the time of testing he had occasional cough and some sputum, but no adventitiae in the lungs; school attendance has been regular and exercise tolerance is good.

Case 10. P.C., a male, aged 11 years 3 months, weighing 64 lb., had had abnormal stools since birth and pneumonia as a baby. Cough and sputum have been present nearly all his life but are well controlled with continuous antibiotics and postural coughing. He attends school regularly, taking part in athletics. He has emphysema of the chest with rales and occasional rhonchi and mild clubbing of the fingers. At the time of testing cough and sputum were present.

Case 11. A.N., a male, aged 15 years, weighing 67 lb., had had abnormal stools and abdominal distension since babyhood. The diagnosis was established at 7½ years when he had his first chest infection associated with purulent sputum. Before that occasional colds had cleared readily but now some cough and sputum is present most of the time. At the time of testing there were crepitations over the right lower lobe posteriorly, and slight clubbing of the fingers. He could produce a small amount of sputum. School attendance is fairly regular and exercise tolerance is moderately good.

Group 3

Case 12. B.M., a male, aged 10 years, weighing 41½ lb., had had abnormal stools together with recurrent bronchitis and bronchopneumonia. The diagnosis was made at 6 years when he was undersized, and had severe cough with sputum. He improved with continuous antibiotic therapy and postural coughing, but at the time of examination had cough and sputum with rales scattered over the chest. He attends school regularly but has only fair exercise tolerance.

Case 13. B.B., a male, aged 13 years 6 months, weighing 68½ lb., had had abnormal stools since birth and a long history of suppurative lung infection with increasing dyspnoea, emphysema and finger clubbing. The diagnosis was made at the age of 9½ years. Since then considerable improvement with continuous antibiotic therapy and postural coughing has occurred but at the time of testing he still had suppurative lung infection, clubbing of the fingers and emphysema. He attends school regularly but his exercise tolerance is only fair.

Case 14. G.M., a male, aged 6 years, weighing 40 lb., had had abnormal stools and distended abdomen since birth with recurrent bronchitis followed by persistent cough and sputum. He has a palpable, firm liver, emphysematous chest, clubbing of the fingers, intermittent rales and rhonchi and persistent cough and sputum. He can be controlled with antibiotics and postural coughing but home care is poor. He attends school but has limited exercise tolerance.

Case 15. P.L., a male, aged 9 years 6 months, weighing 49 lb., had had abnormal stools since birth. The diagnosis was established at 6 months. He was free of chest infection until 5 years of age. Recurrent bronchitis occurred until 6 years when he was involved in a severe car accident with injuries leading to several major surgical operations. Severe suppurative lung infection developed during this period. At the time of testing he was dyspnoeic, and mildly cyanosed with scattered rales in the chest and gross clubbing of the fingers. He attends school intermittently and exercise tolerance is severely limited.

Case 16. M.B., a female, aged 14 years 3 months, weighing 50 lb., had had abnormal stools since the first year of life and severe suppurative lung infection for about 12 years. At the time of testing she had severe dyspnoea and some cyanosis. Signs of emphysema with scattered rhonchi and rales and clubbing of the fingers were present. She does not attend school and exercise tolerance is severely limited.

CONGENITAL BOWING OF THE LONG BONES: REPORT OF A CASE

BY

A. D. BAIN and HELEN S. BARRETT

From the Departments of Pathology and Anatomy, University of Edinburgh, and the Royal Hospital for Sick Children, Edinburgh

(RECEIVED FOR PUBLICATION MAY 8, 1959)

Congenital bowing of many long bones in a single individual is comparatively rare and Angle (1954), in a review of the English literature, found only eight reported cases. On the other hand, bowing of individual long bones occurs with greater frequency, the same author reviewing 12 cases of anterior and 14 cases of posterior tibial angulation and three cases with bilateral involvement of the femora only. The present case is that of a stillborn child who had congenital bowing of several long bones. In order to ascertain the presence or absence of accompanying abnormalities, anatomical and radiological investigations were undertaken, as detailed dissection of the entire skeleton had not previously been reported in these cases.

The diagnosis in this case was based on the presence of typical deformities in the lower limbs, associated with cutaneous dimpling.

Case Report

History. The mother, aged 23, had been well during this pregnancy, and was first seen one month before the estimated date of delivery when she was found to have an acute hydramnios. Radiological examination failed to reveal foetal malformation, but foetal ascites or hydrops foetalis was suspected. The pregnancy continued and the mother was delivered of a mature stillborn female foetus weighing 3,175 g. The mother's blood group was O, Rh+. Blood Wassermann was negative.

Previous maternal history showed that the only notable illness was two attacks of pneumonia contracted at 3 and 4 years of age, but since then she had experienced no trouble with her chest. She had been pregnant on two previous occasions: in 1948 she had a spontaneous delivery of a full-term healthy male infant weighing 8 lb. 12 oz. (3,968 g.); this child is now alive and well. In 1951 she became pregnant again, but aborted spontaneously at the sixth week.

The family history is clear. She has two brothers and one sister, none married and all in good health. There is no history of any babies suffering from congenital abnormalities in either her own or her husband's family.

External Appearance. The lower limbs appeared relatively short in comparison with the trunk and arms (Fig. 1). There was pronounced anterior angulation of the legs immediately above the ankles. At the apex of the protuberance there was a clearly defined cutaneous dimple. The feet showed a bilateral talipes equino-varus. No abnormality was noted in the upper limbs. The head was unusual in shape with considerable protuberance of

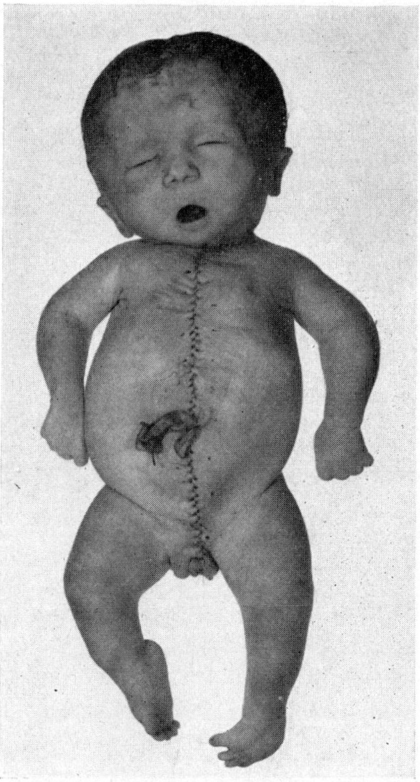

FIG. 1.—Photograph at autopsy showing relative shortness of lower limbs with anterior angulation of tibiae. Note shape of head.

the frontal bones and a widely patent frontal suture. In view of these abnormalities the baby was examined radiologically before the autopsy (Fig. 2).

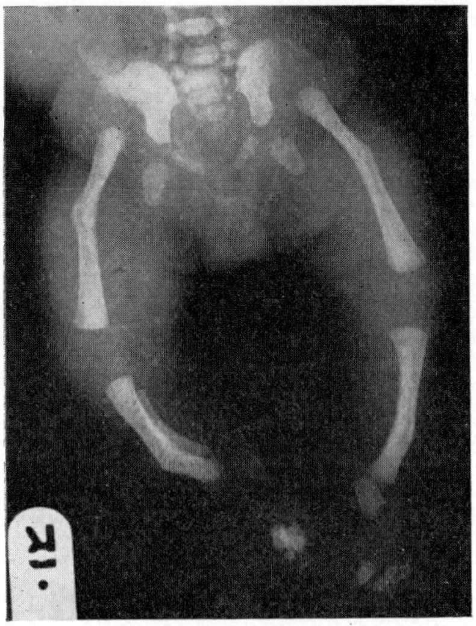

FIG. 2.—Radiograph of lower limbs showing anterior angulation of bones and splaying of ischia.

Autopsy Findings. The subcutaneous tissues were slightly oedematous, and all the serous sacs contained an excess of free fluid. The brain was injected with formalin in order to leave the skull intact for dissection and, when removed at a later stage, showed no pathological abnormality. The pharynx, oesophagus and trachea were normal. The lungs were completely atelectatic and were slightly compressed as a result of the excess free fluid in the pleural sacs. No subpleural haemorrhages were present. The heart, thyroid and thymus showed no abnormality. The alimentary tract was normal. The liver was slightly enlarged and paler than normal but showed no other abnormality. The Prussian blue reaction was negative. The gall bladder, bile ducts, pancreas, spleen, adrenals, ovaries, tubes and uterus showed no pathological changes. The right kidney was enlarged to about one and a half times the normal size on account of a hydronephrosis. The right ureter was moderately dilated, but there was no obstruction at either the pelvi-ureteric or vesico-ureteric junctions to explain the hydronephrosis. The left kidney and left ureter were normal. No abnormality was noted in the bladder or urethra.

Microscopical Findings. The lung parenchyma was mature; the alveoli contained an excess of amniotic débris, compatible with an anoxial state. The liver showed a considerable excess of erythropoiesis, much of this being of primitive type. In the spleen, groups of normoblasts were present throughout the pulp, showing excessive erythropoiesis for a mature foetus. The pancreas, adrenals and heart were normal. The kidneys were mature. Sections were taken from rib, sternum, tibia and fibula. In all of these there was a normal alignment of cartilage cells at the epiphyseal junction, and normal ossification in these regions. Sections of the placenta and membranes failed to reveal any pathological condition.

Further Investigation. Immediately following the autopsy the body was immersed in formalin. The right lower limb together with the ischium and conjoint ramus was amputated for histological examination. After decalcification, serial sagittal sections were made from the right femur and sections were also taken from the right tibia. All were stained with haematoxylin and eosin but fixation was poor and the results were disappointing. The remainder of the body was macerated in potassium hydroxide. The joints of the pelvis, left hip and knee were left intact, as were those of the right shoulder and elbow and most of the vertebral column; the left upper limb and several cervical vertebrae were macerated further to provide dried and separate bones. Radiographs were taken at many stages.

After maceration in potassium hydroxide cartilage remains gelatinous. In this foetus some of the 'cartilage' did not have this gelatinous quality and is described as 'membrane'. Histological examination of this tissue was not possible.

The long bones of the left lower limb and the right humerus were then sectioned longitudinally with a fret-saw and their architecture was compared with that of macerated bones from six normal stillborn foetuses. In the abnormal bones the sections passed through the nutrient foramen and through the convexity of the angulation. The normal bones were cut in similar planes. The bones of the lower limb were thus sectioned in a sagittal plane and the humeri in a coronal plane. When the sections were examined under a hand lens, the direction of the trabeculae which lay longitudinally in the plane of section was easily seen as the trabeculae were outlined by the intervening vascular spaces.

Examination of Skeleton. The bones were all smaller and lighter than normal. The abnormalities noted were bilaterally symmetrical except where otherwise stated. Epiphyseal centres of ossification for the lower ends of the femora and the upper ends of the tibiae were absent. The long bones showed multiple small vascular foramina towards the ends of the shafts. There was no evidence of fracture.

HEAD. A cleft soft palate extended into the posterior part of the hard palate. The base of the skull (chondrocranium) was small in proportion to the vault. The interfrontal suture was wide open and the frontal bones were bulging. The cranial capacity was within normal limits. The individual bones were normal.

VERTEBRAL COLUMN. There were seven cervical, 12 thoracic, six lumbar and four sacral vertebrae. The cervical column was flexed, this flexion being acute between C3 and C4. No bony cause for this flexion was found.

Spina Bifida. Spina bifida was present in the cervical region (C2-C6) and in the lumbosacral region from L1 downwards. The laminar defect was gross in the lumbo-sacral region but was less marked in the cervical region. The defects were bridged across by membrane. The bony laminae of C7 and of T1 had met in the midline and undergone premature synostosis.

Abnormality of Pedicles (Fig. 3). The pedicles in the lumbar region were ossified. The pedicles in the thoracic and cervical column were not ossified but represented by membranous bars uniting the bony neural arch to the body. Each bony neural arch was made up of a lamina with superior and inferior articular processes. The right pedicle of T11 was partly ossified, a spicule of bone being continued forwards from the bony neural arch but failing to reach the body, to which it was attached by membrane. The right pedicle of T12 was almost completely ossified. On the left side the transition from membranous to bony pedicle took place in the same manner but occurred one segment lower.

Neuro-central Joints. These were clearly defined in the lumbar region where the bony neural arches continued forwards beyond the pedicle to form the lateral parts of the body, leaving a normal neuro-central cartilaginous joint between bony neural arch and centrum.

In the cervical and thoracic regions no typical neuro-central joints were present. The cervical bodies were transversely elongated; C3 and C4 showed a small accessory centre of ossification in the right lateral part of the body, and in C6 a knob of bone was incompletely fused to the right side of the body. The thoracic bodies were heart-shaped and transversely elongated. These findings suggested that ossification was present in the anterior ends of some of the neural arches and that the neuro-central synchondroses had undergone premature synostosis in C6 and possibly in the thoracic region as well.

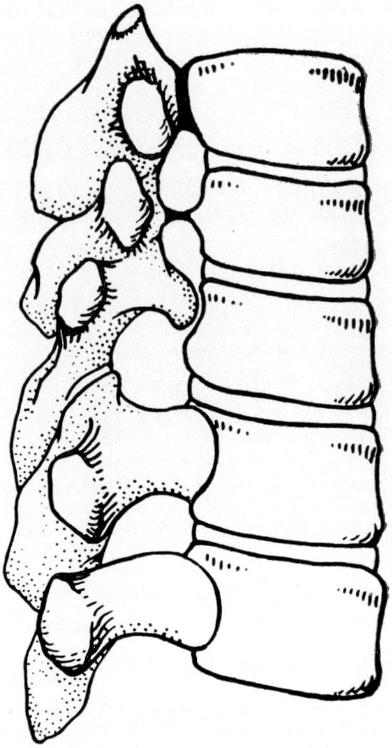

FIG. 3.—Drawing of lateral view of T.10–L.2 showing normal pedicles and neuro-central joints in L.1 and L.2. Pedicle of T.10 is membranous and neuro-central joint is absent. Pedicle of T.11 is partly ossified and pedicle of T.12 almost completely ossified.

Transverse Processes. These were normally ossified in the lumbar region and in the thoracic region where they formed the most anterior part of the bony neural arches. In the cervical region the transverse processes were membranous except in C7 where the transverse element was bony and continuous with the bone forming the upper and lower articular processes. In this vertebra the left costal element was membranous while the right costal element formed the upper head of a two-headed first right rib.

SACRUM. The bodies and pedicles of the sacral vertebrae were normal. The cartilaginous lateral masses were small, thus producing a very narrow sacrum. No centres of ossification were present in the lateral masses.

PELVIS (Fig. 4). The inlet of the pelvis was abnormally long antero-posteriorly and narrow transversely. The decrease in transverse diameter was partly accounted for by the narrowness of the lateral masses of the sacrum. The antero-posterior diameter of the brim was almost twice the greatest transverse diameter.

The outlet of the pelvis was extraordinarily wide. The remaining (left) ischium was splayed forwards and laterally so that the conjoint ramus ran medially to the pubis. This conjoint ramus was membranous.

A normal sacro-iliac joint cavity was present on both sides. The left hip was dislocated, the false socket being above and slightly anterior to the acetabulum. The acetabular rim was normal.

LEFT FEMUR (external form) (Fig. 5). A spine projected forward from the junction of the upper and middle thirds of the shaft. This was the most obvious abnormality. The spine was not attached to the skin and no dimple was present. At the level of the spine the shaft was bent slightly forwards. Above and below the angulation the shaft was straighter than usual, the normal anterior convexity of the shaft being absent. The ends of the shaft were normally expanded. The only nutrient artery entered the upper third of the back of the bone and was directed distally and forwards towards the apex of the angulation.

LEFT AND RIGHT FEMORA (internal structure) (Fig. 6). At the site of angulation the cortical bone was greatly thickened posteriorly and composed of trabeculae converging towards the spine. The nutrient artery ran along the upper of these radiating trabeculae and was directed towards the apex and the angulation. The marrow cavity was displaced anteriorly by this cortical thickening. The cortical bone forming the spine was of normal thickness.

Histological examination of the shaft of the femur (Fig. 7) showed that some bony trabeculae had an acel-

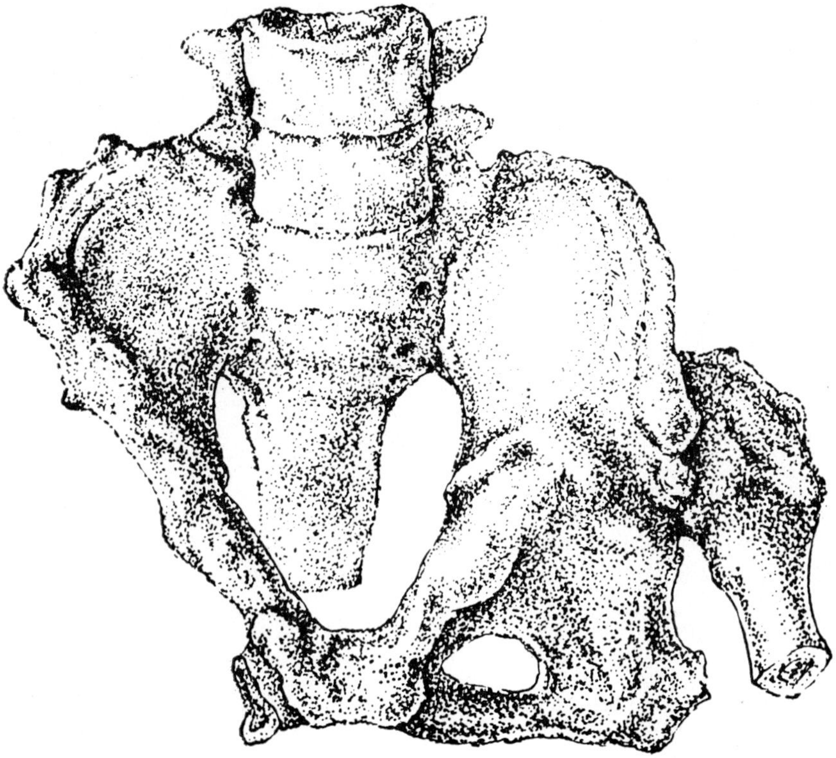

FIG. 4.—Pelvis drawn to scale with L.4, 5 and 6 attached and right ischium removed. Note abnormal shape of pelvic brim; narrowness of lateral masses of sacrum (identifiable on left side between first anterior sacral foramen and sacro-iliac joint); left ischium splayed forward and laterally; dislocation of left hip.

lular cartilaginous core. These cartilaginous cores were more numerous in trabeculae above and below the angulation, more numerous anteriorly than posteriorly, and towards the medullary cavity. At the angulation no cartilage was present in the trabeculae converging towards the spine though cartilage was present in some trabeculae near the medullary cavity in the region of the spine. Subperiosteal trabeculae showed cartilage cores only at the anterior part of the middle of the shaft. The compact bone of the shaft showed many scattered areas of primitive bone, i.e. areas where bone cells were numerous and rounded and separated by a relatively small amount of matrix. The matrix showed lines of irregular density, most numerous in the region of the spine. In the shaft of the bone there were remarkably few osteoblasts and osteoclasts were virtually absent. There were no osteoclasts in the spine. At the metaphysis the bone structure was normal. The periosteum was intact in median sections. The outer fibrous layer was thin over the apex of the spine but normal elsewhere. The inner cellular layer was abnormally thin above and below the spine and absent over the spine where the fibrous layer was in direct contact with the bone. Both layers of periosteum were normal towards the metaphysis and over the concave aspect of the angulation.

LEFT TIBIA (Fig. 5). This showed pronounced anterior angulation at the junction of the middle and lower thirds of the shaft. The apex of this angulation was on the anterior border of the tibia, and the periosteum here was attached by tough fibrous tissue to the overlying skin dimple. The shaft of the tibia above and below the angulation was less curved than normal. As in the femur, the cortical bone on the posterior aspect of the shaft was greatly thickened and composed of trabeculae converging towards the apex of the angulation, this thick cortex narrowing and displacing the medullary cavity forwards. The cortical bone forming the apex of the angulation was slightly thickened. The canal for the nutrient artery ran in the upper part of the thickened posterior cortex and was directed towards the apex of the angulation.

RIGHT TIBIA. Serial sections were unfortunately not available. Examination of sections showed the same abnormalities as those of the femur. The metaphyseal region was normal.

LEFT FIBULA (Fig. 5). This showed a similar degree of

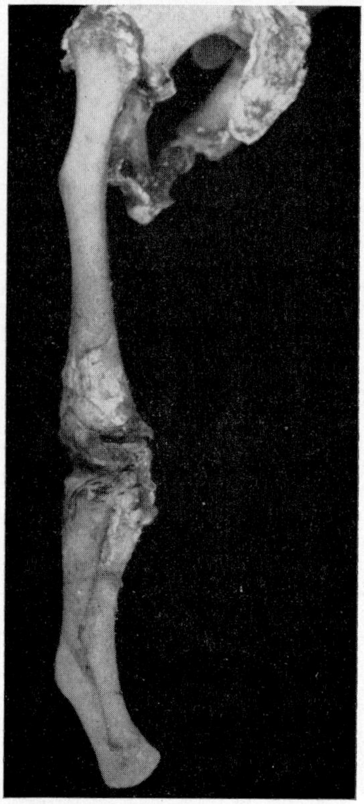

FIG. 5.

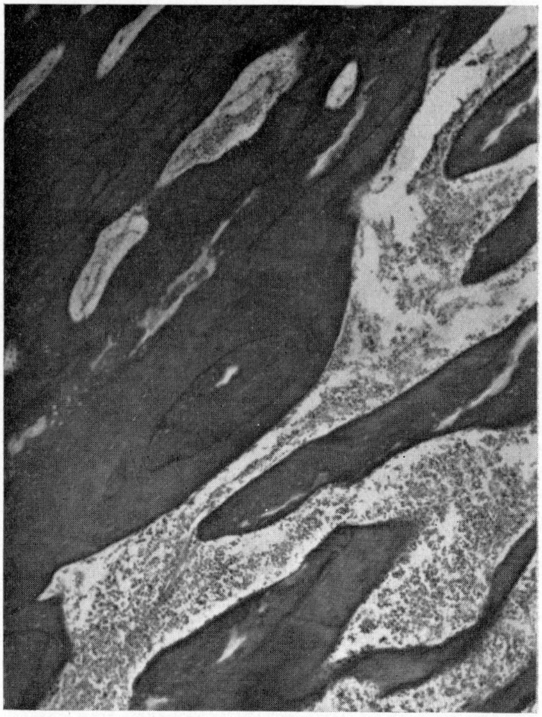

FIG. 7.

FIG. 5.—Lateral view of left lower limb showing angulations.

FIG. 6.—Section through angulation of femur showing thickened posterior cortex, radiating trabeculae and displaced medullary cavity. (H. and E. × 2½).

FIG. 7.—Section of anterior cortex of femur immediately above angulation showing lines of irregular density, cartilage cores in trabeculae and areas of primitive bone. (H. and E. ×48).

FIG. 8.—Abnormal scapula on right; scapula from normal full-term foetus on left. Absence of infraspinous portion of blade is obvious. Note poorly developed spine. Acromion process is absent and coracoid process is clearly seen.

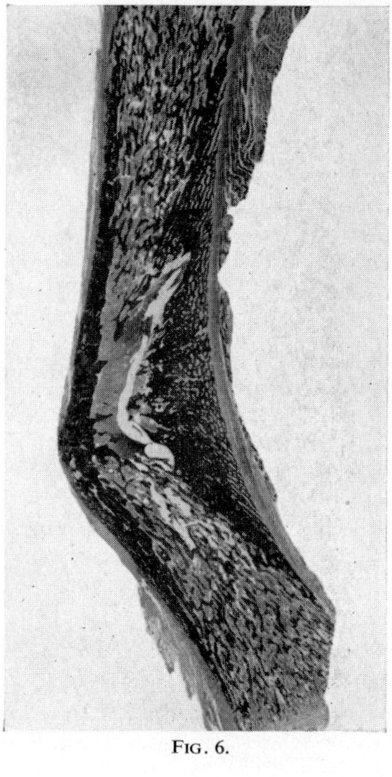

FIG. 6.

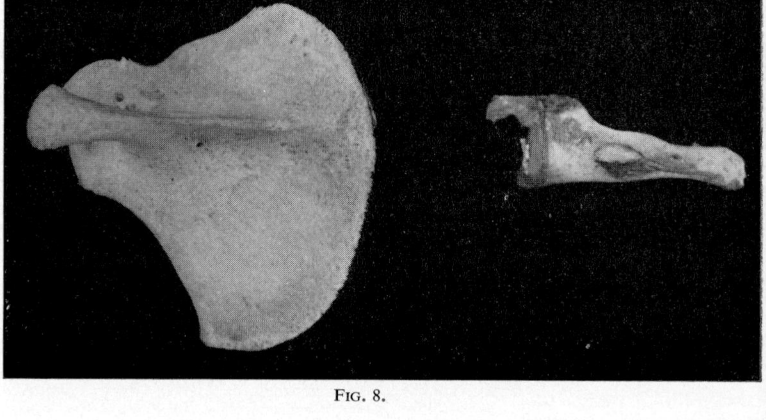

FIG. 8.

angulation, the apex of which was slightly proximal to that of the tibia. The apex was not attached to the skin dimple. Sections showed that the architecture of the bone was similar to that of the tibia. The only nutrient artery entered the middle of the shaft posteriorly and ran in the upper radiating trabeculae towards a point just below the angulation.

CLAVICLES. These were normal.

SCAPULAE (Fig. 8). These were very small, especially the blades, which were virtually absent below the level of the spines and were not represented by cartilage.

HUMERUS. A small spine projected from the postero-lateral aspect of the shaft just above its midpoint. This spine marked the summit of a slight postero-lateral angulation of the shaft.

Section showed that the cortical bone was thickened to form the spine. Below the level of the spine, the cortex on the antero-medial aspect was thickened and composed of trabeculae radiating towards the spine. The nutrient artery ran in the upper border of the thickened cortex towards a point below the spine.

RADIUS AND ULNA. These were normal. Each bone showed two canals for the nutrient arteries.

Discussion

Multiple bowing of the long bones is not necessarily a fatal condition. Caffey (1947) records three cases in living children, and Bound, Finlay and Rose (1952) reported this condition in a child aged 5 months, in whom they noted the easy assumption at this age of the presumed foetal position in which each foot compressed the opposite thigh. Abnormalities accompanying the bowing have been noted by Williams (1943). In a case involving bowing of the femora and anterior angulation of the tibia, he noted incomplete ossification of the body and hypoplasia of the neural arch and spinous processes of the fifth cervical vertebra. In one of the cases of multiple bowing reported by Bound *et al.*, there was micrognathia, cleft palate, plagiocephaly and a marked pigeon-breast deformity. Caffey, on the other hand, found no evidence of other deformities or other skeletal disease in his cases. Angle (1954), in a newly born premature infant, found no radiological evidence of other skeletal deformity except multiple bowing. In the present case the deformities of particular interest, other than the bowing, are those related to the scapula, the vertebrae and the pelvis. Angle (1954) stated that the most widely accepted hypothesis was the mechanical theory. This held that the curvatures in the bones were mechanical in origin resulting from the moulding of long bones over other parts by centripetal forces. Murray (1936) reproduces a photograph of an angulated tibia from a chondrodystrophic chick. The photograph shows bony trabeculae radiating from the concave aspect of the shaft towards the apex of the angulation. Murray attributes the formation of radiating trabeculae to normal ossification, occurring in a cartilage model pathologically soft and unable to resist bending stresses.

In the present case the long bones of the lower limbs were severely affected, the tibia and fibula being more deformed than the femur. The humerus was only slightly deformed and was atypical in that the spine lay above the level of the angulation. This spine might have been interpreted as a secondary marking caused by a fibrous attachment; such markings are not, however, normally present at birth. The slight angulation and cortical thickening on the concave aspect suggest that the humerus was affected in the same way as the lower limb bones but to a lesser extent.

The abnormality of the pelvic brim was similar to that described by Robert (1842), in which there was symmetrical transverse contraction with maldevelopment of the lateral masses of the sacrum and synostosis of the sacro-iliac joint. Robert's pelvis was transversely narrow at all levels, whereas the pelvis of this foetus was transversely narrow at the inlet only and very wide at the outlet. In this foetus the lateral masses of the sacrum were abnormal though the sacro-iliac joints were normal. Little (1958), who described a case of Robert's pelvis, could only find nine reported cases, it being doubtful if all these were indeed true examples of this type of pelvis. The abnormality of the sacrum and the pelvic brim in this case supports the theory that Robert's pelvis is primarily a congenital defect of the lateral masses of the sacrum.

Two-headed first ribs, like congenital dislocation of the hip, are fairly common as isolated abnormalities and these defects need not be further considered.

The abnormalities noted in this foetus were confined to tissues arising from mesoderm. With the exception of the cleft palate and unexplained hydronephrosis, these abnormalities were limited to that part of the skeleton ossified in cartilage, though not all bones ossified in cartilage were abnormal, the radius and ulna being notable exceptions. We have tried to answer the following questions:

(1) **Was the Original Cartilage Model of the Skeleton Normal?** The disproportionately small size of the chondrocranium and of the lateral masses of the sacrum, the spina bifida and the almost complete absence of the cartilaginous precursor of the infraspinous portion of the blade of the scapula indicate either that, in these sites at least, a normal cartilaginous model had failed to develop, or that

having developed, it was partly resorbed. The 'membranous' condition of parts normally cartilaginous at birth, i.e. the pedicles of some vertebrae and the laminae of others, and of the conjoint ramus is not necessarily significant since these parts have a high surface/mass ratio and maceration would therefore proceed more rapidly in these than in other parts. These membranous pedicles and laminae were nevertheless not ossified as they should have been. One possible reason for this could have been an abnormality of the cartilage.

We conclude that the cartilaginous axial skeleton was not normal and hence abnormality of the cartilaginous skeleton of the angulated limb bones cannot be excluded. As chondrification begins just after the end of the first month and is widespread by the end of the second month of gestation, the abnormality could have originated at this early period. Evidence bearing on the normality or abnormality of the precartilage condensations was naturally not available.

(2) Was the Process of Ossification of the Cartilage Models of Angulated Bones Normal? (*a*) Gross structure: Thickening of the cortex on the concave side of the angulated long bones was described by Angle (1954). He described the trabeculae of this cortex as radiating towards the apex of the curvature. It is universally accepted that the cortex of a long bone is very thin over the ends but becomes thick towards the middle of the shaft. Each bone of the six normal foetuses sectioned showed this cortical thickening on the concave aspect of the shaft, a thickening composed of trabeculae converging towards the convexity of the shaft. In every case the nutrient artery or arteries reached the medullary cavity by running between these trabeculae. In longitudinal sections of normal bones the trabeculae formed a triangle, the base of which was along the concave aspect of the shaft, and the apex of which was truncated by the medullary cavity. This triangle was present in both the abnormal and the normal bones. The abnormality in the angulated bones was not the presence of the radiating trabeculae but rather the shortness of the base of the triangle so formed.

The angulated bones showed normal modelling, the metaphysis being expanded and the cartilaginous epiphysis of normal shape. If the angulation of the shafts had been artificially corrected by removing a wedge from the convex side and resetting the upper and lower fragments, the resultant shaft would still have been abnormal because the shaft above and below the angulation was unduly straight and lacked the gentle curvature of the normal bone. Indeed, the angulated portion contained the whole longitudinal curvature of the shaft concentrated into a short length of bone, and the apex of the angulation pointed in the direction of the normal curvature.

The angulation of the long bones was symmetrical in degree, position and direction. We offer the following hypothesis. The primary centre of ossification in a long bone lies near the centre of the cartilage model. The more rapid growth in length of the growing end of the bone results in the gradual displacement of the site of the primary centre of ossification away from the growing end of that bone. The growing ends of the long bones are those at the wrist, shoulder and knee, except in the case of the fibula where it is probably situated in the lower end. Thus the site of the original primary centre of ossification would lie symmetrically in the upper parts of the shafts of the femora, in the lower parts of the shafts of the tibiae, a little higher in fibula than in tibia and in the lower part of the shaft of the humerus. These positions correspond approximately to the sites of angulation (Fig. 5) in the long bones in the present case. In the case of each of these bones the nutrient artery was directed through the thickened bone on the concave side of the angulation and, except in the humerus, towards the apex of the angulation. The abnormal situation and direction of the nutrient artery of the femur was probably of no significance. Indeed, the first two of six full-term normal femora, with which the angulated femur was compared, also showed the same anomaly of the canal for the nutrient artery.

(*b*) Histological examination of the bones was unfortunately limited, but the appearance of the femur and tibia showed that the epiphyseal and metaphyseal regions were normal, in sharp contrast to the shaft. The bony trabeculae in the mid-shaft contained cartilaginous cores. This abnormally situated cartilage could have represented either a new formation of cartilage or a persistence of original cartilage. This latter hypothesis is unlikely as the medullary cavity was not abnormally small and all the bone developed in the original cartilaginous shaft must have been absorbed as the medullary cavity developed. Moreover, some subperiosteal trabeculae (i.e. those most recently formed and normally ossified without an intervening cartilaginous stage) showed cartilaginous cores. These observations suggest that the cartilaginous cores were a new formation. The lack of osteoblasts and osteoclasts noted may have been partly accounted for by the poor preservation of the material sectioned. This lack of cells, especially osteoclasts, was almost complete in the shaft and not evident in the metaphysis which was subjected to the same treatment. The lack of active bone resorption in the region of the spines of the long bones showed that ossification was not proceeding normally in this region at birth.

We conclude that ossification in the shafts of the femur and tibia was abnormal, and that the angulation occurred at approximately the site of the original centre of ossification which develops during the second month of gestation.

(3) **Was the Cause of the Abnormality Extrinsic (Mechanical) or Intrinsic?** Browne (1936) has stated that hydramnios is commonly associated with congenital, mechanically induced abnormalities, and that sparing of the forearm is associated with its protection from pressure by the head in the foetal position. The present foetus showed sparing of the forearm and there was also an associated hydramnios. The association of spina bifida in the second to the sixth cervical vertebrae with premature synostosis in the laminae of the seventh cervical and the first thoracic vertebrae is difficult to explain on a mechanical basis. Likewise, it is difficult to explain the abnormality of the scapula and sacrum on this basis. Any deforming force would have to be symmetrically applied in order to produce bilateral symmetrical deformities and it would also need to be maintained for a considerable period of time, i.e. from at least the second month onwards. Even had the angulation been produced by mechanical factors, the bone, if normal, ought to have shown some tendency to remodel to its normal form. There was no evidence whatsoever of bone resorption in the region of the spine.

We conclude that mechanical factors alone could not account for all the skeletal abnormalities present in this case, and an intrinsic abnormality of ossification in the angulated bones must have been present.

(4) **What might be the Nature of this Intrinsic Defect?** We suggest that the defect might have been located in the perichondrium and periosteum, although the state of the skeleton after maceration and section was unfit for investigations to prove or refute this theory. Ham (1957) states:

> 'The appearance of capillaries in the perichondrium profoundly affects the differentiation of the relatively undifferentiated cells of its inner layer. For, instead of continuing to develop into chondroblasts and chondrocytes, they, in the presence of capillaries, begin to differentiate into osteoblasts and osteocytes, with the result that a thin layer or shell of bone is soon laid down around the model. Since perichondrium thereafter covers bone tissue, its name is changed from perichondrium to periosteum. . . . Indeed, the cells of the inner layer of the periosteum retain their ability to differentiate into chondroblasts and to form cartilage even into adult life. This is easily demonstrated in the repair of broken bones.'

There are thus two essential elements in the perichondrium, vascular and cellular. The perichondrium forms the perichondrial sleeve and gives rise to the periosteal bud which invades the cartilage model to form the primary centre of ossification.

Poor vascularization of the perichondrium of the angulated long bones, especially in the region of the periosteal bud, the capillaries of which become the nutrient artery, could account for the angulations being in the positions of the primary centres of ossification. Poor vascularization could also account for the presence of cartilage cores in some of the trabeculae of the angulated long bones. The normal forearm bones could then be associated with the presence of multiple vascular foramina which were observed in these bones and which probably represented a more adequate blood supply. The apparent normality of the metaphyseal and epiphyseal regions of the angulated bones could also be due to a more adequate blood supply towards the ends of the bones, such a blood supply being derived from the multiple small periosteal vessels.

Deficiency in the other (cellular) element of the perichondrium could be held to account for the paucity of bone cells in the angulated shafts.

Lacroix (1951) suggests that movement of the periosteal sleeve influences the arrangement of the subperiosteal trabeculae of a bone. In an angulated bone such failure of movement, localized to the concave side, might account for the angulation and the trabecular arrangement noted in this and in previously reported cases. This local failure, however, would not necessarily explain the abnormal straightness of the shaft above and below the angulation.

In this foetus we suggest that a perichondrium deficient in both cellular and vascular elements could have caused all the skeletal abnormalities.

Summary

A detailed examination has been made of a stillborn foetus showing multiple bowing of the long bones. In addition to the bowing of the bones other defects were found and those of particular interest were in the scapula, vertebrae and pelvis.

As a result of the studies on this case the following conclusions were reached:

(1) The cartilaginous axial skeleton was abnormal. The cartilaginous skeleton of the angulated bones may likewise have been abnormal.

(2) Ossification in the angulated long bones was abnormal.

(3) The abnormality of ossification in the long bones was intrinsic in nature and situated approximately in the position of the primary centre of ossification.

(4) The basic disorder underlying the angulation was probably a deficiency in both vascular and cellular elements of the perichondrium.

We wish to thank Professor G. J. Romanes, Professor R. W. B. Ellis, Professor G. L. Montgomery and Professor L. H. Wells for their helpful criticism. We are grateful to Dr. J. B. King and Dr. W. Macleod for radiographs and to Dr. Nora Campbell for the drawings. We also wish to thank Mr. T. C. Dodds and Miss C. Brydon for photography.

REFERENCES

Angle, C. R. (1954). *Pediatrics*, **13**, 257.
Bound, J. P., Finlay, H. V. L. and Rose, F. C. (1952). *Arch. Dis. Childh.*, **27**, 179.
Browne, D. (1936). *Proc. roy. Soc. Med.*, **29**, 1409.
Caffey, J. (1947). *Amer. J. Dis. Child.*, **74**, 543.
Ham, A. W. (1957). *Histology*, 3rd ed., p. 278. Lippincott, Philadelphia.
Lacroix, P. (1951). *The Organization of Bones*, trans. S. Gilder, p. 67. Churchill, London.
Little, E. W. (1958). *J. Obstet. Gynaec. Brit. Emp.*, **65**, 465.
Murray, P. D. F. (1936). *Bones: A Study of the Development and Structure of the Vertebrate Skeleton*, p. 34. University Press, Cambridge.
Robert, F. (1842). *Beschreibung eines im höchsten Grade querverengten Beckens.* Karlsruhe.
Williams, E. R. (1943). *Brit. J. Radiol.*, **16**, 371.

BIOCHEMICAL STUDIES IN IDIOPATHIC HYPERCALCAEMIA OF INFANCY

BY

JOHN O. FORFAR, S. L. TOMPSETT and W. FORSHALL

From the Departments of Paediatrics and Biochemistry, Edinburgh Northern Group of Hospitals, and the Departments of Child Life and Health and Clinical Chemistry, University of Edinburgh

(RECEIVED FOR PUBLICATION MAY 21, 1959)

Part I. Serum Calcium and Cholesterol Levels from the First to the Fifteenth Month of Life

Idiopathic hypercalcaemia tends to develop between the first and fifteenth months of life and diagnosis rests primarily on biochemical findings. We have determined for this age period the normal values for serum calcium, serum cholesterol and the serum cholesterol fractions by the methods which we use.

Over a period of four years samples of blood were taken from 110 infants in hospital, or attending hospital, who required venupuncture. None was suffering from idiopathic hypercalcaemia, diabetes, nephrosis or hypothyroidism.

Methods

Serum Calcium. Initially the method of Kramer and Tisdall (1921) and Tisdall (1923) was employed in which calcium is precipitated as calcium oxalate and titrated with potassium permanganate. Two ml. of serum are required. Later Trinder's (1957) method was used in which calcium is precipitated with chloranilic acid; the precipitate is dissolved in a colour reagent consisting of ferric nitrate and sulphuric acid and the result determined colorimetrically by comparison with a similarly treated standard calcium solution. This method requires only 0·5 ml. of serum.

Serum Cholesterol. Total serum cholesterol was determined by the method of Zlatkis, Zak and Boyle (1953), in which a direct colour reaction is obtained by the addition of a ferric chloride/glacial acetic acid/concentrated sulphuric acid mixture. No preliminary extraction is necessary and only 0·1 ml. of serum is required.

Free cholesterol was estimated by the method of Zak, Dickenman, White, Burnett and Chemey (1955) in which free cholesterol is precipitated from an alcohol-acetone extract with digitonin, the resulting digitonide separated and its cholesterol content estimated by the method of Zlatkis *et al.* (1953). One ml. of serum is required.

Cholesterol esters which are not precipitated by digitonin were estimated by difference.

Results

A comparison between the Kramer and Tisdall and Trinder methods of calcium estimation is given in Table 1. Both methods were applied to random

TABLE 1

COMPARISON BETWEEN KRAMER AND TISDALL AND TRINDER METHODS OF ESTIMATING SERUM CALCIUM. CARRIED OUT ON 30 RANDOM SAMPLES OF ADULT BLOOD

Serum Calcium (mg. %)	
Kramer and Tisdall	Trinder
13·9	13·2
7·7	7·6
9·1	9·2
8·3	7·6
8·8	9·1
8·7	8·8
9·0	9·0
7·1	6·6
13·3	13·4
9·4	9·2
14·5	14·5
9·4	9·8
8·8	9·2
9·4	9·5
9·9	9·4
8·9	9·0
9·0	8·8
8·8	8·8
10·2	9·9
9·0	8·5
10·5	10·3
8·6	9·0
8·8	8·7
8·2	8·5
8·7	8·5
10·1	10·1
10·1	9·9
14·5	13·7
9·1	9·0
9·2	9·2
Average 9·7	9·6

TABLE 2

SERUM CALCIUM, TOTAL CHOLESTEROL, FREE CHOLESTEROL AND CHOLESTEROL ESTER ESTIMATIONS IN 110 INFANTS AGED 1–15 MONTHS

No.	Age (mth.)	Weight (lb. oz.)	Sex	Serum Calcium (mg. %)	Total Chol. (mg. %)	Free Chol. (mg. %)	Chol. Ester (mg. %)	Free Chol. / Chol. Ester	Ca × Total Chol.	Ca × Free Chol.	Ca × Chol. Ester
1	6	12·0	M	9·5	162	—	—	—	1,539	—	—
2	9	24·6	M	9·5	106	—	—	—	1,007	—	—
3	10	21·2	M	12·2	165	—	—	—	2,008	—	—
4	7	16·5	F	10·0	133	56	77	·727	1,330	560	770
5	10	14·10	M	8·3	135	35	100	·350	1,120	290	830
6	11	20·8	M	12·5	196	83	113	·735	2,450	1,037	1,412
7	11½	20·9	M	10·6	208	83	125	·664	2,204	879	1,324
8	8½	17·14	F	11·7	233	61	172	·355	2,726	713	2,010
9	9	19·0	F	—	237	67	170	·394	—	—	—
10	5	8·8	M	9·3	144	87	57	1·526	1,340	809	530
11	15	22·0	M	—	183	48	135	·356	—	—	—
12	13	18·0	M	9·8	212	81	131	·618	2,076	794	1,284
13	9	15·5	F	9·4	204	89	115	·775	1,916	837	1,081
14	5½	13·3	M	9·7	139	63	76	·824	1,348	611	737
15	4½	12·4	M	10·7	175	79	96	·823	1,874	846	1,027
16	11	18·2	M	10·2	204	100	104	·962	2,081	1,020	1,060
17	2	7·5	M	10·4	166	71	95	·748	1,725	738	988
18	6	16·12	M	10·2	179	42	137	·307	1,826	428	1,396
19	12	14·9	M	10·0	129	31	98	·316	1,290	310	980
20	6	21·4	M	—	200	52	148	·352	—	—	—
21	13	18·12	F	10·1	162	46	116	·397	1,636	464	1,170
22	12	16·7	F	10·4	157	39	118	·331	1,634	406	1,226
23	15	16·9	M	10·2	208	50	158	·316	2,120	510	1,611
24	11½	20·0	M	10·9	237	79	158	·500	2,582	861	1,722
25	6	11·14	M	11·2	174	46	128	·359	1,950	515	1,434
26	13	21·5	F	8·8	226	58	168	·345	1,988	511	1,478
27	7	14·2	M	10·0	148	38	110	·345	1,480	380	1,100
28	4	10·0	F	10·4	159	41	118	·348	1,654	436	1,227
29	2	9·14	F	10·3	222	59	163	·362	2,286	605	1,677
30	15	18·11	M	10·3	231	59	172	·343	2,376	605	1,770
31	3	8·11	M	9·5	150	38	112	·339	1,424	361	1,063
32	6	12·11	M	10·2	150	34	116	·293	1,529	347	1,182
33	12	21·11	M	10·3	211	47	164	·287	2,172	484	1,688
34	3½	13·2	F	10·9	177	79	98	·806	1,928	861	1,068
35	15	24·5	M	10·1	—	—	—	—	—	—	—
36	12	18·1	M	10·6	218	89	129	·690	2,311	943	1,366
37	9	13·8	F	10·7	258	102	156	·654	2,757	1,091	1,669
38	8	14·12	F	9·5	162	—	—	—	1,538	—	—
39	9	14·4	F	10·7	171	50	121	·413	1,828	535	1,294
40	2½	6·6	F	9·6	164	74	90	·828	1,573	710	864
41	15	24·6	M	10·4	—	—	—	—	—	—	—
42	8	17·0	F	—	289	74	215	·344	—	—	—
43	12	17·8	F	10·4	233	56	177	·316	2,421	582	1,840
44	13	18·0	F	11·0	200	—	—	—	2,200	—	—
45	5	14·0	F	10·4	144	60	84	·715	1,496	624	873
46	3½	12·3	M	11·0	154	16	138	·116	1,694	176	1,518
47	8	17·6	M	9·8	210	35	175	·200	2,056	343	1,715
48	3	6·13	F	10·1	175	21	154	·138	1,768	212	1,554
49	4	10·0	M	10·1	202	33	169	·196	2,040	333	1,705
50	7	12·14	F	9·9	202	—	—	—	2,000	—	—
51	7	16·0	F	10·0	280	73	207	·353	2,800	730	2,070
52	3	7·3	F	11·0	154	38	116	·328	1,694	418	1,276
53	10½	12·12	M	10·0	241	67	174	·385	2,410	670	1,740
54	10½	13·13	M	9·3	—	—	—	—	—	—	—
55	3	12·15	F	10·5	237	23	214	·108	2,488	241	2,246
56	9	15·4	M	9·6	183	54	129	·418	1,756	518	1,238
57	10	13·13	M	10·8	233	79	154	·513	2,515	853	1,663
58	5½	13·8	M	10·6	229	75	154	·487	2,425	795	1,632
59	3	13·0	F	10·5	229	71	158	·444	2,401	745	1,659
60	11	16·3	M	10·0	—	—	—	—	—	—	—
61	9	16·6	M	11·0	171	65	106	·613	1,881	715	1,166
62	9	11·12	M	10·4	192	—	—	—	1,996	—	—
63	8	16·4	F	9·7	217	46	171	·269	2,104	446	1,659
64	4	13·8	M	10·8	200	54	146	·370	2,160	583	1,576
65	2	10·0	F	10·2	133	—	—	—	1,356	—	—
66	3	9·8	M	9·9	183	52	131	·397	1,810	515	1,296
67	6	10·2	M	9·8	142	38	104	·366	1,392	372	1,019
68	1	8·4	F	11·5	188	56	132	·424	2,160	644	1,517
69	1	7·0	F	—	275	—	—	—	—	—	—
70	5	16·0	M	9·9	178	40	138	·290	1,762	396	1,366
71	5	14·1	M	10·0	250	56	194	·289	2,500	560	1,940
72	3	10·12	M	9·7	188	54	134	·403	1,823	523	1,299
73	1	5·12	M	9·3	204	46	158	·291	1,897	428	1,470
74	7	24·13	M	9·6	—	—	—	—	—	—	—
75	5	11·8	M	—	209	47	162	·291	—	—	—
76	6	12·6	M	10·1	149	—	—	—	1,503	—	—
77	3	10·6	F	10·9	217	50	167	·300	2,365	545	1,819
78	5	12·0	F	10·7	192	—	—	—	2,053	—	—
79	2	10·13	F	9·4	217	—	—	—	2,040	—	—
80	7	18·0	M	9·7	158	52	106	·491	1,532	504	1,027

(contd.)

TABLE 2—*contd.*

No.	Age (mth.)	Wt. (lb. oz.)	Sex	Serum Calcium (mg. %)	Total Chol. (mg. %)	Free Chol. (mg. %)	Chol. Ester (mg. %)	Free Chol. / Chol. Ester	Ca × Total Chol.	Ca × Free Chol.	Ca × Chol. Ester
81	7	14·11	M	10·2	171	71	100	·710	1,743	724	1,020
82	2½	9·5	M	9·7	171	42	129	·326	1,659	407	1,250
83	8	10·6	M	8·9	160	33	127	·260	1,424	294	1,130
84	10	14·4	F	9·7	237	—	—	—	2,298	—	—
85	7	18·4	M	10·0	194	42	152	·277	1,940	420	1,520
86	13	21·0	M	9·6	258	104	154	·676	2,475	999	1,478
87	8	13·5	M	9·5	131	34	97	·351	1,244	323	922
88	2	6·8	M	8·9	177	52	125	·416	1,574	463	1,112
89	5½	11·8	F	10·1	155	83	72	1·154	1,564	838	727
90	8	11·8	F	10·3	219	76	143	·532	2,255	783	1,472
91	1	7·7	M	9·9	196	84	112	·751	1,940	832	1,108
92	6	13·2	M	9·8	196	40	156	·256	1,920	392	1,528
93	15	23·0	M	8·5	217	52	165	·316	1,844	442	1,401
94	1	8·15	M	8·9	190	65	125	·520	1,690	578	1,112
95	1½	5·12	M	9·8	196	58	138	·420	1,921	568	1,352
96	13	16·12	M	10·6	233	73	160	·457	2,368	773	1,698
97	14	23·7	M	10·2	279	—	—	—	2,845	—	—
98	9½	22·0	M	11·7	167	—	—	—	1,954	—	—
99	6	11·10	F	9·9	179	56	123	·455	1,771	554	1,217
100	13	17·0	F	9·3	175	46	129	·357	1,627	427	1,199
101	10½	18·3	F	9·3	171	—	—	—	1,590	—	—
102	4	10·3	F	9·9	218	46	172	·267	2,159	455	1,703
103	15	13·7	F	9·9	282	54	228	·237	2,794	535	2,256
104	5	11·11	F	10·7	192	63	129	·489	2,052	674	1,379
105	4	11·0	F	9·0	250	—	—	—	2,250	—	—
106	4	8·0	M	9·8	202	54	148	·365	1,978	529	1,449
107	4	7·14	F	11·1	217	68	149	·456	2,408	755	1,653
108	2	12·8	M	9·1	250	—	—	—	2,274	—	—
109	5½	18·0	M	9·8	225	50	175	·286	2,204	490	1,715
110	4	10·8	M	10·3	—	—	—	—	—	—	—

TABLE 3

SERUM CALCIUM, CHOLESTEROL, FREE CHOLESTEROL, CHOLESTEROL ESTERS, FREE CHOLESTEROL/CHOLESTEROL ESTERS RATIO, CALCIUM × CHOLESTEROL, CALCIUM × FREE CHOLESTEROL, CALCIUM × CHOLESTEROL ESTERS—MEANS, STANDARD DEVIATIONS AND RANGES

Estimation	Observations (no.)	Mean	S.D.	Range Mean ± S.D. × 2 (P = 0·05)	Range Mean ± S.D. × 2·57 (P = 0·01)
Calcium (all results)	104	10·11 mg. %	0·707	8·7–11·5 mg. %	8·3–11·9 mg. %
Calcium (Kramer and Tisdall method)	61	10·26 mg. %	0·693	8·9–11·6 mg. %	8·5–12·0 mg. %
Calcium (Trinder method)	43	9·88 mg. %	0·699	8·5–11·3 mg. %	8·2–11·6 mg. %
Total cholesterol	104	194 mg. %	38·2	118–270 mg. %	96–292 mg. %
Free cholesterol	86	57 mg. %	18·6	20–94 mg. %	9–105 mg. %
Cholesterol esters	86	137 mg. %	33·3	70–204 mg. %	51–223 mg. %
Free cholesterol/cholesterol esters ratio	86	0·453	0·229	0–0·9	0–1·0
Calcium × total cholesterol	98	1,947	403	1,141–2,753	914–2,980
Calcium × free cholesterol	81	583	205	173–993	56–1,110
Calcium × cholesterol esters	81	1,374	348	678–2,070	481–2,267

samples of blood from adult patients. No significant difference was observed in the results obtained by the two methods.

Table 2 gives the results of the estimation of serum calcium, cholesterol, free cholesterol and cholesterol esters in 110 infants aged 1 to 15 months. In each infant these estimations were carried out on the same specimen of blood. In the first 65 infants calcium was estimated by the Kramer and Tisdall method, thereafter by the Trinder method. The Table also gives the age, weight and sex of the infants and the arithmetical products of calcium and total cholesterol, calcium and free cholesterol and calcium and cholesterol esters. These products are included in view of the suggestion that they might be of value in the diagnosis of idiopathic hypercalcaemia of infancy (Forfar, Balf, Maxwell and Tompsett, 1956).

There is no significant sex difference between serum calcium, total cholesterol, free cholesterol and cholesterol esters levels.

Table 3 gives means, standard deviations and ranges for calcium, total cholesterol, free cholesterol, cholesterol esters, free cholesterol/cholesterol esters ratio, calcium × cholesterol, calcium × free cholesterol and calcium × cholesterol esters.

TABLE 4
CORRELATIONS

Correlation	Observations (no.)	Coefficient of Correlations (r)	P
Age: calcium	104	+0·023	0·81
Age: cholesterol	104	+0·116	0·075
Age: free cholesterol . .	86	+0·181	0·095
Age: cholesterol esters . .	86	+0·178	0·10
Age: free cholesterol/ cholesterol esters ratio	86	−0·021	0·85
Calcium: cholesterol . .	98	+0·081	0·42
Calcium: free cholesterol . .	81	+0·199	0·075
Calcium: cholesterol esters	81	+0·044	0·69
Calcium: free cholesterol/ cholesterol esters ratio	86	−0·082	0·45
Free cholesterol: cholesterol esters	86	−0·126	0·245

In Table 4 correlations have been calculated between age, calcium and the various cholesterol fractions.

Discussion

Serum calcium levels quoted by different authors show some variation according to the method used. There is general agreement that the level tends to be higher in infancy than in later life. Jaffe and Bodansky (1943) give a range for infancy (excluding the first week of life) of 10·5–12·0 mg./100 ml. By the two methods we used we found a somewhat wider range but a similar upper limit of normal.

Although there was no significant difference in the results obtained by the Kramer and Tisdall and the Trinder methods when both were carried out on random samples of adult blood it will be observed (Table 3) that at the idiopathic hypercalcaemia age period the 61 results obtained by the Kramer and Tisdall method gave a slightly higher average result (10·3 mg./100 ml.) than the 43 results obtained by the Trinder method (9·9 mg./100 ml.). The difference is significant (P=0·01).

Serum cholesterol levels in the first year of life have been estimated by Hodges, Sperry and Andersen (1943) and by Rafstedt (1955). The former found a mean level of 200 mg./100 ml. for the age period 2–6 months and 207 mg./100 ml. for the period 7–12 months. Their results were thus similar to ours, as too was the range which they observed. Rafstedt (1955) for the period 1–12 months found a mean total cholesterol level of 130 mg./100 ml. with a range of 69–173 mg./100 ml. Rafstedt's results for free and combined cholesterol in infancy were also lower than ours, the mean levels being 40 mg./100 ml. (range 27–66 mg./100 ml.) for free cholesterol and 90 mg./100 ml. (range 51–132 mg./100 ml.) for cholesterol esters. He found the mean free cholesterol/cholesterol ester ratio between 1–12 months to be 0·45, a figure almost identical with ours. His range was narrower (0·31–0·77) but also revealed the considerable variation in the ratio which we found.

As regards the correlations shown in Table 4 it will be observed that none is significant. The probability value of three of these correlations is less than 0·1, however, i.e. age: cholesterol, age: free cholesterol and calcium: free cholesterol. It is possible that with a larger number of estimations these correlations might have become significant. Positive correlation between age and cholesterol would be in keeping with the findings of György (1926) and Rafstedt (1955) (who in childhood observed a rise in total serum cholesterol with increasing age) but not with those of Hodges *et al.* (1943). So far as we are aware it has never been suggested that there might normally be a correlation between serum calcium and serum free cholesterol levels at this age.

Summary

A group of 110 infants aged 1–15 months has been examined.

Estimations of the serum calcium level (using two different methods) showed a range of 8·5–12·0 mg./100 ml. A difference was observed in the mean results obtained by the two methods.

Total serum cholesterol, free cholesterol and cholesterol esters were estimated and mean levels and ranges obtained.

Free cholesterol/cholesterol esters ratios, calcium × total cholesterol, calcium × free cholesterol and calcium × cholesterol esters products, and correlations between age and the cholesterol fractions, calcium and the cholesterol fractions and between the cholesterol fractions themselves have been calculated.

Part II. Serum Calcium and Cholesterol Levels in Idiopathic Hypercalcaemia of Infancy

Idiopathic hypercalcaemia of infancy presents the paediatrician with a particular problem in management and therapy. To him as well as to the biochemist, to those interested in calcium and cholesterol metabolism and to the nutritionist, the disease has even wider implications not least in its possible relationship to vitamin D activity and the light which it may shed on the ill-understood metabolism of this vitamin. As the incidence of idiopathic hypercalcaemia appears to be waning, opportunities for studying the disturbed biochemical relationships which occur may be diminishing.

It is generally accepted, and implied in the title, that the serum calcium level is raised in idiopathic hypercalcaemia. A raised blood cholesterol level

TABLE 1

RESULTS OF SERUM CALCIUM AND CHOLESTEROL ESTIMATIONS CARRIED OUT ON 19 INFANTS IN THE NATURAL STATE OF IDIOPATHIC HYPERCALCAEMIA

Case	Calcium (mg.%)	Chol. (mg.%)	Free Chol. (mg.%)	Chol. Esters (mg.%)	Free Chol./Chol. Ester
1	15·6	281	—	—	—
	10·8	217	—	—	—
	10·4	167	—	—	—
2	12·2	306	—	—	—
	11·4	184	106	78	1·36
	11·9	186	—	—	—
	10·4	197	—	—	—
	11·4	204	52	152	·342
3	11·2	265	—	—	—
	10·0	194	—	—	—
	10·3	198	52	146	·357
4	16·2	243	—	—	—
	15·5	238	141	97	1·454
	12·3	145	—	—	—
	12·5	202	84	118	·712
	14·1	262	127	135	·942
	14·6	256	—	—	—
	13·3	237	—	—	—
	10·2	229	100	129	·776
5	12·1	249	—	—	—
	13·5	213	123	90	1·367
	13·6	158	—	—	—
	10·8	179	75	104	·722
	11·0	196	50	146	·343
	10·6	155	38	117	·325
6	14·8	216	152	64	2·375
	14·0	206	112	94	1·192
	12·9	175	102	73	1·399
	10·7	161	39	122	·320
7	12·5	217	100	117	·855
	11·9	133	37	96	·386
	10·8	126	29	97	·299
	10·6	183	46	137	·336
	13·6	165	41	124	·331
	11·0	230	46	184	·250
	11·0	168	52	116	·449
9	11·0	251	124	127	·997
	11·7	316	126	190	·664
	12·0	370	135	235	·575
	10·7	320	102	218	·468
	10·2	292	28	264	·106
	10·7	229	75	154	·487
10	11·8	267	—	—	—
11	13·0	245	91	154	·591
	11·8	179	67	112	·599
	10·8	188	61	127	·481
	10·4	217	56	161	·348
	12·6	254	100	154	·650
	9·5	198	75	123	·610
12	12·8	229	60	169	·355
	11·1	229	58	171	·339
	10·7	176	63	113	·557
	10·2	225	54	171	·316
	11·9	238	50	188	·266
	12·9	233	104	129	·807
13	12·0	320	130	190	·684
14	12·2	250	54	196	·276
	10·6	192	58	134	·433
	14·1	200	52	148	·352
	12·8	292	188	104	1·810
	11·0	158	42	116	·362
15	13·4	210	63	147	·428
16	13·8	307	—	—	—
	17·5	270	—	—	—
	9·9	160	60	100	·666
	10·3	130	—	—	—
17	12·7	197	59	138	·429
	10·9	116	36	80	·450
	15·2	181	45	136	·331
	12·4	242	71	171	·415
	12·0	200	50	150	·333
18	12·2	233	—	—	—
	11·4	202	55	147	·375
	10·4	221	113	108	1·046
19	15·3	285	85	200	·425
	15·1	257	83	174	·477
20	11·8	250	73	177	·413
	9·6	240	55	185	·298
Mean	12·08	219·4	76·4	140·6	·612
Normal mean	10·1	194	57	137	·453

has also been a frequent finding (Lowe, Henderson, Park and McGreal, 1954; Creery and Neill, 1954; Dawson, Craig and Perera, 1954; Macdonald and Stapleton, 1955; Forfar *et al.*, 1956).

We have studied the relationship between calcium and cholesterol in the blood in 20 infants with idiopathic hypercalcaemia, and in addition have sought to establish certain diagnostic criteria based on calcium and cholesterol levels.

Serum Calcium, Serum Cholesterol and Serum Cholesterol Fractions

Forms of treatment such as a low calcium diet and steroid therapy can significantly lower the serum calcium level in idiopathic hypercalcaemia and may have other biochemical effects. In studying the biochemical relations pertaining in the 'natural' state of the disease therefore it is necessary to exclude estimations made under any treatment which might modify these.

Table 1 gives the results in 19 cases, of serum calcium, serum cholesterol, serum free cholesterol and serum cholesterol esters estimations carried out (on the same specimen of blood) in the 'natural' state of the disease. Any treatment given had been discontinued for at least a week before the specimens were taken.

There is, as expected, a significant rise in the mean serum calcium level and in addition a significant rise in the total cholesterol and free cholesterol levels. The cholesterol esters level, on the other hand, shows no change from normal. The rise in total cholesterol is thus determined by the rise in its free cholesterol component.

The correlation co-efficients between calcium and cholesterol fractions have been calculated as shown in Table 2. There is a significant positive correlation

TABLE 2

CORRELATIONS

Correlation	Observations (no.)	Coefficient of Correlation (r)	P
Calcium: total cholesterol ..	75	+·280	0·015
Calcium: free cholesterol ..	57	+·361	>0·01
Calcium: cholesterol esters..	57	−·118	0·37
Free cholesterol: cholesterol esters	57	−·150	0·26
Calcium: free cholesterol/ cholesterol esters ratio..	57	+·405	>0·01

between calcium and both total cholesterol and free cholesterol levels; also between calcium and the free cholesterol/cholesterol esters ratio. There is no significant correlation between calcium and cholesterol esters or between free cholesterol and cholesterol esters. The critical correlation therefore is that between calcium and free cholesterol.

Calcium and Cholesterol Levels in Diagnosis

The diagnosis of idiopathic hypercalcaemia of infancy is based on clinical, radiological and especially biochemical findings. By the methods employed in our laboratory the upper limits during the age period 1–15 months for various biochemical estimations are as follows (Part I, Table 3):

Estimation	Mean+S.D.×2·57	Mean+S.D.×2
Serum calcium	12·0 mg.%	(11·6) mg.%
Serum cholesterol	292 mg.%	(270) mg.%
Serum free cholesterol ..	105 mg.%	(94) mg.%
Serum cholesterol esters ..	223 mg.%	(204) mg.%
Calcium × cholesterol ..	2,980	(2,753)
Calcium × free cholesterol ..	1,110	(993)

It has been suggested previously (Forfar *et al.*, 1956) that as both serum calcium and cholesterol tend to be raised in idiopathic hypercalcaemia the use of their product might be of value in diagnosis where neither is in itself raised above the upper limit of normal. In addition to the basic estimations of calcium and cholesterol we have used these products as diagnostic criteria as shown in Table 3.

This Table presents the results of simultaneous (on the same specimen of blood) serum calcium, cholesterol and free cholesterol estimations carried out on 131 blood samples at all stages of the disease. It also gives the highest serum calcium level obtained at any time.

In 15 of the 20 cases there would be no doubt on biochemical grounds of the diagnosis of idiopathic hypercalcaemia. Stapleton and Evans (1955) have put the diagnostic level at above 12·5 mg./100 ml. These fifteen cases show serum calcium levels greater than this. Among them it will be observed that in Cases 2 and 5 the serum free cholesterol level and the calcium × free cholesterol product were both raised at a time when the serum calcium level was within normal limits, and in Case 19 that total cholesterol and the calcium × cholesterol product on one occasion, and the free cholesterol and calcium × free cholesterol product on another were raised in the presence of a normal calcium level. Thus the cholesterol and free cholesterol levels and/or their products with calcium may be diagnostic when the serum calcium level itself is not significantly raised.

Turning to the other five cases it will be observed that in two (Cases 10 and 18) the highest serum calcium level was greater than 12·0 mg./100 ml., i.e. above our upper limit of normal, and that in addition the calcium × cholesterol product in Case 10 and the free cholesterol level and calcium × free cholesterol product in Case 18 were above normal.

In two of the remaining three cases the highest serum calcium level reached was 12·0 mg./100 ml. In both of these (Cases 9 and 13) the serum cholesterol level, serum free cholesterol, calcium × cholesterol product and calcium × free cholesterol product were raised.

The remaining case is Case 3 whose highest serum calcium level was 11·2 mg./100 ml. His calcium × cholesterol product reached 2,968, practically the upper limit of normal. He suffered from an illness which, although comparatively short-lived and mild, was clinically suggestive of idiopathic hypercalcaemia and he was the identical twin of Case 2, who undoubtedly suffered from this disease. His serum calcium fell as he recovered.

Serum cholesterol, serum free cholesterol and their products with serum calcium are thus of value in the diagnosis of idiopathic hypercalcaemia where the calcium level itself does not establish diagnosis or on occasion when the serum calcium level has been lowered by treatment (as indicated in Table 3). With a low calcium diet, for instance, the serum calcium level may fall quickly but cholesterol and free cholesterol and their products with calcium may still remain elevated. A raised total or free cholesterol level is also confirmatory of a raised calcium level in this disease.

Of the 131 blood samples taken, 59 were positive in respect of one or more of the five biochemical criteria, yet in 14 (24%) of these positive samples the serum calcium level was not above normal. In four, total cholesterol, free cholesterol, calcium × cholesterol and calcium × free cholesterol conferred positivity; in one, free cholesterol, calcium × cholesterol and calcium × free cholesterol; in two,

TABLE 3

CALCIUM, CHOLESTEROL AND FREE CHOLESTEROL ESTIMATIONS FOR 131 BLOOD SAMPLES FROM 20 CASES OF IDIOPATHIC HYPERCALCAEMIA

Case (Highest Serum Calcium (mg. %))	Serum Calcium (mg. %)	Serum Cholesterol (mg. %)	Serum Free Cholesterol (mg. %)	Calcium × Cholesterol	Calcium × Free Cholesterol	Treatment
1	**15·6**	281	—	**4,384**	—	
(16·4)	10·8	217	—	2,344	—	
	10·4	167	—	1,736	—	
2	**12·2**	**306**	—	**3,732**	—	
(15·6)	11·4	184	**106**	2,095	**1,207**	
	11·9	186	—	2,212	—	
	11·5	156	—	1,793	—	
	15·1	206	—	**3,110**	—	
	10·4	197	—	2,049	—	
	11·4	204	52	2,324	593	
3	11·2	265	—	**2,968**	—	
(11·2)	10·0	194	—	1,940	—	
	10·3	198	52	2,039	534	
4	**16·2**	243	—	**3,936**	—	
(16·2)	15·5	238	**141**	**3,687**	**2,185**	
	12·3	145	—	1,783	—	
	13·4	226	—	**3,026**	—	
	15·5	261	—	**4.047**	—	
	12·5	202	84	2,526	1,050	
	14·1	262	**127**	**3,692**	**1,791**	
	14·6	256	—	**3,735**	—	
	10·7	197	—	2,107	—	Cort.
	13·3	237	—	**3,151**	—	
	10·2	229	100	2,334	1,020	
5	**12·1**	249	—	**3,013**	—	
(13·6)	**13·5**	213	**123**	2,876	**1,661**	
	13·6	158	—	2,148	—	
	9·8	155	71	1,520	696	Pred.
	10·8	179	75	1,932	810	LCD
	11·4	206	**141**	2,346	**1,608**	LCD
	9·8	260	**136**	2,546	**1,333**	LCD
	11·0	196	50	2,156	550	
	10·6	155	38	1,643	404	
6	**14·8**	216	**152**	**3,198**	**2,250**	
(14·8)	**14·0**	206	**112**	2,881	**1,567**	
	12·9	175	102	2,257	**1,315**	
	12·2	171	85	2,085	1,037	
	10·0	196	54	1,960	540	LCD
	9·7	135	45	1,310	437	LCD+Pred.
	9·8	150	50	1,470	490	LCD
	10·5	158	50	1,660	525	
	9·7	162	46	1,570	446	LCD+Pred.
	10·6	166	30	1,759	318	LCD+Pred.
	10·1	240	38	2,423	384	
	10·7	161	39	1,722	417	
7	**12·5**	217	100	2,711	**1,250**	
(13·6)	11·9	133	37	1,582	440	
	10·8	126	29	1,361	313	
	10·6	192	50	2,035	530	Pred.
	10·6	183	46	1,939	487	
	13·6	165	41	2,243	557	
	11·0	230	46	2,530	506	
	11·0	168	52	1,847	572	
8	**15·1**	247	88	**3,728**	**1,328**	LCD
(17·0)	10·9	172	86	1,874	937	LCD
9	11·0	251	**124**	2,760	**1,364**	
(12·0)	11·7	**316**	**126**	**3,700**	**1,475**	
	12·0	**370**	**135**	**4,438**	**1,620**	
	10·7	**320**	102	**3,424**	1,091	
	10·2	292	28	2,975	286	LCD+Cort.
	10·4	283	58	2,941	603	LCD+Cort
	9·9	254	81	2,515	802	LCD
	10·7	229	75	2,448	802	
	11·4	286	**142**	**3,259**	**1,618**	LCD
	9·6	**342**	**131**	**3,282**	**1,257**	LCD
	10·3	272	73	2,832	741	LCD
10	11·8	267	—	**3,150**	—	
(12·2)	10·4	250	60	2,600	624	LCD

(*contd.*)

TABLE 3—*contd.*

Case (Highest Serum Calcium (mg. %)	Serum Calcium (mg. %)	Serum Cholesterol (mg. %)	Serum Free Cholesterol (mg. %)	Calcium × Cholesterol	Calcium × Free Cholesterol	Treatment
11 (13·0)	**13·0**	245	91	**3,184**	**1.182**	
	11·8	179	67	2,112	791	
	10·8	188	61	2,029	659	
	10·4	217	56	2,257	582	
	12·6	254	100	**3,198**	**1,260**	
	10·0	276	83	2,760	830	LCD
	9·5	198	75	1,882	713	
12 (12·9)	**12·8**	229	60	2,928	768	
	11·1	229	58	2,540	644	
	10·7	176	63	1,882	674	
	10·2	225	54	2,295	551	
	11·9	236	50	2,832	595	
	10·4	267	38	2,777	395	
	12·9	233	104	**3,001**	**1,340**	
13 (12·0)	12·0	**320**	**130**	**3,840**	**1,560**	
	10·1	242	46	2,443	464	LCD
14 (14·1)	**12·2**	250	54	**3,050**	659	
	10·6	192	58	2,034	615	
	14·1	200	52	2,820	733	
	12·8	292	**188**	**3,738**	**2,406**	
	11·0	158	42	1,738	464	
	10·5	198	94	2,078	987	LCD
15 (13·4)	**13·4**	210	63	2,812	844	
16 (17·5)	**13·8**	**307**	—	**4,232**	—	
	17·5	270	—	**4,722**	—	
	11·4	220	—	2,507	—	LCD
	11·4	156	—	1,778	—	LCD
	11·5	146	50	1,676	575	
	15·8	160	—	2,527	—	
	16·6	163	63	2,704	1,045	
	14·9	150	50	2,234	745	LCD
	16·6	140	45	2,324	747	LCD
	12·3	156	61	1,919	750	LCD
	12·0	138	50	1,654	600	LCD
	10·2	190	55	1,936	561	LCD
	9·9	160	60	1,584	594	
	10·3	130	—	1,337	—	
17 (15·2)	**12·7**	197	59	2,501	749	
	10·9	116	36	1,263	392	
	15·2	181	45	2,748	684	
	12·4	242	71	**3,000**	880	
	12·0	200	50	2,400	600	
	10·9	174	—	1,896	—	LCD
	10·4	192	50	1,996	520	LCD
	10·3	225	96	2,317	989	LCD
	10·1	232	98	2,343	990	LCD
18 (12·2)	**12·2**	233	—	2,840	—	
	11·4	202	55	2,302	627	
	10·4	221	**113**	2,297	**1,175**	
19 (15·3)	**15·3**	285	85	**4,358**	**1,299**	
	15·1	257	83	**3,880**	**1,252**	
	12·1	178	50	**2,154**	605	LCD
	9·4	283	**158**	2,660	**1,484**	LCD
	12·0	215	50	2,580	600	LCD
	12·1	207	45	2,503	545	LCD+Pred.
	11·2	172	36	1,925	403	LCD+Pred.
	12·0	**320**	—	**3,840**	—	LCD
	10·8	234	68	2,525	734	LCD
	11·2	250	53	2,800	593	LCD
	10·0	228	65	2,280	650	LCD
	11·0	—	78	—	858	
20 (13·4)	11·8	250	73	2,950	862	
	9·6	240	55	2,302	528	

LCD=low calcium diet; Cort.=cortisone; Pred.=prednisolone

cholesterol and calcium × cholesterol; in six, free cholesterol and calcium × free cholesterol, and in one, calcium × cholesterol alone.

We have purposely set our upper limits of normal high at mean + standard deviation × 2·57 (P=0·01). We may in fact have set the limit too high. Had we used the customary upper limit of normal, mean + standard deviation × 2 (as also given above), a considerably greater number of values in Table 3 would have been diagnostic.

Discussion

One of the most fascinating aspects of idiopathic hypercalcaemia concerns aetiology and possible relationship to vitamin D administration. Many reports testify that the dosage of vitamin D has often been no greater than that considered optimal and seldom greater than the average dosage received by the vast majority of healthy infants. The dosage has been in no way comparable to that known to cause frank vitamin D poisoning. Lacking evidence of gross overdosage the concept of undue hypersensitivity to vitamin D has been put forward by Lightwood (1952) and supported by Lowe *et al.* (1954), Bonham Carter, Dent, Fowler and Harper (1955) and Morgan, Mitchell, Stowers and Thomson (1956). On the other hand, administration of increased amounts of vitamin D to infants suffering from idiopathic hypercalcaemia may not cause any worsening or significant biochemical change (Creery and Neill, 1954; Forfar *et al.*, 1956).

Vitamin D poisoning in the adult may cause hypercholesterolaemia but the scanty evidence available on vitamin D poisoning in infancy suggests that at that age period it does not do so. Fanconi and de Chastonay (1950) found that hypocholesterolaemia occurred in three infants aged 9½, 6 and 11 months who had received grossly excessive dosages of vitamin D, but hypercholesterolaemia occurred in a 4½-year-old child in similar circumstances. These authors comment particularly on this age distinction. Jelke (1946) found no hypercholesterolaemia in vitamin D poisoning in an infant.

In view of the apparently increased vitamin D-like activity in idiopathic hypercalcaemia and the fact that some cholesterol derivatives have a vitamin D-like effect (e.g. vitamin D_3 is derived from 7-dehydrocholesterol), it has been suggested that this disease may be related primarily to a disorder of cholesterol metabolism with excess production of a cholesterol derivative with a vitamin D-like effect (Forfar *et al.*, 1956). The recent work of Fellers and Schwartz (1958) has lent some support to this view. They estimated the vitamin D-like activity in two severe cases of idiopathic hypercalcaemia by bio-assay methods and found increased activity which persisted unchanged for periods up to 17 months after all exogenous vitamin D had been withdrawn. The degree of activity was greater than that found in two children receiving 100,000 units of vitamin D daily.

Whether the synthesis or storage of a provitamin can occur in the human is uncertain but it can certainly occur in animals. Glover, Glover and Morton (1952) have shown that provitamin D_3 can be found in the tissues of certain animals even when the animals are fed on a practically sterol-free diet. They concluded that the animal could synthesize provitamin D from cholesterol. In the guinea-pig infection of the liver with *Pasteurella pseudotuberculosis* was found to be associated with an increased concentration of provitamin in the intestinal mucosa, an interesting observation in view of the possible role of infection in idiopathic hypercalcaemia.

While activation of vitamin precursors, such as 7-dehydrocholesterol and ergosterol, is readily effected by irradiation, chemical activation is theoretically possible. Raoul, Le Boulch, Baron, Bazier and Guerilot-Vinet (1956) showed that cholesterol can be transformed to antirachitic compounds by a variety of natural earth, floridin. It has been suggested by Forfar (1958) that calciferol may act as a chemical activator in this disease; that apart from its own vitamin D effect calciferol may activate endogenous vitamin D precursors present in excess. A hypothesis of this sort would explain many of the features of idiopathic hypercalcaemia of infancy. Infants with an increased formation of endogenous vitamin D precursor would be those susceptible. Primarily, activation of that vitamin precursor would cause the disease. The dosage of exogenous vitamin D required to do this may not be large and dosage in excess of the activating amount will presumably merely aggravate the disease. This concept explains the comparatively small intake of vitamin D with which idiopathic hypercalcaemia may be associated and also the absence of a direct quantitative relationship between intake of vitamin D and severity of the disease. This theory could also explain the prolonged vitamin D-like activity which frequently persists in idiopathic hypercalcaemia after withdrawal of all vitamin D. As a corollary, variations in endogenous vitamin D precursor formation might explain the varying vitamin D needs in infancy to which Follis, Park and Jackson (1953) have drawn attention. Infants with low endogenous formation would be those liable to develop rickets, infants with high formation those requiring little or no exogenous vitamin D. It may be not without relevance that hypothyroid children, in whom there is also a disorder of cholesterol metabolism with a tendency to hypercholesterolaemia, are peculiarly resistant to rickets and peculiarly sensitive to vitamin D (Fanconi, 1956). If indeed idiopathic hypercalcaemia is associated with the use of the synthetic substance calciferol, as opposed to natural vitamin D, the advisability of using calciferol in place of natural vitamin may need further consideration.

It is doubtful whether idiopathic hypercalcaemia exists in two distinct types, the severe and the mild, or whether the difference is merely one of degree.

Reviewing the literature, Daeschner and Daeschner (1957) reported that the average interval between the time of onset of symptoms and diagnosis in the severe type of the disease was 13 months. In 52 reported cases of the mild type we have found that the corresponding average interval was less than six months. It seems possible that the severe type of the disease results essentially from delay in diagnosis. The use of total cholesterol and free cholesterol estimations in diagnosis in the manner outlined above may allow earlier positive recognition of the disease and the earlier institution of treatment and may allow recognition where diagnosis cannot be made on the basis of serum calcium estimations alone. Earlier diagnosis and treatment will presumably reduce the risks of mental retardation and permanent renal damage which accompany this disease. The use of the cholesterol factors may also be of some value in assessing progress during treatment.

Summary

An assessment has been made of the calcium, cholesterol, free cholesterol and cholesterol esters fractions of serum in 19 cases of idiopathic hypercalcaemia examined in the 'natural' (untreated) state of the disease.

Serum calcium, cholesterol and free cholesterol levels are significantly raised in the disease. Serum cholesterol esters level is not raised.

Calculation of correlation coefficients shows that there is a significant positive correlation between serum calcium, cholesterol and free cholesterol levels. The critical correlation is that between serum calcium and serum free cholesterol.

The results of simultaneous estimations of serum calcium, cholesterol and free cholesterol at all stages of the disease are presented. The role of the cholesterol fractions on their own and as a product with serum calcium in increasing the accuracy of diagnosis in idiopathic hypercalcaemia is indicated.

Disturbances of cholesterol metabolism are discussed in the light of the possible relationship of the condition to vitamin D, and an aetiological hypothesis is elaborated.

Part III. Blood Citrate Levels and Urinary Citrate Output in Idiopathic Hypercalcaemia of Infancy

Citrate occurs in high concentration in bone, probably 50–100 times the concentration found in other tissues (Dickens, 1941; Dixon, 1956). The general consensus of opinion is that citrate is actively involved in the metabolism of bone. Harrison (1954), for instance, considers that the serum citrate level may be related to the activity of those metabolic processes in skeleton which actively destroy bone matrix and dissolve bone salts. Armstrong and Singer (1956), on the other hand, consider that the concentration of citrate in bone may be merely adventitious, body citrate being attracted to bone in virtue of the peculiar chemical and physical character of the latter.

We have made observations on the serum citrate levels and urinary citrate output at various stages of idiopathic hypercalcaemia. In addition we have assessed the normal serum citrate level in a group of 32 unaffected infants aged 2–15 months.

Methods

The method employed for the determination of citrate in serum and urine was predominantly that of Taylor (1953). Untreated urine and trichloracetic extract of serum were used. Citrate was converted into pentabromoacetone (bromide/bromate/vanadate reagent plus sulphuric acid). After neutralization of the reaction mixture with ferrous sulphate, the pentabromoacetone was extracted with petroleum ether. A yellow colour was produced in the presence of a solution of borax and thiourea (Snell and Snell, 1953), the final estimation being made colorimetrically. Urine for citrate analysis was collected in a bottle containing dilute sulphuric acid to prevent loss of citrate.

Serum calcium was determined by the method of Trinder (1957).

Results

Serum Citrate Levels. The results of 32 serum citrate estimations carried out on controls, aged 2–15 months, are shown in Table 1. Serum calcium was estimated coincidentally with serum citrate. The mean serum citrate level was 2·4 mg./100 ml. and the range (mean ±S.D. ×2) 1·2–3·5 mg./100 ml. For the age range 2 months–2 years Harrison and Harrison (1952) found the mean serum citrate level to be 2·5 mg./100 ml. with range 2·0–3·4 mg./100 ml. There is no evidence of correlation between calcium and citrate levels (correlation coefficient = −0·04).

The results of 28 coincident estimations of serum calcium and serum citrate at various stages of the disease in 11 cases of idiopathic hypercalcaemia in the 'natural' (see Part II) state are shown in Table 2. It will be seen that the mean citrate level is not significantly different from normal. The range however is wider than normal, being (mean ± S.D. ×2) 0·6–4·8 mg./100 ml. Study of individual cases (the levels are in chronological order for individual cases) suggests that the serum citrate level is low in the acute phase of the disease and high in the recovery phase. Indeed the mean serum citrate level on the 10 occasions when the serum calcium was 11·6 mg./

TABLE 1

SERUM CALCIUM AND CITRATE LEVELS IN 32 CONTROL INFANTS AGED 2–15 MONTHS

Age (mth.)	Serum Calcium (mg. %)	Serum Citrate (mg. %)
9	9·4	2·0
5½	9·7	1·8
12	10·4	2·4
15	10·2	2·8
6	11·2	2·8
13	8·8	2·4
7	10·0	3·5
4	10·4	2·0
2	10·3	2·1
15	10·3	1·8
3	9·5	2·3
6	10·2	2·0
12	10·3	2·1
3½	10·9	2·1
15	10·1	2·0
12	10·6	2·4
9	10·7	2·6
8	9·5	1·6
9	10·7	3·0
2	10·2	2·2
7	9·6	3·4
5	10·7	2·5
2	9·4	0·8
8	8·9	3·3
13	9·6	3·4
5½	10·1	2·5
8	10·3	1·9
6	9·9	2·5
13	9·3	1·6
4	9·9	2·3
4	9·8	2·9
4	11·1	1·6
Mean	10·1	2·35

TABLE 2

SERUM CALCIUM AND CITRATE LEVELS IN IDIOPATHIC HYPERCALCAEMIA

Serum Calcium (mg. %)	Serum Citrate (mg. %)
11·4	2·5
10·3	3·1
12·0	1·8
11·6	2·4
13·5	0·7
10·8	1·8
11·0	3·3
10·6	3·7
14·8	0·25
14·0	2·8
12·9	1·3
10·1	4·7
10·7	2·9
12·0	1·9
11·9	2·3
10·8	2·1
10·6	3·5
13·6	2·4
11·0	3·0
11·0	3·0
11·4	2·6
9·6	4·4
10·3	3·4
10·6	2·7
12·4	2·5
10·4	2·4
9·6	5·4
10·0	2·5
Mean 11·4	2·7

100 ml. or above (we have taken 11·6 mg./100 ml. as this is the upper limit of normal for the method of calcium estimation we were using) was 1·8, and on the 18 occasions when the serum calcium level was below 11·6 mg./100 ml. it was 3·1 mg./100 ml.

The correlation coefficient between serum calcium and serum citrate levels for the results shown in Table 2 is $-0·732$ ($P = > 0·01$). There is thus a highly significant negative correlation between calcium and citrate levels in idiopathic hypercalcaemia.

In Fig. 1 the results of all serum citrate levels in 14 cases before, during and after treatment have been charted. Points plotted along the time abscissa have been dated from time of admission to hospital with the object of indicating the pattern of citrate level during the course of the disease. As the early cases were treated less efficiently than the later ones and as some cases were already undergoing some spontaneous improvement by the time of admission to hospital, this method of representing the course of the disease is of necessity somewhat artificial. It does again suggest, however, that the serum citrate level tends to be low in the early stages of the disease and rises with improvement. Recovery indeed seems to be associated with a rise up to or beyond the upper limit of normal with a later fall to average levels.

Urinary Citrate. Seventeen estimations of urinary citrate were made at various stages of the disease on seven patients. These are charted in Fig. 2, indicating that urinary citrate was low in the acute stage of the disease, rose with recovery and later tended to fall. We have taken the lower limit of normal to be in the region of 50 mg./24 hr.

Discussion

Much of our knowledge of citrate metabolism has been derived from animal experiments. It has been established that levels are low in rickets and that citrate will promote healing, that the administration of vitamin D to rats receiving normal or rachitogenic diets increases tissue citrate content including that of blood and that concurrent elevations of serum calcium and serum citrate levels occur under the influence of vitamin D (Armstrong and Singer, 1956). The level of calcium in the diet also appears to have some influence on the citrate content of bones, higher citrate concentrations being observed with high calcium diets as opposed to calcium-deficient diets (Steenbock and Bellin, 1953; Carlsson and Hollunger, 1954).

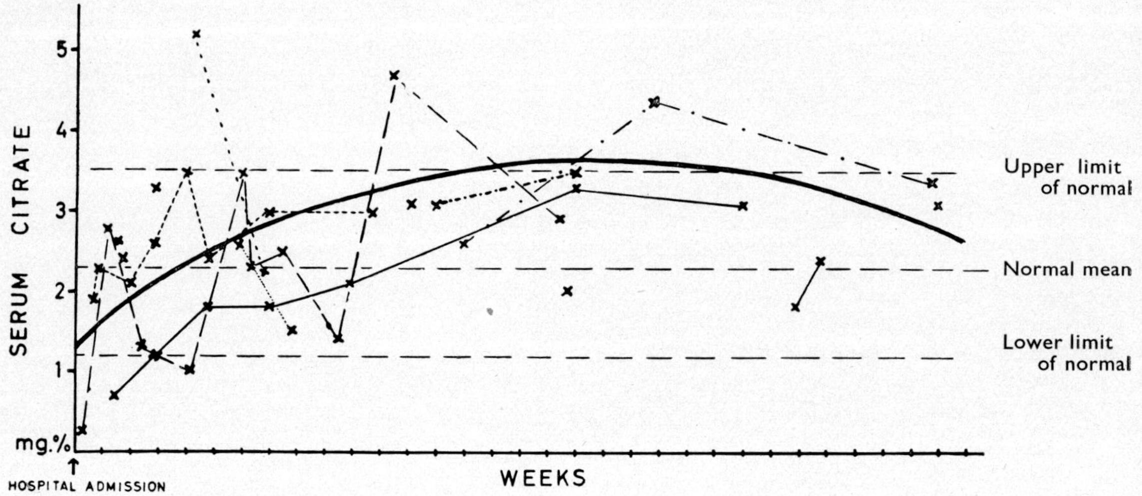

FIG. 1.—Serum citrate levels in 14 patients during the course of idiopathic hypercalcaemia.

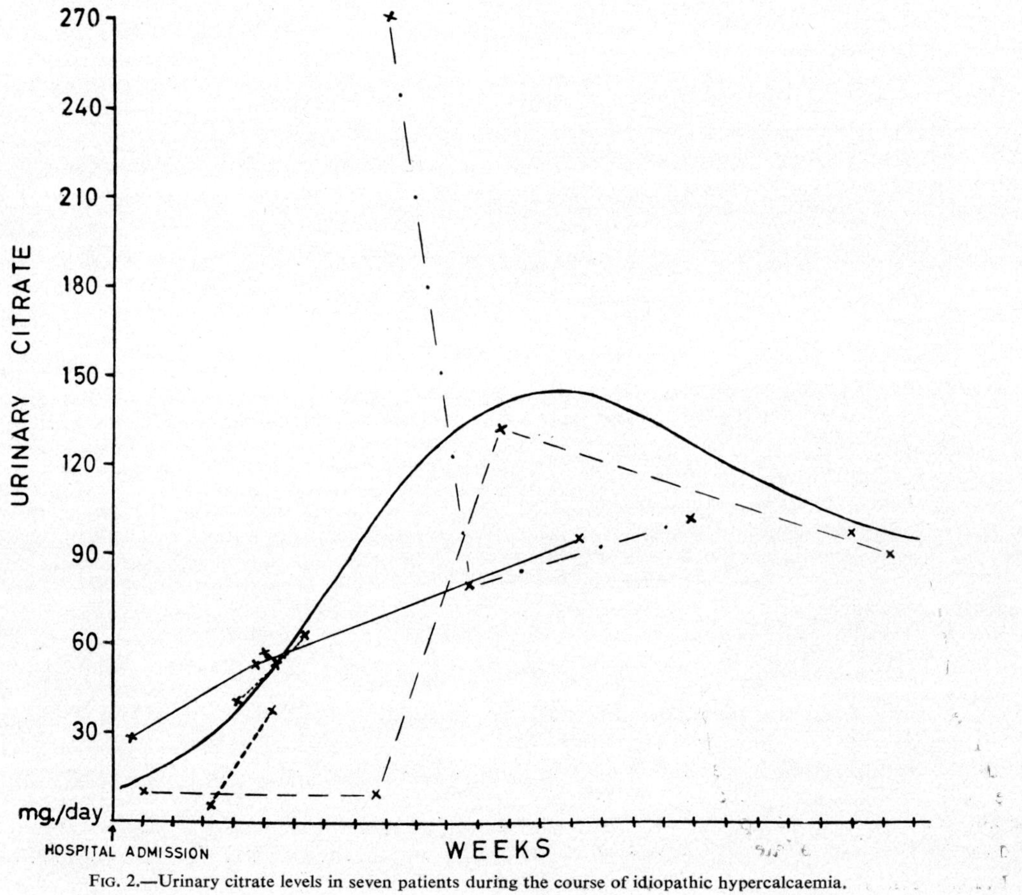

FIG. 2.—Urinary citrate levels in seven patients during the course of idiopathic hypercalcaemia.

In the human, low blood citrate levels and a low urinary output of citrate have been observed in rachitic children. The levels rise with vitamin D administration (Harrison and Harrison, 1952). In hypervitaminosis D raised serum citrate levels up to 6 mg./100 ml. have been observed (Harrison, 1954).

Our findings of lowered serum citrate levels in blood and urine in the acute phase of idiopathic hypercalcaemia with a rise on withdrawal of vitamin D and recovery from the illness, and our evidence that the serum calcium level and serum citrate level are inversely related are thus apparently the reverse of those which would be expected with increased vitamin D activity. They appear to argue against increased vitamin D activity (when there is so much other evidence that it is present) or to suggest that the vitamin D-like action operates differently in respect of citrate metabolism. One should be very cautious, however, about applying to the period of infancy findings relevant to an older age group. Idiopathic hypercalcaemia is a peculiarly age-limited disease. At the age period at which it occurs hypervitaminosis D has indeed been reported to produce lowered serum citrate levels and a lowered urinary citrate output. Winberg and Zetterström (1956) observed these changes in an infant aged 11 months who over a period of five months had received 8,000,000 units of vitamin D and whose serum calcium level had risen to 16 mg./100 ml. It may be that citrate metabolism in infancy and disorders of it conditioned by vitamin D and vitamin D-like substances show a different pattern from that seen at an older age.

Summary

Observations have been made on the normal serum citrate level in infancy (1·2–3·5 mg./100 ml.) and on the serum citrate level and urinary citrate output in idiopathic hypercalcaemia of infancy.

It is concluded that in idiopathic hypercalcaemia the serum citrate is low in the acute phase of the disease and rises up to or beyond the upper limit on recovery with a subsequent fall to average levels.

There is a statistically significant negative correlation between the serum calcium level and the serum citrate level in idiopathic hypercalcaemia.

The urinary output of citrate is low in the acute phase of the disease rising to normal levels with recovery.

We are greatly indebted to Dr. D. N. Nicholson and Dr. D. M. Douglas for allowing us access to patients under their charge and for generously making case records available to us.

References

Armstrong, W. D. and Singer, L. (1956). In *Ciba Foundation Symposium on Bone Structure and Metabolism*, pp. 103-113. Churchill, London.
Bonham Carter, R. E., Dent, C. E., Fowler, D. I. and Harper, C. M. (1955). *Arch. Dis. Childh.*, **30**, 399.
Carlsson, A. and Hollunger, G. (1954). *Acta physiol. scand.*, **31**, 317. Quoted by Nicolaysen, R. and Eeg-Larsen, N. In *Ciba Foundation Symposium on Bone Structure and Metabolism*, p. 181. Churchill, London.
Creery, R. D. G. and Neill, D. W. (1954). *Lancet*, **2**, 110
Daeschner, G. L. and Daeschner, C. W. (1957). *Pediatrics*, **19**, 362.
Dawson, I. M. P., Craig, W. S. and Perera, F. J. C. (1954). *Arch. Dis. Childh.*, **29**, 475.
Dickens, F. (1941). *Biochem. J.*, **35**, 1011.
Dixon, T. F. (1956). In *Ciba Foundation Symposium on Bone Structure and Metabolism*, p. 113. Churchill, London.
Fanconi, G. (1956). In *Ciba Foundation Symposium on Bone Structure and Metabolism*, p. 189. Churchill, London.
—— and de Chastonay, E. (1950). *Helv. paediat. Acta*, **5** Suppl. to no. 4 p. 5.
Fellers, F. X. and Schwartz, R. (1958). *A.M.A. J. Dis. Child.*, **96**, 476.
Follis, R. H., Park, E. A. and Jackson, D. (1953). *Bull. Johns Hopk. Hosp.*, **92**, 426.
Forfar, J. O. (1958). M.D. Thesis. University of St. Andrews.
——, Balf, C. L., Maxwell, G. M. and Tompsett, S. L. (1956). *Lancet*, **1**, 981.
Glover, M., Glover, J. and Morton, R. A. (1952). *Biochem. J.*, **51**, 1.
György, P. (1926). *Jb. Kinderheilk.*, **112**, 283. Quoted by Behrendt, H. (1949). *Diagnostic Tests for Infants and Children.* Interscience, New York.
Harrison, H. E. (1954). *Pediatrics*, **14**, 285.
—— and Harrison, H. C. (1952). *Yale J. Biol. Med.*, **24**, 273.
Hodges, R. G., Sperry, W. M. and Andersen, D. H. (1943). *Amer. J. Dis. Child.*, **65**, 858.
Jaffe, H. L. and Bodansky, A. (1943). *J. Mt Sinai Hosp.*, **9**, 901. Quoted by Behrendt, H. (1949). *Diagnostic Tests for Infants and Children.* Interscience, New York.
Jelke, H. (1946). *Acta med. scand.*, Suppl. 170, p. 345.
Kramer, B. and Tisdall, F. F. (1921). *J. biol. Chem.*, **47**, 475.
Lightwood, R. (1952). *Arch. Dis. Childh.*, **27**, 302.
Lowe, K. G., Henderson, J. L., Park, W. W. and McGreal, D. A. (1954). *Lancet*, **2**, 101.
Macdonald, W. B. and Stapleton, T. (1955). *Acta paediat.* (*Uppsala*), **44**, 559.
Morgan, H. G., Mitchell, R. G., Stowers, J. M. and Thomson, J. (1956). *Lancet*, **1**, 925.
Raoul, Y., Le Boulch, N., Baron, C., Bazier, R. and Guerilot-Vinet, A. (1956). *Bull. Soc. Chim. biol.* (*Paris*), **38**, 495. Quoted by Cook, R. P. (1958). *Cholesterol* Academic Press, New York.
Rafstedt, S. (1955). *Studies on Serum Lipids and Lipoproteins in Infancy and Childhood.* Lund.
Snell, F. D. and Snell, C. T. (1953). *Colorimetric Methods of Analysis*, 3rd ed., Vol. 3, p. 394. Van Nostrand, New York.
Stapleton, T. and Evans, I. W. J. (1955). *Helv. paediat. Acta*, **10**, 149.
Steenbock, H. and Bellin, S. A. (1953) *J. biol. Chem.*, **205**, 985.
Taylor, T. G. (1953). *Biochem. J.*, **54**, 48.
Tisdall, F. F. (1923). *J. biol. Chem.*, **56**, 439.
Trinder, P. Association of Clinical Biochemists, News Letter (No. 15), p. 17, Aug. 1957.
Winberg, J. and Zetterström, R. (1956). *Acta paediat.* (*Uppsala*), **45**, 96.
Zak, B., Dickenman, R. C., White, E. G., Burnett, H. and Chemey, P. J. (1955). Personal communication.
Zlatkis, A., Zak, B. and Boyle, A. J. (1953). *J. Lab. clin. Med.*, **41**, 486.

NARCOLEPSY IN A CHILD UNDER 7 YEARS OLD

BY

D. J. SALFIELD

From the Brambling House Children's Centre, Chesterfield

(RECEIVED FOR PUBLICATION MAY 19, 1959)

Narcolepsy is very rare. It begins almost always after the age of 10 years. Only two cases have been reported, as far as could be ascertained, at the age of 8 years, and this early onset was described as 'remarkable' (Kanner, 1957). It therefore appears justified to report this case.

Case Report

The patient was referred to the school medical officer at the age of 6 years as 'somewhat microcephalic' (head circumference 19 in.) 'and in need of special educational treatment'. Some months before he had been seen by an orthopaedic surgeon because of bad posture; he also had 'weak ankles and knees'. No organic disease was found. The advice that he should do postural exercises was not followed by the parents. Later the child was sent to an educational psychologist for further assessment, but he was variously assessed as having an I.Q. between 75 and 87, i.e. in the 'dull and backward' range. The I.Q. did not quite account for his poor school attainments and, in view of further reports received, my attention was drawn to him.

His mother was thin and harassed-looking, of only moderate intelligence, less than sufficiently understanding of the child's needs, and she appeared inadequate. The health visitor had reported a lack of co-operation over measures suggested to raise the child's standard of well-being. 'She is willing, but does not seem able to get there'; 'has to have all arrangements made for her'. The family is well known to the local health authority. All six children in the family have poor health records. Three of them are of the mother's first marriage. The head teacher thinks they are all equally neglected.

The psychologist's report described the father as 'oafish-looking, contributing little to the conversation. Mother did not talk freely in his presence'. Another report stated: 'There is mismanagement of money. They have sufficient income but seem to be in debt.' Another said that the father is an irresponsible man; he left the mother twice, and she expects him to do so again. They used to live in rooms. Whenever the child cried his mouth had to be pressed with a towel lest the noise should be heard. They were frequently evicted. The Assistance Board used to help when the father went off on his spring-time wanderings, and the family were left without food. The universal verdict of the reports on the boy seemed to be that 'He is shy and timid'.

The head teacher described him as well-behaved because apathetic, sometimes stubborn, occasionally found to bully younger children, having a pinched and cowed look, and being ill-nourished and insufficiently clothed. He fell asleep at school each afternoon, which was thought possibly to be related to his not being sent to bed before the parents.

The family doctor reported, apart from childish ailments, frequent colds and upper respiratory infections. He felt that the home conditions from the matrimonial and psychological points of view were very poor. 'All the children appear pinched and cowed.'

My own examination did not contribute anything new. The child looked pale and in a poor state of nutrition; he was shy, fearful, and unintelligent. His gait was clumsy. He had a marked cervical and upper thoracic kyphosis, and the musculature was of poor tone.

The slowly elicited history contained no mention of illness which could be said to resemble encephalitis. There had been no head injuries. The mother said that during the last two years the boy had been suddenly dropping off to sleep several times a day. He frequently walked about 'half-dazed' at night. No history of cataplexy, etc. was obtained. While I was talking to him and his mother on one occasion the boy sank forward in his chair, his eyes closed, his impassive face becoming completely blank. After about two to three minutes he opened his eyes, was perfectly conscious and orientated, and did not seem to suffer any after-effects. There was no visible change of colour, tonus, etc. He seemed to have been normally asleep. Narcolepsy was then diagnosed.

A neurosurgeon, whose opinion was sought to exclude organic causes for the condition, reported a negative neurological examination. The electroencephalogram was reported to 'show a very slow tracing, mainly of 4 c/s with practically no alpha rhythm, without epileptic bursts'. The impression from the electroencephalogram was of a very immature cortex. Radiographs of the skull showed no abnormality.

Long-acting dexamphetamine (Dexten), 2·5 mg. in the morning, was prescribed but, as might have been expected from the family history, the patient failed to attend again.

Discussion

The criteria for the diagnosis of narcolepsy are ill-established and the classification of the various forms the disease may take is confused. The aetiology is equally uncertain.

Narcolepsy is the irresistible onset of sleep, which is indistinguishable from normal sleep. The sleep lasts sometimes for seconds, sometimes for a few minutes, rarely for hours. Most narcoleptics are said also to have cataplexy, the attacks following a strong emotional stimulus, when all voluntary muscles become flaccid. The patient sinks down but does not undergo an alteration of consciousness. So far the authors seem to be agreed.

Sleep paralysis, hypnagogic hallucinations and vivid dreams are said to be often associated with the two conditions. Yoss and Daly (1957) found, however, that of 241 cases observed during five years only 11% had the 'complete narcoleptic tetrad'; 68% had cataplexy, 24% sleep paralysis and 30% hypnagogic hallucinations. All authors seem agreed that the le sex predominates. Early waking, waking acks, headaches and disturbances of the autonic nervous system have been observed by Heyck 955).

Often a distinction is made between symptomatic d idiopathic narcolepsy; and the psychogenicity of me cases has been postulated (Langworthy and etz, 1944), as also cure by psychotherapy. Williamson (1951) thinks that in children it is nearly always a sequel of encephalitis. Hypoglycaemia has been implicated by Delay (1942). Association between epilepsy and narcolepsy is extremely rare. Kanner (1957) states that 'in the symptomatic attacks which occur chiefly in epidemic encephalitis and further in brain tumours, epilepsy and hysteria, the cataplectic component is absent'; while Coleman (1950) says '. . . in cases of psychogenic origin narcolepsy is seldom accompanied by cataplexy', which is, presumably, his quotation from Lehrman and Weiss (1943).

As to the localization of possible lesions, Heyck (1955) states that tonus and sleep functions depend on the interlaminar areas of the thalamus, the hypothalamus and the mesencephalon. It seems likely that the central reticular formation of the brain stem, which has been shown to exert a desynchronizing (waking) effect on the cortex, could be involved.

The reported E.E.G. findings are contradictory. Most workers seem to have found no abnormality apart from the appearance of a deep sleep pattern. But epileptic-like patterns have been reported by some. Strauss, Ostow and Greenstein (1952) conclude that these 'may be easily taken for bursts of slow activity'.

Conclusion

Our patient is remarkable in regard to the early age, probably 5 years, at which the disturbance began. No organic disease was detected in his present condition or history which would account for it, unless one of his many infectious diseases was accompanied by a subclinical encephalitis.

His electroencephalogram seems consistent with normality, if moderate immaturity. He has typical frequent sleep attacks of short duration. The sleep attack in which he was observed appeared indistinguishable from normal. Although no cataplexy, sleep paralysis or hypnagogic hallucinations have been demonstrated, these do not appear essential for the diagnosis of narcolepsy. The 'half-dazed' state in which he walks about at night may well be the consequence of frightening but not recollected dreams. The psychological state of the family group is consistent with the development in the child of a psychogenic type of narcolepsy. His low intelligence and the poor co-operation of the parents makes a psychotherapeutic approach unpromising. It was not possible to assess the effect of dexamphetamine, which, as well as similar drugs, has been recommended as the only measure, apart from psychotherapy, which alleviates the condition.

Thanks are due to the various writers of reports and particularly to Mr. James Hardman, neurological surgeon to the United Sheffield Hospitals.

References

Coleman, S. M. (1950). In *Recent Progress in Psychiatry*, ed. G. W. T. H. Fleming, Vol. 2, p. 254. Churchill, London.
Delay, J. (1942). *Ann. méd.-psychol.*, **100** (**2**), 375.
Heyck, H. (1955). *Dtsch. med. Wschr.*, **80**, 1524.
Kanner, L. (1957). *Child Psychiatry*, 3rd ed. Thomas, Springfield, Illinois.
Langworthy, O. R. and Betz, B. J. (1944). *Psychosom. Med.*, **6**, 211.
Lehrman, S. R. and Weiss, E. J. (1943). *Psychiat. Quart.*, **17**, 135.
Strauss, H., Ostow, M. and Greenstein, L. (1952). *Diagnostic Electroencephalography*. Grune and Stratton, New York.
Williamson, B. (1951). *A Handbook on Diseases of Children*, 6th ed. Livingstone, Edinburgh.
Yoss, R. E. and Daly, D. D. (1957). *Proc. Mayo Clin.*, **32**, 320. Quoted from *The Year Book of Neurology, Psychiatry and Neurosurgery*, 1957-58, p. 199. The Year Book Publication, Chicago.

Addendum

Since this article was written, the boy has been admitted to a hostel for maladjusted children where he received 2·5 mg. Dexten in the morning for four months. During that time he was observed in two attacks. These have not recurred for two months now since discontinuing the drug, but he is in better physical and mental condition than before.

BOOK REVIEWS

Inborn Errors of Metabolism. By David Yi-Yung Hsia. Foreword by Sydney S. Gellis (Pp. 358; illustrated. 72s.) Chicago: The Year Book Publishers Inc.

It is fitting that a book with this title should be published to mark the fiftieth anniversary of the appearance of Archibald Garrod's classic work bearing the same name, even if the genius and magnitude of Garrod's contributions do not receive quite the recognition they merit. To-day there are many advantages in constructing a book around this central theme. In the first place, many of the conditions that all would agree should be classified as inborn errors of metabolism have had much of their underlying biochemical mechanism elucidated; we are brought close to the primary actions of genes and can perceive the chains of events which follow. In the second place, they tend to be discrete and separable genetic entities so that their genetics in turn tend to be simple and clear-cut. All this facilitates brief and didactic treatment.

As far as is possible Professor Hsia treats each condition under the headings: clinical features, heredity, pathogenesis, diagnosis and treatment, ending with a limited number of key references. Graphically he starts with an illustrative pedigree. Then the primary gene effect (as far back as it can be traced) is stated, followed by the secondary effects, which with well studied conditions may be manifold and complex.

As long as the book deals with manifest or very probable inborn errors of metabolism there is little to criticize. The presentation is succinct yet clear. It is also authoritative and up-to-date. Students, for example those studying for the Diploma in Child Health, will find this a very useful book. It is doubtful whether any other offers so much information in so small a space. The research worker wishing to refresh his memory, or read about an unfamiliar condition, will find an excellent account, which will be a good starting point for further reading.

Yet, even in this, the main part of the book, there are a few lapses, mostly in the genetic field. On page 198 it is estimated that one person in every 16–20 carries the gene for fibrocystic disease of the pancreas. How can so high a frequency of a gene lethal in the homozygote be maintained? Dr. Hsia considers two hypotheses: (1) increased reproductive fitness of the heterozygotes, (2) a high mutation rate. (He does not mention a third possibility, namely, that there may be two or more alternative genes.) He states that as there is no evidence to support the first possibility 'we must assume that the latter is the case'. This is surely wrong. So high a mutation rate is almost unthinkable, whereas there is no evidence at all which could possibly show whether or not heterozygotes enjoy a sufficient advantage in reproductive fitness. It would not have to be large, and the onus of proof rests with those who prefer so unlikely an alternative. In dealing with classical haemophilia (Haemophilia A) it is stated: 'In most instances the defect is transmitted as a sex linked recessive character.' What can this mean? No other form of genetic transmission is known or has even been suggested.

It is when the book turns to conditions which might possibly be attributed to inborn errors of metabolism that difficulties multiply. Of course no two people would agree on the line separating what is (or might be) and what is not an error of metabolism. Probably no one else would agree in detail with Dr. Hsia. As he points out, the limits could be made so wide that everything is included, for of course an apparently morp logical defect might be due, if we but knew it, to sc chemical influence during early development. difficulty is to know where to stop. To give one examı the muscular dystrophies are included. They are different from other conditions that not naturally separate chapter has to be devoted to them, and this where the disadvantages of the brief didactic approacı are especially manifest. For the genetics are not simple, and no one could deal with them, as is attempted here for the severe generalized type, for instance, in seven lines: 'Pseudohypertrophic muscular dystrophy occurs six times as frequently in males as in females. The disease can also be transmitted by affected females. Because of this, it is generally agreed that the condition is transmitted as a sex linked recessive.' These are not the criteria for recognizing sex-linkage. The author is relying on Bell's excellent monograph of 1943. But there have been several admirable and more recent surveys; those of Stevenson and Cheeseman and of Walton, for example, which modify Bell's conclusions. The affected females are due to a mixture of sex-linked and recessive cases, and the separation can now be effected with almost complete efficiency.

A final chapter of four pages is entitled 'The Future of Biochemical Genetics'. Two tables are given. The first is a list of 67 conditions said to be genetic, but for which there is little or no evidence for a biochemical cause. But it includes some conditions which are only very partially genetic, for example, harelip and cleft palate and clubfoot, and at least one which is hardly genetic at all, namely, disseminated sclerosis. The other table is baffling. It purports to give a list of 35 conditions stated to be biochemical, but which 'cannot be classified as among the hereditary diseases in the classical sense', though 'they may be genetic'. Yet the list includes the Laurence-Moon-Biedl syndrome and Milroy's disease, which are genetically determined, and, astonishingly, secretion and non-secretion of the blood group substances, and ability to taste phenylthiocarbamide, which are 100% genetic in their determination. The list also includes epilepsy and psychosis (why not skeletal disease or muscular disease?). One is almost tempted to suppose that something went wrong with the manuscript or the proofs and it is a pity that this chapter was included at all.

As stated at the outset, however, this should prove a useful book to many readers, though some caution is advisable when the author gets beyond the field of the well-studied and well-understood errors of metabolism.

Recent Advances in Cerebral Palsy. Edited by RONALD S. ILLINGWORTH. (Pp. 375; illustrated. 50s.) London: J. & A. Churchill Ltd. 1959.

Professor Illingworth has collected a team of 14 collaborators to review recent thought on cerebral palsy and, though he makes no claim to have edited a textbook on the subject, between them the authors cover an impressive amount of ground. There are three chapters on classification, pathology and diagnosis; four on the ical, psychological and intellectual handicaps of ed children; three on education and the statutory voluntary services available in this country; a chapter on therapy with drugs, physical medicine and speech apy; and finally two surgical chapters, by an orthodic and neuro-surgeon respectively. Professor gworth has chosen his team well, and it is obvious t he has briefed them carefully, so that the book ieves marked unity of purpose even though the styles y considerably from chapter to chapter. The quality high throughout; not only is a tremendous amount of formation available, but to anyone working with a ecial interest in this subject the book provides an outok of informed and intelligent sympathy which work ith these children often brings out. At the same time is free of that kind of uncritical optimism which colours much of the writing on handicapped children. It would be difficult to pick out any chapter for special comment, but Professor Illingworth's opening chapter is a good summary of the scope of the subject, the aetiology and classification, and the chapters on diagnosis, education, treatment of deafness in these children and on drug therapy are perhaps the most immediately useful.

The authors are drawn from England, Australia and America. The English and even the Australian is simple enough to understand, but some of the American is difficult for the English reader, and unfortunately good translations are unobtainable. For instance, 'Far from envisioning static, fixed mechanisms, the neurohumoral orientation views organismic mechanisms as essentially dynamic, ever in flux and, within wide limits, capable of compensatory activity such that noxious influences can be tolerated to a considerable degree without resulting in clinically manifest derangements. Above all, it considers neurohumoral circuits as expressive of relationships that obtain among component parts—relationships not apprehendable by scrutiny limited to the anatomical elements themselves'. The reviewer thinks he understands but is relieved that the author's next sentence begins: 'This rubric appears to be one of the hardest for the student to grasp.' This neo-American medical lingo is tedious reading and spoils an otherwise thoughtful, almost philosophical chapter on neurosurgery.

As usual, the binding and the paper is first-class. Some of the photographs, particularly those of abnormal brains, are helpful, and I would say this book is well worth its 50s. as a book of reference for a practising paediatrician.

Textbook of Paediatrics. 7th ed. By WALDO E. NELSON. (Pp. xxiv+1462; 428 figs. £5 15s. 6d.) Philadelphia and London: W. B. Saunders. 1959.

Griffiths-Mitchell, Mitchell-Nelson to Nelson in seven unfolding editions. A book which a quarter of a century ago set out to be an encyclopaedia of paediatrics in two volumes has now become the accepted text throughout the English-speaking world.

The present volume performs the exceptional feat of including much that is new but at the same time being somewhat shorter than its predecessor. There are new sections on: 'Prenatal Factors in Diseases of Children' by Josef Warkany and F. Clarke Fraser, on 'Diseases of Mesenchymal Tissues', by Ralph J. P. Wedgwood, on 'Behaviour Problems Associated with Organic Brain Damage' by John B. Bartram and an excellent chapter by Clement Smith and C. Davenport Cook on 'Pulmonary Ventilation in Health and Disease'.

Like the aphorism 'which says too much in trying to be too small' the excessive condensation which has enabled so much paediatric information to be distilled into such a small compass extracts its penalties. The book is an impressive compendium of facts and data but it is on the whole humourless and impersonal. One can feel the pressure of the Editor's pen erasing the anecdotes, the historical asides and the individual bigotry which make some smaller text-books memorable. Again the accepted viewpoints are well expounded but the reasoning which has led to their acceptance is frequently lacking. Amid the welter of facts there is little space for opinion and doubt. This may be admirable in a book of reference but in an undergraduate text-book it is liable to breed the student who is too pre-occupied in absorbing facts to have time to think. For this reason the seventh edition is more suited for a place in the practitioner's cupboard than on the student's desk.

In a book with no less than 81 contributors the uniform excellence of each section is remarkable. Since all the writers work in the United States there is in some sections a strong transatlantic emphasis. Certain views on dysplasia of the hip joint, or on allergy to cow's milk may be intriguing rather than acceptable in this country. Perhaps it is more surprising in a book of this magnitude that there is so much agreement with accepted British practice.

The illustrations and production are of the extremely high standard one expects in American text-books. The diagrams are easy to understand and the short selection of references at the end of each chapter provides a useful entrée to the literature of each topic. This edition will do much to maintain and enhance the reputation its predecessors have gained.

Children in Practice. By JOHN PETERSON. (Pp. vii + 227. 25s.) Cambridge University Press. 1959.

At school we could always count on a question in the English paper beginning with the words 'Explain with reference to the context'. Believing that this is a sound principle for medicine, Mr. Peterson tries to open the eyes of his students to the complex but increasingly significant social context in which health and disease arise and medicine is practised. And since many illnesses 'can only be explained by the physician in environmental terms' and since the emphasis in medical education is still on morbid anatomy and the management of organic disease, this is, in intention, a timely book. Mr. Peterson has useful things to say about the need in family practice for new categories of illness and the more sensitive use of prognosis: 'His object (the family doctor's) must be the optimum health of the whole family. He must see that the right questions are asked by members of the family at the right time . . . The fact that a boy cannot make head or tail of, say, arithmetic may be an important factor in his unacceptable conduct . . . The realization that a child has an irremedial handicap places before the family doctor the fact that both he and the parents are presented with a permanent problem'. And since the autthor is actively engaged in trying to remedy the problems of which he speaks, he knows that in dealing with contemporary disorders of personal and family life the doctor cannot remain isolated within a pretended neutrality. 'All these things have to be accomplished by dint of his own efforts' and he must achieve 'confidence in moving about among his own thoughts and feelings'.

Yet as a whole this is an unsatisfactory and disappointing book, and if it is really addressed to medical students it is too long. Mr. Peterson recognizes that the student learns chiefly through contact with patients: 'It is sick men and women and children who present themselves at the surgery', yet his human examples are few, and fail in most instances to offer convincing solutions. He could have protected himself fairly against this charge by admitting that this is the inherent limitation of social medicine at the present stage of its development. It knows that social factors are relevant, but equally that they can rarely be defined with the precision that the student has come to expect from the laboratory. We recognize broad categories of 'social class' or 'family competence' but frequently cannot isolate the particular adverse factor or factors within the complex or devise specific social therapy to correct it. The student must understand and respect this if he is to avoid asking more of social medicine than it can give. 'Changing the ways of an individual or a society is no easy thing.' Perhaps the most serious criticism of this book, and it is not Mr. Peterson's fault, is that although it is about medicine it is not written from within it. It is not enough for medical schools to send students into the east ends of their cities for a brief encounter with a sociologist or social worker and a taste of social medicine. Family doctors and physicians, epidemiologists, sociologists and social workers must work together at the centre of medical education, refining the social concepts involved in health and disease and testing their validity in family practice. Mr. Peterson recognizes this in his pertinent quotation from Dr. Vaughan of the Harvard School of Public Health: 'We have found it extremely difficult to use successfully the existing tools which the social sciences have to offer. Social scientists later, after we have worked for a year or two together, say "You have to tell us what it is you want to know and together we have to develop new concepts and tools to fit that particular problem".'

This book is a gallant failure, since rejecting the simpler role of guide to the social services it attempts an interpretation for which the subject as a whole is not ready and the author's experience is in itself inadequate. I would not recommend it to medical students. I hope it will be read critically by those younger doctors (both in medical schools and in family practice) who want to achieve greater precision in their understanding of relationship of society to medicine.

Status Thymico-Lymphaticus: A Nutritional Endoc Syndrome. By W. N. KEMP. (Pp. 48.) Obtainable from the author, 2414 Main S Vancouver, 10, B.C.

In this monograph, which in form and co resembles the polemical broadsheet of another er author forcibly poses the problem of unexplained s death in infants and children, and then procee explain these and other less sudden neonatal deat terms of a hypothetic dysfunction of the pituit thyroid-adrenal 'axis'. The underlying cause of dysfunction of the 'axis' is said to be maternal iod deficiency. Unfortunately, no evidence is provided support of the claim that maternal iodine deficien occurs.

With some apparent justification, Dr. Kemp challenge the finality of the report of the British Status Lymphaticus Committee of 1931, which firmly denied the existence of status thymicus lymphaticus as a pathological entity. Certainly, since 1931, much new knowledge has accrued; more is known, for instance, of the relation of the ductless glands to environmental stress on the one hand and to lymphoid tissue on the other.

In the historical section of Dr. Kemp's monograph we find the following quotation: 'There can be no doubt that the constitutional disturbance known as status lymphaticus is a real entity . . .' taken from 'Pathology for the Physician' by William Boyd, published as recently as 1958. This appears to be an authoritative enough pronouncement on the subject, except perhaps that the title of the work conveys a warning that there is more than one kind of pathology.

Nevertheless Dr. Kemp has reminded us that the cause of sudden death in infants not infrequently remains an unsolved problem.

INDEX TO VOLUME XXXIV

Addison's disease with hypofunction of parathyroid glands, 498
Adrenal cortex, surgery of, in children, 36
—— haemorrhage, massive, in newborn, 178
African children, tetanus in, 398
Agammaglobulinaemia associated with pneumocystis pneumonia, 338
Alimentary canal, enterogenous cysts and congenital diverticula of, 189
Amino-aciduria in liver disease, 188
Anaemia, acute haemolytic, following ingestion of para-dichlorobenzene, 74
—— and kwashiorkor, 357
——, neonatal, foetomaternal transfusion as a cause of, 471
Anderson, C., *see* Gandevia, B., and Anderson, C.
Anderson, G. S. Congenital goitre due to potassium chlorate, 189
Aneurysm, congenital, of coronary artery, 8
Aortic rings, 35
Arey, J. B., and Di George, A. Gonadal dysgenesis in infants and children, 189
Arneil, G. C. Nephrosis in the early months of life, 357
Arteriolar disease, general, sudden death in asthmatic boy on prednisone therapy, associated with, 189
Arthrogryposis multiplex congenita with lesions in nervous system, 505
Asthmatic boy on prednisone therapy, sudden death in, associated with general arteriolar disease, 189
Atresia, oesophageal, complications after operation for, 24

B

Bain, A. D., and Barrett, H. S. Congenital bowing of the long bones: report of a case, 516
Barrett, H. S., *see* Bain, A. D., *and* Barrett, H. S.
Basu, R. Perforation of the bowel in Henoch-Schönlein purpura, 342
Becker, W., *see* McKenzie, D., Hansen, J. D. L., and Becker, W.
Benson, P. F. A case of calcification of the basal ganglia with osteoporosis and other abnormalities, 120
Berg, J. M. Neurological sequelae of pertussis with particular reference to mental defect, 322
Birch, L. B., *see* Illingworth, R. S., and Birch, L. B.
Birth trauma to vertebral arteries, 436
Black, J.: Renal tubular damage in infantile gastro-enteritis, 158
Blood transfusion, extended exchange, in pre-hydropic infants, 174
—— ——, foetomaternal, as a cause of neonatal anaemia, 471
Bloxsom, A.: The electrical conductivity of electrolytes found in the sweat of patients with fibrocystic disease of the pancreas, 420
Bone lesions of urticaria pigmentosa in childhood, 205
Bones, long, congenital bowing of, 516
Book Reviews: Advances in paediatrics, Vol. 10, 1958, 186; Boudin, G., and Pepin, B.: Dégénérescence hépato-lenticulaire, 1959, 456; Brugsch, J., and Brockmann-Rohne, K.: Untersuchungen zur klinischen Problematik der progressiven Muskeldystrophie, 1958, 360; Chao, D. H.-C., *et al.*: Convulsive disorders of children, 1958, 360; Ciba Foundation Colloquia on Ageing, Vol. 4, 1958, 98; Coirhault, R., *et al.*: Le syndrome de Guillain-Barré, 1958, 360; Collis, W. R. F., *ed.*: Neonatal paediatrics, 1958, 185; Debré, R., and Doumic, A.: Le sommeil de l'enfant, 1959, 456; Dupin, H.: Étude des carences protidiques observées chez l'enfant en pays tropical, 1958, 184; Ergebnisse der Bluttransfusionsforschung, Vol. 4, 1959, 359; François, J.: L'hérédité en ophtalmologie, 1958, 279; Gairdner, D.: Recent advances in paediatrics, 2nd ed., 1958, 184; Gaisford, W., and Lightwood, R.: Paediatrics for the practitioner—Supplement, 1958, 185; Glanzmann, E.: Einführung in die Kinderheilkunde, 4th ed., 1958, 99; Hardy, J. B., and Brailey, M. E.: Tuberculosis in white and negro children, 2 vols., 1958, 183; Hsia, D. Y.-Y.: Inborn errors of metabolism, 540; Illingworth, R. S., *ed.*: Recent advances in cerebral palsy, 1959, 541; Jesserer, H.: Tetanie, 1958, 186; Kemp, W. N.: Status thymico-lymphaticus, 1959, 542; Klein, M.: La psychoanalyse des enfants, 1959, 456; Launay, C., and Duche, D. J.: L'enfant physiquement handicapé, 1958, 98; Lecuyer, R.: Le mongolisme, 1958, 279; Lelong, M., *et al.*: Le nouveau-né thérapeutique médicale, 1958, 280; Lyon, R. A., and Wallinger, E. M.: Nursing of children, 5th ed., 1959, 457; Menger, W.: Häufigkeit und Art meteorotroper Erscheinungen im Kindesalter, 1958, 97; Nelson, W. E.: Textbook of paediatrics, 7th ed., 1959, 541; Nice, C. M., Jr., *et al.*: Roentgen diagnosis of abdominal tumours in childhood, 1957, 184; Oehme, J., *et al.*: Leukämie im Kindesalter, Vol. 4, 1958, 98; Opitz, H., and Rudder, B. de, *eds.*: Pädiatrie, 1957, 99; Parmalee, A. H.: Management of the newborn, 2nd ed., 1959, 279; Patton, E. F.: Pediatric index, 1958, 97; Peiper, A., *ed.*: Krankheiten der Neugeborenen, 1958, 185; Peterson, J.: Children in practice, 1959, 542; Silverthorn, N.: Principal infectious diseases of childhood, 1958, 183; Slobody, L. B.: Survey of clinical paediatrics, 3rd ed., 1959, 457; Streng, A., *et al.*: Hearing therapy for children, 2nd ed., 1958, 99; Watson, E. H., and Lowrey, G. H.: Growth and development of children, 3rd ed., 1958, 359; Wilkes, E. T.: Family guide to teenage health, 1958, 98; Windle, W. F.: Neurological and psychological deficits of asphyxia neonatorum, 1958, 359; Winnicott, D. W.: Collected papers, 1958, 359; Wolf, H. G.: Röntgendiagnostik beim Neugeborenen und Säugling, 1959, 458
Bowel perforation in Henoch-Schönlein purpura, 342
Bower, B. D., and Jeavons, P. M.: The prognosis of infantile spasms, 357
Bowing of long bones, congenital, 516
Brain atrophy in microcephalic cousins, 325
——, calcification of basal ganglia with osteoporosis and other abnormalities, 120
——, defect in Chinese children, 231
Brandon, M. G. W., Kirman, B. H., and Williams, C. E.: Microcephaly in one of monozygous twins, 56
British Association of Paediatric Surgeons, 5th annual meeting, 35
—— Paediatric Association, 30th annual general meeting, proceedings, 354

Bronchiectasis in children, multiple clinical and pathological aspects of, 192
Bronchodilator aerosol, effect of, on ventilatory capacity in fibrocystic disease of pancreas, 511
BROWN, N. J.: Neonatal hepatitis in twins, 187
BUCHANAN, M. C.: Sequestration of the lung, 137

C

Calcium-phosphorus metabolism, the 'Krebs cycle' and steroid metabolism, relationship between, 371
Calomel, effect of, on plasma epinephrine in rat and the relationship to mechanisms in Pink disease, 501
CAMPBELL, S., and MACAFEE, D. A. J.: A case of idiopathic pulmonary haemosiderosis with myocarditis, 218
Cardiovascular problems after birth, 281
CARRÉ, I. J.: The natural history of the partial thoracic stomach (hiatus hernia) in children, 344
Cerebral atrophy in microcephalic cousins, 325
—— defect in Chinese children, 231
—— palsy and mental retardation, congenital anomalies associated with, 228
Ceylon, incidence of rheumatic fever in, 247
CHEEK, D. B., and WU, F.: The effect of calomel on plasma epinephrine in the rat and the relationship to mechanisms in Pink disease, 501
Chest, funnel, effect on cardiac function, 5
CHITRE, R. G., *see* KULKARNI, B. S., *et al.*
Circulation changes after birth, 282
CLAYE, A. M., and CRAIG, W. S.: Pregnancy complicated by diabetes mellitus, 312
Coeliac diet, oats in, 51
Colitis, chronic ulcerative, in childhood, 257
CORLETT, K., *see* LIU, M. C., and CORLETT, K.
Coronary artery, congenital aneurysm of, 8
CRAIG, W. S., *see* CLAYE, A. M., and CRAIG, W. S.
CREVELD, S. VAN: Glycogen disease, 298
CUNNINGHAM, A. A.: Physiological jaundice, 262
Cysts, enterogenous, of alimentary canal, 189

D

DANCASTER, C. P., and JACKSON, W. P. U.: Familial vitamin D-resistant rickets, 383
DAWES, G. S.: Some respiratory and cardiovascular problems after birth, 281
DE SILVA, S.: Incidence of rheumatic fever in Ceylon, 247
Diabetes mellitus, pregnancy complicated by, 312
Diabetes, renal gluco-phospho-amino acid, with renal rickets, 376
Diabetic mother, baby of, 76, 358
DI GEORGE, A., *see* AREY, J. B., and DI GEORGE, A.
DICKSON, W., and WOODCOCK, R. C.: Visceral larva migrans, 63
Diplegic children, fertility of mothers of, and fate of their conceptions, 357
Diverticula, congenital, of alimentary canal, 189
DOUGLAS, D. M.: Spontaneous hyper-insulinism due to benign hyperplasia of islet cells, 171
DRILLIEN, C. M.: A longitudinal study of the growth and development of prematurely and maturely born children, Part III. Mental development, 37; Part IV. Morbidity, 210; Part V. Patterns of maternal care, 487
Ductus arteriosus, patent, surgical treatment during first year of life, 358
DUDGEON, J. A.: Virus aspects of hepatic disease in infancy, 188
DUTTON, G.: The physical development of mongols, 46
——: The size of mental defective boys, 331

E

EDWARDS, F. R.: Aortic rings, 35
Electrolytes found in sweat of patients with fibrocystic disease of pancreas, electrical conductivity of, 420
Encephalitis, varicella, 318
Epinephrine, plasma, effect of calomel on, in rat, and relationship to mechanisms in Pink disease, 501

F

FARQUHAR, J. W.: The child of the diabetic woman, 76
Foetus, female, masculinization of, with oestrogenic effect, 485
FORSHALL, W., *see* FORFAR, J. O., TOMPSETT, S. L., and FORSHALL, W.
FORSYTHE, W. I., MCKEOWN, E. F., and NEILL, D. W.: Three cases of Niemann Pick's disease in children, 406
FOWLER, M.: A case of arthrogryposis multiplex congenita with lesions in nervous system, 505
FRANCE, N. E.: Lung changes in cystic fibrosis of the pancreas, 188
FYFE, W. M.: Treatment of tuberculous meningitis, 334

G

Galactosaemia, congenital, treatment of, 307
GANDEVIA, B., and ANDERSON, C.: The effect of a bronchodilator aerosol on ventilatory capacity in fibrocystic disease of the pancreas, 511
Ganglia, basal, calcification of, with osteoporosis and other abnormalities, 120
GANS, B.: The pupillary membrane in premature infants, 292
Gastro-enteritis, infantile, renal tubular damage in, 158
GEARTY, G.: A review of 25 cases of patent ductus arteriosus diagnosed and treated surgically during the first year of life, 358
GELLMAN, V.: Congenital hydrocephalus in monovular twins, 274
GIBBS, I. E., *see* OPPÉ, T. E., and GIBBS, I. E.
Giggling, micturition induced by, 358
Glycogen disease, 298
Glycosuria, diagnostic importance of, in lead poisoning in childhood, 70
Goitre, congenital, due to potassium chlorate, 189
Gonads, dysgenesis of, in infants and children, 189
GOODLIN, R., *see* KRIVIT, W., *et al.*
GORDON, R. R., *see* O'NEILL, E. M., and GORDON, R. R.
GRIEVE, J.: Subhyoid median ectopic thyroid, 18
GROB, M., and KOLB, E.: Congenital aneurysm of the coronary artery, 8

H

HAAS, L., *see* ROXBURGH, R. C., and HAAS, L.
Haemosiderosis, pulmonary, idiopathic, with myocarditis, 218
HALLOWELL, M.: Acute haemolytic anaemia following ingestion of para-dichlorobenzene, 74
HANSEN, J. D. L., *see* MCKENZIE, D., HANSEN, J. D. L., and BECKER, W.
HART-MERCER, J.: Sudden death in an asthmatic boy on prednisone therapy, 189
HEADY, J. A., *see* MORRISON, S. L., HEADY, J. A., and MORRIS, J. N.
Heart block, congenital, 223
—— defects, congenital, in mongolism, 410
—— disease, congenital, surgical treatment of, analysis of results of, 358
—— function, effect of funnel chest on, 5
——, systolic murmurs in children, 131

Henoch-Schönlein purpura, perforation of bowel in, 342
Hepatic duct, rupture of, in newborn infant, 277
Hepatitis, neonatal, in twins, 187
HEPPLESTON, J. D., PEARCE, K. M., and YATES, P. O.: Varicella encephalitis, 318
Hernia, hiatus, in children, natural history of, 344
——, inguinal, incidence of, in Newcastle children, 482
Herpes simplex virus infection, dissemination in association with malnutrition, 250
HEYMANN, G., *see* MAINZER, W., PINCOVICI, R., and HEYMANN, G.
HILL, E. E., and WILLIAMS, J. A.: Massive adrenal haemorrhage in the newborn, 178
Hip, dislocation, congenital paralytic, 36
HOWARD, R.: Funnel chest: its effect on cardiac function, 5
HURWITT, E. S.: The surgical importance of a persistent left superior vena cava, 1
Hydranencephaly and allied disorders, 231
Hydrocephalus, congenital, in monovular twins, 274
5-Hydroxyindole metabolism, decreased, and mental defect, relationship between, in phenylketonuria, 422
Hypercalcaemia, idiopathic, of infancy, biochemical studies, 525
Hyperinsulinism, spontaneous, due to benign hyperplasia of islet cells, 171
Hyperparathyroidism and steatorrhoea, syndrome of, 302
Hypoglycaemia, idiopathic infantile, 166

I

Ileum, terminal, duplication of, intestinal obstruction in case of, 480
ILLINGWORTH, R. S.: Congenital anomalies associated with cerebral palsy and mental retardation, 228
——, and BIRCH, L. B.: The diagnosis of mental retardation in infancy, 269
Indian newborn infants, electrophoretic studies of serum protein patterns in, 392
Infants, newborn, anaemia in, foetomaternal transfusion as a cause of, 471
——, ——, hepatitis in twin, 187
——, ——, Indian, electrophoretic studies of serum protein patterns in, 392
——, ——, liver disease of, serum lipoprotein electrophoresis patterns in, 187
——, ——, —— function tests in, 187
——, ——, maintenance of stability in, 1. Chemical exchange, 361; 2. Thermal balance, 459
——, ——, massive adrenal haemorrhage in, 178
——, ——, pre-hydropic, extended exchange transfusion in, 174
——, ——, problems of, 35
——, ——, respiratory and cardiovascular problems in, 281
——, ——, rupture of hepatic duct in, 277
——, ——, —— of liver in, 30
——, premature, maternal care of, in Scotland, 487
——, ——, mental development of, 37
——, ——, morbidity of, 210
——, ——, pupillary membrane in, 292
——, ——, sulphobromophthalein excretion in, 125
INGRAM, T. T. S.: A description and classification of the common disorders of speech in children, 444
——: The fertility of mothers of diplegic children and the fate of their conceptions, 357
Intestinal obstruction, acute, due to mesenteric lymphangioma, 442
—— ——, in case of duplication of terminal ileum, 480
Islet cells, benign hyperplasia of, spontaneous hyperinsulinism due to, 171
Isoniazid, acute pellagra in child under treatment with, 68
—— in treatment of tuberculous peripheral lymphadenitis, 36

J

JACKSON, W. P. U., *see* DANCASTER, C. P., and JACKSON, W. P. U.
Jaundice, physiological, 262
JEAVONS, P. M., *see* BOWER, B. D., and JEAVONS, P. M.
JOLLEYS, A.: The value of treatment with I.N.H. and P.A.S. in tuberculous peripheral lymphadenitis, 36
JONES, N. L., and LEAK, D.: The treatment of congenital galactosaemia, 307

K

KATZUNI, E., and SANDBANK, U.: Oxalosis, 60
Kidneys, calcinosis in infants, 115
——, nephrosis, comparison of different forms of therapy in, 357
——, —— in early months of life, 357
——, tubular damage in infantile gastro-enteritis, 158
KING, R. C., LINDNER, A. E., and POLLARD, H. M.: Chronic ulcerative colitis in childhood, 257
KINSBOURNE, M., and WOOLF, L. I.: Idiopathic infantile hypoglycaemia, 166
KIRMAN, B. H., *see* BRANDON, M. G. W., KIRMAN, B. H., and WILLIAMS, C. E.
KOLB, E., *see* GROB, M., and KOLB, E.
KNOX, G.: The incidence of inguinal hernia in Newcastle children, 482
'Krebs cycle', calcium-phosphorus metabolism and steroid metabolism, relationship between, 371
KRIVIT, W., *et al.*: Foetomaternal transfusion as a cause of neonatal anaemia, 471
KULKARNI, B. S., *et al.*: Electrophoretic studies of serum protein patterns in newborn Indian infants, 392
Kwashiorkor and anaemia, 357

L

LANZKOWSKY, P.: Investigation into the aetiology and treatment of pica, 140
Larva migrans, visceral, 63
LAURENCE, K. M.: The natural history of spina bifida, 36
Lead poisoning in childhood, diagnostic importance of glycosuria in, 70
LEAK, D., *see* JONES, N. L., and LEAK, D.
LEES, M. H., and STROUD, C. E.: Bone lesions of urticaria pigmentosa in childhood, 205
Leonard Parsons Lectures, Birmingham, 1959, 361, 459
LIENKE, R., *see* KRIVIT, W., *et al.*
LINDNER, A. E., *see* KING, R. C., LINDNER, A. E., and POLLARD, H. M.
Lipoprotein, serum, electrophoresis patterns in neonatal liver disease, 187
LIU, M. C., and CORLETT, K.: A study of congenital heart defects in mongolism, 410
Liver disease, amino-aciduria in, 188
—— —— in infancy, viral aspects of, 188
—— ——, neonatal, serum lipoprotein electrophoresis patterns in, 187
—— function tests in newborn, 187
——, rupture of, in newborn, 30
Lung changes in cystic fibrosis of pancreas, 188
—— hernia secondary to congenital absence of ribs, 94
——, honeycomb, with pericholangitis, 426
——, sequestration of, 137
Lymphadenitis, tuberculous peripheral, value of I.N.H. and P.A.S., in treatment of, 36

Lymphangioma, mesenteric, acute intestinal obstruction due to, 442
Lymphoedema, primary, 35

M

MACAFEE, C. A. J., *see* CAMPBELL, S., and MACAFEE, C. A. J.
MCCANCE, R. A. The maintenance of stability in the newly born. 1. Chemical exchange, 361; 2. Thermal balance, 459
MACDONALD, A. M., *see* SHANKS, R. A., and MACDONALD, A. M.
MAC KEITH, R. C.: Micturition induced by giggling, 358
MCKENZIE, D., HANSEN, J. D. L., and BECKER, W.: Herpes simplex virus infection: dissemination in association with malnutrition, 250
MCKEOWN, E. F., *see* FORSYTHE, W. I., MCKEOWN, E. F., and NEILL, D. W.
MAINZER, W., PINCOVICI, R., and HEYMANN, G.: Systolic murmurs in children, 131
Malnutrition, dissemination of herpes simplex virus infection in association with, 250
Masculinization of female foetus with oestrogenic effect, 485
Maternal care of prematurely and maturely born children in Scotland, 487
Measles, pre-eruptive illness of, 149
Meningitis, tuberculous, treatment of, 334
Mental defect and decreased 5-hydroxyindole metabolism, relationship between, in phenylketonuria, 422
—— defective boys, size of, 331
—— development of prematurely and maturely born children, 37
—— retardation, congenital anomalies associated with, 228
—— —— in infancy, diagnosis of, 269
MERCER, J. H-., *see* HART-MERCER, J.
Mesenteric lymphangioma, acute intestinal obstruction due to, 442
Microcephalic cousins, cerebral atrophy in, 325
Microcephaly in one of monozygous twins, 56
Micturition induced by giggling, 358
Mongolism, congenital heart disease in, 410
Mongols, physical development of, 46
Morbidity of prematurely and maturely born children, 210
MORRIS, J. N., *see* MORRISON, S. L., HEADY, J. A., and MORRIS, J. N.
MORRISON, S. L., HEADY, J. A., and MORRIS, J. N.: Social and biological factors in infant mortality. VIII. Mortality in the post-neonatal period, 101
Mortality in post-neonatal period, social and biological factors in, 101
MOULTON, A. L. C.: The place of oats in the coeliac diet, 51
MUIR, C. S.: Hydranencephaly and allied disorders, 231
——: Splenic agenesis and multilobulate spleen, 431
Myocarditis with idiopathic pulmonary haemosiderosis, 218

N

Narcolepsy in child under 7 years old, 538
NASH, D. F. E.: Urethral plication in management of urinary incontinence, 33
NEILL, D. W., *see* FORSYTHE, W. I., MCKEOWN, E. F., and NEILL, D. W.
Nephrocalcinosis infantum, 115
Nephrosis, comparison of different forms of therapy in, 357
—— in early months of life, 357
Newborn infants, anaemia in, foetomaternal transfusion as a cause of, 471
—— ——, hepatitis in twin, 187
—— ——, Indian, electrophoretic studies of serum protein patterns in, 392
—— ——, liver disease of, serum lipoprotein electrophoresis patterns in, 187
—— ——, —— function tests in, 187
—— ——, maintenance of stability in. 1. Chemical exchange, 361; 2. Thermal balance, 459
—— ——, massive adrenal haemorrhage in, 178
—— ——, pre-hydropic, extended exchange transfusion in, 174
—— ——, problems of, 35
—— ——, respiratory and cardiovascular problems in, 281
—— ——, rupture of hepatic duct in, 277
—— ——, —— of liver in, 30
Newcastle children, incidence of inguinal hernia in, 482
Niemann Pick's disease in children, 406
NORDIO, S., *see* TONI, E. DE, Jr., and NORDIO, S.

O

Oats in the coeliac diet, 51
Oesophageal atresia, complications after operation for, 24
Oesophago-trachea, 36
Oestrogen excretion in childhood in health and disease, 358
O'NEILL, E. M., and GORDON, R. R.: Extended exchange transfusion in pre-hydropic infants, 174
OPPÉ, T. E., and GIBBS, I. E.: Sulphobromophthalein excretion in premature infants, 125
O'REILLY, R. N., *see* WILLIAMS, H., and O'REILLY, R. N.
Osteoporosis associated with calcification of basal ganglia, 120
OUTON, E. B., *see* SMITHELLS, R. W., and OUTON, E. B.
Oxalosis, 60
Oxygen consumption, changes in, at birth, 283

P

Paediatric Pathology Club, 4th annual meeting, proceedings, 187
Paediatrician, regional, problems of, 358
Pancreas, benign hyperplasia of islet cells, spontaneous hyperinsulinism due to, 171
——, cystic fibrosis of, lung changes in, 188
——, fibrocystic disease of, effect of a bronchodilator aerosol on ventilatory capacity in, 511
——, —— ——, electrical conductivity of electrolytes found in sweat of patients with, 420
Para-aminosalicylic acid in treatment of tuberculous peripheral lymphadenitis, 36
Para-dichlorobenzene, acute haemolytic anaemia following ingestion of, 74
Parathyroid glands, hypofunction of, with Addison's disease, 498
PARE, C. M. B., SANDLER, M., and STACEY, R. S.: The relationship between decreased 5-hydroxyindole metabolism and mental defect in phenylketonuria, 422
PARIKH, M. N., *see* KULKARNI, B. S., *et al.*
PARRY, T. E.: Amino-aciduria in liver disease, 188
Parsons, Leonard, Lectures, Birmingham, 1959, 361, 459
PARTINGTON, M. W.: An English family with Waardenburg's syndrome, 154
——, and QUINTON, J. F. P.: The pre-eruptive illness of measles, 149
PAYNE, W. W.: A comparison of different forms of therapy in nephrosis, 357

PEARCE, K. M., *see* HEPPLESTON, J. D., PEARCE, K. M., and YATES, P. O.
PEEL, J. H.: The baby of the diabetic mother, 358
Pellagra, acute, in child under treatment with isoniazid, 68
Pericholangitis, honeycomb lungs with, 426
Pertussis, neurological sequelae of, with particular reference to mental defect, 322
Phenylketonuria, relationship between decreased 5-hydroxyindole metabolism and mental defect in, 422
PHILPOTT, M. G., and PLAYER, H. P.: Acute pellagra in child under treatment with isoniazid, 69
Pica, aetiology and treatment, 140
PINCOVICI, R., *see* MAINZER, W., PINCOVICI, R., and HEYMANN, G.
Pink disease, effect of calomel on plasma epinephrine and the relationship to mechanisms in, 501
PLAYER, H. P., *see* PHILPOTT, M. G., and PLAYER, H. P.
Pneumonia, pneumocystis, associated with agammaglobulinaemia, 338
POLLARD, H. M., *see* KING, R. C., LINDNER, A. E., and POLLARD, H. M.
PORADOWSKA, W.: Some neonatal problems, 35
Potassium chlorate, congenital goitre due to, 189
Prednisone therapy, sudden death in asthmatic boy on, associated with general arteriolar disease, 189
Pregnancy complicated by diabetes mellitus, 312
Pre-hydropic infants, extended exchange transfusion, in, 174
Premature infants, maternal care of, in Scotland, 487
—— ——, mental development of, 37
—— ——, morbidity of, 210
—— ——, pupillary membrane in, 292
—— ——, sulphobromophthalein excretion in, 125
Protein, serum, patterns in newborn Indian infants, electrophoretic studies of, 392
Pulmonary artery, aberrant, respiratory stridor produced by, 202
—— haemosiderosis, idiopathic, with myocarditis, 218
Pupillary membrane in premature infants, 292
Purpura, Henoch-Schönlein, perforation of bowel in, 342
Pyloric stenosis before and after Ramstedt, 20

Q

QUINTON, J. F. P., *see* PARTINGTON, M. W., and QUINTON, J. F. P.

R

Ramstedt, pyloric stenosis before and after, 20
REES, J.: Anaesthetic methods applied to the treatment of respiratory disease in infancy, 358
REHBEIN, F., and YANAGISWA, F.: Complications after operation for oesophageal atresia, 24
Respiratory disease in infancy, anaesthetic methods applied to treatment of, 358
—— problems after birth, 281
—— stridor produced by aberrant pulmonary artery, 202
RHANEY, K.: Enterogenous cysts and congenital diverticula of the alimentary canal, 189
Rheumatic fever, incidence in Ceylon, 247
Ribs, congenital absence of, lung hernia secondary to, 14
Rickets and sensitivity to vitamin D, 372
—— and steroid metabolism, 375
——, renal, with renal gluco-phospho-amino acid diabetes, 376
——, vitamin D-resistant, familial, 383
RICKHAM, P. P.: Lung hernia secondary to congenital absence of ribs, 14
ROBB, P. M., *see* SCHUTT, W. H., and ROBB, P. M.
ROXBURGH, R. C., and HAAS, L.: The diagnostic importance of glycosuria in lead poisoning in childhood, 70
RUSSELL, J. G. B.: Pneumocystis pneumonia associated with agammaglobulinaemia, 338

S

SALFIELD, D. J.: Narcolepsy in child under 7 years old, 538
SALT, H. B., and WOLFF, O. H.: Serum lipoprotein electrophoresis patterns in neonatal liver disease, 187
SANDBANK, U., *see* KATZUNI, E., and SANDBANK, U.
SANDLER, M., *see* PARE, C. M. B., SANDLER, M., and STACEY, R. S.
SAPIECHA, J., *see* SZCZEPANSKA, H., and SAPIECHA, J.
SATOSKAR, R. S., *see* KULKARNI, B. S., *et al.*
SCHUTT, W. H., and ROBB, P. M.: Respiratory stridor produced by an aberrant pulmonary artery, 202
Scotland, child rearing in, 487
Serum lipoprotein electrophoresis patterns in neonatal liver disease, 187
—— protein patterns in newborn Indian infants, electrophoretic studies of, 392
SHANKS, R. A., and MACDONALD, A. M.: Nephrocalcinosis infantum, 115
SHARRARD, W. J. W.: Congenital paralytic dislocation of hip, 36
SIMPKISS, M. J.: Anaemia and kwashiorkor, 357
SIVANESAN, S.: Honeycomb lungs with pericholangitis, 426
SMITHELLS, R. W., and OUTON, E. B.: Congenital heart block, 223
SNAITH, A. H.: Oestrogen excretion in childhood in health and disease, 358
Spasms, infantile, prognosis of, 357
Speech, common disorders of, in children, 444
Spina bifida, natural history of, 36
Spleen, agenesis of, 431
——, multilobulate, 431
Stability, maintenance of, in newborn: 1. Chemical exchange, 361; 2. Thermal balance, 459
STACEY, R. S., *see* PARE, C. M. B., SANDLER, M., and STACEY, R. S.
Steatorrhoea and hyperparathyroidism, syndrome of, 302
Steroid metabolism and rickets, 375
—— ——, calcium-phosphorus metabolism and the 'Krebs cycle', relationship between, 371
Stomach, thoracic, partial, in children, natural history of, 344
Stridor, respiratory, produced by aberrant pulmonary artery, 202
STROUD, C. E., *see* LEES, M. H., and STROUD, C. E.
Sulphobromophthalein excretion in premature infants, 125
SYLVESTER, P. E.: Cerebral atrophy in microcephalic cousins, 325
SZCZEPANSKA, H., and SAPIECHA, J.: Addison's disease with hypofunction of the parathyroid glands, 498

T

TAYLOR, G. W.: Primary lymphoedema, 35
TAYLOR, S.: Pyloric stenosis before and after Ramstedt, 20
Tetanus in African children, 398
Tetany, rachitogenous, 380
—— with hyperadrenocorticism and (?) hypoparathyroidism, 378
Thermal stability, maintenance of, in newborn, 459
Thyroid, ectopic, subhyoid median, 18
TOMPKINS, A. B.: Tetanus in African children, 398

TOMPSETT, S. L., *see* FORFAR, J. O., TOMPSETT, S. L., and FORSHALL, W.
de Toni-Debré-Fanconi syndrome, 376
TONI, E. DE, Jr., and NORDIO, S.: The relationship between calcium-phosphorus metabolism, the 'Krebs cycle' and steroid metabolism, 371
Transfusion, extended exchange, in pre-hydropic infants, 174
Tuberculous meningitis, treatment of, 334
Twins, monovular, congenital hydrocephalus in, 274
——, monozygous, microcephaly in one of, 56
——, neonatal hepatitis in, 187

U

UNDERHILL, B. M. L.: Acute intestinal obstruction due to mesenteric lymphangioma, 442
Urethral plication in management of urinary incontinence, 33
Urinary incontinence, urethral plication in management of, 33
Urticaria pigmentosa, bone lesions of, in childhood, 205

V

VALENTINE, G. H.: Masculinization of female foetus with oestrogenic effect, 494
Varicella encephalitis, 318
Vena cava, left superior, persistent, surgical importance of, 1
Vertebral arteries, birth trauma to, 436
Virus hepatitis in infancy, 188
Vitamin D, sensitivity to, rickets and, 372

W

Waardenburg's syndrome, English family with, 154
WESTON, H. J.: Analysis of the results of surgical treatment of congenital heart disease, 358
WILKINSON, R. H.: Liver function tests in the newborn, 187
WILLIAMS, C. E., *see* BRANDON, M. G. W., KIRMAN, B. H., and WILLIAMS, C. E.
WILLIAMS, D. I.: Surgery of adrenal cortex in children, 36
WILLIAMS, E., and WOOD, C.: The syndrome of hyperparathyroidism and steatorrhoea, 302
WILLIAMS, H., and O'REILLY, R. N.: Bronchiectasis in children, 192
WILLIAMS, J. A.: Intestinal obstruction in a case of duplication of terminal ileum, 480
——, *see also* HILL, E. E., and WILLIAMS, J. A.
WOLFF, O. H., *see* SALT, H. B., and WOLFF, O. H.
WOLFROM, I.: Rupture of the liver in the newborn, 30
WOOD, C., *see* WILLIAMS, E., and WOOD, C.
WOODCOCK, R. C., *see* DICKSON, W., and WOODCOCK, R. C.
WOOLF, L. I., *see* KINSBOURNE, M., and WOOLF, L. I.
WORSLEY, H. E., *see* WRIGHT, J. P., and WORSLEY, H. E.
WRIGHT, J. P., and WORSLEY, H. E.: A case of rupture of the hepatic duct in a newborn infant, 277
WU, F., *see* CHEEK, D. B., and WU, F.

Y

YANAGISWA, F., *see* REHBEIN, F., and YANAGISWA, F.
YATES, P. O.: Birth trauma to the vertebral arteries, 436
——, *see also* HEPPLESTON, J. D., PEARCE, K. M., and YATES, P. O.

Z

ZACHARY, R. B.: Oesophago-trachea, 36
ZIEGLER, N., *see* KRIVIT, W., *et al.*

PRINTED IN GREAT BRITAIN BY HEADLEY BROTHERS LTD
109 KINGSWAY LONDON WC2 AND ASHFORD KENT